Pediatric Nursing

Pediatric Nursing

As per INC Syllabus

Subrata Sarkar PhD (N) Calcutta Univ.
Visiting Professor
National Institute of Orthopedically Handicapped
Kolkata, West Bengal, India
Charnock College of Nursing
Kolkata, West Bengal, India

Former Principal
Government College of Nursing
RG Kar Medical College and Hospital
Kolkata, West Bengal, India

Former Principal
Tripureswari College of Nursing
Agartala, Tripura, India

Former Reader
West Bengal Government College of Nursing
Institute of Post Graduate Medical Education (IPGMER)
Kolkata, West Bengal, India

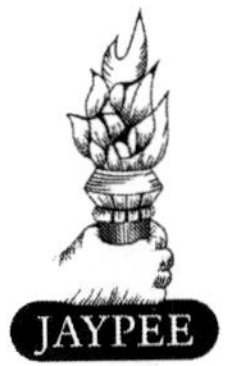

JAYPEE BROTHERS MEDICAL PUBLISHERS
The Health Sciences Publisher
New Delhi | London

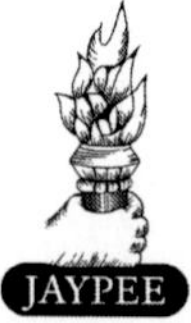

Jaypee Brothers Medical Publishers (P) Ltd

Headquarters
EMCA House
23/23-B, Ansari Road, Daryaganj
New Delhi - 110 002, India
Landline: +91-11-23272143, +91-11-23272703
+91-11-23282021, +91-11-23245672
E-mail: jaypee@jaypeebrothers.com

Corporate Office
4838/24, Ansari Road, Daryaganj
New Delhi - 110 002, India
Phone: +91-11-43574357
Fax: +91-11-43574314
E-mail: jaypee@jaypeebrothers.com

Overseas Office
J.P. Medical Ltd
83 Victoria Street, London
SW1H 0HW (UK)
Phone: +44 20 3170 8910
E-mail: info@jpmedpub.com

EU GPSR Authorised Representative
Logos Europe, 9 rue Nicolas Poussin
17000, La Rochelle, France
Phone: +33 (0) 6 67 93 73 78
E-mail: contact@logoseurope.eu

Website: www.jaypeebrothers.com
Website: www.jaypeedigital.com

Pediatric Nursing

First Edition: 2018
Reprint: **2026**
ISBN: 978-93-86150-87-5
Printed at: Samrat Offset Pvt. Ltd.

Dedication

I respectfully dedicate this book in memoriam of my parents
Lilabati and Narendra Chandra Sarkar
and my parent-in-laws
Shantilata and Krishnapada Bhadra

Preface

Pediatric Nursing is a challenging and rewarding career, where no two days are the same. A pediatric nurse has the chance to work with some of the most precious and unpredictable creatures on the face of the planet—children. Not only do the nursing professionals typically provide help in medical care for youngsters, but they also often get the chance to watch children grow up as well. So the knowledge about their bodies which are still growing and developing, different needs and even different anatomies, their bodies and health issues are often much different than those of adults are important to learn.

The care of children has changed during recent years owing to the rapid expansion of knowledge and technology. Research reports of different disciplines such as psychology, sociology, anthropology, medicine and nursing highlight on understanding the growth and development of children in various cultural and socioeconomic groups, the meaning of parent-child relations, the effects of family disharmony and deprivation on the child, lifestyle diseases and the place of child and adolescent in present day changing of world. While considering the recent research studies, the changing role and responsibilities of child health nurse, and basic principles of teaching and learning, basic growth and development of child (prenatal to adolescence) have been discussed in initial chapters in this book and normal phenomenon with illustration has put up as a basis of care in each chapter.

In this comprehensive edition, the content is so arranged based on syllabuses of various universities in India, though the focus was on postgraduate child health nursing syllabus laid down by Indian Nursing Council. The author hopes the book will be an important asset in advanced knowledge and training in the care of critically ill children who require more frequent and invasive monitoring such as in the pediatric intensive care unit (PICU), educating to recognize early signs of problems and how and when to intervene in intermediate care facilitate transition between the critical and general pediatric units. In addition, this text will be able to influence nursing care outcomes by providing education, anticipatory guidance, expert consultation, and leadership in defining and implementing evidence-based practice for the students and staff in institution and in community. The aim of this work is to make it of value in the learning process of students and later as a reference when they practice nursing or become parents.

The author welcomes all views and suggestions from teachers, students, reviewers, specialists so that this book can further help in developing a genuine care for children and a firm understanding of the common health issues that they face. Above all, however, it will help nurses contribute their best efforts to the care and support of children and their families and find deep personal satisfaction in working with children in well and sickness.

Subrata Sarkar

Acknowledgments

Many professional persons have supported to make the creation of this book possible. A special tribute should be accorded to all of my students who studied different undergraduate and postgraduate nursing courses at West Bengal Government College of Nursing from 1992 to 2007, and worked with me at Alexandra ward of SSKM Hospital, NRSMCH, Singur Health School, Hooghly, West Bengal and Khidirpur Urban Health Centre, Kolkata, West Bengal, India. Their continuous inspiration and persuasion compelled me to undertake this herculean task. On completion of the job my heart melts, and once again I want to convey thanks to you all.

In this book, I honestly do not pretend to claim credit for original contributions in the subject, except my working experience in the field of child health; has taken help from the books, journals, periodicals, newsletters, e-sites; so it is an extension of collaboration and contribution of various experts and authors concerned with the subject. So, I express my heartfelt thanks to all, whose direct or indirect assistance helped me on every step to shape this effort in the form of book.

Present my earnest gratefulness to my husband, Sujato Bhadra, Prof of History and a known Human Right Activist in West Bengal and beyond. Despite of his busy schedule, Prof Bhadra gladly accepted the proposal and has taken the pain to complete the important chapter on 'Rights of Children in India'. I hope students will understand the health of child through a newer perspective and learn to see the child health problems integrating physical, mental and social dimensions of child health including rights of the children.

I express my gratitude to all members of M/s Jaypee Brothers Medical Publishers (P) Ltd, New Delhi, India. A special word of appreciation should be extended to Shri Jitendar P Vij (Group Chairman), Jaypee Brothers Medical Publishers, for giving me the opportunity to put some pinnacle contribution in the domain of child health nursing. The author wishes to express thanks to all members of Kolkata branch of Jaypee Brothers Medical Publishers (P) Ltd. Special thanks goes to Mr Sabyasachi Hazra, Commissioning Editor, Kolkata branch and Ms Ruby Sharma, Project Manager, New Delhi for their intense effort for present publication and promotion of the book.

I would like to acknowledge the help and encouragement given to me by all members of my extended family, and my daughter, Diti; whose constant inspiration has made it possible to complete this huge task. Special indebtedness goes to Diti, as she has given time to edit some of the things of this book, despite her busy schedule of PhD work in USA.

Acknowledgements

INC Syllabus

CLINICAL SPECIALTY I
CHILD HEALTH (PEDIATRIC) NURSING

Placement: Ist Year

Hours of Instruction
Theory: 150 Hours
Practical: 650 Hours
Total: 800 Hours

Course Description

This course is designed to assist students in developing expertise and in depth understanding in the field of Pediatric Nursing. It will help students to appreciate the child as a holistic individual and develop skill to function as neonatal and pediatric nurse specialist. It will further enable the student to function as educator, manager, and researcher in the field of Pediatric Nursing.

Objectives

At the end of the course the students will be able to:

1. Appreciate the history and developments in the field of pediatrics and pediatric nursing as a specialty.
2. Apply the concepts of growth and development in—providing care to the pediatric clients and their families.
3. Appreciate the child as a holistic individual.
4. Perform physical, developmental, and nutritional assessment of pediatric clients.
5. Apply nursing process in providing nursing care to neonates and children.
6. Integrate the concept of family centered pediatric nursing care with related areas such as genetic disorders, congenital malformations and long-term illness.
7. Recognize and manage emergencies in neonates.
8. Describe various recent technologies and treatment modalities in the management of high-risk neonates.
9. Appreciate the legal and ethical issues pertaining to pediatric and neonatal nursing.
10. Prepare a design for layout and management of neonatal units.
11. Incorporate evidence based nursing practice and identify the areas of research in the field of pediatric/neonatal nursing.
12. Recognize the role of pediatric nurse practitioner and as a member of the pediatric and neonatal health team.
13. Teach pediatric nursing to undergraduate students and in-service nurses.

Course Content

Unit	Hours	Content	Chapter
I	10	**Introduction** • Historical development of Pediatrics and Pediatric Nursing in India • Current status of child health in India • Trends in Pediatrics and Pediatric Nursing • Ethical and cultural issues in pediatric care • Rights of children • National health policy for children, special laws and ordinances relating to children • National goals • Five year plans • National health programs related to child health	1, 3, 30

Unit	Hours	Content	Chapter
II	10	**Assessment of pediatric clients** • History taking • Developmental assessment • Physical assessment • Nutritional assessment • Family assessment	7
III	10	**Hospitalized child** • Meaning of hospitalization of the child, preparation for hospitalization, effects of hospitalization on the child and family • Stressors and reactions related to developmental stages, play activities for ill hospitalized child • Nursing care of hospitalized child and family-principles and practices	9
IV	15	**Prenatal Pediatrics** • Embryological and fetal development, Prenatal factors influencing growth and development of fetus • Genetic patterns of common pediatric disorders, chromosomal aberrations, genetic assessment and counseling legal and ethical aspects of genetic, screening and counseling role of nurse in genetic counseling • Importance of prenatal care and role of pediatric nurse	5
V	15	**Growth and Development of children** • Principles of growth and development • Concepts and theories of growth and development • Developmental tasks and special needs from infancy to adolescence, developmental milestones • Assessment of growth and development of pediatric clients • Factors affecting growth and development	4
VI	15	**Behavioral Pediatrics and Pediatric Nursing** • Parent child relationship • Basic behavioral pediatric principles and specific behavioral pediatric concepts/disorders-maternal deprivation, failure to thrive, child abuse, the battered child • Common behavioral problems and their management • Child guidance clinic	6
VII	15	**Preventive Pediatrics and Pediatric Nursing** • Concept, aims and scope of preventive pediatrics • Maternal health and its influence on child health antenatal aspects of preventive pediatrics • Immunization, expanded program on immunization/universal immunization program and cold chain • Nutrition and nutritional requirements of children, changing patterns of feeding, baby-friendly hospital initiative and exclusive breastfeeding • Health education, nutritional education for children • Nutritional programs • National and international organizations related to child health • Role of pediatric nurse in the hospital and community	8
VIII	30	**Neonatal Nursing** • Newborn baby—profile and characteristics of the newborn • Assessment of the newborn • Nursing care of the newborn at birth, care of the newborn and family • High-risk newborn—preterm and term neonate and growth retarded babies • Identification and classification of neonates with infections, HIV and AIDS, Ophthalmia neonatorum, congenital syphilis • High-risk newborn—Identification, classification and nursing management • Organization of neonatal care, services (Levels), transport, neonatal intensive care unit, organization and management of nursing services in NICU	5
IX	30	**IMNCI** (Integrated management of neonatal and childhood illnesses)	10

Practical

Total = 660 Hours
1 Week = 30 Hours

S. No.	Department/Unit	No. of Week	Total Hours
1	Pediatric Medicine Ward	4	120 Hours
2	Pediatric Surgery Ward	4	120 Hours
3	Labor Room/Maternity Ward	2	60 Hours
4	Pediatric OPD	2	60 Hours
5	NICU	4	120 Hours
6	Creche	1	30 Hours
7	Child Guidance Clinic	1	30 Hours
8	Community	4	120 Hours
	Total	**22 Weeks**	**660 Hours**

Student Activities

- Clinical presentations
- Growth and developmental assessment
- Assessment and prescription of nursing interventions for sick children
- Health education related to disease conditions
- Nutritional assessment
- Project work
- Field visits

CLINICAL SPECIALTY II
PEDIATRIC (CHILD HEALTH) NURSING

Placement: IInd Year

Hours of Instruction
Theory: 150 Hours
Practical: 950 Hours
Total: 1100 Hours

Course Description

This course is designed to assist students in developing expertise and in depth understanding in the field of Pediatric Nursing. It will help students to develop advanced skills for nursing intervention in various pediatric medical and surgical conditions. It will enable the student to function as pediatric nurse practitioner/specialist. It will further enable the student to function as educator, manager, and researcher in the field of Pediatric Nursing.

Objectives

At the end of the course the students will be able to:

1. Apply the nursing process in the care of ill infants to pre adolescents in hospital and community
2. Demonstrate advanced skills/competence in nursing management of children with medical and surgical problems
3. Recognize and manage emergencies in children
4. Provide nursing care to critically ill children
5. Utilize the recent technology and various treatment modalities in the management of high-risk children
6. Prepare a design for layout and describe standards for management of pediatric units/hospitals
7. Identify areas of research in the field of pediatric nursing

Course Content

Unit	Hours	Content	Chapter
I	5	**Introduction** • Current principles, practices and trends in Pediatric Nursing • Role of pediatric nurse in various settings—Expanded and extended	
II	35	• Pathophysiology, assessment (including interpretation of various invasive and non-invasive diagnostic procedures), treatment modalities and nursing intervention in selected pediatric medical disorders – Child with respiratory disorders: - Upper respiratory tract: choanal atresia, tonsillitis, epistaxis, aspiration - Lower respiratory tract: Broncheolitis, Bronchopneumonia, Asthma, cystic fibrosis – Child with gastrointestinal disorders: - Diarrheal diseases, gastroesophageal reflux - Hepatic disorders: Hepatitis, Indian childhood cirrhosis, liver transplantation - Malabsorption syndrome, Malnutrition – Child with renal/urinary tract disorders: Nephrotic syndrome, Nephritis, Hydronephrosis, hemolytic-uremic syndrome, kidney transplantation – Child with cardiovascular disorders: - Acquired: Rheumatic fever, Rheumatic heart disease - Congenital: Cynotic and acynotic – Child with endocrine/metabolic disorders: Diabetes insipidus, Diabetes Mellitus—IDDM, NIDDM, hyper and hypothyroidism, phenylketonuria, galactosemia – Child with Neurological disorders: Convulsions, Meningitis, encephalitis, guillian—Barre syndrome – Child with oncological disorders: Leukemias, Lymphomas, Wilms' tumor, nephroblastomas, neuroblastomas, Rhabdomyosarcoma, retinoblastoma, hepatoblastoma, bone tumors – Child with blood disorders: Anemias, thalassemias, hemophilia, polycythemia, thrombocytopenia, and disseminated intravascular coagulation – Child with skin disorders – Common Eye and ENT disorders – Common communicable diseases	13, 12, 16, 19, 14, 18, 17, 15, 21, 22, 31, 20, 11
III	35	• Assessment(including interpretation of various invasive and non-invasive diagnostic procedures), treatment modalities including cosmetic surgery and nursing interventions in selected pediatric surgical problems/Disorders – Gastrointestinal system: Cleft lip, cleft palate and conditions requiring plastic surgery, Tracheoesophageal fistula/atresia, Hirschsprungs' disease/megacolon, malrotation, intestinal obstruction, duodenal atresia, gastrochisis, exomphalus, anorectal malformation, omphafocele, diaphragmatic hernia – Anomalies of the nervous system: Spina bifida, Meningocele, Myelomeningocele, hydrocephalus – Anomalies of the genito-urinary system: Hypospadias, Epispadias, Undescended testes, Exstrophy bladder – Anomalies of the skeletal system – Eye and ENT disorders – Nursing management of the child with traumatic injuries: General principles of managing Pediatric trauma - Head injury, abdominal injury, poisoning, foreign body obstruction, burns and - Bites – Child with oncological disorders: Solid tumors of childhood, Nephroblastoma, Neuroblastoma, Hodgkin's/Non Hodgkin's Lymphoma, Hepatoblastoma, Rhabdomyosarcoma – Management of stomas, catheters and tubes – Management of wounds and drainages	23

Unit	Hours	Content	Chapter
IV	10	**Intensive care for pediatric clients** • Resuscitation, stabilization and monitoring of pediatric patients • Anatomical and physiological basis of critical illness in infancy and childhood • Care of child requiring long-term ventilation • Nutritional needs of critically ill child • Legal and ethical issues in pediatric intensive care • Intensive care procedures, equipment and techniques • Documentation	29
V	20	**High-risk Newborn** • Concept, goals, assessment, principles • Nursing management of – Post-mature infant, and baby of diabetic and substance use mothers – Respiratory conditions, Asphyxia neonatorum, neonatal apnea meconium aspiration syndrome, pneumothorax, pneumomediastinum – Icterus neonatorum – Birth injuries – Hypoxic-ischemic encephelopathy – Congenital anomalies – Neonatal seizures – Neonatal hypocalcaemia, hypoglycemia, hypomagnesaemia – Neonatal heart diseases – Neonatal hemolytic diseases – Neonatal infections, neonatal sepsis, opthalmia neonatorum, cogenital syphilis, HIV/AIDS – Advanced neonatal procedures – Calculation of fluid requirements – Hematological conditions—erythroblastosis fetalis, hemorrhagic disorder in the newborn – Organization of neonatal care, services (Levels), transport, neonatal intensive care unit, organization and management of nursing services in NICU	28
VI	10	**Developmental disturbances and implications for nursing** • Adjustment reaction to school • Learning disabilities • Habit disorders, speech disorders • Conduct disorders • Early infantile autism, Attention deficit hyperactive disorders (ADHD), depression and childhood schizophrenia	24, 2
VII	10	**Challenged child and implications for nursing** • Physically challenged, causes, features, early detection and management • Cerebral palsied child • Mentally challenged child • Training and rehabilitation of challenged children	25
VIII	5	**Crisis and nursing intervention** • The hospitalized child • Terminal illness and death during childhood • Nursing intervention-counseling	26
IX	5	**Drugs used in Pediatrics** • Criteria for dose calculation • Administration of drugs, oxygen and blood • Drug interactions • Adverse effects and their management	27

Unit	Hours	Content	Chapter
X	10	**Administration and management of pediatric care unit** • Design and layout • Staffing • Equipment, supplies • Norms, policies and protocols • Practice standards for pediatric care unit • Documentation	6
XI	5	**Education and training in Pediatric care** • Staff orientation, training and development • In-service education program • Clinical teaching programs	

Practical

Total = 960 Hours
1 Week = 30 Hours

- **Field visits:**

S. No.	Department/Unit	No. of Week	Total Hours
1	Pediatric medicine ICU	4	120 Hours
2	Pediatric surgical ICU	4	120 Hours
3	NICU	4	120 Hours
4	Pediatric OT	2	60 Hours
5	Pediatric medicine ward	6	180 Hours
6	Pediatric surgery ward	6	180 Hours
7	Emergency/ Casualty	4	120 Hours
8	Field visits*	2	60 Hours
	Total	**32**	**960 Hours**

*Child care center, Anganwadi, Play school, Special schools for challenged children, Juvenile Court, UNICEF, Orphanage, Creche, SOS village

Essential

I. **Procedures Observed:**
- Echo cardiogram
- Ultrasound head
- ROP screening (Retinopathy of prematurity)
- Any other

II. **Procedures Assisted:**
- Advanced neonatal life support
- Lumbar Puncture
- Arterial Blood Gas
- ECG Recording
- Umbilical catheterization—arterial and venous
- Arterial BP monitoring
- Blood transfusion—exchange transfusion full and partial
- IV cannulation and therapy
- Arterial catheterization
- Chest tube insertion
- Endotracheal intubation

- Ventilation
- Insertion of long line
- Assist in surgery

III. **Procedures Performed:**

- Airway Management
  - Application of Oropharyngeal Airway
  - Oxygen therapy
  - CPAP (Continuous Positive Airway Pressure)
  - Care of Tracheostomy
  - Endotracheal Intubation
- Neonatal Resuscitation
- Monitoring of Neonates—clinically and with monitors, CRT (Capillary Refill Time), assessment of jaundice, ECG
- Gastric Lavage
- Setting of Ventilators
- Phototherapy
- Assessment of Neonates: Identification and assessment of risk factors, APGAR Score, gestation age, Anthropometric assessment, Weighing the baby, Newborn examination, detection of life threatening congenital abnormalities
- Admission and discharge of neonates
- Feeding—management of breastfeeding, artificial feeding, expression of breast milk, OG (Orogastric) tube insertion, gavage feeding, TPN, Breastfeeding counseling
- Thermoregulation—Axillary temperature, Kangaroo Mother Care (KMC), Use of Radiant warmer, incubators, management of thermoregulation and control
- Administration of Drugs: I/M, IV injection, IV Cannulation and fixation infusion pump, Calculation of dosages, Neonatal formulation of drugs, use of tuberculin/insulin syringes, Monitoring fluid therapy, Blood administration
- Procedures for prevention of infections: Hand washing, disinfections and sterilization, surveillance, fumigation
- Collection of specimens
- Setting, Use and maintenance of basic equipment: Ventilator, O_2 analyzer, monitoring equipment, Photo therapy unit, Flux meter, Infusion pump, Radiant warmer, incubator, Centrifuge machine, Bilimeter, Refractometer, laminar flow

IV. **Other Procedures**

Contents

1. Introduction to Child Health and Child Health Nursing **1**
- Child Health: Concept and Importance *1*
- Historical Background: Child Health *2*
- Indian Perspective: Child Health *3*
- Child Health Nursing *3*
- Family-centered Care *4*
- Cost Containment *6*
- Advanced Preparation of Pediatric Nurse *10*

2. Family-centered Care **12**
- The Family and Child Health Nurse *12*
- Parenting *13*
- Types of Family *16*
- Role of Family in Child Health Promotion and Prevention of Diseases *24*
- Qualities of a Child Health Nurse *25*

3. Child Health Promotion **26**
- Nutrition: Child Health *26*
- Nutritional Policy *33*
- Relevance to Clinical Practice *34*
- Sleep *38*

4. Growth and Development of Child **43**
- Concepts of Growth and Development *43*
- Influences of Heredity on Growth and Development *46*
- Importance of Learning Growth and Development *46*
- Overview of Growth and Development *46*
- Stages of Growth and Development *46*
- Parameters of Growth and Development *48*
- Growth Monitoring and Growth Chart *48*
- Principles of Child Development *50*
- Factors Affect Growth and Development of Child *52*
- Theory of Growth and Development of Child *54*
- Psychoanalytic Theory *54*
- Psychosocial—Developmental Theory *55*
- Cognitive Development Theory *58*
- Summary of Cognitive Development *61*
- Lev Vygotsky's Social Development Theory *63*

5. Stages of Pediatric Life **66**
- Prenatal Pediatrics *67*
- Embryological and Fetal Development *67*
- Fetal Growth and Development *70*
- The Neonate *78*

- Respiratory System *79*
- Circulatory System *80*
- Gastrointestinal (GI) System *83*
- Immune System *84*
- Skin *85*
- Neurologic System *85*
- Sensory Development *86*
- Immediate Post Birth Care *86*
- Assessment of Gestational Age *89*
- Physical Examination of the Newborn *91*
- Thermal Regulation of Newborn *92*
- Breastfeeding and Lactation Management *93*
- To Ensure Safety, Prevent Injury and Infection *100*
- Identification and Early Registration *101*
- To Identify Actual or Potential Problems and Immediate Action *102*
- The Normal Infant *103*
- The Toddler *115*
- General Characteristics of Toddler *115*
- Overview of the Growth and Development *116*
- Cognitive Development *117*
- Physical Growth and Development *119*
- Language Development *121*
- Social Development *122*
- Behavior *122*
- Physical Development and Role of Parent *123*
- Needs of the Toddler *123*
- Injury Prevention *131*
- Injuries and Accidents in Toddlers *132*
- Safe Play *134*
- Preschool Child *135*
- Overview of the Growth and Development *135*
- Role of Parent in Development *139*
- Special Problems of Preschool Child *140*
- Promoting Optimal Health of Preschool Child *144*
- The School Child *147*
- Overview of Emotional Development in School Child *147*
- The School Child, His Family and Friends *147*
- Health Problems During School-age *154*
- Adolescence *155*
- Changes during Adolescence *155*

6. Behavioral Pediatric and Pediatric Nursing **167**
- Behavioral Pediatrics and Pediatric Nursing *167*
- Common Behavioral Problems and their Management *170*
- Temper Tantrums *173*
- Enuresis *175*

- Toilet Training Difficulties 176
- Child Guidance Clinic 176
- Educational Guidance 177
- Role of a Pediatric Nurse in Child Guidance Clinic 178

7. Assessment of Pediatric Patient **180**
- Importance of Assessment in Pediatric Patients 181
- Skills Used for Assessment 181
- Developmental Approach to the Examination 182
- Assessment of Pediatric Patient 184
- Admission Assessment 184
- Developmental Assessment 193
- Assessment of Nutritional Status 193
- Purposes of Nutritional Assessment 193
- Various Techniques with Different Approaches 193

8. Preventive Pediatrics **197**
- Aim 198
- Preventive Pediatrics: Few Related Concepts 198
- Milestones in the History of MCH Care in India 201
- Child Health 202
- ICDS 205
- IMNCI 206
- Handicapped Child Care 208
- Adolescent Health 208
- School Health 209
- Center for International Child Health are WHO, UNICEF, FAO, CARE, USAID 211
- National Organizations 214
- Nurses' Role in Preventive Pediatrics 214

9. Hospitalized Child **217**
- Meaning of Hospitalization 217
- Need for Hospitalization 218
- Modern Concepts of Hospitalization 218
- Effects of Hospitalization on Child and Family 218
- Preparation of the Child for Hospitalization 223
- Nursing Care of the Child Who is Hospitalized 223
- Nursing Management of a Child in the Hospital 224

10. Integrated Management of Neonatal and Childhood Illness (IMNCI) **228**
- The IMNCI Package 229
- Principles of IMNCI Integrated Care 231

11. The Child: A Fluid and Electrolyte Alteration **235**
- Review of Fluid and Electrolytes in Children 235
- Overview of Dyselectrolytemias 237
- Disturbances in Acid-Base Status 242
- Fluid Imbalance 244
- Maintenance of Fluid and Electrolyte Balance: Nursing Responsibilities 248

12. The Child with a Gastrointestinal Disorder **250**
- Review of the Gastrointestinal (GI) System *250*
- Pediatric Differences in the GI System *251*
- Endoscopy *257*
- Colonoscopy *258*
- Disorders of Prenatal Development *259*
- Motility Disorders *260*
- Inflammatory and Infectious Disorders *265*
- Obstructive Disorders *275*
- Malabsorption Disorders *275*
- Hepatic Disorders *279*
- Hepatitis *280*

13. A Child with Respiratory Disorders **288**
- Respiratory System *288*
- Lower Respiratory Tract Disorders *298*
- Allergic Disorders *315*

14. Child with Genitourinary Disorders **324**
- Review of Renal System *324*
- Congenital Abnormalities *328*
- Congenital Abnormalities Related to Bladder and Lower Urinary Tract *331*
- Other Disorders of GU System of Children *336*
- Dialysis *348*

15. The Child with a Hematologic Alteration **349**
- Hematologic System *349*
- Anemia *351*

16. The Child with Neurologic Alterations **372**
- The Axial Skeleton *373*
- The Cranial Nerves *375*
- Approach to the Child with Neurological Problem *376*
- Disorders of CNS *378*
- Acute Flaccid Paralysis (AFP) *383*
- Neural Tube Defects and CSF Circulation Problem *388*
- Seizure Disorder *396*
- Injury *402*

17. The Child with Malignancy **409**
- Review of Cancer *409*
- Leukemia *419*
- Malignant Lymphomas *428*

18. The Child with an Endocrine or Metabolic Disorder **443**
- Review of the Endocrine System *443*
- Inborn Errors of Metabolism *447*
- Psychological Support of Short Stature Child *455*
- Endemic Cretinism (Environmental Diseases) *457*

19. Cardiovascular System **468**

- Review of the Heart and Circulation *468*
- Cyanotic Heart Diseases *471*
- Acyanotic Heart Diseases (Left to Right Shunting Lesions Cause Increased Pulmonary Blood Flow) *475*
- Obstructive Heart Diseases *479*
- Nursing Care of the Family and Child with Congenital Cardiac Diseases *483*
- Acquired Heart Diseases *489*
- Arrhythmias *494*
- Hypertension *497*
- Kawasaki Disease *499*
- Shock *501*

20. Common Communicable Diseases in Children **504**

- Common Viral Infections *505*
- Whooping Cough *506*
- Measles *508*
- Poliomyelitis *510*
- Treatment of Residual Paralysis *514*
- Chickenpox (Varicella-Zoster, Shingles) *516*
- Dengue *518*
- Rabies *519*
- HIV Infection *521*
- Common Bacterial Infection *523*
- Tuberculosis *526*
- Leprosy *529*
- Common Parasitic Infections *532*
- Kala-Azar *535*
- Filariasis *536*
- Helminthiasis *538*
- Echinococcosis (Hydatid Disease) *539*

21. The Child and Skin Conditions **541**

- Review of Structure and Function of the Skin *541*
- Nursing Care of Child with Skin Infection *546*
- Herpes Simplex Virus Infection *547*
- Burns *553*
- Insect Bites and Stings *561*

22. The Child with Sensory Alteration **562**

- Eye and Disorders of the Eye *562*
- Refractive Errors *564*
- Ear and Disorders of the Ear *569*

23. Management of Selected Pediatric Surgical Problems/Disorders **575**

- Hypospadias *575*
- Epispadias *576*
- Undescended Testes *576*
- Nursing Management for Congenital Genitourinary Malformations Preoperative *577*

- Cheilorrhaphy *579*
- Care of the Patient with an Ostomy *585*

24. Developmental Disturbances, Challenged Child and Implications for Nursing **597**
- Developmental Delay *597*
- Behavior Disorder *604*

25. Challenged Child and Implications for Nursing **610**
- Impairment in Motor Development *610*
- Chromosomal/Genetic Disorders *612*

26. Crisis and Nursing Intervention **616**
- Four Phases of Crisis Process *616*
- Effects of Hospitalization on Parents and the Family of Child *620*
- Hospice Care *623*

27. Drugs used in Pediatrics **624**
- Neurologic System *624*
- Cardiovascular System *625*
- Body Composition *625*
- Respiratory System *626*
- Gastrointestinal System *626*
- Endocrine System *626*
- Renal System *626*
- Rational Drug Therapy (RDT) *627*
- Calculation of Drugs in Pediatrics *629*
- Administration of Drug and Fluid: Nursing Responsibilities *631*

28. High-risk Newborn **635**
- Concept, Goal, Assessment, Principles of High-risk Newborn Care *635*
- Apnea *644*

29. Intensive Care for Pediatric Patients **653**
- Resuscitation, Stabilization, and Monitoring of Pediatric Patients *653*
- Bili Lights *660*
- Bili Blanket *661*

30. Rights of Children in India **665**
- Homes *666*
- The Right of Children to Free and Compulsory Education Act, 2009 *667*
- The Child Labor (Prohibition and Regulation) Act, 1986 *667*
- Some Salient Features of Some Acts Related to Children Welfare and Rights *667*

31. The Child with a Musculoskeletal Alteration **669**
- Review of the Musculoskeletal System *669*
- Disorders of Musculoskeletal System *670*

Appendices **687**
- Appendix 1: Birth Registration of Newborn *687*
- Appendix 2: Steps of Newborn Resuscitation *688*

- Appendix 3: Height and Weight Chart of Children *690*
- Appendix 4: Maturational Assessment of Gestational Age (New Ballard Score) *691*
- Appendix 5: Pediatric Vital Signs *693*
- Appendix 6: Some Important Calculations *694*
- Appendix 7: Tooth Eruption of Child *695*
- Appendix 8: Motor Reflexes *696*
- Appendix 9: Normal Development of Child *697*
- Appendix 10: Recommended Dietary Allowances (RDA) *699*
- Appendix 11: Important Maternal and Child Health Indicators—Current Status vs Goals *700*
- Appendix 12: Common Pediatric Medicines and Doses *701*
- Appendix 13: Drugs and Breastfeeding *704*
- Appendix 14: National Health Mission (NHM) *708*
- Appendix 15: The National Policy for Children, 2013 *711*

Index **717**

CHAPTER 1

Introduction to Child Health and Child Health Nursing

Chapter Outline

- Child Health: Concept and Importance
- Historical Background: Child Health
- Indian Perspective: Child Health
- Child Health Nursing
- Family-centered Care
- Cost Containment
- Advanced Preparation of Pediatric Nurse

INTRODUCTION

Pediatrics is commonly known as the branch of medicine that deals with the medical care of infants, children, and adolescents. A medical practitioner who specializes in this area is known as a **pediatrician**. The word *pediatrics* and its cognates mean *healer of children*; they derive from two Greek words, *pais* = child and *iatros* = doctor or healer. Pediatrics is the study and care of children in sickness and health, i.e. preventive, promotive, curative and rehabilitative care of children (Fig. 1.1). In developing countries in the world, this care is extending to children up to 10–12 years of age. In developed countries, children up to adolescence are covered under pediatric care and child health care support.

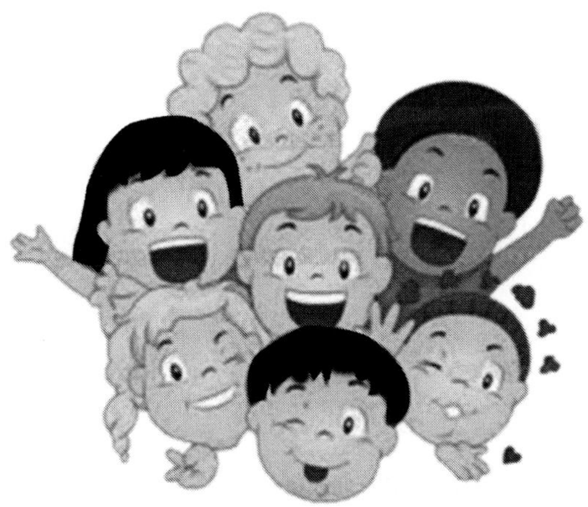

Fig. 1.1: Healthy child healthy world

But the term pediatrics is no more seems to be appropriate to use, as it appears to be doctoring children. Child health concepts and practice have changed. The child health care is most appropriate than pediatric care as it covers multipronged activities in child health care. Child health care is a complex field, requiring an interdisciplinary involvement to meet its needs. This team includes geneticists, pediatrician, biochemists, psychologists, pediatric-surgeons, educationist, pediatric nurse, dietician, dentists. The contribution from these professionals is important for safe journey of our future generation.

CHILD HEALTH: CONCEPT AND IMPORTANCE

Child health refers to a state of complete physical, mental and social well-being and not merely the absence of disease or infirmity in matters relating to growth and development of fetus during antenatal period and from birth of the baby till five-year of age. It implies health care of the fetus during antenatal period which refers to antenatal pediatrics, health care of neonates from birth to 28 days, care of infants up to one year, care of toddler from one year up to two years, care of preschool child from two years to five years of age, and care of the school going children.

The health of the children is also very important not only because they are the asset and future of their families and nation but also because health status, health behavior and lifestyle, thus form during childhood determines quality of life during the following years of life. The health of the children differs from place to place and in the same place. It is assessed in terms of child morbidity and mortality. The factor which affect the health of children include poverty, ignorance, illiteracy, age, sex, environment, size of the family, malnutrition, lack of access to maternal and child health services, etc.

HISTORICAL BACKGROUND: CHILD HEALTH

Pediatric is a relatively new medical specialty. Greek physicians and philosophers; Hippocrates, Aristotle, Celsus, Soraneus, and Galen, understood the differences in growing and maturing organisms that necessitated different treatment. In the first century AD, Celsus was reported to be the first one to state that children require different treatment from adults. A 2nd century AD manuscript by the Greek physician and gynecologist Soraneus of Ephesus dealt with neonatal pediatrics. Soraneus wrote the first known manuscript devoted to pediatrics. Byzantine physicians; *Oribasius, Aëtius of Amida, Alexander Trallianus*, and *Paulus Aegineta* stand out for their contributions to child care. The Byzantines also built *brephotrophia*, 'baby shelters,' or 'children's hospitals.' Islamic writers served as a bridge for Greco-Roman and Byzantine medicine and added ideas of their own especially *Haly Abbas, Serapion, Rhazes, Avicenna*, and *Averroes*, The Persian scholar and doctor *al-Razi* (865–925) published a short treatise on diseases among children. The first printed book on pediatrics was in Italian (1472), Bagallarder's *Little Book on Disease in Children. Paulus Bagellardus a Flumine* (d.1492) *De Infantium Aegritudinibus et Remediis* 1472, *Bartolomaeus Metlinger* (d.1491) *Ein Regiment der Jungerkinder* 1473, *Cornelius Roelans* (1450–1525) no title Buchlein, or Latin compendium, 1483, and *Heinrich von Louffenburg* (1391–1460) *Versehung des Leibs* written 1429 published 1491; together form the *Pediatric Incunabula*, four great medical treatises on children's physiology and pathology.

Industrial revolution brought remarkable changes in the lives of people. New intellectual climate of the Renaissance made people to observe, to ask questions of different aspects of child health in conducting experiments and made to leave findings for others. The recognition of childhood diseases differ from adult diseases led to the establishment of hospital devoted solely for children. In the Western world, the first generally accepted pediatric hospital is the *Hôspital des Enfants Malades* (French: Hospital for Sick Children), which opened in Paris in June 1802 on the site of a previous orphanage. From its beginning, this famous hospital accepted patients up to the age of fifteen years, and it continues to this day as the pediatric division of the Necker-Enfants Malades Hospital, created in 1920 by merging with the physically contiguous *Necker Hospital*, founded in 1778.

This example was only gradually followed in other European countries. The [Charité] (a hospital founded in 1710) in Berlin established a separate Pediatric Pavilion in 1830, followed by similar institutions at [Saint Petersburg] in 1834, and at Vienna and *Breslau* now [Wrocław], both in 1837. The English-speaking world waited until 1852 for its first pediatric hospital, the Hospital for Sick Children, Great Ormond Street, some fifty years after the founding of its namesake in Paris. In the USA, the first similar institutions were the Children's Hospital of Philadelphia, which opened in 1855, and then Boston Children's Hospital (1869).

Pediatrics as a specialized field of medicine developed in the mid-19th century; under the influence of the Persian born Abraham Jacobi (1830–1919). He is known as the father of pediatrics because of his many contributions to the field. He was born in Germany, where he received his medical training, but later practiced in New York City. He was awarded the first professorship in pediatrics in America in 1870. Pediatric department in several hospitals in Newyork were started by Prof. Jacobi and he was one of the founders of American Pediatric Society, 1888.

Throughout the world, about a century and half ago, children were not considered as somebody who should be treated differently when illness occurs. It was in United States of America, for the first time, recognition was given to Pediatrics as a separate subject. Even Great Britain was more than fifty years behind in adopting Pediatrics as a specialty (Fig. 1.2).

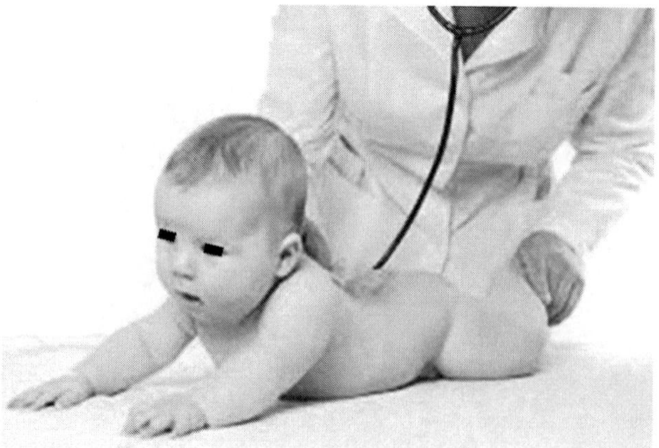

Fig. 1.2: Assessment of baby is an integral part of pediatric care

INDIAN PERSPECTIVE: CHILD HEALTH

In India, Kashyapa Tantra written in BC had a chapter on Koumara Mritya, i.e. service to children. Perhaps this is the first record of pediatrics anywhere in the world. Our rich heritage of Ayurveda has detailed description of maternal and child health care. Sushruta, the Indian Hippocrates in his *Sushruta Samhita*, had devoted a chapter to *Kaumarabrita* (service to children). This was perhaps the first record of pediatrics in ancient India. Pediatrics was called *Kaumarbhritya tantra*. The *Atharva Veda* (1500 BC) describes children's diseases and *Kaushika Sutra* included pediatrics. Kashyapa and Jeevaka (400 BC) were well known pediatricians of ancient India. *Kashyapa Samhita* deals exclusively with pediatrics. Charaka wrote in details about the care and management of newborn in *Sarira–Sthana* and *Ashtanga–Hridaya*. The *Charaka Samhita* in fact mentions an international conference of scholars. *Kaumarbhritya* and *Prasuti tantra* talk of prenatal care, and also lay emphasis on neonatal care, care of the baby including feeding and management of illnesses of children. This includes—maternal care (with respect to food, drink, leisure, restricted work, sleep, etc.), neonatal care (cleaning, dressing, bath, procedure akin to cardiac compression), care of the umbilical cord, breastfeeding (including concept of a wet nurse), *annaprasana* (initial eating of solid food), daily care of eyes and skin, and common symptomatology in childhood illnesses.

Till independence in our country, medical care of children was under professors of adult medicine. The idea that the children are not miniature adults, took some time to dawn on medical profession. Many of the problems seen in young children and neonates are different in nature and approach and treatment were quite different from that of adults. The focus and scope of pediatrics, the health problems of children vary widely among the nations and problems are complex in children of the developing countries. In the developing countries which represent three quarter of humanity, many children suffer due to diseases that are attributable to poverty and poor hygiene.

Our state Tamil Nadu has the honor and pride of having created the first post of Professor of Pediatrics in India at the Madras Medical College even though there were fairly well-developed Pediatric Departments in centers like Mumbai, Patna and Kolkata. The creation of the first Pediatric Department at the Government General Hospital, Madras in the year 1948 with late Prof. ST Achar, a Professor of Medicine turned Pediatrician as the first Professor of Pediatrics, Madras Medical College, paved the way for the birth of the speciality of Pediatrics in Tamil Nadu. Later due to the untiring combined efforts of Dr ST Achar, Dr V Balagopal Raju and Dr MS Ramakrishnan, a separate Hospital for Pediatrics at Egmore was created. Now in all states in India, there are many children's hospital under public sectors and private sectors too. Almost all medical colleges in India offer specialist and super-specialist training for doctors and nurses in the field of pediatrics.

CHILD HEALTH NURSING

Pediatric nursing is 'the practice of nursing with children, youth, and their families across the health continuum, including health promotion, illness management, and health restoration'. Although the pediatric nurse must be knowledgeable about a wide range of medical conditions and treatment options, pediatric nursing is 'not 'med-surg nursing' on little people'. It requires knowledge of both child development and of the physiological differences between children and adults. It also is family-centered, recognizing both the vital role that families play in children's lives, growth, and development and that this must be reflected in children's care when they are ill. Family-centered care involves collaborative partnerships between families and health care professionals, built on respect for diversity and grounded in the family's strengths, choices, and values. In addition to family-centered care, pediatric nurses attempt to provide atraumatic care, that is, therapeutic care that utilizes 'interventions that eliminate or minimize the psychological and physical distress experienced by children and health care system' (Fig. 1.3).

So, pediatric nursing is a medical specialty that promotes the care, both urgent and preventative, of children and youth. Nurses in this field must have a

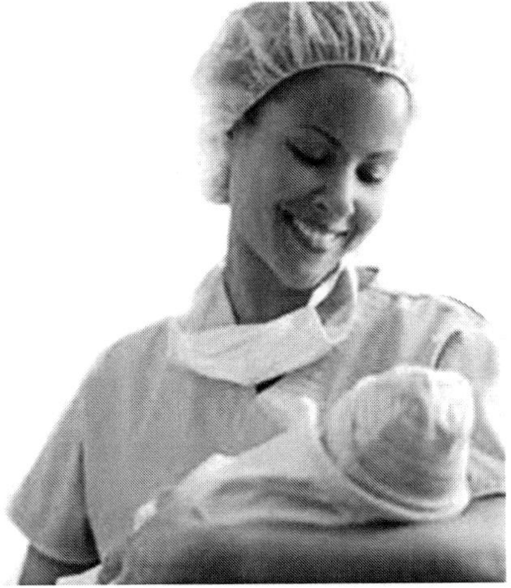

Fig. 1.3: Your child is in caring hands

wide range of knowledge, including the physiological differences between children and adults. This specialized care propels nurses into different roles, including caregiver, health promoter and prevention of infection, advocate and educator, counselor, consultant, advocate, care coordinator, or health systems manager. They may work as researchers or at the advanced practice level as pediatric clinical nurse specialists. Pediatric nurses may practice in many locations, including the home, hospitals, clinics, long-term care facilities, and schools.

Goals of Pediatric Nursing

- Enhance the care of children and adolescents worldwide
- Recognize the rights of the child to promote and advocate for the health, well-being/welfare and development of children
- Encourage communication between pediatric nurses to help further the care of all children.
- Promote a therapeutic relationship between parent and child
- Accomplish family-centered care
- Promote continued growth and development.

Trends in Child Health Nursing

Remarkable changes have occurred in the field of pediatric nursing in recent years. Modern approach of child health care emphasizes on preventive care rather than curative care. Illness is the situations when individual faces physical, physiological, and mental difficulties. So concept of care of 'Whole child' is possible only in normal situation, not in illness. Moreover, most childhood diseases are preventable, and nurses play pivotal role to prevent those diseases and render services at the door step of the families.

Health promotion and holistic care of children is an emerging trend. According to UNICEF, assistance for fulfilling the needs of children should no longer be confined to only one aspect like nutrition or immunization but it should be wide-based and geared to their long-term growth and development ensuing holistic health care of children. Nursing care of children of modern time, highlights health promotion and disease prevention as national attention. Hospital stay of even acutely ill child is made brief, and parents are encouraged to render care with technological support. For example, parents are better able to assess the respiratory status of their asthma child with the support of pick flow meter and can control some exacerbations by nebulization of medications.

Acceptance of family-centered care of children impart more responsibility on pediatric nursing and pediatric nurse. The philosophy of family-centered care is to recognize and respect the pivotal role of family in the lives of both well and ill children. The pediatric nurse maintains liaison between family and health team to set treatment/care plan and thus to prevent psychological trauma or mental stress of both child and family. Family-centered philosophy in health care setting respects choices of family members, provide input, and are given information that are understandable by them. The family's inputs are honored, and its strengths are recognized. Some hospitals have started child life programs to help children and their families cope up with the stress of illness, anxiety due to hospitalization, etc. In family-centered care, not only the needs of the child but the needs of the family members are also considered.

FAMILY-CENTERED CARE

Children's health care needs cannot be identified in the absence of the family. Family-centered care recognizes that the family is the major participant in the prevention of diseases and promotion of health of a child or adolescent. As such, the families have the right and responsibilities to participate individually and collectively in determining and satisfying the health care needs of their children and adolescent. The health care provider realized that the family, community and society surrounding the child have a particular way of life and culture. Being family-centered means that policies regarding access, availability and flexibility take into consideration the various structures, functions, cultural background of family in the community being served. Family-centered care reflects an understanding of the nature, role and understanding of children's health, illness, disability, or injury in the family and the impact of family structure, function and dynamics on both risks to ill health and promotion of health.

Without family, children's health care needs cannot be identified. Children face environmental health hazards as a result of their family's social and economic circumstances and lifestyle. They are vulnerable to particular disease because of their genetic predisposition; and they may suffer physical health consequences of family stress such as unemployment, divorce, parental disability. Furthermore, because children generally are not in a position to seek health care on their own, even when illness symptoms are present, the decision to seek health care is family matter.

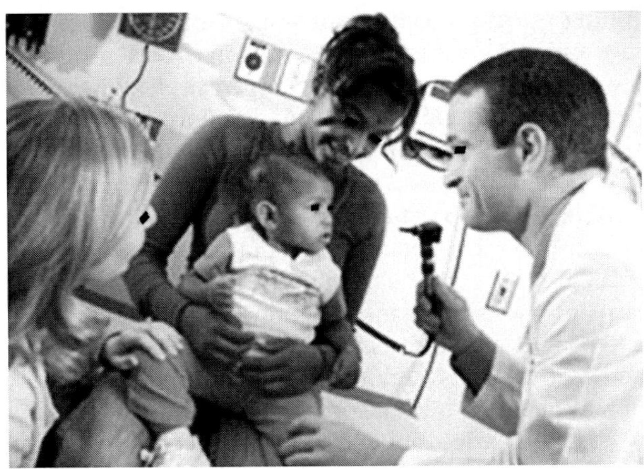

Fig. 1.4: Family-centered care

A community health care provider (primary level) must therefore understand not only physical health risks of a child but also family stress as well as various social, economic, psychological, emotional and cultural factors that influence a family's decision to seek health care for a child. Finally, because compliance with a prescribed treatment for children is likely to be influenced by their family, family impact must also be considered when deciding on a child's plan of care (Fig. 1.4). The issues of guardianship, privacy, legal responsibility and informed consent must always be considered in every pediatric procedure. In a sense, pediatricians and pediatric nurses often have to treat the parents and sometimes, the family, rather than just the child.

High Technology Care

High technology care benefits pediatric nursing care. Advancement in the domain of medical field has created the care of sick children too technologically versatile. 'Telemedicine and tele-monitoring are commonplace now,' as care coordination is made electronically. Electronic medical records allow nurses to immediately access important information of child like prior health history, medications, lab reports and co-existing medical conditions—whether care was provided at the current facility or another location. This provides a more complete and accurate clinical picture, ensuring that the patient receives the appropriate care for his or her condition.

Currently, every hospital tries to offer a specialized intensive care unit exclusively for newborns, children, called Pediatric Intensive Care Unit (NICU, PICU). Children requiring highest level of care during their treatment and recovery receive special care in NICU, PICU. A team of pediatric intensivists works closely with specially trained pediatric nurses, respiratory therapists and other health care professionals to provide round-the-clock, high-tech care in a compassionate environment that supports parents and encourages them to take an active role during their child's hospital stay.

Technological advancement in the working place challenges nurse for continuing nursing education. They need to be oriented on specialized equipment like ventilators, specialized beds and cribs to accommodate patients with special needs, cardio-respiratory monitoring, computer charting and documentation, peritoneal dialysis monitoring and specialized syringe pumps. Day by day this stream of nursing is becoming popular, and student nurses aspire to be a high tech pediatric nurse. They want to be skillful in rendering care in trauma populations, as well as children with a variety of medical/surgical diagnoses.

Evidence-based Practice (EBP)

Trend in evidence-based practice is enriching the domain of pediatric nursing. Scientific enquiry about care and support is an integral part of nursing practice. Research and EBP initiated by nurses, and particularly bedside nurses, are important components to develop a body of knowledge. EBP can be applied to any problem that seeks solution, and nurses need to make decisions on the best available evidences.

Few steps are involved in the process of EBP. The problem seeking solution needs to be framed as question/questions, need to search for evidences in literature, search for evidences assess for evidences make decisions evaluate performance.

Atraumatic Care

There are lot of advances, changes in pediatric care and treatment which is traumatic, painful upsetting and frightening. Children experience both physical and psychological stresses in the pediatric care setting. They experience psychological distress like anxiety, fear, anger, disappointment, sadness, shame, or guilt. They also experience the physical distresses like sensory stimuli such as pain, temperature extremes, loud noises, bright lights or darkness. Health professionals must be aware of the stresses and strive to provide intervention which is safe, effective and helpful.

Atraumatic care is the provision of therapeutic care in environments, by personnel and through the use of interventions that eliminate or minimize the physical and psychological distresses experienced by the children

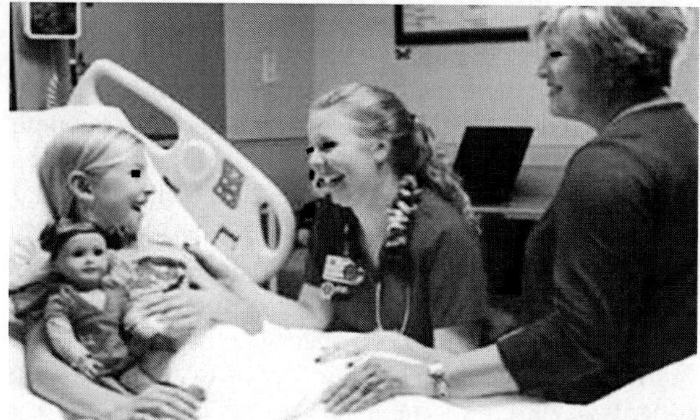

Fig. 1.5: Atraumatic care: First 'DO NO' harm to the child and her family in the health care system

and their families in the health care system (Fig. 1.5). It promote sense of comfort minimize child's separation from family. It prevents injury minimize pain, provide privacy respect religious differences. It helps to cope up stress and prepare the child before procedure. Basic principles involved in atraumatic care are: (i) prevent or minimize the child's separation from the family, (ii) promote sense of comfort and secured, (iii) prevent or minimize bodily injury and pain, and (iv) promote a sense of control.

It is an integral part of pediatric nursing care and needs to include following interventions:

- Maintaining positive, supportive and loving relationship with child
- Foster parent-child relationship during hospitalization
- Physical and mental preparation of child before any procedure
- Prevent injury and minimize pain
- Protect child's sensitivity by providing privacy
- Provide play for free expression of fear and aggression
- Involve parent (if possible) in nursing intervention to obtain child's better cooperation
- Respect cultural and religious differences child and his family.

COST CONTAINMENT

It is a management technique used to control rising cost of medical treatment. In this arrangement, clients need not to pay whatever charges determined by the hospital for their service. Instead, client will agree to pay on in advance a fixed amount of money for necessary services for specially diagnosed conditions. It is achieved in various ways in health care setting by cutting nursing positions, or improving the process of care and minimizing nonlabor resources. Last few years the government, insurance companies, hospitals and health care providers have made concerted effort to reform health care delivery system of our country and control rising cost.

The current practice of child health nursing requires nurses to aware about cost containment of adopting procedures to the specific needs of children and families. By reducing mortality rates, length of stay, cost and complications and by increasing family satisfaction and readiness and ability to function upon discharge, nurses make significant contribution to both the quality of hospital services and the containment of hospital cost.

Statistics Related to Child Health

Children represent the future, and ensuring their healthy growth and development ought to be a prime concern of all societies. Child health status is assessed through measurement of morbidity and mortality. Some recent facts are:

- 17,000 children die every day, mostly from preventable or treatable causes.
- The births of nearly 230 million children under age 5 worldwide (about one in three) have never been officially recorded, depriving them of their right to a name and nationality.
- 2.5 billion people lack access to improved sanitation, including 1 billion who are forced to resort to open defecation for lack of other options.
- Out of an estimated 35 million people living with HIV, over 2 million are 10 to 19 years old, and 56 per cent of them are girls.
- Globally, about one third of women aged 20 to 24 were child brides.
- Every 10 minutes, somewhere in the world, an adolescent girl dies as a result of violence.
- Nearly half of all deaths in children under age 5 are attributable to undernutrition. This translates into the unnecessary loss of about 3 million young lives a year.

The frequently used mortality indicators related to child health are perinatal, neonatal, post neonatal, infant mortality and under five mortality rates.

Perinatal Mortality Rate (PMR): Perinatal mortality includes both late fetal deaths (stillbirths) and early neonatal deaths. According to International Classification of Diseases, the perinatal period lasts from the 28th week of gestation to the seventh day after birth. It is calculated as:

$$PMR = \frac{\text{Late fetal and early neonatal deaths weighing above 1000 g at birth}}{\text{Total live births weighing over 1000 g at birth}} \times 1000$$

PMR has greater significance as it is a yardstick of obstetric and pediatric care before and around the time of birth. The main causes of perinatal death are intrauterine and birth asphyxia, low birth weight, birth trauma, and intrauterine or neonatal infections.

Neonatal Mortality Rate (NMR): Neonatal deaths are deaths occurring during the neonatal period, commencing at birth and ending 28 completed days after birth. NMR is the number of neonatal deaths in a given year per 1000 live births in that year. It is calculated as :

$$NMR = \frac{\text{Number of deaths of children under 28 days of age in a year}}{\text{Total live births in the same year}} \times 1000$$

Neonatal mortality is a measure of intensity with which 'endogenous factors' (i.e low birth weight, birth injuries) infect infant life. Each year, about 4 million newborns die before they are 4 weeks old and half of them die in their first 24 hours. It accounts for 40 percent of under-five mortality. Ninety eight percent of these deaths occur in developing countries. Neonatal mortality is generally related to short gestation and low birth weight, congenital malformations, and conditions originating in the perinatal period, such as maternal complications related to pregnancy or complications experienced by the newborn resulting from birth.

Postneonatal mortality rate: The annual number of deaths of infants ages 28 days to 1 year per 1,000 live births in a given year. Postneonatal mortality rate is the ratio of the number of deaths in a given year of children between the 28th day of life and the first birthday relative to the difference between the number of the live births and neonatal deaths in that year, the denominations sometimes simplified, less correctly, number of live births. The ratio is sometimes approximated as the difference between the infant mortality rate and the neonatal mortality rate.

Whereas neonatal mortality is dominated by endogenous factors, postneonatal mortality is dominated by exogenous (i.e. environmental and social) factors. The main causes of death during postneonatal periods are diarrhea and respiratory infections. Malnutrition is an additional factor, reinforcing the adverse effects of the infections. In developed countries, the main cause of postneonatal mortality is congenital anomalies. Studies show that postneonatal mortality increases steadily with birth order.

Infant mortality rate: The death of a baby before his or her first birthday is called infant mortality. The *infant mortality rate* is an estimate of the number of infant deaths for every 1,000 live births. This rate is often used as an indicator to measure the health and well-being of a nation, because factors affecting the health of entire populations can also impact the mortality rate of infants.

Under 5 mortality rate: Probability of a child born in a specific year or period dying before reaching the age of five years, expressed as a rate per 1000 live births. UNICEF considers this is as the best single indicator of social development and well-being rather than GNP per capita, as the former reflects income, nutrition, health care and basic education. The risk of a child dying before completing five years of age is still highest in the WHO African Region (90 per 1000 live births), about 7 times higher than that in the WHO European Region (12 per 1000 live births).

Reducing child mortality to achieve millennium development goal (MDG) 4: Overall, substantial progress has been made towards achieving MDG 4. The number of under-five deaths worldwide has declined from 12.7 (12.5, 12.9) million in 1990 to 6.3 (6.1, 6.7) million in 2013. This translates into 17 000 fewer children dying every day in 2013 than in 1990. About half of the world's under-five deaths in 2013 still occurred in only five countries: India, Nigeria, Pakistan, Democratic Republic of the Congo, and China. India (21%) and Nigeria (13%) together account for more than a third of under-five deaths worldwide.

Ethical Perspectives in Child Health Nursing

Pediatric nurses are trained in child development, health care and diseases of children. They deal with infants all the way up to adolescent children. These nurses are specialized in examining both the physical and psychosocial well-being of a child and often struggle with ethical and socio-cultural dilemmas. The ethical issues pediatric nurses face can be quite challenging at times, as they must often professionally solve conflicts involving a family's personal values.

Ethics: Ethics refers to well-founded (Fig. 1.6) standards of right and wrong that prescribe what humans ought to do, usually in terms of rights, obligations, benefits to society, fairness, or specific virtues. Ethical standards also include those that enjoin virtues of honesty, compassion, and loyalty. And, ethical standards include

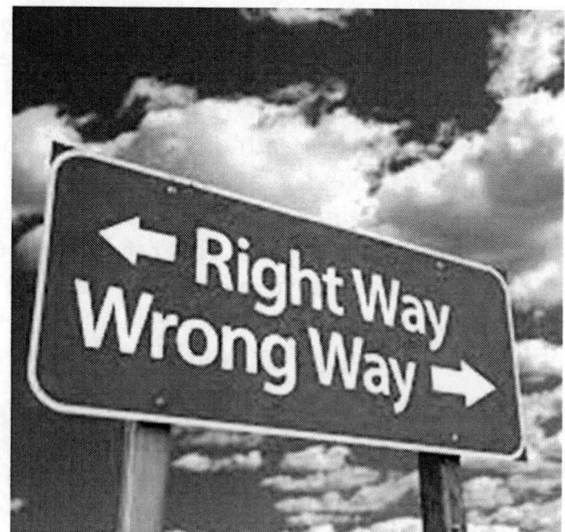

Fig. 1.6: The ethical challenges confronted by pediatric nurses

standards relating to rights, such as the right to life, the right to freedom from injury, and the right to privacy. Such standards are adequate standards of ethics because they are supported by consistent and well-founded reasons.

Nursing ethics: A valuable resource for helping to define nursing ethics is a nursing Code of Ethics. Ethical behavior for nurses is described in various codes, such as American Nurses Association Code for Nurses, Canadian Nurses Association Code for Nurses, etc. A nursing Code of Ethics is usually developed by a nursing organization that has some responsibility for defining nursing standards, explicitly stating the requirements for ethical nursing practice. Despite their various differences, most nursing Codes of Ethics agree highly on various fundamental ethical considerations, such as informed consent, respect for confidentiality, professional competence, and patient safety. The important principal values highlighted in different nursing code of ethics are providing safe, compassionate, competent and ethical care; promoting health and well-being; preserving dignity; promoting and respecting informed decision-making; maintaining privacy and confidentiality; promoting justice; and being accountable.

Bioethics: Bioethics is the application of ethics to health care. Bioethics has been very important toward the development of nursing ethics. Bioethics emerged as a new discipline in the late 1900s and helps to address growing ethical questions in the health sciences.

Ethical principles: The most widely recognized bioethical framework in the health sciences is referred to as principlism. Principlism is based on the view that clinical care has to attend to fundamental ethical principles. The most popular principlist framework in the health sciences, has been published by Beauchamp and Childress.

According to Beauchamp and Childress, four major principles that should define ethical care are autonomy, beneficence, non-maleficence, and justice. These principles are also important in solving ethical dilemmas.

The principle of autonomy is based on the right to self-determination, which is operationalized through the doctrine of informed consent. This requires that patients should be free to choose or refuse health care interventions, without pressure or coercion, and should be given all of the information needed about their condition and possible treatments/interventions, so they can make an informed choice.

The principle of justice requires fairness in determining which resources or services an individual or group will receive.

Beneficence relates to the requirement for clinicians to help others, to actively seek to do good.

Nonmaleficence refers to the Hippocratic Oath: primum non nocere. Clinicians cannot intentionally inflict harm.

Although harm may be a secondary effect of beneficial care, it cannot be desired and it should be minimized. So in some instances the caregivers and parent need to weigh the principle of beneficience against the principle of nonmaleficence.

Some ethicists have developed 'contextualist' frameworks, where 'good and bad' is understood through an analysis of the particular situation in question.

Ethical dilemmas: Ethical dilemmas, also known as a moral dilemmas, are situations in which there are two choices to be made, neither of which resolves the situation in an ethically acceptable fashion. In such cases, societal and personal ethical guidelines can provide no satisfactory outcome for the chooser. It is a situation in which no solution seems completely satisfactory. Ethical dilemmas are among the most difficult situations in nursing practice.

Common Ethical Dilemmas

Nurses need to involve in common issues on ethical decision-making in ethical dilemmas. Such issues are refusal of treatment, euthanasia, prolongation of life, prenatal genetic screening, abortion, in-vitro fertilization, allocation of scarce medical resources and rights of children in health care research, etc.

Moral dilemmas for pediatric nurses arise from power conflicts about treatment in which the nurse may need to decide whether to continue to cooperate with the health team and follow the physicians' directions or not to follow them. Legal issues related to consumer protection act, malpractice and negligence are great challenges in all areas of nursing practice and also in child care.

Ethical Concerns in Child Health Care

It can be envisioned that these problems can be particularly challenging in the context of pediatrics, where patients are commonly incapable of adequately expressing their needs. Parents must be involved in decision-making process and informed about available options. Very little literature has examined the ethical challenges confronted by pediatric nurses. However, to review ethical considerations related to the nursing care of children and their families is necessary.

Focusing on pediatric nursing, nurses practicing as moral agents should be particularly sensitized to the vulnerabilities confronted by children and their families, and actively advocate for improving their well-being.

Two of the most common ethical questions that arise in pediatric health care are: How should health care decisions for children be made? Who should make these decisions? For example, any treatment considered contrary to the child's best interests can be withheld or withdrawn, even if this may result in death (e.g. withdrawal of mechanical ventilation). Developed countries encourage society to engage in a thorough debate about the economic, cultural, social, religious and moral consequences of imposing limits on which patients should receive intensive care.

Accepted standards in palliative sedation can also be practiced with children, as long as this is based on the child's best interests and that the 'principle of double effect' is respected. In other words, sedation and analgesia can be administered in the context of end-stage terminal illness even if this happens to compromise ventilation and results in death, as long as the doses that are used are intended solely for the requirements for sedation and analgesia and not for death. If death resulted as an adverse effect of providing necessary sedation and analgesia to a dying patient, and there was no other way to manage the discomfort and pain, then the unintended death can be legally and ethically excusable.

Although young children may not have a legally recognized right to independently consent to health care, nurses, physicians, and other health care professionals should consider seeking children's assent whenever possible. Assent implies that health care information should be provided to children, adapted to their ability to understand, and their voluntary cooperation should be solicited as much as is reasonably possible. Solicitation of the child's assent would help promote attention and regard for the child's own moral outlook toward proposed health care.

A clinical ethics committee has been developed to assist patients, families, and health care teams. An ethics consultation involves a process of clarification of the principal ethical concerns, an examination of legal and ethical norms relevant for the case, and a reconciliation of these toward a plan of action that is maximally attentive to all of the morally meaningful considerations. It should be highlighted that an ethics consultant or ethics committee should not function as a 'moral police or arbiter'. These should serve as consultation resources for those who are involved with a case where there is an ethical concern. An ethics consultation can be conducted with part or all of the clinical team. This can be helpful for strengthening inter-professional collaboration. An ethics consultation can also include the patient and family, to help reconcile disagreements or conflicts to develop a cohesive plan of care.

Various ethics consultation models have been described in the literature. The rapprochement framework can be helpful in pediatrics. Rapprochement, adapted from the work of Canadian philosopher Charles Taylor, seeks to bridge the various ethical views, values, and preferences involved with the case, through a gradual cultivation of common understandings. These common understandings provide the groundwork for developing treatment agreements while strengthening the quality of the relationship between the patient, family, and health care team.

Given the complex responsibilities that pediatric nurses are required to fulfill, nurses have important insights into considerations of a child's best interests, recognition of parental perspectives and the voice of the child, as well as the particular challenges of providing nursing care in selected clinical cases. Mechanisms should be in place to assist nurses in addressing nursing-specific ethical concerns to ensure they can provide care according to respected pediatric standards. These can include the active inclusion of nurses in inter-professional team meetings to review cases or problems, where the meeting chairperson ensures that nurses have an opportunity to speak and have their concerns treated seriously. Nurses should have access to ethics consultants for discussing their ethical concerns, both privately and within a group discussion, depending on the nature of the concern. Ethics consultants should be sensitized to the moral complexities of nursing responsibility and practice. In some situations, access to a nursing ethics consultant or nursing ethics committee may be particularly important, to ensure nursing-specific concerns are adequately addressed. These ethics review and consultation processes should then seek to reconcile nursing concerns with those of others, such as physicians, patients, and families.

ADVANCED PREPARATION OF PEDIATRIC NURSE

Pediatric Nurse Specialist

Pediatric nurse specialist is another emerging concept. This advanced practice nurses provide direct care to acute and chronically ill children, and participate in the support of systems, education, and consultation in a variety of settings including intensive care units (Fig. 1.7), emergency departments, other inpatient units, as well as ambulatory, rehabilitative and specialty-based clinics. Pediatric clinical nurse specialists are the ones, responsible for any kind of emergency care. Their role involves recognizing the pediatric patients needs, both physical and emotional, and to treat them accordingly. They usually work within hospital settings. They are mostly focused on patient's education. They teach both the patients and their families how to go about the necessary care. So, growth of specialization within the field of pediatric medicine has had an impact on nursing care. Pediatric Clinical Nurse Specialists (PCNS), collaborate with members of the health care team to enhance patient care and provide clinical expertise to patients in the pediatric setting.

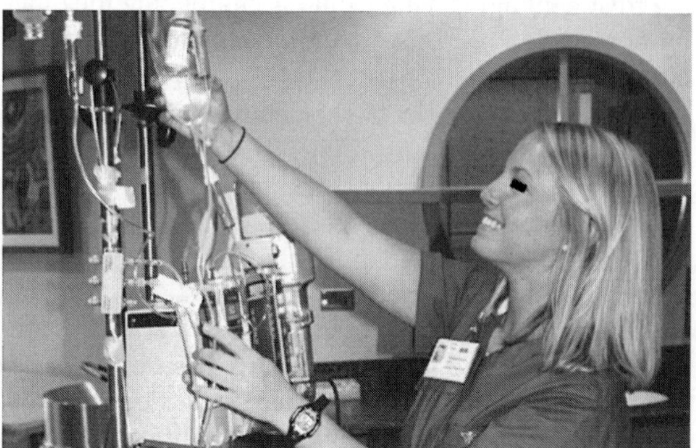

Fig. 1.7: Advanced preparation of pediatric nurse

Pediatric Nurse Practitioners

Pediatric nurse practitioners are recognized and well-accepted in developed countries. They take care of babies, young children and teenagers. This is a rising trend because everywhere nurses shoulder the major responsibilities of pediatric care, e.g. immunization, nutrition, hygienic care, demonstration, health education, etc. To provide therapies and treatments to children, nurses educate them and their families. So yes, they need broad exposure of orienting multitask skill ability training. The curriculum should combine both broad foundational knowledge essential for the care of children as a vulnerable population, as well as specialty knowledge in pediatrics. Attention is given to health promotion, prevention of disease and disability, disease process, treatment, clinical management, and family-centered care provided in a variety of community settings. The pediatric nurses can act as independent practitioner and fulfill an autonomous position as a member of an interdisciplinary health.

Pediatric Nurse Researcher

Child health nursing (CHN) is a complex field, requiring an interdisciplinary involvement and research to meet its needs. Pediatric nursing is 'the practice of nursing with children, youth, and their families across the health continuum, including health promotion, illness management, and health restoration'. Although the pediatric nurse must be knowledgeable about a wide range of medical conditions and treatment options, CHN is 'not 'med-surgical nursing' on little people'. Research in the field of CHN is needed to develop body of knowledge of both child development and safe and evidence-based child care. When PNS practice on the basis of science and research and document their practice outcomes, they validate their contributions not only to the health systems but also for the profession too.

Goal of CHN is to involve nurses in research, quality, and evidence-based practice in order to improve patient and family care outcomes. Research in CHN is important as this discipline needs more and more accuracy and scientific basis for intervention in child's body or mind. So emphasis is given towards documentation on measurable outcomes to determine the efficacy of interventions. It is necessary as pediatric nurses attempt to provide atraumatic care, that is, therapeutic care that utilizes 'interventions that eliminate or minimize the psychological and physical distress experienced by children and their families in the health care system'.

We define excellence in nursing practice as a mindset of continually evaluating care challenges and improvements that result in enhanced outcomes for the patient, the family, and the organization. This includes disseminating findings in ways that benefit the children and families of the world. For example involvement of families in the care of children was studied by different researchers and reflected in the child health nursing curriculum.

In the late nineteenth and the first half of the twentieth century, many nurses in acute care setting 'viewed mothers as unnecessary, bothersome, and at times, even harmful in the care of hospitalized children'. The effects of maternal deprivation were little understood. As a result, hospital visitation policies greatly restricted the frequency and amount of parental visits. However, it took the cumulative effect of research in the 1940s, 1950s, and 1960s on the effects of maternal deprivation to bring about real change in attitudes and policies.

Different studies in CHN established both the vital role that families play in children's lives, growth, and development and in children's care when they are ill. Family-centered care involves collaborative partnerships between families and health care professionals, built on respect for diversity and grounded in the family's strengths, choices, and values.

The child health nursing curriculum has also reflected changing attitudes and research on many issues, including the involvement of families in the care of children. While those involved in community health nursing, thought that mothers were essential for the survival of their children. In addition, the hospitalization period was viewed as a chance to educate poor children about good health habits and inculcate the values of the middle class into them without the interference of their parents.

In India, lot of studies have undertaken in the field of pediatric nursing. The goals of those researches are quality care, and evidence-based practice in order to improve patient and family care outcomes. But there is lacking in utilization of research results in evidence-based practice. The concept of evidence- based practice involves analyzing and translating published clinical research into everyday nursing practice. Moreover in our country, there is scarcity in inter-professional scholarly research in the field of pediatric and disseminating findings in ways that benefit the children and families of the world.

CONCLUSION

Remarkable changes have occurred in the field of pediatric nursing in recent years. Modern approach of child health care emphasizes on preventive care rather than curative care. Growth of specialization within the field of pediatric medicine has had an impact on nursing care of children.

Independent pediatric nurse practitioner can fulfill an autonomous position, she can also act as a member of an interdisciplinary health team. Acceptance of family-centered care of child, impart more responsibilities on pediatric nursing and pediatric nurses. Involving in research and findings newer techniques, pediatric nurses are contributing a lot in nursing sciences. Pediatric care needs specialized education and training of pediatric. Increasing number of HIV infected innocent children create problems in nurse. Problems among children due to unhealthy competition, comparison, single parent and family disruption are rising and it calls for increasing number of psychological pediatric care and nursing practices. With multi-tasking skills and knowledge, pediatric nurses provide therapies and treatments to children and they also educate them and their families.

CHAPTER 2

Family-centered Care

Chapter Outline

- The Family and Child Health Nurse
- Parenting
- Types of Family
- Role of Family in Child Health Promotion and Prevention of Diseases
- Qualities of a Child Health Nurse

The true measure of a nation's standing is how well it attends to its children—their health and safety, their material security, their education and socialization, and their sense of being loved, valued, and included in the families and societies into which they are born.

—**UNICEF**

A family can be defined as an institution where individuals related through biology or enduring commitments, and representing similar or different generations and genders, participate in roles involving mutual socialization, nurturance, and emotional commitment (Lerner, Sparks, and McCubbin, 1999). It has been said that the family is the bedrock of society and can be proven by the fact that all over the world every society is structured by the same pattern. The traditional pattern is, a man and woman marry and form a family. The family has a crucial role in society by being a model of love in three different aspects; love for the children, love between husband and wife, and finally love in promoting moral values. The parents are to be a living model of patience and kindness, showing love through their intimate relationship with his children (Fig. 2.1). The role of family is to protect and promote children's growth and development, health and well-being until the children reach maturity. Children need stable families to grow into happy and functioning adults.

Knowledge of the intricacies of child growth and development and the complexities of family and community dynamics are invaluable for an adequate appraisal of the health needs of the child and for a responsible discharge of professional service.

THE FAMILY AND CHILD HEALTH NURSE

A family is a system in which each member had a role to play and rules to respect. Members of the system are expected to respond to each other in a certain way according to their role, which is determined by relationship agreements. Within the boundaries of the system, there are subsystems, i.e. individuals. Inputs occur intrafamilial and extrafamilial which affects the whole systems means functioning of the family. For example, a newborn comes to a family affects the husband and the older child in addition to the mother. The change in roles may maintain the stability in the relationship, but it may also push the family towards a different equilibrium. So, all members of the family who

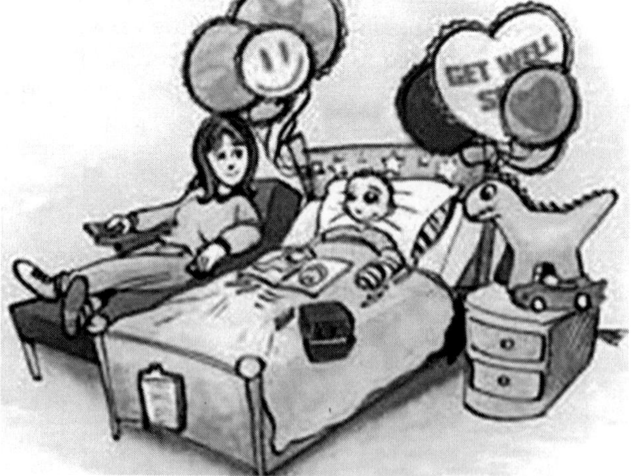

Fig. 2.1: Acceptance of newborn by parents and family

are affected by the pregnancy and child birth, must be added in a consideration of nursing interventions.

The nurses are prepared to provide care for all members of the family, including children. They play an important role in preparation of parenthood, adjustment of family with new born, or to guide them to handle different crises. But this is not an isolated work, nursing of infants and children is intimately involved with care of the child and the family. For nurses, caring for children, the whole family is the client, nurses must be aware of the dynamics of the family, various types of family structures, parenting styles, and theories that provide a basis for understanding the changes within a basis for understanding the changes within a family and for directing family-oriented interventions.

PARENTING

According to Steinberg 'There is no more important job in any society than raising children, and there is no more important influence on how children develop than their parents.' **Parenting** practices around the world share three major goals: ensuring children's health and safety, preparing children for life as productive adults and transmitting cultural values. A high-quality parent-child relationship is critical for healthy development. Good parenting, says Steinberg, is 'parenting that fosters psychological adjustment—elements like honesty, empathy, self-reliance, kindness, cooperation, self-control and cheerfulness.

Good parenting is parenting that helps children succeed in school. It promotes the development of intellectual curiosity, motivation to learn and desire to achieve. It deters children from anti-social behavior, delinquency, and drug and alcohol use. And good parenting is parenting that helps protect children against the development of anxiety, depression, eating disorders and other types of psychological distress.

Motivation for Parenthood

In all societies there is a dominant characteristic that adults are expected as parents. Usually individuals try to conform to the social role expectations which results in a generational continuity. Parents are expected to promote the physical survival and health of the children. For comfortable parenting, they need to learn the growth and development of child, interpersonal communication and basic child care skill.

Preparation for Parenthood

A new baby brings joys and challenges to a family. Parents are excited but they are also nervous because raising a child from birth do adulthood is no easy task. When parents look at it all at once it is overwhelmingly daunting. The most important things are to always, love the children, the unconditional love. The unconditional love is what will always keep the children close to parent in everything that parents do with, for, or to their children. Parents should do it out of love for them. Because raising children requires great sacrifice from the parents, be it financial sacrifices, offerings of vast amounts of time, relinquishment of freedom from responsibility or drastically changing the life plans of parent. But the best part about those sacrifices is that they are easy to make when parents love their children.

When pregnancy occurs mother needs good family support for her good health care to prevent harm to her and her baby. The family must understand the importance of thorough physical examination and detection and treatment of anemia, diabetes, tuberculosis, cardiac or renal diseases of mother. Gynecological examinations are necessary to obtain pelvic measurements and to note the growth of the fetus, so that a safe delivery can be planned. The laboratory screening must include determination of the Rh type of the mother's blood. If mother is Rh negative necessary steps are to be taken during delivery to prevent sensitization to the Rh factor. The mother should be protected from all viral and bacterial infections.

During pregnancy proper diet, rest and cleanliness are important. Diet containing essential nutrients including proteins and vitamins contributes to the well-being of the mother and promotes optimum growth in the fetus. Mothers need to avoid cigarete smoking as it reduces her oxygen supply and thus that of the fetus.

Families make health decisions for their children everyday. Ideally, they know the importance of immunizations and regular check-ups. They understand that good health depends on family routines, including healthy meals, physical activity, and discipline. And, families work with health care professionals to build the strong partnerships that are so important in supporting healthy children.

Transition to Parenthood

The transition to parenthood is one of the most common experiences in adult life. In fact, over 90% of married couples end up having children at some point in their lives. Maybe this is the reason why the experience of parents has been, at best, trivialized if not completely ignored. A baby can bring a lot of joy and happiness to their parents (Fig. 2.2A). However, caring for a baby may put a significant strain on the parents, especially on the main caretaker. Lack of sleep, difficulties with breastfeeding, lack of time for self-care, little time to connect with their partner, frustrations with the baby's routine or lack thereof can all contribute to exhaustion, irritability and a feeling of lack of control and of being overwhelmed. When the main caretaker has no help or support, the situation may be worse; the parent's mood may be adversely affected and they can develop depression. In fact, around 15% of new mothers become depressed during the first year postpartum. A baby may enrich and challenge the couple relationship in ways they may not have anticipated. Many couples that have a good relationship believe that a baby will deepen and strengthen their relationship as well as make it more complete. Some couples, whose relationship is distressed, believe that a baby will fix their relationship and make the problems go away. Indeed, some couple experience these positive changes in their relationship when they first have a baby, but many others feel that, more than anything else, the baby, who they absolutely love and adore, has put a strain on their relationship. In fact, research indicates that marital satisfaction drops significantly following the birth of a baby. Why is that?

Most importantly, when a new baby arrives, a dramatic shift in the focus of attention and energy occurs. As a childless couple, the partners could direct a lot of their attention and energy toward one another. However, when they become parents they naturally invest themselves in taking care of the baby. This is especially true for the main caretaker, which, in most cases, is the mother. As a result, one or both partners may feel neglected, unimportant or even, unloved. Fathers often complain that their partners completely immerse themselves in taking care of the baby, to the point that they feel almost completely ignored. Similarly, some mothers feel that a lot of the love, pampering and attention that they used to get from their partner is now directed exclusively toward the baby. These feelings may result in mutual resentment and emotional alienation. To make things worse, many postpartum women experience a marked decreased in sexual desire and interest that may last for a few months. It may be that fatigue and exhaustion are at least partially responsible for this phenomenon. Regardless of the reasons for the drop in desire, the reality is, that when a woman rejects her partner's sexual advances, there is a good chance that her partner will feel rejected, unloved and frustrated and may become less cooperative and more irritable and impatient. These processes may start a vicious cycle that may take its toll on the relationship.

Responsible Parenthood

A parent must:

- Protect his/her young from physical harm, even from the parent.
- Provide physical necessities, such as food, water, clothing protection from the elements.
- Provide emotional necessities, such as a nurturing home environment.
- Assist with education in preparation for the child to become a productive adult.
- Provide moral guidance so that the child can turn out to be a responsible adult.
- *Irresponsible Parenthood:* Spoiling a child is never the result of showing too much love. It is usually the consequence of giving a child things in place of love—things like leniency, lowered expectations, or material possessions.

Newborn and Adjustment of Family

Through their childbearing years, individuals decide whether or not to have children or a larger family than two. Many factors influence their decisions. Many families try to anticipate the best time for a child to come into the family. They consider job security or career levels. Some couples have financial goals they

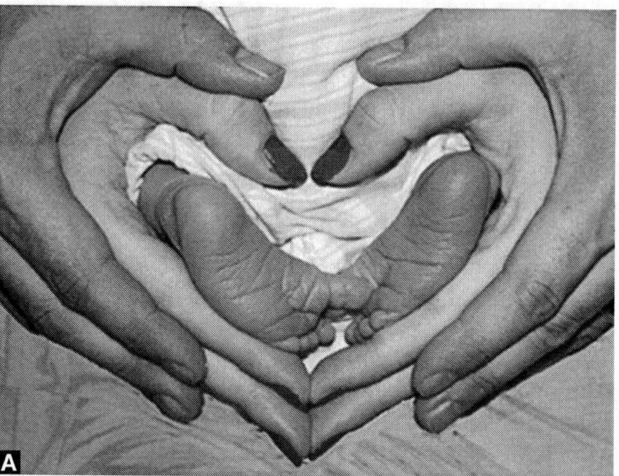

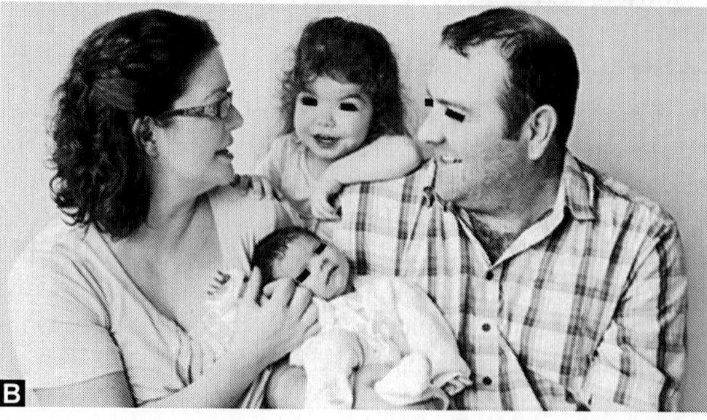

Figs 2.2A and B: Acceptance of newborn by parents and family. **A.** Acceptance of newborn by parents; **B.** Older child needs special attention from parents

would like to reach before having a child. Having a new member of the family is typically an exciting, welcomed event. Often, though, the transition from nonparent to parent is a very stressful one. Responsibilities change overnight and never change back to the way they were prior to a child. Many factors can influence how a new baby impacts a family's life, whether it is the first baby or not.

A first child may have an especially large impact on the family's routine because the couple only had themselves to worry about before the baby. With time and experience, parents learn to adjust.

Mothers and fathers may differ in some of the ways they accommodate a new infant. On the average, for example, mothers respond more frequently to their baby's signals and learn the baby's needs. Fathers are more likely to disregard cues and direct the baby's attention to other things. Fathers are also more likely to continue their leisure activities, such as reading or watching television, while the baby is present. Mothers tend to interact with the baby more. Each of these results in different relationships between parent and child.

Social support beyond the baby's other parent can increase the quality of parenting and family life. This support may come from grandparents, other family members, and friends. Using a social network helps parents not to be isolated while developing parenting skills. Others are often able to help identify and interpret child-rearing problems.

If the parent has previous experience with children, either through siblings or job experience, he or she is more likely to be efficient at problem-solving. The faster a minor problem is taken care of, the les s impact that child has on a family adapting to the new role.

Infants provide a certain amount of stress on the family, although they also may provide a guard against loneliness. This impact on family life may occur throughout the life of the child and parent. Research has shown that babies definitely impact the family in different way which *needs specific considerations.*

During the first few months after a child is born, both parents are usually exhausted from lack of sleep. They are often inexperienced in the care of a baby and have a new schedule. The constant search for answers or help from friends, family, pediatricians and books can create tension between marriage partners. Child-rearing practices can also create tension between parents. Even if the parents have discussed how a baby will be raised and disciplined, these tensions may occur. The husband-wife relationship is likely to take second priority to the ever-present needs of the new infant. There is less time for the couple to be together without the baby. Occasionally there may be feelings of resentment towards the new family member due to the lack of time for self or spouse. The parents' experiences as a child influence the way they react in the parenting role. If either parent had a difficult childhood, for example, the baby might remind the parent of negative aspects of their own experiences. As the parents adjust to the new role in the early months of the baby's life, the family may strengthen. Over time, parents are likely to be better able to define their parental role and its importance in family life.

Role of Family on Adjustment of Older Child with Newcomer

The child does not understand how to share mother with others. The child also may be very sensitive to change and may feel threatened by the idea of a new family member. Few steps may help ease the child into being a big brother or big sister:

- Parents should tell the child before he hears about the new baby from someone else. Proper explanation regarding new comer is important.
- Reassurance about love and affection is necessary for older child. The child is to be told that the baby will take a lot of parent's time and attention, before he can play with the new baby.
- The older child is to be involved in planning for the new comer, which will make him less jealous. Let him shop with parents for baby items. His own baby pictures can be shown to him. If the parents are going to use some of his old baby things, let him play with them a bit before they get them ready for the new baby. The child (boy or girl) can be given a doll so he can take care of 'his' baby.
- Older child may show regressive behavior a little. For example, the toilet-trained child might suddenly start having 'accidents,' or he might want to take a bottle. This is normal and is older child's way of making sure he still has parent's love and attention. Instead of telling him to act his age, let him have the attention he needs. Praise him when he acts more grown-up.
- The child is to be prepared for hospitalization of mother. He may be confused when mother leaves for the hospital. Explain that she will be back with the new baby in a few days.
- Older child needs special time. Read, play games, listen to music, or simply talk together. Show him that father loves him and wants to do things with him. Also, make him feel a part of things by having him cuddle next to mother when she feeds the baby.

- Older child needs special attention from others when they come to see the new baby. This will help him feel special and not left out of all the excitement. They might also give him a small gift when they bring gifts for the baby.
- Older child helps get things ready for the new baby by fixing up the baby's room, picking out clothes, or buying diapers.
- Older child can be allowed to the hospital soon after the baby is born, so she feels part of the growing family.
- *Role of older child:* The older child must feel that she has a role in caring for the baby when the new baby comes to home. Tell her she can hold the baby, although she must ask parent first. Praise her when she is gentle and loving toward the baby.
- Taking care of older child's needs and activities is important. The child will develop trust on love and affection of parents and to remind her how special she is (Fig. 2.2B).

TYPES OF FAMILY

According to family system theory, the family is considered as a system whose members continually interact with each other. An action of one family member affects other members. Different family structures can produce varying stressors. For example, the stress faced by single parent for resources is different than two parents. Nurses must have knowledge about different family structures and its function. So they will be able to meet the needs of children from many diverse family structures and home situations.

Traditional Families

Nuclear Families

In 21st century where nuclear family is a common thing. Add to this, both husband and wife are working and here comes a small baby who needs to be taken care of. Spouses or partners can role model a loving, caring and supportive relationship for their children. This will translate into future success by teaching children how to seek out positive relationships and interact well with others. Children will also benefit from watching partners work together to solve problems, delegate household responsibilities and support one another through positive and negative issues. The nuclear family can provide children with consistency, in addition to stability and can provide children with luxuries and opportunities in life. Children may be able to attend dance, gymnastics, music or other types of classes, especially both partners work outside the home. Children who are provided with these types of opportunities are more likely do better academically and socially, as well as develop confidence and time management skills.

However, the nuclear family unit can also isolate people from other relatives and relationships. This can break down the extended family unit, which can be beneficial in hard times. Grandparents, aunts and uncles should have a place within a family, but the nuclear family does not always create one for them. Conflict is a part of life, and conflict resolution skills are beneficial in school, in the community and in the workplace. While independence is a big take away from a nuclear family, it brings along with it a stream of other problems. Kids are left at daycare or at the mercy of a maid while the parents are away at work. In a joint family setup, they are looked after by a trusted family member, under whose supervision the children feel protected, loved and nurtured. When finances are on the downslide, there are always people to bail you out. But in a nuclear setup, couples problems, whether financial or emotional, are their alone. But then again, they win some and they lose some.

Extended Families

Having the support of an extended family can help parents through many of the tougher times with child raising. Extended families play an important part in at least three areas of parenting. The extended family can assist with childcare needs on a limited or full-time basis. They can come to the rescue when parents cannot see solutions to problems that they face with their children. In this case, twenty heads can be much better than two. The extended family can give a greater sense of the importance of the family reputation and name than just a single set of parents could ever do.

Many parents suffer through finding childcare providers for their small children. When these parents are attached to a strong extended family unit, childcare is rarely a problem. Often, permanent childcare solutions can be found within the extended family that will give dependable care at a large monetary savings to young parents. Because of the availability of childcare, parents will have far fewer absences from work due to problems in this area.

In an extended family that spans multiple generations, parenting help is easy to find. Questions that arise about situations in children's lives often have already been faced and answered by previous generations of family members. Having a lot of such people also means that the family will have influence in the school and other public venues that will help keep young lives out of trouble.

Extended families also can give children a sense of depth and importance that a nuclear family cannot achieve. Children can see the value of a good name extending back through multiple generations. This builds a sense of family pride and self-esteem into the child. The feeling of being with your own kind and having a place to belong cannot be overstated. The family becomes the place where you go to be accepted unconditionally.

Multigenerational Families

Many families around the world live in multigenerational household, which are defined as spanning three or more generations. There are several cultures, particularly in developing countries (Fig. 2.3). The practice has its pros and cons. It would force more of the old family continuity. But it needs very well planning. The toughest part would be the parent/grandparent clash, over the children.

It is noted in different studies, that the total care time children receive strongly differs by household structure, multigenerational households generate more care time for children than nuclear households. This difference is largely driven by grandparents who provide additional care time. Since parents' time on childcare did not differ between multigenerational and nuclear households, the childcare time generated by grandparents represent the additional time. That is, grandparents are not substituting the child care time of the parents but supplementing it. Therefore, children of multigenerational household benefit from the presence of grandparents.

Nontraditional Families

Nontraditional families like single parent families, same sex parent families, blended families and adoptive families have been emerging in society more and more. The requirements of children of these families are different, and need special care for growth and development of their children.

Single Parent Families

In modern society, single parenting can result from death, separation, child abuse/neglect, or divorce. A single parent is usually considered the primary caregiver, and who has most of the day-to-day responsibilities in raising the child or children (Fig. 2.4). If the parents are separated or divorced, children live with their custodial parent and have visitation or secondary residence with their noncustodial parent. Custody battles, awarded by the court or rationalized in other terms, determine who the child will spend majority of their time with. This affects children in many ways, and counseling is suggested for them.

A mother is typically the primary caregiver in a single parent family structure as a result of divorce or unplanned pregnancy. Single parent families in today's society have their corresponding daily struggles and long-term disadvantages. The issues of expensive day care, shortage of quality time with children, balance between work and home duties and economic struggle

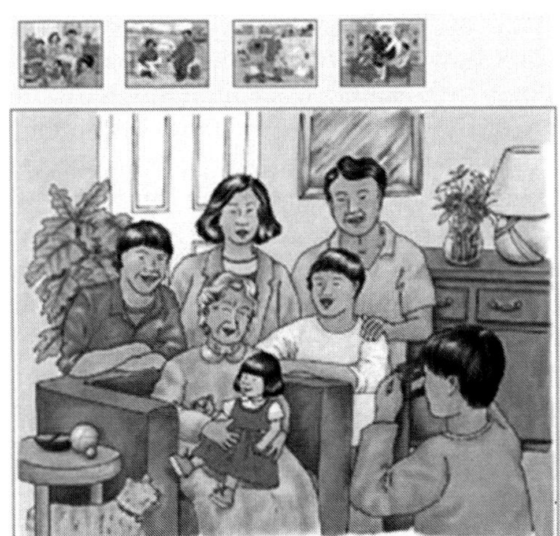

Fig. 2.3: Multi-generational family, which are defined as spanning three or more generations

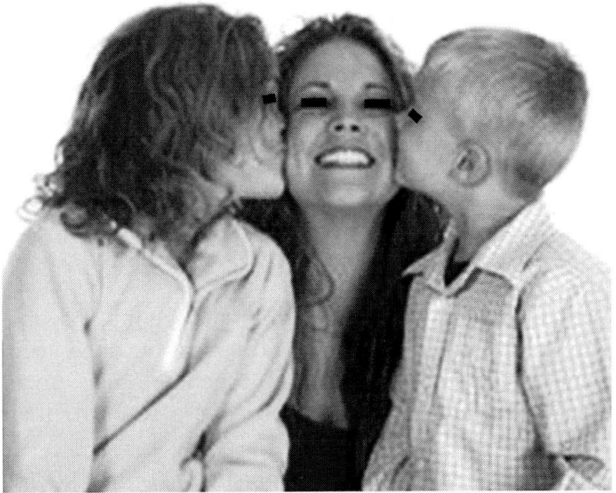

Fig. 2.4: Loving single mother with her children

are seemingly endless problems these families have to solve. Single mothers often to do over shift hours to meet up the economic burden of the family, as a result child care gets neglected. Government subsidized day care is not yet a realized dream, and many single mothers pay large amount of money for this service.

Same Sex Families

In some countries, as the social visibility and legal status of same sex families has emerged, three major concerns about the influence of lesbian and gay parents on children have been often voiced, one is that the children of lesbian and gay parents will experience more difficulties in the area of sexual identity than children of heterosexual parents. For instance, one such concern is that children brought up by lesbian mothers or gay fathers will show disturbances in gender identity and/or in gender role behavior. A second category of concerns involves aspects of children's personal development other than sexual identity. For example, some observers have expressed fears that children in the custody of gay or lesbian parents would be more vulnerable to mental breakdown, would exhibit more adjustment difficulties and behavior problems, or would be less psychologically healthy than other children. A third category of concerns is that children of lesbian and gay parents will experience difficulty in social relationships. For example, some observers have expressed concern that children living with lesbian mothers or gay fathers will be stigmatized, teased, or otherwise victimized by peers. Another common fear is that children living with gay or lesbian parents will be more likely to be sexually abused by the parent or by the parent's friends or acquaintances.

Fears about children of lesbian or gay parents being sexually abused by adults, ostracized by peers, or isolated in single-sex lesbian or gay communities have received no scientific support. Overall, results of research suggest that the development, adjustment, and well-being of children with lesbian and gay parents do not differ markedly from that of children with heterosexual parents.

Blended Families

In this family structure the children have more people in their lives that love them and care about their well-being. Parents also believe that in general, they are all more open-minded and accepting as a result of their 'untraditional' family lives.

At least one step parent, step sibling, or half sibling includes a blended family or household. A step parent is the spouse of a child's biologic parent but is not the child's biologic parent. Step siblings do not share a common biologic parent. The step parent of one child is the biologic parent of the other. This type of family structure is emerging in the society. Nurses must have knowledge about blended family for better interaction and care.

Adoptive Families

There has also been a major increase in the number of children in care placed with foster parents, which is seen as a key step towards adoption under the government's reforms. Raising healthy, happy, well-adjusted children is not easy. In fact, people wanting to parent a child who needs a home likely begin with a heart full of love and optimism. Choosing adoption is a way for many women to regain their identities as responsible, caring adults. This allows them to feel they are making up for their past failures by doing the best they can for their babies whom they feel are the innocent parties in the situation. By acting responsibly and giving their babies to loving families, these women are able to see themselves as responsible and unselfish. They feel good about themselves because they are able to see beyond their own desires and strong emotional urges to keep the children regardless of what is actually the best thing to do. But sometimes couple return home with their child and the excitement dies down and the troubles begin because they cannot handle their child, their dreams turn to muck. They find themselves alone, frightened, bereft and full of regret. They become helpless and do not know how to behave under those circumstances.

Theory of Family

The family systems theory is a theory introduced by Dr Murray Bowen suggests that individuals cannot be understood in isolation from one another, but rather as a part of their family, as the family is an emotional unit. Families are systems of interconnected and interdependent individuals, none of whom can be understood in isolation from the system. People do not exist in a vacuum. They live, interact, play, go to school, and work with other people. The social group that seems to be most universal and pervasive in the way, it shapes human behavior is the family. For social workers, counselors, community health nurses, the growing awareness of the crucial impact of families on their clients has led to the development of family systems theory.

Family systems theory is more than a therapeutic technique. It is a philosophy that searches for the causes of behavior, not in the individual alone, but in the interactions among the members of a group. The basic rationale is that all parts of the family are interrelated. Further, the family has properties of its own that can be known only by looking at the relationships and interactions among all members.

The family systems approach is based on several basic assumptions: each family is unique, due to the infinite variations in personal characteristics and cultural and ideological styles; the family is an interactional system whose component parts have constantly shifting boundaries and varying degrees of resistance to change; families must fulfill a variety of functions for each member, both collectively and individually, if each member is to grow and develop; and families pass through developmental and nondevelopmental changes that produce varying amounts of stress affecting all members, a change in the family situation means readjustment of the total system and can pose problems and challenges for every single member, a family has an invisible boundary that helps to define it as separate and different from other systems.

Table 2.1: Principles of Parenting
• *The privilege of parenting:* Children are not a possession of parents. Parenting is a privilege, not a right.
• *Children come first:* If needs of the children are taken care of, the rest falls into place.
• *Harmony conquers conflict:* Children are traumatized by conflict between their parents, not divorce.
• *Family matters:* The family does not disappear, it is redefined.
• *Stack their corner:* Parents should embrace all those who are part of their children's lives and who want the best for them.
• *Positive energy, strong energy:* A strong mental, emotional and physical strength come from a positive attitude, which all parents need.
• *Happy parent, good parent:* Parents need to take good care of themselves, to do things that make them happy and create the best life possible for them. Their children will benefit from it.
• *Self care:* Taking good care of self (parents) can help to take care of their child. They should make time for nurturing own spirit and balancing own emotions. Concept of HALT is important. Being hungry, angry, lonely or tired (HALT) impacts decisions and actions.

Parenting Style

Developmental psychologists have long been interested in how parents impact child development (Table 2.1). However, finding actual cause-and-effect links between specific actions of parents and later behavior of children is very difficult. Some children raised in dramatically different environments can later grow up to have remarkably similar personalities. Conversely, children who share a home and are raised in the same environment can grow up to have astonishingly different personalities than one another. Despite these challenges, researchers have uncovered convincing links between parenting styles and the effects these styles have on children.

Parents have definite approach to their children which is unique, as unique as they are. Parenting is not only a collection of skills, rules, and tricks of the trade. It is who parents are, what their family culture is, and how they transmit the most personal aspects of their values to their child. Parenting is challenging enough. Key factors associated with child-rearing styles include warmth, rules, behavior control, supportive responsiveness and expectations. Parenting styles affect children's traits such as achievement, independence, curiosity, self-reliance, self-control and friendliness.

But here are the facts: Nearly 50 years of research have found that some parenting styles are more effective than others and show far better outcomes for children. Studies have identified four major parenting styles, i.e. authoritarian, authoritative, permissive and hands off. Each of these parenting styles appears to have certain influences on children's behavior. However, culture also influences the outcome, especially for school success. The majority of parents fall into one of these categories most of the time. When parents are inconsistent in their parenting approach, it is very damaging to their children because they do not know what to expect. Nurses are in good position to help parents with information on effective parenting style technique through different platforms, such as parenthood classes, well baby clinic, mental health clinic, etc.

Authoritarian

Authoritarian child-rearing emphasizes obedience above all else. Sensitivity to the individual child or circumstances is not part of the authoritarian approach. Authoritarian parents aim to control children's behavior through constant direction and swift consequences. In this style children are expected to obey parents regardless of the situation, and negotiation and discussion are not tolerated. This style is also characterized by rigid adherence to rules, regardless of whether those expectations are realistic. Children raised in this style tend to rely on authority figures to make decisions for them, and they also have higher rates of depression, anxiety and poor self-esteem. The use of punitive and forceful measures to enforce proper behavior causes anger, resentment, and deceit and impairs wholesome parent-child relationships. In Baumrind's 1967 research, preschoolers with authoritarian parents are withdrawn and unhappy. They appear anxious and insecure with peers and react hostilely if frustrated. Baumrind's 1971 research shows girls to be dependent and lacking in motivation and boys much more likely to be angry and defiant.

Authoritative

Authoritative child-rearing emphasizes warmth and responsiveness to children's needs, but parents also maintain high behavioral expectations. Parents who are nurturing and set, discuss, and enforce developmentally appropriate limits are the most successful in helping their children become autonomous, independent, self-controlled, self-confident, and cooperative. These children also are more likely to have high levels of competence and high self-esteem during middle childhood and adolescence. They also internalize moral standards and their academic performance in high school is superior to that of children from either authoritarian or permissive homes.

Different studies show, parents who raise their children in this style, set limits and allow natural consequences as a means of modifying behavior. They are sensitive to their child's point of view and temperament, and they may adjust consequences or expectations accordingly. Parents also explain why certain rules are important rather than citing their authority as the reason why children should obey. According to different peer-reviewed psychology publications, authoritative parenting is considered the 'gold standard' and typically produces independent, confident children who are well-adjusted, creative and cooperative.

Permissive

Permissive or indulgent child-rearing involves lots of love, support and sensitivity, but parents have few expectations and make few demands of the child. Limits and rules are poorly enforced, and children are given significant freedom to do as they like. Parents do not correct poor behavior through discipline or instruction, and they frequently indulge the child's demands regardless of behavior. Maintaining control over the child's behavior is not as important as it is in authoritarian and authoritative child-rearing.

Children raised in this style tend to have very high self-esteem, but they are also less achievement-oriented and more likely to encounter problems with drugs and alcohol. Parents who are non-punitive, loving, and accepting of the child often have children who lack independence and are selfish because they are not taught how their actions affect others. These children tend to be impulsive, aggressive, and low in taking responsibility (Flowchart 2.1).

Uninvolved

Uninvolved child-rearing is most harmful. Not only is parental warmth and responsiveness absent, but few expectations or demands are placed on the child. Children learn not to rely on parents for anything; in extreme cases, this can include basic needs such as food and clean clothing. Parents remain unresponsive to their children, showing little to no affection or encouragement. The lack of limits also means children receive no guidance or examples of appropriate behavior. Such children are most likely to have poor self-esteem and lack the ability to cooperate. Most juvenile offenders were raised in this style of parenting. The combination of permissiveness and indifference or rejection in varying degrees has detrimental effects on children.

Positive Parenting

According to Dr Laura Markham, positive parenting means discipline, gentle guidance, or loving guidance. It is simply guidance that keeps kids on the right path, offered in a positive way that resists any temptation to be punitive. Studies show that is what helps kids learn consideration and responsibility, and makes for happier kids and parents.

Day by day the concept of positive parenting is emerging in our social psyche because study after study shows that children who are physically disciplined are more aggressive toward other children, more rebellious as teenagers, and more prone to depression and violent acting out as adults. So parents are realizing that a change must be made in child rearing practices, because all parents possess a tremendous power to make a child's life miserable or joyous.

Positive parenting is a belief, a way of living, wherein children should be treated with respect, free from fear of violence and shame, and guided with loving encouragement which encourages healthy development. Secure attachment builds resilience, paves the way for how well the child will function as an adult in a relationship, and have a positive impact on brain development.

Children are not born knowing elders rules. Punishing them for bad behavior does not teach them good behavior. Parents have to give them the tools to do better before they can expect them to do better. The

Flowchart 2.1: Child outcomes result from each parenting style

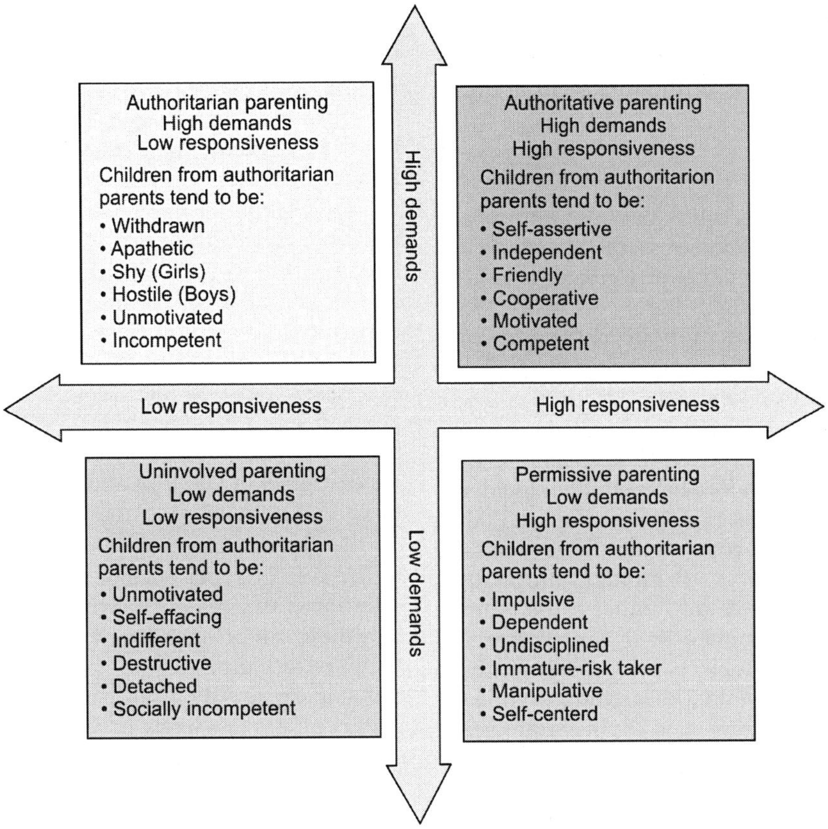

High demands

Low responsiveness

High responsiveness

Low demands

Authoritarian parenting
High demands
Low responsiveness

Children from authoritarian parents tend to be:
- Withdrawn
- Apathetic
- Shy (Girls)
- Hostile (Boys)
- Unmotivated
- Incompetent

Authoritative parenting
High demands
High responsiveness

Children from authoritarion parents tend to be:
- Self-assertive
- Independent
- Friendly
- Cooperative
- Motivated
- Competent

Uninvolved parenting
Low demands
Low responsiveness

Children from authoritarian parents tend to be:
- Unmotivated
- Self-effacing
- Indifferent
- Destructive
- Detached
- Socially incompetent

Permissive parenting
Low demands
High responsiveness

Children from authoritarian parents tend to be:
- Impulsive
- Dependent
- Undisciplined
- Immature-risk taker
- Manipulative
- Self-centerd

best parenting tools are connection, example, teaching, respect, empathy, love.

Stressors of Family Affect Child Care

Stress and chronic stress is bad for body and for the brain. Stress hormones end up swamping human bodies for days, weeks, months. Research shows that cortisol, specifically, chews up the brain if it loiters there long-term. It kills brain cells in their hippocampus region, leaving them depressed, anxious, fearful, immature, needy, and unable to learn new behaviors (e.g. stuck in the same old 'rat race'). Newer studies suggest it is not only extreme kinds of stress that can affect kids' ability to learn and think. They frequently experience school problems, have difficulty making friends, and lag behind their peers in psychosocial development. They are more likely than other children to bully and to be bullied. In 2009, Virginia Polytechnic Institute and State University scientists found that kids exposed to 'household chaos' had lower IQ and more conduct problems. A joint study between Harvard Medical School/McLean Hospital and Catholic University of Korea in 2009 found that children who experienced maternal verbal abuse had lowered verbal IQs and less white matter in their brains. (White matter affects learning by coordinating communication between different regions of the brain). Research indicates that the negative impact of stress is more profound on children who are younger than age 10, have a genetic temperament that is 'slow-to-warm-up' or 'difficult,' were born premature, are male, have limited cognitive capacity, or have experienced prenatal stress.

Our increasing knowledge about the importance and impact of stress on young children should be put to good use in reducing stress factors for young children and in assisting children to increase coping strategies and healthy responses to the unavoidable stresses in their lives.

Sickness

When serious illness or disability strikes a person, the family as a whole is affected by the disease process and by the entire health care experience. Long-term illness, even in the most stable and supportive families, brings changes in family relationships. When a mother is sick, she is unable to carry on the mothering role for her children. This illness produces disequilibrium in the family structures and affects child care a lot. If pediatric nurses do not recognize the change, what might mean to the child and family, and how it might affect the child's acceptance and ability to carry out health care recommendations, the goals of the treatment and care will be diminished.

Poverty

There exist a well-established link between poor health and low socioeconomic. The stress of poverty is not simply worries about money, poverty creates a 'context of stress', in which conflict, family violence, food insecurity and residential mobility (to name a few) are also common. This negative context is not helpful in psycho-physiological development of children.

It was hypothesized that individuals of low socioeconomic status are exposed to a greater number of stressful events and therefore have a higher incidence of psychological disorders. However, the way they interpret, evaluate and cope with these stressful situations within a context of limited information, social support, and resources may either cause them to maintain, intensify or eliminate their overall stress. It was found that non-poor subjects use problem-focused coping methods more than the other groups, while the poor use more emotionally-focused coping strategies.

Poverty affects the well-being of children, contributing to low self-worth and increased risky behavior while detracting from educational orientation and engagement in home life. The strongest negative effect appears to be on home life, followed by that on educational orientation.

Migration

Children are the most vulnerable to risk when being left behind by one or both parents, migrating with the family or alone. The well-being of children affects their development into adulthood. Migration has a serious effect on the mental health of the children regarding the process of migration, which causes stress due to the loss of family, friends, and habitual surroundings. Questions about their identity and sense of belonging, the fear of deportation, and discrimination cause problems that are taken into adulthood. The negative effect due to the lack of parental contact with children associated with long-term parental absence is poor academic other performances. Children with strong parental support do better in school and develop mature psychological traits. They aspire to do good work, experience pleasure in one's work.

Death: Death in the family affects everyone. Children, in particular, need to be thought about even if it is a difficult time for the whole family. Being aware of how children normally respond to death makes it easier for an adult to help. It also makes it easier to identify that a child is finding it particularly hard to cope with. Experience shows that children benefit from knowing the truth at an early stage. They may even want to see the dead relative. The closer the relationship, the more important this is.

The child's age and level of understanding and how the death affects their life. Children from about the age of 5 are able to understand basic facts about death; it happens to all living things; it has a cause; it involves permanent separation. They can also understand that dead people do not need to eat or drink and do not see, hear, speak or feel. Most children get angry and worried, as well as sad, about death. Anger is a natural reaction to the loss of someone who was essential to the child's sense of stability and safety. A child may show this anger in boisterous play.

Adults can also help children to cope by listening to the child's experience of the death, answering their questions, and reassuring them. Children often worry that they will be abandoned by loved ones, or fear that they are to blame for the death. If they can talk about this, and express themselves through play, they can cope better and are less likely to have emotional disturbances later in life.

Abuse

Child abuse is the physical, sexual or emotional maltreatment or neglect of a child or children. There are four major categories of child abuse: neglect, physical abuse, psychological or emotional abuse and sexual abuse. Physical abuse means shaking, hitting, beating, burning, or biting a child; in emotional or psychological abuse the child is constantly blamed or put down; excessive yelling, shaming. Sexual abuse means incest, any forced sexual activity, exposure to sexual stimulation not appropriate for the child's age. Failure to provide for the child's physical needs, such as food, clothing, shelter, and medical care is called neglect. It is also a pattern of failure to provide for the child's emotional needs, such as affection, attention, and supervision.

Children are deeply affected by abuse and find various ways to deal with their feelings of unworthiness, inadequacy, and hopelessness. Child mistrusts adults, refuses to be touched by adults. He/she shows destructive behavior, avoids the company of others. Child becomes aggressive and goes out looking for trouble, develops a habit of running away from home, school, or place of care. Child wants to kill herself (common among teenage girls).

As caregivers, nurses need to know how to help children cope as well as possible with the abuse that has happened to them. When they think of helping children or how they are coping nurses need to know in which area or areas they need help. **The potential areas are health, emotions, learning, personal relationships (HELP).**

Family Coping with Stress

In studies, it was found that parents who are obese are more likely than those who are normal weight to have children who are obese. In addition, overweight children are more likely than normal-weight children to report that their parents are often worried and stressed.

Children model their parents' behaviors, including those related to managing stress. Parents who deal with stress in unhealthy ways risk passing those behaviors on to their children. Alternatively, parents who cope with stress in healthy ways can not only promote better adjustment and happiness for themselves, but also promote the formation of critically important habits and skills in children.

Parents know that changing a child's behavior, let alone their own, can be challenging. By taking small, manageable steps to a healthier lifestyle, families can work toward meeting their goals to be psychologically and physically fit. Families can adopt following steps for a healthy path.

Evaluate Own Lifestyle

The model healthy behavior of parents has a great impact on their own children. Children are more likely to lead a healthy lifestyle and less likely to associate stress with unhealthy behaviors if the whole family practices healthy living and good stress management techniques. So, parents should ask themselves, how do they respond to stress? Do they tend to overreact or engage in other unhealthy behaviors, such as smoking and drinking alcohol, when they feel stressed? In what ways could their stress coping skills be improved?

Talk about it: If parents notice that their children are looking worried or stressed, ask them what is on their minds. Having regular conversations can help a family work together to better understand and address any stressors children are experiencing. Low levels of parental communication have been associated with poor decision-making among children and teens. Talking to your children and promoting open communication and problem-solving is just as important as eating well and getting enough exercise and sleep.

Create a healthy environment: Home, work place and even social environment can influence individual behaviors. Altering environment can help individual to alleviate stress. Clearing up own home space for the family is something parents and their children can control, and it teaches children to focus on those things they can control when feeling stressed.

Focus on one's self: The correlation between health, obesity and unhealthy choices is strong. When the parents and their family are experiencing stress, make a conscious decision to take care of family members. Get adequate doses of nutrients, physical activity and sleep. When they feel overwhelmed, it is easy sometimes to fall into cycles such as eating fast food, plugging into sedentary electronic activities like playing video games or watching TV, or not getting enough sleep. Research shows that children who are sleep-deficient are more likely to have behavioral problems, and, parents have an extraordinary amount of influence on their children's food choices. A healthy dinner followed by an activity with family, such as walking, bike riding, playing catch or a board game, and topped off with a good night's sleep can do a lot to manage or to lessen the negative effects of stress.

Change one habit at a time: Parents may aspire for their family to make multiple important changes at once such as eating healthier foods, being more physically active, getting a better night's sleep or spending more time together. However, if they are already overextended from juggling many different responsibilities, doing all of this at once can feel overwhelming. Changing behaviors usually takes time. By starting with changing one behavior, parents and their family are more likely to experience success, which can then encourage their family to tackle other challenges and to continue making additional healthy changes.

If parent or a family member continues to struggle with changing unhealthy behaviors or feels overwhelmed by stress, consider seeking help from a health professional, such as a psychologist. Psychologists are licensed and trained to help individual develop strategies to manage stress effectively and make behavioral changes to help improve their overall health.

Facilitating Parent Child Relationship

Everything children want are not to be given, or they would not appreciate any thing they have. Give them everything they *need*, but only some of what they *want*.

Teach them by example. Do not go by the old 'Do as I say, not as I do' adage.

They need praise when they do well. Positive reinforcement is the best way to teach and encourage child to want to do well. For every harsh or unfair criticism they get, it takes many, many more praises to undo the damage the harsh and unfair criticisms cause.

Screaming and yelling at them is not helpful, raising voice serves no purpose other than making *parents* feel better for the moment. And while it may make parents feel better, it can be devastating and quite destructive to a child's self-esteem. Speaking in a calm, yet firm voice can convey parents' anger. Parents have to remember they are children, and they are going to mess up from time to time, just as adults do.

Deliberate humiliation of child is to be avoided. The things that are said and done to a child can literally stay with them for the rest of their life. If they do something stupid, it is fine to call the *behavior* stupid, but *not the child*.

Criticizing children in front of their friends or in public places brings harm to them. Kids have it hard enough trying to fit in with other kids as it is, without being publicly humiliated.

Parents can say 'sorry', if realize they were wrong. Children need to realize parents are people too, and make mistakes, just as everyone else does.

Responsibilities around the house are to be given to the children, which should be age appropriate. Children learn the meaning of team work, responsibility, and get a sense of being part of the better good when they do participate in the daily chores of the household.

Parents should not make an issue of every little thing they do that annoys them, or their childhood will be one long battle. The big issues are to be tackled, but let the little ones go.

Teach them the value of money, and start early while they are young.

However, when parent has prepared a new dish children have never tasted before and they do not want to even try it, they will be strongly suggested to have them try *just one bite*. Then, if they do not like it, do not make them eat it. It would be surprised at how often they realize they *do* like it, after all. And if they never tried it, they would have never found out they actually like it. It also teaches them not to be so quick to judge something based on how it looks.

Parents should be consistent; children really do want rules and boundaries. Otherwise, they get confused and do not know what is expected of them.

Parents need to say **'I love you'** to their child every day.

ROLE OF FAMILY IN CHILD HEALTH PROMOTION AND PREVENTION OF DISEASES

Securing the health and wider well-being of children and young people is of fundamental importance. Good health makes an active and enjoyable life possible, as well as underpinning achievement in school and in due course in the work place. That is why promoting health is an integral part of care planning.

Nurses work within a primary health care model with families, their infants and young children. Primary health care aims to promote the health of individuals, families, communities and populations, and promote an environment that supports health. Nursing practice is based on a unique understanding of how the environmental context influences health, nursing theory and knowledge, social sciences and public health science with primary health care. Nurses use a strength-based, wellness focused interaction and view disease prevention, health protection and health promotion as the goals of nursing practice. Their collaborate role with individuals, families, groups, communities, other health professionals and populations help to design, implement and evaluate community development, health promotion and disease prevention strategies that build on the capacity of the individual or community. Nurses play a key role in the provision of specialist primary, secondary and tertiary level child *and family health services.*

Not only do parents have much to learn from community health nurses but nurses also can learn from families. In addition to discussing questions and problems, families should share what is going well. They can offer real-life feedback about which health recommendations were useful and which were not. Since parents are caregivers themselves, they often have learned things that might help health care professionals or other families. Nurses who encourage parents to contribute information and ideas verbally, on bulletin boards, or in other ways will find an increasing wealth of ideas to benefit children and families. And, families will be reinforced in their roles as partners in their children's health care. Communication is vital in this partnership to raise healthy children. Communication empowers families, promotes cooperation, and creates a comfortable environment where patients, families, and health care professionals can discuss any issue.

How can Parents and Their Family Foster Communication in Health Care Partnership?

Strong communication with health care professionals does not happen in one visit, but develops with work and over time. Parents need to share information with their child's health care professionals. Health care professional goes to the families for promotion of child health and their proper growth and development, and prevention of diseases. Parents want to discuss, ask questions, and they should not be afraid to take notes on what their child's health care professional says during the visit. Get more information. Often, health care professionals will have handouts and will be able to guide the families to other materials or community resources. Parents can ask what is likely to happen in the next phase of their child's development. They need to find out how and when to contact their health care professional between visits.

Different studies had explored the work of public health nurses, means the knowledge, skills, and decision-making of public health nurses in the context of their efforts to maintain and promote child and family welfare. The results indicate that the nurses' knowledge basis and skills cover the scientific concepts of health promotion and prevention of diseases. The nurses tackle existing situations in the lives of children and their family, attempt to solve the current problems, and together with parents, *make collaborative decisions*.

QUALITIES OF A CHILD HEALTH NURSE

The WHO (2000) encourages advocacy role of nurses and also encourages its expansion to work directly towards family-related support structures that influence broad social, economic and policy changes (Fig. 2.5).

The role of the nurse in family health promotion is as an advocate in dealing with complex social systems, as an identifier of community-based resources and as a direct liaison between family and community systems.

As an advocate for health promotion within the family, the nurse should give priority to the following realities:

- Safety as part of family health
- Lifestyles as part of health
- Role of family's social networks
- Coping strategies

Talking: Expressing feelings

- Positive attitude to life
- Comparisons

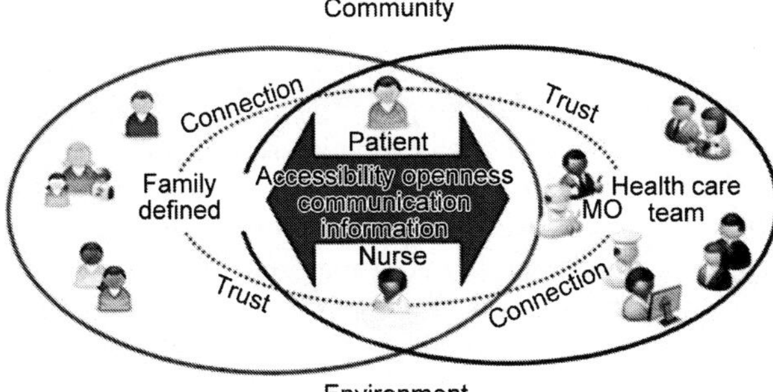

Fig. 2.5: Family-centered care and advocacy role of nurse

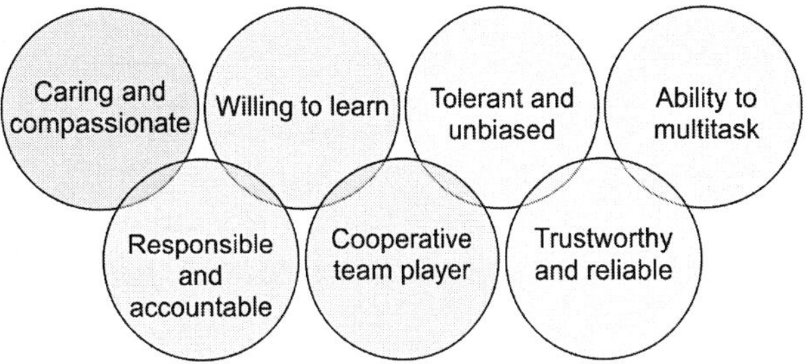

Fig. 2.6: Qualities of a child health nurse

- Common rules and agreements
- Independence of parents
- Humor
- Recognition of own limits

A nurse who is monitoring the children will become an important, trustworthy advisor for the staff, students and families treating them and guiding them for proper care wherever required (Fig. 2.6). The constant supervision by the same nurse will help people open up more since the nurse is familiar with the situations and practices there. If there is a new nurse again and again it will take time to explain, to open up, where important details can be missed out. The students will be open to clear their misconceptions, be free to express their health concerns to a known qualified health personal. The nurse monitoring the accidental cases and records can advise about areas that require improvements.

Children from families offering open communication and emotional support are linked with following healthier diets, while couples who share in decision-making and tasks while participating in common activities also have healthier lifestyles.

CONCLUSION

The success of child health programs always depend on family involvement of the child. Family-centered care is best understood by explaining the elements of this care that work together to move an individual or an institution toward providing a family-centered approach. These elements recognize each family's uniqueness and explain the influence of the family as a constant in the child's life. Health team should be flexible and creative in caring for the child within his family as their intervention are based on the needs of parent and child and on their coping resources. Although the family is the ultimate coordinator of its own care, the nurse can help establish a positive environment for family members and help them accept and utilize the care provided. She can guide family members through the unknown of new experiences in seeking holistic heal.

CHAPTER 3

Child Health Promotion

Chapter Outline

- Nutrition: Child Health
- Nutritional Policy
- Relevance to Clinical Practice
- Sleep

Children represent the future, and ensuring their healthy growth and development ought to be a prime concern of all societies.

Health promotion is the process of enabling children and families to increase control over, and to improve, their health (Fig. 3.1). It includes measures taken at the population and individual level to promote the health of children through personal skills development, building healthy public policy, and creating supportive environments. Child health promotion focuses on health rather than disease prevention and requires the active participation of individuals or families. Health promoting measures seek to ensure that children and their parents have the opportunity to adopt healthy lifestyles through the provision of education and information and health supportive environments (for example, with legislation). Therefore, health promotion is not just the responsibility of the health sector, but goes beyond health lifestyles to well-being.

There is an established body of evidence to show that what happens in the early years of a child's life has a profound impact on their future health, development and well-being. Children who have a poor start in life are more likely to develop learning, behavioral or emotional problems which may have far-reaching consequences throughout their lives and in turn, the lives of their children. These problems accrue to the whole society in the form of increased social inequality, reduced productivity and high costs associated with entrenched intergenerational disadvantage.

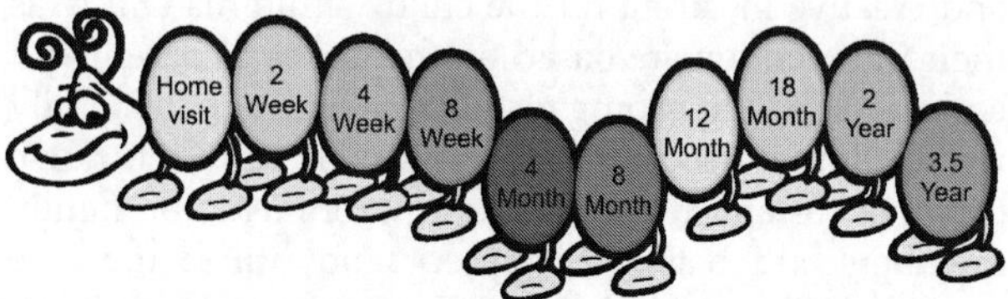

Fig. 3.1: Health promotion of child is a process

The evidence is clear that supporting and nurturing all children's development from birth is crucial to long-term health, educational, social and economic outcomes. Child health promotion also has important benefits for optimal development and education. Child health promotion includes nutrition, immunization, play, sleep, growth monitoring, etc. These health promotional aspects help in reducing infections and avoiding illness while also benefiting growth and development of children.

NUTRITION: CHILD HEALTH

Growth and development of child require the supply of adequate food from conception to maturity (Table 3.1). Food supplies the energy for physical activity and other metabolic needs of the body. The nutritional status of women when becoming pregnant and during pregnancy can have significant influence on both infant and maternal health outcomes. Pregnant women require additional supplements of energy giving foods (about 150–350 kcals/day) for the growth of the fetus and the deposition of fat which is used during lactation to meet the additional energy needs for milk secretion. Micronutrient deficiencies such as calcium, iron, vitamin A and iodine can lead to poor maternal health outcomes and pregnancy complications which put the mother and baby at risk. Poor maternal weight gain in pregnancy due to an inadequate diet, increases the risk of premature delivery, low birth weight and birth defects.

Table 3.1: Daily estimated calories and recommended servings for grains, fruits, vegetables, and milk/dairy by age and gender					
	1 Year (kcal)	*2–3 Years (kcal)*	*4–8 Years (kcal)*	*9–13 Years (kcal)*	*14–18 Years (kcal)*
Calories	900	1000			
Female			1200	1600	1800
Male			1400	1800	2200
Fat	30–40%	30–35%	25–35%	25–35%	25–35%
Milk/Dairy	2 cups	2 cups	2 cups	3 cups	3 cups
Lean Meat/Beans	1.5 oz	2 oz		5 oz	
Female			3 oz		5 oz
Male			4 oz		6 oz
Fruits	1 cup	1 cup	1.5 cups	1.5 cups	
Female					1.5 cups
Male					2 cups
Vegetables	3/4 cup	1 cup			
Female			1 cup	2 cups	2.5 cups
Male			1.5 cup	2.5 cups	3 cups
Grains	2 oz	3 oz			
Female			4 oz	5 oz	6 oz
Male			5 oz	6 oz	7 oz

The six classes of nutrients found in foods are carbohydrates, lipids (mostly fats and oils), proteins, vitamins, minerals, and water. Carbohydrates, lipids, and proteins constitute the bulk of the diet, amounting together to about 500 grams (just over one pound) per day in actual weight. These macronutrients provide raw materials for tissue building and maintenance as well as fuel to run the myriad of physiological and metabolic activities that sustain life. In contrast are the micronutrients, which are not themselves energy sources but facilitate metabolic processes throughout the body: vitamins, of which humans need about 300 milligrams per day in the diet, and minerals, of which about 20 grams per day are needed. The last nutrient category is water, which provides the medium in which all the body's metabolic processes occur.

Nutrients are needed for maintaining growth of the individual, and for repair of the worn out and ageing tissues. Food is necessary for synthesis of basic constituents of digestive juices, enzymes and hormones. Inappropriate infant and young child-feeding practices (breastfeeding and complementary feeding) can cause a major cause of malnutrition. Accelerating interventions aimed at improving infant and young child feeding at community level is a key priority in the effort to improve survival, growth, and development of children with equity (Table 3.2).

Energy

The amount of energy that food and drink contains is measured in both kilojoules (kJ) and kilocalories (kcal) and is commonly referred to as calories. Body needs calorie for energy and it depends on the person's age, sex, height, weight and level of physical activity. Children

Table 3.2: Daily requirement for water and calorie		
Age range	*Water requirement (mL/kg)*	*Calorie requirement (cals/kg)*
First 3 days	80–100	120
3 to 10 days	125–150	120
15 days to 3 m	140–160	120
3 months to 1 year	150	110–115
1 year to 3 years	125	100
4 years to 6 years	100	90
7 to 9 years	75	80
10 to 12 years and above	50	70

Table 3.3: Calories needed each day for boys and men

Age	*Not active*	*Somewhat active*	*Very active*
2–3 years	1,000–1,200 calories	1,000–1,400 calories	1,000–1,400 calories
4–8 years	1,200–1,400 calories	1,400–1,600 calories	1,600–2,000 calories
9–13 years	1,600–2,000 calories	1,800–2,200 calories	2,000–2,600 calories
14–18 years	2,000–2,400 calories	2,400–2,800 calories	2,800–3,200 calories
Calories needed each day for girls and women			
2–3 years	1,000 calories	1,000–1,200 calories	1,000–1,400 calories
4–8 years	1,200–1,400 calories	1,400–1,600 calories	1,400–1,800 calories
9–13 years	1,400–1,600 calories	1,600–2,000 calories	1,800–2,200 calories
14–18 years	1,800 calories	2,000 calories	2,400 calories

(*Source:* HHS/USDA Dietary Guidelines for Americans, 2010)

need sufficient calories to support rapid growth. Any health promotion counseling during childhood and adolescence needs to include an emphasis on energy and calories requirement, food selection and its servings (Table. 3.3).

It is important to keep in mind that although all calorie-containing foods provide energy, food must also provide children with a banquet of essential nutrients. Choosing a diet based on the Food Guide Pyramid (Fig. 3.2) is one of the best ways for children to get all the nutrients they need to grow healthy and strong while avoiding excess calories.

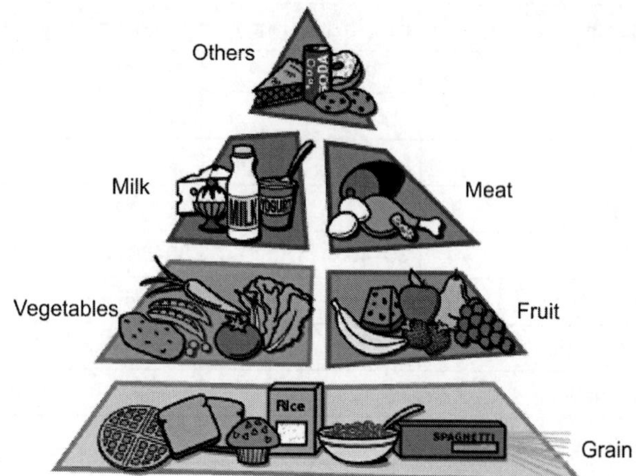

Fig. 3.2: Food groups needed for child

Breastfeeding (BF)

BF is the feeding of the infant or young child with breast milk directly from female breast rather than a baby bottle or container.

WHO recommendations:

- Initiation of BF within one hour after birth
- Exclusive BF for 6 months
- Continue BF up to first 2 years or more

(Discussed in Chapter 5: Stages of Pediatric Life)

Formula Feeding

Infant formula is 'a food which purports to be or is represented for special dietary use solely as a food for infants by reason of its simulation of human milk or its suitability as a complete or partial substitute for human milk' (Federal Food, Drug, and Cosmetic Act, US). Infant formula is a manufactured food designed and marketed for feeding to babies and infants under 12 months of age, usually prepared for bottle-feeding or cup-feeding from powder (mixed with water) or liquid (with or without additional water).

In 2003, the WHO and UNICEF published their *Global Strategy for Infant and Young Child Feeding*, which restated that 'processed-food products for infants and young children should, when sold or otherwise distributed, meet applicable standards recommended by the Codex Alimentarius Commission', and also warned that 'lack of breastfeeding—and especially lack of exclusive breastfeeding during the first half-year of life—are important risk factors for infant and childhood morbidity and mortality'. In particular, the use of infant formula in less economically developed countries is linked to poorer health outcomes because of the prevalence of unsanitary preparation conditions, including lack of clean water and lack of sanitizing equipment. Infant formula does not have the immunologic properties and digestibility of human milk, but it does meet the energy and nutrient requirements of infants.

Formula feeding is used due to some physiologic and other reasons like the mother is infected with HIV or has active tuberculosis. She is malnourished, extremely ill or has had certain kinds of breast surgery. She is taking any kind of drug that could harm the baby, or drinks unsafe levels of alcohol. The baby is unable to breastfeed as she/he has a birth defect or inborn error of metabolism such as galactosemia that makes breastfeeding difficult or impossible.

The mother may dislike breastfeeding or think it inconvenient. In addition, breastfeeding can be difficult for victims of rape or sexual abuse; for example, it may be a trigger for posttraumatic stress disorder. Many families bottle feed to increase the father's role in parenting his child. The child is adopted, orphaned, abandoned, or in the sole custody of a man. The mother is separated from her child by being in prison or a mental hospital. The mother has left the child in the care of another person for an extended period of time, such as while traveling or working abroad.

Use of infant formula has been cited for numerous increased health risks. Studies have found infants in developed countries who consume formula are at increased risk for acute otitis media, gastroenteritis, severe lower respiratory tract infections, atopic dermatitis, asthma, obesity, type 1 and 2 diabetes, eczema and necrotizing enterocolitis when compared to infants who are breastfed. Some studies have found an association between infant formula and lower cognitive development, including iron supplementation in baby formula being linked to lowered IQ and other neurodevelopmental delays, however, other studies have found no correlation.

In addition, mothers who forego breastfeeding in favor of formula feeding are reported more likely to develop certain types of cancer.

Formula Feeding and Responsibility of the Health Professional

The health professional has a responsibility to meet the WHO recommendations for infant feeding, Article 4:2. The health professional's responsibilities to women who choose to artificially feed their babies are to:

- Ensure they have made an informed choice and are aware of the benefits of breast milk/breastfeeding.
- Ensure they are aware of the financial costs for providing feeding equipment and providing formula until the infant is 12 months old.
- Document in the infant's clinical records the feeding choice of the mother.
- Initiate a documented feeding plan that includes the appropriate volume and frequency of feeds for age and weight of the baby.
- Provide one-on-one education on the safe administration of artificial feeding including the correct preparation of formula, safe storage, sterilization techniques, and how to bottle-feed.
- The opportunity exists for the mother to provide her own feeding equipment for the infant.
- No feeding equipment or formula is to be given to a mother or family unless it is specialized and or prescribed.

Cow's milk: In the first 12 months, cow's milk is not recommended as it is hard curd is difficult to digest and contains too little iron. Moreover its high renal solute load and unmodified derivatives can put small infants at risk of dehydration. The infants on cow's milk show more incidences of allergy and iron deficiency anemia than in those who receive breast milk or formula.

Human milk contains, on average, 1.1% protein, 4.2% fat, 7.0% lactose (a sugar), and supplies 72 kcal of energy per 100 grams.

Cow milk contains, on average, 3.4% protein, 3.6% fat, and 4.6% lactose, 0.7% minerals and supplies 66 kcal of energy per 100 grams. See also nutritional value further on.

Types of Formulas

Formula can be available in different forms, like ready to use preparations, concentrated liquid, powdered formula. Most commonly used formula is powdered formula. It is most convenient and economical as it can be mixed one bottle at a time without waste. Powdered formula is prepared as per direction of manufacturer, mixed with warm water and usually one scoop milk (21 cals) is added to 30 mL of water. Some formulas are designed for feeding low birth weight or ill infants. These include high calorie formula (24 cal) and pre-digested formula. In a day newborn infants consume 2 to 3 ounces of formula per feeding in six to eight feedings.

Formula feeding is based on scientific principles of nutrition and sterilization. An adequate fluid intake should be 100 mL per kg of the expected body weight of infant.

- Always hold the baby close to you and look into his eyes when feeding. This helps the baby feel safe and loved.
- Try to hold the baby fairly upright, with his head supported in a comfortable, neutral position.
- Hold the bottle horizontal to the ground, tilting it just enough to ensure that the baby is taking milk, not air, through the teat. Babies feed in bursts of sucking with short pauses to rest. In this position, when your baby pauses for a rest, the milk will stop flowing, allowing him to have a short rest before starting to suck again.
- Brush the teat against his lips and when he opens his mouth wide with his tongue down, help him draw the teat in.

- Baby may need short breaks during the feed; he may also need to burp sometimes.
- Interrupting the feed from time to time also gives the baby a chance to register how 'full' he is, and thus control his intake. Baby needs to be able to relate to those caring for him. Aim to keep the number of people who feed him as small as possible. The baby should always be held and never be left unattended while feeding from a bottle.

Complementary Feeding/Weaning

It is well recognized that the period from birth to two years of age is the 'critical window' for the promotion of optimal growth, health, and development. The transition from exclusive breastfeeding to family foods, referred to as complementary feeding, typically covers the period from 6 to 18–24 months of age, and is a very vulnerable period. Insufficient quantities and inadequate quality of complementary foods, poor child-feeding practices and high rates of infections have a detrimental impact on health and growth in these important years. It is the time when malnutrition starts in many infants, contributing significantly to the high prevalence of malnutrition in children under five years of age world-wide. WHO estimates that 2 out of 5 children are stunted in low-income countries. Even with optimum breastfeeding children will become stunted, if they do not receive sufficient quantities of quality complementary foods after six months of age (Lancet 2008). An estimated six per cent or six hundred thousand under-five deaths can be prevented by ensuring optimal complementary feeding.

Definition

The transition from exclusive breastfeeding to family foods, referred to as complementary feeding, typically covers the period from 6 to 18–24 months of age. Complementary feeding (commonly known as **weaning**) means introducing a variety of foods gradually to a baby, alongside the usual milk feeds, until he or she is eating the same healthy foods as the rest of the family (Fig. 3.3). The weaning stage is an opportunity to emphasize healthy eating and help parents set up good eating habits and a healthy diet for life for their children.

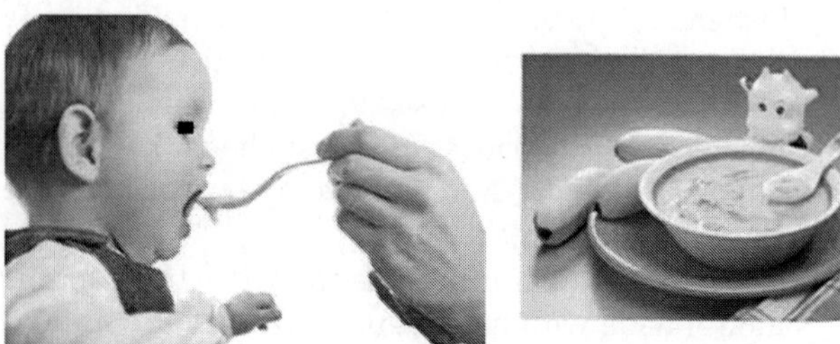

Fig. 3.3: Complementary feeding of a child

Appropriate complementary feeding is:

- *Timely:* Meaning that foods are introduced when the need for energy and nutrients
- Exceeds what can be provided through exclusive and frequent breastfeeding
- *Adequate:* Meaning that foods provide sufficient energy, protein, and micronutrients
- To meet a growing child's nutritional needs
- *Safe:* Meaning that foods are hygienically stored and prepared, and fed with clean
- Hands using clean utensils and not bottles and teats;
- *Properly fed:* Meaning that foods are given consistent with a child's signals of appetite and satiety, and that meal frequency and feeding method actively encouraging the child to consume sufficient food using fingers, spoon or self-feeding, are suitable for age.

Principles

Improving complementary feeding requires attention to foods as well as to feeding behavior of caregivers. Infants and young children need assistance that is appropriate for their age and developmental needs to ensure that they consume adequate amounts of complementary food.

WHO recommends that infants start receiving complementary foods at 6 months of age in addition to breast milk. This is due to the developmental readiness of babies' digestive systems and their kidneys and in the first six months of life. It is best for a baby to get all their nutritional needs from breast milk.

Gradually increasing food consistency and variety as the child gets older: Feed mashed and semi-solid (thick gruel) foods by 6 months of age. Feed energy-dense soft foods to 6–11 months. Introduce snacks that can be eaten by children alone by 8 months and family foods by 12 months.

Diversifying the diet to improve quality and micronutrient intake: Feed vitamin A rich fruits and vegetables daily. Feed meat, poultry, or fish daily or as often as possible. Use fortified foods or other staples, when available. Vitamin-mineral supplements are needed when animal products and/or fortified foods are not available.

Infant feeding is to be done directly and assist older children when they feed themselves, being sensitive to their hunger and satiety cues; feeding should be done slowly and patiently, and encourage children to eat, but do not force them; if children refuse many foods, experiment with different food combinations, tastes, textures and methods of encouragement; minimize distractions during meals if the child loses interest easily; remember that feeding times are periods of learning and love—talk to children during feeding, with eye to eye contact.

Food Preparation and Food Hygiene

Practicing good hygiene and proper handling of foods: Wash caregivers and children's hands before and after food preparation and feeding. Serve food immediately after preparation. Use clean utensils to prepare and serve food. Serve using clean cups and bowls, and never use feeding bottles which difficult to clean.

Feeding Technique

Complementary Feeding at Different Age

Increase the number of times that the child is fed complementary foods as he/she gets older (Fig. 3.4). The appropriate number of feedings depends on the energy density of the local foods and the usual amounts consumed at each feeding. For the average healthy breastfed infant, meals of complementary foods should be provided 2–3 times per day at 6–8 months of age and 3–4 times per day at 9–11 and 12–24 months of age. Additional nutritious snacks (such as a piece of fruit or bread or chapatti with nut paste) may be offered 1–2 times per day, as desired. Snacks are defined as foods eaten between meals, usually self-fed (Fig. 3.5), convenient and easy to prepare. If energy density or amount of food per meal is low, or the child is no longer breastfed, more frequent meals may be required.

Feeding Problems

A pediatric feeding disorder is a condition in which a child does not eat enough to provide adequate nutrition, calories or hydration. Feeding problems are considered to

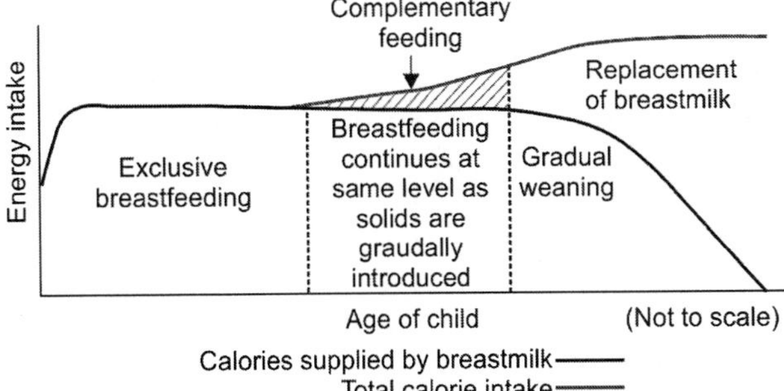

Fig. 3.4: The *complementary feeding*—meaning the period between exclusive breastfeeding and complete weaning

WEANING FOODS

- By 8 months, most infants can also eat 'finger foods' (snacks that can be eaten by children alone)
- By 12 months, most children can eat the same types of foods as consumed by the rest of the family
- Avoid foods that my cause choking (i.e. items that have shape and/or consistency that nuts, grapes, raw carrots)
- Avoid giving drinks with low nutrient value, such as tea, coffee and sugary drinks such as soda
- Limit the amount of juice offered so that to avoid displacing more nutrient-rich foods

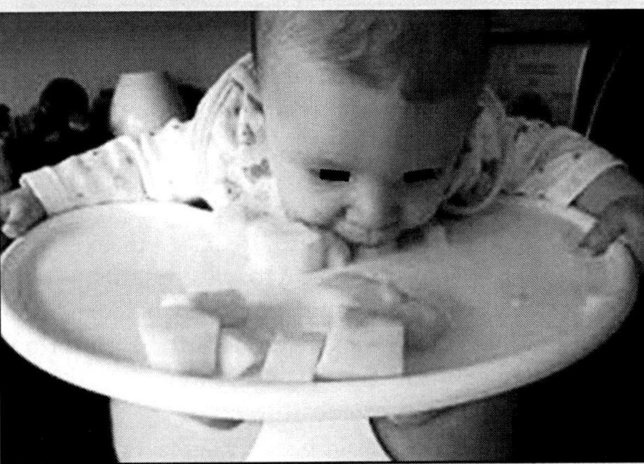

Fig. 3.5: Snacks are defined as foods eaten between meals and child learns to take it on her own

be pediatric feeding/eating disorders only if a child is safe to eat by mouth. The identification of feeding problems in infancy and early childhood is no simple task because there is no universally accepted definition or classification system. If the child is experiencing physiological issues, which make eating or drinking unsafe, the feeding problem is not considered to be feeding disorder, rather neuro-developmental disabilities.

One common definition of feeding problems is the inability or refusal to eat certain foods. Problems with feeding may lead to significant negative nutritional, developmental and psychological sequelae. Because the severity of these sequelae is related to the age at onset, degree and duration of the feeding problem, early recognition and management are important.

An in-depth feeding history is necessary for information about present feeding habits but also to understand the feeding patterns of the child from birth. A review of growth parameters–height and weight– is an essential part of any comprehensive assessment of feeding problems because it can help to identify children with growth failure. Meal time observation of child is also important. Observation should focus on child-feeder interactions, the child's oral motor skills and behaviors, the caregiver's responses to adaptive and maladaptive feeding behaviors, and the feeding's surroundings.

Balanced Diet for Children

A balanced diet is a description of food combination, consists of the five major food groups the proteins, carbohydrates, vitamins, fats and minerals. The food groups should be taken in portions in a meal so as to attain a balanced diet. A balanced **diet** is one that helps maintain or improve general health. It provides the body with essential nutrition: fluid, adequate essential amino acids from protein, essential fatty acids, vitamins, minerals, and adequate calories (Figs 3.6A and B). The requirements for this diet can be met from a variety of plant-based and animal-based foods. A healthy diet supports energy needs and provides for human nutrition without exposure to toxicity or excessive weight gain from consuming excessive amounts. Where lack of calories is not an issue, a properly balanced diet (in addition to exercise) is also thought to be important for lowering health risks, such as obesity, heart disease, type 2 diabetes, hypertension and cancer.

Infancy is the most rapid period of growth in human life. Infants are expected to triple their weight by age one, according to the Academy of Nutrition and Dietetics. In addition, early childhood is an important period for cognitive, behavioral, and physical development. A balanced diet is one of the most important factors for ensuring that a child reaches optimal development. It means that his body needs all kinds of food for proper growth which are only present in balanced diet. A balanced diet keeps children fit and healthy so they can have fun and enjoy life.

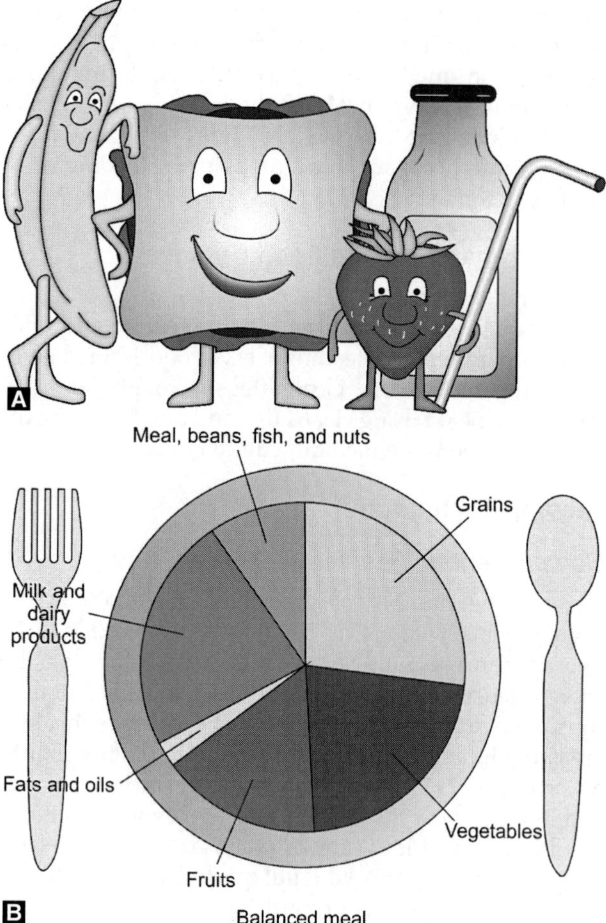

Figs 3.6A and B: Balanced diet for children

Children who eat a variety of healthy foods feel better and are able to enjoy a better quality of life; eating a balanced diet also can prevent serious health problems as children grow into adulthood. Child's overall development depends upon his/her dietary habits. A stipulated amount of oils, the essential fatty acids aid in proper functioning of the brain and help in maintaining mental health. Folates refers to vitamin B which helps produce red blood cells. Green leafy vegetables and citrus fruits are good sources of folate. Vitamin A is required for the proper growth and development of cells and is good for the eyes. Carrots, pumpkin are rich sources of vitamin A and vitamin C, an antioxidant, helps in iron absorption. Fruits like apples, grapes, oranges are rich in vitamin C. Deficiency of vitamin D causes rickets in children. Eggs and oily fish contain vitamin D. Fibers should be incorporated in the diet to prevent constipation. Fibers help in proper digestion and body metabolism. Proper water intake is needed to prevent dehydration.

A balanced diet for children is necessary to boost their energy levels. What children eat affects their growth, their behavior, their performance in schools their self-esteem, their mood, eyesight, motor skills and can either lower the risk of osteoporosis and other diseases. Nutrition is especially important to children under the age of six because that is when their brain is developing. A proper diet can keep child fit and healthy, while processed food and junk food may tickle the taste buds. The eating habits children learn at an early age will often stay with them through adulthood, which is why it is necessary to develop healthy eating habits. Along with a balanced meal of vegetables, lean meats, fruits and dairy, child should also exercise regularly. Children older than the age of 2 should get at least

30 minutes of daily rigorous physical activity, according to the American Heart Association.

Assessment of Nutritional Status

Health and development are intimately interconnected. Meeting primary health care needs and the nutritional requirement of children are fundamental to the achievement of sustainable development. Anthropometric measurements to assess growth and development of children, are the most widely used indicators of nutritional status in a community (Discussed detail in Chapter 7: Assessment of Pediatric Patient).

Counseling for Nutrition

Nutrition counseling of young families offers a tangible means to implement preventive measures for lifestyle-related chronic diseases. Nurses in health clinics are at prime position to execute this preventive work, which demands knowledge of current nutrition research as well as skill in counseling.

Nurses considered nutrition counseling an important but challenging task in the clinics. In addition to promotion of health, they had counseled clients in the management of various disorders ranging from constipation to coeliac disease. Variability was noted in the extent to which nurses had adopted nutrition guidelines. As means to improve counseling, better collaboration with both families and health care professionals and an increase in resources, including time available for counseling, up-to-date educational material and clinical guidelines, as well as increased education in nutrition were suggested.

By training health workers to assess nutritional status and feeding problems, to provide appropriate feeding counseling and to give follow-up recommendations, caretaker knowledge and behavior is expected to improve. Consequently, the child's intake of energy and other nutrients should improve, with an impact on nutritional status and morbidity.

NUTRITIONAL POLICY

Every child has a right to adequate nutrition and to be safeguarded against hunger, deprivation and malnutrition. The State commits to securing this right for all children through access, provision and promotion of required services and supports for holistic nurturing, well-being with nutritive attainment of all children, keeping in view their individual needs at different stages of life in a life cycle approach.

'National Nutrition Policy' was adopted by the Government of India in 1993 under the aegis of the Department of Women and Child Development. It advocated a multi-sectoral strategy for eradicating malnutrition and achieving optimum nutrition for all. The policy advocates the monitoring the nutrition levels across the country and sensitizing government machinery on the need for good nutrition and prevention of malnutrition. The National Nutrition Policy also includes the Food and Nutrition Board, which develops posters, audio jingles and video spots for disseminating correct facts about breastfeeding and complementary feeding.

In India, undernutrition levels remain persistently and unacceptably high—especially in utero and in the first two years of life, in adolescent girls and in women across the life cycle, in disadvantaged/excluded community groups and those living in areas or conditions of nutritional vulnerability. Taking cognizance of the problem of hunger and malnutrition in the country, different nutritional programs have been undertaken by Government of India (ICDS program, Mid-day meal program, NRHM, Food Security Program, **Nutrition Programme for Adolescent Girls (NPAG) National Iodine Deficiency Disorder Control Programme, etc).** The highest priority is being accorded to combating malnutrition, through concerted multisectoral action to address the immediate, underlying and basic determinants of under nutrition.

What is the relationship between child nutrition and school outcomes?

Recent research has shown that poor health and nutrition among children reduces their time in school and their learning during that time. This implies that programs or policies that increase children's health status could also improve their education outcomes. Good nutrition helps students show up at school prepared to learn. Because improvements in nutrition make students healthier, students are likely to have fewer absences and attend class more frequently. Studies show that malnutrition leads to behavior problems (Fig. 3.7). However, these effects can be counteracted when children consume a balanced diet that includes protein, fat, complex carbohydrates, and fiber. Thus students will have more time in class, and students will have fewer interruptions in learning over the course of the school year. Additionally, students' behavior may improve and cause fewer disruptions in the classroom, creating a better learning environment for each student in the class. Every student has the potential to do well in school. Failing to provide good nutrition puts them at risk for missing out on meeting that potential. However, taking action today to provide healthier choices in schools can help to set students up for a successful future full of possibilities.

Role of Nurse in Nutritional Counseling

The results demonstrated a need and a readiness amongst nurses to develop nutrition counseling in

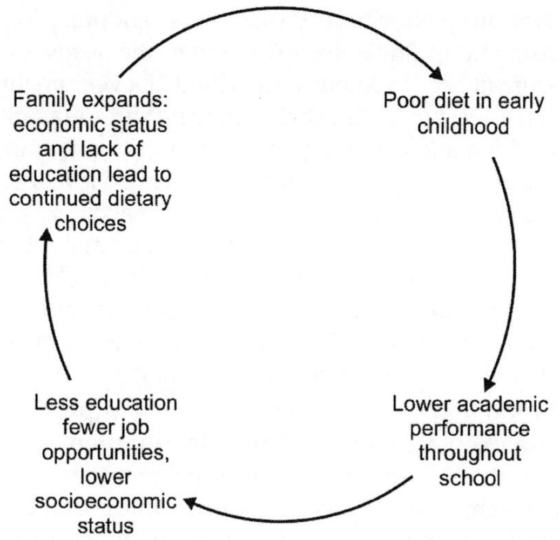

Fig. 3.7: Cycle shows relationship between nutrition and academic performance

health clinics. Given the health benefits presumably deriving from nutrition counseling, investments in operational counseling, comprising advancement of both knowledge and skills in the health clinics, are clearly warranted.

RELEVANCE TO CLINICAL PRACTICE

Immunization

Immunization is one of the safest and most effective methods of preventing childhood diseases. Under the Universal Immunization Programme (UIP), significant achievements have been made in preventing and controlling Vaccine Preventable Diseases (VPDs). Immunization has to be sustained has a high priority to further reduce the incidence of all VPDs, control measles, eliminate tetanus and eradicate poliomyelitis. Full immunization (i.e. received one dose of BCG, three doses of DPT, Hep B and OPV each and one dose of Measles before one year of age) gives a child the best chance for a healthy life. Preventing diseases before it occurs saves money, energy, and lives. Immunization is a key strategy to child survival (Figs 3.8A to C). By protecting infants from VPDs, immunization significantly lowers morbidity and mortality rates in children. The security provided to families can lead to lower birth rates. Immunization is an indicator of a strong primary health care system.

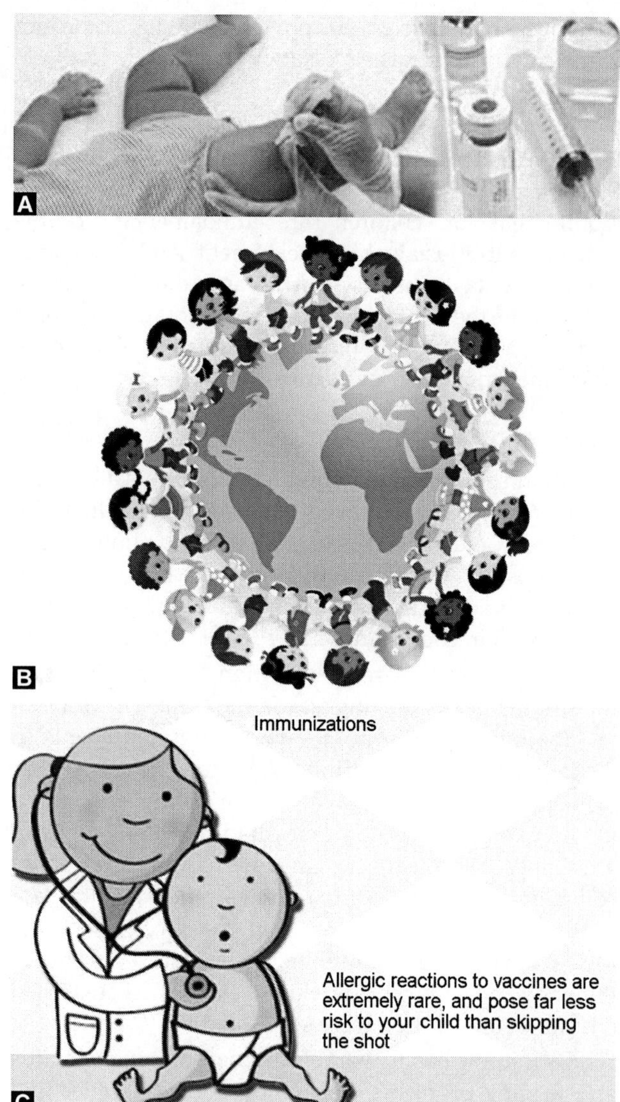

Figs 3.8A to C: Immunization of children

Immunization Coverage

Although health for all by 2000 has not been achieved in many countries including India, improving child health remains one of the top priorities since signing of the World Summit for Children 1990. Immunization is recognized as one of the most cost-effective interventions to achieve Millennium Development Goal 4—the reduction of under-five mortality rates by two-thirds in 2015. To know the immunization coverage is important to eradicate, eliminate or reduce six most common vaccine-preventable diseases. Immunization coverage can be defined as the percent of people who receive one or more vaccine(s) of interest in relation to the overall population. Monitoring trends in coverage is important in order to identify the potential for outbreaks of vaccine-preventable diseases (i.e. when coverage rates drop in a population, that population has increased chances of having a vaccine-preventable disease outbreak). In addition, monitoring also guides the authority to recommend where public health should allocate its resources, such as to improving access to immunization services or to public education efforts.

Vaccine preventable diseases are responsible for about 25% of the 10 million deaths occurring annually among children under 5 years of age.

Immunization coverage is decided by various determinants including, demographic and including government and many non-governmental organizations. Some assessments are done on a regular timely basis and some are cross-sectional studies (standalone events). These assessments provide valuable information about the impact of immunization, reach, logistic and programmatic issues. Hence, it is important to ensure that these coverage surveys are conducted to optimum standards. Socioeconomic characteristics like child's sex, mother's education, place of residence, religion, caste, culture and tradition. The other important set of determinants includes availability, accessibility and quality of services.

Immunization coverage is assessed using rigorous research methods by various agencies.

Vaccine Prevented Diseases

Tuberculosis (TB) is caused by a bacteria (*Mycobacterium tuberculosis*). It is highly contagious disease that affects the lungs but can also affect the intestine, bones and joints, lymph glands, meninges, and other tissue of the body.

Polio is a viral infection that affects the nervous system can cause severe illness, paralysis and even death. Due to intensive immunization campaigns, there has been a very significant decline of polio cases in the country.

Diphtheria is caused by bacteria (*Corynebacterium diphtheriae*). Diphtheria is an infectious disease that commonly infects the tonsils and pharynx, forming a membrane that can lead to obstructed breathing and death.

Pertussis, commonly known as (Whooping cough), is caused by bacteria (*Bordetella pertussis*). Pertussis is a highly contagious bacterial disease, involving the respiratory tract. It is characterized by repeated cough that may lead to aspiration and possible death, in a few cases.

Tetanus is caused by bacteria (*clostridium tetani*). People of all ages can become infected with tetanus.

Measles is a highly infectious illness caused by a virus that can be found in the nose, mouth or throat of an infected person. Infection is characterized by fever, cough and spreading rash that may lead to death due to secondary infections like diarrhea and pneumonia.

Hepatitis B is a highly infectious disease (40–100 times more infectious than HIV) and is the leading cause of jaundice, fulminant liver disease, cirrhosis and liver cancer.

Expanded Program of Immunization (EPI) and Universal Immunization Program (UIP)

Following the WHO recommendation, India introduced six vaccines under the expanded EP) in 1978 to reduce child mortality. [Bacillus Calmette-Guerin (BCG), TT, DPT, DT, polio, and typhoid] in its EPI.

Subsequently, in 1985 the Indian government included measles vaccination and launched the UIP and a mission to achieve immunization coverage of all infants and pregnant women by the 1990's. Diseases protected by vaccination under UIP are 1. Diphtheria 2. Pertussis 3. Tetanus 4. Polio 5. Tuberculosis 6. Measles 7. Hepatitis B 8. Japanese Encephalitis (commonly known as brain fever) 9. Meningitis and Pneumonia caused by *Haemophilus Influenzae* type B.

Pentavalent vaccines: A pentavalent vaccine is five individual vaccines conjugated in one intended to actively protect infant children from 5 potentially deadly diseases: whooping cough, tetanus, diphtheria, hepatitis B and *Haemophilus Influenza* type B (a bacteria that causes meningitis, pneumonia and otitis).

Pentavalent vaccine introduced in several states in India, i.e. Tamil Nadu, Kerala, Haryana, J & K, Gujarat, Karnataka, Goa, Puducherry, Andhra Pradesh, Telengana, etc.

National Immunization Schedule

The national immunization schedule comprises of those vaccines that are given free of cost to all children of the country under EPI (Table 3.4).

What is AEFI surveillance?

Adverse event following immunization (AEFI) surveillance in India started in 1988. The WHO defines AEFI as 'a medical incident that takes place after an immunization, causes concern, and believed to be caused by immunization'. There is an evolving AEFI surveillance system in India for the vaccines delivered through universal immunization program (UIP) of government sector. AEFI surveillance in country monitors immunization safety, detects and responds to adverse events following immunization; corrects unsafe immunization practices, reduces the negative impact of the event on health and contributes to the quality of immunization activities.

Table 3.4: National immunization schedule

Age	*Vaccines*
Birth	BCG, OPV0 (for institutional deliveries)
6 weeks	DTwP1, OPV1, HepB1, (BCG if not given at birth)
10 weeks	DTwP2, OPV2, HepB2, Hib2
14 weeks	DTwP3, POV3, HepB3, Hib3
9–12 months	Measles
16–24 months	DTwP B1, OPV4, MMR
5–6 years	DTwP
10 years	TT**
16 years	TT
Pregnant women	TT1 (early in pregnancy)
	TT2 (1 month later)
	TT booster (if vaccinated in past 3 years)
	Vitamin A 9, 18, 24, 30 and 36 months
Other immunization Japanese Encephalitis (JE) vaccination (in selected high disease burden districts) Lyophilized vaccine Japanese Encephalitis	Subcutaneous 2 doses. 9-12 months of age and 2nd dose at 16-24 months (6 month after vaccination drive)
Hib containing Pentavalent vaccine DPT + HepB + Hib (pneumonia and meningitis)	3 Intramuscular doses. 6, 10 and 14 week of age

*A second dose of DTwP vaccine should be given at an interval of one month if there is no clear history or documented evidence of previous immunization with DTwP

**A second dose of TT vaccine should be given at an interval of one month if there is no clear history or documented evidence of previous immunization with DTwP, DT or TT vaccines

Growth Monitoring

Growth monitoring is a screening tool to diagnose nutritional, chronic systemic and endocrine disease at an early stage. It is necessary to identify children with growth deviation, i.e. undernutrition and over nutrition and to identify diseases and conditions that manifest through abnormal growth. Monitoring the growth of a child requires taking the same measurements at regular intervals, approximately at the same time of the day, and seeing how they change (Discussed in Chapter 4: Growth and Development of Child).

Play

Physical activity can have an impact on child health and development, and may be affected by access to local recreational facilities such as sporting clubs; sufficient time for children to engage in physical activities; and positive parental and sporting role models.

Play is essential to development because it contributes to the cognitive, physical, social, and emotional well-being of children and youth. Play is so important to optimal child development that it has been recognized by the United Nations High Commission for Human Rights as a right of every child. Play allows children to use their creativity while developing their imagination, dexterity, and physical, cognitive, and emotional strength. Play is important to healthy brain development. It is through play that children at a very early age engage and interact in the world around them. Play allows children to create and explore a world they can master, conquering their fears while practicing adult roles, sometimes in conjunction with other children. So the every child deserves the opportunity to develop to their unique potential, child advocates must consider all factors that interfere with optimal development and press for circumstances that allow each child to fully reap the advantages associated with play (Figs 3.9A and B).

Communication Development

Play provides opportunities for children to develop and also to practice listening. Children practice both verbal and nonverbal communication skills by negotiating roles, trying to gain access to ongoing play, and appreciating the feelings of others. Whether their play is companion-based with a sibling, peer, or parent, or solo play using imagination, children talk and listen while playing. Parent can be excited to hear their child sitting in the corner of room interacting with toys and hearing her play one character, then another, as the toys interact. It can be invigorating to watch male child dresses up and act as a superhero.

Play Helps with Relationship

Play promotes social interaction, and social skills and competence. Children who play, both with parents and peers, learn how relationships work through their play experiences. The number of friendships and the quality of their friendships will also usually increase as play becomes more prevalent.

Boosts Cognitive Development

Imaginative play and role-playing are particularly powerful kinds of play that help the brain develop in more functional and positive ways. Children who engage in these kinds of play have a more sophisticated level of interaction with others and with their environment

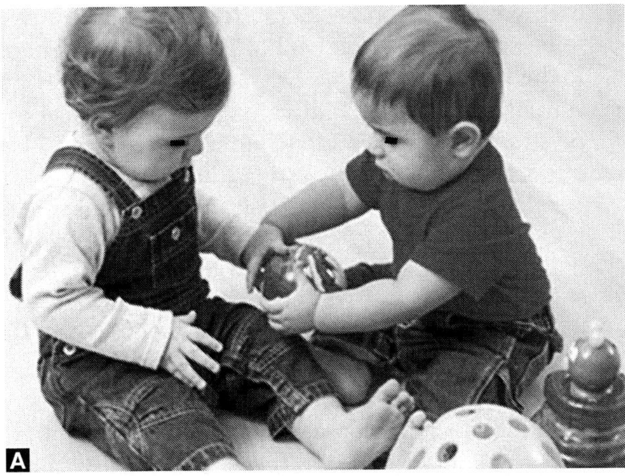

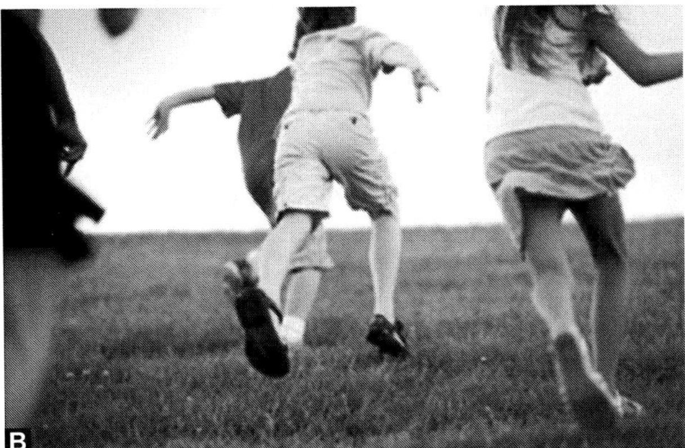

Figs 3.9A and B: A. Development and social interaction of toddlers; **B.** Play in different levels

than those who do not. This is particularly evident in studies of children who watch high levels of television in comparison to children who spend more time playing.

Social and Emotional Development

Children express their feelings in play. They also learn to cope with their feelings as they act out being angry, sad, or worried in a situation they control (Erikson, 1963). Pretend play allows them to think out loud about experiences charged with both pleasant and unpleasant. When play is allowed to be child driven, children practice decision-making skills, move at their own pace, discover their own areas of interest, and ultimately engage fully in the passions they wish to pursue.

For some children, the hurried lifestyle is a source of stress and anxiety and may even contribute to depression. Increased pressure to achieve is likely to manifest in school avoidance and somatic symptoms. The challenge for society, schools, and parents is to strike the balance that allows all children to reach their potential without pushing them beyond their personal comfort limits and while allowing them personal free playtime.

Role of Nurse

Play, the birthright of children, is challenged by forces including child labor and exploitation practices, neighborhood violence, and the limited resources available to children living in poverty. However, even those children who are fortunate enough to have abundant available resources and who live in relative peace may not be receiving the full benefits of play. Many of these children are being raised in an increasingly hurried and pressured style that may limit the protective benefits they would gain from child-driven play. The overriding premise is that play (or some available free time) is essential to the cognitive, physical, social, and emotional well-being of children and youth.

Moreover, so many conflicting messages about what parents should do to prepare their child for what is perceived to be an increasingly complicated, competitive world, child health/community health nurses have a natural role to serve as caring, objective child professionals with whom parents can discuss their approach to child rearing and reflect on their own desires for their children. Because nurses have a unique and important role in promoting the physical, emotional, and social well-being of children and adolescents, it is important that they promote strategies that will support children to be flexible and to reduce excessive stressors in their lives.

- Child health nurse can promote free play as a healthy, essential part of childhood. They should recommend that all children are afforded ample, unscheduled, independent, non-screen time to be creative, to reflect, and to decompress. They should emphasize that although parents can certainly monitor play for safety, a large proportion of play should be child-driven rather than adult-directed.
- Advantages of active play and discourage parents from the overuse of passive entertainment (e.g. television and computer games).
- Nurses should emphasize the importance of physical activities/play on growth and development of child.
- The benefits of 'true toys' such as blocks and dolls, with which children use their imagination fully, over passive toys that require limited imagination, should be explained to parents.
- Nurses can educate families regarding the protective assets and increased resiliency developed through free play and some unscheduled time.

- Nurses can aware about play and role of parent. It has observed that parent who share unscheduled spontaneous time with their children and who play with their children are being wonderfully supportive, nurturing, and productive.
- Nurses can discuss that, although very well intentioned, arranging the finest opportunities for their children may not be parents' best opportunity for influence and that shuttling their children between numerous activities may not be the best quality time. Children will be poised for success, basking in the knowledge that their parents absolutely and unconditionally love them. This love and attention is the best demonstrated when parents serve as role models and family members make time to cherish one another: time to be together, to listen, and to talk, nothing more and nothing less.
- Nurses can help the parents to understand that the most valuable and useful character traits that will prepare their children for success arise not from extracurricular or academic commitments but from a firm grounding in parental love, role modeling, and guidance.
- Nurses can reinforce the parents that the cornerstones of parenting—listening, caring, and guiding through effective and developmentally appropriate discipline—and sharing pleasurable time together are the true predictors of childhood, and they serve as a springboard toward a happy, successful adulthood.
- Parents can seek help to evaluate the claims made by marketers and advertisers about the products or interventions designed to produce super-children. So, nurses must be oriented about the products and can suggest parents the age appropriate toys for children.
- Nurses should emphasize the proven benefits of reading to their children, even at very early ages. They can give information to parents about available community resources (school, library, play facilities) after school hours and on weekends.
- Nurses can be available to parents as sounding boards to help parents evaluate the specific needs of their child in terms of promoting resiliency, developing confidence and competence, and ultimately enhancing that child's trajectory toward a successful future.
- To explore a variety of interests in a balanced way without feeling pressured to excel in each area can be done. But nurses should encourage parents to avoid conveying the unrealistic expectation that each young person needs to excel in multiple areas to be considered successful or prepared to compete in the world
- As parents choose child care and early education programs for their children, nurses can reinforce the importance of choosing settings that offer more than 'academic preparedness.' They should be guided to also pay attention to whether the settings attend to the social and emotional developmental needs of the children.
- Nurses can join with other child professionals and parents to advocate for educational settings that promote optimal academic, cognitive, physical, social, and emotional development for children and youth.
- Nurses should assess their patients for the manifestations of stress, anxiety, and depression in family-centered interviews for children and privately conducted interviews with adolescents.

National Institute for Play

The National Institute for Play is a non-profit public benefit corporation committed to bringing the unrealized knowledge, practices and benefits of play into public life. It is gathering research from diverse play scientists and practitioners, initiating projects to expand the clinical scientific knowledge of human play and translating this emerging body of knowledge into programs and resources which deliver the transformative power of play to all segments of society.

SLEEP

Every living creature needs to sleep. It is the primary activity of the brain during early development. Circadian rhythms, or the sleep-wake cycle, are regulated by light and dark and these rhythms take time to develop, resulting in the irregular sleep schedules of newborns. The rhythms begin to develop at about six weeks, and by three to six months most infants have a regular sleep-wake cycle. Sleep is especially important for children as it directly impacts mental and physical development. A protein hormone secreted by the pituitary gland called growth hormone (or 'human growth hormone') is a key player in these events. Several factors affect its production, including nutrition, stress, and exercise. In young children, though, the most important factor is sleep.

Sleep is a vital need, essential to a child's health and growth. Sleep promotes alertness, memory and performance. A child needs uninterrupted sufficient amount of sleep with age appropriate naps. Healthy sleep allows optimal alertness, a child remains calm

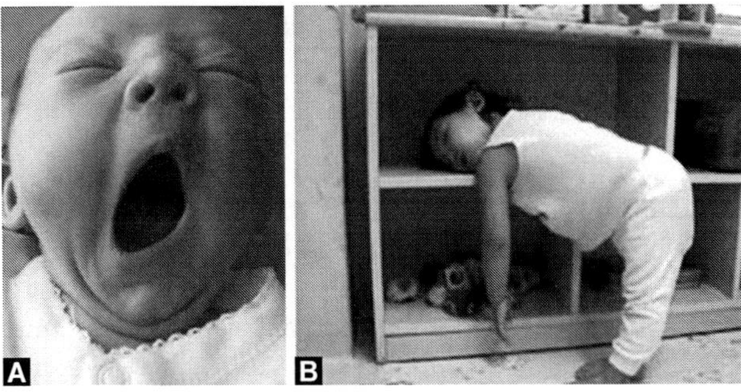

Figs 3.10A and B: Child and sleep

Table 3.5: Child and Sleep

Age	*Hours of sleep*
2 months	10.5–18
2–12 months	14–15
1–3 years	12–14
3–5 years	11–13
5–12 years	10–11

and attentive, pleasant, with wide eyes looking around, absorbing everything in the environment. Children simply must have a sufficient amount of sleep to grow, develop, and function optimally (Figs 3.10A and B). Children who get enough sleep are more likely to function better and are less prone to behavioral problems and moodiness. That is why it is important for parents to start early and help their children develop good sleep habits. Each child is different and has different sleep needs. This chart presents recommended hours of sleep that includes naps for children up to five years of age (Table 3.5).

When man slowly falls asleep, he/she begins to enter the five different stages of sleep:

Stage 1: In this stage, your brain gives the signal to your muscles to relax. It also tells your heart to beat a little slower, and your body temperature drops a bit.

Stage 2: After a little while, you enter stage 2, which is a light sleep. You can still be woken up easily during this stage. For example, if your sister pokes you or you hear a car horn outside, you will probably wake up.

Stage 3: When you are in this stage, you are in a deeper sleep, also called slow-wave sleep. Your brain sends a message to your blood pressure to get lower. Your body is not sensitive to the temperature of the air around you, which means that you would not notice if it's a little hot or cold in your room. It is much harder to be awakened when you are in this stage, but some people may sleepwalk or talk in their sleep at this point.

Stage 4: This is the deepest sleep yet and is also considered slow-wave sleep. It is very hard to wake up from this stage of sleep, and if you do wake up, you are sure to be out of it and confused for at least a few minutes. Like they do in stage 3, some people may sleepwalk or talk in their sleep when going from stage 4 to a lighter stage of sleep.

Rapid eye movement (REM): Even though the muscles in the rest of your body are totally relaxed, your eyes move back and forth very quickly beneath your eyelids. The REM stage is when your heart beats faster and your breathing is less regular. This is also the stage when people dream!

The stages 2, 3, 4, and REM are repeated about every 90 minutes until man wakes up in the morning. For most kids, that is about four or five times a night. 'Sleep is the power source that keeps human mind alert and calm. Every night and at every nap, sleep recharges the brain's battery. Sleeping well increases brainpower just as weight lifting builds stronger muscles, because sleeping well increases attention span and allows human being to be physically relaxed and mentally alert at the same time. Then man is at his/her personal best.'

Safety of Children

Children are our nation's most precious resource, but as children, they often lack the skills to protect themselves. All children are at risk for injury because of their normal curiosity, impulsiveness, and impatience. It is elders' responsibility, as parents and teachers, neighbors, friends to guard children and to teach them the skills to be safe. Injury risks are different around the world, but all children, whether rich or poor, living in an industrialized nation or living in rural poverty, have the right to grow up healthy and safe.

- Working with families to teach them how to keep their kids safe from injuries
- Social stories to discuss with children
- Basic 'people safety' skills for protecting emotional and physical well-being
- Solutions to potential problems such as bullying and stranger safety
- Researching what injuries are causing the most harm and how to prevent them
- Advocating for laws and regulations that will protect children

- Providing lifesaving devices such as child safety seats, helmets and smoke alarms to families in need
- Bringing together communities and governments, NGOs, clubs to save children's lives.

Directions for Adults on how to Introduce Personal Safety to Children 3 to 10 Years

Prevention of Injury

Everyday more than 2000 children and teenagers die from unintentional injury like road traffic injuries, drowning, burns, falls and poisoning, which could have been prevented. There is a plea to keep kids safe by promoting evidence-based injury prevention interventions and sustained investment by all sectors (WHO/UNICEF Report).

Mechanisms of injury are rooted in a complex web of social, economic, environmental, criminal, and behavioral factors that necessitate a multifaceted, systemic of injury prevention approach. This is a largely neglected area of public health and account for a significant health burden for all populations. Nurses need to hold positive attitudes and to become proactive towards injury prevention activities in the home and in the institution. The activities most commonly undertaken employ an educational model on safety education. Different experiences emphasize a more integrated approach to injury prevention and thus to increase the awareness of the children and adults. It has been observed that injury counseling is a cost-effective method of preventing childhood injuries and should be more widely adopted.

Safety for Children—Teaching Strategies

Injury prevention is a relatively new concept of child health promotion. The term accident, has its implied meaning of an avoidable situation or set of circumstances over which one has control or is able to exercise control but fails to do so due to ignorance, lack of understanding or intelligence, behavioral based actions or inaction and is normally caused either by one person or another. So this term has been replaced by injury, and primary focus goes to injury prevention through safety education.

Family Rules

Establishing a system of 'family rules' about personal safety is a good way to teach children the difference between safe and unsafe situations. Many families already have rules about bedtime, TV watching, chores, and the like. By adopting rules about personal safety, parents can teach good habits through reinforcement and repetition without generating excessive fear. The following suggestions for personal safety rules can be incorporated into a family routine.

Inside Rules

- Children should know their complete home address, telephone number including area code, and parents' first and last names.
- If children are old enough to answer the telephone, they should be taught how to dial emergency number.
- Children should be taught not to reveal any personal information about themselves or their family (their name, address, school) over the phone or to a stranger without a parent's permission.
- If children are home alone and answer the telephone, teach them to say that the parent cannot come to the phone right now and take a message, or ask the person to call again later.
- Have a 'code' worked out with your children if you do not want them to answer any telephone calls but yours when they are home alone.
- Teach your children not to open the door until they know the identity of the person knocking. Then teach them to whom they are allowed to open the door to. Just because they know the person at the door does not mean they should open the door to them.
- Children should be taught how to lock and unlock the doors in the home.

Other Rules

- Establish a system of accountability. Learn the full names, addresses, and telephone numbers of your children's friends and parents. Verify the information with the parents of your child's friend. Learn the 'rules' of the friends' houses. Who will be there when your child is there? The parents? Other children? Other neighbors? Will the children be alone?
- Know your children's routes to and from school, the playground, best friends' houses. Insist that the children stick to that route, NO SHORTCUTS! If you have to look for the children, you will know where to begin.
- Children need to be taught never to go anywhere with anyone, on foot or in a vehicle, without parent permission. This includes getting permission a second time if plans change and calling home for permission to go to a different friend's houses or play location.

- Teach children not to play in isolated areas of parks and playgrounds. The 'buddy' system should be used to enter public restrooms.
- Teach your children what to do if they are walking to school or to a friend's house and they are being bothered or followed. Walk these common routes with your children and point out safe locations. A safe location can be a school, library, police station, store, or neighbor's house, anywhere that they can find a responsible adult or lots of people.
- Knocking on the door of a stranger is a last resort. If the child has no other choice because someone is bothering or following them, teach them to select a house with lights on at night or a house with children's toys visible. Teach the child to ask the person who answers the door to phone the police because they are being followed or bothered, but teach them NOT to go inside a stranger's house.
- If there is no safe place for your child to receive help, teach your child to run away as fast as possible, screaming and yelling for help to attract as much attention as possible.
- Teach your child not to take ride from unknown person. If the car follows them or anyone gets out of the car and approaches them, teach them to run to a safe place screaming and yelling as fast as they can.

Bad Guy Rules

- Teach children that bad guys might act nice and even offer gifts of toys or money. Make sure that they know NOT to accept gifts from strangers.
- Teach children that bad guys lie and that they should not believe them. Especially if the stranger tells them things like, 'Your mom told me to pick you up after school,' or 'Can you help me find my lost puppy?'
- Bad guys even use threats like, 'I will hurt your mother if you do not come with me right now.'
- Teach children that bad guys are people who ask them to violate family rules, including someone telling your child that they do not need permission to get a ride home, or that it is okay to come into a house without mom's permission, or, 'Let's keep this a secret.'

Injury Prevention and Attainment of Child Health

The prevention of accidents of children requires an understanding of growth and development of children. The causes and types of injury are closely related to the child's level of growth and development at the time of accident. Once the child is able to move around, his mobility and in addition to innate curiosity may put the child in extreme danger. They lack the ability to perceive potential dangers and also lack the physical coordination to protect his/her from danger. Nurses need to educate the parents about injury prevention in one to one, or one to many sessions (Fig. 3.11).

Child injury prevention can be integrated with broader child and adolescent health promotion strategies. Healthy public policy—a key health promotion tool–is an essential component of child injury prevention, as indicated by the impact of enforced legislation and regulations. Health-promoting initiatives in schools can incorporate injury prevention and safety promotion in policies designed to create a healthy school environment and also in the curricula of school health programs aimed at students. Similarly, child-injury prevention can be taken up by 'healthy cities' programs in areas where the burden is large but not currently on the agenda. Community-led approaches to child injury prevention can work well and make a good match with the community-based approaches at the foundation of many health promotion initiatives. Finally, education, skills development and behavior change approaches to child injury prevention can be integrated with health

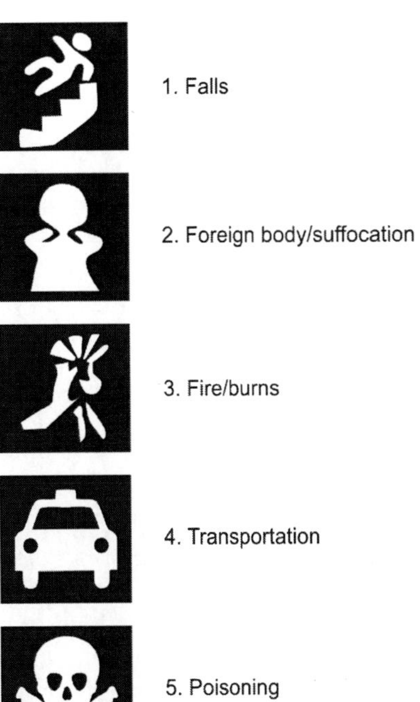

Fig. 3.11: Leading causes of injury/hospitalization (0–5 years)

promotion campaigns designed to change child and adolescent behavior (WHO Report on Injury Prevention of Children).

CONCLUSION

Children have the right to health, a safe environment and protection from injury. Countries that have signed the Convention on the Rights of the Child are obliged to take legislative, administrative, social and educational measures to ensure to the maximum extent the survival and development of the child; this obligation includes proper nutrition, immunization, play, safe environment and protecting children from injury. Unless the multisectoral initiatives are disseminated and implemented in a timely manner worldwide, the burden of children's morbidity and mortality will increase. The obstacles that currently hinder progress in child health can be partially overcome by integrating child health in the larger health agenda of the country, both in policy and in practice.

CHAPTER 4

Growth and Development of Child

Chapter Outline

- Concepts of Growth and Development
- Influences of Heredity on Growth and Development
- Importance of Learning Growth and Development
- Overview of Growth and Development
- Stages of Growth and Development
- Parameters of Growth and Development
- Growth Monitoring and Growth Chart
- Principles of Child Development
- Factors Affect Growth and Development of Child
- Theory of Growth and Development of Child
- Psychoanalytic Theory
- Psychosocial—Developmental Theory
- Cognitive Development Theory
- Summary of Cognitive Development
- Lev Vygotsky's Social Development Theory

CONCEPTS OF GROWTH AND DEVELOPMENT

Human development is a lifelong process of physical, behavioral, cognitive, and emotional growth and change (Fig. 4.1). The period of growth and development extends throughout the life cycle; however, the period in which the principal changes occur is in the early stages of life—from conception to childhood, childhood to adolescence, and adolescence to adulthood—enormous changes take place. Throughout the process, each person develops attitudes and values that guide choices, relationships, and understanding. Growth and development are interdependent, inter-related process. Growth generally takes place during the first 20 years of life; development continues beyond that.

Generally, people think that the two terms 'growth' and 'development' are the same. People use these two terms interchangeably. However, in the field of physical education it is not so. They are both different terms with different meanings.

Growth

Growth refers to an increase in physical size of the whole or any of its part. Growth is the growth of the organs of an individual and indicators of growth include height, weight, bone size, and dentition. The change, i.e. in form of size, height or growth can be measured in centimeters or inches, or in pounds or kilograms.

Growth rates vary during different stages of growth and development. The growth rate is rapid during the prenatal, neonatal, infancy and adolescent stages and slows during childhood. Physical growth is minimal during adulthood.

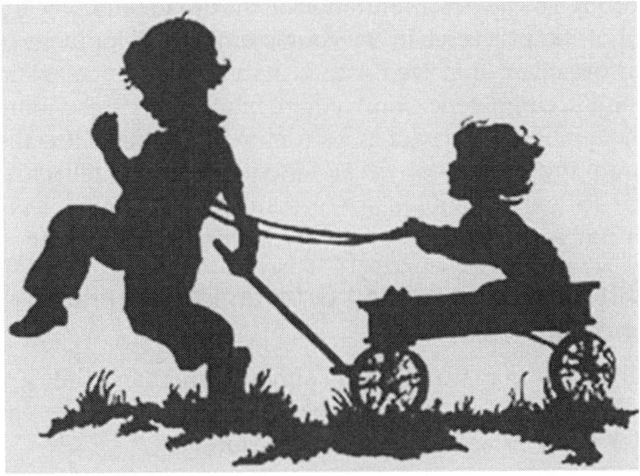

Fig. 4.1: 'Liberty, when it begins to take root, is a plant of rapid growth' —George Washington

According to Watson and Lowery growth means an increase in physical size of the whole or any of its parts and synthesizes new proteins, results in increased size and weight of the whole or any of its parts.

Juan Comas defines it is the objective manifestation of hypertrophy and hyperplasia of the organism constituent tissues and is determined by post-natal body size'. The increase in body size is limited by predetermined constitutional and hereditary factors. It is however influenced by exogenous factors like diet, environment factor, race, etc.

Development

'Development means the qualitative changes.'

—**Harlock**

'Development is that direction, which is continuously revealed in individual in the form of improving changes. This occurs in all individuals from their embryonic stage to old age stage.'

—**James Drever**

Development refers to progressive increase in skill and capacity of function. It can also be described as the improvement of series of sequential changes. It is an increase in the complexity of function and skill progression. For example, a baby first learns to sit, to stand and then to walk and run. It is the capacity and skill of a child to adapt the environment. Development is the behavioral aspect of growth.

Maturation

The term 'maturation' is often used as a synonym for development. It has the more limited application, however, of referring to the development of traits carried through the genes. Maturation, in the broad sense, means all of the processes in the course of the development of an organism that lead it to a mature state. Increase in child's competence and adaptability. It is describing the qualitative change in a structure. In humans it is the unfolding of full physical, emotional, and intellectual capacities that enable a person to function at a higher level of competency and adaptability within the environment.

Differentiation among Growth, Development and Maturation

Growth and maturation are almost similar and they are related to nature, means genetically controlled whereas development is involved with nurture.

Growth refers to the physical and orderly changes in the body with age; on the other hand, development includes experience as well that how your different aspects of life developed with the passage of time.

Table 4.1: Difference between growth and development

Growth	*Development*
It is increase in size, height/length or weight	It is improvement in ability or quality
It is part of development	Growth is part of it
It is a narrow concept	It is a broader concept
Growth is irreversible	
Growth occurs in its own pace	Development is orderly, not haphazard; there is a direct relation between each of its stages and the next.
It takes place till a certain age	It is a life-long process, and does not stop at any age
Its measurement is easy	Its measurement is tough
Can be measured quantitatively	Qualitative change
Growth is genetically controlled	Development depends on environmental domains as well.

Growth is somewhat physical and development covers vast range of life (Table 4.1).

Maturation or growth is genetically controlled; development involves environmental domains as well.

The growth stops with the start of maturation. Maturity is the point of life when no more true growth occurs. An increase in the number of cells at this stage is solely used for regeneration processes. Whereas the development continues in many different forms of life.

Domains of Development

The first few years of life are a time of significant growth and development. Children all develop at different rates, but most young children will reach certain milestones by specific ages. Basic principles of child development is multidimensional. Children develop in certain broad areas, which refer to as 'domains' of development:

- *Physical development:* Physical development includes changes in body size, shape, appearance, functioning of body systems, perceptual and motor capacities, and physical health of child. Development of child proceeds from the head downward. This is called the cephalocaudal principle. This principle describes the direction of growth and development. This is particularly evident during the period of gestation and the 1st year of life. According to this principle, the child gains control of the head first, then the arms, and then the legs. Infants develop control of the head and face movements within the first two months after birth. In the next few months, they are able to lift themselves up by using their arms. By 6 to

12 months of age, infants start to gain leg control and may be able to crawl, stand, or walk. Coordination of arms always precedes coordination of legs.

- *Social/emotional development:* Changes in a child's unique way of dealing with the world (e.g. understanding and expression of emotions, knowledge about others, interpersonal skills, self-awareness, friendships, moral reasoning and behavior). Emotion and behavior are based on the child's developmental stage and temperament. Every child has an individual temperament, or mood. Some children may be cheerful and adaptable and easily develop regular routines of sleeping, waking, eating, and other daily activities. These children tend to respond positively to new situations. Other children are not very adaptable and may have great irregularities in their routine. These children tend to respond negatively to new situations. Still other children are in between.

  Social development can actually impact many of the other forms of development a child experiences. A child's ability to interact in a healthy way with the people around her can impact everything from learning new words as a toddler, to being able to resist peer pressure as a high school student, to successfully navigating the challenges of adulthood. Healthy social development can help child to develop language skills, to build self-esteem, to strengthen learning skills, to resolve conflicts, and to establish positive attitude. Emotional growth and the acquisition of social skills are assessed by watching children interact with others in everyday situations. When children acquire speech, the understanding of their emotional state becomes much more accurate.
- *Cognitive development:* Cognitive development refers to the intellectual maturation of children. Changes in intellectual abilities, including learning, memory, reasoning, thinking, problem-solving, creativity and language development.

  Increasingly, appropriate attachments and nurturing in infancy and early childhood are recognized as critical factors in cognitive growth and emotional health. For example, reading to children from an early age, providing intellectually stimulating experiences, and providing warm and nurturing relationships all have a major impact on growth in these domains. Intellect is appraised in young children by observations of language skills, curiosity, and problem-solving abilities. As children become more verbal, intellectual functioning becomes easier to assess using a number of specialized clinical tools. Once children start school, they undergo constant monitoring as part of the academic process.
- *Language development:* There is perhaps nothing more remarkable than the emergence of language in children. Children go through a number of different stages as language develop, from the earliest stage of producing cooing sounds through being able to produce complex multiword sentences. Researchers have proposed several different theories to explain how and why language development occurs. For example, the behaviorist theory of BF Skinner suggests that the emergence of language is the result of imitation and reinforcement. According to Noam Chomsky's nativist theory language is an inherent human quality and that children are born with a language acquisition device that allows them to produce language once they have learned the necessary vocabulary.

The pre-linguistic, babbling or cooing stage is known as first stage of language development, which typically lasts from the age of three to nine months. Babies begin to make vowel sounds such as *oooooo* and *aaaaaaa* and by five months, infants typically begin to babble and add consonant sounds to their sounds such as *ba-ba-ba, ma-ma-ma* or *da-da-da*. The second stage is known as the one-word or holophrase stage of language development. Around the age of 10 to 13 months, children will begin to produce their first real words and capable of producing a few single words at this point. Infants begin to comprehend language about twice as fast as they are able to produce it. At the age of 18 months children begin to use two word sentences. These sentences usually consist of just nouns and verbs, such as 'Where mummy?' and 'Puppy big!'. Children begin to produce short, multi-word sentences that have a subject and predicate around the age of two years. For example, a child might say 'Daddy is tall' or 'Want more icecream.' As children age, they continue to learn more new words every day. By the time they enter school around the age of five, children typically have a vocabulary of 10,000 words or more.

The ability to understand language precedes the ability to speak; children with few words usually can understand a great deal. Generally delays in expressive speech are not accompanied by other developmental delays, still all children with excessive language delays should be evaluated for the presence of other delays in development. Children who have delays in both receptive and expressive speech more often have additional developmental problems. Hearing test is done at first to assess any delay in language acquisition.

It has been observed that most children who experience speech delay have normal intelligence. In contrast, children with accelerated speech development are often of above-average intelligence.

These domains of development overlap and often interact with each other. What happens in one domain can have a major influence on another domain. For example, the toddler's newly acquired physical development (ability to walk) can influence his or her potential to learn about new aspects of the environment (cognitive development). On the other hand, if a child has a physical impairment, such as the inability to hear, it can affect his or her language acquisition (social/ emotional and cognitive development). In addition, development can occur unevenly across the various domains. In some children, physical development outpaces social/emotional development, or vice-versa.

INFLUENCES OF HEREDITY ON GROWTH AND DEVELOPMENT

Heredity is a biological process through which the transmission of physical and social characteristics takes place from parents to off-springs. It greatly influences the different aspects of growth and development. Heredity and genes certainly play an important role in the transmission of physical and social characteristics from parents to off-springs. Different characteristics of growth and development like intelligence, aptitudes, body structure, height, weight, color of hair and eyes are highly influenced by heredity.

IMPORTANCE OF LEARNING GROWTH AND DEVELOPMENT

The nurse must have knowledge about growth and development of the child. She can use this knowledge to observe and to assess each child in terms of norms for specific levels of development. A child may be guided into more mature behavior if the sequence of developmental behavior is understood.

The knowledge regarding the sequence of developmental behavior throughout childhood and adolescence is necessary, as it helps in preparing nursing process for each child.

The knowledge of growth and development is important to the nurse in order to better understand the reason for particular conditions and sickness which occurs in various age groups.

Parents of a child often ask questions regarding developmental progress of the child. The knowledge of growth and development helps the nurse to meet up those queries.

OVERVIEW OF GROWTH AND DEVELOPMENT

Between the big growth stages of infancy and adolescence, boys and girls grow in height and weight at about the same slow-but-steady rate. There are not notable differences between the sexes until late elementary school, when girls start to grow taller faster, although boys catch up and exceed them within a few years. Girls typically grow close to 3 inches per year, or a bit more. Boys grow 3 to almost 4 inches per year.

On average, girls begin puberty at ages 10–11; boys at ages 11–12. Girls usually complete puberty by ages 15–17, while boys usually complete puberty by ages 16–17. The major landmark of puberty for females is menarche, the onset of menstruation, which occurs on average between ages 12–13; for males, it is the first ejaculation, which occurs on average at age 13.

In the 21st century, the average age at which children, especially girls, reach puberty is lower compared to the 19th century, when it was 15 for girls and 16 for boys. This can be due to any number of factors, including improved nutrition resulting in rapid body growth, increased weight and fat deposition, or exposure to endocrine disruptors such as xenoestrogens, which can at times be due to food consumption or other environmental factors.

Girls begin to show the first changes of puberty, which usually take place between ages 9 and 12. They precede a growth spurt, which is followed eventually by menstruation.

STAGES OF GROWTH AND DEVELOPMENT

Children go through distinct periods of growth and development as they move from infants to young adult (Table 4.2). Child development stages are the theoretical milestones of child development, during each of these stages multiple changes in the development of the brain are taking place. There exists a wide variation in terms of what is considered 'normal,' caused by variation in genetic, cognitive, physical, family, cultural, nutritional, educational, and environmental factors. Developmental norms are sometimes called milestones—they define the recognized pattern of development that children are expected to follow. Each child develops in a unique way; however, using norms helps in understanding these general patterns of development while recognizing the

Table 4.2: Overview of child development			
Stage	*Physical and Language*	*Emotional*	*Social*
Birth to 1 month	• *Feedings:* 5-8 per day • *Sleep:* 20 hrs per day. • *Sensory capacities:* Makes basic distinctions in vision, hearing, smelling, tasting, touch, temperature, and perception of pain.	Generalized	• Tension, helpless asocial • Fed by mother
2–3 months	• *Sensory capacities:* Color perception, visual exploration, oral exploration. • *Sounds:* Smiling and cooing, cries, grunts. • *Motor ability:* start turning their head and even hold it up, while sleeping on his/her tummy, eye muscles,	Distress	Visually fixates at a face, smiles at a face, may be soothed by rocking.
4–6 months	• *Sensory capacities:* Localizes sounds. • *Sounds:* Babbling, makes most vowels and about half of the consonants. • *Feedings:* 3-5 per day. Gains more motor control, rolls over from tummy to back, child can do head and arm movements, purposive grasping. He/she may be able to sit for a small time with support.	• Enjoys being cuddled • Recognizes his mother	Smiles more spontaneously and can distinguish between familiar persons and strangers. Expects feeding, dressing, and bathing.
7–9 months	Child will be able to control of trunk and hands, sits without support, crawls about, even pull himself/herself up with a little support from objects around house.	Specific emotional attachment to mother	Protests separation from mother. Enjoys 'peek-a-boo'
10–12 months	• *Motor ability:* Control of legs and feet, stands and even walk alone, creeps, apposition of thumb and fore-finger. Language: says one or two words such as 'mummy' or 'daddy', imitates sounds, respond to simple commands. • *Feedings:* 3 meals, 2 snacks. • *Sleep:* 12 hours, 2 naps.	• Affection • Fear of strangers • Curiosity, exploration	Responsive to own name. They will communicate with simple gestures like waving their hand to say 'bye' shaking their head to say 'no'. Gives and takes objects. Plays imitative games such as pretending to use the phone
1–2 years	• *Motor ability:* Creeps up stairs, walks alone (10-20 min), makes lines on paper with crayon. Dependent behavior. • *Motor ability:* runs, kicks a ball, can build 6 cubes tower, hold his/her cup to drink and even eat with a spoon. He /she is able to control bowel and bladder. • *Language:* vocabulary of more than 200 words. • *Sleep:* 12 hours at night, 1-2 hr nap	• Very upset when separated from mother. • Temper tantrums.	Obeys limited commands. Repeats a few words. Interested in his mirror image. Feeds himself (1-3 yrs). Resentment of new baby, does opposite of what he is told (18 months).
2–3 years	• *Motor ability:* Jumps off a step, moves around the house, rides a tricycle, uses crayons, builds a 9-10 cube tower. • *Language:* Starts to use short sentences controls and explores world with language, stuttering may appear briefly. Fear of separation.	Negativistic (2½ yrs) Violent emotions, anger. Differentiates facial expressions of anger, sorrow, and joy. Sense of humor (Plays tricks)	Talks, uses 'I' 'me' 'you'. Copies parents' actions. Dependent, clinging, possessive about toys, enjoys playing alongside another child. Negativism (2½ yrs). Resists parental demands. Gives orders. Rigid insistence on sameness of routine. Inability to make decisions.
3–4 years	*Motor ability:* Stands on one leg, jumps up and down, draws a circle and a cross (4 yrs) Jealousy of same-sex parent. Imaginary fears of dark, injury, etc. (3 to 5 years)	Self-sufficient in many self care. Affectionate toward parents. Enjoys manipulation of genitalia. Romantic attachment to parent of opposite sex (3 to 5 yrs)	Likes to share, uses 'we'. Cooperative play with other children, nursery school. Imitates parents. Beginning of identification with same-sex parent, practices sex-role activities. Intense curiosity and interest in other children's bodies. Imaginary friend.

Contd...

Contd...

Stage	*Physical and Language*	*Emotional*	*Social*
4–5 years	• *Motor ability:* Mature motor control, skips, broad jumps, dresses himself, copies a square and a triangle. • *Language:* Talks clearly, uses adult speech sounds, has mastered basic grammar, relates a story, knows over 2,000 words (5 yrs)	Responsibility and guilt. Feels pride in accomplish-ment	Prefers to play with other children, becomes competitive prefers sex-appropriate activities
5–9 years	*Steady growth stage:* Learning to use small and large muscles. Steady to rapid growth rate as puberty commences. Small muscles rapidly developing. Size, vision balance, Coordination. Small size - will tend to climb over or step out to see around things. Poor side vision. Have balance problems and slow reaction times.	Seeks parental approval and wants to be seen as competent. Tries to master more complex skills but may and take on tasks without adult supervision beyond their capability.	Often doesn't hear what is said to them (not an active listener). May question authority and refuse cooperation. Tries to find fault of parents.
10–14 years	Steady to rapid growth rate as puberty commences. Small muscles rapidly developing. Increasing size can be a misleading sign of maturity and strength. Similar coordination to adults.	Desire to learn and try out new skills without constant adult supervision. Thinks logically and capable of more abstract thinking processes. Can find solutions to own problems with some adult guidance.	Easily distracted and caught up by peers. Often affords safety a low priority compared to group needs and sense of self-competency and invincibility.

Table 4.3: Stages in growth and development of male and female in years up to adulthood

	Females																						
Females (age)	0	1	2	3	4	5	6	7	8	10	11	12	13	14	15	16	17	18	19	20	21	22	23
Females (stage)	Infancy			Childhood						Puberty			Adolescence						Adulthood				
Males (stage)	Infancy			Childhood								Puberty			Adolescence					Adulthood			
Males (age)	0	1	2	3	4	5	6	7	8	10	11	12	13	14	15	16	17	18	19	20	21	22	23
	Males																						

wide variation between individuals. Many children reach some or most of these milestones at different times from the norm (Table 4.3).

PARAMETERS OF GROWTH AND DEVELOPMENT

Physical growth includes attainment of full height and appropriate weight and an increase in size of organs. Growth from birth to adolescence occurs in 2 distinct phases. The 1st phase (from birth to about age 1 to 2 year) is one of rapid growth. At puberty, a 2nd growth spurt occurs, affecting boys and girls slightly differently.

GROWTH MONITORING AND GROWTH CHART

Growth, a positive change in the size of a growing individual, is a dynamic measure of health, the best available indicator of nutrition status. Growth monitoring has gained popularity in the last two to three decades and has been practiced in over 80 countries. The most widely promoted method of growth monitoring is weighing and charting growth (Fig. 4.2), since weight gain is believed to be the most sensitive indicator of growth and is universally applicable. This method is favored by UNICEF. Among other techniques, measuring arm circumference is claimed to be the easiest and cheapest alternative to weighing and has been recommended for use at the home and village levels whenever regular and frequent weighing is not possible.

Growth monitoring has been advocated worldwide as one of the key elements of child-survival and primary health care strategies and as an excellent tool for assessing the growth and development of a child in order to detect the earliest changes and bring about appropriate responses to ensure that growth continues uninterrupted.

Growth monitoring and nutritional status: The role of growth monitoring in bringing about a remarkable

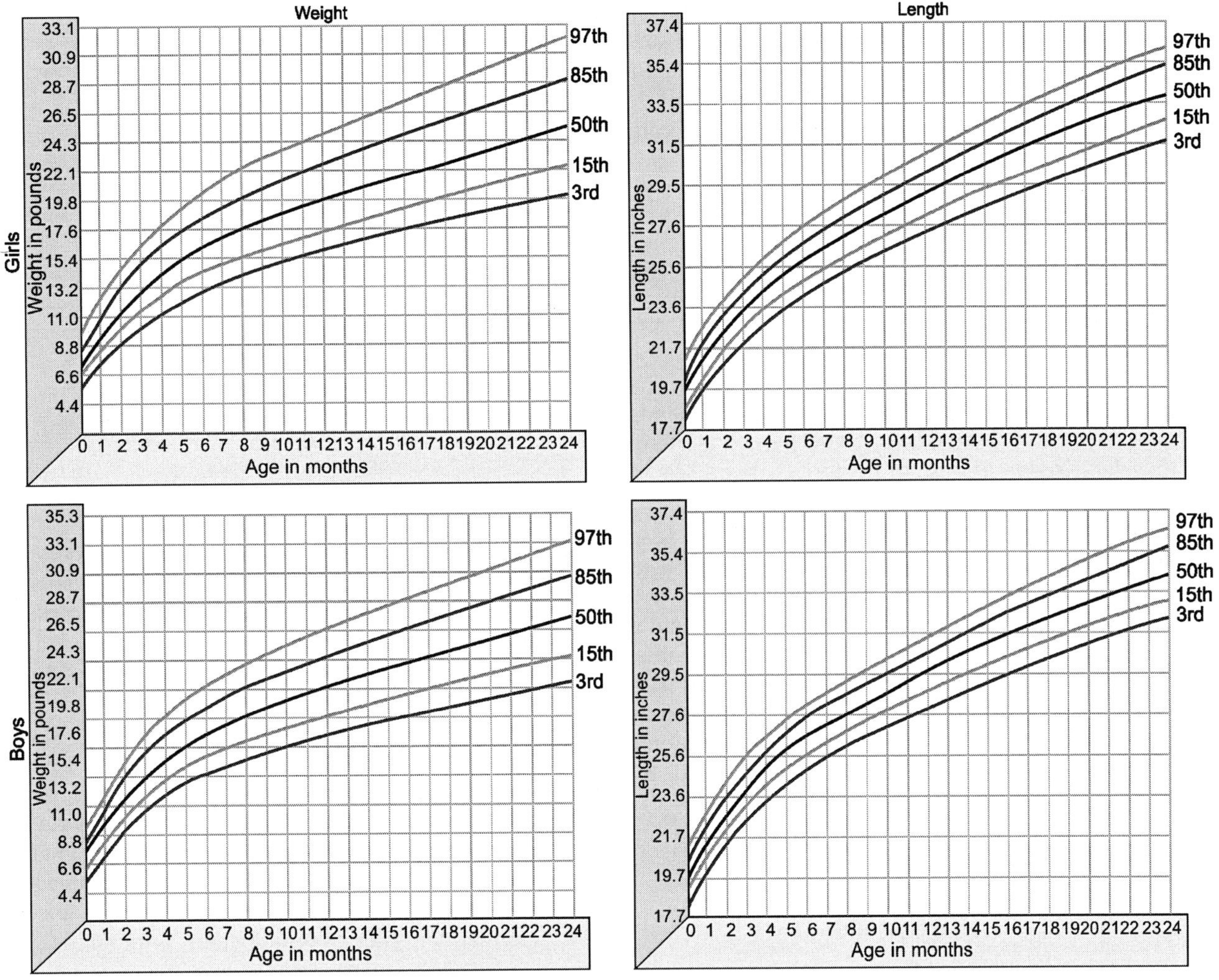

Fig. 4.2: Growth monitoring chart

improvement in nutritional status is practiced in implementing regular growth monitoring using growth charts.

Growth monitoring and the use of primary health care: Growth-monitoring programmes have been shown to increase the use of primary health care services.

Growth monitoring and nutrition education: Data from Thailand has indicated that growth monitoring per se was ineffective in changing nutritional status but that it was effective when combined with nutrition education. The growth charts serve as an educational tool, as most mothers can interpret the trends of the growth lines and seem to be able to relate a downward trend with an illness, especially diarrhoea. It has been discussed that growth charts can be practical and powerful in teaching mothers how to protect children from malnutrition and foster better nutrition through simple messages and discussions.

Growth monitoring and nutrition surveillance: Nutrition surveillance emphasizes the detection of malnutrition among children. Generally the weight cards used in growth monitoring, is used in nutrition surveillance program.

Growth Chart

During the first year of life, an infant's weight and length are charted at each well baby clinic/doctor's visit to make sure that growth is proceeding at a steady rate. Percentiles are a way of comparing infants of the same age. For an infant at the 10th percentile for weight, 10%

of infants weigh less and 90% weigh more. For an infant at the 90th percentile, 90% of infants weigh less and 10% weigh more. For an infant at the 50th percentile, 50% of infants weigh less and 50% weigh more. Of more significance than the actual percentile is any significant change in percentile between doctor's visits.

PRINCIPLES OF CHILD DEVELOPMENT

Development proceeds from the center of the body to outward of the body. This is the principle of proximodistal development that also describes the direction of development (Fig. 4.3). This means that the spinal cord develops before outer parts of the body. The child's arms develop before the hands and the hands and feet develop before the fingers and toes. Finger and toe muscles (used in fine motor dexterity) are the last to develop in physical development.

Motor development includes fine motor (e.g. picking up small objects, drawing) and gross motor (e.g. walking, climbing stairs) skills. It is a continuous process that depends on familial patterns, environmental factors. Children typically begin to walk at 12 months, can climb stairs holding on at 18 months, and run well at 2 years, but the age at which these milestones are achieved by normal children varies widely. Motor development cannot be significantly accelerated by applying increased stimulation.

Children's development occurs in a predictable (orderly) sequence - While there are always exceptions, children's growth and development normally occurs in a predictable manner across the various domains (i.e., children tend to go through similar changes at certain intervals). Children's later abilities, skills and knowledge are built upon those acquired at an earlier age. This does not mean, however, that all children will develop in the same way or achieve certain developmental milestones at the same time. Every child is a unique person, with a unique personality, temperament, learning style and family background. There will always be variations in development from child to child. Developmental charts that identify key milestones for children at different ages and stages of development are not intended to be viewed in a rigid manner. They provide parents with an idea of what tends to happen in a child's life within a particular age range (Fig. 4.4). However, parents should be aware that if a child has not reached a certain developmental milestone at the expected time, it could be a sign of a problem that should be assessed by a pediatrician or specialist.

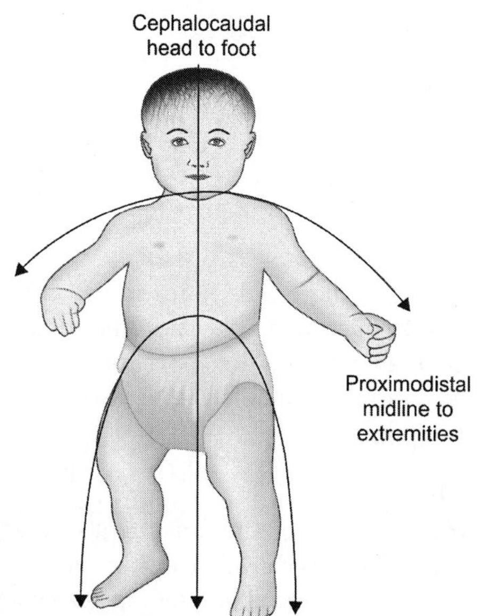

Fig. 4.3: Chephalocaudal and Proximodistal growth

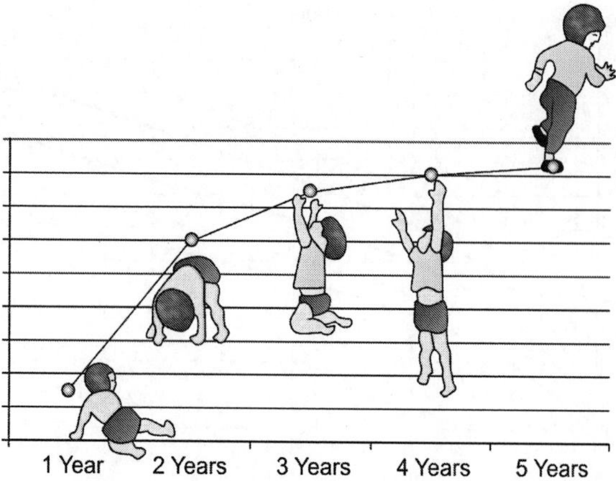

Fig. 4.4: Phases of growth and development of child from 1–5 years

Children's development is affected by early experiences. It is well established that children's early experiences can have a decisive effect on their later development. Those experiences, depending on whether they are positive or negative, can facilitate or hinder healthy development. It has impact on child's early brain development. Researchers have discovered that there are optimal periods, also known as 'sensitive periods' or 'windows of opportunity,' for acquiring certain kinds of knowledge and skills (e.g. language development). Good prenatal care, warm and loving parent-child attachments, and positive stimulation from the time of birth provide children with an optimal environment for development.

A longitudinal study conducted by the National Institute of Child Health and Human Development (NICHD, 2006) found that good quality care in the early years, from parents and other caregivers, is associated with better social and thinking skills, better language ability, better math skills, higher levels of school readiness, and fewer reports of behavior problems.

Children's development occurs in a broader context. Parents are the most influential people in the lives of their children. At the same time, it is important to recognize that outside forces can also play a prominent role. For example, as children grow older, their peers become increasingly influential. Parents must actively monitor and supervise their children at all times, which includes knowing where they are and who they are with. This does not mean that a child's desire for independence should be squelched; however, parents must find a balance between allowing their children more independence as they grow older and maintaining their own parental authority.

Children's development depends on the interplay between genes and environment. *For decades, researchers and practitioners were at odds over which plays a more prominent role in a child's development—heredity (genes) or the environment. Today, there seems to be broad consensus that child development depends on the interplay between genes and environment. Genes obviously set limits and boundaries on certain aspects of development (e.g. height, weight and other physical characteristics), whereas, the environment is thought to influence the entire process of development. A child's environment includes prenatal nutrition, the quality of the parent-child relationship, family structure, neighborhood safety, etc. In fact, a child's genetic makeup and the environment in which he or she is raised are so intertwined that it is very difficult, if not impossible, to determine the precise effect of each.*

Development depends on **maturation and learning.** Maturation refers to the sequential characteristic of biological growth and development. The biological changes occur in sequential order and give children new abilities. Changes in the brain and nervous system account largely for maturation. These changes in the brain and nervous system help children to improve in thinking (cognitive) and motor (physical) skills. Also, children must mature to a certain point before they can progress to new skills (Readiness). For example, a four-month-old cannot use language because the infant's brain has not matured enough to allow the child to talk. By two years old, the brain has developed further and with help from others, the child will have the capacity to say and understand words. Also, a child can not write or draw until he has developed the motor control to hold a pencil or crayon. Maturational patterns are innate, that is, genetically programmed. The child's environment and the learning that occurs as a result of the child's experiences largely determine whether the child will reach optimal development. A stimulating environment and varied experiences allow a child to develop to his or her potential.

Development proceeds from the **simple (concrete) to the more complex**. Children use their cognitive and language skills to reason and solve problems. For example, learning relationships between things (how things are similar), or classification, is an important ability in cognitive development. The cognitive process of learning how an apple and orange are alike begins with the most simplistic or concrete thought of describing the two. Seeing no relationship, a preschool child will describe the objects according to some property of the object, such as color. Such a response would be, 'An apple is red (or green) and an orange is orange.' The first level of thinking about how objects are alike is to give a description or functional relationship (both concrete thoughts) between the two objects. 'An apple and orange are round' and 'An apple and orange are alike because you eat them' are typical responses of three, four and five year olds. As children develop further in cognitive skills, they are able to understand a higher and more complex relationship between objects and things; that is, that an apple and orange exist in a class called fruit. The child cognitively is then capable of classification.

Growth and development is a **continuous process.** As a child develops, he or she adds to the skills already acquired and the new skills become the basis for further achievement and mastery of skills. Most children follow a similar pattern. Also, one stage of development lays the foundation for the next stage of development. For example, in motor development, there is a predictable sequence of developments that occur before walking. The infant lifts and turns the head before he or she can turn over. Infants can move their limbs (arms and legs) before grasping an object. Mastery of climbing stairs involves increasing skills from holding on to walking alone. By the age of four, most children can walk up and down stairs with alternating feet. As in maturation, in order for children to write or draw, they must have developed the manual (hand) control to hold a pencil and crayon.

Growth and development proceed from the **general to specific**. In motor development, the infant will be able to grasp an object with the whole hand before using only the thumb and forefinger. The infant's first motor movements are very generalized, undirected, and reflexive, waving arms or kicking before being able to reach or creep toward an object. Growth occurs from large muscle movements to more refined (smaller) muscle movements.

There are **individual rates** of growth and development. Each child is different and the rates at which individual children grow is different. Although the patterns and sequences for growth and development are usually the same for all children, the rates at which individual children reach developmental stages will be different. Rates of development also are not uniform within an individual child. For example, a child's intellectual development may progress faster than his emotional or social development.

FACTORS AFFECT GROWTH AND DEVELOPMENT OF CHILD

Many factors play a role in child's growth and development, including internal and external factors called as 'nature' and 'nurture'. Development is not determined solely by genetics (nature), nor is the child only a product of the environment (nurture). Rather, bio-psychosocial models recognize the importance of both intrinsic and extrinsic forces. Height, for example, is a function of a child's genetic endowment (biologic), personal habits of eating (psychologic), and access to nutritious food (social). Research demonstrating the profound impact of early experience on the development of the brain has illuminated the interaction of nature and nurture.

The combination of factors responsible for growth and development are:

Genetics: Genetics have an enormous influence on how a child develops. Embryonic life begins with the cytoplasm and the nucleus of the fertilized ovum, genetically determined by both parents. The sperm and ovum each contain chromosomes that act as a blueprint for human life. The genes contained in these chromosomes are made up of a chemical structure known as DNA that contains the genetic code, which make up all life. Except for the sperm and ova, all cells in the body contain 46 chromosomes. The sperm and ova each contains only 23 chromosomes and when the two cells meet, the resulting new organism has the correct 46 chromosomes.

Genetic expressions pass down from both parents to a child are described as genotype (genetic inheritance) and actual expression of those genes (phenotype). These traits are classified according to whether they are dominant and recessive and whether the gene is located on one of the auto-some pairs or on the sex chromosomes. Whether or not a gene is expressed depends on two different things: the interaction of the gene with other genes and the continual interaction between the genotype and the environment. While our genotype may represent a blueprint for how children grow up, the way that these building blocks are put together determines how these genes will be expressed.

Environment: The environment a child is exposed to both in utero and throughout the rest of his or her life can also impact how genes are expressed. For example, exposure to harmful drugs while in utero can have a dramatic impact on later child development. Height is a good example of a genetic trait that can be influenced by environmental factors. While a child's genetic code may provide instructions for tallness, the expression of this height might be suppressed if the child has poor nutrition or a chronic illness.

The way a child is treated by others, has an impact on how she/he grows and develops. A loving and supportive environment helps children focus on learning and growing instead of having to worry about gaining acceptance and praise. Helping children solve problems and learn new things and spending quality time together are effective ways to nurture children and help them develop. Adequate learning opportunities are one of the biggest contributors to an optimal development of child. According to WHO, playing with open-ended toys, dramatic play, arts and crafts, reading and playing games as a way to promote healthy development in young children. As kids get older, parents/elders need to continue to encourage a love of reading, play games together and help their child solve problems.

In addition, the early childhood group environment has a very crucial role in children's learning and development. The young children are in the process of rapid brain development. In the early years, the brain develops more synapses or connections than it can possibly use. Those that are used by the child form strong connections, while the synapses that are not used are pruned away. The development of the brain is compared with construction of a house stating, 'Just as a lack of the right materials can result in blueprints that change, the lack of appropriate experiences can lead to alterations in genetic plans.' It is also stated, 'Building more advanced cognitive, social, and emotional skills on a weak initial foundation of brain architecture is far more difficult and less effective than getting things right from the beginning'. Because children's experiences are limited by their surroundings, the environment elders provide for them has a crucial impact on the way the child's brain develops.

Children who are surrounded, both at home and at school/day care facilities, by a strong learning environment that is both informative and supportive may improve their development.

Culture: Culture matters in child development because culture is the way of life of a people, including their habits, beliefs, language, customs and values. So, understanding how childhood is supported, constrained, and constructed in any community is a part of understanding child development.

Nutrition: Proper nutrition can have a direct impact on a child's development both physically and psychologically and it plays a vital role in a child's growth and development (Fig. 4.5). Lack of proper nutrition can interfere with the maturation of your child's brain and body. Good nutrition should start before a baby is even born and should continue throughout her life. Children need a variety of foods from each food group to ensure that they are getting enough of the nutrients that are vital to growth. The safest course for ensuring cognitive and behavioral development is to meet all nutrient needs with natural or fortified foods prepared appropriately for young children. The benefits of breastfeeding also must be considered in fostering growth and development. This includes calcium, protein, magnesium, carbohydrates and vitamins A, C, D and E. Children who are malnourished are at a disadvantage when it comes to cognitive and physical development because their brains and bodies do not have the nutrition they need to grow. The effect of undernutrition on young children (ages 0–8) can be devastating and enduring. It can impede behavioral and cognitive development, educability, and reproductive health, thereby undermining future work productivity.

Health status: Chronic illness or other special needs in children can also affect growth. Children who are sick often or have special needs should be closely monitored by their doctor (*See* Chapter 7).

Family: Families are considered the first or primary agent of socialization because most children are raised from infancy to adulthood with parents and siblings (Figs 4.6A and B). Families may affect child development directly through their parenting styles, for instance, but

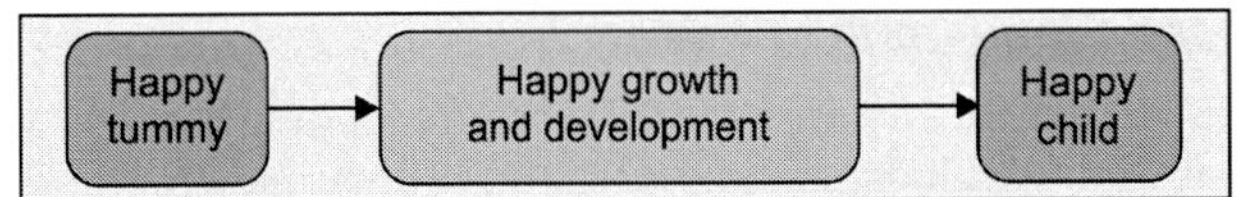

Fig. 4.5: Nutrition and development of child

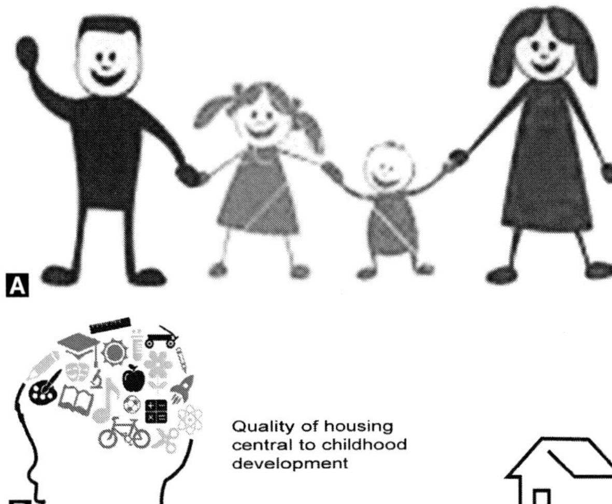

Figs 4.6A and B: Quality of family enviroment central to childhood development

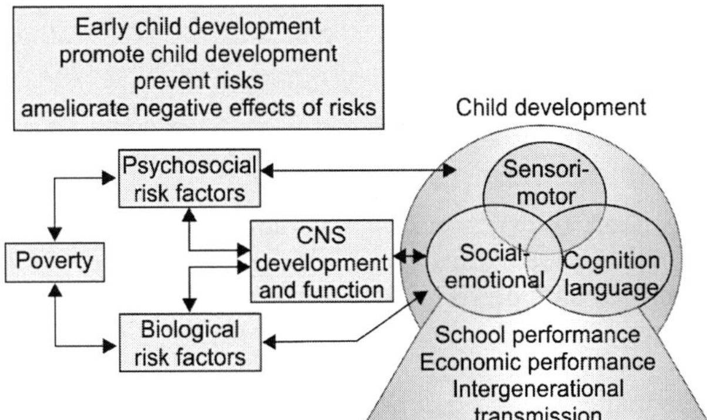

Fig. 4.7: The overall context of development of child and its outcome

those techniques often reflect larger cultural patterns. Family structures also affect the development of child (Discussed detail in Chapter 2).

Children who come from families with adequate finances are more likely to grow and develop to optimal levels, according to the Annual Review of Psychology. Parents who have more money can provide enough food, pay for an education and supply their child with stimulating toys, books and activities. Children who come from the lower economic strata might not get enough nutrition or opportunities to learn, which can interfere negatively with development.

Early child development sets the foundation for lifelong learning, behavior, and health (Fig. 4.7). Interaction and positive relationship between family and community strengthen the ability of early childhood settings to meet the needs of young children. Respect for diversity, equity and inclusion are prerequisites for honoring child's rights, optimal development, and learning.

THEORY OF GROWTH AND DEVELOPMENT OF CHILD

Psychologists and development researchers have proposed a number of different theories to describe and explain the process and stages that children go through as they develop. Some tend to focus on the developmental milestones, or specific achievements that children reach by a certain age. Others focus on specific aspects of child development such as personality, cognition, and moral growth (Fig 4.8). Theories have been devised to study the development of children.

PSYCHOANALYTIC THEORY

Sigismund Schlomo Freud; (6 May 1856 – 23 September 1939) was an Austrian neurologist, known as the 'Father of Psychoanalysis.'

Psychoanalytic Theories (Sigmund Freud,1961) (Fig 4.9)

The theory of psychosexual development was proposed by the famous psychoanalyst Sigmund Freud and described how personality developed over the course of childhood. His theories were in vogue for many years and provided basis for other theories. This theory of personality argued that human behavior was the result of the interaction of three component parts of the mind; the id, ego and superego. The psychoanalytic view holds that there are inner forces outside of our awareness that are directing our behavior.

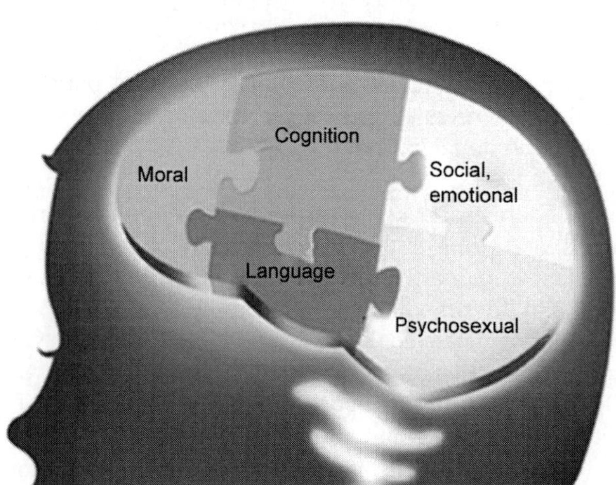

Fig. 4.8: Overall development of child

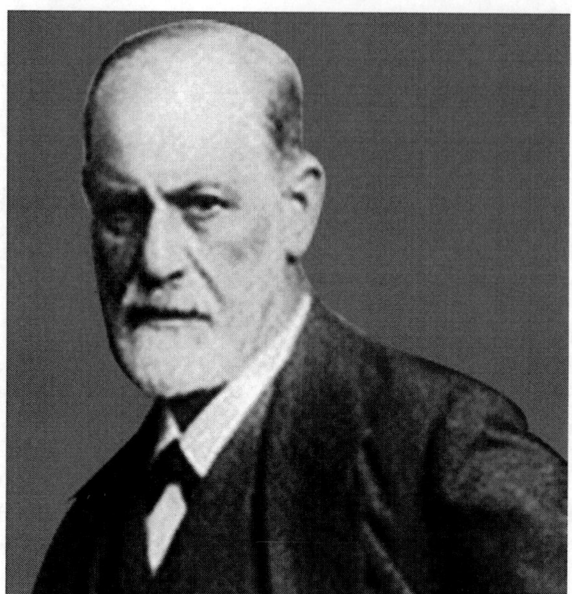

Fig. 4.9: Sigismund Schlomo Freud

Freud believed that personality developed through a series of childhood stages in which the pleasure-seeking energies of the 'id' become focused on certain foci (erogenous areas). This psychosexual energy, or libido, was described as the driving force behind behavior. This work may help to explain normal behavior that others may confuse with abnormal behavior, and it also may provide a good foundation for sexual health education.

According to Freud sexual feelings do not suddenly emerge during puberty and adolescence. They are present from infancy and gradually change from one form to another until adult sexual life is achieved. Development of child was described by Freud as a series of 'psychosexual stages.' Freud postulated that early childhood experiences provide unconscious motivation for actions later in life. Each stage requires mastery for a human to develop properly and move on to the next stage successfully. Each stage involves the satisfaction of a libidinal desire and can later play a role in adult personality. The psychoanalytic theory is explained in following ways:

Oral Stage (birth to 1 year)

In infancy the major source of pleasure seeking is centerd on oral activities such as sucking, biting, chewing and vocalizing.

Children who did not master this stage would develop an oral fixation that might lead to drinking, smoking and nail biting or other mouth-based aggressive behaviors.

Anal Stage (1 to 3 years)

During early childhood, one of the first impulses that a baby must learn is to control his/her excretion system. Toilet training becomes a major developmental task of the child and sensations seem to shift from mouth to anal region. According to psychoanalytical theory, this the time of holding on or letting go. The child develops the sense of autonomy as she/he is able to control body functions. Freud believed that positive experiences during this stage served as the basis for people to become competent, productive, and creative adults.

At this stage the climate surrounding toilet training can have lasting effects on children's personalities. This might lead to anal retentive or anal expulsive personalities in which one is overly tidy, stringent, orderly, rigid, and obsessive, and the other overly messy, wasteful, or destructive personality.

Phallic Stage (3 to 6 years)

This stage begins at 3 years old and ends when the child reaches six years of age. The phallic stage focuses on the genitals as pleasure seeking areas of the body. Children recognize difference between the sexes and become curious about the dissimilarities, childbirth and sexuality.

Boys in this stage experience the Oedipus complex while girls experience the Electra complex. In both cases the child develops incestuous feelings for the parent of the opposite sex. Children tend to develop characteristics of the same-sex parent during this stage. Due to the possessiveness for the opposite sex parent, the child become aggressive towards same sex parent, is considered as normal behavior, as is a heightened interest in sex. To overcome these disturbing sexual feelings, the preschooler identifies with or becomes more like the same sex parent.

Latency Period (6 to 11 years)

The fourth stage is the latency stage which begins at the age of six and continues until the age of eleven. During this stage there is no pleasure seeking region of the body; instead all sexual feelings are repressed. Physical and psychic energy are channelized into acquisition of knowledge and vigorous play. Thus, children are able to elaborate the previously acquired traits and skills, and find comfort through peer and family interaction. Best friends and same sex peer groups are influential in the school-age child's life.

Genital Stage (12 years and older)

The final stage of psychosexual development is the genital stage. This stage commences at the age of eleven, lasts through puberty, and ends when one reaches adulthood at the age of eighteen. Maturation of the reproductive system and production of sex hormones occur at puberty, and the genital organs become the major source of sexual tensions and pleasures. The onset of puberty reflects a strong interest from one person to another of the opposite sex. The interest in sex again flourishes as children search for identity during adolescence. If one does not experience fixation in any of the psychosexual stages, once he or she has reached the genital stage, he or she will grow into a well-balanced human being.

There have been many revisions and additions to psychoanalytic theories since Freud's time.

Freud's theories explains the concepts of love, hate, childhood, family relations, civilization, sexuality, fantasy, conflicting emotions, etc. A gender role or sexual identity is not established at birth, but learned gradually through experiences and instructions during the years of development.

It is important that people who guide and work with children have a basic knowledge of the development of sexuality from infancy to adolescence. One of the key developmental tasks faced by all children is learning how to interact with others and engage in socially appropriate behaviors. These are abilities that we are not born with. Young children are in the process of developing gender identity (the realization that they are either a boy or a girl) and gender role (adopting social characteristics typical of girls or boys). Children are also developing their understanding of relationships and values. We generally do not think of these things as sexually related but these important achievements in early child development lay the foundation for how our sexuality will develop and evolve as children become teenagers and teenagers become adults. Parents and caregivers indirectly teach infants and toddlers about sexuality when they interact with them on a number of levels including the way they speak to children, and cuddle and play with them.

Freud's ideas have since been met with criticism, because of his singular focus on sexuality as the main driver of human personality development.

PSYCHOSOCIAL—DEVELOPMENTAL THEORY

Erik Homburger Erikson (15 June, 1902–12, May 1994) was a German-born American developmental psychologist and psychoanalyst known for his theory on psychosocial development of human beings. He is certainly a key figure in the study of children and development of the modern era. He may be most famous for coining the phrase identity crisis.

Erikson's theory

- Stages involve psychosocial crises
- Each crisis can be ***resolved*** in one of two ways
- The way earlier crises were resolved influences how subsequent crises are resolves

Psychosocial Development (Erik Erikson, 1963) (Fig. 4.10).

Like those of Freud and Piaget, the Erikson's theory of human development states that life is a series of stages, through which a healthily developing human should pass from infancy to late adulthood (Table 4.4). In each stage, the person confronts, and hopefully masters, new challenges. A stage is a period during which certain changes occur. Each stage builds upon the successful completion of earlier stages. The challenges of stages not successfully completed may be expected to reappear as problems in the future. What one achieves in each stage is based on the developments of the previous stages. Centering on basic crises at each stage of development, the theory of psychosocial development proposes that these conflicts are part of the life process and that successful handling of these issues can give a person the

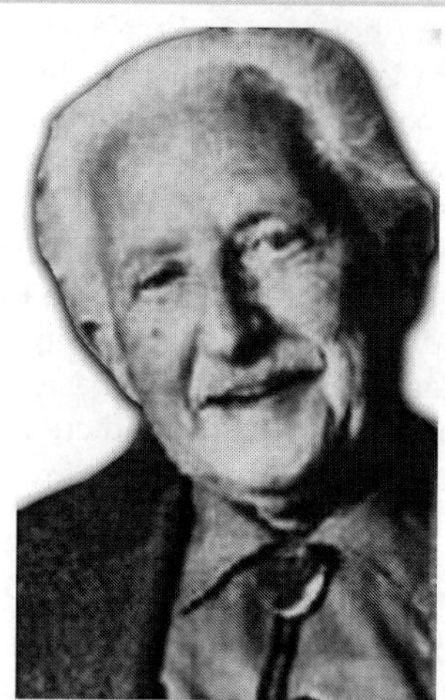

Fig. 4.10: Erik Homburger Erikson

Table 4.4: Erikson's life span approach to personality development related to childhood

Description/ Approximate age	*Significant relationship*	*Challenges*	*Strength*	*Existential questions and outcome*
Oral-sensory, birth–2 years	Mother	Trust vs. mistrust	Hopes	• Can I trust the world? • A sense of trust is developed in child when caregivers provide reliability, care, and affection. A lack of this will lead to mistrust.
Muscular-anal, 2–4 years	Parents	Autonomy vs. shame and doubt	Will power	• Is it okay to be me? • A sense of personal control over physical skills and a sense of independence developed. Success leads to feelings of autonomy, failure results in feelings of shame and doubt.
Locomotor-genital, preschool, 4–5 years	Family	Initiative vs. guilt	Purpose	• Is it okay for me to do, move and act? • Children need to begin asserting control and power over the environment. Success in this stage leads to a sense of purpose. Children who try to exert too much power experience disapproval, resulting in a sense of guilt.
Latency 5–12 years	Neighbors, school	Industry vs. inferiority	Competence	• Can I make it in the world of people and things? • Children need to cope with new social and academic demands. Success leads to a sense of competence, while failure results in feelings of inferiority
Adolescence 13–19 years	Peers, role-models	Identity vs. role confusion	Fidelity	• Who am I? Who can I be? • Teens need to develop a sense of self and personal identity. Success leads to an ability to stay true to yourself, while failure leads to role confusion and a weak sense of self.

'ego strength' to face life positively. For example, the primary conflict during the adolescent period involves establishing a sense of personal identity. Success or failure in dealing with the conflicts at each stage can impact overall functioning. During the adolescent stage, for example, failure to develop an identity results in role confusion.

Trust vs Mistrust (Birth to 1 year)

First and most important attribute to develop a healthy personality is basic trust which dominates the first year of life and describes all of the child's satisfying experiences at this age. It is a time of 'getting' and 'taking in' through all the senses (Figs 4.11A and B). It exists only in relation to something or someone—a mothering person is essential for development of trust. Mistrust develops when trust promoting experiences are deficient or lacking or when basic needs are inconsistently or inadequately met.

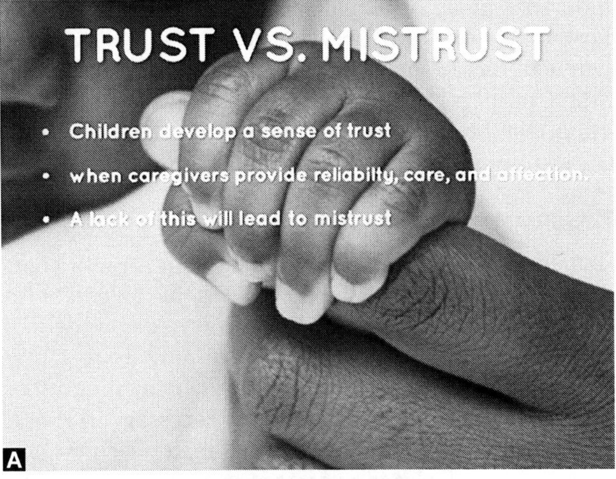

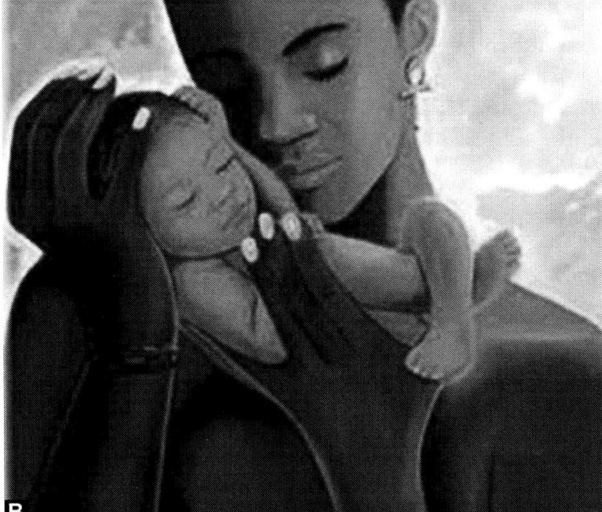

Figs 4.11A and B: Trust Vs Mistrust (Basis of Psychological Development by Eric Erikson)

Autonomy vs Shame and Doubt (1 to 3 years)

The goal of this stage is to gain courage and independence while minimizing shame and doubt. Children in this stage want to do things for themselves, using their newly acquired motor skills of walking, climbing and manipulating and mental powers of selecting and decision-making. Much of their learning is acquired by imitating the activities and behavior of others. The parents are supposed to give freedom and courage to their kids. They should allow kids to try new things and not to be overprotective. Negative feelings of doubt and shame arise when children are forced to be dependent in areas in which they are capable of assuming control. The favorable outcomes are self-control and willpower. But if parents give too much freedom to the kids become careless they can become impulsive and not care for their actions. Children who develop autonomy will feel confident about their self while the children who do not will feel shame and guilt.

Initiative vs Guilt (3 to 6 years)

Initiative vs guilt is the psychological conflict of early childhood which is characterized by vigorous, intrusive behavior, enterprise and strong imagination. Children explore the physical world with all their senses and powers. It is resolved positively through play experiences that foster a healthy sense of initiative and through development of a conscience that is not overly strict. When parents are supportive of a child's efforts to show initiative, then children develop purpose and set goals and act in ways to reach them. But too much purpose and no guilt can lead to ruthlessness. When parents punish children when they try to show initiative, then children are likely to develop a sense of guilt. Excessive guilt can lead to inhibition.

Guilt is defined in Erikson's theory as 'the capacity for self-condemnation'. It implies both cognitive reflective ability, and also the ego strength to be able to tolerate that inner disapproval. True guilt is healthy. Children become curious about people and imitate adults. Erickson, like Freud, believed children do attempt to possess the opposite sex parent and experience rivalry toward the same sex parent.

They develop a conscience, they have an inner voice that warns and threatens. Children sometimes undertake goals or activities that are in conflict with those of parents or others and being made to feel that their activities or imagining are bad, produces a sense of guilt. Children must learn to retain a sense of initiative without impinging on the rights and privileges of others. The lasting outcomes are direction and purpose.

Industry vs Inferiority (6 to 12 years)

This stage is based on early school from 5 to 10 years of age. Industry refers to a child's involvement in situations where long, patient work is demanded of them. They learn concepts of space and time, moral values, cause and effect, reading and writing and other crucial elements and skills that are necessary in life. If the children are encouraged from their teachers and parents, they feel sense of competence and develop belief on their own abilities. Children feel pride on their accomplishment and abilities when they interact with other in the society. On the other hand, if children are not encouraged they cannot develop belief on their own abilities. Inferiority is the feeling created when a child gets a feeling of failure when they cannot finish or master their school work (Fig. 4.12).

Children want to engage in tasks and activities that they can carry through to completion; they need and want real achievement. Children learn to complete and cooperate with others, they can learn rules. It is a decisive period in their social relationships with others, feelings of inadequacy and inferiority may develop if too much is expected of them or if they believe that they cannot measure up to the standards set for them by others. The ego quality developed from a sense of industry is competence.

Identity vs Role Confusion (12 to 18 years)

This stage of development is characterized by rapid and marked physical changes. Previous trust in their body is shaken, and children become overly preoccupied with the way they appear in the eyes of others as compared with their own self-concept. The concern for teens during this period is how people perceive them/view them in society (their identity). The questions that arise in their minds are 'Who am I' and ' What am I going to do with my life?' This is where teens pull away from their parents; feel more independent. The outcome of successful mastery is devotion and fidelity to others and values and to values and ideologies.

Inability to solve the core conflict results in the role confusion. Role confusion is basically failure. If children fail to resolve the crisis, they develop identity diffusion; their sense of self is unstable and threatened; too little identity and they may join hate groups, too much identity and they may show fanaticism (Figs 4.13A and B).

Industry vs. inferiority

- Development of self-confidence
- Industry = hard working, sacrificing play for work
- Inferiority = ridiculed or punished for lack of ability
- Development of individual talents
- Not doing so can lead to poor self- esteem

Fig. 4.12: Industry vs. Inferiority (Psychological Development of child 6-12 years)

COGNITIVE DEVELOPMENT THEORY

Jean Piaget (French, 9 August 1896–16 September 1980) was a Swiss developmental psychologist and philosopher known for his epistemological studies

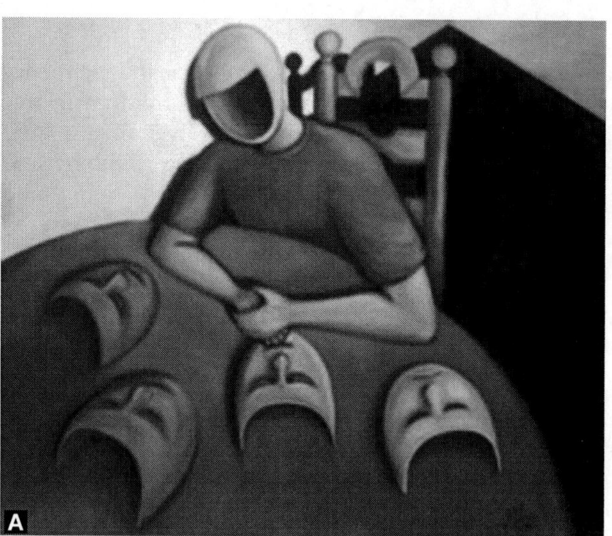

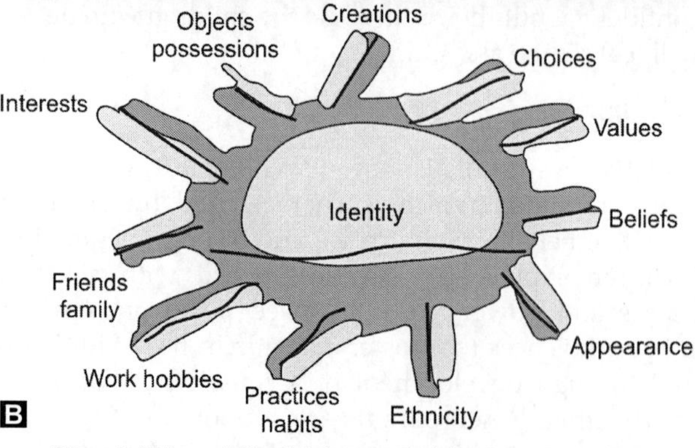

Figs 4.13A and B: Adolescent's identity crises and identity formation

with children. His theory of cognitive development and epistemological view are together called 'genetic epistemology'. Einstein called Piaget's discovery 'so simple only a genius could have thought of it.'

Piaget created a theory of cognitive development that described the basic stages that children go through as they mentally mature. He believed that children are like 'little scientists,' actively trying to make sense of the world rather than simply soaking up information passively.

Piaget's Theory of Cognitive Development (1969)

One of the key concepts in Piaget's theory is the use of schemas. According to Piaget (Fig. 4.14), schemas are cognitive frameworks or concepts that help people organize and interpret information. As experiences happen, this new information is used to modify, add to or completely change previously existing schemas.

It is a comprehensive theory about the nature and development of human intelligence. Early childhood is not only a period of amazing physical growth, it is also a time of remarkable mental development. Cognitive abilities associated with memory, reasoning, problem-solving and thinking continue to emerge throughout childhood. Piaget believed that one's childhood plays a vital and active role to the growth of intelligence, and that the child learns through doing and actively exploring. The theory of intellectual development focuses on perception, adaptation and manipulation of the environment around them. It is primarily known as a developmental stage theory, but, in fact, it deals with the nature of knowledge itself and how humans come gradually to acquire, construct, and use it.

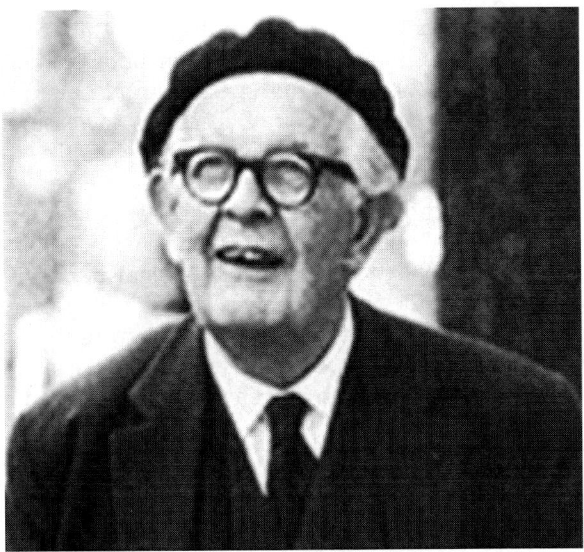

Fig. 4.14: Jean Piaget

Theorist Jean Piaget suggested that children think differently than adults and proposed a stage theory of cognitive development. He was the first to note that children play an active role in gaining knowledge of the world. He claimed that cognitive development is at the center of the human organism, and language is contingent on knowledge and understanding acquired through cognitive development. To Piaget, cognitive development was a progressive reorganization of mental processes resulting from biological maturation and environmental experience. Accordingly, he believed that children construct an understanding of the world around them, after that experience discrepancies between what they already know and what they discover in their environment. It consists of age-related changes that occur in mental activities (Fig. 4.15). Many parents have been encouraged to provide a rich, supportive environment for their child's natural propensity to grow and learn. Child-centerd classrooms and 'open education' are direct applications of Piaget's views.

Mental development is demonstrated in problem-solving and in a general understanding of what to do in a given situation. It is important to let children solve the problems that they can by themselves and to teach them how to solve the problems that are within their abilities but for which they lack the necessary experience and practice. By the time children are one-year old they should be in the process of learning decision-making.

Cognitive development refers to the development of the ability to think and reason. Children (typically 6 to 12 years old) develop the ability to think in concrete ways (concrete operations) such as how to combine (addition), separate (subtract or divide), order (alphabetize and sort), and transform (change things such as two 50 paisa coins = 1 rupee). objects and actions. These processes are called concrete because they are performed in the presence of the objects and events being thought about.

Adolescence marks the beginning development of more complex thinking processes (also called formal logical operations) including abstract thinking (thinking about possibilities), the ability to reason from known principles (form own new ideas or questions), the ability to consider many points of view according to varying criteria (compare or debate ideas or opinions), and the ability to consider the process of thinking.

Piaget proposed three stages of reasoning—**intuitive, concrete operational and formal operational.** The course of intellectual development is both maturational and invariant and is divided into the following stages:

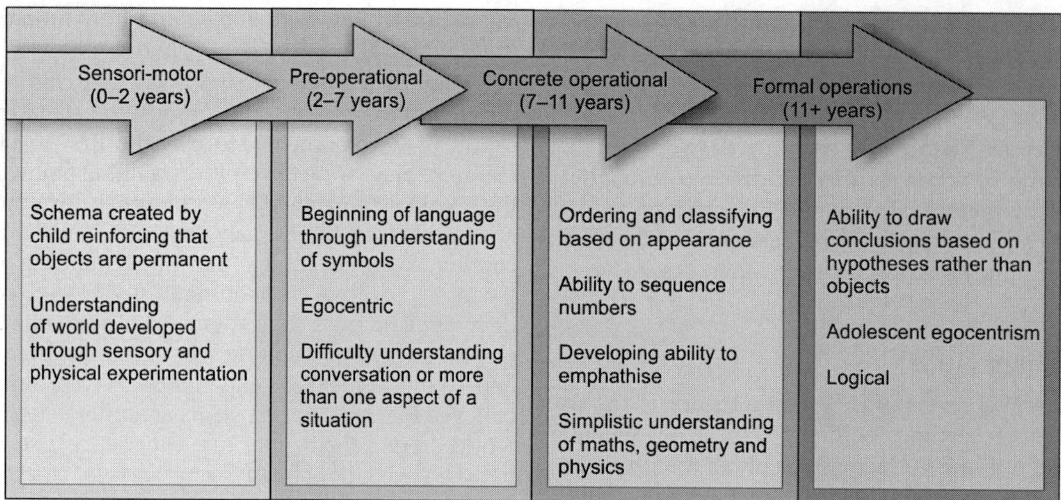

Fig. 4.15: Development of child and proposed three stages of reasoning by Piaget

Sensorimotor (Birth to 2 years)

This stage consists of 6 sub-stages that are governed by sensations in which simple learning takes place. Children progress from reflex activity through simple repetitive behavior to imitative behavior. Behaviors are limited to simple motor responses caused by sensory stimuli. They show coordination of senses with motor response, and sensory curiosity about the world. They develop a sense of cause and effect as they direct behavior toward objects. Problem-solving is primarily by trial and error. They display a high-level curiosity, experimentation, and enjoyment of novelty and begin to develop a sense of self as they are able to differentiate themselves from their environment. They become aware that object have permanence–that an object exists even though it is no longer visible. Toward the end of the sensorimotor period, language is used for demands and cataloguing.

Preoperational (2 to 7 years)

During this stage, children learn to use language, but do not yet understand concrete logic, cannot mentally manipulate information and are unable to take the point of view of other people. Children develop symbolic thinking, can use proper syntax and grammar to express full concepts.

The predominant characteristics of the preoperational stage of intellectual development is egocentrism, which in the sense does not mean selfishness or self-centeredness, but the inability to put oneself in the place of another. Children interpret objects according to their own perception not in the view of others. Preoperational thinking is concrete and tangible. Children cannot reason beyond their observation and they lack generalization. Thought is dominated by what they see, hear or otherwise experience. In the later stage of this period their reasoning is intuitive (e.g. the stars have to go bed as they do) and they are beginning to deal with problems of weight, height, size and time. Reasoning is also transductive (two events occur together, they cause each other, e.g. all women with big bellies have babies). Imagination and intuition are strong, but complex abstract thought still difficult.

Concrete Operation (7 to 11 years)

In this stage, children gain a better understanding of mental operations. They begin to think logically about concrete events, but have difficulty in understanding abstract or hypothetical concepts. Concepts attached to concrete situations. Thought becomes increasingly logical and coherent. Time, space, and quantity are understood and can be applied, but not as independent concepts. Children are able to classify, sort, order, and organize facts about the world to use in problem-solving. They solve problem in a concrete, systematic fashion based on what they can perceive. Through progressive changes in thought process and relationships with others, they become less self-centered. They can consider others point of view. Thinking has become socialized.

Formal Operations (11+ years)

Theoretically, child develop hypothetical, and counterfactual thinking and abstract logic and reasoning. Strategy and planning become possible. Concepts learned in one context can be applied to others.

The skills such as logical thought, deductive reasoning and systematic planning also emerge during this stage. Thought is characterized by adaptability and flexibility. Adolescents can think in abstract symbols and draw logical conclusions from a set of observations. They can make hypothesis and test them. They can consider abstract, theoretic and philosophic matters.

SUMMARY OF COGNITIVE DEVELOPMENT

Theory of Moral Development

Lawrence Kohlberg (October 25, 1927–January 19, 1987) was a psychologist best known for his theory of stages of moral development. He served as a professor in the psychology department at the University of Chicago and at the Graduate School of Education at Harvard University.

Moral development: It is the process through which children develop proper attitudes and behaviors toward other people in society, based on social and cultural norms, rules, and laws. Moral development focuses on the emergence, change, and understanding of morality from infancy through adulthood. In the field of moral development, morality is defined as principles for how individuals ought to treat one another, with respect to justice, others' welfare, and rights (Table 4.5).

Moral Development (Kohlberg,1968) (Fig. 4.16)

Morality is our ability to learn the difference between right and wrong and understand how to make the right choices. As with other facets of development, morality does not form independently. Children's experiences at home, the environment around them, and their physical, cognitive, emotional, and social skills influence their developing sense of right vs. wrong.

Children also acquire moral reasoning in a developmental sequence. Moral development described by Kohlberg in 1968, is based on cognitive developmental theory. The theory holds that moral reasoning, the basis for ethical behavior, has six identifiable developmental stages, each more adequate at responding to moral dilemmas than its predecessor. Kohlberg followed the development of moral judgment far beyond the ages studied earlier by Piaget, who also claimed that logic and morality develop through constructive stages. Kohlberg and Piaget, both viewed moral development as a result of a deliberate attempt to increase the coordination and integration of one's orientation to the world.

Expanding on Piaget's work, Kohlberg determined that the process of moral development was principally concerned with justice, and that it continued throughout the individual's lifetime. He discussed moral development as a complicated process involving

Table 4.5: Kohlberg's moral stages level and age of child

Stage	*Age*	*Characteristics*	*Developmental changes*
Sensorimotor stage	Birth to 2 years	The infant knows the world through their movements and sensations.	Infants learn that things continue to exist even though they cannot be seen (object permanence). They are separate beings from the people and objects around them. They realize that their actions can cause things to happen in the world around them. Learning occurs through assimilation and accommodation.
Preoperational stage	2–7 years	Children begin to think symbolically and learn to use words and pictures to represent objects. They also tend to be very egocentric, and see things only from their point of view.	Children at this stage tend to be egocentric and struggle to see things from the perspective of others. While they are getting better with language and thinking, they still tend to think about things in very concrete terms.
Concrete operational stage	7–11 years	During this stage, children begin to thinking logically about concrete events.	They begin to understand the concept of conservation; the amount of liquid in a short, wide cup is equal to that in a tall, skinny glass. Thinking becomes more logical and organized, but still very concrete. Begin using inductive logic, or reasoning from specific information to a general principle.
Formal operational stage	12 years and up	At this stage, the adolescent or young adult begins to think abstractly and reason about hypothetical problems.	Abstract thought emerges. Teens begin to think more about moral, philosophical, ethical, social, and political issues that require theoretical and abstract reasoning. Begin to use deductive logic, or reasoning from a general principle to specific information.

Kohlberg's Stages

Preconventional level
- **Stage 1:** The punishment and obedience orientation
- **Stage 2:** The instrumental purpose orientation

Conventional level
- **Stage 3:** The 'good boy-good girl' orientation
- **Stage 4:** The social-order-maintaining orientation

Postconventional level
- **Stage 5:** The social-contract orientation
- **Stage 6:** The universal ethical principle orientation

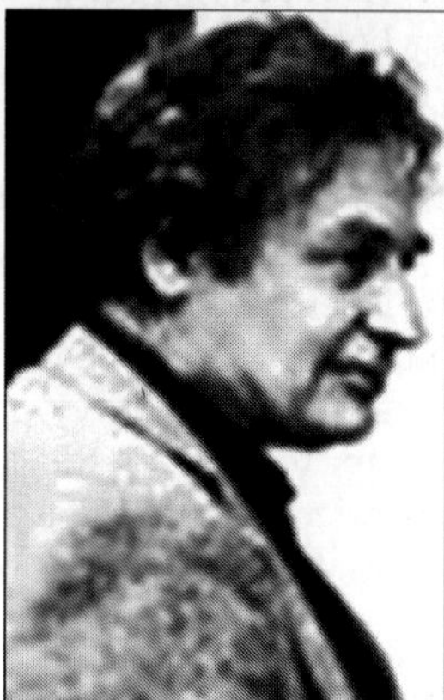

Fig. 4.16: Lawrence Kohlberg

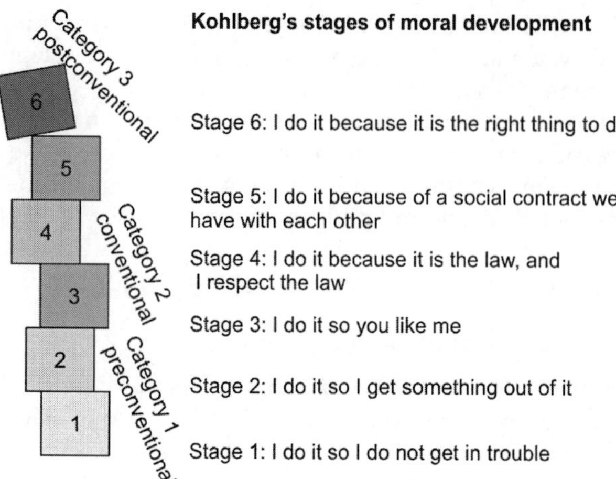

Fig. 4.17: Moral development stages explained by Kohlberg,1968

the acceptance of the values and rules of society in a way that shapes behavior. Kohlberg's studies and research provided a systematic 3-level, and 6-stage sequence reflecting changes in moral judgment throughout the lifespan. Specifically, Kohlberg argued that development proceeds from a selfish desire to avoid punishment (personal), to a concern for group functioning (societal), to a concern for the consistent application of universal ethical. An emotion closely tied to moral reasoning is 'Guilt', and it is expressed as self-criticism and remorse. Most children 12 years age and above, react to misbehavior with guilt. Guilt helps them realize when their moral judgement fails. Furthermore, Kohlberg believed that in order for a child to advance to a more developed level of morality, he or she must develop an equivalent level of intellectual ability.

Pre-conventional Level (Pre-conventional Morality)

Preconvention level of moral development (Fig. 4.17) is parallel to the preoperational level of cognitive development and intuitive thought, and it has three substages. Children oriented to good/bad, right/wrong and express it in physical or pleasurable actions. They demonstrate acceptable behavior, obey superior force (who have the power to determine and enforce the rules and labels) without question, as children want to avoid punishment. This stage is known as the Punishment-Obedience stage. Children at this stage are not able to see someone else's side. At this stage of cognitive and moral development, children cannot reason as a mature member of the society because they have no concept of the basic moral order that supports these consequences. They view the world in a selfish, egocentric way, with no real understanding of right and wrong. To them morality is an external thing, an external locus of control. So, he will not steal sister's money because his mother will spank him. It is not his internal drive to do the right thing.

Later they determine the right behavior consists of that which satisfies their own needs (and sometime the need of others). Although the elements of fairness, give and take, and equal sharing are evident, they are interpreted in a practical, concrete manner without loyalty, gratitude or justice.

Conventional Level (Morality of Conventional Role Conformity)

This level broadens the scope of human wants and needs. Children in this level are concerned about being accepted by others and living up to their expectations. This stage begins around age 10 but lasts well into adulthood, and is the stage most adults remain at throughout their lives. At this stage children are concerned with conformity and loyalty which is often called as the 'good boy/good girl' stage. They understand the concepts of trust, loyalty, and gratitude. They abide by the Golden Rule as it applies to people around them every day. Morality is acting in accordance to what the social group says is right and moral.

They still have an external locus of control, but they value the maintenance of family, group or national expectation regardless of consequences. Behavior that meets with approval and 'please' or helps others is emerged and replace the more egocentric thinking of the earlier stage. One earns approval by being 'nice'. The child has increased awareness of others' feeling. In the child's view obeying the rules, doing one's duty, showing respect for authority and maintaining the social order are the correct behavior. The child feels guilty, if his/her behavior is not accepted. This level is correlated with the stage of concrete operations in cognitive development.

At the next stage, the child's world become wide (family, peers, society as a whole), his/her cognitive capacities increase and internal sense of right and wrong emerges. Along with this locus of control comes the ability to consider circumstances when judging behavior.

Postconventional, Autonomous (Morality of Self-accepted Moral Principles)

At this level individual has reached the cognitive stage of formal operations. Correct behavior tends to be defined in terms of general individual rights and standards that have been examined and agreed on by the entire society. Although procedural rules for reaching consensus become important, with emphasis on the legal point of view, there is also emphasis on the possibility for changing law in terms of societal needs and rational consideration.

The most advanced level of moral development is one in which self-chosen ethical principles guide decisions of conscience (Fig. 4.17). These are abstract and ethical but universal principles of justice and human rights with respect for the dignity of persons as individual. It is believed that few persons reach this stage of moral reasoning.

LEV VYGOTSKY'S SOCIAL DEVELOPMENT THEORY

Lev Semyonovich Vygotsky (November 17, 1896 – June 11, 1934) was a Soviet psychologist, the founder of an original holistic theory of human cultural and biosocial development commonly referred to as cultural-historical psychology.

Social Development

The development of the social and emotional health of a child is essential to his appropriate behavior, understanding of life and transition to adulthood. It involves learning the values, knowledge and skills that enable children to relate to others effectively and to contribute in positive ways to family, school and the community. Social emotional development helps shape a child into what he will become later in life by teaching proper reactions to emotional matters. This kind of learning occurs through children's participation in the culture around them, through their relationships with others and their growing awareness of social values and expectations. Children build a sense of who they are and of the social roles available to them. As children develop socially, they both respond to the influences around them and play an active part in shaping their relationships (Fig. 4.18). Social skills are all about a child's ability to cooperate and play with others, paying attention to adults and teachers, and making reasonable transitions from activity to activity.

Social Development Theory of Lev Vygotsky

In the field of education, Vygotsky is famous for his theories of child development and how children learn. The major theme of Vygotsky's theoretical framework is that social interaction plays a fundamental role in the development of cognition. He worked on ideas about cognitive development, particularly the relationship between language and thought. His writings

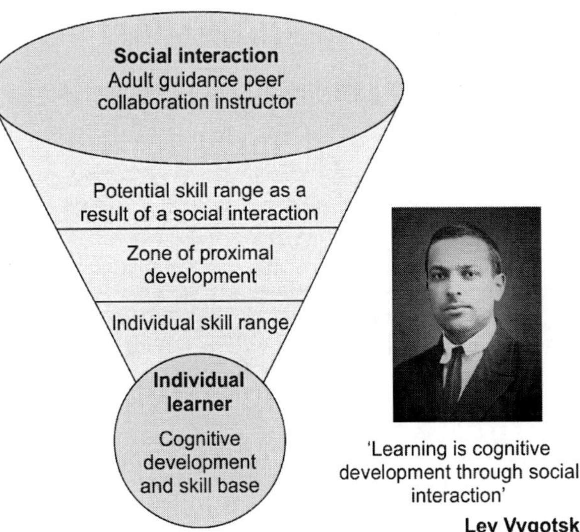

Fig. 4.18: Vygotsky: Developmental perspectives

emphasized the roles of historical, cultural, and social factors in cognition and he argued that language was the most important symbolic tool provided by society.

Vygotsky believed development, to be a lifelong process dependent on social interaction and that social learning actually leads to cognitive development. Through these interactions, children come to learn the habits of his/her culture, written language and other knowledge through which children obtain meaning that affects his/her understanding of knowledge (Fig. 4.18).

Vygotsky also recognized the value of play as a tool for learning and development, he also acknowledged the development of social rules and language skills are consciously acquired through play. Vygotsky's social development theory facilitates cognitive development.

As a child grows and matures, his language skills improve, making social emotional development and social interactions with peers an important part of his life, as he becomes more involved with other children and adults around him (Fig. 4.19). When the child reaches preschool, friendships become increasingly important. At this stage of social development, children often prefer to play with same-sex friends, and often start forming 'best friend' relationship with selected peers.

Friendships, attention and approval of his or her peers and significant adults become increasingly important to a preschool child. At this age, children become focused on seeking approval from their parents and friends. They often prefer playing with their friends or alone, apart from their parents. They begin to show a strong desire for independence and often insist on making their own choices and preferences in clothing, food, activities and so on. Most preschoolers at this stage of social development, however, still often need an adult assistance and supervision in order help them settle arguments or get necessary supplies. Many social development skills are acquired at this age as children learn to compromise, share and take turns.

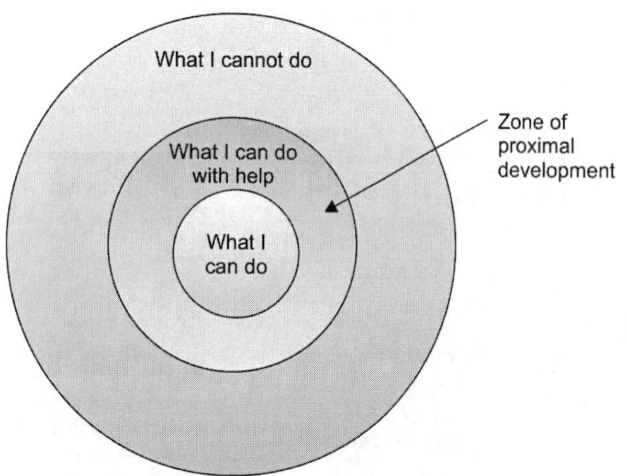

Fig. 4.19: Vygotsky: Zone of proximal development

Every function in the child's cultural development appears twice: first, on the social level, and later, on the individual level; first, between people (interpsychological) and then inside the child (intrapsychological). A second aspect of Vygotsky's theory is the idea that the potential for cognitive development depends upon the 'zone of proximal development' (ZPD): a level of development attained when children engage in social behavior. Full development of the ZPD depends upon full social interaction. The range of skill that can be developed with adult guidance or peer collaboration exceeds what can be attained alone.

Vygotsky's theory was an attempt to explain consciousness as the end product of socialization. For example, in the learning of language, our first utterances with peers or adults are for the purpose of communication but once mastered they become internalized and allow 'inner speech'.

The social development theory includes three major concepts. These are comprised of the role of social interaction in cognitive development, the more knowledgeable other and the zone of proximal development.

Summary of Different Psychosocial Development

Psychoanalytic theory by Sigmund Freud: A controversial theory was proposed by psychologist Sigmun Freud. In psychoanalytic theory, he suggested that the energy of the libido was focused on specific erogenous zones at specific stages. Failure to progress through a stage can result in a fixation at that point in development, which Freud believed could have an influence on adult behavior.

Emotional development by Erik Erikson: Unlike many other developmental theories, Erikson's theory focuses on development across the entire life span. At each stage, children face a development crisis that serves as a major turning point.

Intellectual development by Jean Piaget: Psychologist Jean Piaget proposed a theory centred on the intellectual development of children. Concepts such as schemas, egocentrism, and assimilation are central to Piaget's theory.

Moral development by Lawrence Kohlberg: Psychologist Lawrence Kohlberg proposed a stage theory focused specifically on the moral development of children. The theory describes three overall levels of moral development that can then be broken down further into six stages.

Social development theory by Lev Vygotskys: Every function in the child's cultural development appears twice: first, on the social level, and later, on the individual level; first, between people (interpsychological) and then inside the child (intra psychological). This applies equally to voluntary attention, to logical memory, and to the formation of concepts. All the higher functions originate as actual relationships between individuals.'

- *Role of social Interaction in cognitive development*: The Social development theory (SDT) mainly asserts that social interaction has a vital role in the cognitive development process. With this concept, Vygotsky's theory opposes that of Jean Piaget's cognitive development theory because Piaget explains that a person undergoes development first before he achieves learning, whereas Vygotsky argues that social learning comes first before development. Through the social development theory, Vygotsky states that the cultural development of a child is firstly on the social level called interpsychological, and secondly on the individual or personal level called intrapsychological.
- *The more Knowledgeable other (MKO)*: The MKO is any person who has a higher level of ability or understanding than the learner in terms of the task, process or concept at hand. Normally, when we think of an MKO, we refer to an older adult, a teacher or an expert. For example, a child learns multiplication of numbers because his tutor teaches him well. The traditional MKO is an older person; however, MKOs could also refer to our friends, younger people and even electronic devices like computers and cellphones. For instance, you learn how to skate because your daughter taught you this skill.
- *The zone of proximal development (ZPD):* The ZPD is the distance between what is known and what is unknown by the learner. It is the difference between the ability of learner to performer a specific task under the guidance of his MKO and the learner`s ability to do that task independently. Basically, the theory explains that learning occurs in ZPD.

Relevance to Nursing Practice

- Being able to recognize behaviors associated with the id, ego, and superego will assist in the assessment of clients' developmental level.
- Understanding the use of ego-defense mechanisms is important in making determinations about maladaptive behaviors and in planning care for clients to assist in creating change.
  - To assess a person's condition better
  - To provide proper guidance according to developmental history.
  - For early detection of deviation in child's pattern of development
  - Simple and time-efficient mechanism to ensure adequate surveillance of developmental progress
  - *Helps to assess domain*: Cognitive, motor, language, social/behavioral and adaptive.

CONCLUSION

We know that certain characteristics are typical in certain ages, but these are not set rules, all these are guide only to assess normal growth and development of a child. Each child grows in his own way. One child may progress slower than another and still he/she is perfectly healthy and within the range of development appropriate for his/her age.

CHAPTER 5

Stages of Pediatric Life

Chapter Outline

- Prenatal Pediatrics
- Fetal Growth and Development
- The Neonate
- Respiratory System
- Circulatory System
- Gastrointestinal (GI) System
- Immune System
- Skin
- Neurologic System
- Sensory Development
- Immediate Post Birth Care
- Assessment of Gestational Age
- Physical Examination of the Newborn
- Thermal Regulation of Newborn
- Breastfeeding and Lactation Management
- To Ensure Safety, Prevent Injury and Infection
- Identification and Early Registration
- To Identify Actual or Potential Problems and Immediate Action
- The Normal Infant
- The Toddler
- General Characteristics of Toddler
- Overview of the Growth and Development
- Cognitive Development
- Physical Growth and Development
- Language Development
- Social Development
- Behavior
- Physical Development and Role of Parent
- Needs of the Toddler
- Injury Prevention
- Injuries and Accidents in Toddlers
- Safe Play
- Preschool Child
- Overview of the Growth and Development
- Role of Parent in Development
- Special Problems of Preschool Child
- Promoting Optimal Health of Preschool Child
- The School Child
- Overview of Emotional Development in School Child
- The School Child, his Family and Friends
- Health Problems During School-age
- Adolescence
- Changes During Adolescence

'Children are all human beings. Just at different stages of life'.

Children go through distinct periods of development as they move from infants to young adults. During each of these stages multiple changes in the development of the brain are taking place. What occurs and approximately when these growth and developments take place are genetically determined. However, environmental circumstances and exchanges with key individuals within that environment have significant influence on how each child benefits from each growth and developmental event.

Stages of pediatric life are used to broadly outline key periods in the human development timeline. During each stage growth and development occur in the primary developmental domains including physical, intellectual, language and social-emotional.

Stages of pediatric life (Fig. 5.1) are discussed in this chapters.

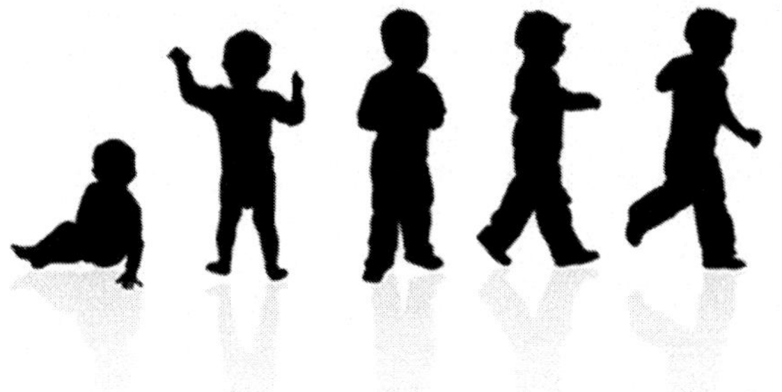

Fig. 5.1: Stages of pediatric life

Prenatal Pediatrics

Did You Know?
'Fetus' Means 'Little One' and 'Offspring'

INTRODUCTION

In their role of advocacy for children and families, pediatric nurses are in position to support and guide parents during their visits during prenatal period. During these visits nurses gather basic information from parents, provide information and counsel them, and identify high-risk situations in which parents may need to be referred to appropriate resources (e.g. counselors, support groups, geneticist) and prepared for potential problems with the child. In addition, a relationship between pediatric nurse and prospective parents and their family can help parents develop parenting skills. Medical and social risks for families and infants are decreased by an early and comprehensive prenatal visit.

Prenatal pediatrics focuses on the assessment, management, support and education of the woman and family experiencing a high-risk pregnancy. Nurses manage a variety of high-risk issues, such as; preterm labor, gestational diabetes, prevention and early detection of toxemia and other medical problems, hyperemesis gravidarum, malnutrition, teen pregnancy, etc.

The goal of prenatal nursing is to prevent or reduce the chance of a troubled maternal life course. To accomplish this goal, prenatal nurses educate and support mothers and fathers during and after the course of their pregnancy. As a result, parents avoid pregnancy related stress and health issues. Moreover, they feel a sense of empowered to begin parenthood on the right track.

EMBRYOLOGICAL AND FETAL DEVELOPMENT

Human fertilization is the union of the ***sperm***atozoon with the ovum, usually occurs in the ***ampulla of the uterine tube***. During sexual intercourse, 2 to 5 mL of semen, usually containing more than 300 million sperm, is ejaculated into the female's vagina. By flagellar (wiggly) movement, the sperm make their way through the fluids of the cervical mucus, across the endometrium, and into the fallopian tube to meet the descending ovum in the ampulla of the fallopian tube. The union between ovum and sperm occurs in the outer third of the fallopian tube. The process of ***fertilization*** involves a sperm fusing with an ovum. The most common sequence begins with ***ejaculation*** during ***copulation***, follows with ***ovulation***, and finishes with fertilization (Figs 5.2A and B).

Scientists discovered the dynamics of ***human*** fertilization in the nineteenth century. The result of this union is the production of a ***zygote***, or fertilized egg, initiating ***prenatal development***. Further that the early stages of development occurs in the tube, whilst the young embryo is on its way to the uterus.

The human fertilized ovum attains some degree of development before it enters the uterus, as it is able to begin to embed itself at once.

The combined ovum and sperm, referred to as the zygote, begins segmentation probably at once, whilst the ovum still in the fallopian tube. The first segmentation naturally divides the egg cell into two, then into four,

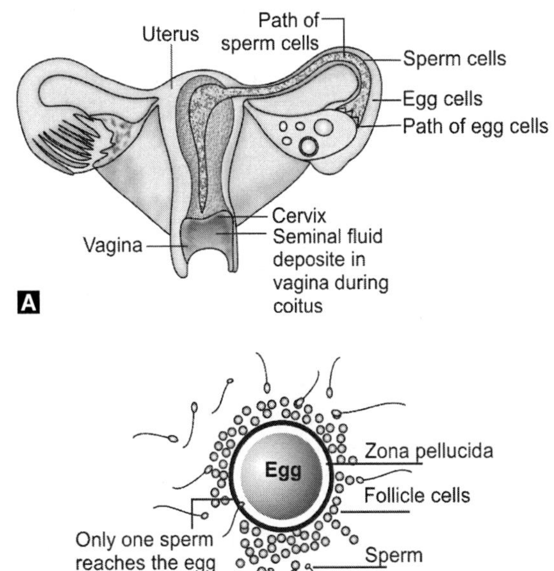

Figs 5.2A and B: A. Travel of sperm to ovum; **B.** Sperm and ovum

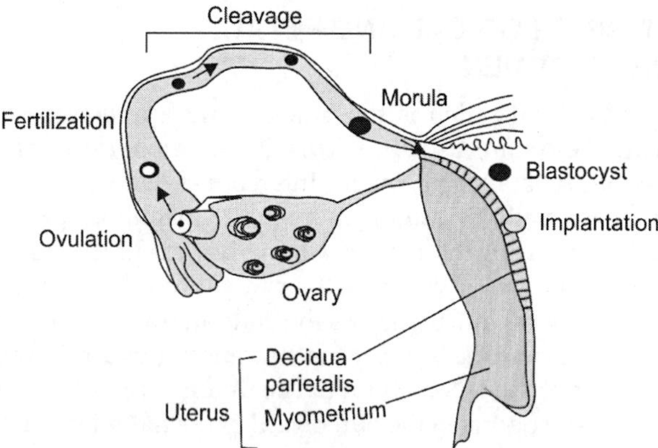

Fig. 5.3: Events of fertilization and implantation

sixteen, thirty-two, etc. until a solid mass of cells is produced in 2–3 days which may be termed the morula stage. The morula is a rapidly growing structure and it floats in the uterus for 3 to 4 days, gaining in size and weight. At this time, the hollow fluid-filled morula, now called blastocyst burrows into the uterine lining (Fig. 5.3).

The outer surface of the blastocyst becomes covered with finger-like projections called chorionic villi. Chorionic villi aid in the process of implantation into the endometrium (decidua). Villi also manufacture human chorionic gonadotropin (HCG) which signal the corpus luteum within the ovaries to continue production of progesterone and estrogen to prevent menstruation.

Implantation normally occurs in the upper, posterior wall of the uterus. The point of implantation becomes the origin for the placenta and umbilical cord.

The zygote contains all of the genetic information (DNA) needed to become a baby. Half the DNA comes from the mother's egg and half from the father's sperm. A blastocyst is made up of an inner group of cells with an outer shell. The inner group of cells will become the embryo and will develop into baby. The outer group of cells will become structures, called membranes, which nourish and protect the embryo. Once the blastocyst reaches the uterus, it buries itself in the uterine wall. At this point in the mother's menstrual cycle, the lining of the uterus is thick with blood and ready to support a baby. The blastocyst sticks tightly to the wall of the uterus and receives nourishment from the mother's blood.

Sex Determination

Chromosomes are small, thread-like structures within each cell that contain genes, which carry genetic instructions. Children inherit some traits like color of eyes, sex, height and skin color from their parents and genes control these physical and chemical traits.

For example, in humans, there are 23 'pairs' of chromosomes: 22 autosomal pairs, and one 'pair' of sex chromosomes. The female has 23 pairs of chromosomes. The pair of chromosomes that determined her sex are named 'XX.' The ovum can only carry an 'X' sex chromosome from each of the female's pairs (23 chromosomes). Females are determined by two identical sex chromosomes: their genotype is XX.

The male has 23 pairs of chromosomes. Males, on the other hand, are determined by a single X in combination with the second kind of sex chromosome, a Y. Therefore, a male's genotype is XY. The sperm carries one chromosome from each of the male's pairs (23 chromosomes). The sperm can carry either an 'X' or a 'Y' sex chromosome. Humans are born with 46 chromosomes in 23 pairs. The X and Y chromosomes determine a person's sex. Most women are 46XX and most men are 46XY (Figs 5.4A and B).

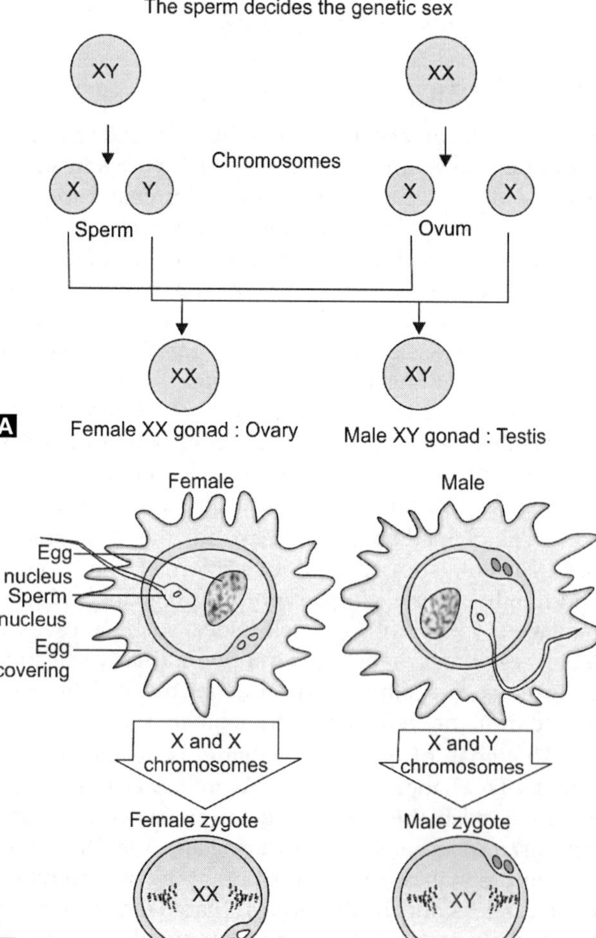

Figs 5.4A and B: Genetic determination of sex of offspring

If the ovum is fertilized by a sperm carrying an 'X' chromosome, the child is a girl. If the ovum is fertilized by a sperm carrying a 'Y' chromosome, the child is a boy. The sperm of the father always determines the child's sex.

Placental Development

The placenta is a fleshy disk like organ. The fully developed placenta (afterbirth) is reddish in color. It is formed from the outer layers of the blastocyst. It is completely formed by the third month of pregnancy. The placenta functions as a transport mechanism between the developing *fetus* to the mother (*uterine* wall) to allow transportation of oxygen, nutrients and antibodies to the fetus by means of the umbilical vein; removes carbon dioxide and metabolic wastes from the fetus by the two umbilical arteries. It serves as a protective barrier against harmful effects of certain drugs and microorganisms (Fig. 5.5).

The umbilical cord (lifeline) connects the fetus to the placenta and is normally 20 inches in length and 3/4 inch in diameter. It contains one umbilical vein and two umbilical arteries (AVA). Placenta acts as a partial barrier between the mother and fetus to prevent fetal and maternal blood from mixing; and produces hormones essential for maintaining the pregnancy. (The hormones are estrogen, progesterone, and human chorionic gonadotropin (HCG)).

Fetal Membranes (Fig. 5.6)

Two closely applied but separate membranes the amnion (inner membrane) and the chorion (outer membrane), line the uterine cavity and surround the developing embryo-fetus (Fig. 5.7). Both membrane,

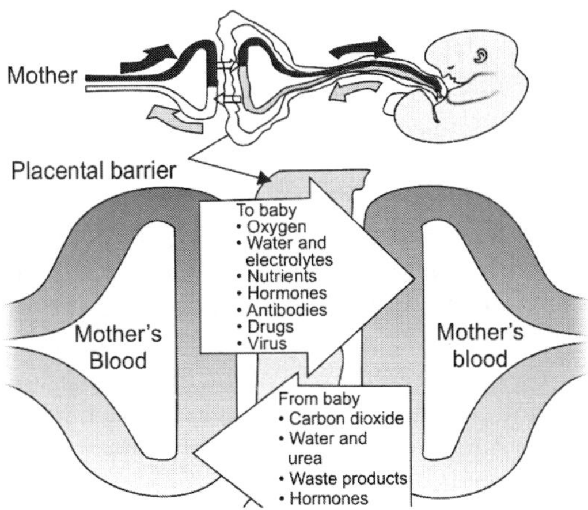

Fig. 5.5: The placental circulation

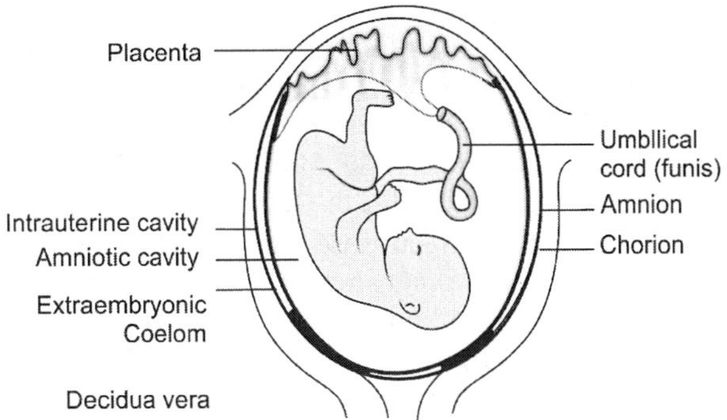

Fig. 5.6: Fetal membranes

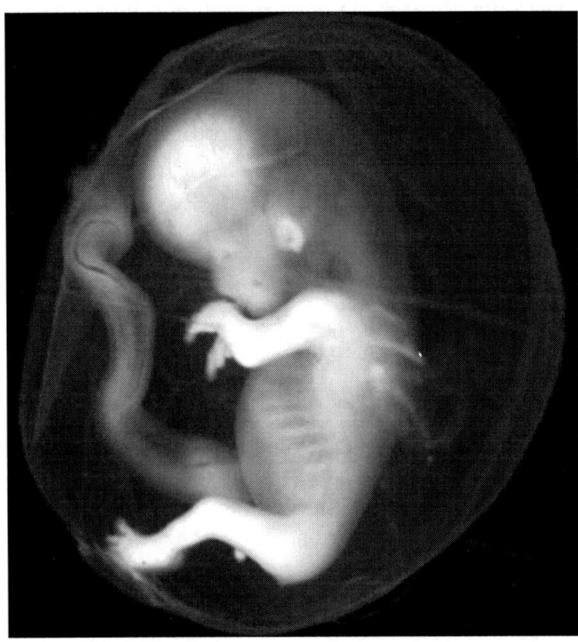

Fig. 5.7: A fetus inside womb

arise from the zygote. As the chorion develops, it blends with the fetal portion of the placenta; the amnion blends with the fetal umbilical cord. These deceptively strong, translucent membranes contain not only the fetus but also the amniotic fluid, and they are continuous with the margins of the placenta.

Amnion and chorion are part of the extraembryonic membranes which function in an embryo's overall development. They also play important roles in the embryo's nourishment, breathing, and see page.

Amnion is the thin, smooth, slippery and glistening, tough innermost membrane that covers an embryo. The membrane is made up of tresodeum on the outside and ectoderm on the inside which has specific cells with specific functions. It is filled with fluid and is often called the 'bag of water.' The fetus floats and moves in the amniotic cavity. At full term, this cavity normally contains 500 cc to 1000 cc of fluid (water). This fluid provides many functions for the fetus.

The amnion's main purpose is to protect the embryo during the months of pregnancy. It helps in reducing the risk of injuries to the unborn embryo and its development in the womb. Basically, the amnion is one of the defenses against any fetal damage during the development. Any injuries or harm can further lead to fetal death. Allow freedom of fetal movement and permits musculoskeletal development and symmetric growth and development of the fetus. Protect the fetus from the loss of heat and maintains a relative and constant fetal body temperature. Serves as a source of oral fluid for the fetus and acts as an excretion and collection system. Separate the fetus from the fetal membranes. The rupture of the amnion and the release of the amniotic fluid is a signal for the start of the pregnancy's delivery stage.

The chorion, on the other hand, is the outer membrane that surrounds the amnion, the embryo and other membranes and entities in the womb. It is considered as the support platform of the fetus and the aminon. It contributes to the growth of the placenta.

The chorion is formed by two layers, trophoblast as the outer layer and mesoderm as the inner layer. The mesoderm is the one in contact with the amnion. The trophoblast provides the nutrients for the fetus during its confinement while the ectoderm further develops into many parts of the embryo's body like teeth, and the nervous system.

The chorion provides additional protection for the embryo but it also used to promote exchange of nutrients and other necessary fluids from mother to embryo and vice-versa.

The chorion also has a special feature called chorion villi. The villi sprout from the chorion in order to reach more maternal blood, which is the main fluid that carries nutrients from the mother's food and meals. They also serve as a fence between the fetal blood and the maternal blood during the time of the fetal development.

FETAL GROWTH AND DEVELOPMENT

Growth refers to an increase in size (Fig. 5.8).

Development is the continuous process by which an individual changes from one life phase to another. These phases include the prenatal period and the postnatal period. Fetal maturation takes place in an orderly and predictable pattern.

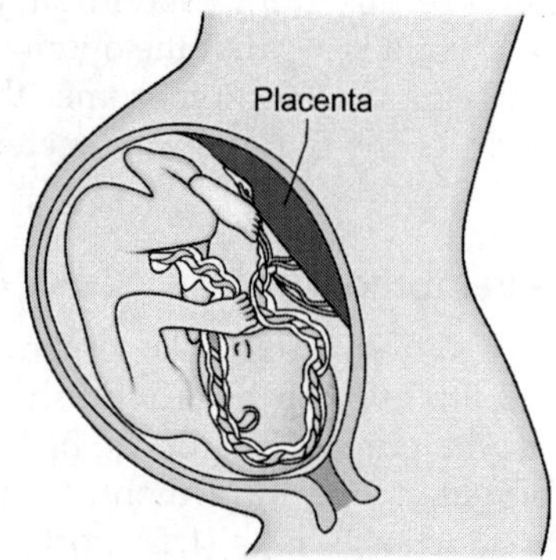

Fig. 5.8: The final stage of development is called the fetal period of development

The age of a pregnancy is referred as lunar months, which corresponds to the usual length of the menstrual cycle, in this respect, it is easier to calculate. A lunar month is a period of four weeks (28 days) and a trimester is a time period of 3 months.

- *First trimester:* During the first three months of pregnancy, the product of conception grows from the just-visible speck to the fertilized ovum to a lively embryo. At the end of the first trimester, the following changes have or are occurring:
  - The fetus is about 2.9 inches long and weighs about 14 grams and all organs are formed, facial features are forming and the fetus becomes human in appearance. External sex organs are visible, but positive sex identification is difficult. Well-defined neck, nail beds beginning, and tooth buds form, rudimentary kidneys excrete small amounts of urine into the amniotic sac. There is movement but just not strong enough to be felt. The fetus becomes less vulnerable to the effects of most drugs, most infections, and radiation.
- *Second trimester:* During these months (4th, 5th, and 6th) the fetus grows fast. Fetal heart tone (FHT) can be heard with a stethoscope, at the end of the second trimester. The skin of the fetus is wrinkled, translucent, and appears pink. Fetus looks like a miniature baby, whose skeleton is calcified and sex is obvious. Birth survival is possible, but the fetus is seriously at risk.
- *Third trimester:* At the end of the third trimester (7th, 8th, and 9th month), the fetus skin is whitish pink, hair in single strands, testes are in the scrotum, if a male child, bones of the skull are firmer, comes closer at the suture lines, lightening occurs, fetus is about 20 inches long and weighs about 2.5 to 3.5 kg.

Prenatal factors influencing growth and development of fetus.

Fetal growth and differentiation may be modified by internal and external factors. Many factors can affect the development of a fetus. Environmental agents that can negatively affect prenatal development are called teratogens. Teratogen exposure tends to be most detrimental during the first trimester of pregnancy, when formation of the organs and brain occurs.

A spontaneous abortion, or *miscarriage*, in the first trimester of pregnancy is usually due to major genetic mistakes or abnormalities in the developing embryo. During this critical period, most of the *first trimester*, the developing embryo is also susceptible to toxic exposures, such as *alcohol*, certain *drugs*, and other *toxins* that cause *birth defects*, such as *fetal alcohol syndrome*.

Biological Factors

Mothers who have their first child when they are over 35 or under 15 are likely to experience more problems during pregnancy and difficulties during delivery than women between these ages. The risks are related to maternal health are seen in both the groups. Young adolescents are less likely to eat properly or to get prenatal care; older women are more likely to have hypertension, diabetes, alcoholism, and other problems related to age. With the advancement in the age of mother (more than 35 years of age), there is increased risk of chromosomal errors like incidence of trisomy birth (Down syndrome); autosomal dominant disorder such as skeletal dysplasia, etc.

Regarding maternal height, weight, nutrition, and parity, there is a good correlation between the maternal weight and the placental and fetal size. The pregnancy diet should include all sorts of nutrients and adequate calories (both for mother and fetus). Deficiencies in maternal diet are related to increased rates of prematurity, stillbirth, infant mortality, physical and neural defects, and small size. If the diet during the last trimester of pregnancy is inadequate, the fetal birth weight, length, and head circumference will be smaller. Nutritional deficiencies in prenatal stage such as lack of folate, contributes to spina bifida. If the caloric intake is less than 400 cal/day, the gestational period will be shortened. In multiple gestations, the weight of newborns is usually decreased in multiple gestations. In relation to the placental weight, twins are lighter than singletons. Placental size (active surface) seems to be a determinant of fetal growth. Growth-retarded fetuses tend to be heavier in relation to the weight of the placenta (i.e. have a higher fetal to placental weight ratio than normal fetuses).

Mothers who smoke cigarettes or drink alcohol are more likely to bear premature or low birth-weight babies than women who do not smoke or drink. Full-term newborns of smoking mothers are approximately 200 g lighter than newborns of non-smokers. Regarding smokers and non-smokers there are, however, also differences in socioeconomic status and other factors, such as maternal alcohol drinking and drug intake. Moreover, maternal drinking is related to **fetal alcohol syndrome**, which results in facial abnormalities, short stature, and mental retardation. Even modest amounts of alcohol and passive smoking have been related to negative effects in the offspring. Moreover, genetic effects of fathers' smoking and drinking may be passed to their offspring.

Drugs taken by the mother during pregnancy, whether legal or illegal, may have a negative impact on the developing fetus. The use of drug in pregnant and lactating women requires a thorough understanding of the unique understanding between the mother, fetus, and the pharmacologic agents that are used in therapy. Sometimes, as in the case of **thalidomide** and **diethylstilbestrol**, the effects of the prescription drug on the infant are not known until much later.

A baby, out of consanguineous marriage is common in different countries. The offspring of consanguineous relationships are at greater risk of certain genetic disorders. Autosomal recessive disorders occur in individuals who are homozygous for a particular recessive gene mutation.

Exposure to infection such as ***rubella*** or ***cytomegalovirus***, toxoplasmosis, chicken pox, syphilis, HIV has serious implication on newborn child. For example, prenatal rubella is a well-known central nervous system teratogen, toxoplasmosis causes hepato-spleenomegaly, retinitis, brain cysts with consequent retardation and epilepsy; syphilis infection causes CNS retardation, blindness, hypoplastic nose, limb deformities, anemia, etc.

Radiation from ***X-rays*** or ***radiation therapy:*** Deleterious effects of radiation include carcinogenicity, mutagenicity and organ system toxicity. For this reason, obstetric X-ray examination in pregnancy has been largely superceded by ultrasound examination.

Genetic Patterns of Common Pediatric Disorders

Children with chromosome abnormalities are born with an irregular number of chromosomes (more than or fewer than 46) or with one or more chromosomes that have irregular structures (deletions from or duplications to parts of an individual chromosome, or with a part of one chromosome moved to another location).

Down Syndrome

Incidence is 1 per 700–1,000 births. Children with Down syndrome have one extra copy of chromosome 21 (trisomy 21). Physical characteristics growth retardation which include a protruding tongue, thick lips, flat nose, short neck, wide gaps between toes, short fingers, specific health problems, and risks for heart problems and hearing loss. Mental retardation can range from mild to severe. Children often have good visual discrimination skills and may be better at understanding verbal language than producing it. About 75% of fetus with trisomy 21 aborts spontaneously. (*See* Chapter 25 of this edition).

Klinefelter Syndrome (Fig. 5.9)

Incidence is 1 per 500–1,000 boys. It is a male Karyotype with an extra X-chrosome (47 XXY). Only boys have Klinefelter syndrome. The extra 'X' chromosome is maternal in origin in 67% and paternal in 33%. Rarely XXXY, XXXXY, or XY/XXY mosaic are seen.

Diagnosis may not occur until adolescence, when testes fail to enlarge. Affected boys tend to have long legs, to grow modest breast tissue, and remain sterile. They tend to show lower than average verbal ability and some speech and language delays. The greater the number of X-chromosome (XXXY, XXY) the more severe are the mental retardation and other clinical features. (*See* Chapter 25).

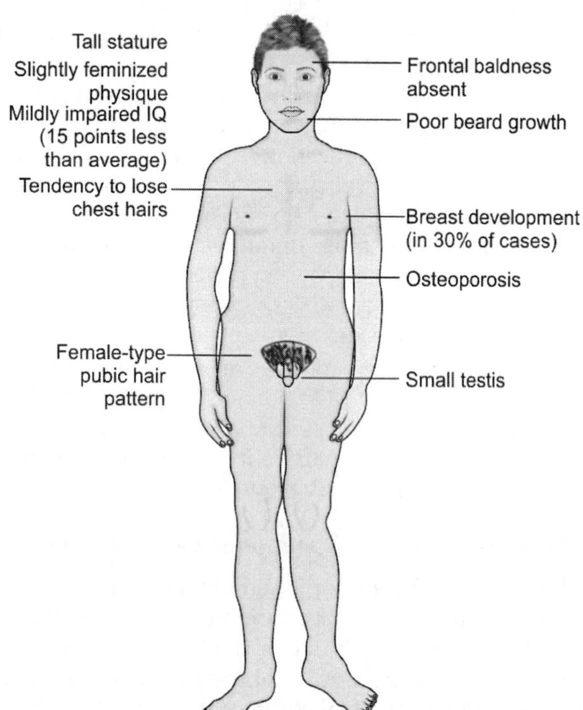

Fig. 5.9: Features of Klinefelter syndrome

Turner Syndrome

Incidence of Turner syndrome is 1 per 2,500 girls. Turner syndrome is of female phenotype; they have one X chromosome and are missing the second sex chromosome. Affected girls have broad chests, webbed necks, short stature, and specific health problems. They do not show normal sexual development. They may show normal verbal ability but lower than average ability in processing visual and spatial information. (*See* Chapter 25 of this edition).

Prader-Willi Syndrome

Incidence of Prader-Willi syndrome is 1 per 10,000–25,000 births. A deletion from a gene segment on chromosome 15 is inherited from the father. Children with this syndrome tend to become obese and show mental retardation; they also have small hands and feet and are short in stature. They may develop maladaptive behaviors such as throwing frequent temper tantrums and picking at their own skin. Beginning at ages 1–6, children may eat excessively, hoard food, and eat unappealing substances.

It needs developmentally appropriate plans to help children regulate eating, decrease inappropriate behaviors, and increase acceptable emotional expression. Seek medical care as necessary.

Mechanism of Genetic Inheritance

Inheritance refers to how genetic information is passed down from parent to child. Gregor Mendel, who is often called the founder of modern genetics, performed many experiments and established 'classic' inheritance rules and patterns which are still followed to this day. Genetic disorders due to traditional modes of inheritance is classified as (Fig. 5.10):

- *Mendelian disorders (single gene, mono gene):*
  - Autosomal dominant (AD)
  - Autosomol recessive (AR)
  - X- linked recessive (XLR)
  - X- linked dominant (XLD)
- *Chromosal disorders:* Numerical disorder
  - Structural abnormalities
- *Multifactorial disorders:* Complex disease traits.

Autosomal Dominant Inheritance

Autosomal dominant inheritance refers to conditions caused by changes ('mutations') in genes located on

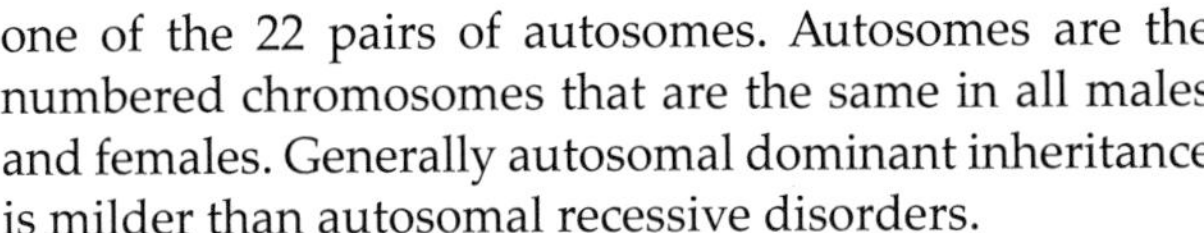

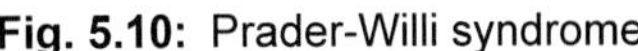

Fig. 5.10: Prader-Willi syndrome

one of the 22 pairs of autosomes. Autosomes are the numbered chromosomes that are the same in all males and females. Generally autosomal dominant inheritance is milder than autosomal recessive disorders.

This aberration is manifested even if only one of the alleles of the abnormal gene is affected. For example, one of father's chromosomes has an allele without a mutation and one of his chromosomes has an allele with mutations, but mother's both chromosomes have alleles without mutations. Abnormal gene is passed from one generation to another in a vertical fashion. Therefore, if one parent is affected with an autosomal dominant genetic condition and the other is not, there is 50% probability of passing the traits with every pregnancy a child will be affected and a 2 in 4 (50%) (Fig. 5.11).

In an autosomal dominant pattern of inheritance (Figs 5.12A and B), a child inherits a normal copy of a gene from one parent and an abnormal gene from the other parent. The abnormal gene dominates the normal gene, so one copy of an abnormal gene is enough to cause an autosomal dominant disorder. Waardenburg syndrome is the most common cause of autosomal dominant syndromic hearing loss, affecting 1 in 42,000 people. Waardenburg syndrome accounts for approximately 2% of cases of profound congenital hearing loss.

Examples of autosomal dominant disorders are mental retardation, Huntington's chorea, Noonan syndrome, tuberous sclerosis, osteogenesis imperfecta, optic glioma, etc.

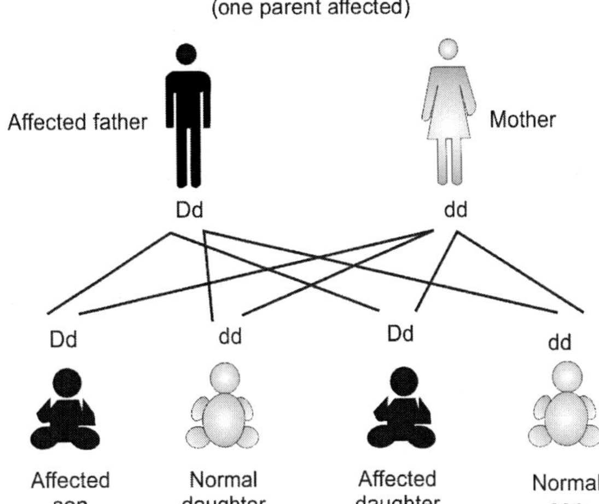

Fig. 5.11: Autosomal dominant inheritance (one parent is affected)

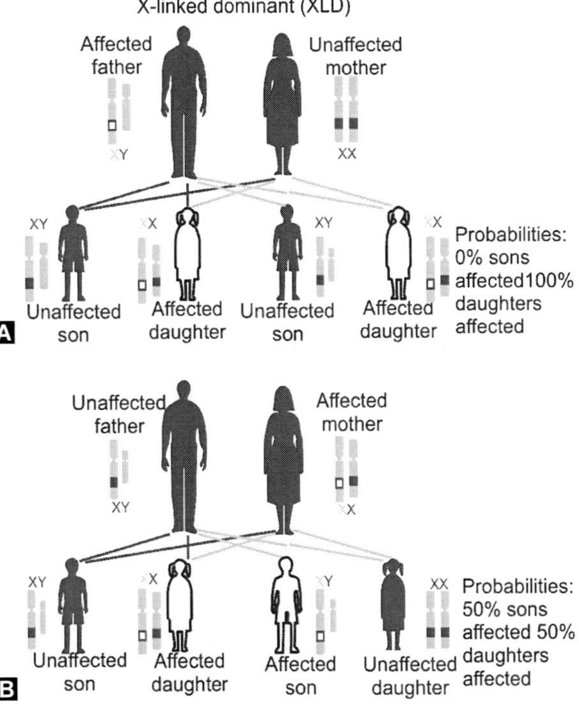

Figs 5.12A and B: A. X-linked dominant, affected father; **B.** X-linked dominant, affected mother

Autosomal Recessive Inheritance

When a disorder is passed on in an **autosomal recessive** fashion, two copies of the abnormal gene are required to cause the disorder. Individuals who inherit only one abnormal gene and one normal gene are referred to as *carriers* and are not affected by the disorder. Carriers frequently are unaware of their carrier status until they have an affected child. Individuals affected by

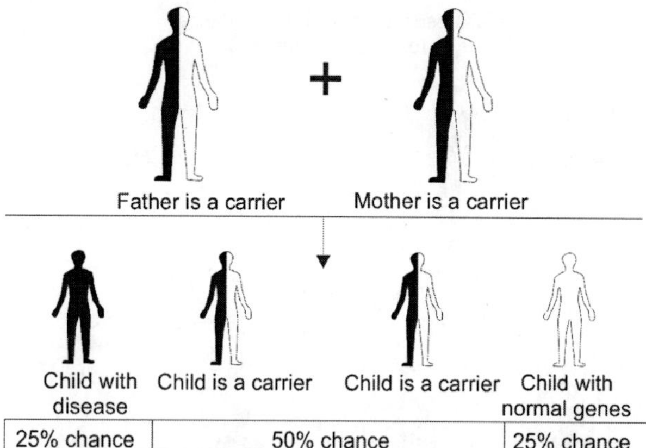

Fig. 5.13: Autosomal dominant inheritance (both parents are carrier and unaffected)

an autosomal recessive disorder usually are the result of matings between two carriers. The above figure demonstrates potential outcomes of such a mating, whereby 25% of offspring are affected by the disorder in question, 50% are unaffected carriers, and 25% are free of the disorder and the abnormal gene (Fig. 5.13). The risk of an autosomal recessive disorder is more in *consanguinity*, or the presence of a common ancestor between mates . Usher syndrome demonstrates an autosomal recessive pattern of inheritance, which is characterized by congenital profound sensorineural hearing loss and progressive vision loss (Fig. 5.14).

Eamples of autosomal recessive disorders are phenyl ketonuria, beta-halassemia, Hurler syndrome, etc.

X-linked Recessive (XLR)

X-linked inheritance means that the gene causing the trait or the disorder is located on the X chromosome (Figs 5.15A and B). It is a mode of *inheritance* in which a mutation in a *gene* on the *X chromosome* causes the phenotype to be expressed (1) in males (who are necessarily *heterozygous* for the gene mutation because they have only one X chromosome) and (2) in females who are *homozygous* for the gene mutation (*i.e.* they have a copy of the gene mutation on each of their two X chromosomes). Example of X-linked recessive inheritance disorders are red-green color blindness, hemophilia A, Duchenne muscular dystrophy, etc.

Chromosomal Disorders

About 50% of abortions occur during the first trimester are with chromosomal abnormalities. Chromosomal abnormalities can affect any chromosome, including the sex chromosomes. Chromosomal abnormalities affect the number or structure of chromosomes and may be visible with a microscope in a test called karyotype analysis. It may be either numeric disorder (quantitative), structural anomalies (qualitative).

Numerical Disorder

When an individual is missing one of the chromosomes from a pair, the condition is called monosomy (Turner syndrome). When an individual has more than two chromosomes instead of a pair, the condition is called trisomy (Down syndrome) (Fig. 5.16).

Mosaicism occurs during mitosis and due to non-disjunction, two new cells are formed, one with 47 chromosomes and the other with 45 chromosomes (may occur in same individual).

Structural Abnormalities

A chromosome's structure can be altered in several ways. Different types of structural abnormalities are:

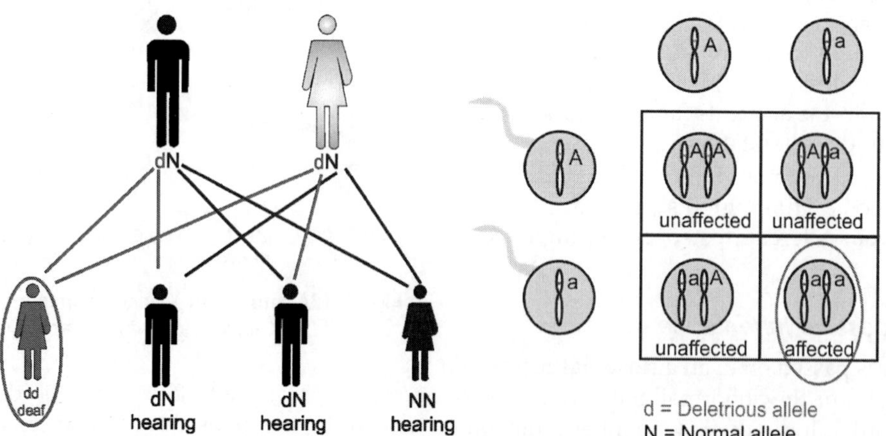

Fig. 5.14: Autosomal recessive inheritance (both parents are carrier and unaffected)

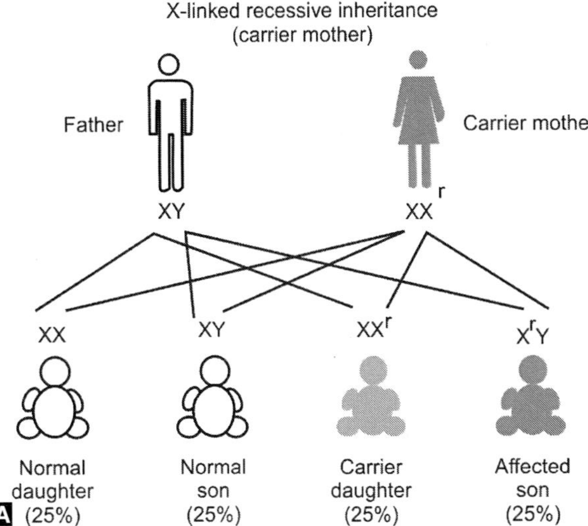

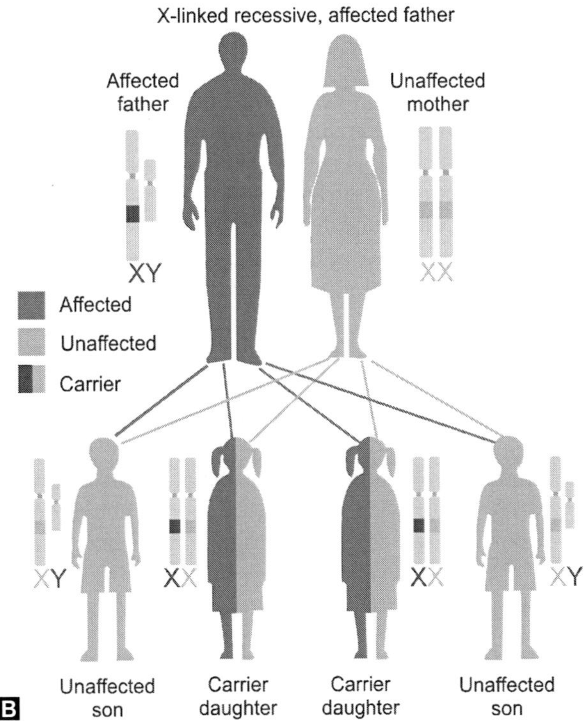

Figs 5.15A and B: Examples of X-linked recessive inheritance

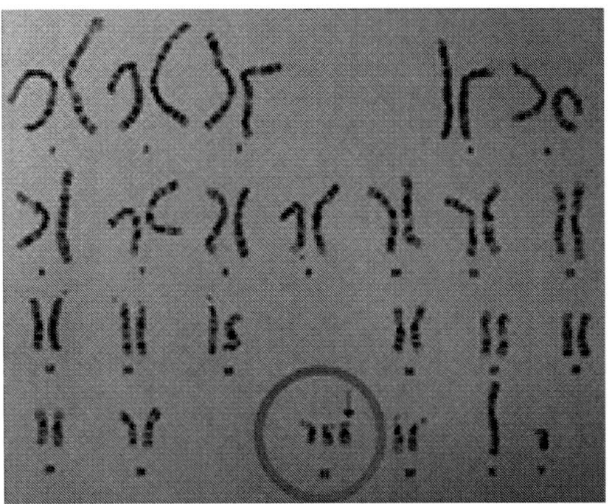

Fig. 5.16: Chromosome pattern of Down syndrome; Trisomy 21 showing three 'X' chromosomes instead of the usual two

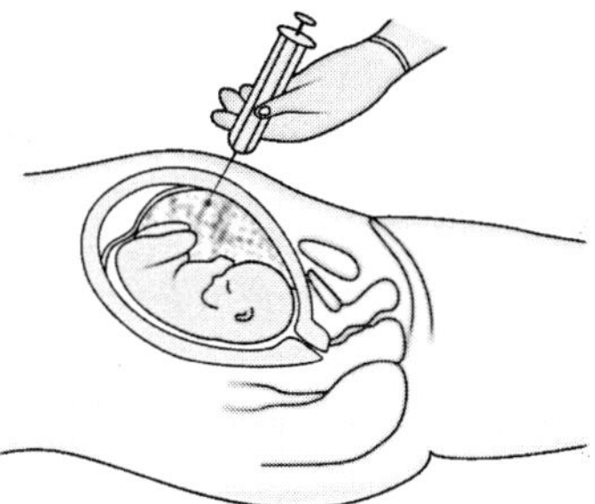

Fig. 5.17: Amniocentesis. A method for assessing fetal maturity and well-being. It is a diagnostic test that detects chromosome abnormalities, neural tube defects and genetic disorders

Deletions: A portion of the chromosome is missing or deleted.

Duplications: A portion of the chromosome is duplicated, resulting in extra genetic material.

Translocations: These are the most common structural chromosomal aberration where two chromosomes are involved. A portion of one chromosome may break off from the parent chromosome and be transferred to another chromosome and vice versa. There are two main types of translocation. In a reciprocal translocation, segments from two different chromosomes have been exchanged. In a Robertsonian translocation, an entire chromosome has attached to another at the centromere.

Inversions: A portion of the chromosome has broken off, turned upside down, and reattached. As a result, the genetic material is inverted.

Rings: A portion of a chromosome has broken off and formed a circle or ring. This can happen with or without loss of genetic material.

Multifactorial Disorders

Multiple factors are involved in this type of disorders. About 60% of birth defects are due to this kind inheritance.

Chromosome abnormalities usually occur when there is an error in cell division. There are two kinds of cell division, mitosis and meiosis.

- Mitosis results in two cells that are duplicates of the original cell. One cell with 46 chromosomes divides and becomes two cells with 46 chromosomes each. This kind of cell division occurs throughout the body, except in the reproductive organs. This is the way most of the cells that make up our body are made and replaced.
- Meiosis results in cells with half the number of chromosomes 23, instead of the normal 46. This is the type of cell division that occurs in the reproductive organs, resulting in the eggs and sperm.

In both processes, the correct number of chromosomes is supposed to end up in the resulting cells. However, errors in cell division can result in cells with too few or too many copies of a chromosome. Errors can also occur when the chromosomes are being duplicated.

Other factors that can increase the risk of chromosome abnormalities are:

- *Maternal Age:* Women are born with all the eggs they will ever have. Some researchers believe that errors can crop up in the eggs' genetic material as they age. Older women are at higher risk of giving birth to babies with chromosome abnormalities than younger women. Because men produce new sperm throughout their lives, paternal age does not increase risk of chromosome abnormalities.
- *Environment:* Although there is no conclusive evidence that specific environmental factors cause chromosome abnormalities, it is still possible that the environment may play a role in the occurrence of genetic errors.

Prevention of Genetic Disorders

- Carrier screening detects the carrier state in case of large number of autosomal recessive or X-linked recessive disorders
- *Metabolic screening:* The handicap can be prevented or minimized by early treatment, i.e. phenylketonuria, galactosemia, congenital hypothyroidism
- Intrauterine diagnosis (USG, amniocentesis, cordocentesis, fetoscopy, chorionic villus sampling).
- Micronutrient sampling (folic acid) prevents neural tube defect.

Genetic Counseling

Task force of the national society of genetic counselors (NSGC) developed the following definition of genetic counseling that was approved by the NSGC Board of Directors: Genetic counseling is the process of helping people understand and adapt to the medical, psychological and familial implications of genetic contributions to disease. Inherited or genetic concerns lead some parents to choose amniocentesis to determine if specific genetic disorders may be present in their babies (Fig 5.17). This process integrates the following: Interpretation of family and medical histories to assess the chance of disease occurrence or recurrence. Education is given about inheritance, testing, management, prevention, resources and research. Counseling aims to promote informed choices and adaptation to the risk or condition.

So, genetic counseling is the process of:

- Evaluating family history and medical records
- Suggesting genetic tests
- Evaluating the results of this investigation
- Counseling to promote informed choices in view of risk assessment, family goals, ethical and religious values
- Support to encourage the best possible adjustment to the disorder in an affected family member and/or to the risk of recurrence of that disorder
- Helping parents understand and reach decisions about what to do next.

Genes are made up of DNA molecules, which are the building blocks of heredity. They are grouped together in specific patterns within a person's chromosomes, forming the unique 'blueprint' for every physical and biological characteristic of that person.

Humans have 46 chromosomes, arranged in pairs in every living cell of our bodies. When the egg and sperm join at conception, half of each chromosomal pair is inherited from each parent. This newly formed combination of chromosomes then copies itself again and again during fetal growth and development, passing identical genetic information to each new cell in the growing fetus.

Current science suggests that every human has about 25,000 genes per cell. An error in just one gene (and in some instances, even the alteration of a single piece of DNA) can sometimes be the cause for a serious medical condition.

Legal and Ethical Aspects of Genetic Testing and Screening

Genetic testing is gaining popularity for the many advantages it has to offer in the prevention, management and treatment of disease. These tests most commonly present an opportunity for individuals to become informed about their genetic predisposition to disease, and for couples to be aware of the possible genetic characteristics of their unborn children. Some critical ethical, legal and social issues have been emerged to the forefront, as genetic testing is stemmed from the informative potential. In order for genetic testing to be used safely and appropriately, these issues should be discussed with clients so that they are aware of risks and benefits.

The Individual's Right to Choose

In many communities, couples are encouraged to perform genetic testing prior to marriage as well as on the fetus during pregnancy, to reduce genetic diseases. While this strategy has effectively reduced the prevalence of some genetic diseases like thalassemia, for which there is still no cure, still couples are not to be coerced to do it. On the other hand genetic tests may provide individuals, who seek them freely, with information needed to make important decisions about their future, therefore supporting their right to make a informed choice. Before taking consent, following issues are to be taken care of:

- Testing is voluntary
- Risks, limitations, and benefits of testing or not testing
- Alternatives to genetic testing
- Details of the testing process (for example, what type of sample is required, accuracy of test, turn-around time, etc.)
- Confidentiality and privacy of test results
- Potential consequences related to results including
  - Impact on health
  - Possible emotional and psychological reactions
  - Treatment/prevention options
- Ramifications for family.

Stigmatization and Discrimination

When considering genetic testing, a major concern often raised is the potential of discrimination based on genetic information. Knowledge of genetic risks can lead to potential social and psychological consequences for the individual. Socially, knowledge from genetic tests may lead to stigmatization and discrimination within the community. Refusing to undergo genetic testing as well as choosing to undergo genetic testing can both lead to discrimination and stigmatization depending on the prevalent social norms regarding acceptance and use of the technology.

In addition, members of minority communities often fear that genetic information will be used to stigmatize them, the test results may lead to the marginalization of the individual from mainstream society by virtue of the health risks identified. Discrimination can be in the form of denial of health insurance, employment or simply social acceptance, benefits and allowances and medical coverage or health insurance. This is especially worrisome in communities that rely heavily on private insurance systems as a source of funding for necessary medical treatments.

On the other hand, within the context of a well-informed community integrated clinical and social support systems which include counseling services for patients and their families, knowledge of genetic disease or predisposition can lead to better care and management of the patient and ultimately to improved quality of life.

Communicating Test Results

Genetic tests give an assessment of an individual's inherent risk for disease and disability. This predictive power makes genetic testing particularly liable for misuse. Genetic test results should be released only to those individuals for whom the test recipient has given consent, and discussion is to be done in an understandable manner. As many genetic tests will not provide simple positive/negative results, but potentially inconclusive results or risk estimates, it is important that patients understand the extent of the information actually provided from a genetic test. Under no circumstances should results with identifiers be provided to any outside parties, including employers, insurers, or government agencies, without the test recipient's written consent.

Respecting a patient's confidentiality by not disclosing the results of a genetic test to third parties can therefore conflict with the well-being of family members, who could benefit from this knowledge. Finding the right balance between the patient's privacy and confidentiality of her genetic information, and what is in the best interests of family members, is an ongoing ethical and social challenge.

Limitations: Genetic testing creates important opportunities for assessment of genetic risk and diagnosis. However, some genetic tests do not identify all of the possible gene mutations that can cause a particular condition, or they have limited predictive value. Because some genetic tests may not provide all the information that families may want, the test may subsequently require difficult decisions without providing full information. This can lead to uncertainties for patients and clinicians. Few questions on impact of genetic information which come to the health care professional are:

- How does a person's genetic information affect that individual and society's perception of that individual?

- How does genetic and genomic information affect members of minority communities?

Role of Pediatric Nurse in Genetic Testing and Genetic Screening

Nurses are on the forefront of care, and therefore will participate fully in genetic based, genomic-based activities such as collecting family history, obtaining informed consent about genetic testing, and administration of gene-based therapy. This new direction in health care calls for all nurses to be able to effectively translate genetic and genomic information to patients with an understanding of associated ethical issues.

Nurses practicing in primary health care settings and specialty care, such as oncology, will continue to be involved in obtaining and reviewing patient family histories and as well collection of medical information from patients and their relatives. She can also encourage the families for genetic screening (thalassemia), give information regarding available service facilities, and outcome of the test and test results. She can protect the child and family from stigma and discrimination.

Nurses in all practice areas will be increasingly involved in the genetic testing process, helping the patient understand the purpose and also the risks and benefits of the genetic test, as part of the informed, decision-making and consent process. The nurse may also obtain written consent for the use of a patient's biological samples for research purposes, and for the purpose of sharing the results of the testing with other family members.

To protect patients from additional distress, nurses should be aware of the relevant ethical, legal, and social issues related to genetics in health care. Genetic counseling provides couples with information that can help them make decisions about future pregnancies. Nurse should provide support and also gives couples additional time to emotionally prepare if a disorder is detected in the fetus.

During pregnancy, nurse can aware pregnant women to reduce exposure to unnatural chemicals, particularly pesticides in food, smoking and consuming alcohol consumption, avoiding environmental hazards including radiation, etc. She can also stress on basic principles and elements of prenatal care which can prevent and minimize genetic disorders. For example many people now eat organic produce, which is grown without chemicals. The simplest precaution to take before consuming vegetables or fruits is to wash them thoroughly. Also, removing the outer surface of vegetables can be helpful since most pesticides will rest on the outside of the vegetable or fruit.

Nurses will therefore have a critical role advocating for, educating, counseling, and supporting patients and families who are making gene-based health care decisions.

The Neonate

INTRODUCTION

Birth is associated with the most drastic changes that ever be fall a person. The nurse is in a unique position to aid the newborn infant in the stressful transition from a warm, dark, fluid-filled environment to an outside world filled with light, sound, and novel tactile stimuli. During this period of the newborn adjusting from intrauterine to extrauterine life, the nurse must be knowledgeable about a newborn's normal biopsychosocial adaptations to recognize any deviations. After birth the newborn must continue the vital activities of intrauterine life and he must also initiate other extrauterine processes which his mother performed for him. These radical and rapid changes are crucial to the maintenance of life. All other neonatal body systems change their functions or establish themselves over a longer period of time. The nurse performs an initial assessment to evaluate the neonate, its immediate post birth adaptations, and the need for further support. The physical and mental well-being of an individual depends on the correct management of events in the perinatal period.

DEFINITION

Neonate: From birth to under four weeks of age (< 28 days), the infant is called newborn or neonate (Fig. 5.18). First seven days of life of birth is called early neonate. Late neonatal period extends from 7th to < 28 day.

Live-born: Product of conception, irrespective of weight and gestational age, that shows an evidence of life like breathing, heartbeat, and pulsation of umbilical cord or definite movements of voluntary muscles after separation from the mother, is called live-born.

Low birth weight (LBW): LBW is defined as a birth weight of a live born infant of less than 2,500 g (5.5 pounds) regardless of gestational age. LBW is either caused by preterm birth (that is, a low gestational age at birth, commonly defined as younger than 37 weeks of gestation) or the infant being small for gestational a preterm birth.

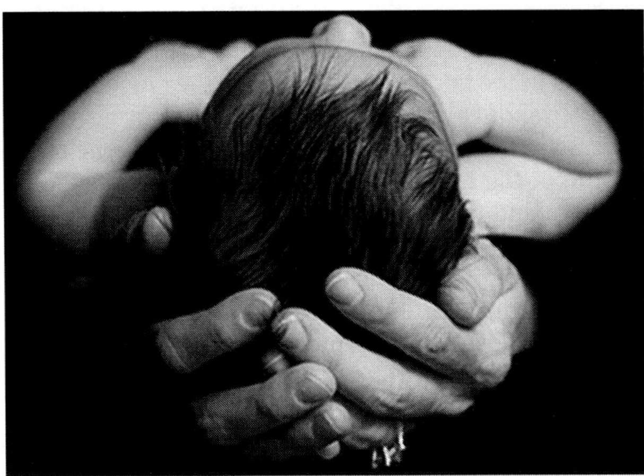

Fig. 5.18: A great joy has come ....

Preterm: Any neonate born before 37 weeks (< 259 days) of pregnancy irrespective of the birth weight is called preterm baby. Four different pathways have been identified that can result in preterm birth and have considerable evidence: Precocious fetal endocrine activation, uterine over-distension, decidual bleeding, and intrauterine inflammation/infection.

Small for gestational age: Being small for gestational age can be constitutional, that is, without an underlying pathological cause, or it can be secondary to intrauterine growth restriction, which, in turn, can be secondary to many possible factors. For example, babies with congenital anomalies or chromosomal abnormalities are often associated with LBW. Problems with the placenta can prevent it from providing adequate oxygen and nutrients to the fetus. Infections during pregnancy that affect the fetus, such as rubella, cytomegalovirus, toxoplasmosis, and syphilis, may also affect the baby's weight.

Postterm baby: Post-maturity is the condition of a baby that has not yet been born after 42 weeks of gestation, two weeks beyond the normal 40 weeks. Postterm, post-maturity, prolonged pregnancy, and post-dates pregnancy all refer to post-mature birth. Post-mature births do not have any harmful effects on the mother; however, the fetus can begin to suffer from malnutrition. After the 42nd week of gestation, the placenta, which supplies the baby with nutrients and oxygen from the mother, starts aging and will eventually fail. If the fetus passes fecal matter, which is not typical until after birth, and the child breathes it in, then the baby could become sick with pneumonia. Postterm pregnancy may be a reason to induce labor (that is, a slow prenatal growth rate), or a combination of both.

Stillborn: A fetal death is a product of conception that does not show any evidence of life, after separation from the mother. A fetal death at a gestational age of 20 weeks or more, or weighing more than 500 gm is designated as still birth or stillborn.

Birth asphyxia: Globally, about one quarter of all neonatal deaths are caused by birth asphyxia. Birth asphyxia is defined simply as the failure to initiate and sustain breathing at birth. Effective resuscitation at birth can prevent a large proportion of these deaths. The need for clinical guidelines on basic newborn resuscitation, suitable for settings with limited resources, is universally recognized.

Neonatal resuscitation: They apply primarily to newly born infants undergoing transition from intrauterine to extra-uterine life. It involves much more than possessing an ordered list of technical skills and having a resuscitation team; it requires excellent assessment skills and a grounded understanding of physiology. Neonatal resuscitation is intervention after a baby is born to help it breathe and to help its heart beat.

Before a baby is born, the placenta provides oxygen and nutrition to the blood and removes carbon dioxide. After a baby is born, the lungs provide oxygen to the blood and remove carbon dioxide. The transition from using the placenta to using the lungs for gas exchange begins when the umbilical cord is clamped or tied off, and the baby has its first breath. Many babies go through this transition without needing intervention. Some babies need help with establishing their air flow, breathing, or circulation. Resuscitation is helping with airway, breathing, and circulation, also known as the ABCs.

Physiologic Resilience of Newborn

The transition from fetal to extra-uterine life is characterized by a series of unique physiological events: the lungs change from fluid-filled to air-filled, pulmonary blood flow increases dramatically, and intra-cardiac and extra-cardiac shunts (foramen ovale and ductus arteriosus) initially reverse direction and subsequently close.

RESPIRATORY SYSTEM

The most critical and profound physiologic change required of the newborn is the onset of breathing. Perfusing its body by breathing independently instead of utilizing placental oxygen is the first challenge of a newborn. At birth, the baby's lungs are filled with fetal lung fluid (which is not amniotic fluid) and are not inflated. The stimuli that help initiate the first respiration are primarily thermal and chemical.

Chemical factors in the blood like low oxygen, increased carbon dioxide and low pH initiate impulses that excite the respiratory center in the medulla. The newborn is expelled from the birth canal to a relatively cooler atmosphere. Its central nervous system reacts to the sudden change in temperature and environment through the sensory impulses of skin. This triggers it to take the first breath, within about 10 seconds after delivery. With the first breaths, there is a fall in pulmonary vascular resistance, and an increase in the surface area available for gas exchange. Over the next 30 seconds, the pulmonary blood flow increases and is oxygenated as it flows through the alveoli of the lungs. Oxygenated blood now reaches the left atrium and ventricle, and through the descending aorta reaches the umbilical arteries.

Oxygenated blood now stimulates constriction of the umbilical arteries resulting in a reduction in placental blood flow. As the pulmonary circulation increases, there is an equivalent reduction in the placental blood flow which normally ceases completely after about three minutes. These two changes result in a rapid redirection of blood flow into the pulmonary vascular bed, from approximately 4 to 100% of cardiac output. The increase in pulmonary venous return results in left atrial pressure being slightly higher than right atrial pressure, which closes the *foramen ovale*. The flow pattern changes results in a drop in blood flow across the *ductus arteriosus* and the higher blood oxygen content of blood **within the aorta stimulates the constriction and ultimately the closure of this fetal circulatory shunt.**

Following birth, the expression and re-uptake of surfactant, which begins to be produced by the fetus at 20 weeks gestation, is accelerated. Expression of surfactant into the alveoli is necessary to prevent alveolar closure (atelectasis). At this point, rhythmic breathing movements also commence. If there are any problems with breathing, management can include stimulation, bag and mask ventilation, intubation and ventilation.

CIRCULATORY SYSTEM

The supply of blood from placenta via the venous duct into the baby's body is disrupted with the cutting through of the umbilical cord. Initiation of respiration allows blood to flow through the lungs. Thereby the blood supply in the right cardiac atrium is decreased and the pressure in the right atrium is reduced. At the same time, through the first couple of breaths of the newborn, the pressure in the small circulatory system is massively attenuated. The result of these **pressure changes** in the body is a reduction of the blood flow via the arterial duct and through the foramen ovale and an increase of the blood flow through the lungs. The **reflex closure of the arterial duct** after the first breaths of the newborn and the elevation of the pressure in the large circulation system are subsidiary mechanisms. The transition from fetal to postnatal circulation involves the functional closures of fetal shunts: the foramen ovale, ductus arteriosus, and eventually the ductus venosus.

The sudden drop in right atrial pressure pushes the septum primum against the septum secundum, closing the **foramen ovale**. Closure of ductus arteriosus is by smooth muscle contraction. The **ductus arteriosus** begins to close almost immediately, and may be kept open by the administration of **prostaglandins**. Smooth muscle on ductus arteriosus occurs to close the blood flow completely in 1–8 days. It is further replaced by fibrous tissue, called *ligamentum arteriosum*. This contraction of smooth muscle occurs because of the increase in availability of oxygen. At birth, opposite direction of blood flow from aorta to pulmonary artery supplies more oxyginated blood than before. The partial pressure of oxygen is used to be 15–20 mmHg before, but now it is 100 mmHg. It is confirmed that the degree of smooth muscle contraction is highly dependent on more availability of oxygen. Closure of ductus venosus is also caused by strong contraction of muscle wall of ductus venosus, but the cause of this contraction is not revealed yet. This structure is changed into fibrous *ligamentum venosum*. It is sometimes continuous with the round ligament of the liver. Other embryonic circulatory vessels are slowly obliterated and remain in the adult only as fibrous remnants.

The sudden pressure differences cause the blood flowing to the lungs and liver to increase and the blood flowing through the bypass channels to decrease. Increased blood flow dilates the pulmonary vessels, pulmonary vascular resistance decreases, and systemic resistance increases, thus maintaining blood pressure.

Blood volume: The blood volume of the full-term infant is about 80–85 mL/kg of body weight. Immediately after birth total blood volume averages about 300 mL (75–100 mL additional blood from umbilical cord – if it's still attached).

Cardiac Output: In average 500 mL/min.

Arterial Pressure: 70/50, but it increases slowly during next several months to about 90/60.

Summary of the Circulatory Changes

Newborn takes breaths which increases uptake of oxygen by lungs (first and subsequent breaths) induces a vasoconstriction of ductus venosus and ductus arteriosis.

Summary of the Circulatory Adjustments

Aeration of the lungs at birth is associated with:

- A dramatic fall in pulmonary vascular resistance due to lung expansion
- A marked increase in pulmonary blood flow (thus raising the left atrial pressure above that of IVC)
- A progressive thinning of the walls of the pulmonary arteries (due to stretching as lungs increase in size with first few breaths).

The first breath: The pulmonary alveoli open up:

- Pressure in the pulmonary tissues decreases
- Blood from the right heart rushes to fill the alveolar capillaries
- Pressure in the right side of the heart decreases
- Pressure in the left side of the heart increases as more blood is returned from the well-vascularized pulmonary tissue via the pulmonary veins to the left atrium.

Resulting circulatory changes include: Blood pressure is now high in the aorta and systemic circulation is well established.

Control of circulation is a reflex function regulated: Peripherally by the baroreceptors in the aortic arch and carotid sinus.

Centrally by baroreceptors in the cardiovascular center of the medulla (in close proximity of the chemoreceptors that regulate respiration). Respiratory and circulatory reflexes are usually strong in the healthy full-term newborn, but their efficiency in controlling cardiovascular function is susceptible to environmental factors.

Changes in Shunts at Birth

Foramen ovale: Before birth the foramen ovale allows most of the oxygenated blood entering the right atrium from the IVC to pass into the left atrium, prevents the opposite direction circulation as the septum primum closes against the relatively rigid septum secundum. Foramen ovale closes at birth due to decreased flow from placenta and IVC to hold open foramen.

Moreover because of increased pulmonary blood flow and pulmonary venous return to left heart causing the pressure in the left atrium to be higher than in the right atrium.

The increased left atrial pressure then closes the foramen ovale against the septum segundum from the right ventricle now flows entirely into the pulmonary circulation.

Other Changes in the Heart

The right ventricular wall is thicker than the left ventricular wall in fetuses and newborn infants because the right ventricle has been working harder. By the end of the first month the left ventricular wall is thicker than the right because it is now working harder than the right one. The right ventricular wall becomes thinner because of atrophy associated with its lighter workload.

Ductus Arteriosus (DA)

The DA constricts at birth, but there is often a small shunt of blood from the aorta to the left pulmonary artery for a few days in a healthy, full-term infant.

In premature infants and in those with persistent hypoxia the DA may remain open for much longer.

Oxygen is the most important factor in controlling closure of the DA in full-term infants. Closure of the DA appears to be mediated by bradykinin, a substance released by the lungs upon initial inflation.

Bradykinin has potent contractile effects on smooth muscle. Action depends upon the high oxygen content of the aortic blood resulting from aeration of the lungs at birth.

When the PO_2 of blood passing through the DA reaches about 50 mmHg, the wall of the DA constricts. As a result of reduced pulmonary vascular resistance, the pulmonary arterial pressure falls below the systemic level and the blood flow through the ductus arteriosis is diminished.

Umbilical Arteries Constrict at Birth

To prevent loss of infants blood, umbilical cord is not tied for 30–60 seconds so that blood flow through umbilical vein continues, transferring fetal blood from placenta to the infant. Blood change from fetal to adult pattern of circulation is not a sudden occurrence in some changes occur during the first breath, others over hours and days. During the transitional stage right to left flow may occur through the foramen ovale. The closure of the fetal vessels and the foramen ovale is initially a functional change; later anatomic closure results from proliferation of endothelial and fibrous tissues.

- *Blood flow:* When the umbilical blood stops flowing at birth, sudden pressure differences occur within the circulatory system. These differences cause the

blood flowing to the lungs and liver to increase and the blood flowing through the bypass channels to decrease. Peripheral circulation refers to residual cyanosis in hands and feet. This may be apparent for one to two hours after birth and is due to sluggish circulation. Blood is shunted to vital organs immediately after birth.
- *Blood coagulation:* During the first few days of life, the prothrombin level decreases and clotting time in all infants is prolonged. This process is most acute between the second and fifth postnatal days. It can be prevented to a large extent by giving vitamin K to the infant after birth. With the ingestion of food, establishment of digestion, and maturation of the liver, vitamin K is manufactured by the baby and clotting time stabilizes within a week to ten days.

Thermoregulation

The importance of maintaining the temperature of the newborn baby has been known for centuries. Heat regulation is most critical to the newborn's survival. Although the newborn's capacity for heat production is adequate, still thermal stress has been associated with an increase in morbidity and mortality. After delivery the newborn must adapt to its relatively cool environment by production of heat metabolically as they are not able to generate heat by an adequate shivering response. Thus, it is important to know about thermoregulation in newborn. Thermoregulation plays a unique and crucial role in the nurturing and development of neonates.

Following factors predispose the new born to excessive heat loss:

- Large skin surface area, for the weight of the newborn.
- Decrease in subcutaneous fat and thus less insulation.
- Less well-developed brown fat store.

A term infant has specialized tissue called brown fat which is highly vascularized and innervated by sympathetic nerves. This brown fat is laid down during the third trimester of pregnancy and is located at the nape of the neck, inter scapular region, axillae, groin and around the kidneys and adrenals.

A typical brown fat cell is characterized by round nucleus and granular cytoplasm with large number of mitochondria and fat vacuoles. When the skin of the baby becomes cold, afferent nerves convey this message to heat regulation center in the hypothalamus. In reply, the neurogenic efferent supplying the brown fat triggers the local release of noradrenalin. This results in oxidation of triglycerides to glycerol and fatty acids. These fatty acids are locally consumed for the generation of heat. Thus, this area of brown fat becomes warmer and heated. Consequently this heat is distributed through the blood stream to the various parts of the body of the neonate.

This process needs more O_2 and glucose. It is therefore obvious that the cold baby will need extra O_2 and glucose for this metabolic activity in order to keep warm. Thus effective metabolic thermogenesis depends upon the integrity of CNS, adequacy of brown fat and availability of O_2 and glucose.

When babies are cold-stressed, they use energy and oxygen to generate warmth. If skin temperatures drop just one degree from the ideal 97.7 °F (36.5 °C), a baby's oxygen use can increase by 10%. By keeping babies at optimal temperatures, neither too hot or cold, they can conserve energy and build up reserves. This is especially important when babies are sick or premature.

Energy Metabolism

Energy metabolism in the fetus must be converted from a continuous placental supply of glucose to intermittent feeding. While the fetus is dependent on maternal glucose as the main source of energy, it can use lactate, free-fatty acids, and ketone bodies under some conditions. Plasma glucose is maintained by glycogenolysis.

Glycogen synthesis in the liver and muscle begins in the late second trimester of pregnancy, and storage is completed in the third trimester. Glycogen stores are maximal at term, but even then, the fetus only has enough glycogen available to meet energy needs for 8–10 hours, which can be depleted even more quickly if demand is high. Newborns will then rely on gluconeogenesis for energy, which requires integration, and is normal at 2–4 days of life.

Fat stores are the largest storage source of energy. At 27 weeks gestation, only 1% of a fetus body weight is fat. At 40 weeks, that number increases to 16%.

Fluid Balance

Fluid balance for a newborn, infant, children or adults is based on the water content in the cells, interstitial spaces and blood. Body water is related to non-fat body weight. Approximately 70% of an infant's body is comprised of water distributed between intracellular and extracellular spaces. Sixty percent of the fluid is found in the intracellular spaces.

The developing baby's kidneys begin producing urine by 9–12 weeks into the pregnancy. After birth, there is a sudden movement of fluid from the intracellular space to the extracellular space, and changes occur in the total body water volume. There is proportionately higher ratio of extracellular fluid in infant than adult, and consequently has a higher level of total body sodium and chloride and a lower level of potassium, magnesium, and phosphate. The increased fluid leads to a salt and water loss resulting in a 10% loss of body weight in the first week of life. Fluid loss also occurs through the skin and respiratory system.

All structural components of renal system are present in newborn. But the kidneys of a newborn have a limited capacity to excrete excess water and sodium, which can adversely affect the fluid balance in their bodies. The rate at which blood filters through the kidneys (glomerular filtration rate) increases sharply after birth and in the first 2 weeks of life. Still, it takes some time for the kidneys to get up to speed. Newborns have less ability to remove excess salt (sodium) or to concentrate or dilute the urine compared to adults. The rate of fluid exchange is seven times greater in the infant than in the adult, and the infant's rate of metabolism is twice as great in relation to body weight. As a result, acid formation is higher and it leads to more rapid development of acidosis in the body of the infant. Moreover, the immature kidneys cannot sufficiently concentrate urine to conserve body water. The infants are more prone to dehydration, acidosis, over hydration or water intoxication due to these three factors. Usual signs and symptoms of dehydration are unreliable in newborns. And, since dehydration is a significant negative risk for newborns, testing and correction is essential.

- By the end of the first week of life total volume of urine per 24 hours is 200 to 300 mL.
- The bladder voluntarily empties as it is stretched by a volume of 15 mL
- Newborn voids as many as 20 times per day
- The first voiding should occur within 24 hours
- *Urine:* Colorless, odorless, Specific gravity—about 1.020

The neonatal kidney has a limited capacity both to excrete and to conserve sodium. Normally there is a salt and water diuresis in the first 48–72 hours of life. After parturition, there is a sudden efflux of fluid from the intracellular fluid (ICF) to the extracellular fluid (ECF) compartment. This increase in the ECF compartment floods the neonatal kidneys eventually resulting in a salt and water diuresis by 48–72 hours. Loss of this excess ECW results in physiological weight loss in the first week of life. Since the ECW compartment is larger in more preterm neonates, the weight loss is greater in preterm neonates. Term infants are expected to lose 10% as compared to 15% weight loss in premature neonates.

GASTROINTESTINAL (GI) SYSTEM

During gestation, baby receives nutrients and disposes of waste products through the placenta. At birth, this changed abruptly, but newborn's digestive system is still very immature. The capacity of the infant's stomach is about **one to two ounces (30 to 60 mL)** at birth, but increases rapidly. Milk passes through the infant's stomach almost immediately. The newborn is capable of digesting simple carbohydrates and proteins, but has a limited ability to digests fats. After birth the baby can digest, absorb, and metabolize food stuff like protein, simple carbohydrate (monosaccharides, disaccharides). But deficient production of pancreatic amylase impairs the digestion of complex carbohydrates polysaccharides. Absorption of fats is limited due to deficient production of pancreatic lipase, especially with ingestion of foods with high saturated fatty acid content such as cow's milk.

Infants have an excessive amount of bilirubin in the blood after birth. The deficient activity of the hepatic enzyme glucuronyl transferase at birth may contribute to physiologic jaundice.

Physiological Jaundice (PJ)

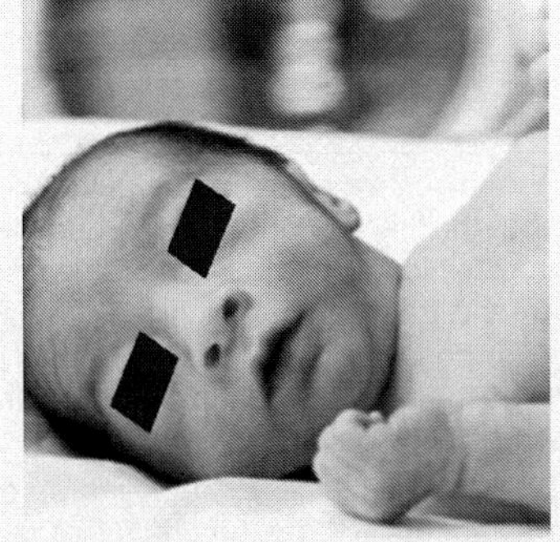

Fig. 5.19: A newborn with jaundice

Physiological jaundice in newborn babies is caused by impaired bilirubin uptake and conjugation. There is increased bilirubin load, due to increased number of RBCs in circulation, shorter duration of life span of erythrocytes and the inability of the immature neonatal liver to conjugate bilirubin out of the blood stream.

The liver is also deficient in forming plasma proteins. Probably the decreased plasma proteins concentration plays a role in the edema usually seen at birth. Prothrombin and other coagulating factors are low during the first few days of life, thus the clotting time is prolonged. Glycogen storage in the liver is low at birth than later in live. As a result the new born is prone to hypoglycemia, which may be prevented by early feeding especially breastfeeding.

Some salivary glands of newborn infant are functioning, but the majority do not start to secrete saliva until about the age of two to three months, when drooling is frequent. The capacity of the infant's stomach is about one to two ounces (30 to 60 mL) at birth, but increases rapidly. Milk passes through the infant's stomach almost immediately. The infant is capable of digesting simple carbohydrates and proteins, but has a limited ability to digest fats.

The intestinal tract functions as an outlet for amniotic fluid as early as the fifth month of intrauterine life. The normal GI tract assumes its function readily after birth. The infant's intestine is longer in relation to body size than that of the adult. Irregularity in peristaltic motility slows stomach emptying. Peristaltic increases in the lower ileum, which results in one to six stools a day. The first stools after birth and for three to four days afterwards are called meconium. Meconium is stringy, tenacious, and black and has a tarry texture. With the ingestion of colostrum or formula, a gradual transition occurs. There may be few greenish stools and the stools will gradually become more yellow. Formula stools are lemon yellow and curdy. Breast milk stools are yellow-orange, soft, and more frequent. Progressive changes in the pattern of stool indicate a properly functioning GI tract.

Before birth, the digestive tract of the fetus is sterile, but within hours of birth, the baby acquires a complex collection of microorganisms which populate the mouth—then eventually the full length of the tract will be colonized. The development of specific microorganisms is influenced by the exposure to certain factors such as maternal microbiota, environmental contact, mode of delivery and the infant's diet.

The human digestive system has a layer of mucous that protects the gastrointestinal tract from microbes and other contaminants that may be present in food or liquids. In infants, this protective barrier is immature, which puts the baby at risk of infection. Antibodies in breast milk help protect the baby until his digestive mucosal lining matures and he increases his ability to produce his own antibodies, which happens around the age of six months.

Meconium: Meconium is a tarry green or black waste substance that is produced in the intestine of a fetus before birth. Meconium is composed of amniotic fluid, mucus, lanugo, bile, and cells that have been shed from the skin and intestinal tract. In some cases, stress baby experiences before or during birth may cause expulsion of meconium into the amniotic fluid. If meconium is present in the amniotic fluid, this is known as meconium aspiration syndrome.

Are there actual anatomical differences in the GI system between infants and adults?
Yes! Let's start with the differences in the head and neck. In the infant, the tongue is larger in relation to the oral cavity and they have extra fat pads on the sides of the tongue that help with sucking. Also, in an infant, the larynx, or voice box, is situated higher and the epiglottis lies over the soft palate to supply extra airway protection.
In a newborn baby, the esophagus is about 11 centimeters long (versus 9 1/2 inches long in adults) and the lower esophageal sphincter is around 1 centimeter. Quite often at birth, a thin suction tube is passed through the esophagus to guarantee that it is open. Esophageal defects can be atresia and fistulas.
Now, the newborn stomach can only hold about 60 to 90 milliliters of fluid whereas adult capacity is about 2–3 liters. The digestive activity of the stomach is the same in both babies and adults. The gastric glands of the stomach include parietal cells, which produce hydrochloric acid and intrinsic factor. The chief cells in these glands secrete pepsinogen, which is changed into pepsin, breaking down proteins in the gastric juice. Amazingly, bowel sounds are already existent one hour after birth and the parietal cells start to work directly after birth. The gastric pH is less than 4 for the first 7 to 10 days of life.
There are anatomical differences in the small intestine as well: It measures 250 to 300 centimeters in newborns and at 10 years 500 cm, and at 20 years 575 cm.
And how about the colon? It is sterile at birth, but within a few hours *E. Coli*, *Clostridium* and *Streptococcus* are established—the gathering of bacteria in the GI tract is essential for digestion and formation of Vitamin K.
Finally, the first stools passed are called meconium. Meconium is thick, sticky and tarlike. It is black or dark green in color and made up of mucus, vernix, lanugo, hormones and carbohydrates. It is extremely necessary that a newborn baby passes stool within 24 hours of birth.

IMMUNE SYSTEM

The immune system begins to develop in the fetus, and continues to mature through the child's first few years of life. The womb is a relatively sterile environment. But as soon as the baby is born, he or she is exposed to a variety of bacteria and other potential disease-causing substances. Although newborn infants are more vulnerable to infection, their immune system can respond to infectious organisms.

Newborns do carry some antibodies from their mother, which provide protection against infection. Breastfeeding also helps improve a newborn's immunity. Moreover they have following defenses against infection:

- The first line of defense is skin and mucous membrane, which prevents infection
- The second line of defense is cellular elements of the immunologic system

- Neutrophils and monocytes are phagocytic cells
- Eosinophils also probably have phagocytic property
- The lymphocytes (T cells and B cells) which are capable of being converted to other cell types, such as monocytes and antibodies.

The third line of defense is the formation of specific antibodies to an antigen. The baby has some immunoglobulins at birth, but the sheltered intra-uterine existence limits the need for learned immune responses to specific antigens. There are three main immunoglobulins, IgG, IgA and IgM, and of these only IgG is small enough to cross the placental barrier. It affords immunity to specific viral infections. At birth the baby's levels of IgG are equal to or slightly higher than those of the mother. This provides passive immunity during the first few months of life. IgM and IgA do not cross the placental barrier but can be manufactured by the fetus. Levels of IgM at term are 20% those of the adult, taking 2 years to attain adult levels.

This relatively low level of IgM is thought to render the infant more susceptible to enteric infections. IgA levels are very low and produced slowly although secretory salivary levels attain adult values within 2 months. IgA protects against infection of the respiratory tract, GI tract and eyes. Breast milk, and especially colostrum, provides the infant with passive immunity in the form of *lactobacillus bifidus*, lactoferrin, lysozymes and secretory IgA among others.

Neonate and Infection

Neonates demonstrate a marked susceptibility to infections, particularly those gaining entry through the mucosa of the respiratory and GI systems. The phagocytic properties of the blood are present in the infant, the inflammatory response of the tissues to localize an infection is poor. As a result, localization of infection is poor, 'minor' infections having the potential to become generalized very easily.

SKIN

Newborn skin will vary depending on the length of the pregnancy. Premature infants have thin, transparent skin. The skin of a full-term infant is thicker. At birth all the structures within the skin are present, but functionally they are immature. The epidermis and dermis of skin are loosely bound to each other and very thin. Rete pegs (the epithelial extensions that project into the underlying connective tissue in both skin and mucous membranes), which anchor epidermis and dermis, are not developed. The infant has delicate skin at birth that appears dark red because it is thin and layers of subcutaneous fat have not yet covered the capillary beds. This redness can be seen through heavily pigmented skin and becomes even more flushed when the baby cries.

Characteristics of Newborn Skin

- A fine hair called lanugo might cover the newborn's skin, especially in preterm babies. The hair should disappear within the first few weeks of the baby's life.
- A thick, waxy substance called vernix may cover the skin. This substance protects the fetus while floating in amniotic fluid in the womb. The sebaceous glands are highly active in late pregnancy due to high levels of maternal androgen, and produce vernix caseosa that covers the infant at birth.
- The sweat producing glands, eccrine glands are functional at birth. The glands are active in response to heat and emotional stimulus, palmer sweating is seen on crying.
- Melanin production is low at birth.
- The growth phase of hair follicles usually occurs simultaneously at birth. But there is temporary disharmony between hair growth and hair fall, so there may be overgrowth of hair or temporary alopecia.

The skin might be cracking, peeling, or blotchy, but this should improve over time. The skin is the largest organ of the human body and has a variety of functions. It is the body's first line of defense providing a protective barrier against infection and environmental toxins. It has pigmentation or melanin provided by melanocytes, which absorb some of the potentially dangerous ultraviolet radiation in sunlight. It also has an important role to play in protecting the internal organs, in insulation and thermoregulation of the body. It discharges electrolytes and prevents excessive fluid loss and syntheses vitamins D and B. The skin also provides tactile perception and is instrumental in the initial bonding attachment phase between a mother and her baby.

NEUROLOGIC SYSTEM

A newborn's nervous system is still maturing. Newborn infants are bundles of endless energy and movement. The central nervous system of a newborn is still immature, and baby does not really have control over his body's movements. Bodily functions and responses to external stimuli of newborn are carried on chiefly by the midbrain and the reflexes of the spinal cord. The autonomic nervous system is crucial during transition, because it stimulates initial respirations, helps maintain acid-base balance, and partially regulates temperature control. Baby is born with several innate reflexes, including sucking reflex.

The nerve fibers become myelinated and make the necessary connections with one another, control from the higher cerebral centers begins, and increasingly fine and gross motor skills developed. Myelin is necessary for rapid and efficient transmission of some, but not all, nerve impulses along the neural pathway. Myelination of the nervous system follows the cephalo-caudal-proximodistal laws of development. Earliest myelination occurs along the pathway of the sensory, cerebellar, and extra pyramidal tracts which accounts for the acute senses of taste, smell, hearing and pain. Except for the optic and alfactory nerves, all cranial nerves are present and myelinated. As soon as myelination occurs and control from the higher cerebral centers begins, more complex and purposeful behavior is possible.

SENSORY DEVELOPMENT

- *Hearing:* Begins before birth, and is mature at birth. The infant prefers the human voice. After draining of the amniotic fluid from the ears, the infant probably has auditory acuity similar to that of an adult. The startle reflex occurs in newborns when they react to a loud sound of about 90 decibels. The internal and middle ear are large at birth, but the external canal is small and bony part of external canal have not yet been developed. Inner ear (vestibular) senses—the infant responds to rocking and changes of position.
- *Vision:* Structurally eye is incomplete at birth. The pupils react to light, blink reflex is seen in minimal stimulus, but the immature ciliary muscles of eyes are not able to focus on an object for any length of time. Babies are born with very fuzzy eyesight. Newborns are very nearsighted. They can see objects and people most clearly when they are just 8 to 12 inches away, and in the midline of the visual field. Color vision develops between 4–6 months. By 2 months, can track moving objects up to 180 degrees, and prefers faces.
- Touch, taste, smell sensations are mature at birth; newborns have the ability to distinguish between tastes and prefer sweet taste. Their taste buds are not yet mature enough to distinguish bitter and sour. The taste buds are distributed mostly on the tip of the tongue. They have a well-developed sense of smell, and can already pick out the scent of their mother's nipple, and breast milk, within the first few days of life.

Newborn can perceive the tactile sensation in any part of the body, especially, the mouth, hands, and soles of feet are seem to be most sensible area. The calming response from the infant is seen by gentle patting of the back or rubbing of the abdomen.

Nursing Management of Newborn

During the immediate postpartum period as well as the early days of birth, care and support must be equally balanced among three critical areas: assessment, monitoring and support of the baby's health and well-being. It is important to ensure that the newborn baby is adapting appropriately to the extra uterine life.

- *Immediate post birth care:* Establish, maintain and support respiration of the newborn
- Assessment using the Apgar scoring system
- Transitional assessment during the period of reactivity
- Assessment of gestational age
- Systematic physical examination
- Thermal protection in newborn
- Breastfeeding and lactation management
- To ensure safety, prevent injury and infection
- Identification and early registration
- To identify actual or potential problems that may require immediate attention.

IMMEDIATE POST BIRTH CARE

Shortly after the baby's birth, the baby will be evaluated for its ability to adapt and transition normally to life outside the uterus. Approximately 85 to 90% of infants make the transition from intrauterine to extrauterine life with no assistance necessary. The most important need for the newborn immediately after birth is a clear airway to enable the newborn to breathe effectively since the placenta has ceased to function as an organ of gas exchange. It is in the maintenance of adequate oxygen supply through effective respiration that the survival of the newborn greatly depends. However, for the remaining 10 to 15% of newborns, some assistance may be required, ranging from simple stimulation to complete resuscitation.

All nurses should be familiar with the ABCs of resuscitation: Airway, breathing, and circulation. Because newborns are wet when they are born, they can suffer rapid heat loss if a warm environment is not maintained. Therefore, it is critical to maintain a warm, or thermoneutral, environment for the infant throughout the first hours and days of life. This can be accomplished by placing the infant on the mother's abdomen, with warm blankets placed over them both to maintain body heat. Alternatively, if the need for further intervention is anticipated, or if the caregiver prefers, the infant should be placed on a preheated radiant warmer.

As the infant is being dried with warm blankets, the nurse should also be evaluating the infant's airway, breathing, muscle tone, color, and gestational age. All of these things should be evaluated within the first 30 seconds of life. The airway should be cleared with a bulb syringe or mechanical suction, and the infant should be positioned in such a manner as to facilitate an obstruction-free airway. If, in the initial evaluation, the infant is found to be clear of meconium, is breathing or crying, has good tone, is pink, and appears to be term gestation, then routine care need only be provided. Routine care is comprised of assuring that the infant is warm and dry and keeping the airway clear. According to Neonatal Resuscitation Program standards, further care is warranted if the newborn fails to respond to birth in this positive manner.

Care needed to establish, maintain and support respiration of the newborn.

To establish and maintain respirations:

- Wipe mouth and nose of secretions after delivery of the head.
- Suction secretions from mouth and nose.
  - Compress bulb syringe before inserting
  - Suction mouth first, then, the nose
  - Insert bulb syringe in one side of the mouth
- A crying infant is a breathing infant. Stimulate the baby to cry if baby does not cry spontaneously, or if the cry is weak.
  - Do not slap the buttocks rather rub the soles of the feet.
  - Stimulate to cry after secretions are removed.
  - The normal infant cry is loud and husky. Observe for the following abnormal cry:
    - High, pitched cry—indicates hypoglycemia, increased intracranial pressure
    - Weak cry—prematurity
    - Hoarse cry—laryngeal stridor.
- Oral mucous may cause the newborn, to choke, cough or gag during the first 12 to 18 hours of life. Place the infant in a position that would promote drainage of secretions.
  - *Trendelenburg position:* Head lower than the body
  - *Side lying position:* If trendelenburg position is contraindicated, place infant in side lying position to permit drainage of mucus from the mouth. Place a small pillow or rolled towel at the back to prevent newborn from rolling back to supine position.
- Keep the nares patent. Remove mucus and other particles that may be cause of obstruction (Fig. 5.20). Newborns are obligatory nose breathers until they are about 3 weeks old.

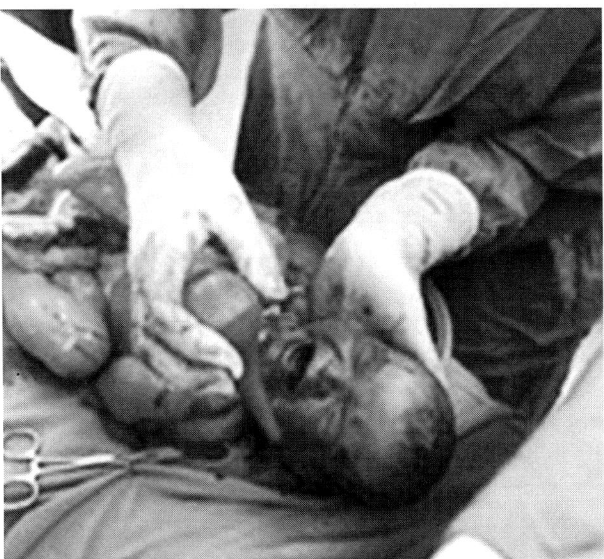

Fig. 5.20: Application of mucus sucker after delivery

Newborns are obligatory nose breathers. The reflex response to nasal obstruction, opening the mouth to maintain airway, is not present in most newborns until 3 weeks after birth.

Common characteristics of newborn respirations:

- *Nose breathers:* Sleeps with mouth closed, does not have to interrupt feedings to breathe.
- Irregular rate.
- Usually abdominal or diaphragmatic in character.
- Ranges from 40 to 60 breathers per minute.
- Breathing is quiet and shallow.
- Easily altered by external stimuli.
- Periods of apnea less than 15 seconds is normal.
- Acrocyanosis may occur during periods of crying. **Acrocyanosis** refers to cyanotic look of the baby's hands and feet when he is crying. When the baby stops crying, his hands and feet get pink again.

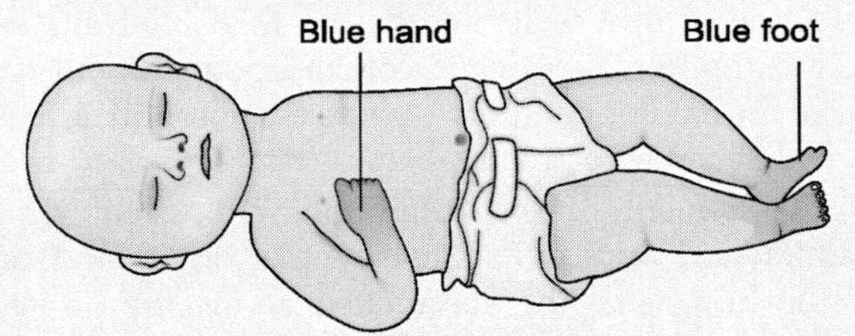

Fig. 5.21: Blue discolored hands and foot in acrocyanosis in newborn

Assessment Using the Apgar Scoring System

In 1953, an anesthesiologist named Virginia Apgar designed a tool for evaluating newborn infants. The

Table 5.1: Apgar scoring

Criteria	*0*	*1*	*2*	*1 minute*	*5 minutes*
Respiration	Absent	Slow, irregular	Good crying		
Heart rate	absent	Slow, irregular (below 100)	More than 100		
Muscle tone	Flaccid	Some flexion of extremities	Active body movements		
Reflex response	No response	Grimace	Cry		
Skin color		Body pink, extremities blue	Completely pink		

Total score = 10

I. No depression 7–10
II. Mild depression 4–6
III. Severe depression 0–3

Apgar scores grade the infant's response to extrauterine life in five categories (Table 5.1):

- Heart rate
- Respiratory effort
- Muscle tone
- Reflex irritability
- Color.

There are a maximum of 2 points possible in each category, for a total of 10 possible points. The Apgar determination is completed at 1 and 5 minutes of life. It is important to note that resuscitative measures should not be delayed while awaiting the 1- and 5-minute marks for Apgar determination.

Morbidity and mortality findings have been found to correlate with the 5-minute Apgar score. The 1-minute Apgar score correlates with the pH of cord blood. The lower the score, the more acidotic the infant; in addition, infants with lower scores have worsening cardiorespiratory depression. Some studies have suggested that the Apgar score loses clinical significance for infants of 23 to 25 weeks gestation who survive their first 24 hours of life.

Heart rate can be determined either through auscultation of the apical pulsation or by palpating the umbilical cord. A heart rate greater than 100 beats per minute (bpm) is awarded a score of 2 points. A pulse of less than 100 bpm garners 1 point. An absent heartbeat would obtain zero points.

Assessment of the respiratory effort requires a multifaceted approach. Movement of air in and out of the lungs may be auscultated at the time that a respiratory rate is obtained. An infant with a good cry is awarded 2 points for respiratory effort. An infant that is making some attempt at breathing but may be categorized as slow or irregular will obtain only 1 point. An irregular breathing pattern, also known as periodic breathing, is a normal finding in some newborns. However, if periodic breathing is associated with nasal flaring, grunting, retractions, cyanosis, or decreased rate, further assessment and intervention may be required. A newborn with an absent respiratory drive will receive zero points.

The nurse considers muscle tone acceptable if the infant's elbows, hips, and knees are flexed and allow active extension of extremities. The infant should return to the gently flexed position after examination. An attitude of flexion is necessary to obtain 2 points. An infant with some flexion should be assigned 1 point. A limp infant would receive zero points.

Reflex irritability is noted as the infant reacts to noxious stimulation. An appropriate response to stimuli, such as suctioning or rubbing the soles of the feet, would be for the infant to cry. This response would be awarded 2 points. If the newborn grimaces in response to such stimuli, 1 point would be awarded for effort. If the infant shows no response, then zero points would be awarded.

Color can be assessed by noting the color of mucous membranes, the trunk, and the soles of the feet. The infant should be pink and not dusky. An infant that is completely pink, including the hands and feet, would be awarded 2 points in this category. An infant that is pink but is acrocyanotic (i.e. has blue hands and/or feet) would receive 1 point. An infant that is blue, gray, or dusky would receive zero points.

Transitional Assessment During the Period of Reactivity

All the newborns go through predictable periods of alertness and sleep that should be assessed and taken into consideration when performing the comprehensive physical examination. Distressed infants also progress through these stages but at a much slower rate. These stages are called the first and second periods of reactivity.

Transitional assessment is usually done in institutional delivery, on the first day of birth (within 24 hours), daily clinical assessment and at the time of discharge. Adaptation to the extra-uterine life or daily clinical evaluation should be done by a careful examination of the baby's respiration, heart rate, perfusion color and axillary temperature, as the newborn baby gets various changes in the vital functions during first 24 hours of life. It is known as period of reactivity.

The first period of reactivity generally lasts 6 to 8 hours. For the first 30 minutes after birth, the newborn is generally very alert and active. The infant will usually have a vigorous suck reflex during this time, and it is generally an excellent time to begin breastfeeding. The infant will have open eyes and will be interested in looking around. Physiologically, the infant's respiratory rate may be increased and the lungs will sound quite wet. The heart rate may be increased (over 60 per minute). The heart rate is 160 per minute, bowel sounds are active, mucous production is increased, and body temperature may be slightly decreased.

After this initial period of alertness, the newborn will go into a deep sleep that generally lasts from 2 to 4 hours, though it may continue much longer. During this period, the infant is very calm. Attempts to stimulate the infant will generally be unsuccessful. Ideally, the physical examination should be completed before this time and the infant can then be left alone to sleep. Physiologically, the infant will experience a decrease in respiratory rate, mucous production, and temperature and will likely not void or stool.

The second period of reactivity, which usually lasts 2 to 5 hours, begins when the newborn wakes from this deep sleep state. The infant is generally very active and alert, responsive once again and showing signs of hunger. This is an excellent opportunity for the infant and family to interact with each other and for the nurse to begin some teaching regarding hunger cues and other ways that the infant may communicate needs. Physiologically, the newborn's heart and respiratory rates increase, the gag reflex is active, and the production of mucous and meconium resumes.

The pediatric nurse should have the knowledge about the normal changes and characteristics of newborn. She can find out the deviation from the normal related to neurological, respiratory, and cardiovascular system of the newborn and take immediate action.

ASSESSMENT OF GESTATIONAL AGE

Over the course of gestation, babies develop a wide range of characteristics that can be measured through simple examinations. As the baby develops muscle tone, distinct posture ensues, as well as measurable angles of resistance in key muscle groups. Maturity of newborn can be identified through physical assessment. But only physical assessments are of limited value before 36 weeks of maturity. Physical and neurological examinations are done to detect the gestational maturity. Assessing a baby's physical maturity is an important part of care. Maturity assessment is (Fig. 5.22) helpful in meeting a baby's needs if the dates of a pregnancy are uncertain. For example, a very small baby may actually be more mature than it appears by size, and may need different care than premature baby.

Following fundamental observations are included in neurological assessment:

- *The muscle tone:* Posture or attitude, passive tone (popliteal angle or scarf sign) and active tone (traction response and recoil) are included to assess the muscle tone of newborn.
- *The joint mobility:* A full-term baby has more flexed and relaxed joints. The degree of flexion at wrist and ankles are (square-windows) is less due to stiffness of joints in early gestation. This mobility is less in preterm baby.
- Certain automatic reflexes like moro reflex, papillary response to light, blink response to glebbella, grasp response, rooting reflex with coordinated suckling efforts are assessed to detect the specific age of gestational maturity based on appearance of these reflexes.
- The fundus examination for disappearance of anterior vascular capsule of the lens is done to assess the gestational age. In infants less than 28 weeks, the anterior capsule is completely vascularized and after 34 weeks of gestational life, the vessels are almost atrophied. This examination is difficult due to non-cooperation and photophobia of the neonate.
- An examination called the Dubowitz/Ballard Examination for Gestational Age often is used. A baby's gestational age often can be closely estimated using this examination. The Dubowitz/Ballard Examination evaluates a baby's appearance, skin texture, motor function and reflexes. The physical maturity part of the examination is done in the first two hours of birth. The neuromuscular maturity examination is completed within 24 hours after delivery.

How is Physical Maturity Assessed?

The physical assessment part of the Dubowitz/Ballard Examination examines physical characteristics that look different at various stages of a baby's gestational maturity. Babies who are physically mature usually have higher scores than premature babies.

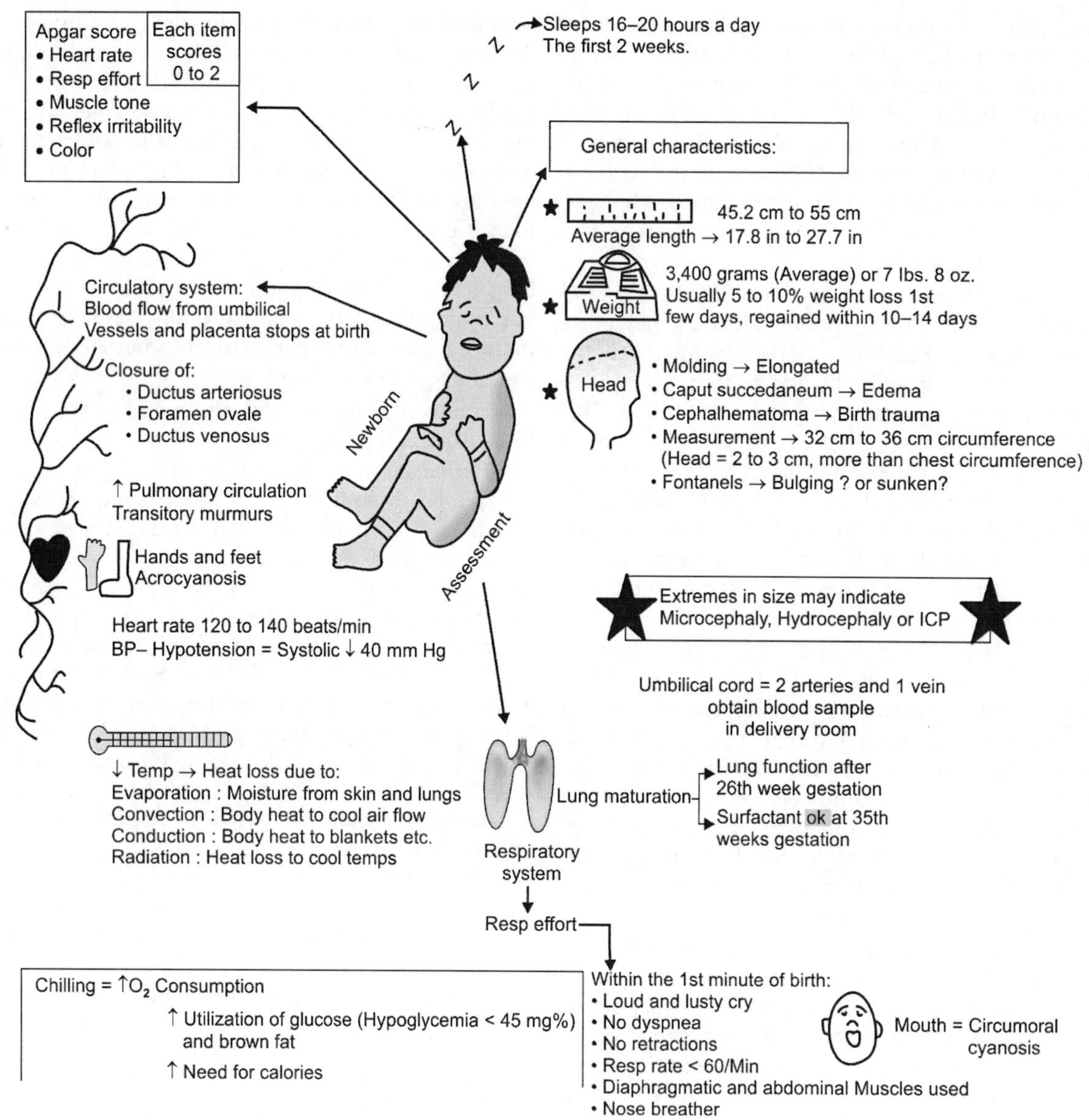

Fig. 5.22: Newborn assessment

Points are given for each area of assessment, with a low of 1 or 2 for extreme immaturity to as high as 4 or 5 for postmaturity. The following physical characteristics are assessed:

- *Skin:* Ranges from sticky and red to smooth to cracking or peeling.

  Lanugo (the soft downy hair on a baby's body) is absent in immature babies, then appears with maturity, and then disappears again with post-maturity.
- *Plantar creases:* These creases on the soles of the feet range from absent to covering the entire foot depending on the maturity.
- *Breast:* The thickness and size of breast tissue and areola (the darkened ring around each nipple) are assessed.
- *Eyes and ears:* Eyes fused or open and amount of cartilage and stiffness of the ear tissue.
- *Genitals, male:* Presence of testes and appearance of scrotum, from smooth to wrinkled.

- *Genitals, female:* Appearance and size of the clitoris and the labia.

How is Neuromuscular Maturity Assessed?

Six evaluations of the baby's neuromuscular system are performed. These include:

1. *Posture:* How does the baby hold his/her arms and legs?
2. *Square window:* How much can the baby's hands be flexed toward the wrist?
3. *Arm recoil:* How much do the baby's arms 'spring back' to a flexed position?
4. *Popliteal angle:* How far do the baby's knees extend?
5. *Scarf sign:* How far can the elbows be moved across the baby's chest?
6. *Heel to ear:* How close can the baby's feet be moved to the ear?

A score is assigned to each assessment area. Typically, the more neurologically mature the baby, the higher the score.

When the physical assessment score and the neuromuscular score are added together, the gestational age can be estimated. Scores range from very low for immature babies (less than 26 to 28 weeks) to very high scores for mature and postmature babies. All of these examinations are important ways to learn about your baby's well-being at birth. By identifying any problems, your baby's physician can plan the best possible care.

Neuromuscular maturity assessment of newborn can be done by Ballard Maturational Assessment of Gestational age. (*See* annexure of this edition).

PHYSICAL EXAMINATION OF THE NEWBORN

The purpose of the newborn physical examination is to assess the baby's transition from intrauterine line to extrauterine existence and to detect congenital malformations and actual or potential disease.

The baby should be examined briefly immediately after birth. This should be confined to quick assessment of respiration, circulation, temperature, neurological status, and screening for anomalies or disease that might mandate emergency treatment. The initial examination should be done with minimal disturbance to the baby, taking particular care to prevent excessive cooling from exposure.

A complete examination should be performed within the first 24 hours and again at discharge from the nursery. The full examination should be performed when the baby is quiet. The baby should be observed from a distance before being touched since a great deal can be learned by observing the infant's spontaneous activity. See, then touch.

Physical examination should be done in the orderly manner. Some principles to be followed in doing physical examination of newborn baby.

Auscultate the heart and chest and feel the pulses before the baby begins to cry, and then proceed systematically to the rest of the examination.

Examination of nose, throat and mouth should be done when the baby is in crying or in very active condition because that time these will be very easily accessible.

Attributes of newborn baby at birth:

General appearance: Mostly neonate lies in flexed position. Activity of newborn baby can be increased with any stimulation.

- *Cry:* Cry of the neonate is vigorous. It is loud and lusty cry.
- *Length:* 45.2 cm to 55 cm, average 50 cm
- *Posture:* The full-term baby lies in an attitude of flexion similar to the position assumed in uterus.
- *Head:* 32 cm to 36 cm circumference. Elongated molding of the skull, the parietal bones slightly overriding the occipital and the frontal bones during vaginal delivery.
- *Fontanels:* Diamond-shaped anterior fontanel is called 'bregma'. It is normally soft and pulsates with each heart beat. The triangular shaped posterior fontanel is called 'lambda'.
- *Hair:* Texture, color, sparseness are observed
- *Face:* It is observed for symmetry and shape
- *Chest:* Normally it is barrel-shaped circumference
- *Weight:* 2.5 kg to 3.4 kg, average loses about 7–8% of the birth weight (not exceeding 10%) during the first week of life. Regained the weight within 10 to 14 days and then continues to gain weight at the rate of 25–30 gm per day (about 10% of birth weight) for the next three months
- *Umbilical cord:* 2 arteries 1 vein
- *Heart rate:* 120–140 per minute
- *Respiratory rate:* Stabilizes at about 35–40. Peripheral cyanosis (acrocyanosis) may be present for a short while after birth even in normal term baby.
- *Sleep:* Normal newborn spends 80% of the time in sleeping. Sleeps 16–20 hours a day during first two weeks of life.
- *Feed:* The neonate is ready to feed within half hour of birth. Colostrum feeding is must. Exclusive breast-feeding is the natural normal nutrition of the baby.

Most babies regularize their feeding pattern by the end of first week and demand feed every 3–4 hours.

- *Elimination:* The neonates usually pass urine during or shortly after birth. About 94% of newborn babies pass urine within 24 hours of birth. The babies pass first stool called meconium, which is black, thick and vicid.

Neonatal Reflexes

Reflexes are involuntary movements or actions. Some movements are spontaneous, occurring as part of your baby's usual activity. Others are responses to certain actions.

Reflexes help identify a baby's normal brain and nerve activity. Some reflexes occur only in specific periods of development. The following are some of the normal reflexes seen in newborn babies:

- *Root reflex:* This reflex begins when the corner of your baby's mouth is stroked or touched. Your baby will turn his head and open his mouth to follow and 'root' in the direction of the stroking. This helps your baby find the breast or bottle to begin feeding.
- *Suck reflex:* Rooting helps your baby become ready to suck. When the roof of your baby's mouth is touched, your baby will begin to suck.
- *Moro reflex:* The Moro reflex is often called a startle reflex because it usually occurs when a baby is startled by a loud sound or movement. In response to the sound, the baby throws back his head, extends out the arms and legs, cries, then pulls the arms and legs back in. A baby's own cry can startle him and begin this reflex. This reflex lasts about five to six months.
- *Tonic neck reflex:* When a baby's head is turned to one side, the arm on that side stretches out and the opposite arm bends up at the elbow. This is often called the 'fencing' position. The tonic neck reflex lasts about six to seven months.
- *Grasp reflex:* Stroking the palm of a baby's hand causes a baby to close his/her fingers in a grasp. The grasp reflex lasts only a couple of months and is stronger in premature babies.
- *Babinski reflex:* When the sole of the foot is firmly stroked, the big toe bends back toward the top of the foot and the other toes fan out. This is a normal reflex up to about 2 years of age.
- *Step reflex:* This reflex is also called the walking or dance reflex because a baby appears to take steps or dance when held upright with his feet touching a solid surface.

Reflex	*Age when reflex appears*	*Age when reflex disappears*
Moro reflex	Birth	2 months
Walking/Stepping	Birth	2 months
Rooting	Birth	4 months
Tonic neck reflex	Birth	5–7 months
Palmar grasp	Birth	5–6 months
Plantar grasp	Birth	9–12 Months

THERMAL REGULATION OF NEWBORN

Newborn is homeotherm. They are equipped with sophisticated mechanisms of body temperature regulation. Neonatal thermoregulation is a critical function for newborn survival, regulated in the hypothalamus and mediated by endocrine pathways. Hypothermia activates cellular metabolism through shivering and non-shivering thermogenesis. In newborns, optimal temperature ranges are narrow and thermoregulatory mechanisms easily overwhelmed, particularly in premature and low-birth weight infants. The lack of thermal protection promptly leads to hypothermia, which is associated with detrimental metabolic and other pathophysiological processes. The smaller is the newborn, the greater the risk. Thermal stability improves gradually as the baby increases in weight.

Appropriate thermal protection of the newborn prevents hypothermia and its associated burden of morbidity and mortality. Thermal protection of the newborn is the series of measures taken at birth and in the first day of life to ensure that the newborn does not become either cold or overheated and maintains a normal body temperature of 36.5–37.5 °C consumption.

The temperature inside the mother's womb is 38 °C, leaving the warmth of the womb at birth; the wet newborn finds itself in a much colder environment and immediately starts losing heat in four different ways. Soon after birth newborn loses heat mainly due to evaporation of amniotic fluid from skin surface. But loss of body heat also occurs by conduction if the baby is placed naked on a cold surface (e.g. a table, a receiving tray, weighing scale or cold mattress); by convection if the naked newborn is exposed to cooler surrounding air (by air current in which cold air replaces warm air around baby); and by radiation from the baby to cooler objects in the vicinity (e.g. a cold wall or a window) even if the baby is not actually touching them (Fig. 5.23). Heat loss increases with air movement (open window,

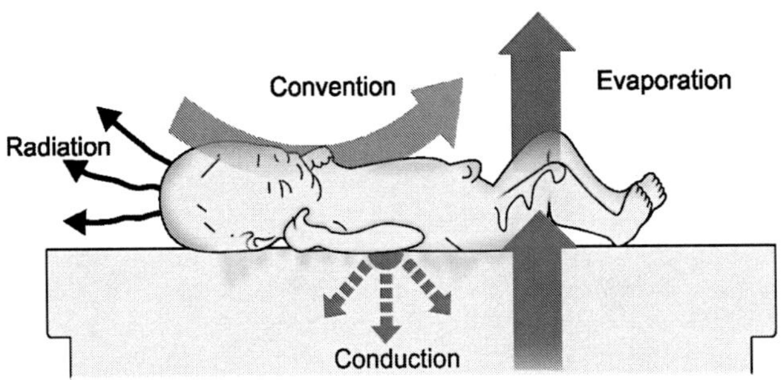

Fig. 5.23: The ways a baby loses heat soon after birth

running fan, etc.) and a baby risks getting cold even at a room temperature of 30 °C if there is a draught.

A naked baby exposed to an environmental temperature of 23 °C at birth, suffers the same heat loss as does a naked adult at 0 °C.

Most cooling of the newborn occurs during the first minutes after birth. In the first 10–20 minutes, the newborn who is not thermally protected may lose enough heat for the body temperature to fall by 2–4 °C, with even greater falls in the following hours if proper care is not given. If heat loss is not prevented and is allowed to continue, the baby will develop hypothermia.

Thermal protection of newborns is very important and not difficult. The basic principles are the same whether the baby is born at home or in an institution. As most cooling of the newborn occurs during the first minutes after birth, it is important to act quickly to prevent heat loss.

The 'warm chain' is a set of interlinked procedures to be taken at birth and during the next few hours and days in order to minimize heat loss in all newborns. Failure to implement any one of these procedures will break the chain and put the newborn baby at risk of getting cold.

Why newborn is prone to hypothermia?

Large body surface area: This area facilitates heat loss to the environment, although this is partially compensated for the newborn's usual position of flexion. This position decreases the amount of surface area to the environment.

Less brown fat: The baby's thin layer of subcutaneous fat provides poor insulation for conservation of heat.

High metabolism rate: Because the newborn's mechanism for producing heat is different from that of the adult, the adult can produce heat through shivering. But the chilled neonate cannot shiver but produces heat through non-shivering thermogenesis, which involves increased metabolism and oxygen consumption.

The 10 steps of the 'Warm Chain'

- Warm delivery room 25–28 °C
- Immediate drying
- Skin-to-skin contact
- Breastfeeding
- Bathing and weighing postponed
- Appropriate clothing/bedding
- Mother and baby together
- Warm transportation
- Warm resuscitation
- Training and awareness raising.

BREASTFEEDING AND LACTATION MANAGEMENT

Most women will make the decision about how they wish to feed their baby well before the birth. Some may find this choice easy, others are unsure and may take a 'wait and see' approach. The decision-making process is usually influenced by many factors. It often reflects the woman's cultural, social, and personal beliefs, past experiences, her perception of her body and breasts, the society she lives in, her plans to return to work, how her mother fed her babies, as well as her partner's preferences. Ideally breastfeeding should start soon after baby is born. Babies tend to be very alert right after birth, so that is a good time to begin breastfeeding. In fact, the American Academy of Pediatrics (AAP) recommends that healthy full-term infants 'be placed and remain in direct skin-to-skin contact with their mothers immediately after delivery until the first feeding is accomplished (Figs 5.24 to 5.26).'

Breast milk is widely acknowledged as the most complete form of nutrition for infants, with a range of benefits for infants' health, growth, immunity and development. Infants are fragile and susceptible to disease, partly because their bodies are not fully developed. They must be treated with special care and given adequate nourishment. Infant formulas are able to mimic a few of the nutritional components of breast milk, but formula cannot hope to duplicate the vast and constantly changing array of essential nutrients in human milk. WHO recommends exclusive breastfeeding for the first six months of life, breastfeeding should begin within one hour of birth. Breastfeeding should be 'on demand', as often as the child wants day and night; and bottles or pacifiers should be avoided.

The Composition of Breast Milk

Breast milk, which is 90% water, consists of—fat, lactose and protein.

- *Carbohydrates:* Lactose is a source of energy and is contained the largest proportion (among fat, lactose

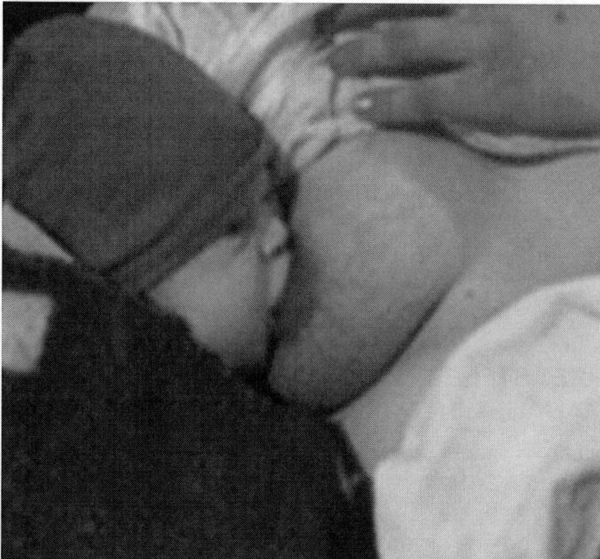

Fig. 5.24: Holding and positioning of baby during breastfeeding

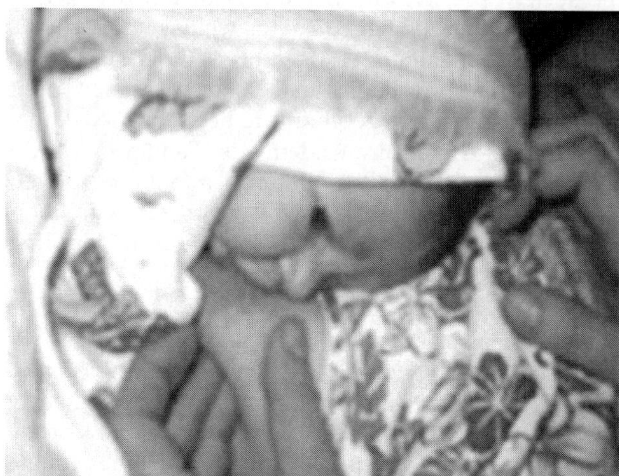

Fig. 5.25: Mother can maintain skin to skin contact during breastfeeding

Suggestions for comfortable feeding positions

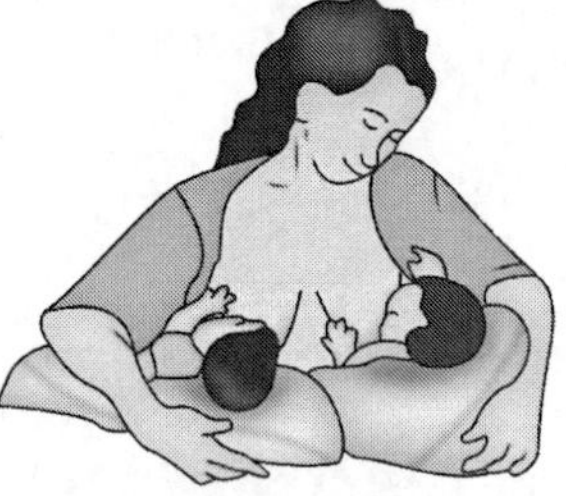

'Football hold': heads on pillows, legs behind

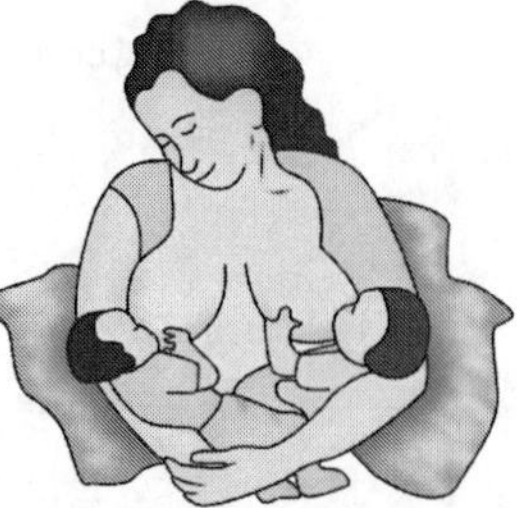

Babies criss - crossed and supported by pillows and mother's arms

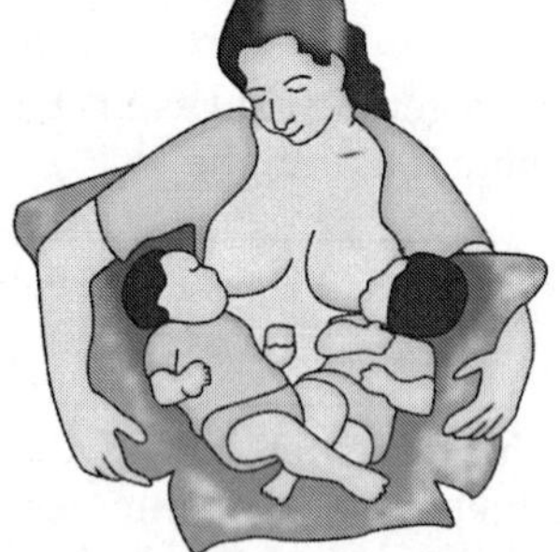

Babies parallel as mother's body

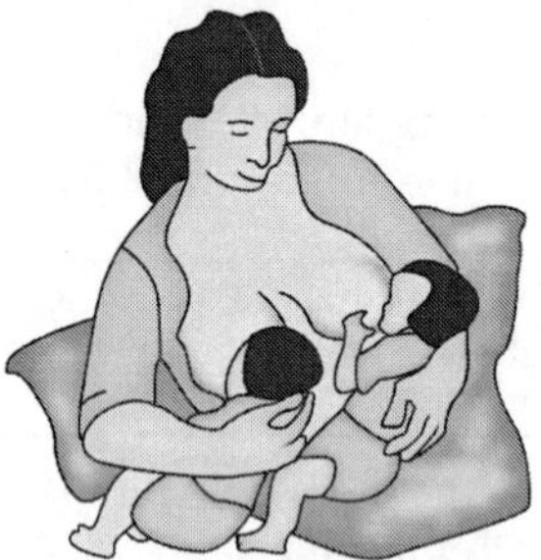

Babies facing the same directions

Fig. 5.26: Giving breastfeeding to twin babies is a challenge to mother

and protein) in breast milk. Lactose is in a high concentrations (6–7g/dL) in breast milk. It helps in the absorption of calcium and enhances the growth of lactobacilli in the intestine.

- *Proteins:* Breast milk contains low protein (.09–1.1 g/dL) as the baby cannot effectively metabolize a high protein load. Protein is broken down into amino acids when it is absorbed into baby's body, and becomes a source for building muscles. Most of the protein is lactalbumin and lactoglobulin (60%), which is easily digested. Human milk contains amino acids like taurine and cysteine which are necessary for neurotransmission and neuromodulation. These are lacking in cow's milk and formula.
- *Fats:* Fat is an important ingredient in the development of your baby's brain and in the maintenance of the body structure. Breast milk is rich in polyunsaturated fatty acids, necessary for the myelination of the nervous system. It also contains omega 2 and omega 6 (very long chain) fatty acids which are important for the formation of prostaglandins and cholesterol, required as a base for steroid hormones.
- Protein is broken down into amino acids when it is absorbed into baby's body, and becomes a source for building muscles.
- *Vitamins and minerals:* The quantity and bioavailability of vitamins and minerals is sufficient for the needs of the baby in the first 4–6 months of life.
- *Water and electrolytes:* The water contain of breast milk is 88%, hence a breastfed baby does not require additional water in the first few months of life even in summer months. The osmolality of breast milk is low, presenting a low solute load to neonatal kidney.

- *Immunological superiority:* It also contains important immune-proteins such as lactoferrin and IgA, lysozyme, macrophages, lymphocytes, bifidus factor (promotes growth of good, protective intestinal bacteria), interferon and other protective substances.

This breast milk looks yellow because it contains β-carotene, which is also found in carrots and other vegetables.

Breast Milk Production Mechanism

The breast is a gland consisting primarily of connective and fatty tissues that support and protect the milk producing areas of the breast. The milk is produced in small clusters of cells called alveoli. The milk travels down along 20 ducts to the nipples. Before reaching the nipple, the ducts widen to form 10–15 lactiferous sinuses which store milk. The lactiferous sinuses lie beneath the circle of dark skin around the nipple called the areola. The areola and nipples are extremely sensitive as they are supplied with a rich network of nerve endings. The nipple and areola (the dark area around the nipple) enlarge and darken during pregnancy. This may help the newborn baby latch on by providing a clear 'target.' The small bumps on the areola are called Montgomery glands. They produce a natural oil that cleans, lubricates, and protects the nipple during pregnancy and breastfeeding. This oil contains an enzyme that kills bacteria and makes breast creams unnecessary.

Breastfeeding success has nothing to do with the size of breasts or nipples. Breast size is an inherited trait and determined by the number of fat cells you have. The breasts will enlarge with pregnancy and breastfeeding. **Breastfeeding is a supply-and-demand process. Therefore, the more women nurse, the more milk they produce!**

Human milk is produced as a result of the interaction between hormones and reflexes.

The let-down reflex in—let-down, also referred to as milk-ejection, is a reflex or natural involuntary reaction that occurs when baby breastfeeds. The action of the infant suckling at breast sends a message to mother's brain to release the hormones prolactin and oxytocin. While prolactin is responsible for making more breast milk, it is the oxytocin that lets milk leave the milk ducts. Prolactin causes alveoli to take nutrients (proteins, sugars) from mother's blood supply and turn them into breast milk. Oxytocin causes the myoepithelial cells around the alveoli to contract and eject milk down the milk ducts. This passing of the milk down the ducts is called the 'let-down' (milk ejection) reflex. This hormone is also produced in response to stimulation by the thought, sight, or sound of the baby.

Let-down is the key to successful breastfeeding: It allows milk supply to flow out of mother's breasts to her baby. Without a good let-down, the baby will only receive a small amount of foremilk, so he may not grow at a healthy pace—or he may become frustrated and refuse to breastfeed.

What Does Let-down Feel Like?

Let-down occurs many times during a feeding. The first release is usually the only one that is noticeable. It may feel like pins and needles, tingling, burning, or pressure, and it could be a little uncomfortable or even mildly painful. Some women feel the sensations very strongly, while others do not feel anything at all.

The hormone oxytocin is associated with love and bonding. It is released during childbirth, when women nurse their baby, and during sex and can bring about feelings of peace, calmness and relaxation. When let-down occurs, the oxytocin causes contractions in the uterus, so you may feel cramping: a good sign that breastfeeding is going well. Other effects of oxytocin that you may feel when you are nursing could include sleepiness, thirst, headache, nausea and vomiting, hot flashes and night sweats.

If you do not feel any of these sensations, it does not necessarily mean that something is wrong. As long as mother can see the signs that her baby is getting enough milk and well, she does not need to be concerned. But if she does not feel let-down, or she has stopped feeling it and she does not see any of the signs listed above, it could indicate that her milk supply is low.

Interference with let-down: Emotions such as embarrassment, anger, irritation, fear or resentment. Fatigue, poor suckling from improper positioning, not enough time baby is actively nursing, stress, negative remarks from relatives or friends. Pain in your breasts or uterus (i.e. sore nipples or afterbirth pains), breast engorgement in the first few days.

Typical Milk Volume

- From birth to 24 hours, colostrum averages about 37 mL
- From 24 to 96 hours, there is a slow rise in volume
- *Day 5:* Approximately 500 mL/day
- *3 to 5 months:* 750 mL/day
- *6 months:* 800 mL/day.

Milk Content is Changed by

- Stage of lactation
- Baby's gestation period

- Mother's age
- Time of feeding
- Baby's feeding patterns.

The Varying Composition of Breast Milk

Breast milk is ever changing, and it adapts to the needs of the growing baby. Its content fluctuates during the day and over the months. From the beginning it is just right for the baby.

There are three main stages that your milk goes through: Colostrum, Transitional milk and Mature milk.

Colostrum

Colostrum is a thick, yellowish milk that is secreted by a woman's breast in the first several days after delivery. It has increased concentration of calcium, potassium, proteins, fat-soluble vitamins, minerals and antibodies. *Colostrum contains large quantities of protective substances and growth factors and has more protein and Vitamins A and K than mature milk.*

It enhances the development and maturation of the baby's gastrointestinal tract. The anti-infective proteins and white cells provide the first immunization against the diseases that a baby encounters after delivery. Although colostrum is secreted in small quantities (30–90 mL), it is sufficient to meet the caloric needs of a normal newborn in the first few days of life.

Colostrum also has a mild purgative effect, which helps to clear baby's gut of meconium (the first, very dark stools) and helps to prevent jaundice by clearing the bilirubin from the gut.

It stimulates the baby's immature intestine to develop in order to digest and absorb milk and to prevent the absorption of undigested protein. If a baby is given any other milk or food before colostrum, it should be known that it can damage the intestine and is a potential cause of allergies.

Colostrum Feeding is Important, It

- Gives immune factors
- Prevents hospital/maternity home infections
- Prevents diarrhea, pneumonia, nosocomial infections, NEC, etc.

Transitional Milk

During the following two weeks, the milk increases in quantity and changes in appearance and composition. The immunoglobulins and protein contents decrease whereas fat and sugar contents increase. At this time, the breasts feel full, hard and heavy. Some people call this as breast milk 'coming in'.

Mature Milk

Mature milk looks thinner and more watery than cow's milk which might be sometimes confusing. But it contains all the nutrients needed for healthy development of the baby. Breast milk is never 'too thin'. Mature milk changes during the length of a single feed to exactly suit the needs of a baby.

The milk that flows at the beginning of a feed is low in fat and high in lactose, sugar, protein, vitamin, minerals and water. As the feed goes on, the milk changes to contain more fat and less sugar.

Foremilk

The milk that comes at the start of a feed is called foremilk. Foremilk, which is watery and bluish in color, has a low level of fat and is high in lactose, sugar, protein, vitamins, minerals and water. It satisfies the baby's thirst and is produced in larger amounts than hindmilk. Mothers sometimes worry that their milk is too thin in the beginning. Milk is never 'too thin', it is important for a baby to have foremilk and hindmilk to get a complete meal and all the water that the baby needs.

Hindmilk

Hindmilk, which comes later in a feed, is richer in fat and this extra fat makes it look whiter than foremilk. It satisfies the baby's hunger and supplies much of the energy of a breastfeed. Therefore, it is important not to take a baby off the breast too quickly. Babies who are fed fore and hindmilk sleep well and grow healthy. There is, however, no sudden change from foremilk to hindmilk. The fat content increases gradually from the beginning to the end of a feed.

The baby needs both the foremilk and the hindmilk for appropriate weight gain.

Preterm Milk

Milk produced by a woman who has delivered prematurely is called preterm milk. This milk has more protein; minerals, immunoglobulins and lactoferrin than mature milk, making it more suited for the needs of a preterm baby. Preterm milk is essential and best suited for the survival and growth of a preterm baby. The breast milk of preterm mothers contains more proteins to suit the fast growing needs of a premature baby. The preterm milk is ideal food for these low birth weight babies.

Term Milk

The composition of milk changes according to the gestational age or maturity of the baby. So, the milk produced by a woman who has a full-term delivery varies in composition to the milk produced by a woman who has a premature delivery.

Why breastfeeding is important within the first or so after birth?

It makes the mother more confident that she can breastfeed.

The baby can receive the immunological effects of colostrums which provides protection against infection and disease.

The baby's digestion and bowels are stimulated.

Suckling difficulties may be avoided if the baby feeds properly at this age.

The bond between mother and baby is enhanced.

Difference between breast milk and other body fluids: The most amazing aspect of breast milk is that it is actually live. It is not a consistent body fluid such as blood—it is a secretion of the mammary gland—and it is constantly changing its composition, dependent, of course, on the interaction with the baby.

Benefits of Breastfeeding

Infants are fragile and susceptible to disease, partly because their bodies are not fully developed. They must be treated with special care and given adequate nourishment. Infant formulas are able to mimic a few of the nutritional components of breast milk, but formula cannot hope to duplicate the vast and constantly changing array of essential nutrients in human milk.

Studies have demonstrated a number of important health benefits to breastfeeding. Among them:

- Breastfed children are more resistant to disease and infection early in life than formula-fed children
- Breastfed children are less likely to contract a number of diseases later in life, including juvenile diabetes, multiple sclerosis, heart disease, and cancer before the age of 15
- Mothers who breastfeed are less likely to develop osteoporosis later in life, are able to lose weight gained during pregnancy more easily and have a lower risk of breast, uterine and ovarian cancer.

Breastfeeding also has economic advantages: it is cheaper than buying formula and helps avoid medical bills later because it helps equip the baby to fight off disease and infection. See below for more information on the benefits of breastfeeding.

Benefits to the Child in the First Year of Life

Breast milk is a unique combination of nutrients essential to a child's health, and cannot be duplicated by any laboratory formula. It provides a number of health advantages beginning at birth and continuing throughout a child's life. In fact, a large number of the health problems today's children face might be decreased, or even prevented, by breastfeeding the infant exclusively for at least the first six months of life. The longer the mother breastfeeds, the more likely her child will get the health benefits of breastfeeding.

The American Academy of Pediatrics (AAP) recommends that mothers breastfeed for at least the first year of a child's life and continue until they both feel they are ready to stop. In the first six months, the baby should be nourished exclusively by breast milk. The slow introduction of iron-enriched foods may complement the breastfeeding in the second half of the first year. Breast milk without supplements during the first six months reduces the possibility of food contamination due to tainted water or malnutrition as a result of over-diluted formula. Therefore, the child should be nursed without the interference of water, sugar water, juices, or formulas, unless a specific medical condition indicates otherwise. The AAP asserts that breast milk has the perfect balance of nutrients for the infant. It is by itself enough sustenance for approximately the first six months of life and should follow as the child's staple throughout the first year.

A variety of studies have demonstrated that breastfeeding increases a child's immunity to disease and infection:

- Many studies show that breastfeeding strengthens the immune system. During nursing, the mother passes antibodies to the child, which help the child resist diseases and help improve the normal immune response to certain vaccines.
- Respiratory illness is far more common among formula-fed children. In fact, an analysis of many different research studies concluded that infants fed formula face a threefold greater risk of being hospitalized with a severe respiratory infection than do infants breast-fed for a minimum of four months.
- Diarrheal disease is three to four times more likely to occur in infants fed formula than those fed breast milk.
- Breastfeeding has been shown to reduce the likelihood of ear infections, and to prevent recurrent ear infections. Ear infections are a major reason that infants take multiple courses of antibiotics.
- In developing countries, differences in infection rates can seriously affect an infant's chances for

survival. For example, in Brazil, a formula-fed baby is 14 times more likely to die than an exclusively breast-fed baby.
- Researchers have observed a decrease in the probability of Sudden Infant Death Syndrome (SIDS) in breast-fed infants.
- Another apparent benefit from breastfeeding may be protection from allergies. Eczema, an allergic reaction, is significantly rarer in breast-fed babies. A review of 132 studies on allergy and breastfeeding concluded that breastfeeding appears to help protect children from developing allergies, and that the effect seems to be particularly strong among children whose parents have allergies.

Benefits to the Child Later in Life

Some benefits of breastfeeding become apparent as the child grows older. Among the benefits demonstrated by research:
- Infants who are breast-fed longer have fewer dental cavities throughout their lives.
- Several recent studies have shown that children who were breast-fed are significantly less likely to become obese later in childhood. Formula feeding is linked to about a 20 to 30% greater likelihood that the child will become obese.
- Children who are exclusively breast-fed during the first three months of their lives are 34% less likely to develop juvenile, insulin-dependent diabetes than children who are fed formula.
- Breastfeeding may also decrease the risk of childhood cancer in children under 15 years of age. Formula-fed children are eight times more likely to develop cancer than children who are nursed for more than six months. (It is important to note that children who are breast-fed for less than six months do not appear to have any decreased cancer risk compared to bottle-fed children.)
- As children grow into adults, several studies have shown that people who were breast-fed as infants have lower blood pressure on average than those who were formula-fed. Thus, it is not surprising that other studies have shown that heart disease is less likely to develop in adults who were breast-fed in infancy.
- Significant evidence suggests that breast-fed children develop fewer psychological, behavioral and learning problems as they grow older. Studies also indicate that cognitive development is increased among children whose mothers choose to breastfeed.
- In researching the psychological benefits of breast milk, one researcher found that breast-fed children were, on average, more mature, assertive and secure with themselves as they developed.

Benefits to the Mother

Studies indicate that breastfeeding helps improve mothers' health, as well as their children's. A woman grows both physically and emotionally from the relationship she forms with her baby. Just as a woman's breast milk is designed specifically to nourish the body of an infant, the production and delivery of this milk aids her own health. For example:
- Breastfeeding helps a woman to lose weight after birth. Mothers burn many calories during lactation as their bodies produce milk. In fact, some of the weight gained during pregnancy serves as an energy source for lactation.
- Breastfeeding releases a hormone in the mother (oxytocin) that causes the uterus to return to its normal size more quickly.
- When a woman gives birth and proceeds to nurse her baby, she protects herself from becoming pregnant again too soon, a form of birth control found to be 98% effective—more effective than a diaphragm or condom. Scientists believe this process prevents more births worldwide than all forms of contraception combined. In Africa, breastfeeding prevents an estimated average of four births per woman, and in Bangladesh it prevents an estimated average of 6.5 births per woman.
- Breastfeeding appears to reduce the mother's risk of developing osteoporosis in later years. Although mothers experience bone-mineral loss during breastfeeding, their mineral density is replenished and even increased after lactation.
- Diabetic women improve their health by breastfeeding. Not only do nursing infants have increased protection from juvenile diabetes, the amount of insulin that the mother requires postpartum goes down.
- Women who lactate for a total of two or more years reduce their chances of developing breast cancer by 24%.
- Women who breastfeed their children have been shown to be less likely to develop uterine, endometrial or ovarian cancer.
- The emotional health of the mother may be enhanced by the relationship she develops with her infant during breastfeeding, resulting in fewer feelings of anxiety and a stronger sense of connection with her baby.
- A woman's ability to produce all of the nutrients that her child needs can provide her with a sense

of confidence. Researchers have pointed out that the bond of a nursing mother and child is stronger than any other human contact. Holding the child to her breast provides most mothers with a more powerful psychological experience than carrying the fetus inside her uterus. The relationship between mother and child is rooted in the interactions of breastfeeding. This feeling sets the health and psychological foundation for years to come.

Social and Economic Benefits of Breastfeeding

The benefits of breastfeeding go beyond health considerations. Mothers who nurse their children enjoy social and economic advantages as well. For example:

- Women who breastfeed avoid the financial burden of buying infant formula, an average expense of $800 per year.
- Breast-fed babies are less likely to need excessive medical attention as they grow. In one study, a group of formula-fed infants had $68,000 in health care costs in a six-month period, while an equal number of nursing babies had only $4,000 of similar expenses.

Breastfeeding Protects the Baby from a Long List of Illnesses

Numerous studies from around the world have shown that stomach viruses, lower respiratory illnesses, ear infections, and meningitis occur less often in breastfed babies and are less severe when they do happen. Exclusive breastfeeding (meaning no solid food, formula, or water) for at least six months seems to offer the most protection.

Drug Safety During Breastfeeding

Many drugs that are prescribed for the mother pass into the milk. So breastfeeding mothers should avoid taking drugs if possible. The type of medication (characteristics such as the molecular weight, protein binding ability, how fat soluble the drug is, and how long it takes for it to be eliminated from mother's system, or it is half-life, all affect how much of the drug is transferred into milk). Usually, if the drug's lipid solubility is high and its protein binding capacity is low (and since human milk has a lower pH than the mother's serum, the chance of its passing into the milk is greater if the drug has a weaker base. Only give a medication if she really needs it. Consider alternative, non-drug therapies if possible. If she has a choice, delay starting the drug until the baby is older. A drug which might cause problems for a newborn may be fine for an older, larger, more mature infant. Give the lowest possible dose for the shortest possible time. When drug therapy is necessary, the mother should check the reference book and avoid contraindicated drugs. Some drugs such as antithyroid, oral anticoagulants, oral contraceptives, cathartic medications should not be taken by breastfed mothers.

When drug treatment is necessary, the safest known alternative should be used; when possible, most drugs should be taken immediately after breastfeeding or before the infant's longest sleep period, although this strategy is less helpful with neonates who nurse frequently and exclusively. Knowledge of the adverse effects of most drugs comes from case reports and small studies. Safety of some (e.g. acetaminophen, ibuprofen, cephalosporins, insulin) has been determined by extensive research, but others are considered safe only because there are no case reports of adverse effects. Drugs with a long history of use are generally safer than newer drugs for which few data exist. If a particular drug is absolutely essential to the health of the mother, she can temporarily discontinue breastfeeding for safety sake of her baby (*See* annexure – Drug and breastfeeding)

Formula Feeding

One of the most frustrating battles in the mommy war is that of **breast vs. bottle**. New research saying that shy moms are less likely to breastfeed should turn up the heat another notch.

According to the results of the study, which was published in the *Journal of Advanced Nursing*, mothers involved in the research who were **introverts** or had anxious tendencies were more likely to formula feed or breastfeed for a shorter period of time. Moms who described themselves as being **extroverts** and 'emotionally stable,' on the other hand, continued breastfeeding for a longer duration.

In the real world, there are plenty of reasons women choose formula. Among them are having a baby with a poor sucking reflex (common in premature babies), prolonged mother-infant separation, painful nursing, the fear that your baby is not getting enough milk, the need to return to work, a health problem that requires medication that's not safe for a nursing infant, and a desire to let other family members help feed the baby.

The composition of infant formula is designed to be roughly based on a human milk at approximately one to three months postpartum, however, there are significant differences in the nutrient content of these products. The most commonly used infant formulas contain purified cow's milk whey and casein as a protein source, a blend of vegetable oil as a fat source, lactose as a carbohydrate source, a vitamin-mineral mix, and other ingredients depending on the manufacturer. In addition, there are infant formulas using soybean as a protein source in place of cow's milk and formulas using protein hydrolyzed into its component amino acids for infants who are allergic to other proteins. An upswing in breastfeeding in many countries has been accompanied by a deferment in the average age of introduction of baby foods (including cow's milk), resulting in both increased breastfeeding and increased use of infant formula between the ages of 3 and 12 months.

In particular, the use of infant formula in less economically developed countries is linked to poorer health outcomes because of the prevalence of unsanitary preparation conditions, including lack of clean water and lack of sanitizing equipment. UNICEF estimates that a formula-fed child living in unhygienic conditions is between 6 and 25 times more likely to die of diarrhea and four times more likely to die of pneumonia than a breastfed child. Rarely, use of powdered infant formula (PIF) has been associated with serious illness, and even death, due to infection with *Enterobacter sakazakii* and other microorganisms that can be introduced to PIF during its production. Although *E sakazakii* can cause illness in all age groups, infants are believed to be at greatest risk of infection. Between 1958 and 2006, there have been several dozen reported cases of *E. sakazakii* infection worldwide. The WHO believes that such infections are under-reported.

TO ENSURE SAFETY, PREVENT INJURY AND INFECTION

The passage from the safety of the uterus to the outside world is made hazardous by the following:

- The skull has to mould to facilitate passage through the pelvis and there may be cephalopelvic disproportion (CPD)—a mismatch between the size of the fetal head and the capacity of the maternal pelvis. It may represent a large head in a normal pelvis or a normal head in a restricted pelvis.
- Mal-position increases risk, whilst mal-presentation necessitates caesarean section.
- Contractions tax the reserve of the placenta.
- The lungs and circulation undergo great changes.

Difficulties in delivery may compound the situation. Delivery may need to be expedited because of fetal distress. This may present as fetal hypoxia and as acidosis on fetal blood sampling.

Injuries may be caused by a combination of mechanical trauma and hypoxia. Birth injuries may be minor and transient but they can produce serious and permanent effect as well as being fatal. Previously it was assumed that most cases of cerebral palsy were due to obstetric mismanagement, but now the figure for those caused by obstetric trauma is put at around 5%.

Baby cannot understand and recognize danger. Baby's immune system is not fully developed. This makes it more likely that the baby will get bacterial and viral infections and more likely that these infections will be dangerous. Newborn babies have very little protection against infection, so it is important to provide a clean, hygienic environment. One of the most important things can be done is to make sure that anyone who handles the baby, has washed their hands first.

People who have infections, for example, colds, flu or herpes simplex, should not come in contact with baby. Cold sores can be particularly dangerous to a newborn baby. Vaccinations are available to protect baby against some infectious diseases.

The steps needed to ensure safety of babies are:

- The baby's environment should be kept as clean as possible, and thorough handwashing is must before handling the baby.
- Prompt detection and management of any infection (umbilicus, eye, ear) to be done.
- Supervise young children whenever they are near the baby.
- Keep animals away from the baby. The change in the household when there is a new baby may upset some pets.
- To avoid serious scald burns, do not drink hot drinks when holding the baby.
- Put the baby down in a safe place during changing, for example, on a change table with raised edges to prevent the baby rolling off. Remember to keep one hand on the baby at all times. Never leave the baby alone on the change table. To prevent falls, some parents choose to change the baby on the floor.
- Keep one hand on baby whenever baby is on an elevated surface, such as a change table or bed. This will stop baby falling or wriggling off.
- Always test that bath water temperature is approximately 36 °C before placing baby in the bath. Stay with baby the whole time.
- Check that baby is in a safe sleeping position and environment, whether at home or out and about, with no risk of suffocation or strangulation.
- Give baby a safe environment for any car travel, with a properly fitted baby restraint that you use at all times.

Use clothes without ribbons, strings or ties around the neck. Take off any bibs or hooded clothes before putting baby to bed.

- Avoid cooking when holding the baby, either in your arms or in a sling. Baby could easily be burned.
- Smoking and nursing a baby is dangerous. As well as the risk of burns, the smoke can damage baby's health, and smoking around babies has been linked to increased risk of SIDS.

How can stress level of caregiver affect baby's safety?

Taking care of oneself is a vital part of keeping the child safe. Most injuries to children occur when parents or caregivers are tired, hungry, or emotionally drained or are having relationship problems. Other common causes of family stress include changes in daily routines, moving to a new house, or expecting another child.

IDENTIFICATION AND EARLY REGISTRATION

A new mother may worry about a mix-up occurring when she delivers. If a question arises about the baby's identity, the most reliable way to be sure he or she has not been switched in the hospital is for the mother and child to undergo a maternity DNA test.

Newborn Identification

Newborn identification varies from hospital to hospital, but one of the most common methods is the use of corresponding identification tags/bracelets between mothers and their babies. These tags typically list the mothers' names and a matching code between the two (for example, if the mother's code is '67,' her child's code will be '67').

Despite advancements in ID tag technology, infant-mother mix-ups often occur in health set up. The leading cause of these mix-ups is human error. The common causes of mix ups are:

- Misreading infant or mother bracelet information
- Bracelets falling off the infants' ankles or wrists, which is particularly common in newborns, whose arms and legs may shrink after birth due to water loss
- Bed mix-ups, in which a child is removed for bathing or treatment and then returned to the wrong bed
- Mix-ups of babies with similar or identical names
- Inadequate physical security mechanisms
- Parents who are not fluent in the staff's native language.

Hospitals also employ fingerprinting and/or foot printing of the infant at birth for identification. Foot printing and fingerprinting require consistent and careful procedures, and if a staff member is not highly experienced in these techniques, the chance of less complete and clear footprints and fingerprints is greater.

In light of some of the shortcomings these forms of identification may have, maternity DNA testing is becoming more popular when doubt arises. Maternity DNA tests compare the genetic information of the mother with the child to identify matches. Because the DNA of a child comes directly from his or her parents, half of the DNA should match the mother's DNA. DNA samples are painlessly collected through buccal swabs–the process of rubbing the inside of one's cheeks to pick up cheek (buccal) cells that contain DNA–and submitted to a laboratory for analysis. In as little as a day, the laboratory can determine if the child and mother are biologically related.

Hospital Security Measures to Prevent Baby Swaps

The maternal instinct may curb some of the baby-switching anxiety. US researchers discovered that postpartum mothers have natural cues that can help them to recognize the crying sounds and smells of their babies. 65.9% of mothers tested recognized their babies from recorded crying, and 52.3% recognized their babies by smell, according to the *British Journal of Nursing*.

Hospital nurseries have implemented security measures such as video surveillance in the nursery and computerized chips in bracelets that cause an alarm to go off if they leave without authorization. When touring the maternity ward before their child's birth, new parents are encouraged to ask if their hospital has these kinds of precautions in place, along with learning the identification protocol of newborns. During this tour, parents can ask questions such as:

- What are the security precautions in the maternity ward?
- What is the procedure for infant identification?
- Where will the baby be when he or she is not with mother?

If parents are unable to choose the hospital where the birth will take place, their birthing coach can ask these questions during labor.

Some hospitals allow for the baby to stay in the room with the mother at all times. If the mother needs to leave the room for any reason, she is advised to find a authorized care provider to watch over the baby. Other hospitals still keep the baby separated from the mother, but the mother is encouraged to choose a family member or friend to keep guard outside the nursery in these settings.

Registration of birth of child: Registration of birth of child is a legal requirement done by some administrative branch of government. It is a permanent and official record of a child's existence. The birth registration should be done no later than three months after his/her birth. The right to birth registration is enshrined in the 1989 Convention on the Rights of the Child (CRC), which applies to every human being under the age of 18 years. If the child is not registered at birth is in danger of being shut out of society—denied the right to an official identity, a recognized name and a nationality. In 2000, according to UNICEF an estimated 50 million babies—more than two fifths of those born—were unregistered. These children have no birth certificate, the 'membership card' for society that should open the door to the enjoyment of a whole range of their rights including education and health care, participation and protection. If the children are not visible to the system, it is more likely that the discrimination, neglect and abuse they experience will remain unnoticed.

But the importance of registration or the lack of it not only an individual phenomenon, it goes beyond of that. Without proper birth registration, a country cannot even be certain of its own birth or death rate. The effective planning and development strategies of country are not possible without strong civil registration system. Unregistered children who do not show up in the data are often overlooked in social development planning. They are completely invisible when important policy and budget decisions are made.

A birth certificate is needed to enroll the child in school, to avail other benefits of the country, to apply for passport, etc. It gives national identity of a child. The birth certificate will contain the information on the child and the parents that is given at the time of registration, so it is important that the information given is accurate. It is difficult to change the details after the initial registration.

The information are needed to register a birth are: The baby's date of birth, the baby's first, middle and last names, his/her parental information, the name of the hospital or birthing center, the name of the person at the birth (physician, midwife or other), the baby's weight, the length of pregnancy in weeks.

TO IDENTIFY ACTUAL OR POTENTIAL PROBLEMS AND IMMEDIATE ACTION

The tiniest humans can create big challenges for their parents. So parents need to know about their newborn babies, why babies cry, their sleeping habits, immunization, clothing, etc. It is helpful for them if they can learn some common problems faced by newborns.

Umbilical Cord

The umbilical cord was baby's lifeline when he was in his mother's womb. It is through the umbilical cord that a baby receives nourishment and oxygen. However, after birth, the baby no longer needs it.

After baby is born, the cord is cut as closely as possible, leaving a little stump that is clamped off by care provider. Once mother takes the baby home, she should remember to keep this area as clean and dry as possible. No need to cover it with the diaper or dress.

In less than a month, the umbilical stump will shrivel and dry and fall off. The mother needs to keep the navel area as dry as possible for a few more days.

Many young parents tend to panic at the slightest 'change' in their bundle of joy. But there is seldom any need to worry. Here are some common problems babies may face in the first three months.

Colic: Some babies cry incessantly for hours, especially in the evenings. They may be suffering from colic. In simple language, this means the baby has swallowed some air during his feed and has not been burped adequately. The air passes from the stomach into the intestine, giving rise to pain and discomfort. This results in colic. For relief, hold the baby in the 'burping' position. Do not give any kind of medication (including gripe water).

Vomiting: A slight trickle of milk from the side of the mouth after a feed is quite common among well-fed babies. Do not worry about it.

Jaundice

On the third day of birth, a number of babies develop a yellow skin color and yellowishness in eyes due to jaundice. Babies get jaundice when they have too much bilirubin in their blood. Bilirubin forms when red blood cells break down; this is part of the body's normal wear and tear process and is nothing to worry about. Red blood cells break down to form fat-soluble indirect bilirubin, which cannot be excreted by kidneys. Indirect bilirubin is turned to direct bilirubin by the action of hepatic enzyme glucuronyl transferase and thus it becomes water soluble and excreted through kidneys. In most cases, a baby's liver is not mature enough to process the bilirubin and ensure it gets excreted from the blood. This is how a baby develops jaundice.

It may increase over the following two to three days and subsides by the seventh or 10th day. This kind of infant jaundice is nothing to worry about. The mother needs to expose her baby to the rays of the early morning sun.

- *Thrush:* Oral candidiasis (thrush) is characterized by white patches that coat the inside of the cheeks, tongue, palate and cannot be easily wiped off. It is caused by a very mild yeast infection, is often difficult to distinguish from coagulated milk. The condition tends to be acute in newborn and the baby refuses to suck due to pain in the mouth. Topical application of 1 mL nystatin (Mycostatin) four times a day or every six hours in the oral cavity prevents the spread of the disease.

- Thrush appears when the oral flora is altered due to antibiotic therapy, or poor handwashing by the baby's caregiver. The disease is treated with good hygiene, fungicide and correction of any underlying cause.
- *Dry skin:* Usually normal, but you can use a mild soap and a moisturizer once or twice a day.
- *Spitting up:* Many babies spit up (reflux) after eating due to overfeeding or because the valve that closes the upper part of the stomach is immature. It is usually not a concern as long as the baby is gaining weight and it is not causing him to cough or choke. Some steps to take to improve this problem are slow feeding with smaller amounts, more frequent burping during feeds, avoiding pressure on his belly or vigorous activity after eating. It improves with age, usually without treatment.
- *Watery eyes:* This is usually caused by a blocked tear duct and is not a concern unless the eyes become infected (let your pediatrician know so that they can prescribe antibiotic eye drops). It usually clears up on its own before the baby is 12 months old.
- *Diaper rashes:* It is common and characterized by bright red and surrounded by red dots in the buttocks. Diaper rashes can be prevented by frequent diaper changes, increasing air exposure by keeping the diaper off as much as possible, and using a mild soap only after bowel movements (rinse with just warm water at other times).
- *Upper respiratory infections:* These are very common and include symptoms of a clear or green runny nose and cough and are usually caused by cold viruses. The best treatment is to use salt water nasal drops and a bulb suctioner to keep their nose clear. Pediatrician is to be contacted if the child has high temperature, difficulty breathing or is not improving in 7–10 days.

Warning or 'Alarm Signs' of Potentially Serious Problems—When to Seek Immediate Medical Attention

When a new born baby is unwell, there are often warning signs. If the baby has any of the following symptoms, medical attention is to be sought right away:

- Does not pass a greenish-black stool within 36 hours after birth
- Skin or whites of the eyes appear to be turning yellow
- Vomits forcefully or more frequently than usual (more than just spitting up)
- Refuses feedings for more than 6 to 8 hours
- Has a fever before 6 weeks of age
- Has a persistent cough
- Is excessively or uncharacteristically fussy or irritable
- Is unusually lethargic or sleepy
- Has color changes in the lips or face
- Has bad diarrhea or unusually frequent and very watery stools
- Appears dehydrated
- Or has any other unusual symptoms.

The Normal Infant

'An empty book is like infant's soul, in which anything may be written'.
'It is capable of all things, but contain nothing. I have a mind to fill this, with profitable wonders'.

—T Traherne

The term *infant* has come from the Latin word *infans*, meaning 'unable to speak' or 'speechless'. Children between the ages of 1 month and 12 months are called infants. Infancy is a plateau in development. During the prenatal period the rapid growth and development took place but suddenly come to stop with birth. There is a slight regression such as loss of weight, less strong and healthy than it was at the time of birth. This characteristic of plateau is due to the necessity for radical adjustments to the postnatal environment. Once the adjustments are made the infant resumes its growth and development (Fig. 5.27).

During infancy, a great deal of initial learning occurs. This learning is provided through environmental cues, such as a parents' behavior. Very basic skills are mastered during this time period, such as crying, nursing, co-ordination and the ability to represent images and objects with words. In this first year of an infant's life, the parents must learn the cues of their child, what he/she is trying to tell them to adjust to environment, and then act on their observations. The parents must learn to observe their infant's behavior and to act toward fulfilling his/her need.

An important influence in the child's life at this stage is the parents. It is very common to see a child at

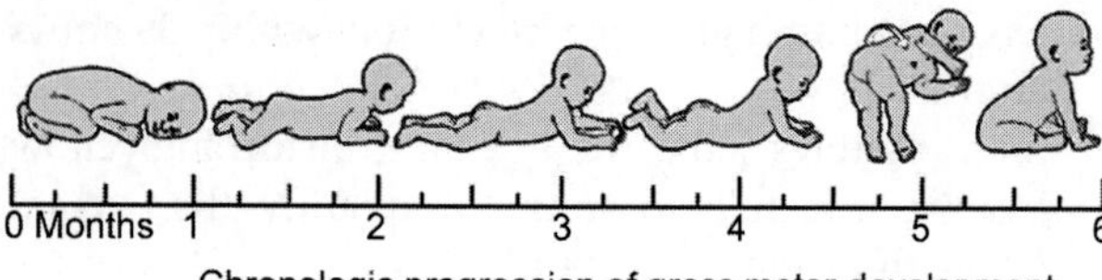

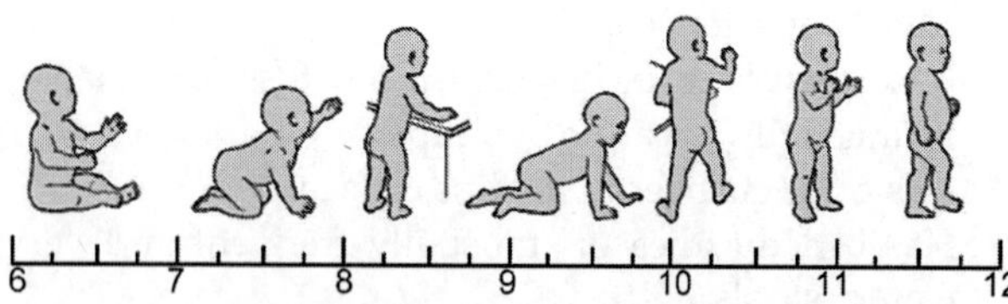

Fig. 5.27: Normal growth and development during infancy

the age of 7–9 months old become upset when they are separated from their parents/primary caregiver. This phenomenon is known as attachment, and is important in determining how a child will behave in future relationships as they mature.

Infancy is a preview of the later development. It is not possible to predict exactly what the future development of the individual will be on the basis of the development at birth. We notice only a clue of what to expect later on. Sometimes it has been observed that parents are not aware about the emotional development needed in relation to their child's development and may need help in this regard. Many times nurses can interpret this process to parents and thus alleviate much of their misunderstandings.

Overview of the Physical and Mental Growth and Development

The first year is characterized by rapid physical growth. A normal baby doubles its birth weight in six months and triples it in a year. During that time, there is great expansion of the head and chest, thus permitting development of the brain, heart, and lungs, the organs most vital to survival. The bones, which are relatively soft at birth, begin to harden, and the fontanelles, the soft parts of the newborn skull, begin to calcify, the small one at the back of the head at about 3 months, the larger one in front at varying ages up to 18 months. Brain weight also increases rapidly during infancy: by the end of the second year, the brain has already reached 75% of its adult weight.

Growth and size depend on environmental conditions as well as genetic endowment. For example, severe nutritional deficiency during the mother's pregnancy and in infancy are likely to result in an irreversible impairment of growth and intellectual development, while overfed, fat infants are predisposed to become obese later in life. Human milk provides the basic nutritional elements necessary for growth; however, weaning, (supplemental foods) are generally added to the diet during the first year.

Healthy infants come in a range of sizes. Still, infant growth tends to follow a fairly predictable path. Consider these general guidelines for infant growth in the first year:

- *Length/height:* In general, length in normal-term infants increases about 30% by age 5 months and more than 50% by age 12 months. From birth to age 6 months, a baby may grow 1/2 to 1 inch (about 1.5 to 2.5 cm) a month. From ages 6 to 12 months, a baby may grow 3/8 inch (about 1 cm) a month and gain 3 to 5 ounces (about 85 to 140 gm) a week. Expect your baby to triple his or her birth weight by about age 1 year. Infants typically grow about. 10 inches (25 cm) during the first year, and height at 5 years is about double the birth length. In boys, half the adult height is attained by about age 2. In girls, height at 19 months is about half the adult height.
- *Weight:* Newborns normally lose 5 to 8% of their birth weight during the first few days of life. They regain this weight by the end of the first 2 weeks. After this period of time, newborns typically gain about 1 ounce per day (about 200 gm/week), during the first 2 months, and 1 pound per month after that. This weight gain typically results in a doubling of birth weight by age 5 months and a tripling by 1 year. By the age of 2, a baby's weight will have quadrupled.
- The best way to estimate a child's physical maturity is to use *skeletal age*, a measure of bone development. This is done by having a X-ray of the long bones of the body to see the extent to which soft, pliable cartilage has hardened into bone.
- *Changes in body proportions:* Cephalocaudal trend means that growth occurs from head to tail. The head develops more rapidly than the lower part of the body. At birth the head takes up to one fourth of the total body length and legs only one third. The lower body catches up by age 2 and the head accounts for only one fifth and legs for nearly one half of the body length. Proximodistal trend means that head growth proceeds literally from near to far or from center of the body outward.
- *The brain development:* At birth the brain is nearer its adult shape and size than any other physical structure. The brain continues to develop at an astounding pace

throughout infancy and toddlerhood. The neurons of infants and adults differ in 2 significant ways, i.e. growth of neural fibers and synapses increases connective structures. When synapses are formed, many surrounding neurons die. This occurs in 20 to 80% of the brain region.

- *Dendrites synapses:* Synapses are tiny gaps between neurons where fiber from different neurons come close together but do not touch. Neurons release chemicals that cross the synapses sending messages to one another. During the prenatal period, the neural tube produces far more neurons than the brain will ever need. Myelination: The coating of neural fibers with a fatty sheath called myelin that improves the efficiency of message transfer. Multi-layered lipid cholesterol and protein covering produced by neuralgia cause a rapid gain in overall size of brain due to neural fibers and myelination.
- *Synaptic pruning:* Neurons seldom stimulated soon loose their synapses. Neurons not needed at the moment return to an uncommitted state so they can support future development. However, if synaptic pruning occurs in old age neurons will lose their synapses. If neurons are stimulated at a young age, even though neurons were pruned, they will be stimulated again.
- *Cerebral cortex:* Surrounding the brain, it is the largest most complex brain structure. The cortex is divided into four major lobes: Occipital lobe, parietal lobe, temporal lobe, and frontal lobe which is the last to develop.
- *Brain plasticity:* The brain is highly plastic. Many areas are not yet committed to specific functions. If a part of the brain is damaged, other parts can take over tasks that they would not normally have handled.
- *Changing states of arousal:* The newborn infant sleeps almost constantly, awakening only for feedings, but the number and length of waking periods gradually increases. Child sleeps about 16 hours each day for the first 3 months. From 3 months until 6 months, he will sleep about 13 to 14 hours each day. Sleep patterns are more developed as the brain develops. It is not until the first year of life that the secretion of *melatonin*, a hormone produced in the brain, affects more drowsiness in the night than in the day. In addition, he will sleep more at night and less during the day as he gets older.
- By the age of three months, most infants have acquired a fairly regular schedule for sleeping, feeding, and bowel movements. By the end of the first year, sleeping and waking hours are divided about equally.
- *Teeth:* The timing of tooth eruption varies, mainly for hereditary reasons. However, tooth eruption may also be delayed by disorders such as rickets, hypopituitarism, hypothyroidism, or Down syndrome.

Lower front teeth usually begin to appear by the age of 5 to 9 months. Upper front teeth usually begin to appear by 8 to 12 months. On average, infants should have 6 teeth by age 12 months, 12 teeth by 18 months, 16 teeth by 2 years, and all 20 of their baby (deciduous) teeth by 2½ years (Fig. 5.28). Baby teeth are replaced by permanent (adult) teeth between the ages of 5 years and 13 years. Permanent teeth tend to appear earlier in girls.

- *Respiratory system:* The respiratory system continues to mature over the first year of life. During this period the lungs increases three times their weight and six times their volume at birth. In comparison with the adults, in the infants.
  - The bronchus and bronchioles are shorter and narrower, leave infants vulnerable to respiratory difficulties caused by infection and foreign bodies
  - In the newborn infant, alveoli number approximately 20 million, increases to the adult number of 300 million by the age of 8 years
  - The trachea remains small and supported by only soft cartilage
  - The eustachian tube is short and relatively horizontal, and increases the risk for middle ear infection.
  - The respiratory rate slows from an average of 30–60 breaths in newborn to about 20–30 in the 12 month old. As the infant matures, the respiratory pattern becomes more regular and rhythmic.

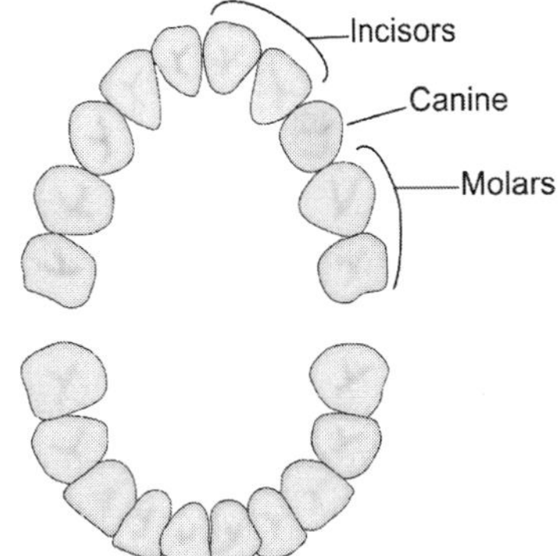

Fig. 5.28: First teeth—sometimes called 'Baby teeth'

- *Cardiovascular system:* A dramatic changes takes place during the fetal to extrauterine circulation (*See* newborn chapter).
  During infancy the heart doubles in size and weight, the heart rate gradually slows and blood pressure increases.
- *Gastrointestinal system:* 10–20 mL capacity stomach at birth increases in size with feedings and reaches to approximately 200 mL capacity at one year of age. The human digestive system has a layer of mucous that protects the gastrointestinal tract from microbes and other contaminants that may be present in food or liquids. In infants, this protective barrier is immature, which puts baby at risk of infection. Antibodies in breast milk help protect baby until his digestive mucosal lining matures and he increases his ability to produce his own antibodies, which happens around the age of six months. Although a newborn can digest carbohydrates and proteins as well as fat, her pancreas is not fully developed, baby produces much lower levels of digestive enzymes than an older child. Enzymes in breast milk and baby's saliva, help make up for this shortcoming. The newborn's digestive system is capable of digesting protein and lactase, the ability to digest and absorb fat does not reach adult levels until approximately 6 to 9 months of age.

In addition, the esophageal valve, which controls the entry of food into infant's stomach, is underdeveloped. This is why babies frequently spit up. These digestive shortcomings, along with the immature state of the infant kidney, can put baby at risk for dehydration, electrolyte imbalance and insufficient absorption of nutrients.

- *Immune system:* Trans-placental transfer of maternal antibody IgG confer immunity to the child approximately 4–6 months of age. The infant starts synthesizing immunoglobulins soon after birth, by one year reaches 40–60 of adult levels of IgG, 75% of the adult levels IgM and about 20% of the adult IgA level. The activity of T lymphocytes also increases after birth. Protection against infection is not achieved until early childhood, though the immune system matures during infancy. This state of immature immune system places the infant at risk for infection.
- *Renal system:* During first year of life, the kidney mass increases in three fold. The glomeruli enlarges but the glomerular filtration rate remain low. The kidney is not so mature in concentrating urine until after the first year of life. The infant is at great risk for fluid and electrolyte imbalance as the functioning of the renal system is immature.
- *Motor development:* Infants need to learn how to move and to use their bodies to perform various tasks, a process better known as motor development. Over time, babies learn to move their body parts voluntarily to perform both gross (large) and fine (small) motor skills. The term 'gross motor skills' refers to those which uses large muscles (i.e. holding head, rolling body, sitting, walking). In general, they begin developing motor skills from the center of the body outward and from head to tail. They learn to control their head and neck before they learn to maneuver their arms; they learn to maneuver their arms before they learn to manipulate their fingers. Babies learn to move their torso before they learn how to move their arms and legs.

When babies are born, they are equipped with a set of reflexes, or automatic actions. Some reflexes help them perform basic tasks (respiration, feeding), while other reflexes seem to have no real purpose. All of these reflexes can help to assess babies for any neurological problems at birth and as they grow. As infants mature in the first few months of life and begin developing the ability to voluntarily move and use their bodies, most of these reflexes gradually and naturally fade away.

Fine motor skills develop alongside gross motor skills. Beyond just learning how to use and manipulate their bodies in large movements, babies are learning how to use their hands and how to coordinate smaller movements with their senses, such as sight. Like the gross motor skill development, fine motor development comes gradually as infants build one skill on top of previous skills. (the motor development of infant in detail is given in box).

- *Cognitive development:* Babies are growing physically as well as mentally (cognitively) during the first 2 years of life. Every day while they interact with and learn about their environment they are creating new connections and pathways between nerve cells both within their brains, and between their brains and bodies. While physical growth and change is easily observed and measured in precise terms such as in inches and pounds, cognitive change and development is a little harder to determine as clearly. Therefore, much about what experts know about mental and cognitive development is based on the careful observation of developmental theorists and their theories, such as Piaget's theory of cognitive development and Erickson's psychosocial stages helps explain infant mental growth to some extent (*See* Chapter 4).

- *Sensory development:* Though hearing should be developed at birth, the other senses to continue to develop as the child matures. The senses like sight, smell, taste and touch starts to develop at different rates after birth.
- Infant reflexes like Moro's reflex, tonic neck reflex, dancing reflex (discussed above)

During their first year, babies start to develop skills they will use for the rest of their lives. The normal growth of babies can be broken down into the following areas:

- *Gross motor:* Controlling the head, sitting, crawling, may be even starting to walk
- *Fine motor:* Holding a spoon, picking up a piece of cereal between thumb and finger
- *Sensory:* Seeing, hearing, tasting, touching and smelling
- *Language:* Starting to make sounds, learning some words, understanding what people say
- *Social:* The ability to play with family members and other children.

Babies do not develop skills at the same rate. There is a wide range of what is considered 'normal.' The baby may be ahead in some areas and slightly behind in others. If parents are worried about possible delays, the nurse has to examine the child and give guidance to the parents. The average achievements levels of infants are given below:

Average achievement levels of infants: 1 Month to 1 Year			
0–3 months			
Motor	*Sensory*	*Communication*	*Feeding*
• Lifts and holds head up in mid position • Pushes up on arms while lying on tummy (Fig. 5.29) • Able to move fists from open to fist • Able to bring hands to mouth • Moves legs and arms off of surface when excited	• Moves eyes to visually track objects • Attempts to reach for a toy held above their chest • Keeps head centered to watch faces or toys • Able to calm with rocking, touching, and gentle sounds • Is not upset by everyday sounds • Enjoys a variety of movements	• Turns head towards sound or voice • Quiets or smiles when spoken to • Shows interest in faces • Makes eye contact • Cries differently for different needs (e.g. hungry vs. tired) • Coos and smiles	• Turns head toward nipple or bottle • Tongue moves forward and back to suck • Drinks 2 oz. to 6 oz. of liquid per feeding, 6 times per day • Sucks and swallows well during feeding

Warning signs to watch for:

- Poor suckling at the breast or refusing to suckle
- Little movement of arms and legs
- Little or no reaction to loud sounds or bright lights
- Crying for long periods for no apparent reason
- Vomiting and diarrhea, which can lead to dehydration.

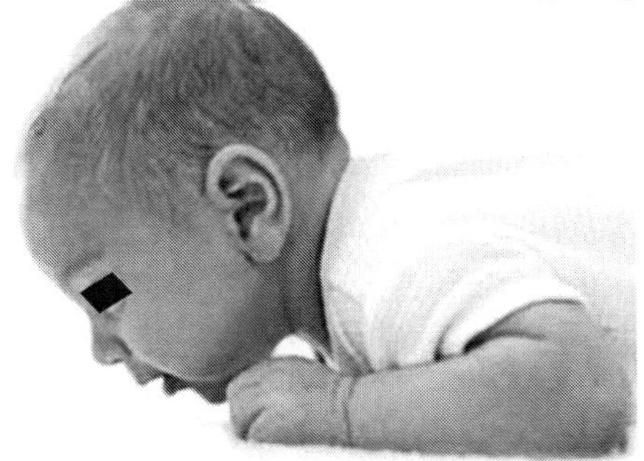

Fig. 5.29: Two-month-old infant can hold the head erect in mid position when lying on abdomen

Average achievement levels of infants: 1 Month To 1 Year			
4–6 months (Figs 5.30A to C)			
Motor	*Sensory*	*Communication*	*Feeding*
• Uses hands to support self while sitting • Rolls from back to tummy and tummy to back • While standing with support, accepts entire weight with legs • Reaches for toys while on tummy • Reaches both hands to play with feet • Uses both hands to explore toys	• Reaches for toys and transfers them from hand to hand • Reaches both hands to play with feet • Brings hands and objects to mouth • Generally happy when not hungry or tired • Able to calm with rocking, touching, and gentle sounds • Is not upset by everyday sounds • Enjoys a variety of movements	• Fears loud or unexpected noises • Listens and responds when spoken to • Begins to babble with p, b, and m sounds • Begins to babble with constant sounds • Uses babbling to get attention • Makes different kinds of sounds to express feelings • Imitates sounds and facial expressions • Notices toys that make sounds	• Shows interest in food • Begins to eat cereals and pureed foods • Opens mouth as spoon approaches • Moves pureed food from front of mouth to back

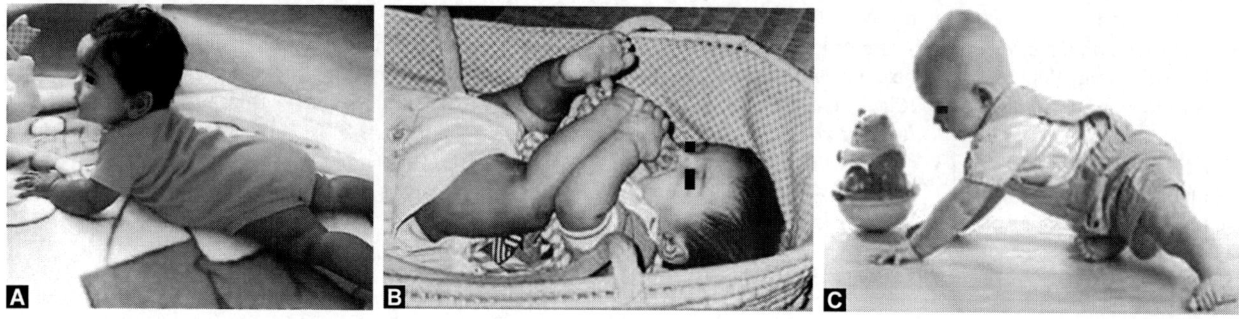

Figs 5.30A to C: A. The 4-month-old infant lifts head and shoulders at a 90° angle when on abdomen and looks around; **B.** The 5-month-old infant grasps object with whole hand and carries them to the mouth; **C.** The 6-month-old infant uses both hands to explore toys

Warning signs to watch for:

- Stiffness or difficulty moving limbs
- Constant moving of the head (this might indicate an ear infection, which could lead to deafness if not treated)
- Little or no response to sounds, familiar faces or the breast
- Refusing the breast or other foods.

Average achievement levels of infants: 1 Month To 1 Year			
7–9 months (Figs 5.31A to C)			
Motor	*Sensory*	*Communication*	*Feeding*
• Sits and reaches for toys without falling • Moves from tummy or back into sitting • Creeps on hands and knees with alternate leg movement • Uses both hands to explore toys • Picks up head and pushes through elbows during tummy time • Turns head to visually track objects • Shows more control while rolling, sitting, and scooting • Starts to crawl and pull to a stand • Enjoys a variety of movements – bouncing up and down, rocking back and forth • Picks up small objects with thumbs and fingers • Tries to lean towards, reach for, and throw toys • In simple play imitates others	• Explores and examines an object using both hands and mouth • Turns several pages of a chunky board book at once • Experiments with the amount of force needed to pick up different objects • Focuses on objects near and far • Investigates shapes, sizes, and textures of toys and surroundings • Observes environment from a variety of positions—while lying on back or tummy, sitting, crawling, and standing with assistance	• Uses increased variety of sounds and syllable combinations in babbling • Looks at familiar objects and people when named • Recognizes sound of their name • Participates in two-way communication • Begins using hand movements to communicate wants and needs, e.g. reaches to be picked up • Follows some routine commands when paired with gestures • Distinguishes between familiar and unfamiliar voices • Shows recognition of commonly used words • Mimics facial expressions and gestures • Shows interest when looking or pointing • Responds to name	• Holds and drinks from a bottle • Places pacifier in mouth • Begins transition from milk or formula to infant cereal • Begins to eat junior and mashed table foods • Enjoys chew toys that can massage sore and swollen gums during teething • Feels full longer after eating more solid foods • Starts to look and reach for food that is nearby • Shows strong reaction to new smells and tastes • Begins to form associations with familiar smells and tastes

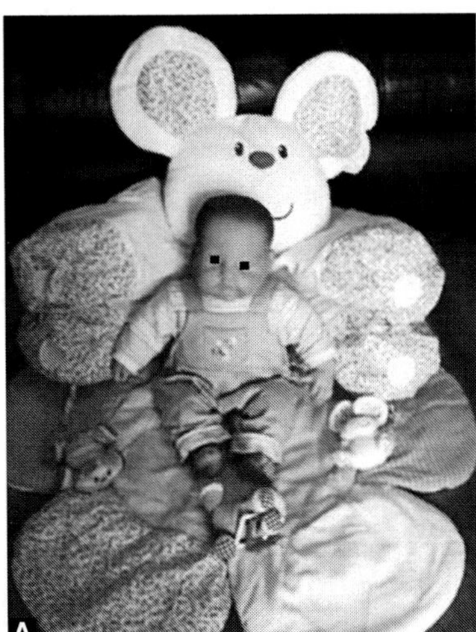

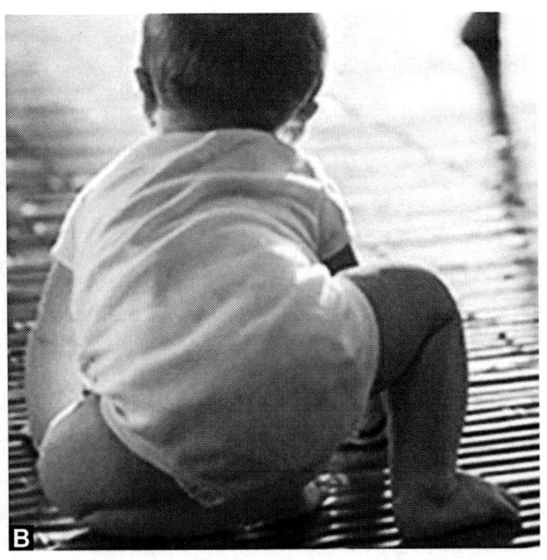

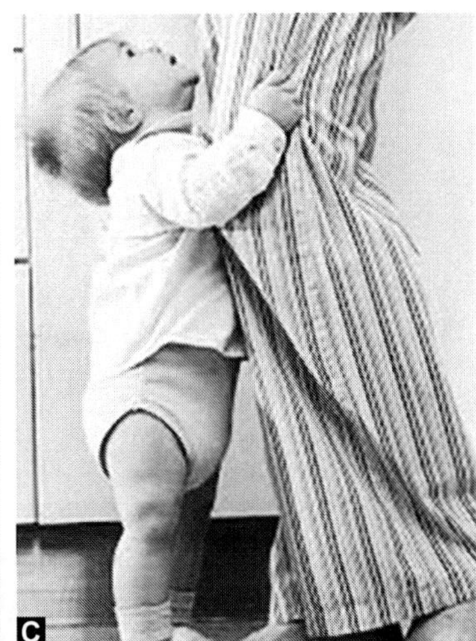

Figs 5.31A to C: A. The 7-month infant sits alone steadily; **B.** The 8-month-old infant can creep, carries trunk above the floor; **C.** The 9-month-old infant can pull self to feet if assisted

Warning signs to watch for:

- Does not make sounds in response to others
- Does not look at objects that move
- Listlessness and lack of response to the caregiver
- Lack of appetite or refusal of food.

Average achievement levels of infants: 1 Month to 1 Year			
10–12 months (Figs 5.32A to C)			
Motor	*Sensory*	*Communication*	*Feeding*
• Pulls to stand and cruises along furniture • Stands alone and takes several steps with independent steps • May start to walk independently • Moves in and out of various positions to explore environment and get desired toys • Sits unsupported and is able to turn head to look at objects without losing balance • Maintains balance when throwing objects • Claps hands • Looks around while body is in motion • Cranes neck to see around a corner or other obstacle • Releases objects into a container with a large opening • Uses thumb and pointer finger to pick up tiny objects	• Enjoys listening to songs • Enjoys different textures from food, blankets, mud, paint etc. • Explores toys with fingers and mouth • Crawls to or away from sounds coming from a distance • Crawls to or away from objects baby sees in the distance	• Meaningfully uses 'mama' or 'dada' • Responds to simple directions, e.g. 'Come here' • Produces long strings of gibberish (called jargoning) in social communication • Says one or two words • Imitates speech sounds • Babbling has sounds and rhythms of speech • Understands up to 50 words • Pays attention to where you are looking and pointing • Cries and notices when hurt	• Finger feeds self • Eating an increasing variety of food • Ready to try soft-cooked vegetables, soft fruits, and finger foods (teething biscuits, cooked pasta) • Might be ready to start self-spoon feeding • Enjoys a greater variety of smells and tastes • Is developing more teeth and better control of tongue and lips • Begins to use an open cup

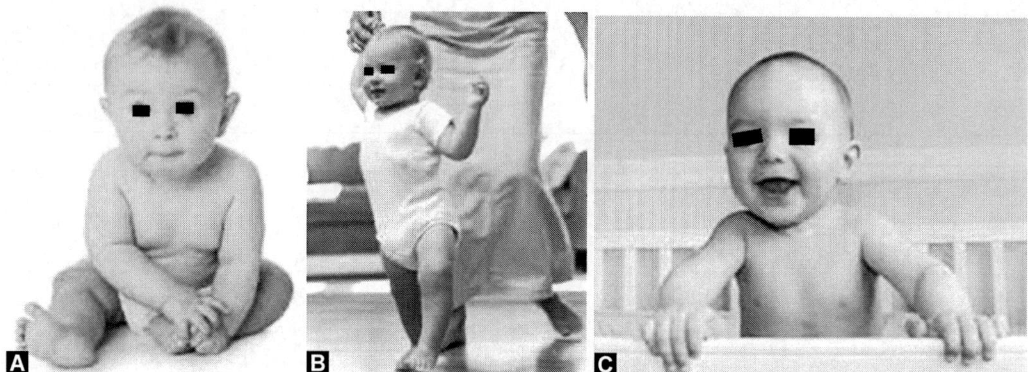

Figs 5.32A to C: A. The 10-month old infant sits steadily for an indefinite time; **B.** Pulls self to feet, holding on the side of the crib; **C.** The 11-month old infant stands erect with the help of mother's hand

Major Adjustments of Infancy

- Change in temperature requires adjustment. There is a constant temperature of 100 °F in the uterine sac and it is 60 to 70 °F in the hospital or home.
- Breathing by own starts. When the umbilical cord is cut the infant must begin to breathe on its own.
- Sucking and swallowing starts. When the umbilical cord is cut off, the child gets nourishment by the reflexes of sucking and swallowing instead of receiving it from the mother through umbilical cord.
- Elimination of waste products begins. Letting out urine and stools is not a matter of adjustment. But some infants are seen to have trouble shooting with elimination matters.

Needs During the First Year

Infants put everything into their mouth and later to bite was given priority among his essential needs because of its great psychologic importance. They have five other needs which must be met if they have to learn to trust the people about him are feeding, sucking pleasure, warmth and comfort, both love and security, and sensory stimulation.

Need for feeding: The infant's world is small, he/she lives entirely in the moment and responds to the physiologic mechanism. To him hunger means tension and his cue is nothing but crying. He/she soon learns that people around him can satisfy this need and reduce his tension, make him comfortable—and that is done with varying emotional attitudes on their part. This is the time for showing love and affection to the child.

During feeding his mother holds him closely and the baby gets warmth and comfort. The mother's attitude is expressed in voice, touch, and handling the infant while she/he is nursing. This is also important in case of hospitalized child. The nurses must be aware about the importance of this attitude and show emotional attachment when feeding hospitalized infants.

Need for sucking pleasure: Infants put fingers and toys into their mouth and get pleasure in sucking. During infancy, the mouth is the area of pleasure and the child enjoys sucking thoroughly apart from the need for food. If she does not get the opportunity for sucking, it results tension. So, giving him something to suck on relieves the tension, and he promptly relaxes. The intensity of the sucking urge varies and is an example of individual differences in children.

During the second six months the child may bite upon the nipple, when he/she is on breastfeeding. This hurts the mother even if his teeth have not erupted. If the baby wants to bite, he/she should be given a suitable toy. The intensity of the urge for oral satisfaction through sucking and biting gradually decreases as other gratifications become available.

Need for warmth and comfort: Mother holds her baby in her arms and the infant enjoys the warmth and softness of his mother's body. Every child has real hunger for this pleasant experience. He/she enjoys rhythmic rocking, being handled, and the comfort of having his position changed.

'Warmth' is the most powerful personality trait in social judgment, and attachment theorists have stressed the importance of warm physical contact with caregivers during infancy for healthy relationships in adulthood. Intriguingly, recent research in humans points to the involvement of the insula in the processing of both physical temperature and interpersonal warmth (trust) information. Because of these frequent early life experiences with the trustworthy caregiver, a close mental association should develop between the concepts of physical warmth and psychological warmth. Indeed, recent research on the neuro-biology of attachment has added further support for the proposed link between tactile temperature sensation and feelings of psychological warmth and trust.

Meeting for love and security: Encouraging emotional bonding. Baby needs to be close to mother and to anticipate that she will respond to his or her needs. Stimulating learning and communication, newborn learns through bonding and interaction.

The secure attachment bond is the nonverbal emotional relationship between an infant and parents or primary caregiver, defined by emotional responses to the baby's cues, as expressed through movements, gestures, and sounds. Although baby's needs are basic, it is important to respond promptly to his or her cues and to recognize safety issues. The success of this wordless interactive emotional relationship enables a child to feel secure enough to develop fully, and affects how he or she will interact, communicate, and form relationships throughout life. This emotional exchange draws the parents and child together, ensuring that infant will feel safe and be calm enough to experience optimal development of their nervous system. The attachment bond is a key factor in the way infant's brain organizes itself and influences child's social, emotional, intellectual, and physical development.

However, children need something more than love and care-giving in order for their brains and nervous systems to develop in the best way possible. Children need to be able to engage in a nonverbal emotional exchange with their parents and others in a way that communicates their needs and makes them feel understood, secure, and balanced. The quality of the attachment bond varies. A *secure* bond provides the baby with an optimal foundation for life: eagerness to learn, healthy self-awareness, trust, and consideration for others. An *insecure* attachment bond, one that fails to meet infant's need for safety and understanding, can lead to confusion about his or her own identity and difficulties in learning and relating to others in later life. Children who feel emotionally disconnected from their primary caregiver are likely to feel confused, misunderstood, and insecure.

Need for sensory stimulation: At birth, an infant's brain is not fully developed, and the size of a newborn baby's brain is only about one-quarter of that of an adult. It has recently been researched, that genetics no longer play the only role in infant brain development; a sensory stimulation and neural pathway connections are major factors that lead to healthy brain function in babies. Parents and others can help change or influence the child's nervous system development while it is most malleable, particularly in the first five to seven years of life. It is now known that sensory stimulation and neural pathway connections are major factors that lead to healthy brain function in babies.

Billions of brain cells, or neurons, are formed throughout the first stages of fetal development and through birth. When an infant is born, the only developed part of the brain is the brain stem. The functions such as kicking, sleeping, rooting, crying and feeding are controlled by this part of the brain. Right after birth, an infant's brain begins making over a trillion neuron connections, or synapses which are used to transmit information based on various life experiences. Stimulation from the environment through the senses of touch, hearing, seeing, smelling, and tasting; directly affect the sensory neurons and help in establishing these connections.

This process occurs mostly with the neurons and synapses that control a baby's sensory areas such as the eyes, ears, nose, mouth, and skin. Many of these 'new' connections help infants to reach important milestones such as color vision, develop a pincer grasp, or strive for parent attachment.

The more frequently the neuron connections are used, the more they retain information and the stronger they become. If some of the neural pathways are not used, they will end up in pruning (dying out). This is a necessary step in the brain development process for it prevents 'overload' so to speak. Once these synapses gain strength and are noted by the brain that these are the pathways of important information, they become protected by a myelin sheath that helps in sending messages to the brain even faster.

The development of an infant's brain is essential to the life-long learning process and through proper sensory stimulation. During this developmental phase, it will be easier for parents to understand the needs of their babies. By providing them with physical, emotional, and cognitive experiences, they will gain much more knowledge to use in the future (Fig. 5.33). However, there are negative forms of stimulation that can lead to life-long developmental delays. The negative stimuli like neglect, stress, trauma, and abuse are all can have a tragic effect on brain growth. Studies show, that those infants or children that receive little to no attention and are not exposed to positive, purposeful stimuli by their parents, end up with brains 20 to 30% smaller than those who have had those 'good' sensory experiences.

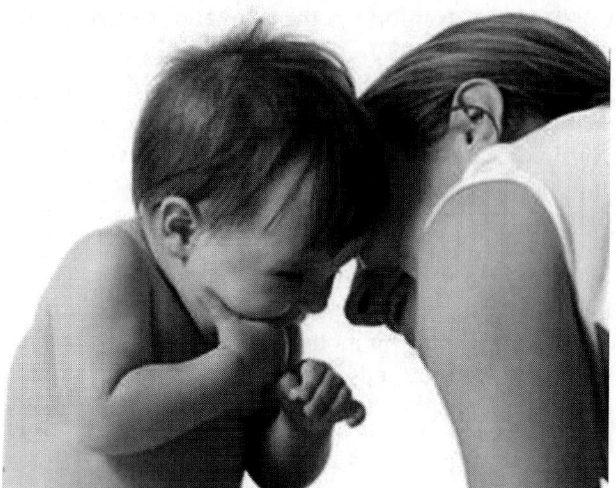

Fig. 5.33: A nonverbal emotional exchange between mother and child

Health Promotion for the Infant and Family

For healthy growth and development, newborns need physical and emotional care. Nurses can provide valuable information and specific guidance to the parents for health promotion for the infants such as feeding, cry, sleep, immunization, etc. Nurses can offer support to new parents by identifying strategies for coping with the first few months with an infant. At each well baby visit the nurse does the following:

- A physical examination and testing the reflexes
- Weigh and measure the baby to see how the baby compares to other babies of the same age.
- Growth chart is maintained. Length, weight, and head circumference measurements are taken. These measurements are plotted on a growth chart and are compared to previous and later markings to make sure the baby is growing as expected.
- Review of the child's immunization record. Needed immunizations are given or scheduled
- Elicit about how the family and the baby are doing
- Health education based on child's need and care.
- This is a good time to talk to health professional about any concerns parents have.

Babies need routine checkups every 2 to 3 months from age 1 month to 12 months. These visits are important to check for problems and to make sure that baby is growing and developing as expected. Between visits, parents can be told to write down any questions they want to ask the doctor/nurse next time.

Feeding and nutrition: Responding to baby's hunger cues, no matter how frequent it is, called feeding on demand. As infancy is a period of rapid growth, nutritional needs are of special significance. Nutrition and nurturing during the first years of life are both crucial for life-long health and well-being. In infancy, no gift is more precious than breastfeeding; yet barely one in three infants is exclusively breastfed during the first six months of life.

During infancy, the nutritional needs are of special importance as it is a period of rapid growth. The World Health Organization recommends that infants start breastfeeding within one hour of life, are exclusively breastfed for six months, with timely introduction of adequate, safe and properly fed complementary foods while continuing breastfeeding for up to two years of age or beyond.

Malnutrition is responsible, directly or indirectly for about one third of deaths among children under five. Well above two thirds of these deaths, often associated with inappropriate feeding practices, occur during the first year of life.

In this period, eating progresses from a principally reflex activity to relatively sophisticated, yet messy, attempts at self-feeding. Because the child's gastrointestinal system continues to mature throughout the first year, the changes in diet, the introduction of new foods, and even upsets in routines can result in feeding problems. The nurse must have a clear understanding of gastrointestinal maturation, and knowledge about breastfeeding and various infant formulas and foods, as well as familial and cultural background of the infant, before giving anticipatory guidance regarding feeding and nutrition of child (*See* Chapter 3).

Immunization: Prevention of disease is one of the most important goals in child care. During infancy and childhood preventive measures can be carried out against certain infectious diseases. Infants are particularly vulnerable to infectious diseases; that is why it is critical to protect them through immunization. The recommended immunization schedule is designed to protect infants and children early in life, when they are most vulnerable and before they are exposed to potentially life-threatening diseases. Immunization is one of the most important things a parent can do to protect their children's health. Today we can protect children from 14 serious diseases. Failure to vaccinate may mean putting children at risk for serious diseases.

Immunization is a healthy choice that saves lives. The following vaccines are available for children, free vaccines are provided through national immunization program to protect children against these vaccine-preventable diseases:

- Diphtheria
- Tetanus
- Pertussis
- Hepatitis B
- Polio
- *Haemophilus influenzae* type B (Hib)
- Meningococcal disease
- Pneumococcal disease
- Rotavirus
- Measles
- Mumps
- Rubella (German Measles)
- Varicella (Chickenpox)
- Influenza

(*See* Chapter 8)

Skin care: A newborn baby is born with wrinkly skin and a protective covering called vernix that naturally peels off during the first week. There is no need to rush it, rub it, or treat it with lotions or creams. Newborn skin is delicate, and so is the baby's immune system. Chemicals, fragrances, and dyes in clothing, detergents, and baby products can cause newborn skin irritation, dryness, chafing, and rashes. However, there is much parents can do to protect baby from these skin problems.

It is important to provide proper care for the portion of remaining cord at the baby's navel until it heals and separates from the umbilicus—usually within two weeks after birth. Keep the stump dry, and expose the stump to air as much as possible to help dry out the base. Some research suggests that the stump may heal faster if left alone and nothing applied on it. Sponge baths are often the best way to wash the infant until the cord falls off.

Too-frequent bathing during the first year of life can remove the natural oils that protect baby's skin. That leaves baby's skin vulnerable, so it may react to any potential allergen and can trigger a reaction like eczema. Wash baby clothes, bedding, and blankets separately from the family's laundry.

Touching on newborn's skin has a soothing, nurturing effect and is critical to baby's development. Giving newborn a massage is important one-on-one time. Like cuddling, a massage is a way to convey love and affection for baby. In fact, research shows that a baby's very survival depends on being touched by others as touch triggers hormones, boosts immunity, and helps fight disease. Also, massaged babies are calmer, sleep better, and cry less.

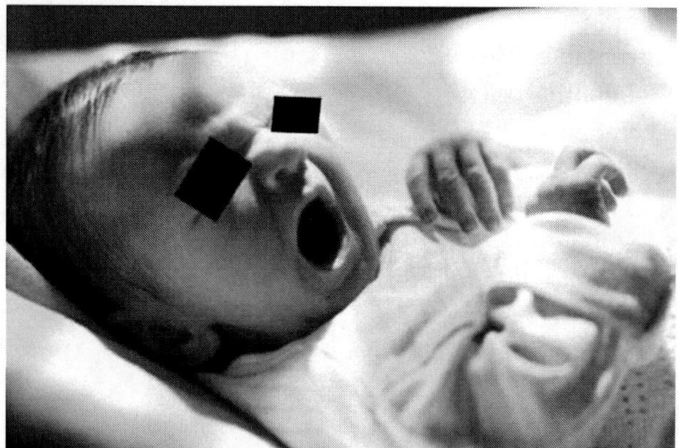

Fig. 5.34: The infant needs rest for his rapid growth, and his energy output

Sleep, rest and crying: The greater part of an infant's time is spent in sleep. The infant needs rest for his rapid growth, and his energy output (Fig. 5.34). The amount of sleep he/she takes depends upon his/her need, which vary from day to day. During first few months of life, infants sleep about 15–18 hours a day. Signs of increasing maturity in relation to sleep are a reduction in the total sleeping hour and longer interval between sleeping periods. At six months the average amount of sleep is about 12 hours at night and 3–4 hours during the day (*See* Chapter 4).

Rest: All children have individual sleep and rest requirements. Children need a comfortable relaxing environment to enable their bodies to rest. This environment must be safe and well supervised to ensure children are safe, healthy and secure in their environment. A relaxing atmosphere for resting children can be created by playing relaxation music, reading stories, cultural reflection, turning off lights and ensuring children are comfortably clothed. The environment should be tranquil and calm for both parents and children.

Communications with families are to be maintained to encourage a consistent approach in responding appropriately and respectfully to children's sleep and rest needs. Safe sleeping practices are followed to minimize the risk of harm to children and babies.

Cry: Baby cannot do anything for herself and relies on parents to provide her with the food, warmth and comfort that she needs. Crying is baby's way of communicating any or all of those needs and ensuring a response from parents/primary caregiver. The common reasons of infant crying are:

- *Hunger:* Hunger is one of the most common reasons that newborn baby will cry. The younger baby is, the more likely it is that she is hungry. Baby's small stomach cannot hold very much, so if she cries, feed to be given. She may be hungry, even if her last feed does not seem very long ago.
- *Colic:* Persistent and inconsolable crying in an otherwise healthy baby is traditionally called colic. Some people also associate colic with wind and tummy or digestive problems. These may be due to an allergy or intolerance to certain substances in feeding.
- *The child needs to be held:* Baby need lots of cuddling, physical contact and reassurance to comfort her. So it may be that she just wants to be held. Mother can try a baby sling to keep her close to her, perhaps swaying and singing to her while mother holds her.

Mother may be worried about spoiling her baby if she holds her too much. But during the first few months of her life that is not possible. Small babies need lots of physical comfort. If mother holds the baby close she may be soothed by hearing mother's heartbeat.

Baby is tired and need a rest: Often, babies find it hard to get to sleep, particularly if they are over-tired. You will soon become aware of your baby's sleep cues. Whining and crying at the slightest thing, staring blankly into space, and going quiet and still are just three examples.

If baby has received a lot of attention and cuddles from doting visitors, she may become over-stimulated. Then, when it comes to sleeping, she will find it hard to switch off and settle. The baby is to be taken somewhere calm and quiet to help her to settle down.

Baby is too cold or too hot: Baby may hate having her nappy changed or being bathed. She may not be used to the feeling of cold air on her skin and would rather be bundled up and warm. Parents will soon learn how to perform a quick nappy change if this is the case.

Take care not to overdress baby, or she may become too hot. She will generally need to wear one more layer of clothing than parents to be comfortable.

Use sheets and cellular blankets as bedding in baby's cot. Parents can check whether their baby is too hot or too cold by feeling her tummy. If her tummy feels too hot, remove a blanket, and if it feels cold, add one.

Usually baby protests if her clothes are too tight or if a wet or soiled nappy is bothering her. Or she may not mind if her nappy is full and may actually enjoy the warm and comfortable feeling. But if baby's tender skin is being irritated she will most likely cry.

Be aware of changes in baby. If she is unwell, she will probably cry in a different tone to her usual cry. It may be weaker, more urgent, continuous, or high-pitched. And if, baby usually cries a lot but has become unusually quiet, it may be a sign that she is not well.

If baby has difficulty breathing through the crying, or if the crying is accompanied by a fever, vomiting, diarrhea or constipation, inform health professionals to take concerns seriously.

Safety measures: Infancy is a hazardous period both physically and psychologically. Physically the infant finds it difficult in making adjustments to the new environment. Psychologically the infant suffers a little when the attitudes of significant people towards the infant radically changes. Since accidents are a principal cause of death in infants and children of all ages, great emphasis should be placed on accident prevention.

Most newborn accidents in the home involve falls. Be sure that baby is not left alone on high surfaces unless proper barriers are in place to prevent baby from rolling off. The safest place for a newborn when not being held, is on the floor or in a crib with the sides up and no pillows or toys inside. Never leave baby alone on the table or counter top! Keep a hand on baby at all times.

- Keep toys, stuffed animals and pillows out of the crib.
- Do not leave baby alone with pets until they have adjusted to each other.

Reduce the risk of sudden infant death syndrome (SIDS) by always placing baby to sleep on his or her back (not on the stomach). Make sure that the crib mattress is firm and covered by a sheet and that there are no pillows or blankets that could block the baby's mouth or nose.

Play: Through play infants learn so many things. In play they practice motor skills, acquire control of the body, and gain in general coordination of movements and specific coordination of hand-eye movements. Infants learn to relate to objects and to people, to express their feelings, and to work of frustrations through play. Play then, is all important in the development of the child's personality; it occupies almost all his waking hours.

Summary of the Contribution of the Nurse to Child Health

The nurse can contribute in many ways to improving the physical and mental health of infants and children.

- Observation of children
- Parental education and anticipatory guidance
- Emotional support of parent
- The improvement of child health care.

The Toddler

GENERAL CHARACTERISTICS OF TODDLER

The toddler period extends from age 1 year to approximately 3 years of age. Those curious little creatures known as toddlers are leaving the immature infant stage, but not yet ready for the more precocious preschool phase. The word toddler is derived from 'to toddle', which means to walk unsteadily, like a child of this age (Fig. 5.35). Typical toddler development includes a leap forward in motor development, increases in mental reasoning skills and the budding beginnings of social and emotional growth.

The toddler stage is very important in a child's life. As the child moves from passive dependency to active interaction with those about him, society or his family—guides him/her in conformity with social norm. Most children learn to walk, talk, solve problems, relate to others, and more during this stage. The most important demand made upon him during the toddler period is that of toilet training. Everything that happens to the toddler is meaningful. With each stage or skill the child masters, a new stage begins. This growth is different for each child. Children have their own timetable. The toddler is discovering that they are a separate being from their parent and are testing their boundaries in learning the way the world around them works.

One major task for the toddler is to learn to be independent. That is why toddlers want to do things for themselves, have their own ideas about how things should happen, and use 'NO' many times each day. This

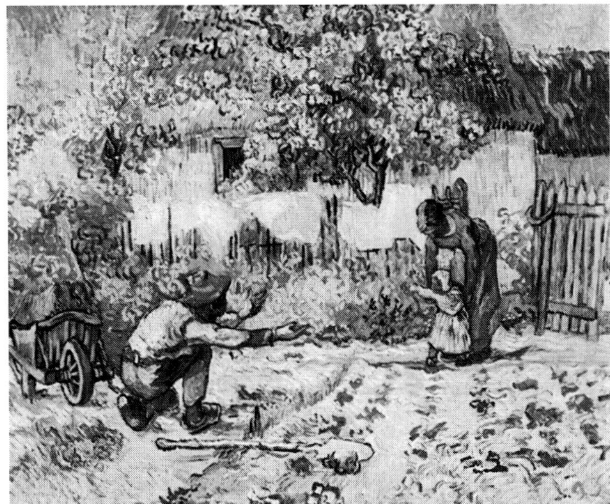

Fig. 5.35: Vincent van Gogh—first steps

stage is characterized by much growth and change, mood swings and some negativity. Toddlers are long on will and short on skill. This is why they are often frustrated and 'misbehave.' Some adults call the toddler stage 'the terrible twos.' Toddlers bursting with energy and ideas need to explore their environment. Parents need to make sure that they can explore in an environment that is safe for them. They want to be independent, and yet, they are still very dependent. During the toddler period parents must learn to accept the child's new wish for freedom to explore and to become a person in his/her own right.

OVERVIEW OF THE GROWTH AND DEVELOPMENT

The renowned child psychologist Erik Erikson described how the physical development of a child in his second year of life serves as the foundation for cognitive, personality and social development. As a result of the muscularization of the legs, the child is now able to walk and explore on his own. With the gross motor skill abilities to walk, run and climb, as well as the fine motor skills of grasping and manipulating objects, a toddler experiences less dependence on his parents and an increased sense of autonomy.

Sense of Autonomy

As children grow older, they like to explore and push boundaries and look for a sense of autonomy and self-confidence, which is an important cog in the wheel of development. The way parents handle this is crucial for the child's development. It is important to note that a **'sense' of autonomy** of children is discussed here, not autonomy itself. Having a sense of autonomy does not mean that a child gets to do what he likes and runs the home, making decisions on behalf of the parents. It is not permissiveness. Erikson, the child psychologist believed, that is essential that parents give their children a chance to seek for this 'sense' and make it stronger than the feelings of shame and doubt.

Understanding love for the child of his/her age is shown by giving him/her all the freedom he/she can safely use, by giving him/her all the love and help he needs to keep him safe in the environment which he/she is unable to control and in which he is dependent upon others for the satisfaction of bodily drives, and by giving him guidance in avoiding hazards in the changing social situations in which he feels himself to be the focal point. So, autonomy is best promoted in a safe, learning environment free of danger. This calls for a child proof home that allows children to explore, to test what they can do and develop such activities as holding on and letting go. Understanding this and reacting to it appropriately usually means that abstract concepts such as 'no' and smacking are deemed as useless and inappropriate. Moreover if restrictions are imposed on child, the side effect of this is lack of intellectual stimulation; which could be a hampering of brain and muscle development, so essential in the first three years. The promotion of autonomy helps to develop the life skills needed when parents are no longer around.

By the end of toddler period, if the child learns to accept and utilize guidance, he has gained a new level of self-control without losing his self-esteem. If he does not learn to be self helpful within the limits of his ability, not able to accept adult direction in situations in which he cannot carry on alone, he is likely to be feel insecure in ability to meet physical and social problem in future. A sense of doubt will emerge and the child will be withdrawn from the reality and a sense of what an adult would feel as shame. He lacks newer skills as he avoids newer experiences than has the child with an outgoing personality.

A sense of autonomy allows toddlers to explore the surrounding, to be independent, do things for themselves, and make decisions. Their earlier developed sense of trust (in their parents or other adults) allows them to feel safe enough to try new things. They may say 'no' a lot, but this is a way to test limits, rather than intentional misbehavior. Toddlers are struggling with their conflicting needs to be cared for and to do things for themselves. *Parents or caregiver are be kind but firm. Another factor here is respect.* Toddlers develop a sense of autonomy when their parents and other caregivers:

- Teach the child by doing. This means less talk, fewer lectures and more action. For example, most toddlers like to hit either the parents, other children or pets. Adults often make the mistake of telling them not to hit or hitting them back. This behavior is often just exploration. Modelling appropriate behavior would mean taking the child's hand and saying and doing repeatedly 'touch nicely'.
- Help them learn how to control their own behavior
- Respond quickly and calmly to their cries
- Allow them to make decisions (what color shirt to wear, an apple or a mango for snack)
- Provide a safe environment for exploration; protect the child from plug points
- Encourage the child to think. Involve him in his environment by allowing to ask 'how' and 'what' questions
- Allow them to make mistakes when they are learning to do things for themselves (such as using the toilet)

- Continue providing lots of support, while at the same time allowing for toddlers' need to do things for themselves.

COGNITIVE DEVELOPMENT

In infancy and early toddler months, a child learns about the world by touching, looking, manipulating, and listening. Toddlers have a greater understanding of the world around them by this stage. Their cognitive development (also known as intellectual development and thinking skills) continues to increase during this period. Exploration of the environment increases in parallel with improved dexterity (reaching, grasping, releasing) and mobility (Figs 5.36A and B). The ability to learn new skills, understanding of concepts, begins to make sense of current events, solve problems and use of memory steadily improves. Toddlers will begin to interpret the meanings of their experiences and they also have a vivid imagination.

When he is two-year-old, his learning processes become more thoughtful. His grasp of language is increasing, and he is beginning to form mental images for things, actions, and concepts. He also can solve some problems in his head, performing mental trial-and-error instead of having to manipulate objects physically. And as his memory and intellectual abilities develop, he will begin to understand simple time concepts, such as 'You can play *after* you finish eating.'

Learning follows the precepts of Piaget's sensory-motor stage. Toddlers manipulate objects in novel ways to create interesting effects, such as stacking blocks or putting things into a computer disk drive. Playthings are also more likely to be used for their intended purposes (combs for hair, cups for drinking). Imitation of parents and older children is an important mode of learning. Make-believe (symbolic) play centers on the child's own body (pretending to drink from an empty cup).

Generally toddler uses a combination of different forms of attention, including selective attention where she chooses to focus on one thing, there by ignoring other things to do so, as well as dividing her attention so she can pay attention to multiple things and will also maintain periods of sustained attention where she can block everything out and concentrate solely on certain tasks for a few minutes at a time.

According to the Swiss child psychologist Jean Piaget, children between the ages of 1 and 3 begin to be able to represent objects with words. Children of this age are able to think symbolically and to refer to objects that are not immediately present, however, they are unable to see from the point of view of others. This 'egocentrism,' as described by Piaget, is evident when asking the toddler what someone standing opposite his viewpoint can see. The typical 3-year-old can only describe what he sees.

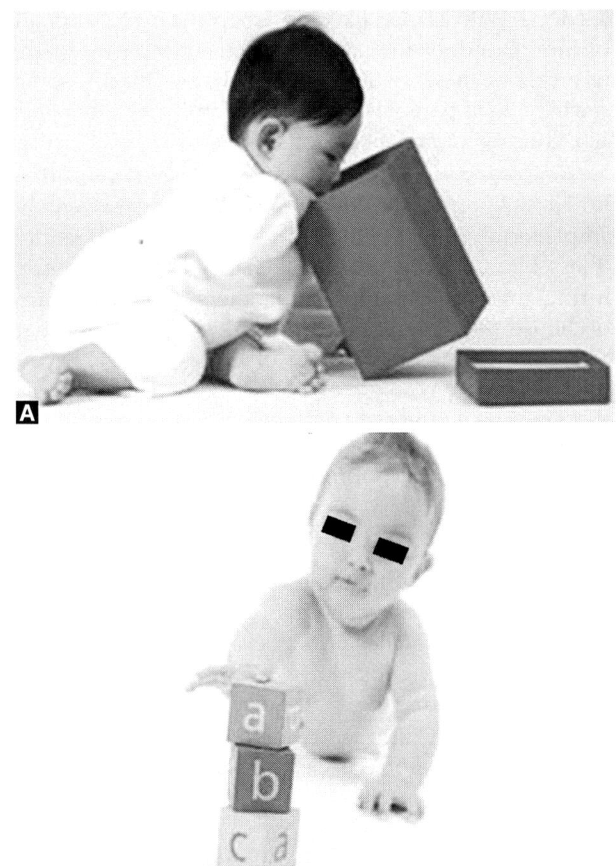

Figs 5.36A and B: Exploration of the environment increases in toddler, parallel with improved dexterity (reaching, grasping, releasing) and mobility

Toddlers of this age may also seem totally absorbed in play at times because they have no sense of time and giving your toddler plenty of warnings to help her make the transition to a new task more easily will lead to less resistance to other activities that interrupt play, such as baths and bedtime. She will still need help in finishing activities. She starts and taking the time necessary to do this enables her to be completely engaged in what she is doing as a way of building concentration and allowing her to develop interests by being exposed to a wide range of experiences.

If it is to single out the major intellectual limitation at this age, it would be the child's feeling that everything that happens in his world is the result of something he has done. With a belief like this, it becomes very difficult for him to understand correctly such concepts as death, divorce, or illness, without feeling that he played some role in it. So, if parents separate or a family member gets sick, children often feel responsible.

Reasoning with a two-year-old child is often difficult. After all, he views everything in extremely simple terms. He still often confuses fantasy with reality unless he is actively playing make-believe. Therefore, during this stage, parents and others should be sure to choose their own words carefully: Comments that parent may think are funny or playful—such as 'If you eat more cereal, you will explode'—actually may panic him, since he would not know parent is joking.

Cognitive Development Milestones

- Groups objects according to specific characteristics (color, size, shape, etc.)
- Name and identifies objects in pictures, interested in looking through books, enjoys simple stories and songs. Matches an object in hand or room to a picture in a book, sorts objects by color, enjoys drawing pictures
- Completes puzzles with 3 or 4 pieces, builds tower of five to seven objects
- Points to body parts when asked
- Can repeat two numbers in a row
- Relates what they are doing to others
- Observe and imitate adult actions, for example pretending to drive a car, understands consequences of their actions
- Plays make-believe with dolls, animals, and people
- Lines up objects in 'train' fashion
- Recognizes and identifies common objects and pictures by pointing
- Enjoys playing with sand, water, dough; explores what these materials can do more than making things with them
- Uses symbolic play, e.g. use a block as a car
- Shows knowledge of gender-role stereotypes, identifies picture as a boy or girl
- Begins to count with numbers
- Recognizes similarities and differences
- Imitates rhythms and animal movements
- Can follow two or more directions
- Understands concept of 'two'
- Matches objects and pictures one to one
- Plays make believe play (pretending to be batman or snow white
- Able to complete simple puzzles and play simple board games
- Begins to understand the concept that two halves make a 1 whole
- Gives brief details of what is happening in a picture
- Places objects in a certain logical order, e.g. stack blocks from largest to smallest
- Tries to obtain more information through 'why' and 'what' questions
- Pays attention to an activity between 5–15 minutes at a time.

Primarily, toddler learns through a combination of methods, from the sensual to the higher level techniques of problem-solving. The methods and techniques used to gain knowledge and learning skills are:

- *Using senses:* When he feels wind blow through the window, when he compares the texture of a ball made of rubber to one made of sponge, when he smells a flower, listens to a song, or sees the color of a tree, the toddler is categorizing his experiences in ways that help him make sense of the world around him.
- *Experimenting:* A toddler may drop a spoon on the floor over and over again, not to annoy mother, but to memorize the cause and effect of things. She will also vary an action slightly to see if the change affects the outcome. 'What will happen if I drop the spoon and the fork together? What if I toss the spoon onto a cushion instead of the floor? Will it make a different sound?' All of these experiments prove that the world follows certain physical rules and enables her to make reasonable predictions. This knowledge gives her the safety to venture out, with the firm knowledge, for instance, that the floor is solid and will support her attempt to walk across it.
- *Manipulating objects:* Toddler learns a great deal by 'accident' as he handles objects and learns how one object interacts with another. For example, he may try to push a toy through the bars of his crib and find that, in the position he is holding the toy, it does not fit through. Eventually, by chance, he may rotate the toy and succeed at sliding it through the bars this time. The next time he tries the same action, he will remember to turn the toy so it fits through easily. He learns the correct position by accident, and is able to retain this bit of information to use the next time. This accidental learning, a form of experimentation, is the beginning of problem-solving.

Exploring with Questions

- The toddler's curiosity knows no limits.
- Even if his body is quiet, his eyes and mind are busy. He is getting better and better at talking and listening. He is watching other people. He is exploring by asking questions about everything he

sees. When parents hear 'Why? Why? Why?' from their child, remember how young children learn.

- Children ask questions in bits and pieces because they need time to make sense of the answers they get. They seem to know what they can manage, and they stop asking when they have had enough. Try to keep a balance by giving the child enough information but not too much.

PHYSICAL GROWTH AND DEVELOPMENT

Physical development in early childhood encompasses both physical growth and motor skill development. Both parents and health providers keep a close eye on physical development to ensure that children are meeting certain physical developmental milestones as they progress through the first five years of life. Physical growth and motor development are slower between one and three years than during infancy. The toddler period is marked primarily by increasing strength and skill in performance.

Physical Growth

Weight and Height

By the age two, toddler probably weighs four times more than the day he was born. From the age two years to until puberty parents can expect their child to gain about 4 1/2 lbs per year (Fig. 5.37).

In 3-year-olds, growth is still slow compared to the first year. Most children have become slimmer and lost

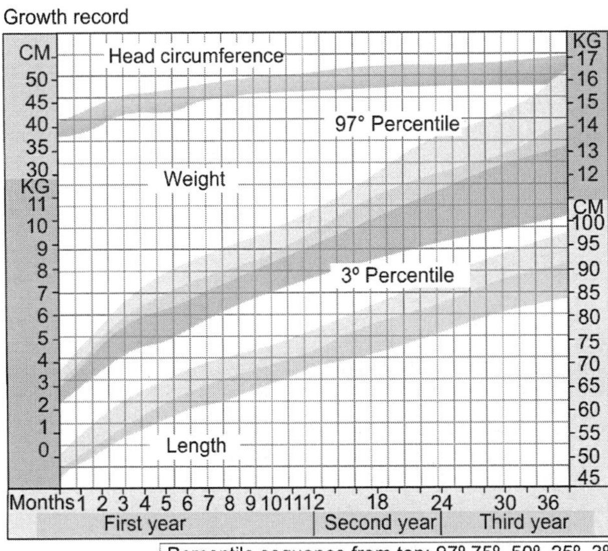

Fig. 5.37: IAP chart on length, weight and head circumference for girls from 0–36 months

the rounded tummy of a toddler. While all children may grow at a different rate, the following indicate the average for 3-year-old boys and girls:

Weight: Average gain of about 1.8 to 2.7 kg (4 to 6) pounds per year.

Height: Slow and steady growth at 2 to 3 inches per year. Adults height is about twice the height of 2 year old child height.

After age two, children of the same age can noticeably vary in height and weight (Fig. 5.38). As long as the child is maintaining his or her own rate of growth, there should be no reason to worry.

Anterior fontanel: Closes between 12 and 18 months.

Head circumference: The rate of increase head circumference slows somewhat by the end of infancy and head circumference is usually equal to chest circumference by 1 to 2 years of age. The usual total increase of head circumference during 2nd year is 2.5 cm. then the rate of increase slows until the age of 5 years and the increase is 1.25 cm per year.

Chest circumference: Exceeds head circumference in toddler years.

Dentition: Full set of twenty deciduous teeth appear.

Increases in Motor Skills

Physical development during the toddler years includes some *major advances in gross motor skill and fine motor skill.* Between ages 2 and 3 years, young children stop 'toddling,' or using the awkward, wide-legged robot-like stance that is the hallmark of new walkers. Walking, obviously, is one of the most significant physical milestones. As they develop a smoother gait, they also develop the ability to run, jump, hop and riding tricycle. Children of this age can participate in throwing and catching games with larger balls. They can also push themselves around with their feet while sitting on a riding toy.

Toddlers also become more adapts at activities that require fine motor movements such as scribbling, stacking blocks, using a spoon, and drinking from a cup. During this period the child creeps up stairs, walks (10–20 min), makes lines on paper with crayon, runs, kicks a ball, builds 6 cube tower (2 years), jumps off a step, uses crayons, capable of bowel and bladder control.

Self-feeding: Toddlers also become much more skilled at feeding themselves, and may insist on eating meals without assistance from an adult. Self-feeding is important for many reasons. Not only does it help a child practice using their hands and fingers, it also helps foster independence. The self-feeding process

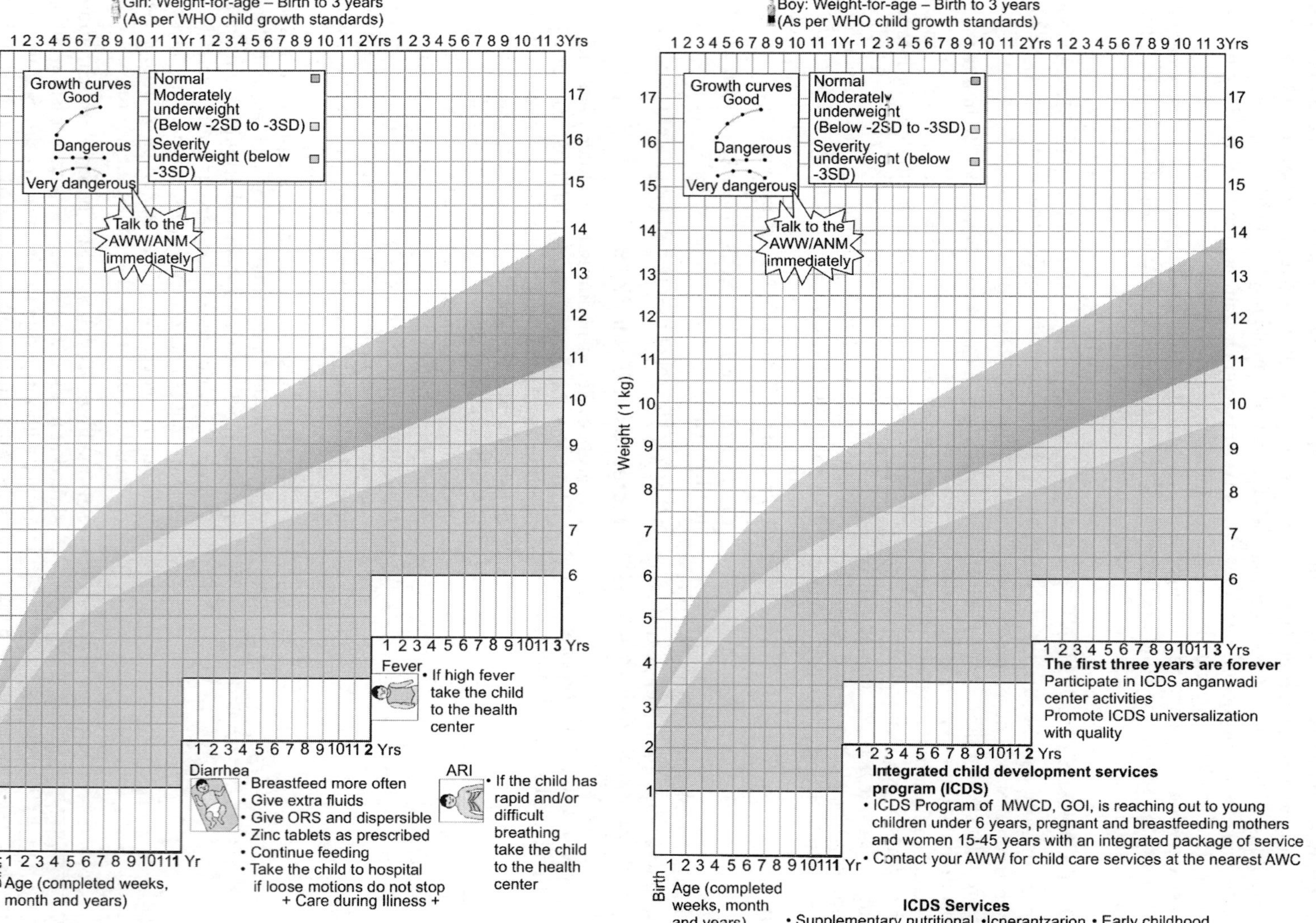

Fig. 5.38: Growth chart of toddler

usually begins with the introduction of finger foods, or small bites of food that she can pick up on her own. It can be messy, but once a child begins to pick up and feed herself small bites of food, it might be time to start introducing utensils to the process. While mealtimes may take longer and will certainly be much messier, this is an important step in development.

Development of Gross Motor Skills (in Brief)

- Stands alone well by 12 months
- Walks well by 12–15 months (if the child is not walking by 18 months, he or she should be evaluated by a health care provider)
- Learns to walk backwards and up steps with help at about 16–18 months
- Throws a ball overhand and kicks a ball forward at about 18–24 months
- Jumps in place by about 24 months
- Rides a tricycle and stands briefly on one foot by about 36 months.

Fine Motor Skills

- Makes tower of three cubes by around 15 months
- Scribbles by 15–18 months
- Can use spoon and drink from a cup by 24 months
- Can copy a circle by 36 months.

Sensory Development

By the time children reach the toddler stage, they have learned to use of their senses—particularly hearing, seeing and touching—to help them understand the world around them. Parents should be aware, however, that children's integration of sensory skills is a particularly important marker in their development.

Sight

Although a newborn baby's eye is only 75% of the size of an adult's, a toddler's eyes and vision are fully developed. Toddlers begin to develop eye-hand coordination and depth perception.

Hearing/Speech

Toddlers are usually able to change the way they speak according to the audience. They have been able to pick up cues when listening that show them how to speak differently to a friend, a younger child or a parent.

Tactile

Toddlers are sensitive to the texture of the clothes they wear, and sticky fingers often bother them as do soiled diapers—an aid to toilet training.

Sensory Integration

By the time children are three, they are learning to integrate the senses and, in doing so, to be able to do such combined activities as sing while scrubbing in the tub, or draw a picture while listening to music.

LANGUAGE DEVELOPMENT

Learning to talk takes a long time. Between the ages of one and three years the child is increasingly able to understand others and to express his feelings and ideas in words. Often their sentences do not make sense to parents, but clearly the more successful the toddler is in getting their message across, the more they will want to communicate.

Characteristics include:

- By two, many children are naming lots of things and, by the end of this year, most are saying short sentences.
- By three, most children can follow complex instructions.
- They will still get 'you' and 'me' mixed up sometimes.
- Most children of this age will not be able to say all of their words clearly.
- Uses 2–3 words (other than Mama or Dada) at 12–15 months
- Understands and follows simple commands ('bring to Mommy') at 14–16 months
- Names pictures of items and animals at 18–24 months
- Points to named body parts at 18–24 months
- Begins to say his or her own name at 22–24 months
- Combines 2 words at 16 to 24 months—there is a range of ages at which children are first able to combine words into sentences; if a toddler cannot do so by 24 months, parents should consult their health care provider
- Knows gender and age by 36 months.

The first words child learns are nouns of one syllable, nouns like the sounds he has babbled ('ma-ma, da-da'). He next learns verbs that mean some form of action which he sees about him and whose meaning he understands (such as give, take, run). From 18 months onward child learns adjectives. Usually 'good' and 'bad' are the adjectives, child learns first, as hears them frequently. 'Here' and 'where' are the adverbs child usually learns and uses first, as his mother uses these words in speaking to him. He starts to use short sentences controls and explores world with language, stuttering may appear briefly and vocabulary of more than 200 words.

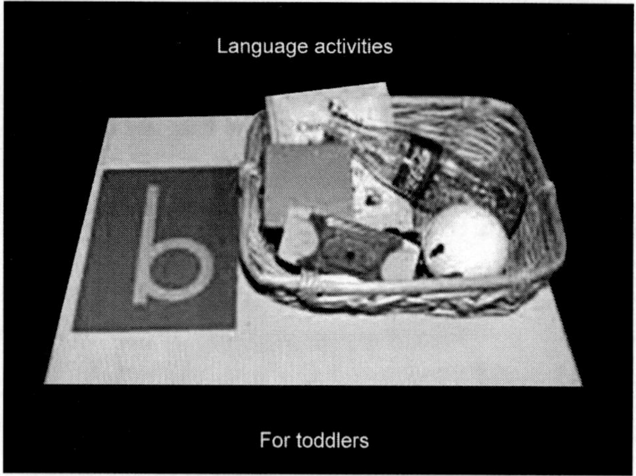

Fig. 5.39: A child gets motivated to speak through language activities

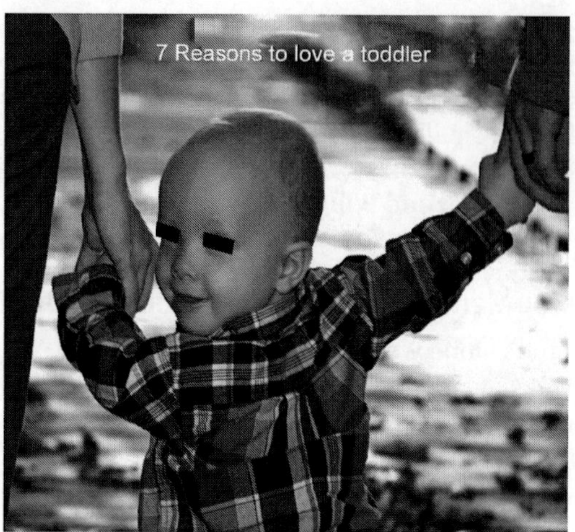

Fig. 5.40: In nurturing relationship toddlers learn how to form friendships, how to communicate emotions, and how to deal with challenges

A young child must have a good model or she will not learn to speak correctly. If an adult uses baby talk in speaking to him, the child has no model for learning the correct words for objects, experiences and attitudes. Moreover, if all his needs are supplied without his asking, he is poorly motivated to speak until he feels the need for words to express attitudes, ideas and emotions (Fig. 5.39).

SOCIAL DEVELOPMENT

This area of development involves learning to interact with other people, and to understand and control own emotions. Babies start to develop relationships with the people around them right from birth, but the process of learning to communicate, share, and interact with others takes many years to develop. Developing the ability to control own emotions and behavior is also a long process. Children continue to develop their social-emotional skills well into their teenage years, or even young adulthood. Between the ages of 1–3 years, child will:

- Recognize herself in the mirror or photograph and smile or make faces at herself
- Begin to say 'no' to bedtime and other requests
- Looks for help when in trouble by 18 months
- Helps to undress and put things away by 18–24 months
- Imitate adults' actions and words (e.g. chores)
- Understand words and commands, and respond to them
- Hug and kiss parents, familiar people and pets
- Bring things to 'show' other people
- Begin to feel jealousy when she is not the center of attention
- Show frustration easily
- May play next to another child, but will not really share until 3 or 4 years of age
- Be able to play alone for a few minutes
- Share a piece of food
- Listens to stories when shown pictures and can tell about immediate experiences by 24 months
- Can engage in pretend play and simple games by 24–36 months
- Develop a range of emotions (may have tantrums, show aggression by biting, etc.)
- Start to assert independence by preferring to try do things 'by myself', without help.

Children get a sense of comfort, safety, confidence, and encouragement through loving relationship. If toddlers live in nurturing connections he/she learns how to form friendships, how to communicate emotions, and how to deal with challenges (Fig. 5.40). Supportive relationships with parents, friends, and caregivers also help children develop trust, empathy, compassion, and a sense of right and wrong (a conscience).

BEHAVIOR

Toddlers are always trying to be more independent. This creates not only special safety concerns, but discipline challenges. The child must be taught—in a consistent manner—the limits of appropriate vs. inappropriate behavior.

When toddlers try out activities they cannot quite do yet, they can get frustrated and angry. Breath-holding, crying, screaming, and temper tantrums may be daily occurrences.

It is important for a child to learn from experiences and to be able to rely on consistent boundaries between acceptable and unacceptable behavior.

PHYSICAL DEVELOPMENT AND ROLE OF PARENT

Once the toddler is up and walking, parenting gets a whole lot more challenging and parents and their home will never be the same again. The child is much more confident with her physical abilities but does not have a good idea of when to stop. They often test limits. They cannot keep themselves safe, so parents need to set and enforce the limits for them. It can help them develop their skill by providing safe chances for them to play, while parents supervise.

Suggestions on encouraging and supporting parents for development include:

Help the toddler to become a confident problem-solver

- They need individual attention whenever possible
- Praise the process, not just the result
- Establish routines and transitions
- Parents need to read aloud to them and talk about the pictures.
- Talking with child and asking questions about what they are doing are important. A real interest is to be shown in them.
- Toys are to be provided for stacking, things for pulling apart, blocks, simple jigsaws, toy cars, animals, dolls and so on.
- Opportunities for fun on playground equipment, such as slides, sand pits and slippery dips are needed
- Toddler needs encouragement in their attempts to explore the world, but a firm eye on safety issues cannot be ignored.
- The most important thing to remember is that two or three year old is still a baby.
- They may play with other children for a short time, but are not yet capable of true sharing.
- By two, many children are naming lots of things and, by the end of this period, most are saying short sentences.

NEEDS OF THE TODDLER

The basic needs of infant and toddler are same. The toddler needs security and love and he/she also needs graded independence.

Love and Attachment

Attachment theory is based on the idea that the bond between a child and his or her primary caregiver is the crucial and primary influence in development and as such forms the basis of coping, the development of relationships, and the formation of personality. In an attached relationship, toddlers rely on their parents/primary caregiver to help them navigate the world. The parents/primary caregiver serve as a secure base that is used for exploration and learning. At the same time, the child forms the necessary skills of self-protection and intimacy (Figs 5.41A to C).

According to a growing body of scientific evidence, children with responsive parents/caregivers during the initial years of life develop a stronger ability to manage stress, form healthier relationships, perform better in school, and enjoy higher self-worth. Overall, they have a greater shot at a well-balanced and fulfilling life.

Graded Independence

Independence is learned gradually and is given the child only in situations in which she/he can protect herself/himself from physical and emotional trauma. When the child is too young, independence must be denied as he will not be able to use it successfully. A painful experience might make him afraid to try out

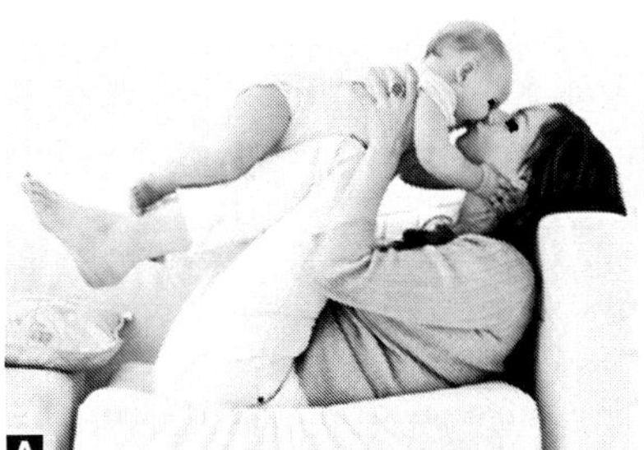

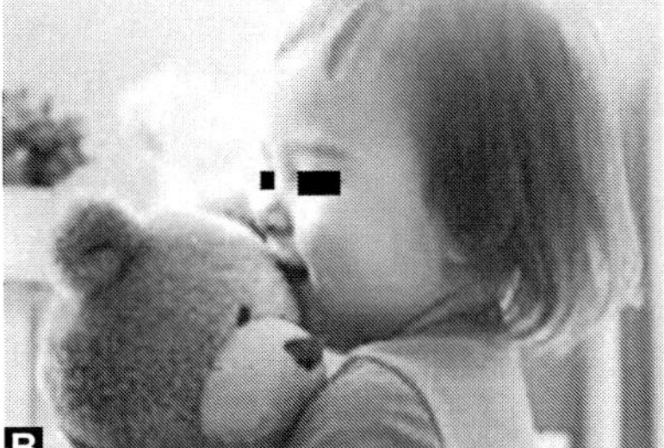

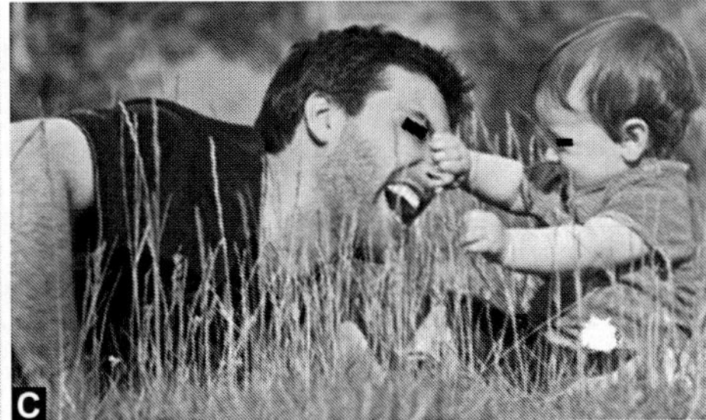

Figs 5.41A to C: In an attached relationship, toddlers rely on their parents to help them navigate the world

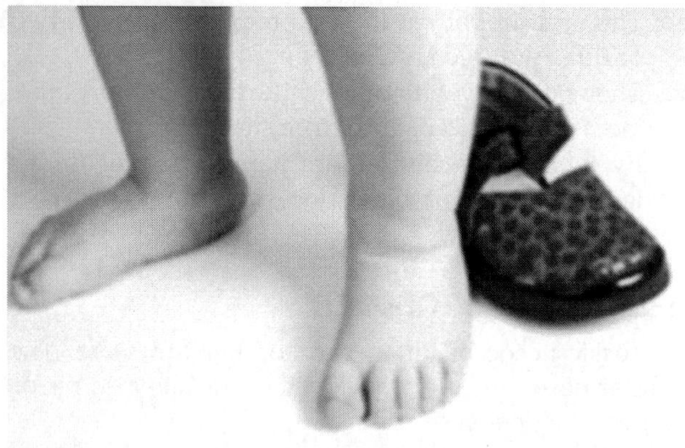

Fig. 5.42: Toddler: Steps of independence and thus to explore own world

new skills. Graded independence brings pleasurable results, develops a sense of self-reliance and adequacy, of autonomy (Fig. 5.42). The child finds that he may make choices under the guidance of his parents.

Safe Environment

Children between one and three years of age have loads of energy and want to try lots of new things. But their behavior can be difficult to manage. Very big changes are happening for them, and if we understand these changes we can often work around them, so there are fewer problems.

This is a time when toddlers become more independent. They are now little people with their own way of doing things. They find out that they can make things happen. They touch, explore, run away. They like doing things their way and doing things for themselves. They say 'No', 'I won't', 'Give me' and 'Me do'.

Toddler needs a safe environment to explore his world. They are too young to know how or remember to behave safely. Telling them and teaching them about danger does not keep them safe. Keeping the toddler safe is parents and others responsibility.

Though it can be hard to keep up with an exploring toddler, exploring is good! It helps children grow in important ways. First is the **growth of intelligence**. A toddler's interest in learning about the world encourages him to use his senses—tasting, touching, seeing, and smelling. His senses help him understand how things are different from each other and how they work. By trying new ways to handle objects and by asking questions, a toddler begins to learn how to solve problems. Imagine your toddler exploring with his 'sippy cup' of milk. By banging it on the high chair tray, he hears what sound the cup makes. By shaking it, he learns how to tell whether it is empty. And by turning it upside down, he discovers he can make a mess!

Another result of exploring is social and emotional growth. When a toddler knows that she can explore her environment and yet return to a parent when she needs help, she becomes secure and confident. Exploring is also vital for physical growth. Toddlers develop coordination in the large muscles used to walk, run, climb and jump. In addition, toddlers gain eye-hand coordination as they learn to manipulate objects. Toddlers must move around to learn about their world.

Helping the Child to Explore Safely

Parents of toddlers often feel tired, day and night. Just watching your active little person zoom around the house can be exhausting!

Keeping a toddler safe requires constant attention, and sometimes it seems parents cannot relax for a minute. It is surprising how many dangerous places and objects toddlers can discover. But the extra work it takes to encourage child as he explores and learns is worth it. Sometimes parents may want to stop their child's need to explore, but remember: **exploring is necessary for a growing child**. Parents need to focus energy on providing safe places for their child to learn about his world.

Parents would not have to go running after their toddler so often if they get rid of some of the dangers at home. Their toddler is just too young and too active to think about safety. She ignores things that are in the way. Bumps and falls do not stop her (Fig. 5.43). Parents can never leave a child of this age unsupervised. However, their job will be easier if they take the following steps:

- Put away anything that your child can easily damage or that can hurt him.
- Make sure furniture is stable and will not topple over easily.
- Use safety gates on stairways and porches.
- Block the way to open, unguarded windows.
- Cover electric plugs.
- Keep all medicines and poisons (like cleaning products) in a locked cabinet.
- Teach the child how to climb up and go down stairs safely.
- Make safe play areas and provide safe toys.
- Understand that the words of the parents would not always stop the child from doing something unsafe. When that happens, take firm action to stop the toddler. Then tell her why it was done.

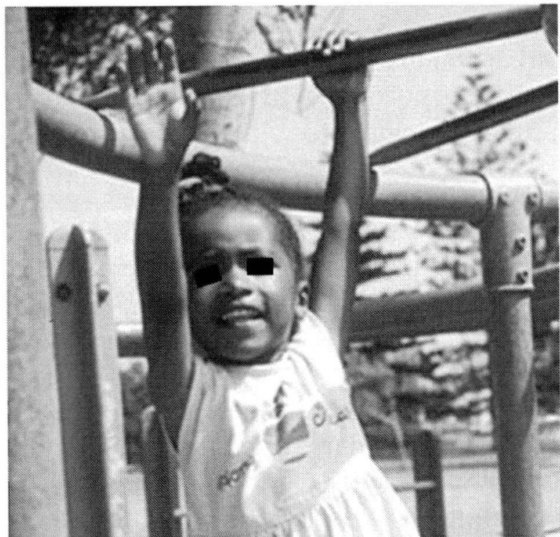

Fig. 5.43: Toddlers try to get into everything

Control of Bodily Functions (of Urination and Defecation)

In infancy child receives all care, love, attention; now he is asked to assume the responsibility of giving up his comfort and to contribute to the comfort of others. In more technical terms, the infant lives according to *pleasure principle*, the toddler must begin to accept the *reality principle*. The child would like to continue emptying bladder and bowels whenever he is conscious of pressure from tension in these organs. But he must learn to excrete urine and feces only at the appropriate time and place, although he cannot understand the necessity for this. So, gradually the toddler must learn to face the frustration of retention, and gain control of defecation and urination with the help of those he loves.

Toilet Training: Most people advise that toilet training is a mutual task, requiring cooperation, agreement and understanding between the child and the caregiver, and the best potty training techniques emphasize consistency and positive reinforcement over punishment, making it enjoyable for the child. Generally, signs that child is ready for toilet training appear from about two years on though the vast majority of studies concentrate on children 18 months old and older. For that time frame, research suggests that children over 24 months train faster and girls train slightly faster than boys.

When parents stay positive and calm, child will be more likely to settle into things. The secret is to wait for signs that the child is ready for toilet training. Child shows some signs of being ready if he:

- Is walking and can sit for short periods of time
- Has dry nappies for up to two hours—this shows he is able to hold urine
- Tells his mother before it happens, he is ready for toilet training
- Begins to dislike wearing a nappy, perhaps trying to pull it off when it is wet or soiled
- Has regular, soft, formed bowel movements
- Can pull his pants up and down
- Can follow simple instructions, such as 'Give the book to daddy'
- Shows understanding about things having their place around the home.

Not all these signs need to be present when child is ready. A general trend will let parents know it is time to start.

Emotional issues that can profoundly affect toilet training include a desire for independence and self-mastery, the child's need to control some aspects of his environment, testing of limits and rules, his desire to win his parents' approval, fears associated with toilet use, and the desire to mimic or conform to other children's behavior.

The best way to determine the emotional state child is in, and how conducive this is to toilet training, is to observe both his general behavior and his responses to any suggestions about potty use. If he clearly enjoys sitting on his potty or talking about potty use, his urge toward self-mastery will probably support his training (Fig. 5.44). If he resists the idea or cries when parent mentions the potty, he may be experiencing conflict and parent need to wait for a more opportune time (*See* Chapter 4).

Promoting Optimal Health During Toddlerhood

Nutrition

Nutrition is important in the maintenance of the toddler's health and normal growth and development. It is normal for toddlers to be less interested in food than they were as babies. Because toddlers grow more slowly than babies and their appetites are smaller, they want to be independent, so they like saying 'no' to food and this is normal. Toddlers are developing their movement skills, and they want to spend more time exploring and this leaves less time for eating and drinking. To them the world is becoming a very exciting place and there are lots more interesting things to do than eat! Getting into battles with toddlers about food is not meaningful and struggling for feeding can only make life miserable for everyone.

- Diets with essential nutrients are necessary for maintenance, replacement and increase of tissue and for energy. Children can share family meals, by the time, they are two years old. The meal times should be relaxed and happy, and parents need to know that

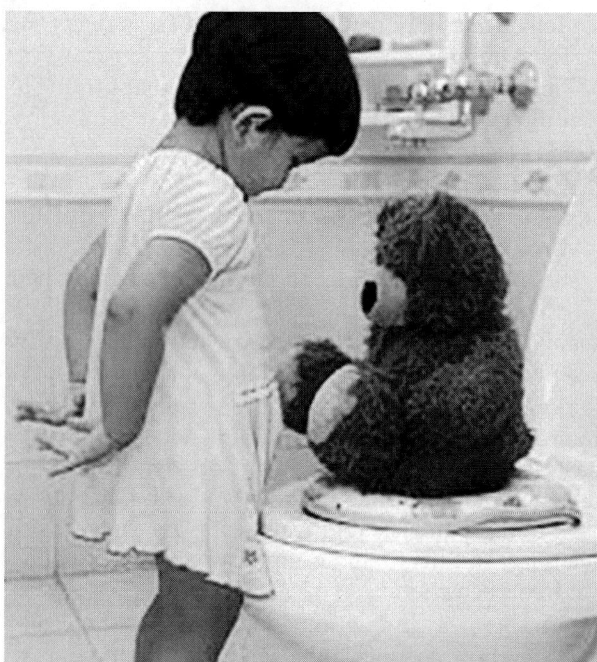

Fig. 5.44: Toilet training: The child teaches her teddy

healthy children will eat when they are hungry and usually not before. They are to be prepared for mess, as it is normal part of toddler eating. A plate piled high with food can put a toddler off eating so he is to offer a small serve first. Most toddlers are easily get distracted, the TV is to be turned off, pets will remain outside and tidy away toys so they can focus on the meal.

Few alternatives may be needed, when the family makes highly spiced food. It is advisable to keep foods, which are too fatty or too sweet out of the child's menu. Such foods may fill his limited space, without providing the nutrients needed. The child may be encouraged to eat sweets towards the end of the meal, so that he/she may not eat these to the exclusion of other foods. It is good to give appetizing beverages such as fruit juices and milk to the children. Usually they need three well-spaced meals with nutritious snacks between meals. It is good to serve part of his milk needs in the form of soups, kheer, custard or ice-cream. Fruits are ideal snacks. Crisp crackers or toast are liked and the child can eat these without help, which helps him to feel independent.

Sample Menu Plan

Typical menu for toddlers aged two to three years:

Breakfast
- 40 mL fruit juice
- 1/4 cup oats porridge with 1 tablespoon honey
- 1/2 cup full cream milk

Mid-morning snack
- 1/2 cup yoghurt
- 1/2 mashed, ripe banana

Lunch
- 1 boiled egg
- 1/2–1 slice whole wheat bread with 1 tablespoon polyunsaturated margarine
- 1/2 apple
- 1/2 cup full cream milk

Mid-afternoon snack
- 15 g sweet milk or Gouda cheese
- 1/2 slice wholewheat bread with 1 tablespoon polyunsaturated margarine
- 40 mL fruit juice

Supper
- 30 g cooked, mince-meat
- Mashed potato 2 tablespoon
- Cooked butternut 1 tablespoon
- 1/4 cup custard

Bed-time snack

1/4 cup full cream milk.

Influence of Growth and Development on Eating Behavior

Child need less food during his second year of life than during infancy, as he is no longer growing so rapidly. Moreover he has greater interest in physical and social environment. Food should not be forced upon him. If food is forced upon him when he refuses his meals, he is likely to rebel, and a feeding problem will develop.

Dietary Guideline

India is home to more than a third of the world's undernourished children. In 1999, the National Family Health Survey (NFHS II) found that 47% of all children under age three were under weight. Data from NFHS-3 (2006) shows only a very small decline, with under-nutrition level remaining around 45% for children below three. Despite vast improvements in the country's economy, under nutrition remains a challenge in India.

By the end of 2007, the nutritional achievement results were not satisfactory. Reasons for this include the inadequate knowledge of caregivers regarding correct infant and young child feeding, frequent infections, high population pressure, low social and nutritional status of girls and women, suboptimal delivery of social services and lack of more viable guidelines.

The first National guidelines on infant and young child feeding (IYCF) were formulated by Ministry of Women and Child Development (Food and Nutrition Board) in 2004, and the same guidelines were revised in 2006. India is committed to halving the prevalence of under weight children by 2015 as one of the key indicators of progress towards the millennium development goals (MDG). By the end of 2009 nutritional achievement goals did not make for happy reading. So, there was need to revise the existing guidelines and to have more viable and scientifically accepted national guidelines on Infant and young child feeding.

Optimal infant and young child feeding (Table 5.2): Early initiation of breastfeeding, exclusive breastfeeding for the first six month of life followed by continued breastfeeding for up to two years and beyond with adequate complementary foods is the most appropriate feeding strategy for infants and young children.

Sleep and Activity

Toddlers need about 12–14 hours of sleep in a 24-hour period. When they reach about 18 months of age their naptimes will decrease to once a day lasting about one to three hours. Naps should not occur too close to bedtime as they may delay sleep at night.

Many toddlers experience sleep problems including resisting going to bed and night time awakenings. Night time fears and nightmares are also common.

Many factors can lead to sleep problems. Toddlers' drive for independence and an increase in their motor, cognitive and social abilities can interfere with sleep. In addition, their ability to get out of bed, separation anxiety, the need for autonomy and the development of the child's imagination can lead to sleep problems. Daytime sleepiness and behavior problems may signal poor sleep or a sleep problem.

Sleep Tips for Toddlers

- Maintain a daily sleep schedule and consistent bedtime routine.
- Make the bedroom environment the same every night and throughout the night.
- Set limits that are consistent, communicated and enforced. Encourage use of a security object such as a blanket or stuffed animal.

There is a connection between poor sleeping patterns in children and inferior school performance. It is also linked to an increased risk of overweight and obesity. The children, who were physically active during the day, fell asleep more rapidly than their more sedentary peers. The more vigorous activity they did, the faster they fell asleep. In addition, every hour of the day spent in sedentary activity increased sleep latency by three minutes. Shorter sleep latency was also associated to longer duration of sleep. It fell by more than 11 minutes for each additional hour of sleep. Tiring out a child with plenty of physical activity will increase the

Table 5.2: Portion sizes and foods for toddlers aged two to three years

Food	*Portions size*	*Number of servings per day*
Milk and dairy products	1/2 cup of milk or yoghurt or 15 g cheese	4–5
Meat, fish, poultry, eggs, peanut butter or cooked legumes	30–60 g meat, fish or poultry, 1 egg, 2 tablespoons peanut butter or 4 tablespoons cooked legumes like baked beans	2
Fruit and vegetables		4–5
Vegetables, cooked	2–3 tablespoons	
Vegetables, raw	A few pieces—only if child can chew well	
Fruit, raw	1/2-1 small fruit	
Fruit, canned	2–4 tablespoons	
Fruit juice	90–120 mL (less than 1/2 cup)	
Bread and cereals		3
Wholewheat or vitamin and mineral fortified bread	1/2–1 slice	
Cooked porridge	1/4–1/2 cup	
Dry breakfast cereal	1/2–1 cup	

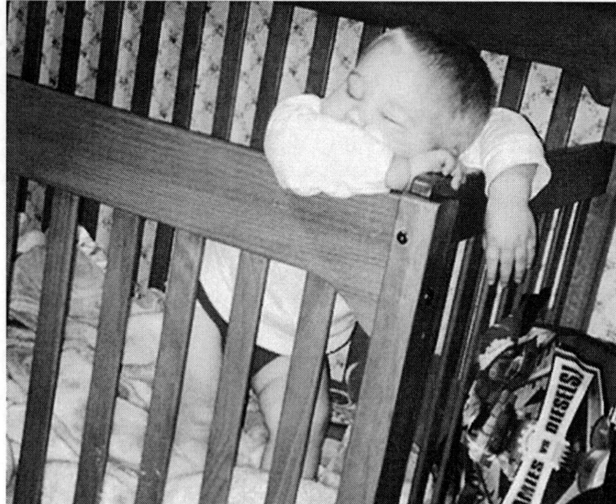

Fig. 5.45: Just resting on eyes

likelihood that she or he will sleep well. The importance of physical activity for children is not only for fitness, cardiovascular health and weight control, but also for sleep (Fig. 5.45).

Dental Health

Teething

Children have their own schedule for teething (Fig. 5.46). Most children begin teething at about 6 months of age. Child should have all of his or her first set of teeth–or 'baby' teeth—by 3 years of age. The bottom front teeth usually appear first, followed by the top front teeth. In total, 20 teeth should appear—10 in the top jaw and 10 in the bottom jaw.

Teething may cause some discomfort, making baby fussy. Baby may also not want to eat.

Baby may feel better if allowed to chew on a clean, chilled teething ring, teething toy, or clean wet face cloth.

Teething cookies or biscuits are not a good choice because these can stick to baby's teeth and cause tooth decay.

Check with dentist or health care provider before using teething ointments, gels or tablets, or any other teething items.

Teething does not cause fevers. If baby has a fever or diarrhea while teething, treat it as any other time.

Nutritional Advice for Building Strong Teeth

Children need food from all the major food groups to grow properly and stay healthy. Too many

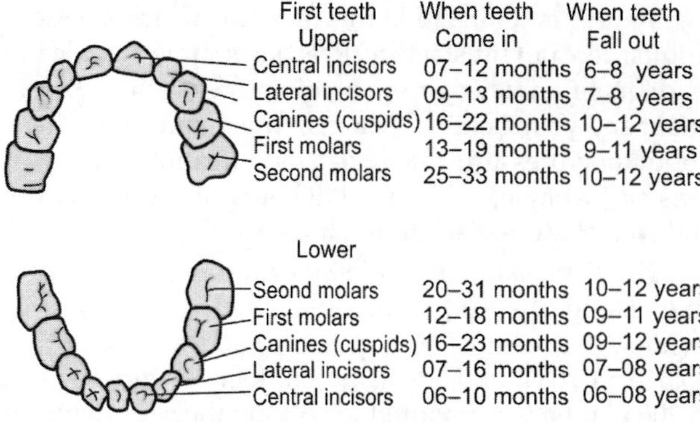

Fig. 5.46: Teething schedule of children

carbohydrates, sugars (for example from cake, cookies, candies, milk, fruit juice, and other sugary foods and beverages), and savory foods and starches (for example potato chips) can cause tooth decay. Carbohydrates remain on the teeth is the main culprit that leads to tooth decay.

Keep fruits and vegetables in house to offer as 'healthy snacks' instead of carbohydrates. Choose fruits and vegetables that contain a high volume of water, such as pears, melons, celery, and cucumbers. Limit bananas and raisins, as these contain concentrated sugar. Brush immediately after these fruits is eaten. Avoid sticky, chewy foods. Raisins, oatmeal or peanut butter cookies, jelly beans, caramel, honey, molasses, and syrup stick to teeth, making it difficult for saliva to wash away. If child consumes these types of products, have him or her to rinse the mouth, if possible brush their teeth immediately after eating.

Give child any sweets as desserts immediately following the meal. There is usually an increased amount of saliva in the mouth around mealtime, making it easier to wash food away from teeth. The mealtime beverage also helps to wash away food particles on teeth.

Get children in the habit of eating as few snacks as possible. The frequency of snacking is far more important than the quantity consumed. Time between meals allows saliva to wash away food particles that bacteria would otherwise feast on. Frequent snacking, without brushing immediately afterwards, provides constant fuel to feed bacteria, which leads to plaque development and tooth decay. Try to limit snacks as much as possible and to no more than one or two a day. Brush teeth immediately after consuming the snack, if possible.

Avoid sugary foods that linger on the teeth. Lollipops, hard candies, cough drops, and mints all contribute to tooth decay because they continuously coat the teeth with sugar. Never put baby to bed with a bottle filled with milk, formula, juice, or soda. If baby needs a bottle at bedtime, fill it with plain water. Offer child plain water instead of juice or soda. Juices, sodas, and even milk contain sugar. Water does not harm the teeth and aids in washing away any food particles that may be clinging to teeth.

Include good sources of calcium in child's diet to build strong teeth. Good sources include milk, broccoli, and yogurt.

Use fluoride and brush and floss child's teeth. The best way to prevent tooth decay is to use a fluoride toothpaste every day after the age of 2 or once child can spit and not swallow toothpaste. Fluoride reverses early decay. Once the tooth is formed, fluoride application remineralizes the surface. This means returning minerals to the teeth. Minerals help keep teeth strong, which, in turn, helps prevent tooth decay. Brush child's teeth at least twice a day and after each meal or snack if possible. If brushing between meals is not possible, at least rinse the mouth with water several times. Floss child's teeth at least once a day to help remove particles between teeth and below the gum line.

Be sure to brush child's teeth after giving him or her medicine. Medicines such as cough syrups contain sugar that bacteria in the mouth use to make acids. These acids can eat away at the enamel—the protective top layer of the tooth.

Visit the dentist regularly. Child should make his or her first visit to the dentist by the age of 1 or within 6 months of the first tooth breaking through the gums.

Play and Exercise

Regular physical activity is good for everyone.

For babies and young children regular physical activity is important for healthy growth and development (Fig. 5.47).

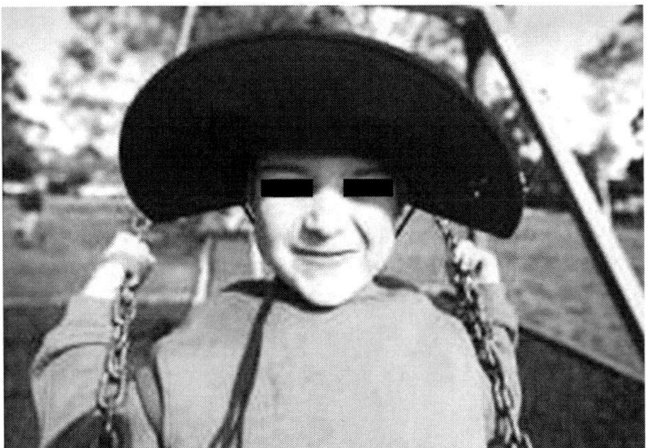

Fig. 5.47: Regular physical activity is important for healthy growth and development

From childhood onwards, regular physical activity is important for:

- Maintaining good health.
- Preventing the development of health risk factors or poor health.
- Enhancing self-confidence and social skills.

Proven benefits of regular physical activity across the lifespan include:

- Healthy growth and development
- Building strong hearts, muscles and bones
- Acquisition of fundamental motor skills
- Improved movement, balance, coordination and reaction time
- Increased mental awareness
- Improved social skills, self-esteem and confidence.
- Healthy weight management
- Prevention of cardiovascular disease
- Prevention of Type II diabetes
- Prevention of some forms of cancer.

Selection of Toys

- Large, sturdy toys to push or pull on the floor
- Toys that can be pushed or pulled along as baby's walking increases
- Tricycle that can be pushed along without pedaling or even one without pedals
- Large truck toys (dump truck, fire truck) that have storage space to load other smaller toys into simple train sets and small planes
- Construction toys like stacking blocks. Blocks that use interlocking mechanisms may be too difficult to use
- Puzzles with 2 to 4 large pieces
- Stacking cups, rings
- Activity boxes (or busy boxes) where doing something makes something else happen
- Shape sorters
- A lightweight multi-colored beach ball or other soft, light, large balls.
- Large crayons that are easily held in baby's tiny fingers and paper
- Dolls and some simple accessories for the doll like a bottle or a blanket or a bed for the doll

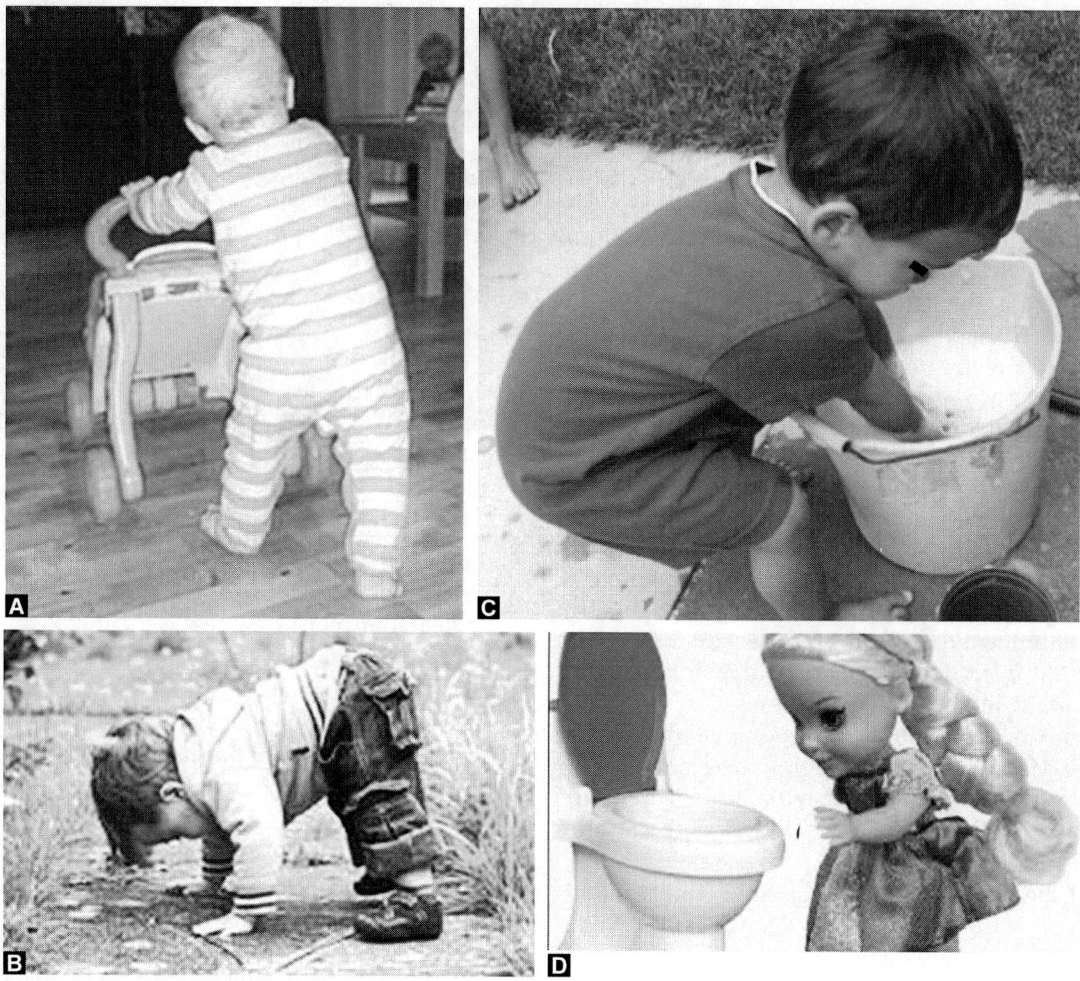

Figs 5.48A to D: Play materials and household items toddlers love to play with

- Mid-size stuffed toys
- Toys that help children imitate adult activities like a toy telephone, a wooden or plastic tool set with large easily liftable tool replicas
- Nursery rhyme CDs may be a good way to help your child go to sleep
- Cloth books, board books with pictures or objects to touch.

Role of Parent in Toddlers Play and Development (Figs 5.48A to D)

- Toddlers are very active between the ages 1 and 3. She will be using her new physical and verbal skills to explore everything around her. As he/she grows, the toddler will spend less time exploring and more time playing. Play is the 'Work' of child as he/she practices and masters new mental, physical and social skills. Parents need to aware about specific need of toddler.
- Parents or adults need to plan interesting things (new play ideas involving shapes. color, sizes) at home and in neighborhood which will help in development of child.
- Take the child to new places like playground, parks, or a zoo. Talk about what they find there. Provide safe places to crawl into, hide in, climb and explore. For example parents can make a pretend cave by draping a table with bed sheet.
- Parent can talk about nature as they take a walk with their toddler. They can be shown the colors of the leaves and grass, and allow them to feel the texture of the grass.

- Talk about what you see and hear while walking, riding the bus, or driving in the car.
- Let the child wash plastic dishes with parent, or give her toys to play with in the bathtub. (And be ready to mop up a mess!).
- Let the child to help her mother to prepare simple food to explore all the textures, shapes, flavors, and colors. (Again, be prepared for a mess).
- Books can also be helpful in helping children learn about their world. Parents can read books with toddler and allow the child to do things (like touch a special place on the page). Others encourage children to explore with the characters. Both types can be enjoyed by children for a long time.

Personality Traits of Toddlers

Tantrums

The need for independence also grows during the toddler years, so kids this age become increasingly determined to do things on their own. The problem, obviously, is that while they might have the desire to do things independently, they very often do not have the skills to do so. Because kids often lack the ability or knowledge to do the things they would like to do, they often become very frustrated when they find themselves unable to accomplish tasks such as buttoning up a shirt. Temper tantrums are quite common at this age, and parents of toddlers usually become quite accustomed to hearing 'No' used numerous times each day. Parents should help foster independence and motor skills by giving children tasks that they are capable of accomplishing either independently or with adult assistance. Tantrums are usually of two general types:

1. Overload/over-tiredness. Too much is happening and the toddler just cannot cope with it all.
2. Demanding attention/anger. Here the child wants to have something or do something the parent does not want him to have or do.

Two ways of handling a tantrum are:

1. Hold the child from behind. When the tantrum finishes the toddler can relax safely into your arms. This is good when your toddler is tired.
2. Stay near but do not pay attention to the tantrum except to say 'I would not give you what you want. When you finish we can have a cuddle and you can tell me about it'. But do not leave—this is too frightening for a toddler.

Toddlers can be scared by their tantrums. They need to know that an adult is there in control who will accept and love them when it is over.

Children are more likely to have tantrums when they are bored, tired, hungry, unwell or overwhelmed by events.

Anger and Aggression

Some anger is normal and healthy. But some children are often angry; they hit, bite, kick or punch for no obvious reason. They need extra help.

- Teach them to be aware of their feelings and put the feelings into words. 'I know you are cross with your little brother. Instead of hitting him can you say to me "I feel cross with him because...?'
- Play active and expressive play. Hammering, play dough, water play, sand play, painting, cutting and tearing paper, etc.
- Watch when they play with other children. Set limits. Let them know it is not OK to hurt others. Children feel more secure if they know someone is there who can control their angry behavior.
- Reward cooperative and non-aggressive behavior with a hug.

Smacking and yelling often make children fearful or angry and can keep the behavior going.

Clinging and Grizzling

All toddlers cling and grizzle to some extent.

A toddler who is clinging, whining and very demanding may be showing a need for more attention and security.

- If your toddler is doing it more than usual it might be a sign that your child is unwell or is more stressed than usual (perhaps being in a new, unfamiliar place or has been expected to separate too early).
- But clinging and whining may make you feel angry and want to push them away just when they need more of you.
- This makes them more insecure and they may cling more.

Let children know that they can ask you for a cuddle when they want one. Try not to push them away.

When they are playing by themselves make sure that you notice and give a hug or some attention. With reassurance of love and security they are more likely to play alone for longer periods of time.

If children whinge you can ignore it or ask them to say it again with a smile.

INJURY PREVENTION

Toddlers are active, curious, and very mobile. Because they can now climb, slide, swing, open doors, and move very quickly, they are much more likely to get into dangerous situations. As they are impulsive by nature, you cannot rely on them to always remember or follow safety rules; they need active supervision. Active supervision means being within an arm's reach at all time, paying close attention and anticipating hazards when child is playing or exploring.

Every day more than 2000 children and teenagers die from an injury which could have been prevented. This joint WHO/UNICEF report is a plea to keep kids safe by promoting evidence-based injury prevention interventions and sustained investment by all sectors. The report presents the current knowledge about the five most important causes of unintentional injury – road traffic injuries, drowning, burns, falls and poisoning.

Injury is a leading cause of death and disability in young children. Injuries in children (such as from burns and scalds, poisonings, falls and near drowning) can have many lasting effects including disability and disfigurement and can impair a child's development and future well-being. Most child injuries occur at home or in the yard. However, child injury is not a normal or inevitable part of growing up, with most child injuries being predictable and preventable.

INJURIES AND ACCIDENTS IN TODDLERS

Accidental injuries are a leading cause of hospitalization and death for young children. Because many childhood injuries happen in or around the home, it is the parents who must assume responsibility for making the home a safe place. Injury prevention, like parenting, is an ongoing process. Sometimes, it seems, the job is never done. Parents must constantly be on the lookout for potential dangers in and around the home. Children are at risk for injury from the moment they are born. Therefore, injury prevention strategies must be implemented even before newborns come home from the hospital. As children grow, they become more mobile. With this mobility comes a greater risk for injury. The more ground children can cover, the more potential dangers they will come into contact with. It is especially important, therefore, for the parents of children who can crawl, toddle, walk, and run to pay close attention to injury prevention.

The Major Causes of Injury

- Falls
- Suffocation or choking
- Poisoning
- Scalds and burns
- Motor vehicle accidents.

Injury Prevention Strategies

Falls

- Never leave infants or toddlers on a raised surface, such as a changing table or a counter top, unattended. Even if parents turn their backs for only a second, that is enough time for children to roll over and fall to the floor.
- Change children's diapers on a crib instead of a changing table. This way, if parents have to leave their children for a minute, they can protect their children from falling simply by pulling up the crib side.
- Always pull the crib side all the way up when children are in the crib. This way, children would not be able to climb out.
- Do not leave large stuffed animals in children's cribs or play pens. Children will quickly learn to use such toys to stand on to get out.
- When using infant seats, always strap children into them.
- Never leave infant seats on narrow raised surfaces such as a chair or a counter top. Sudden movements by infants can easily cause the seat (with baby in it) to fall.
- Do not allow children to stand on high chairs or regular chairs. They can easily fall.
- Lock all windows or screens, or install safety stops so they will only open a few inches.
- Do not allow children to sit on counter tops
- Do not allow children to play on balconies unsupervised.
- Use safety gates at the top and bottom of all stairways in the home. Do not rely on doors. Eventually one will be left open.
- Provide rubber soled shoe, canvas shoes when children start walking. Stiff leather shoes are hard to walk in and may cause more frequent falls.
- Discourage running in the house, especially in rooms that have a lot of furniture.
- Cover all sharp furniture edges with corner guards and edge covers.
- Make sure all play areas are free of falling hazards such as deep holes, glass, and rusty and/or sharp objects.

Suffocation or Choking

- Do not cover mattresses or pillows with plastic.
- Tie knots in plastic bags before throwing them away
- Store all plastic bags (garbage bags, sandwich bags, grocery bags) out of reach.

- Use baby powder cautiously. It can be dangerous if large amounts are inhaled.
- After meals, remove bibs before taking children out of their high chairs.
- Never pin or tie pacifiers to children. The strings can easily wrap around children's necks.
- Fasten the restraining straps on children's high chairs close to the body.
- Make sure crib mattresses fit tightly in the crib. If the mattress is too small, children are at risk for getting their heads, legs, or arms stuck between the mattress and the side of the crib.
- Make sure all mobiles are hung beyond children's reach.
- Never prop bottles or pacifiers in children's mouths.
- Make sure all sheets and bedcovers are loose so children cannot get stuck underneath them.
- Be wary of certain finger foods, especially for children under five years of age. Foods that are most frequently a choking hazard are nuts and popcorn. Grapes, hot dogs, hard candy and carrots can also be dangerous. Make sure they are cut into very small pieces before children attempt to eat them.
- Use balloons with extreme caution. They are especially dangerous if swallowed.
- Never leave infants or toddlers unsupervised near water. This includes bath tubs, wading pools, and swimming pools. A good rule to follow with infants in the bathtub is to keep one hand on them at all times. Keep bathroom doors shut at all times, and make sure the lids to all toilets are down when not in use.
- Keep the doors to all household appliances shut at all times.
- If there is an unused refrigerator or freezer in or around the house, remove the door, or lock it shut.
- As soon as children are old enough to crawl, make sure the floor of the home and any area that is within children's reach is free of small objects that can fit into children's mouths. Since, young children do a lot of exploring with their mouths, they are at risk of choking on small objects that can become lodged in their throats. Frequent vacuuming or sweeping will limit the risk. Also make sure that all toys are free of small parts that can be pulled off and swallowed. Check clothing frequently for loose buttons and fasteners.
- Take an infant/child CPR course. The knowledge gained will be invaluable if a life threatening situation, such as a choking or a loss of consciousness, should arise.

Poisoning

- Keep all toxic materials, including household cleaners, medications, and chemicals out of the reach of children in cabinets that are locked or that have childproof latches.
- Throw out all medication, household cleaners, and other toxic substances that have not been used in the last year. The fewer poisonous substances there are in your house, the less the risk for accidental poisoning.
- Lock up all medications. Unfortunately, children sometimes figure out how to open bottles that have childproof caps.
- Avoid carrying medications in purses or briefcases. Children love to go through them and may mistake the medication for candy.
- When giving medication to a child, avoid calling it candy or making a game of it.
- Make sure that all medications and chemicals in the home are correctly labeled. Parents will need to know exactly what their children have swallowed in the event of a poisoning.
- Try to store all non-edible substances in a place other than the kitchen.
- Never store chemicals or cleaners in food containers.
- Teach children to recognize and to avoid dangerous products.
- Rinse empty chemical containers before throwing them away. Make sure they are discarded in a place where they cannot be retrieved by children.
- Use insect and rodent poisons very carefully. Make sure they are placed only in areas where children cannot find them.
- Treat alcoholic beverages as poisons. Lock them up out of the reach of children.
- Make sure that all paint in the home is lead free. Paint manufactured before 1976 contains lead. If there is any sanding and stripping of old paint going on in the home, remove children from the premises. Exposure to even paint dust can cause lead poisoning.
- Many house plants are poisonous. Keep them out of the reach of children.
- Keep the telephone number of the local poison control center on or near the telephone.
- Make sure a bottle of syrup of ipecac is in the home at all times to induce vomiting. NEVER use it unless instructed to do so by a physician or poison control center.

Scalds and Burns

- Use fire resistant clothing for infants. Wash them according to the manufacturer's instructions.
- Keep children away from all hot appliances, including stoves, light bulbs, toasters, portable heaters, grills, irons, and curling irons.
- Do not leave cups of hot liquid (coffee, tea, soup) within the reach of children. Never carry children while pouring or carrying a cup of hot liquid.
- Always check the temperature of bath water before bathing children.
- When children begin to understand words, teach them the meaning of 'hot.'
- Use safety plugs or outlet caps on all unused electrical outlets in the home.
- Turn all pot handles away from the edge of the stove while cooking.
- Avoid using tablecloths. Toddlers often use them to pull themselves up, and if hot food is on the table, it can come down on top of them.
- Make sure the cords to all appliances used in the home do not dangle within the reach of children.
- Tape extension cords together to prevent children from pulling them apart.
- Make sure all matches and cigarette lighters are kept out of the reach of children.
- If there is a fireplace in the home, make sure it is well screened.

Motor Vehicle Accidents

- Always restrain children in automobile safety seats. Use safety seats until children no longer fit in one, and are big enough to use standard adult seat belts (usually about 60 pounds, or five years of age).
- Make sure the seat belts and/or harnesses used to secure children into the safety seats are tight enough.
- Do not allow children to play in driveways.
- Teach traffic safety as early as possible.
- Do not allow children to play outdoors unsupervised.

SAFE PLAY

- Playgrounds are designed for children of all ages. Find one with equipment that is right for your toddler's age and size. This includes easy climbers, low stairs and platforms, small slides and tunnels, activity panels and playhouses. If your child cannot reach equipment, it is too advanced for her.
- Toddlers and preschoolers are still developing their strength, balance, coordination and climbing skills. They sometimes try things they are not quite ready to do, especially when playing around older children and with adults. They may soon be ready for a tricycle. By law in Alberta, anyone under the age of 18 (toddlers and babies included) must wear a helmet in a bike trailer or on a bicycle or tricycle. When you wear a helmet too, your toddler is more likely to adopt this habit for life.
- **Prevention of falls**
  - Falls are the leading cause of hospital visits for childhood injuries. The most serious falls for children aged 1 to 4 years are down stairs, from windows, balconies, or other high spots.
  - Use protective devices such as stair gates and safety straps. They are designed to keep child from falling.
  - Move furniture and beds away from windows. Window screens will not protect toddler from falling out. Safety devices can prevent children from opening windows. Make sure, however, that an adult can still open them in case of emergency.
  - Put outdoor play equipment on a soft surface such as sand, pea gravel, a rubber surface, or wood chips so that if child falls, they have a safe landing. Toddlers need constant supervision on play equipment.
- **Preventing scalds**
  - Scalds and burns can happen in an instant, parents need to be alert and protect the child.
  - Keep toddler safely out of the way when the stove or oven is being used. Be careful with microwaves as they often heat and cook food unevenly, leaving hot spots in throughout the food. Stir food thoroughly before serving.
  - Use lids on hot drinks and keep them away from child, as their sudden movements can cause spills. The child is to be kept safely out of the way when mother is cooking.
- **Playing safe**
  - Toys should be age appropriate with no small parts. Do not let child have latex balloons. Children can choke very quickly if they get a piece in their mouth.
  - Make wearing a helmet an automatic part of riding in bike trailers or on tricycles. Remove helmets before playing (for example, on playground equipment). Always supervise toddler's play.
- **Removing dangerous items**
  - Choking and poisoning are real hazards to children under the age of 5 because they explore by putting things in their mouths. They do not understand that this can be dangerous. Toys

should be suited to child's age and have no small parts. Latex balloons are not toys-a piece of broken balloon can choke a child.
  - Cleaning solutions, matches, and medications are to be kept in locked cupboards out of baby's reach.
- **Travelling smart**
  - To use an approved, forward-facing child safety seat is needed every time toddler is in a vehicle until they are 18 kg (40 lbs.). Make sure it is secured with a tether strap.
- **Teaching safety rules**
  - Help toddler to learn to hold parent's hand and stay close to parent when he/she is walking along roads or in parking lots. Teach toddler's never to play in the driveway, garage, or street. The safety rules they learn now will help them make safer choices when they are older.
  - Having fun and staying healthy while playing outside
  - While outside, children need protection from the sun, insects, heat, and cold. Insect bites are irritating and can cause disease. Children's small bodies are at greater risk of becoming too hot or too cold, putting them at risk of heat stroke or hypothermia.

As parents and children begin their lives together as a family, parents embark on a significant new challenge, that of promoting their babies' healthy growth and development. Nurse will see, the care that parents provide for their babies impacts all areas of their early and later development. During assessment of the child and family, nurses' responsibility is to identify the areas and aware the parents/caregiver about age-specific developmental tasks of toddlers and prevention of hazards.

Preschool Child

Let's go out and play on the preschool playground
'Play is the answer to how anything new comes about.'

—Jean Piaget

OVERVIEW OF THE GROWTH AND DEVELOPMENT

The preschool years are a time when the child's unique personality begins to emerge more dramatically, which can include willful and contradictory behavior. Like infants and toddlers, preschoolers grow quickly—both physically and cognitively (Figs 5.49A and B).

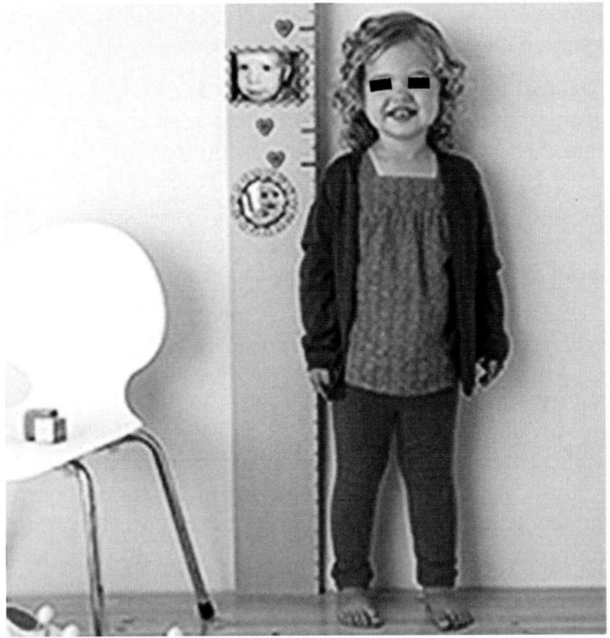

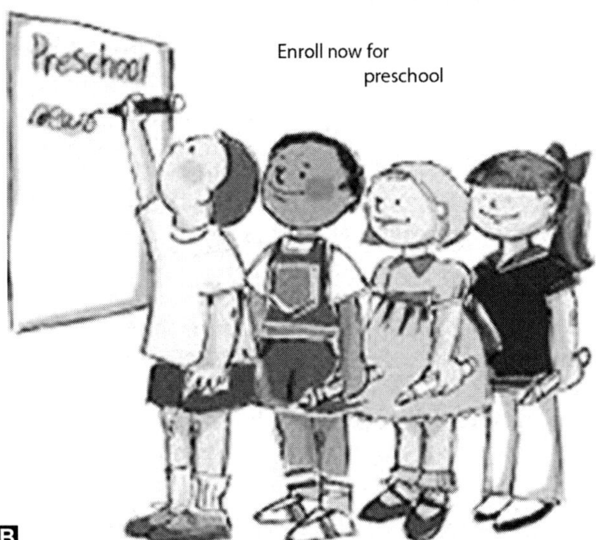

Figs 5.49A and B: A. Like infants and toddlers, preschoolers grow quickly; **B.** Preschool stage: Time for school enrollment

A short chubby toddler who can barely talk suddenly becomes a taller, leaner child who talks incessantly. Especially evident during early childhood is the fact that development is truly **integrated,** i.e. the biological, psychological, and social changes occurring at this time (as well as throughout the rest of the life span) are interrelated. Children are learning new rules of behavior and modes of self-expression and widening their social universe. A youngster may vacillate from clinging demands for attention to rebellious independence, testing a caregiver's limits and patience.

Physical development: In these years, a child becomes stronger and starts to look longer and leaner. During this period child starts to shed the baby fat from his face and looks lankier, since kids' limbs grow more by the time they are preschoolers. A preschooler will grow about 3 inches and gain 4–6 pounds each year. Boys may weigh about 29 to 40 pounds during this time. They may be 35 to 42 inches tall. Girls may weigh 27 to 39 pounds. They may be 34 to 42 inches tall.

Three-four- and five-year-olds are filled with energy and are constantly moving. As they grow, they are developing and refining their gross and fine motor skills. Three-year-olds experience considerable growth in the area of physical development as they acquire the coordination of everyday movement. Running, jumping, and climbing becomes more automatic and less a conscious, purposeful act. Three-year-olds are still a bit unsteady on their feet and will often fall and get back up and try again.

Motor development: Three-, four-, and five-year-olds are filled with energy and are constantly moving. As they grow, they are developing and refining their gross and fine motor skills. Three-year-olds experience considerable growth in the area of physical development as they acquire the coordination of everyday movement. Running, jumping, and climbing become more automatic and less a conscious, purposeful act.

Three-year-olds are learning to run with more dexterity and coordination, as they transition from slow, stiff running to a more playful pace. Three-year-olds mount small tricycles, but are learning how to coordinate pedaling and will often use their feet to move. As three-year-olds grow, they progress from climbing steps with two feet on a step to using alternating feet. Throwing a ball often requires the use of two hands and uses both forearms to push.

Child's balance will continue to improve. He will be able to stand on one foot, can kick a ball. He will also learn to walk up and down the stairs alternating his feet. He may also be able to skip and throw a ball. During these years, he learns to dress and feed himself and to use the toilet on his own. Child will improve his fine motor skills. He will learn to hold a book and turn the pages. He will learn to hold a pen and write his name, and draw simple strokes with a pencil. By age 5, most can dress and undress themselves and write some lowercase and capital letters. So gross motor and fine motor skills achieved by preschool child are:

Gross Motor Skills

- Walks with agility, good balance, and steady gait
- Run at a comfortable speed in one direction and around obstacles; she can also stop, restart, and turn while running
- Aim and throw a large ball or beanbag, or catch one thrown to her
- Hop several times on each foot
- Walk along and jump over a low object, such as a line, string, or balance beam
- Bounce a large ball several times
- Kick a stationary ball
- Pedal and steer a tricycle.

Fine Motor Skills

- Brush teeth, comb hair, and get dressed with little help
- Skillfully use eating utensils
- Use (child-sized) scissors to cut along a line
- Pick up small items such as coins, toothpicks, and paperclips
- Assemble simple puzzles
- Copy simple shapes, like a circle or square
- Print some letters of the alphabet
- Stack objects so they do not fall.

Moving

Your preschooler loves moving and being active. He is getting better at walking up stairs, pedaling a tricycle, throwing, catching and kicking a ball, running, climbing, jumping, hopping and balancing on one foot.

When it comes to using her hands, your preschooler might have the skills to draw a circle or square, build big towers of up to 10 blocks and use scissors. She will love using crayons, pencils and paintbrushes, which is great because drawing and painting fire up your child's imagination.

Other things your preschooler might do at this age are:

- Unscrewing a lid from a jar
- Knowing his own gender and age
- Starting to understand time
- Knowing the names of some shapes and colors
- Holding a pencil in the writing position and by four years, copying some letters
- Dressing and undressing himself.

Brain Development

Brain and nervous system developments during early childhood also continue to be dramatic. The better developed the brain and nervous systems are, the more complex behavioral and cognitive abilities children are capable of.

The brain is comprised of two halves, the right and left **cerebral hemispheres. Lateralization** refers to the localization of assorted functions, competencies, and skills in either or both hemispheres. Specifically, language, writing, logic, and mathematical skills seem to be located in the left hemisphere, while creativity, fantasy, artistic, and musical skills seem to be located in the right hemisphere. Although the hemispheres may have separate functions, these brain masses almost always coordinate their functions and work together.

The two cerebral hemispheres develop at different rates, with the left hemisphere developing more fully in early childhood (ages 2 to 6), and the right hemisphere developing more fully in middle childhood (ages 7 to 11). The left hemisphere predominates earlier and longer, which may explain why children acquire language so early and quickly.

Another aspect of brain development is **handedness,** or preference for using one hand over the other. Handedness appears to be strongly established by middle childhood. About 90% of the general population is right-handed, while the rest of the population is left-handed and/or **ambidextrous.** A person is ambidextrous if he or she shows no preference for one hand over the other. Typically, right-handedness is associated with left-cerebral dominance and left-handedness with right-cerebral dominance.

The nervous system undergoes changes in early childhood, too. The majority of a child's **neurons,** form prenatally. However, the **glial cells,** (nervous system support cells surrounding neurons) that nourish, insulate, and remove waste from the neurons without actually transmitting information themselves, develop most rapidly during infancy, toddlerhood, and early childhood. The **myelin sheaths** that surround, insulate, and increase the efficiency of neurons (by speeding up the action potential along the axon) also form rapidly during the first few years of life. The postnatal developments of glial cells and myelin sheaths help to explain why older children may perform behaviors that younger children are not capable of.

Cognitive

A child this age makes great strides in being able to think and reason. In these years, children learn their letters, counting, and colors.

Preschooler is seen **fascinated by the world around her** and will ask 'who', 'what' and 'why' questions as she tries to understand more about her world. Child understands opposites like big/small and more/less and concepts like 'on', 'in' and 'under'. He loves telling stories and can remember and recite nursery rhymes. He will start to identify letters and numbers when you name them, and can count up to four objects and sort them by color and shape.

Four and five-year-olds experience important changes in cognitive growth. In general, four- and five-year-olds are beginning to problem solve, think about cause-and-effect relationships, and express these ideas to others. As four- and five-year-olds' cognition matures, they begin to make the distinction between private thoughts and public expressions.

Language

By age 2, most children can say at least 50 words. By age 5, a child may know thousands of words and be able to carry on conversations and tell stories. Child's vocabulary increases. He may use 4 or more words to make sentences. He may use basic rules of grammar, such as talking in the past tense. Language of the child will develop a lot this year. She will show more interest in communicating and might show interest in telling stories and having conversations.

He will learn **hundreds and hundreds of new words** this year. He learns words by listening to parents and other adults and by guessing from context. He also learns from new experiences and from listening to stories read the out loud. He will still understand many more words than he says. Around three years, child will understand hundreds of words and use sentences of 3–5 words, or even more. Other people will understand what she is saying most of the time. She will point to parts of pictures, e.g. the nose of a dog, and name common objects.

By four, he will speak in longer sentences of around 5–6 words or more. Other people will understand him all the time. He understands most things you say and will follow instructions with 2–3 steps, as long as they are about familiar things, e.g. 'Close the book, and give it to Mum'. He will understand adjectives such as 'long' or 'thin', and use 'feeling' words like 'happy' or 'sad'. Preschool child is busy talking, exploring and playing. All of these activities are important for his or her growth and development—and for learning communication skills.

Children of this age will need well-developed communication skills when it's time to start going to school—to make friends, learn new things, and start learning to read and write. Communication skills are critical to child's future success.

Play is an important part in child's ongoing communication development. Talking, listening and playing with child will help to build the skills he or she needs to succeed in school and in life. About one in ten children needs help developing normal speech and language skills. Without help, it's a struggle to listen and talk, it's difficult to learn to read, and it's hard to play with other children.

Emotional and Social Development

This is an important period in emotional and social development for preschooler. Parents have the biggest influence on child's emotional and social development. Preschooler loves family meal together. She understands family routine and appreciates special events, like birthdays.

Child will become more independent. She will probably be toilet trained and can do some daily hygiene tasks on her own, like going to the toilet alone, wiping urine from her bottom and washing her hands and face. She will still need help and supervision with tasks like brushing teeth. Simple tasks, such as dressing himself, will help boost his self-confidence. He will learn how to handle his emotions better and the frustration and temper tantrums will improve. He will start to be interested in playing with other children.

Between the ages of 2 and 5, children gradually learn how to manage their feelings. By age 5, friends become important. During this year child really starts to understand that her body, mind and feelings are her own. She is much better at recognizing her own feelings—such as happiness, sadness, fear or anger.

Child in this age also shows a wide range of feelings, including fear of imaginary things, concern about how others act and affection for familiar people. As his self-esteem develops, he will learn to reassure himself that things are OK and he will get better at handling his emotions. Your child will start to form real friendships now and develop more social skills (Fig. 5.50).

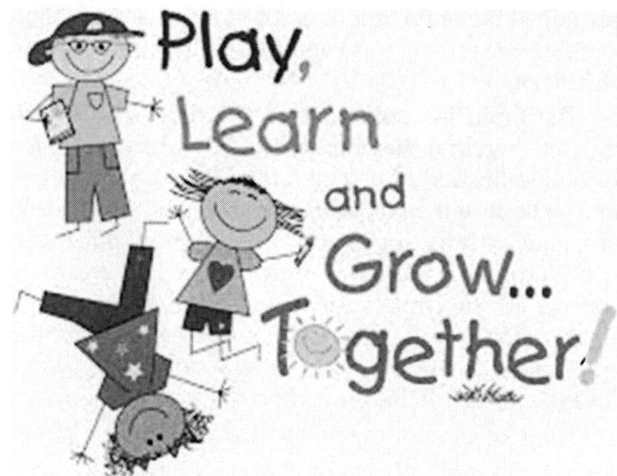

Fig. 5.50: Preschool children's characteristic is to play together

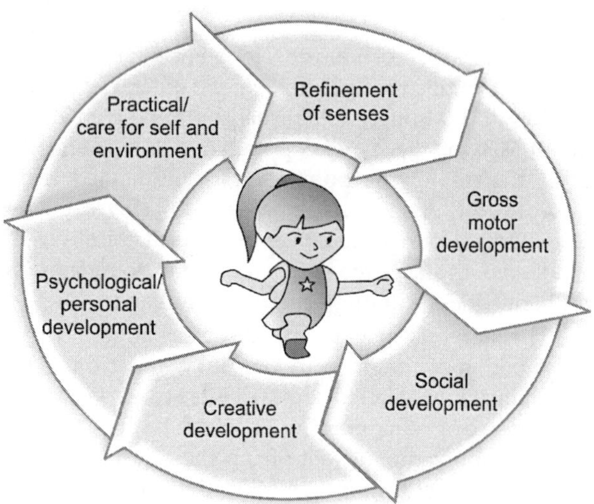

Fig. 5.51: Overall development of preschool child

Mental Development

Child has a very active imagination. He may be afraid of the dark and may fear monsters or ghosts. He may pretend to be another character when he plays. He will learn his colors and letters. He will start to learn the idea of time. He will be able to retell familiar stories and follow complex directions.

Each child grows and gains skills at his or her own pace. It is common for a child to be ahead in one area, such as language, but a little behind in another.

Learning what is normal for children this age can help you spot problems early or feel better about how your child is doing (Fig. 5.51).

Play of Preschool Child

Young children are learning at a very fast rate. They are learning language skills, developing opinions and interests and coping with change as well as learning about themselves and their abilities. **Playing and learning** goes on because it is still how child learns and explores feelings. She is becoming more interested in playing with other children and might start to play more cooperatively in small groups. She understands the concept of 'mine' and 'his/hers' so sharing starts to get easier. Preschool friends become more important, and it is common for preschoolers to have imaginary friends too. Child is interested in new experiences and is becoming more creative during play such as, he might play pretend games with imaginary friends or toys, such as having a tea party with his toys. At this age, he can probably tell the difference between real and fantasy. They need lots of playtime, play space: Messy play—in sand or mud or with paints—play with plenty of safe and appropriate equipment, i.e. puppets or toys, puzzle and outdoor play–with plenty of running, tumbling and rolling—are all great ways for preschoolers to express feelings, particularly if they are upset or angry.

By four, child might enjoy tricking others and describing what happened, for example, 'Mum thought I was asleep!' At the same time, she will also worry about being tricked by others.

In this age, preschooler might be very curious about bodies—his own and other people's. He will try different roles and behavior, and might play 'doctors' or 'mums and dads'. This combination of natural curiosity and role-playing sometimes leads to childhood sex play, e.g. looking at his/her own and other children's genitals.

As young children make sense of their world through active exploration and interaction, it is important to give children real and authentic experiences with quality objects and materials. Plastic equipment, while cheap, easily accessible and attractive to children, is often poor imitations of real objects. For example, a plastic hammer, plastic spanner and plastic carpentry bench have little educational value for carpentry play. By using a real hammer or spanner successfully, a child can learn a lot of carpentry skills as well as gain useful knowledge about these objects and their uses. With adult support, children will also learn about important issues relating to the safe use of real equipment.

ROLE OF PARENT IN DEVELOPMENT

The best thing parents can do for their child is to show love and affection. But there are also many other ways they can help preschooler to grow and learn like:

- *Offering healthy foods to the child:* Keep lots of fruits, vegetables, and healthy snacks in the house. Child needs adequate sleep and nutrition to fuel her overall development and activity.
- *Make time for child to be active:* Limit TV and computer time to 2 hours a day or less.
- *Read and talk to child:* This helps children learn language and opens them up to new ideas. Nurture her love for books by taking her to the library or bookstore. Help child develop good language skills by speaking to him in complete sentences and using 'grown up' words. Help him to use the correct words and phrases.
- *Help child get enough rest:* Between the age of 2 and 5, children need about 11 to 13 hours of sleep each day.
- *Help child play with other children:* Preschool or play groups can be a great way for children to learn to interact. This helps him to learn the value of sharing and friendship. Encourage child to play with other children. Be clear and consistent when disciplining child. Explain and show the behavior that is expected from her. Whenever tell her no, follow-up with what he should be doing instead.
- *Encouraging physical development at home:* Parents need to reinforce child's development and foster further progress where necessary. It is easy and fun to practice physical skills with child in the family. They need a space and freedom to use large muscles, through activities such as running, climbing and swinging on playground equipment. Toys and equipment that child can use to help her develop large muscles are to be supplied. (For example: skipping rope, bean bags, tricycle, large beach balls and a child-sized basketball hoop). Active play with child is important, such as play catch, tag, or set up a simple obstacle course.
- Teach skills, such as how to get dressed and how to use the toilet. Help child through the steps to solve problems when she is upset. Give child a limited number of simple choices (for example, deciding what to wear, when to play, and what to eat for snack).
- Set limits that help child feel safe and secure but that also allow child to explore.

  Raising a preschooler can be challenging task to parents. What works are right for a 3-year-old may not be right for a 5-year-old.
- Regular well-child examination is to be done to have her vision and hearing checked. Even small problems, caught and addressed at this age, can greatly enhance motor skill development and confidence.

Parents own physical and mental health is an important part of being a parent. But with all the focus on looking after a child, lots of parents forget or run out of time to look after themselves. Looking themselves will help parents with the understanding, patience, imagination and energy they need to be a parent.

If parents do feel frustrated, upset or cannot cope situation, they need to put their preschooler somewhere safe and take some time out until parent feels calmer. Or ask someone else to look after the child for a while. **Never shake a preschooler.** It can cause bleeding inside the brain and likely permanent brain damage.

In fact, as a parent, people always learn. Every parent makes mistakes and learns through experience. It is OK to feel confident about what they know. And it is also OK to admit that some of the things parents don't know and ask questions–often the 'dumb' questions are the best kind!

SPECIAL PROBLEMS OF PRESCHOOL CHILD (FIGS 5.52A TO C)

Over the past several years, a number of studies have shown a rise in behavior problems among preschoolers. Investigators say that these problems include 'prolonged tantrums, thumb sucking, enuresis, physical and verbal aggression, disruptive vocal and motor behavior, destructiveness, self-injury, noncompliance, and withdrawal.

Thumb Sucking

Babies have a natural urge to suck. This urge usually decreases after the age of 6 months. But many babies continue to suck their thumbs to soothe themselves. Thumb-sucking can become a habit in babies and young children, who use it to comfort themselves when they feel hungry, afraid, restless, quiet, sleepy, or bored. Thumb-sucking in children younger than 4 is usually not a problem. Children who suck their thumbs often or with great intensity around age 4 or 5, or those who are still sucking their thumbs at age 6, are at risk for dental or speech problems. It causes the teeth to become improperly aligned (malocclusion) or push the teeth outward. This usually corrects itself when the child stops thumb-sucking. But the longer thumb-sucking continues, the more likely it is that *orthodontic treatment* will be needed. Speech problems caused by thumb-sucking can include not being able to say Ts and Ds, lisping, and thrusting out the tongue when talking.

Children who suck their thumbs may need treatment when they:

- Continue to suck a thumb often or with great intensity around age 4 or older. (A callus on the thumb is one sign of intense sucking).
- Cause infections to develop around fingernails to spread infectious diseases.
- Ask for help to stop.

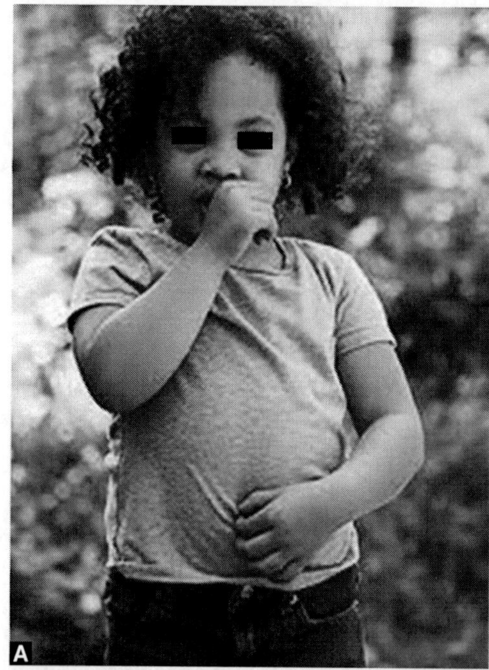

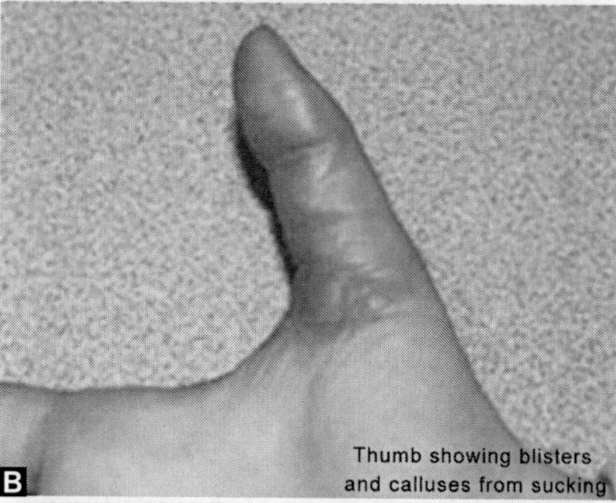

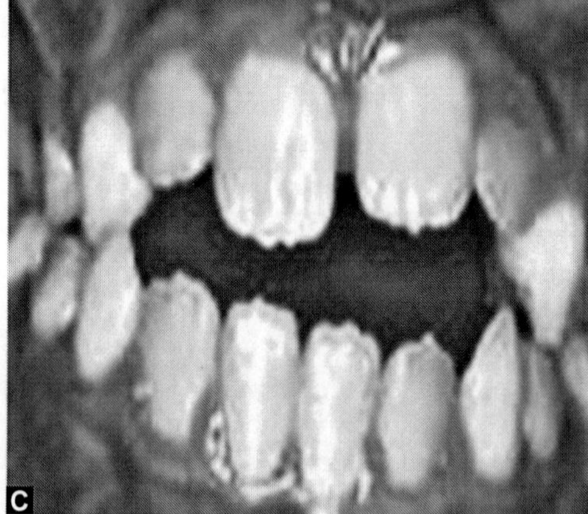

Figs 5.52A to C: A. Thumb sucking child; **B.** Callus on the thumb is one sign of intense sucking; **C.** Deformity in gums and dental structures due to thumb sucking

- Develop dental or speech problems as a result of sucking their thumbs.
- Feel embarrassed or are teased or shamed by other people.

Enuresis

Nocturnal enuresis is the medical term for bedwetting. Bedwetting is a common problem among preschoolers and may persist through (or even beyond) child's fifth year (Fig. 5.53). Indeed, it should not even be considered a 'bad habit,' because child cannot control it. Bedwetting in children is often simply a result of immaturity. The age at which children become able to control their bladders during sleep is variable. Bladder control is a complex process that involves coordinated action of the muscles, nerves, spinal cord and brain. In this case, the problem will resolve in time. On the other hand, it may be an indication of an underlying medical condition, such as obstruction of the urinary tract, an irritable bladder which cannot hold large quantities of urine, or he may have a neurogenic defect or urinary tract infection. If bedwetting persists beyond the age of 6 or 7, seeking medical help from pediatrician and psychiatrist may be necessary.

Whatever the cause of bedwetting and no matter how frequent it is, the fault certainly does not lie on child. A sudden rise in the frequency of bedwetting may indicate stress in preschooler's daily life. The causes of a preschooler's stress are many: The arrival of a new baby, an extended or unanticipated separation from either or both of the parents, getting lost in the department store, an illness or hospital stay, a death in the family, and so on. If parents can recognize the source of stress, they need to talk to the child about it as kindly and openly as possible. If they pamper their child for a while, chances are that the bedwetting frequency will revert to normal.

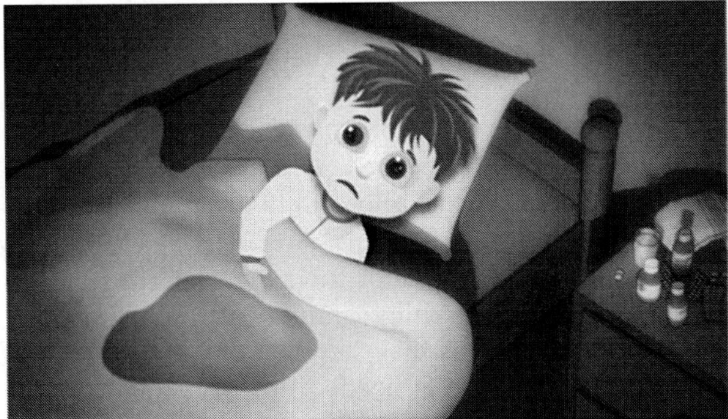

Figs 5.53: Enuresis is a common problem among preschool children

There are both primary and secondary forms of bedwetting. With primary bedwetting, the child has never had nighttime control over urination. The secondary form is less common and refers to bedwetting that occurs after the child has been dry during sleep for 6 or more months. Secondary bedwetting may be caused by psychological stress but may be the result of an underlying medical condition such as constipation or urinary tract obstruction. With secondary bedwetting, an evaluation about the child is important. Commonly prescribed behavioral methods for treating the problem include:

- Establishing a regular *bedtime routine* that includes going to the bathroom
- Waking the child during the night before he/she typically wets the bed and taking him/her to the bathroom
- Developing a reward system to encourage child, such as stickers for dry nights
- Limiting beverages and water in the evening
- Using a 'bell-and-pad' which incorporates an alarm that goes off whenever child's garments or bed become wet during an accident. These systems teach the child to eventually wake-up before the bedwetting occurs.

As a last resort, medication is prescribed for bedwetting, either for short or long-term use. Some examples are imipramine (an antidepressant), which relaxes the bladder, and desmopressin. Although medication usually helps, bedwetting typically resumes once the child stops taking the medicine. As with any drug, it is important to monitor your child's response to the medication.

Encopresis

Encopresis has been defined as 'the repetitive, voluntary or involuntary, passage of stool in inappropriate places by children 4 years of age and older, at which time a child may be reasonably expected to have completed toilet training and to exercise bowel control.'

Most children with encopresis have underlying constipation. Why some children develop encopresis does not seem to reflect differences in either physiology or psychology. Pediatric GI specialists have noted three areas of intestinal maturation that may set the stage (in some children) for the onset of constipation and (in some, ultimately) encopresis. These areas include the following:

- *Introduction of solid foods at proper age:* The increase in solid foods promotes an increase in stool volume and consistency that may require greater effort for stool expulsion.

- *The process of toilet training:* Children who refuse to toilet train develop chronic constipation and are at a substantially higher likelihood of developing encopresis.
- *Not passing urine/stool at school:* Children refuse to use the school toilet for either urinating or bowel movements, due to the lack of privacy, taunting, and often noisy chaos is just too intimidating when compared with the home environment.

Regardless of the cause, many children with constipation will ultimately pass either an overly large and/or hard stool, resulting in a painful experience. The rational step (from the child's perspective) is to avoid stooling and thus avoid further pain. Consequently, stool accumulates in the rectum and becomes desiccated and thus more difficult and more painful to pass. This recurrent cycle reinforces the child's behavior to avoid stooling at all costs. Children who develop encopresis may develop abnormal stretching and enlargement of the rectal area that reduces the reflex urge to stool. As a consequence, the impacted stool mass may allow 'upstream' semisolid stool to leak around the 'downstream' stool obstruction, causing soiling in clothes as well as occasional chunks of stool to also be passed without the child's knowledge or desire.

Bad Language

Preschool is a time when children are making great strides in building their vocabularies. They practice language skills by repeating the sounds and words they hear around them, and often they do not even know/aware of the meaning of many of the words and phrases they are using (Figs 5.54A and B). However, parents can sometimes feel embarrassed, frustrated or angry when 'bad words' come out of their young child's mouth.

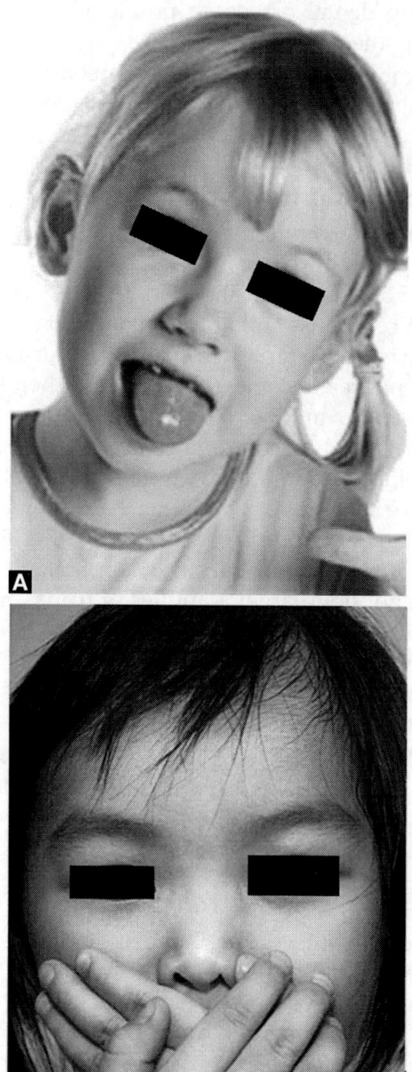

Figs 5.54A and B: A child's reaction after using bad language

So how can parents react constructively to 'bad words'? Simply demanding that a child stop a behavior without teaching her why, no matter what that behavior is, rarely works. In fact, this strategy often backfires, as prohibiting something without explaining why it is prohibited only adds to the allure of the behavior. Therefore, parents have to focus on teaching children how to communicate in a polite and positive manner. Here are some effective ways for dealing with a preschooler who is testing out the use of bad word:

- The most important thing to do is to be relaxed and treat the bad word as if it is no big deal. The child is to be told in a calm voice that he used a word that might make some people feel bad or uncomfortable.
- Parents can turn the use of a bad word into a lesson, instead of a time for punishment. Instead of just banning the use of a particular word, teach the child a few replacement words. Say that a big kid uses these words instead of the one he just used. It is helpful to be prepared. When the child uses the replacement words, a lot of attention and praise is to be given.
- Adults need to monitor their own language. Even if they think their child cannot hear them, they may avoid those words that they do not want their child to use. Extra care is needed not to use bad words when they are angry or frustrated, as parents do not want their child to copy this behavior. If they

do use inappropriate language at any time, admit it right away. Say that even adults make mistakes sometimes, but parents will be careful to choose their words more carefully next time. Ask the child to help parent think of ways that they could have expressed themselves differently.

- Help children learn to control their behavior within different settings, which is a very important foundation for later academic and social development. Instead of banning a word completely, tell the child that the word can make others feel bad, so if he really feels the need to say the word, that is okay. However, he should go into the bathroom or in his room, say the word as many times as he wants, and then return to the group when he is ready to use other words instead.
- The correct names for body parts and functions should not be considered bad words. Teach child how to talk about body parts and functions openly and accurately. Telling children that certain body parts should not be talked about or should not be called by their real names only teaches children that they should be uncomfortable with certain parts of their body. Parents will also be making these words even more appealing to use because children will learn that they upsetting to adults.
- Parents can observe when/in what situation their child use these words. What kinds of situations? Right when he comes home from school or daycare? When his siblings are playing with his things? Only around a group of children? When parents have been busy for the last ten minutes? Fifteen minutes? When he faces a transition? Try to figure out what the situations are that make him feel separate, lonely, or disconnected enough to act harshly. There are clues to places where he loses his confidence in the timing of his behavior. Once parents understand the situations that strain their child's confidence, try offering support.

Destructiveness

Preschool-age children are highly active, often moody, and aggressive. Much of the child's accidental destructiveness is the result of his boundless energy and endless curiosity. Moreover, typical preschoolers disobey 25 to 50% of their parents' commands. To avoid accidental destruction at home, the valuable objects are to be protected and they should provide space for play.

An intentionally destructive child is usually an unhappy child unable to control his feelings of helplessness, jealousy, aggression. Disruptive behavior refers to a wide range of conduct problems, such as oppositional, stubborn, aggressive, and impulsive behaviors, that cluster together and occur at higher rates than usual for preschoolers of the same age (Figs 5.55A and B). With such frequent negative behavior typical of young children, how can parents decide if the 'bad' behavior they are seeing in their preschooler signifies a significant concern or is within normal limits? Parents need to understand the cause of the destructiveness and appropriate treatment given. The child may have a feeling of rejection, unloved, disliked by peers, or bored by inadequate playthings. Sometimes such children seem to want to be punished, means to get attention in other way. Scolding and punishing the child is to be avoided. Parents/care providers should help him to direct his energy into appropriate activities and play. It is important to remember that effective treatment of disruptive behavior prior to school entry may prevent the associated problems with academic performance and peer relationships.

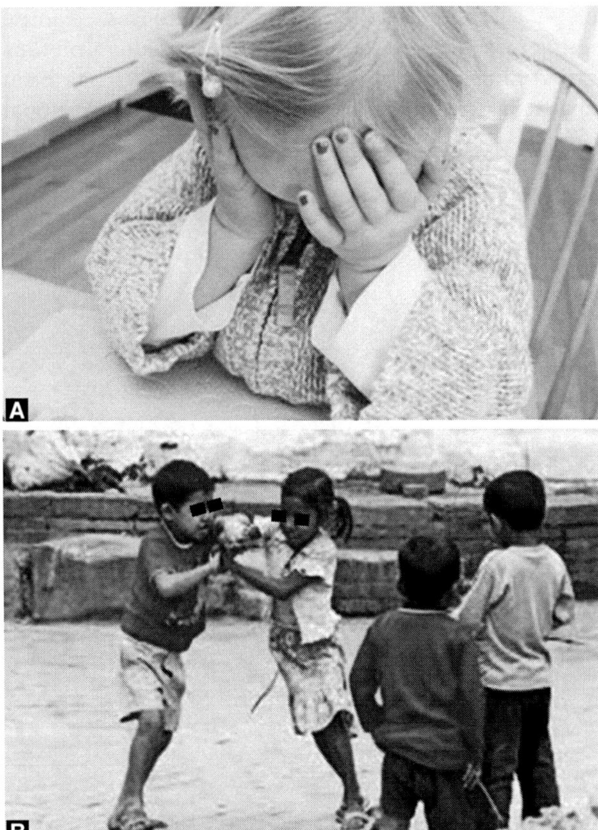

Figs 5.55A and B: Unhappy preschoolers cannot control their emotion–shows withdrawn or disruptive, aggressive behavior

PROMOTING OPTIMAL HEALTH OF PRESCHOOL CHILD

Physical Care

Physical activity habits learned in early childhood can last a lifetime. More and more evidence shows that children who are active tend to have fewer behavioral and disciplinary problems, do better in school, and have longer attention spans in class. Physical activity helps children to build confidence, decrease stress and depression, develop motor skills and build strength, flexibility and endurance, improve social skills and brain development and stay at a healthy weight.

The preschool child is gaining competency in self-care (Figs 5.56A and B). He/she become independent in self-care but he does not take full responsibility for stopping his play and going to the toilet before urgency makes him unable to control elimination.

Nutrition

The preschool years are a critically important period for developing healthy food preferences. Family setting or child-care settings need to provide numerous opportunities to promote healthy eating. It has been identified the opportunities to improve the nutritional quality of foods provided to preschool children, their mealtime behaviors, and the provision of nutrition education.

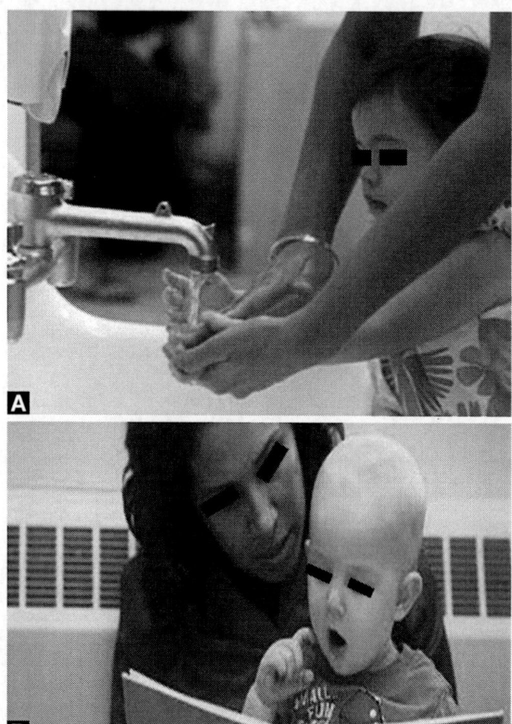

Figs 5.56A and B: Promoting optimal health of preschool child

These children are less interested in eating as they have the interest to explore his environment and because of her relatively slow growth rate than previous years. Forcing, bribing and coaxing for food is to be avoided as it may be persistent eating problems. His appetite will increase as he nears school-age. Few measures can be adopted to maintain nutrition of preschool child:

- Meal is to be served in a quiet environment with few distractions. Sitting arrangements should be comfortable, using pretty dishes, and giving small servings in attractive ways (Fig. 5.57).
- New food should be added gradually. If he refuses the new food, it should be offered again after he has forgotten its taste.
- Preschool children can eat a simple adult diet (*See* the annexures of this edition). In an atmosphere in which everyone enjoying the meal, children are likely to eat more.
- The child should be allowed sufficient time to eat without having attention paid to what he has and has not eaten.
- Teaching the child about handwashing before taking food.
- Older children can be allowed to set the table and helping mother to wash and fix plates. It may result in the child's taking more interest in food and eating more wholesome food.

Some children use poor eating habits as a means of getting attention or expressing sibling rivalry or other reason. These causes are likely to be manifested in other behavior than simply refusal to eat. So cause of

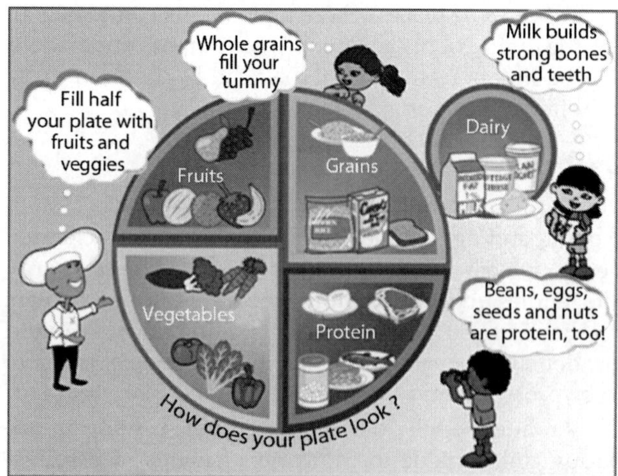

Fig. 5.57: Recommended daily diet of preschoolers

the child's problem is to be explored to prevent trauma to the child's physical and mental health. He needs reassurance that he is loved.

Dental Care

Dental care is important at the preschool-age (Figs 5.58A and B). At the ages of three and six, carries of the deciduous teeth commonly begin and tend to spread rapidly. It is known that the deciduous teeth act as pathfinders for the growth of permanent teeth, so it is essential that the deciduous teeth be kept in good condition until the permanent teeth erupt. The child's intake of refined sugar should be limited because sugar that is not removed by brushing teeth can cause cavities on the tooth enamel.

The way to clean child's teeth: Parent might like to try the following routine when brushing her child's teeth:

- She has to stand or sit behind her child so she feels secure. Being in front of a mirror is good too, because it lets the mother to see her child's mouth.

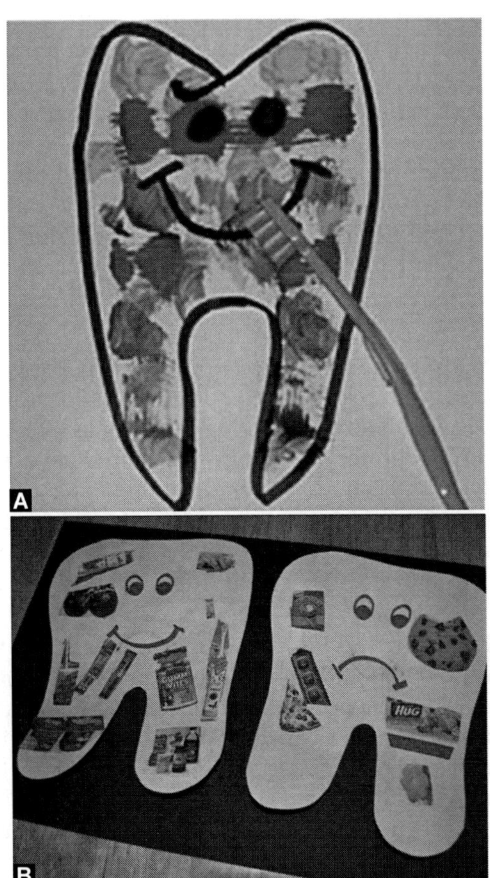

Figs 5.58A and B: Optimum dental health needs proper brushing and healthy nutrition

- Mother will cup her child's chin in her hands, with child's head resting against her body.
- She angles the bristles of the toothbrush towards the gum. She moves the brush in gentle circles to clean the outer and inner sides of the teeth and gums. Lifts her child's lips to brush the front and back of the teeth and at the gum line and brush back and forth on the chewing surfaces of the teeth.

Sleep

Preschoolers need about 11 to 12 hours of sleep each day, which can include a nap. Most preschoolers do still need naps during the day. They are normally so interested in whatever he is doing that running around, playing, going to school, and exploring their surroundings, so it is a good idea to give them a special opportunity to slow down. Even if the child cannot fall asleep, some quiet time during the day for relaxing can be set aside for the child.

Preschool child needs a private place not only for sleeping but also for social, sexual, gender identity, fantasy and individuation development. Favorite objects like stuffed animals and blankets also can help kids feel safe. Establish a bedtime routine that is the same every night and includes calm and enjoyable activities, such as a bath and bedtime stories. The activities occurring closest to 'lights out' should occur in the room where the preschooler sleeps. **Setting up a soothing sleep environment is important.** Child's bedroom should be comfortable, dark, cool, and quiet. A nightlight is fine; a television is not. Sleep of three-year-old is frequently disturbed at night due to frightening dreams. These children may not stay in their beds and want to sleep with parents.

Some parents get into the habit of lying down next to their preschoolers until they fall asleep. While this may do the trick temporarily, it would not help sleeping patterns in the long run. It is important to give comfort and reassurance, but kids need to learn how to fall asleep independently. By the time the child is five years old he usually sleeps quietly and peacefully through the night, but he still may have nightmares. Sleep problems are common during the preschool years, including night time fears and nightmares. Night time fears and nightmares are a part of normal development. Sleepwalking and sleep terrors are also common during the preschool years and peak in this age group.

Sleep is important for your preschooler's health, growth and development. When children sleep well, they are more settled and happy during the day. Getting the right amount of sleep also strengthens your child's immune system and reduces the risk of infection and illness.

Safety Measures

The causes of accidents in this age group are increased initiative and the desire to imitate the behavior of adults, which lead children into situations hazardous for them. Home-related injuries are a major threat to the health of preschool children. Many risk situations can only be avoided through parental safety behavior, especially with measures taken to structure the child's environment. The children in the home/preschool where they play/congregate are monitored at all times by parents/care providers. Balancing supervision with safety precautions will help prevent accidents and injuries as well as allow children to explore. Adults can help protect child from accidents and injuries by taking general safety measures around home.

Checking the play area is to be done regularly. Cleaning and sanitizing of toys are needed at the end of every day. Broken toy pieces, which can be sharp and dangerous should be thrown immediately. Child can choke on things smaller than 1.25 in. (3.2 cm) in diameter and 2.25 in. (5.7 cm) long. These include button batteries and coins. So, items like these should be kept out of child's reach. If a child who is choking cannot talk, cry, breathe, or cough—parents/adults should learn these symptoms of choking.

Keep high traffic areas clear of anything that may cause preschoolers to trip and fall. For example, clean up spills as soon as they happen, and keep toys that are not being played with in designated toy bins.

The classroom is to be arranged in a way that allows the teacher/care provider to see all of the children, at all times. Make sure there are no blind spots where children can get lost from supervisor's sight. It is better to arrange chairs, desks and work tables in circles.

There are a number of precautions in preparing, storing and serving food, in play school. The guidelines of food safety are to be followed, to ensure day-care safety.

Play and Play Area Safety

In a preschool environment, cleaners, insecticides, first aid solutions, medications and all other toxic substances should be kept in a high, flame-resistant and safety-locked cabinet.

Prevent household fires by having and maintaining smoke detectors, planning and practicing escape routes, and teaching child basic fire safety skills. Children ages 2 to 5 are often curious about fire. Warn the child about the dangers of fire, and explain why only grown-ups are allowed to use it.

Children should learn to behave with the pets. Teach them to never tease animals or bother them while they are eating. Explain that animals can sometimes hurt him/her. Also be sure to train own pets and keep them healthy.

Health Supervision

Children are the most vulnerable and dependent members of society, and their well-being is an important measure of the overall health of a society. Investing in early child health promotion can result in health benefits to young children, health improvements across the life span, and economic returns to society in the form of reduced health care costs and increased economic productivity. Making conscious choices about preschool children's health today can lead to good habits and good behavior throughout childhood. After all, teaching preschooler to make healthy food choices now sets the stage for a lifelong healthy diet. Dental supervision is a part of general health supervision, and guidance is given regarding dental care and care of the mouth. Putting childhood bedtime problems to rest can ensure good sleep for both parents and child for years to come. And understanding typical preschool developmental milestones can help parents to monitor their preschooler's growth and development.

Regular child health visits are important where health professional (nurse/doctor) record the growth, gives advice about nutrition, immunization, and any problems which occur in management of the child and instructs the parents on essential safety factors. Tests for visual and auditory perception are important before sending the child to school.

Preschoolers love to explore and discover; parents need to capitalize on this innate curiosity in many ways. The objective of caring preschool child is to provide a warm, safe and secure learning environment for every child, in order for a child to develop intellectually, socially, physically and emotionally. The parents/caregivers must provide a variety of experiences to enhance a sense of pride in child's own achievements and the achievements of skills appropriate in this stage of life.

Monitoring child development is important to ensure that children meet their developmental milestones. Developmental milestone checklist/charts are used as a guide as to what is normal for a particular age range and can be used to highlight any areas that a child may be delayed in. However, it is important to be aware that while child development has a predictable sequence all children are unique in their development and the course in which each child follows to reach each milestone can vary.

The School Child

'Education is teaching our children to desire the right things.'

— Plato

The school years are a very important time in every child's life. While toddlers and preschoolers need constant supervision, school-age children become gradually ready for more independence (Fig. 5.59). But learning to make good choices and exercise self-discipline does not come easily for many children. Parents need to impart a moral code that the child gradually internalizes. When they will equipped, parents can be excellent coaches for their child no matter what the endeavor.

Raising school-age children can be awesome. Watching them try new activities, cheering them on at athletic events and applauding their accomplishments at recitals are usually some of the high points for most parents. All parents want to see their children do well in school and most parents do all they can to provide them with the best educational opportunities.

OVERVIEW OF EMOTIONAL DEVELOPMENT IN SCHOOL CHILD

This area of development involves learning to interact with other people, and to understand and control own emotions. Babies start to develop relationships with the people around them right from birth, but the process of learning to communicate, share, and interact with others takes many years to develop. Developing the ability to control own emotions and behavior is also a long process. As children enter the school-age years, they begin to show signs of a budding independence. This period of growth is also marked by the active pursuit of, and genuine appreciation for, new relationships. Be able to communicate with others without parent's help.

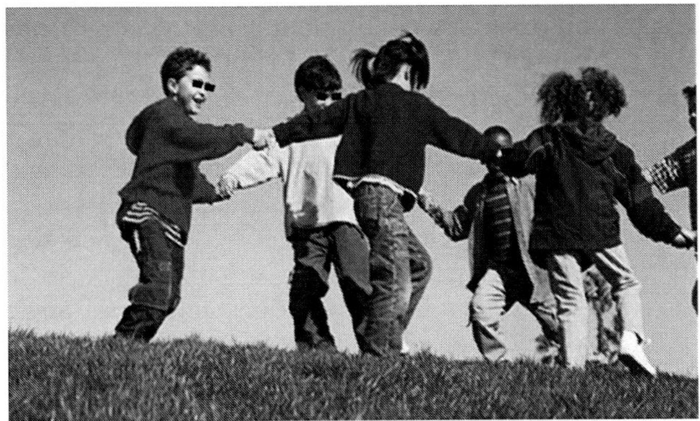

Fig. 5.59: School age is the period of more independence

Parents, or primary caregivers, continue to be the most important people in their child's life, but relationships with peers become increasingly important.

The child at school-age can measure his performance against others. Continue to develop her social skills by playing with other children in a variety of situations. Other significant, and often defining, characteristics of this phase of development are a child's capacity to control their urges and conform to an appropriate standard of behavior without direct supervision. Collectively, this is known as self-regulation. They start to feel sensitive about how other children feel about him. Moreover, the appearance of a 'best friend' is considered a universal feature of the school-age years.

At the age of 5 to 6 years, children enjoy playing alone, but prefer to play with friends, they are willing to play cooperatively, take turns, and share. Understand their own feelings, are able to use words to describe their own feelings. They understand the consequences of their actions. They may show jealousy toward siblings, but show empathy and offer to help when they see another in distress.

At the age of 7 to 8 years, children show a competitive spirit when playing games, show an interest in joining a club or sports team. Form a sense of humor and enjoy telling jokes, they try to be friend children of the opposite gender. School going children help out with chores at home, such as clearing the table after a meal or tidying up personal belongings. An important part of children's emotional development is they strive toward competence, this means they want to be more self-sufficient and independent, and they seek the approval of parents, teachers and peers to confirm their competence.

THE SCHOOL CHILD, HIS FAMILY AND FRIENDS

Family

The child between six and twelve years is more independent than before, better able to care for herself, and more capable of contributing to chores and other household responsibilities. Most families discover that routines can be established, and in many ways life seems more settled. However, youngsters still need parental supervision and guidance (Fig. 5.60). He is still dependent upon his parents' love, companionship with his peers and adults outside the home becomes of increasing importance.

During the middle childhood years, parents have to understand that the child's social horizon has expanded,

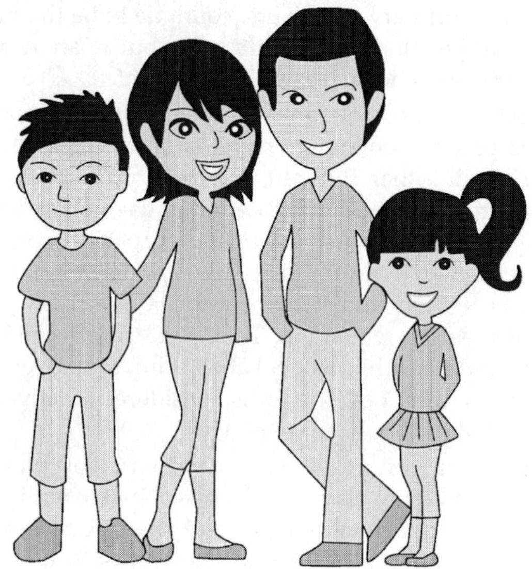

Fig. 5.60: A school child and family

as parents they have two tasks that are especially important. The first is learning to allow and encourage the child to enter the new world of school and friends alone. The second is learning to be parents at a distance. Once children enter school, parents spend less than half as much time with them as they did before. Children gain increasing ideological as well as physical and emotional independence from their parents. Parents thus need to be more efficient, more vigilant, and still very much involved in their children's lives in order to monitor, guide, and support them effectively.

The child's relation with the parent of opposite sex which existed during her preschool years has been resolved. She has come to respect and love that parent of the same sex. By imitating that parent's role she learns her own social role.

Children of large family find adjusting to children outside the family and sharing with the group easier than does the only child. When an only child goes outside the family to make friends in his peer group, he still expects to be the center of the group and becomes upset/frightened when he learns that he is not. On the other hand, sibling jealousy is a problem even in families in which all the members love one another. So being an only child or one of a group of siblings has more and more effect upon personality development of the child.

The school child learns to think of himself as a person of own right. During the school years, youngster may develop more self-confidence, overcome fears and self-doubts, test the limits of her autonomy, find role models, and learn and internalize moral and spiritual values. Parents and the rest of the family should pay particular attention to the following areas, which will become increasingly significant during this time of life:

- Parents should invite the confidence of their child as a parent, not as a buddy
- Parents can leave a space to talk, to discuss different matters, but they should never intrude on the privacy of a child
- Parent can set a good example for their child to follow in building character traits such as honesty and loyalty
- Parents need to set consistent limits on their child's behavior
- Parents can try to their child as others see him, not as an idealized extension of themselves
- Parents are not supposed to compare one child with the another in the family.

Friends

Developing friendships is a vital part of emotional growth of school-age child as the child psychologically moves slowly away from home. It is normal for children to have one or several best friends and also an enemy, though those roles may change frequently. They learn to take his place as members of a group, and their social life begins. They also prefer same-sex friendships and think of the opposite sex as weird. Some children begin to like taking care of or playing with younger children. During this stage, school-age children have developed an increasing need of independence and become more socially accepting of peers. Play becomes more complex, with rules being established in group games and games are focused on having a 'winning' team or being called the 'winner' at the end of a game. Competitiveness begins to emerge as school-age children continue to compare themselves with school peers. It is also common at this age, for school-age children to have unstable friendships as they start to be unkind towards each other.

As important as child's family is to her, friends and acquaintances will become increasingly significant during middle childhood. Children of school-age begin to define themselves in terms of their appearance, possessions and activities. Children of each sex tend to develop its own fashion, language and its own activities and behavior. This can be exacerbated due to peer pressure or advertising, as children begin to judge themselves by the expectations and appearances of those around them. This can lead to them being self-conscious and feeling as if other people notice even small differences in their looks or actions. She will spend more time with her peers, both in and out of school. These playmates will provide companionship, and your youngster will probably become preoccupied with being socially accepted by her friends. She will feel a strong need for both conformity (to be just like the others) and recognition (to be seen as unique).

Children of school-age can be exceedingly cruel to each other. From time to time she may have conflicts with friends, which can undermine her self-esteem. She may be excluded from a circle that she really wants to be a part of, leading to unhappiness and loneliness. Parents and family will also have to deal with the stresses associated with their child's peer relationships.

During these years, parents need to monitor their child's choice of friends and supervise, but do not interfere with, her play activities. Parents of different children can talk and share observations among themselves about the children's activities. Offer support, understanding, and guidance to the child when problems arise in her peer relationships. When a conflict occurs, try to understand how the child feels about it, and what she sees as the factors contributing to it. Then discuss how the other child might view the problem, and together work out ways to resolve the conflict. At the same time keep in mind that the family cannot solve every peer-related difficult.

Toward the end of the school-period children will learn how to get along with their own and other groups and to follow the rules of the larger society. So, parents can offer support and guidance, conveying their own values and expectations along with giving independence to the child when it is needed.

School

School assumes a central role in youngster's life when she reaches the age of five or six, drawing much of her attention and energy away from the family unit. The school is the institution in society specifically designed as the formal instrument for educating its children. Children's elementary-school years can become a time of enormous satisfaction and excitement. As she learns to read and master other academic skills, she will develop a love of learning and a pride in her achievements. This can contribute to her self-esteem, not only because of her accomplishments in the classroom but also as she separates successfully from the home environment. In the process her teacher can become a source of support and an important role model in her life.

The extent to which a child acquires a good self-concept, a sense of personal worth, and a respect for the contribution of others is an important measure of the effectiveness of the school program. The purpose of school is to help each child to develop his potential to the fullest. This includes helping each child develop his sense of industry. The communication skills and the arithmetic fundamentals are the basic tools for achieving this objective. In the school child learns to think critically, to make judgments based on reasons, to accept criticism, to cooperate, and to be both a leader and a follower as the occasion warrants. They also learn the 'rules' of displaying emotion, which is a form of social and emotional development too. The ability to suppress negative emotions is a factor of normal development, as well as other influences, such as gender, the specific situation, cultural influences, and the person likely to receive the expressed emotion.

For some children, however, school may cause frustration and stress. Learning disabilities can interfere with the joy of learning. Poor study habits and/or a lack of motivation can create academic difficulties. Sometimes youngsters may have a poor relationship with their teachers, or they may experience separation anxiety that can interfere with their school attendance.

To make own child's education as positive and productive as possible, parents can closely monitor her academic progress and social adjustment, and get to know her teacher. Discussing with the child what she is learning in the classroom and how she feels about school can be explored by parents. The child can be encouraged to demonstrate her newly learned skills and to practice them in home. Supervising child's homework (but parent should not do it for her), and make sure she is preparing herself well for tests. Parents can set limit on the amount of television she watches and encourage her to read, write, and express herself creatively through hobbies and sports. If she (or her teacher) reports any problem areas, parents can communicate openly with school personnel, and try to figure out how best to help the youngster overcome her difficulties.

School-age children will have many experiences in different social contexts. Whether in the classroom or while playing with friends, a school-age child will experience a roller coaster of emotions. It is important that to re-assure a school-age child through positive interactions, giving them a certain amount of freedom and not to become over critical. This is an important stage in their social and emotional development as they start to explore their social awareness.

Physical, Social, Mental Development

The school-age years are a time of steady growth and development. In contrast to the rapid physical growth and development experienced during infancy and

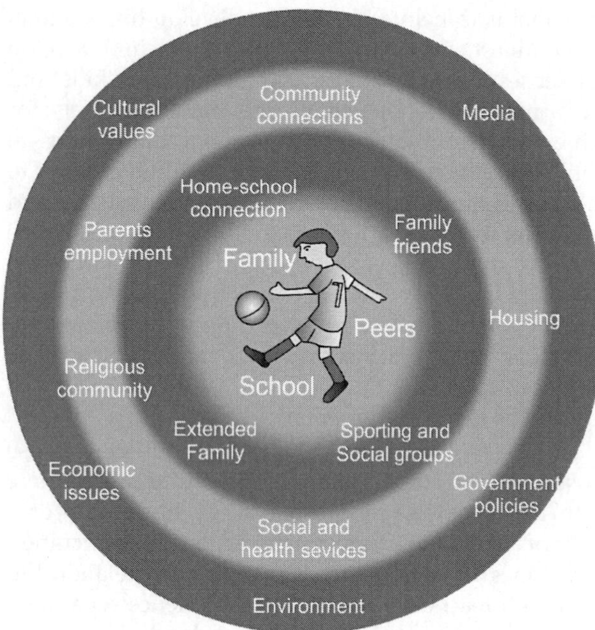

Fig. 5.61: A diagram showing influences of family, school and peers on social development

adolescence, the childhood years, loosely defined as the years between 2 and 11, are typically characterized by much slower and more stable physical growth. He tends to lose the thin, wiry appearance of the earlier years. On average, children gain 4 to 7 pounds and gain 1 to 4 inches per year. At approximately age 10 or 11 the rate of growth once again begins to increase, an indication that the child will soon enter puberty. Muscular coordination improves steadily, previous 'lordosis' posture changes to good posture, the eruption of permanent teeth starts, the vital signs approach to adult norms. The physical changes which indicate pubescence may begin to appear toward the end of the school-age.

Staying physically active during this developmental phase will strengthen the fundamental skills needed to lead a healthy and active life as an adult (Fig. 5.61). Learning and developing these skills will also have a tremendous impact on the children's confidence and self-esteem, as well as providing them with an ongoing sense of accomplishment and independence.

Milestones

5 to 6-year-olds

- Gain up to 2.3 kilograms (five pounds) per year
- Grow approximately 8 centimeters (three inches) per year
- Demonstrate a preference for being right-handed or left-handed
- Can color between the lines, print name legibly, and manage fasteners like zippers, buttons, and snaps independently
- Can catch and throw a medium-sized ball from 1.5 meters (five feet) away
- Can manage playground equipment independently, such as pumping legs on a swing
- Develop enough muscle coordination to climb, swim, and skate.

7 to 8-year-olds

- Weight gain speeds up
- Sleep up to 11 hours a night
- Begin riding a two-wheeler bicycle without training wheels
- Can use a pair of scissors to cut out complex shapes
- Permanent teeth begin to appear
- Improved hand-eye coordination (can bounce and catch a tennis ball).

Social Development

Social and emotional developments are strongly linked with so many things. Parents and other caregivers play an important role in emotional development, but as a child's world expands, other people in the social context also play a part in emotional development.

In school the child has an opportunity to widen his social contacts while he develops his mental abilities. He communicates needs and emotions to others under supportive and fairly positive situations; may be explosive under stress. Demonstrates the ability to work with a peer, and can both lead and follow. In play activities, may be bossy and demand own way, as well as tease or be critical of others and participates in simple group games and board games.

The school hours of the six-year-old in many places are shorter than those of older school children. This makes the transition from home to school life and the adjustment to new experiences easier for the child. They identify close friends on the basis of proximity and frequency of interaction (e.g. neighbors, school peers). Shares food and toys with friends. Friendships at this age have little permanent status and are easily established and terminated. There is little sense of liking or disliking the stable personal traits of another child. The children of this age are aware that other people have different perspectives, thoughts and feelings about ideas and circumstances. They develop the ability to resolve conflict in socially-acceptable ways, want to make up with others when there is a fight. Most conflict resolution at this age typically involves adult help or separation from peers.

Cognitive Development

Piaget referred to the cognitive development occurring between ages 7 and 11 as the **concrete operations stage.** During school-age, the child gives up to a large extent his earlier preoperational egocentricity. Transition into the school-age years coincides with a shift from an egocentric way of thinking(which is not to be confused with selfishness, but rather a child's inability to put themselves in other people's shoes), to a more mature, perceptive, and imaginative way of thinking. The child will demonstrate a genuine enthusiasm for learning new concepts, make strides in gaining self-confidence, and develop the necessary skills to understand the world and people around them, throughout this developmental phase. At age 5, usually children enter kindergarten, their first taste of the world of school. And by age 8, they will function on a higher level to properly articulate their feelings, a range of ideas, and effectively solve problems through dialogue.

School-age children think systematically about multiple topics more easily than preschoolers. Older children have keener **metacognition**, a sense of their own inner world. These children become increasingly skilled at problem-solving. Piaget noted that children's thinking processes change significantly during the concrete operations stage. School-age children can engage in **classification,** or the ability to group according to features, and **serial ordering,** or the ability to group according to logical progression. Older children come to understand cause-and-effect relationships and become adept at mathematics and science. He is thus able to solve an abstract problem when it deals with concrete objects. Comprehending the concept of **stable identity**—that one's self remains consistent even when circumstances change—is another concept grasped by older children. For example, older children understand the stable identity concept of a father maintaining a male identity regardless of what he wears or how old he becomes. Their mental ability permit them to explore more facets of objects and situations beyond their environment. They are able to do **thinking and reasoning,** and a new world of logical operations opens before them.

Development of Sexuality in the School-age Child

Children's sexual awareness starts in infancy and continues to strengthen throughout preschool and school-age years. All aspects of children's development—including cognitive, language, motor, social, emotional, and sexual development—are linked to each other. During the beginning of the school-age period the child has emerged from or is in the process of resolving his oedipal situation. The child is moving away from the intense psychosexual upheaval of the genital period and into a somewhat quieter period, termed latency. In the latency period, it is important for the child to have the parent of the same sex in the home in order for proper identification to occur. During the early latency period children associate with same sex peers and tend to ignore members of the opposite sex.

School-age children may play sexual games with friends of their same sex, touching each other's genitals and/or masturbating together. Most sex play at this age happens because of curiosity. Girls become more hesitant about participation in these activities. But boys tend to surpass girls in their level of sexual activity, may be caused by social pressure from the group.

Sexual development and sexual play are natural and healthy processes in children, from toddlers through childhood and into adolescence. For infants and toddlers, this usually involves body sensations, cuddling and touch, and playing with toys. Puberty, the time when the body matures, begins between the ages of nine and 12 for most children. Girls begin to grow breast buds and public hair as early as nine or 10. Boys' development of penis and testicles usually begins between 10 and 11. Children become more self-conscious about their bodies at this age and often feel uncomfortable undressing in front of others, even a same-sex parent.

Every day, parents around the world are faced with situations like young children's self-exploration and curiosity about body parts and sexual issues is one of the uncomfortable realities of parenting and can raise troubling questions, such as, 'Is my child normal?' 'Should I be worried?' 'What should I say?' In these situations, parents may feel awkward to talk with children about bodily changes and sexual matters. But providing children with accurate, age-appropriate information is one of the most important things parents can do to make sure children grow up safe, healthy, and secure in their bodies.

Promoting Optimal Health of School Child

Parents/care provider, can meet child's physical and biological needs by providing nutritious and healthy food, a regular wake and sleep routine, cleanliness with baths or showers, health with regular medical checkups and making sure the child gets enough exercise to remain physically fit.

Physical Care

Children in this age are fairly self-sufficient in bathing, dressing, and toileting, but need some help in maintaining neatness, cleanliness, etc. They may still need reminders to brush their teeth or wash their hands thoroughly. There are children who resent if their mother try to clean ears, comb hair or brush teeth. Sex differences are apparent, and girls are more careful of their appearance than boys are.

Nutrient Needs

School-age children are capable of understanding the role of nutrition in health. As a result, nutrition education messages provided at school can help children understand the importance of good nutrition. It is important for school-age children to meet the recommended intake levels of all essential vitamins and minerals. The nutrients highlighted below are of special importance:

Calories: Caloric needs vary depending on the child's current rate of growth, the amount of physical activity, and the child's metabolism. It is important that children consume enough calories to ensure proper growth and to spare protein from being used for energy. However, many children, especially those who are not physically active, tend to consume too many calories. Children aged 2 to 3 years, 4 to 6 years, and 7 to 10 years require approximately 1300, 1800, and 2000 calories, respectively.

Protein: The amount of protein needed per kilogram of body weight decreases after infancy and early childhood, from 1.2 gram/kg at 3 years to 1 gram/kg at 10 years.

Fat: Many children consume too much dietary fat, which can lead to excessive calorie consumption and weight gain. As a result, nutrition experts believe that by the age of 5, children should follow adult recommendations for the consumption of fat. These recommendations suggest that total fat intake not exceed 30% of calories and saturated fat should account for no more than 10% of total calories. In addition, cholesterol intake should not exceed 300 mg per day.

Fiber: With the growing recognition of the importance of dietary fiber to health, children, like adults, are encouraged to increase their dietary fiber intake. Children should consume their age plus 5 grams of fiber per day.

Calcium: Calcium is necessary for proper bone growth and maintenance of bone density. For school-age children need calcium from 500 mg per day to 1300 mg per day. This has been recognized on the basis of the fact that childhood is an important time for increasing bone density, and increasing bone density during childhood can help prevent osteoporosis later in life.

Parents/primary caregivers can go through the dietary principles.

- Allow the child to respond to their internal cues for hunger. Prepare healthy snacks and meals, but do not demand that child eat a certain amount of food at one sitting. Forcing a child to clean his/her plate, is a mistake, which can set the child up for a lifetime of overeating.
- High-calorie, high-fat, and sugary snacks is to be minimized. These foods lack essential nutrients and will diminish the child's desire to eat at mealtime.
- A child is to be encouraged to try new foods and continue to make available those foods that are not well-liked. The child may respond to these foods more favorably if they are given when the child is hungry. So the child's least favorite foods should be served at the beginning of the meal.
- The mealtime environment should be full of fun and relaxing, and allow the child to eat at his/her own pace. It will be easier for the child to stay focused on eating if parents can limit distractions and stressful situations during mealtimes, such as television, family arguments, and discipline.
- Many children like to work in the kitchen. A child can be allowed to help prepare snacks and meals.

It is an understatement to say that television influences the food choices of children. On average, today's children spend more time watching television than they spend at school, or doing any other activity besides sleeping. Consequently, children are bombarded with commercials, many of which advertise food.

During the school-age years, children begin to spend more time away from home, either at school or at the homes of their friends. Consequently, factors outside of the home start to influence food choices, which can have either a negative or positive impact on nutrition.

In many cases, peers reinforce poor food choices and contribute to negative body image. In fact, research suggests that the preoccupation with weight and body shape that is typically characteristic of the adolescent years may actually begin in elementary school.

The eating habits and attitudes about food displayed by parents have tremendous influence on the food choices of children. In fact, the food likes and dislikes that become firmly established during childhood are, to a large extent, shaped by the food likes and dislikes of parents.

Sleep

School-aged children need between 10 and 11 hours of sleep per night. Not getting enough sleep is common in this age group for variety of reasons such as, increasing school homework, evening activities, and later bedtimes. Sleep deprivation may cause school-aged child to be moody, irritable, and cranky. In addition, he may have a difficult time regulating his mood, such as by getting frustrated or upset more easily. Sleep-deprived kids can become hyper or irritable, and may have a hard time paying attention in school. Inadequate sleep may result in problems with attention, memory, decision-making, reaction time, and creativity, all which are important in school.

The sleep of the school child is rarely quiescent. Common sleep problems are sleepwalking, sleep terrors, night time fears, snoring, and noisy breathing. The bed time hour should be a quiet time. It is still important to have a consistent bedtime, especially on school nights. Leave enough technology-free time before bed to allow the child to unwind before lights-out. A good rule of thumb is switching off the electronics at least an hour before bed and keeping TVs, computers, and mobile devices out of kids' bedrooms. School-aged children continue to benefit from a bedtime routine that is the same every night and includes calm and enjoyable activities. Including one-on-one time with a parent is helpful in maintaining communication with child and having a clear connection every day.

Exercise

Children who are physically active are more likely to be academically motivated and alert in school, according to the National Association for Sport and Physical Education. To be active is a key part of good health for all school-age kids (Fig. 5.62). Exercise strengthens their muscles and bones and ensures that their bodies are capable of doing normal kid stuff, like lifting a backpack or running a race. It also helps control their weight and decreases their risk of chronic illnesses, such as high blood pressure and type 2 diabetes. There are several hypothesized mechanisms for why exercise is beneficial for cognition, including (Table 5.3):

- Increased blood and oxygen flow to the brain
- Increased levels of norepinephrine and endorphins resulting in a reduction of stress and an improvement of mood
- Increased growth factors that help to create new nerve cells and support synaptic plasticity.

But as children get older, increasing demands on their time can make getting that hour of exercise a challenge. Some of them get caught up in sedentary pursuits like watching TV, playing video games, and surfing the internet. Doing a lot of studying and reading, while important, but it can add to a lack of physical activity.

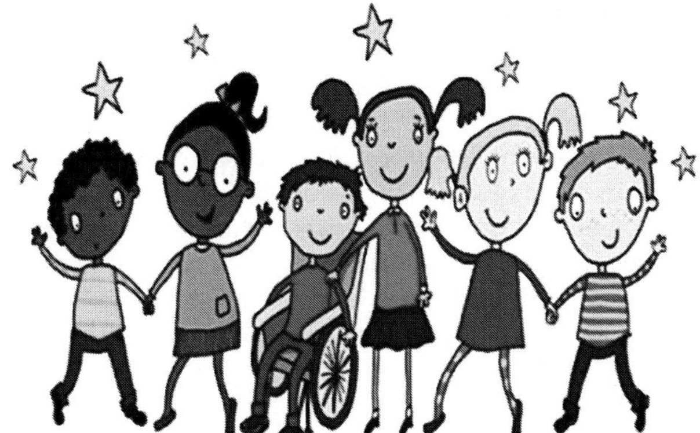

Fig. 5.62: Group activity in school

Table 5.3: Benefits of exercises in children

Reduce risk of metabolic disease: Diabetes and prediabetes	Improve sleep	Stronger bones	Reduce restlessness or hyperactivity; helps decrease symptoms of ADHD
Improve immune system function	Improve mood	Weight loss	Increase energy levels

Abbreviation: ADHD = Attention deficit hyperactivity disorder

Children and young people aged 5 to 18 should do at least 60 minutes of aerobic activity everyday. This should include moderate intensity and vigorous intensity activities. Parents can help by encouraging child to find activities they enjoy, and by building physical activity into family life. Child may like team sports, such as football, basket ball and volleyball, they can also be in other activities like dance, martial arts, or it may be simply running around a park/playground.

Health Check-up

Developmental monitoring and screening of children are done by a number of professionals in health care, community, and school settings.

Early identification of developmental disorders is critical to the well-being of children and their families. It is an integral function of the school health program and other mother and child health programs to provide primary care for children. The school health program is a national program and the main purpose of the program is to maintain, improve and promote the health of every school child. A coordinated school health program consists of comprehensive school health education, physical education, families and community involvement in school health, school health services, school nutrition services, school psychological counseling, healthy school environment and health promotion of staff. It is an approach where the health care team works in partnership with members of educational team and a child and a child's family, to assure that all of the medical and non-medical needs of the child are met.

It recommends that developmental surveillance, which is the process of recognizing children who might be at risk for developmental delays or having different challenges be incorporated at every routine school health program and well-child preventive care visit. This surveillance should include asking about parents' concerns, obtaining a developmental history, making observations of the child, identifying risk and protective factors, and documenting the findings. Any concerns should be addressed promptly with developmental screening tests, i.e. standardized tools to identify and refine any risk or concern that has been noticed.

If a potential developmental problem is noted on the screening test, further developmental and medical evaluation needs to follow. The more detailed evaluation will show whether the child has a developmental disorder or delay and needs treatment, including early developmental intervention services. Children diagnosed with developmental disorders are considered to be children with special health care needs, and their care needs to be managed like the care of children with other chronic conditions (*See* Chapter 6).

HEALTH PROBLEMS DURING SCHOOL-AGE

Child may have a health condition that does not last long but still interferes with her functioning at school. This kind of problem should be brought to the attention of the school nurse, the teacher, or the principal. For instance:

Hearing loss related to an ear infection could require a temporary change of seats to the front of the classroom.

Some infections—especially an ear infection, strep throat, bronchitis, and sinusitis—may necessitate the administration of medication for a week after the child is well enough to return to school.

If any child has a readily visible problem—like a rash, conjunctivitis, or unusual bruises—that has already been evaluated by family physician, let the school staff know about the doctor's diagnosis and treatment. Thus, school personnel will not have to pursue further evaluation of the youngster, which may disrupt her classroom work and unnecessarily concern her.

Exposure to communicable diseases is an important health problem of the school child (*See* Chapter 20). The parents must be informed about of the school regulations to keep the child at home and thus to prevent exposing others.

If any child has an injury or illness that requires immobilization or limitations on physical activity, the school is to decide about alternative activities available during physical education classes and recess.

To meet the needs of the handicapped child in the school is another challenge for school personnel. They are kept informed of the total rehabilitation program being carried out and their specific part in it.

Older school children need orientation about the physical changes they will experience at puberty. Both sexes are informed about this to lessen their stress and anxiety. Parents can talk over this matters to keep good parent child relationships. The school health nurse, or a teacher may also discuss them individually or in class. Sometimes parents seek help from the school nurse or pediatrician in order to help them educate their own children.

Schools can have a major effect on children's health. Schools can teach children about health, and promote healthy behaviors (Figs 5.63A and B). Schools work to prevent risky behaviors such as *alcohol* and *tobacco* use, or *bullying,* encourage healthy habits like exercise and healthy eating, deal with specific health problems in students, such as asthma, obesity and infectious diseases.

In all countries, poverty presents a chronic stress for children and families that may interfere with successful adjustment to developmental tasks, including school achievement. Children raised in low-income families are at risk for academic and social problems as well as poor health and well-being, which can in turn undermine educational achievement.

Poverty and Development of School Child

In all countries, poverty presents a chronic stress for children and families that may interfere with successful adjustment to developmental tasks, including school achievement. Children in poverty are at much greater risk of never attending school. Children are raised in low-income families are at risk for academic and social problems as well as poor health and well-being, which can in turn undermine educational achievement.

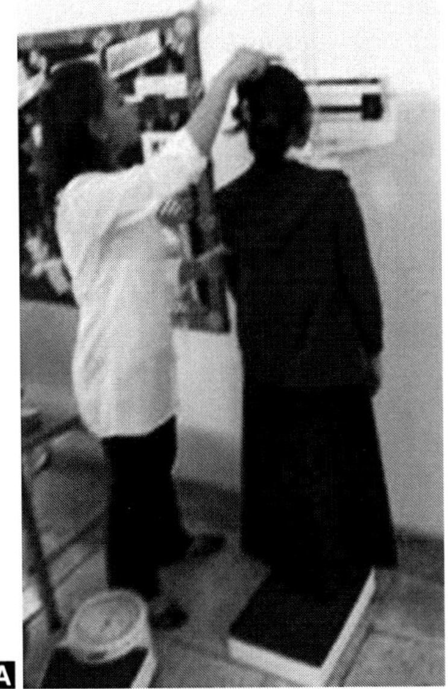

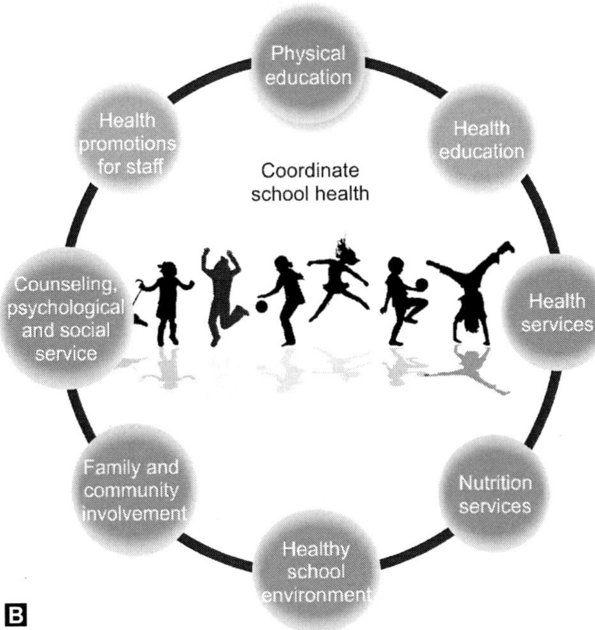

Figs 5.63A and B: A. Health check-up in school; **B.** Coordinated school health program

Poverty is clearly a risk factor for children's poor development and limited educational outcomes, and it may be that risk in the early years will continue to have an effect even if the family moves out of poverty later in the child's life.

Adolescence

Adolescence is considered as a period of transition from childhood to adulthood involving multiple physical, intellectual, personality, and social developmental changes. Adolescence, these years from puberty to adulthood, may be roughly divided into three stages: *early* adolescence, generally ages eleven to fourteen; *middle* adolescence, ages fifteen to seventeen; and *late* adolescence, ages eighteen to twenty-one. In addition to physiological growth, seven key intellectual, psychological and social *developmental tasks* are squeezed into these years. The fundamental purpose of these tasks is to form one's own identity and to prepare for adulthood.

Adolescence: Importance and Impace
• Adolescent population in India—22 to 23% • A large number of them lack formal/informal educate • Many reject schooling and work in unsuperivised unsafe conditions • Many suffer from malnutrition • Early marriage and impact on demography • Habits and behavior picked up-lifelong impact • Sexual experimentation push in vulnerable condition. **Safe and supportive environment needed for development**

CHANGES DURING ADOLESCENCE (FIG. 5.64)

Social Changes

The physical, cognitive, and socio-emotional changes are universal in adolescence. However, the context in which they occur is different from one adolescent to the other and greatly influenced by culture, family, school, peers, etc.

Puberty in Girls and Boys

Puberty is the period of sexual maturation and achievement of fertility. Puberty begins when the pituitary gland begins to stimulate the production of the male sex hormone *testosterone* in boys and the female sex hormones *estrogen* and *progesterone* in girls. The release of these sex hormones triggers the development of the *primary sex characteristics, the sex organs concerned with reproduction*. Puberty is associated with the development of secondary sex characteristics and rapid growth. Teenage bodies undergo dramatic changes, though the time when puberty begins varies greatly among individuals; however, puberty usually occurs in girls

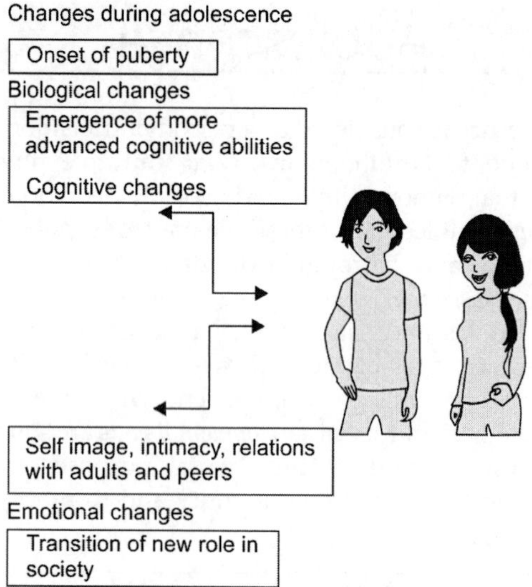

Fig. 5.64: Changes during adolescence

between the ages of 10 and 14 and between the ages of 12 and 16 in boys. Both genetic and environmental factors are likely involved in the timing of puberty. Body fat and/or body composition may play a role in regulating the onset of puberty. By mid-adolescence, if not sooner, most youngsters' physiological growth is complete; they are at or close to their adult height and weight, and are now physically capable of reproduction.

In 1962, James Tanner published a sexual maturity rating system. The scale ranges from prepubertal (stage I) to adult (stage V). For girls, the stages of puberty are based on breast size (B) and shape, and pubic hair (P) development and distribution. For boys, the stages of puberty are based on the genitalia (G) (size and shape of the penis and scrotum) and on pubic hair (P) development and distribution.

Changes in Girls

The onset of sexual maturation in girls usually begins about two years earlier than it does in boys (between 10 to 14 years). An increase in height usually begins at age 10 to 11 and continues to age 15 to 16. Breast development usually begins at age 10 to 11, but it may start as early as 8 or may not occur until age 14 or 15. One breast may start to develop before the other. The emergence of body hair usually begins in the pubic area about the same time as breast development, usually starting at age 10 or 11. Underarm and leg hair appears a year to two later. In general the color, thickness, and pattern of body hair is quite variable.

Menstrual periods usually begin between ages 11 and 14, about one year after breasts begin to develop. On average, a menstrual period occurs every 28 days and lasts 4 days, although periods occurring 23 to 35 days apart and lasting 2 to 7 days are still considered normal. Painful menstrual cramps, or dysmenorrhea, are unusual during the first year or two of menstruation but may occur in later adolescence.

During the first year or two after menarche (the first menstrual period), an adolescent girl may experience irregular periods, skipping one or many months between periods. It can take a while for the hypothalamus, to coordinate the release of the various hormones that control the menstrual cycle.

An increase in weight and body fat begins at ages 10 to 11, when female hormones trigger an increase in fat in the breasts, hips, thighs, and buttocks. Fat makes up about 25% of total body weight in girls, compared to 15 to 20% in boys.

The development of sweat glands, which are responsible for increased perspiration, usually begins at age 12 to 13. These glands can cause underarm odor (which is not present in young children), and pimples in adolescent girls.

Changes in Boys

Growth in teenage boys occurs in spurts, generally over four to five years. The first growth spurt may start anytime between ages 10 and 14. The following changes occur in a boy's physical development.

- *Secondary sex characteristics:* The testicles, penis, and scrotum enlarge, starting at about age 12 to 13. The skin of the scrotum and penis also darkens, and about a year after the penis begins to lengthen, most boys are able to ejaculate semen for the first time. Genital growth is usually completed by age 17
- Breasts can get 'lumps' and become tender
- *Height and weight increase:* An increase in height usually begins at age 12 or 13 and continues until age 17 or 18.
- Muscles develop
- Wet dreams occur
- *Voice cracks and gets deeper:* The larynx, or voice box, begins to grow at age 13 or 14; approximately a year later the voice begins to deepen.
- Skin and hair become more oily
- The development of sweat glands, which are responsible for increased perspiration, usually begins at ages 13 to 15. These glands can cause underarm odor (which is not present in younger children). Pimples may appear

- *Body hair:* Body hair appears, usually beginning in the pubic area at ages 11 to 12. Hair is first visible on skin around the base of the penis, then thickens and extends to the scrotum. Underarm hair subsequently develops at age 13 to 15, along with the first appearance of facial hair (which generally develops more slowly than other body hair). The color, pattern, and thickness of body hair varies considerably from person to person.

Cognitive Development

Cognitive Development
• It is the emergence of the ability to think, reason and understand. • And it is said that 'Adolescene marks the beginning development of more complex thinking processes called formal logical operations'. • Jean Piaget's theory has become one of the most influential theories of cognitive development.

Cognitive development refers to the development of the ability to think and reason. Children (6 to 12 years old) develop the ability to think in concrete ways (concrete operations), such as how to add, subtract, transform, etc. As the body changes and grows during adolescence, the brain undergoes significant changes as well. Rapid cognitive changes occur during childhood, the brain continues to develop throughout adolescence. Specifically, certain areas of the brain grow and develop independent of one another during adolescence. Recent brain imaging studies have shown that the amygdala, which is influential in emotion regulation, develops earlier in adolescence and the cortex, which is influential in thinking and decision-making, occurs later in adolescence (Fig. 5.65).

The developing teenager acquires the ability to think systematically about all logical relationships within a problem. The transition from concrete thinking to formal logical operations occurs over time.

Developmental psychologist, Jean Piaget (*See* Chapter 4), posited that the hallmark of adolescence, from a cognitive perspective, is the ability to engage in formal operational thinking. In general, formal operational thinking involves the ability to understand abstract concepts and the ability to make predictions about future events. In the eyes of cognitive developmental psychologists, the ability to perform functions requiring formal operational thinking, such as developing theories and solving abstract problems, marks the transition into adolescence.

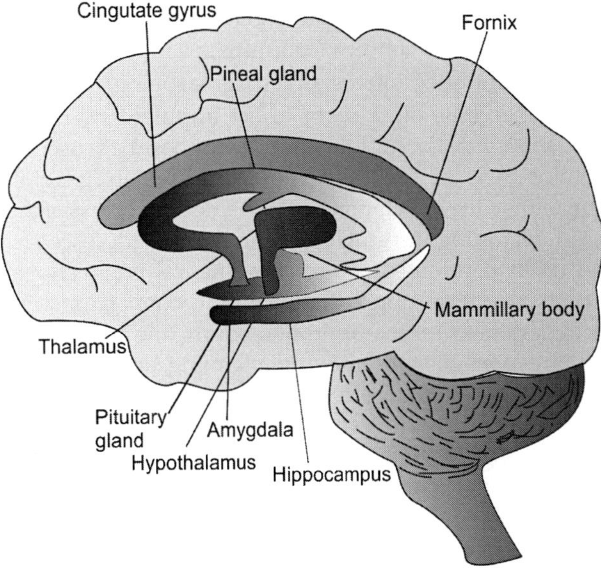

Fig. 5.65: The limbic system

Early adolescence: During early adolescence, the use of more complex thinking is focused on personal decision-making in school and home environments, including the following:

- Begin to demonstrate use of formal logical operations in schoolwork.
- Capacity for abstract thought grows in adolescence
- Mostly interested in present with limited thought to the future
- Intellectual interests expand and become more important
- The early adolescent begins to question authority and society standards
- Deeper moral thinking.

Middle adolescence: With some experience in using more complex thinking processes, the focus of middle adolescence often expands to include more philosophical and futuristic concerns, including the following:

- Continued growth of capacity for abstract thought
- Greater capacity for setting goals
- Interest in moral reasoning
- Thinking about the meaning of life.

Late adolescence: During late adolescence, complex thinking processes are used to focus on less self-centered concepts as well as personal decision-making, including the following:

- Ability to think ideas through
  - Ability to delay gratification
  - Examination of inner experiences
  - Increased concern for future
  - Continued interest in moral reasoning.

Adolescents often seem to act impulsively, rather than thoughtfully, and this may be in part because the development of the prefrontal cortex is, in general, slower than the development of the emotional parts of the brain, including the limbic system. During adolescence, the brain continues to form new neural connections, but also casts off unused neurons and connections. As teenagers mature, the prefrontal cortex, the area of the brain responsible for reasoning, planning, and problem-solving, also continues to develop; and myelin, the fatty tissue that forms around axons and neurons and helps speed transmissions between different regions of the brain, also continues to grow.

Furthermore, the hormonal surge that is associated with puberty, which primarily influences emotional responses, may create strong emotions and lead to impulsive behavior. It has been hypothesized that adolescents may engage in risky behavior, such as smoking, drug use, dangerous driving, and unprotected sex in part because they have not yet fully acquired the mental ability to curb impulsive behavior or to make entirely rational judgment.

The new cognitive abilities that are attained during adolescence may also give rise to new feelings of egocentrism, in which adolescents believe that they can do anything and that they know better than anyone else, including their parents. Teenagers are likely to be highly self-conscious, often creating an *imaginary audience* in which they feel that everyone is constantly watching them (Fig. 5.66). Because teens think so much about themselves, they mistakenly believe that others must be thinking about them, too. It is no wonder that everything a teen's parents do suddenly feels embarrassing to them when they are in public.

Healthy Cognitive Development During Adolescence

For positive and healthy cognitive development of adolescents few things are needed, like:

- Adolescents are to be included in discussions about a variety of topics, issues, and current events.
- Encourage adolescents to share ideas and thoughts with significant adults.

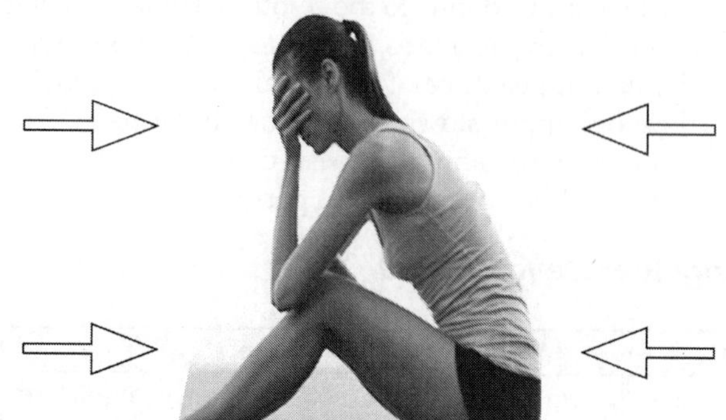

Fig. 5.66: Adolescents are highly sensitive to their immediate environment

- Encourage adolescents to think independently and develop their own ideas.
- Assist adolescents in setting their own goals.
- Stimulate adolescents to think about possibilities for the future.
- Compliment and praise adolescents for well-thought-out decisions.
- Assist adolescents in re-evaluating poorly made decisions for themselves.

The brain continues to develop throughout adolescence. Young people's ability for complex thought, specialized learning, risk assessment and behavior control is growing. These abilities are often sensitive to stress. Reasoning skills are maturing and adolescents may start to question their beliefs.

Emotional/Social Development

Emotional development during adolescence involves establishing a realistic sense of identity in the context of relating to others and learning to cope with stress and manage emotions, processes that are life-long issues for most people. Identity development is a stage in the adolescent life cycle. For most, the search for identity begins in the adolescent years. During these years, adolescents are more open to 'trying on' different behaviors and appearances to discover who they are. The social development of adolescents is best considered in the contexts in which it occurs; that is, relating to peers, family, school, work, and community.

Early Adolescence

- *Struggle with sense of identity:* Busy working out who they are and where they fit in the world. This search can be influenced by gender, peer group, cultural background and family expectations.

- *Body image:* Feel awkward about one's self and one's body; worry about being normal. They are more self-conscious, especially about physical appearance and changes. Teenage self-esteem is often affected by appearance, or by how teenagers think they look. As they develop, children might compare their bodies with those of friends and peers.
- Realize that parents are not perfect; increased conflict with parents; show more independence from parents.
- *Increased influence of peer group:* Spend less time with parents and more time with friends. Peer groups provide a temporary reference point for a developing sense of identity. Through identification with peers, adolescents begin to develop moral judgment and values.
- *Desire for independence:* He/she seeks more independence. This is likely to influence the decisions the child makes and the relationships the child has with family and friends.
- Tendency to return to 'childish' behavior, particularly when stressed.
- *Moodiness:* Adolescents show strong feelings and intense emotions at different times. Moods might seem unpredictable. These emotional ups and downs can lead to increased conflict. The child's brain is still learning how to control and express emotions in a grown-up way.
- *Rule and limit-testing:* Adolescent generally looks for new experiences. The nature of teenage brain development means that teenagers are likely to seek out new experiences and engage in more risk-taking behavior. But they are still developing control over their impulses.
- *Greater interest in privacy:* Adolescents like to stay alone, and fantasy becomes important element in their life.

Middle Adolescence

- Intense self-involvement, changing between high expectations and poor self-concept
- Continued adjustment to changing body, worries about being normal
- Tendency to distance selves from parents, continued drive for independence
- Driven to make friends and greater reliance on them, popularity can be an important issue. Feelings of love and passion. Dating typically begins in middle adolescence, usually between the ages of 14 and 16 years.

Late Adolescence

- Firmer sense of identity is developed
- Increased emotional stability
- Increased concern for others
- Increased independence and self-reliance
- Peer relationships remain important
- Development of more serious relationships
- Social and cultural traditions regain some of their importance.

Important Developmental Issues in Adolescence

Sense of Identity and the Sense of Intimacy

Identity refers to the sense of who they are as individuals and as members of social groups. The development of a strong and stable sense of self is widely considered to be one of the central tasks of adolescence. Egocentrism in adolescents forms a self-conscious desire to feel important in their peer groups and enjoy social acceptance. The adolescents must learn who they are and must modify their conscience for their adult role in life. Identity represents a coherent sense of self-stable across circumstances and including past experiences and future goals. Identity is dynamic and complex, and changes over time.

- Self-identity refers to how people define themselves. Self-identity forms the basis of person's self-esteem. In adolescence, the way they see themselves changes in response to peers, family, and school, among other social environments. Their self-identities shape their perceptions of belonging.
- Social identity is constructed by others, and may differ from self-identity. Typically, people categorize individuals according to broad, socially-defined labels.

Developing a sense of identity
Self-concept
• The cognitive aspect in which individuals have a perception about themselves, such as 'I am good at Math'.
Self-esteem
• The affective aspect in which an indivudual evaluates components of him/herself, such as 'I feel good about my math skills'.

After developing a sense of identity during early adolescence, they need to develop a sense of intimacy with selves and people of both sexes. Once the psychosocial crisis of this period has been handled successfully, the young person is capable of entering into a truly intimate relationship. Close relationships play an important role in psychosocial development in adolescence. Intimacy is the capacity to commit to one's self to another or to others and to continue the commitment. This increasing emphasis on intimacy in relationships is supported by the adolescent's social cognitive capabilities and the young person's growing independence. Adolescents, who report having at least one close friendship report higher levels of self-esteem than ones who do not.

Achievement of Autonomy/Independence from Parents

Autonomy refers to an individual's growing ability to think, feel, make decisions and act on his/her own. This is one of the most important tasks for all adolescents is learning the skills that will help them manage their own lives and make positive and healthy choices. Autonomy can be categorized as emotional autonomy, behavioral autonomy and value autonomy. It has special meaning during teen period as it signifies that an adolescent is a unique, capable, independent individual who depends less on parents and other adults.

Achieving independence is an essential part of child's journey to adulthood. To make this journey successfully, children need freedom to try new things. But they still need parents' guidance and support too. Adolescent-parental separation is part of the natural course of the life cycle. To become a capable adult, the child must learn to depend on parents less and take on more responsibility; make decisions and solve problems; work out life values; form his/her own identity.

Peer Group Identity

The peer group becomes an important part of socialization of children. A peer group is both a social group and a primary group of people who have similar interests (homophily), age, background, or social status. The members of this group are likely to influence the person's beliefs and behavior. Peer relationships provide a unique context for social and emotional development of a person enhancing persons' reasoning abilities, concern for others, cooperating with people. During adolescence, peer groups tend to face dramatic changes. Adolescents tend to spend more time with their peers and have less adult supervision. Adolescents' communication shifts during this time as well. They prefer to talk about school and their careers with their parents, and they enjoy talking about sex and other interpersonal relationships with their peers. Children look to join peer groups who accept them, even if the group is involved in negative activities. Children are less likely to accept those who are different from them.

Attributes of Peer Group

- The peer group becomes an important part of socialization
- Teach gender role
- Serve as a practicing venue to adulthood
- Teach unity and collective behavior in life
- Identity formation.

Negative Attributes

- Peer pressure
- Future problem
- Risky behavior
- Aggression and prosocial behavior
- Sexual promiscuity.

Body Image

Body image is the dynamic perception of one's body. It means how it looks, feels, and moves. It is shaped by perception, emotions, physical sensations, and is not static, but can change in relation to mood, physical experience, and environment.

Some people struggle with their self-esteem and body image when they begin puberty because it is a time when the body goes through many changes. These changes, combined with wanting to feel accepted by their friends, means it can be tempting to compare themselves with others. The trouble with that is, not everyone grows or develops at the same time or in the same way (Figs 5.67A to C).

During adolescence, young people often think a lot about how their bodies look. They also compare their bodies with others. A positive teenage body image is an important part of healthy self-esteem, and parents can help their child think and feel positively about his/her body.

Adolescence marks a time of rapid and intense emotional and physical changes. There is an increased value placed on peer acceptance and approval, and a heightened attention to external influences and social messages about cultural norms. Body image and related self-concept emerge as significant factors associated with health and well-being during this developmental phase, as youths begin to focus more on their physical appearance. How adolescents formulate and define their body image ideals and subsequent self-comparisons is

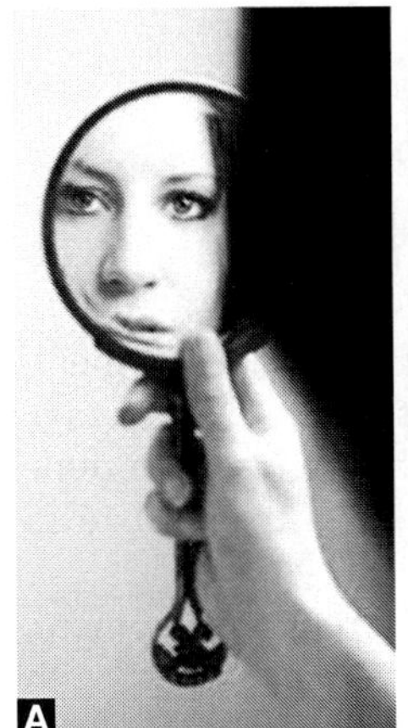

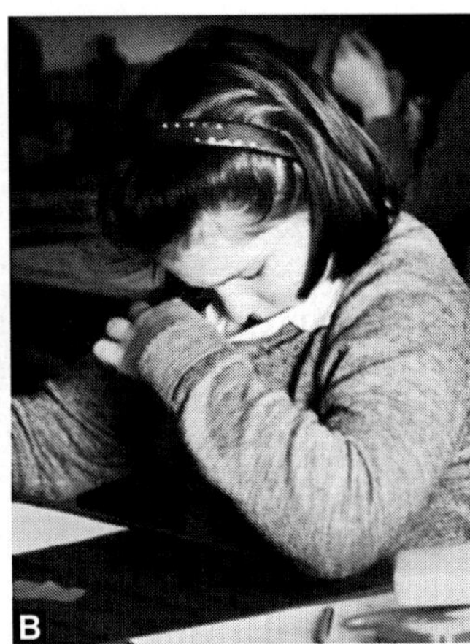

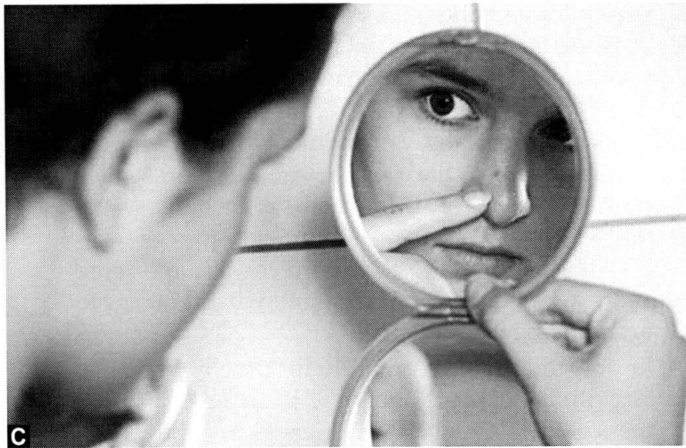

Figs 5.67A to C: Body image issues among young are influenced by peers, television. **A.** The child is concerned about look; **B.** She is worried regarding breast size; **C.** Adolescents are anxious about acne

strongly influenced by personal, familial, and cultural factors. A healthy body image in childhood can lay the foundations for good physical and mental health later in life. An unhealthy body image in childhood can have long-lasting consequences. Feeling of inferiority because of being unable to meet the expectations of peers can result in a distorted body image.

Whirlpool Emotion

Adolescents often seem to act impulsively, rather than thoughtfully, and this may be in part because the development of the prefrontal cortex is, in general, slower than the development of the emotional parts of the brain, including the limbic system. During adolescence, the brain continues to form new neural connections, but also casts off unused neurons and connections. As teenagers mature, the prefrontal cortex, the area of the brain responsible for reasoning, planning, and problem-solving, also continues to develop; and myelin, the fatty tissue that forms around axons and neurons and helps speed transmissions between different regions of the brain, also continues to grow.

Furthermore, the hormonal surge that is associated with puberty, which primarily influences emotional responses, may create strong emotions and lead to impulsive behavior. It has been hypothesized that adolescents may engage in risky behavior, such as smoking, drug use, dangerous driving, and unprotected sex in part because they have not yet fully acquired the mental ability to curb impulsive behavior or to make entirely rational judgment.

The new cognitive abilities that are attained during adolescence may also give rise to new feelings of egocentrism, in which adolescents believe that they can do anything and that they know better than anyone else, including their parents. Teenagers are likely to be highly self-conscious, often creating an *imaginary audience* in which they feel that everyone is constantly watching them. Because teens think so much about themselves, they mistakenly believe that others must be thinking about them, too. It is no wonder that everything a teen's parents do suddenly feels embarrassing to them when they are in public.

Sexual Identity and Roles

Sexual identity is a matter of forming an enduring recognition of the meaning of one's sexual feelings, attractions, and behaviors. Healthy sexual development involves biological, psychological, and sociocultural processes. Like all aspects of adolescent development, sexual development occurs both within an individual and through interaction with the environment. For example, the biological triggers of puberty are genetic, and are also affected by the other factors such as food, exercise. Psychological and social processes occur through interactions with family, peers, cultural institutions, and are also affected by brain development. Adolescent sexual development is likely to be healthy, and to lead to positive sexual health, when each of these processes is appropriately supported in a young person's environment.

Adolescent sexuality is sexual feelings, behavior and development in adolescents and a stage of human sexuality. The sexual behavior of adolescents is, in most cases, influenced by their culture's norms and mores, their sexual orientation, and the issues of social control such as age of consent laws.

Sexual orientation refers to whether a person's physical and emotional arousal is to people of the same or opposite sex. One does not have to be sexually active to have a sexual orientation. Sexual and affectional preferences are not always congruent. Those who are attracted primarily to the opposite sex are heterosexual, those attracted primarily to the same sex are homosexual (gay or lesbian) and those who are attracted to both sexes are bisexual. During adolescence, teens become more and more aware of their sexuality and what it means to be part of their gender.

In humans, mature sexual desire usually begins to appear with the onset of puberty. All adolescents are in a process of learning to relate to peers as friends, as well as potential romantic and sexual partners (Figs 5.68A to C). Sexual expression can take the form of masturbation or sex with a partner.

Sexual interests among adolescents can vary greatly, and they can adopt different risk taking behavior. The risks are elevated for young adolescents because their brains are not neurally mature; several brain regions in the frontal lobe of the cerebral cortex and in the hypothalamus important for self-control, delayed gratification, and risk analysis and appreciation are not fully mature. The creases in the brain continue to become more complex until the late teens, and the brain is not fully mature until age 25.

Putting all of these factors together, healthy adolescent sexual development occurs not along a single path, but through many trajectories. It involves much more than a teenager avoiding sexually transmitted infections or an unintended pregnancy between childhood and adulthood. Healthy adolescent sexual development trajectories prepare a person for a meaningful, productive, and happy life.

Sexual Behaviors

There are a variety of common behaviors that, in and of themselves, have no negative health effects, and that many consider elements of healthy adolescent sexual development, preparing youth for positive sexual lives.

- *Masturbation:* Touching one's own genitals in masturbation is a normal part of sexual development. Overall, more adolescents masturbate than engage in sexual intercourse. Although it tends to be done alone in privacy, males sometimes masturbate in groups.
- *Same-sex touching:* Early in adolescent development, sexual exploratory behavior often occurs with members of the same sex. This behavior does not predict being gay or lesbian in the future.
- *Genital touching:* As adolescents get older, they are more likely to engage in genital touching.

Sexual intercourse is a common behavior among adolescents, but whether it represents healthy sexual development or not depends on a number of factors. Nonconsensual sex of any kind can never be considered healthy. Use of contraception decreases the risk of pregnancy, and use of condoms or dental dams (in oral, vaginal, and anal sex) decreases the risk of disease, including HIV. Anal intercourse, whether heterosexual or homosexual, carries an especially high risk of disease transmission.

The adolescents, to function as effective and well-adjusted adults need to have clear, accurate information to understand the various aspects of sexuality, sexual roles and responsibilities. They need to learn negotiation skills to handle sexual demands that may be put on them or they may put on others. Other factors affecting the health consequences of sexual activity may include an individual's ability to access health care services,

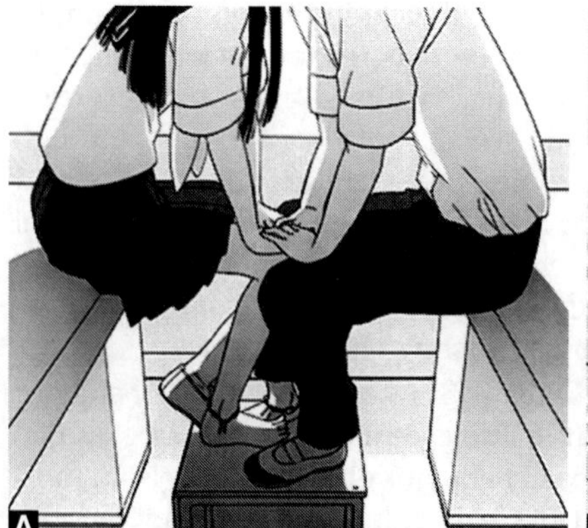

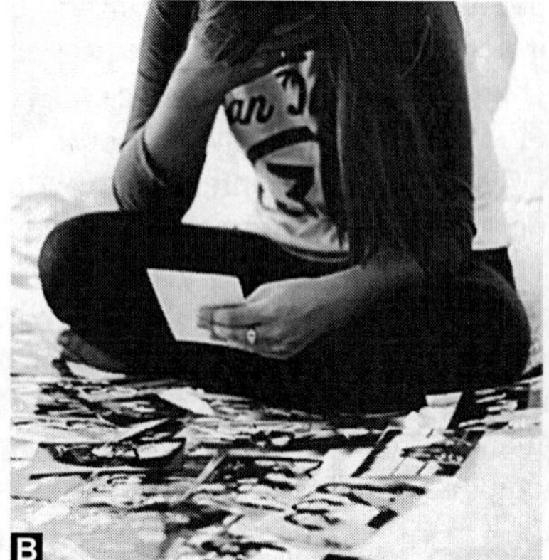

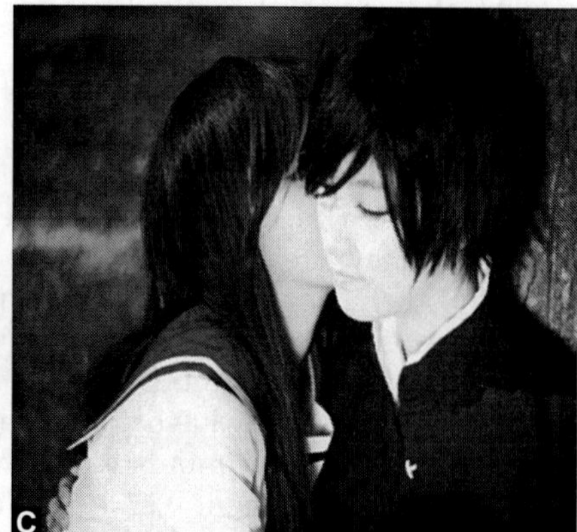

Figs 5.68A to C: All adolescents are in a process of learning to relate to peers as friends, as well as potential romantic and sexual partners

cultural and familial contexts, motivations and self-awareness, risk behaviors, mental health, relationships, personal values, maturity, and capacity for coping with the possible consequences of sex.

Theories of Adolescence

Primary theorist James Tanner: Focus of the period is physical/biological and sexual development determined by genes and biology.

Psychologist Sigmund Freud: Focus on adolescence as a period of sexual excitement and anxiety. ʻ

Psychosocialist Erik Erikson: Focus is on identity formation; adolescents struggle between achieving identity and identity diffusion.

Cognitive Jean Piaget: Focus is on formal operational thought; moving beyond concrete, actual experiences and beginning to think in logical and abstract terms.

U Bronfenbrenner: Focus is ecological (on the context in which between individual adolescents develop; adolescents are and environment) influenced by family, peers, religion, schools, the media, community, and world events.

Social cognitive Albert Bandura: Focus is on the relationship between learning social and environmental factors and their influence on behavior. Children learn through modeling (*See* Chapter 4).

Health Promotion and Anticipatory Guidance

Adolescents in our country are the least likely to access preventative health care; typically their visits are for illness that miss the components of a well-child exam. Several studies have shown that adolescents are interested and very willing to talk with health care providers about selective screening topics and anticipatory guidance, especially when completed within a private, confidential environment.

Unintentional injuries such as automobile crashes, intentional injuries such as homicide and suicide, depression and isolation; and reproductive health issues such as unintended pregnancy and sexually transmitted infections remain the leading causes of adolescent morbidity and mortality. Alcohol and drug use contribute to many of these injuries and deaths. Obesity has become a major cause of adolescent morbidity and is a contributor to a dramatic increase in the number of youth with type 2 diabetes mellitus. The common denominator in this list is that most adolescent morbidity and mortality is related to personal behavior and, as such, is preventable.

Adolescent frequently cannot find a place to receive care in the traditional health care delivery system. The challenge is to integrate preventive services into routine medical care. Practitioners can use clinic visits for routine examinations, such as pre-participation athletic evaluations and chronic disease management, to provide a range of preventive services. These clinical encounters offer an opportunity for early identification of risk behavior and disease, updating immunizations, and offering health guidance. Clinical preventive services are an adjunct to preventive interventions provided through schools and in the community.

Communication Method

With onset of adolescence the push for more independence, parent/child communication becomes more complicated than before. Young adolescents often are not great communicators, particularly with their parents and other adults who love them. Still family-centered, the child values the closeness with parents which talking with one another can create. More peer-centered, the adolescent wants more social independence which distance from parents can help establish.

Where the young child, to enjoy togetherness with them, usually wants a lot of communication and companionship with parents; the adolescent, to create more separation, usually wants significantly less.

Still family-centered, the child values the closeness with parents, in which talking with one another can create. More peer-centered, the adolescent wants more social independence which distance from parents and communication can become more complicated than before.

Psychologists have found that when parents know where their children are and what they are doing (and when the adolescent knows this monitoring), adolescents are at a lower risk for a range of bad experiences, including drug, alcohol and tobacco use; sexual behavior and pregnancy; and delinquency and violence. The key, according to psychologists, is to be inquisitive but **not interfering**, working to respect child's privacy as parents establish trust and closeness.

Guidance for Communication with Adolescents

- *No fixed rule for successful communication:* What works for getting one child to talk about what's important does not always work with another one. Parents should understand liking and attraction of the child, and foster it. It can encourage her/him to open up.
- *Listen:* To listen, means to avoid interrupting and it means to pay close attention. This is best done in a

quiet place with no distractions. Often just talking with child about a problem or an issue helps to clarify things. Sometimes the less parents offer advice, the more, young teen may ask parent for it. Listening can also be the best way to uncover a more serious problem that requires elders' attention.

- *Create opportunities to talk:* To communicate with child need to make parents/elders available. Young adolescents resist 'scheduled' talks; they do not open up when you tell them to, but when they want to. Many of the best conversations grow out of shared activities. It is observed that parents try to grab odd moments and have this deep communication with their child. It results in frustration because it does not happen.
- *Talk over differences:* Communication breaks down for some parents because they find it hard to manage differences with their child. It is often easiest to limit these differences when parents have put in place clear expectations. If a 13-year-old daughter knows she is to be home by 9:30 PM—and if she knows the consequences for not meeting this curfew—the likelihood that she will be home on time increases.

When differences arise, parents should tell the child about their concerns firmly but calmly. It can prevent differences from becoming battles. Explaining why the child made or wants to make a poor choice is more constructive: 'Dropping out of your algebra class will cut off lots of choices for you in the future. Some colleges would not admit you without two years of algebra, plus geometry and some trigonometry. Let's get you some help with algebra.'

- *Avoid over-reacting:* Responding too strongly can lead to yelling and screaming and it can shut down conversation. Parents should keep anxiety and emotions out of the conversation, then children will open up. Instead of getting riled up, it is better to ask, 'What do you think about what you did? Let's talk about this.

Kids are more likely to be open if they look at parent/teacher as somebody who is not going to spread their secrets or get extremely upset if they confess something to him/her. If the child says, 'I have got to tell you something. Friday night I tried beer,' and if the parent/teacher goes off the deep end, the kid would not tell it again.

At a time when they are already judging themselves critically, adolescents make themselves vulnerable when they open up to parents. We know that the best way to encourage a behavior is to reward it. If parents are critical when the teenager talks to them, what he sees is that his openness gets punished rather than rewarded.

- *Talk about things that are important to the young teen:* Different youngsters like to talk about different things. Some of the things they talk about may not seem important to parents, but they need to show interest by asking questions and listening, however, they can show respect his feelings and opinions.
- *Communicate with kindness and respect:* Young teens can say or do things that are outrageous or mean-spirited or both. However, hard child pushes parents buttons, it is best to respond calmly. The respect and self-control that parents display in talks with child may someday be reflected in her conversations with others. Kindness goes hand-in-hand with respect. Communicating with respect also requires not talking down to adolescents. They are becoming more socially conscious and aware of events in the world and they appreciate thoughtful conversations.

Physical Examination

Physical examination includes the adolescent's height and weight, and body mass index (BMI); which need to plot on chart. Share the information with the adolescent and family. As part of the complete physical examination, the following should be particularly noted:

- Sexual Maturity Rating (SMR) or Tanner stage. Evaluate if onset of puberty has not occurred in females by age 13 or in males by age 14.
- Scoliosis or kyphosis (screen males and females annually).
- Evidence of possible abuse or neglect.
- Evidence of eating disorders (e.g. extreme weight loss or gain, erosion of tooth enamel).
- Caries, developmental dental anomalies, malocclusion, gingivitis, pathologic conditions, or dental injuries.
- Acne and common dermatitis.
- Tattoos, piercing.

Excessive body hair (hirsutism). An external genital exam should be performed.

For females: Teach breast self-examination. Examine genitals for normal development. Check for condyloma/ lesions, vulvovaginitis. If adolescent is sexually active or has primary amenorrhea or menstrual complaints, perform a pelvic exam and evaluate.

For males: Teach testicular self-examination. Examine genitals for normal development. Check for varicoceles, hernias, condyloma/lesions, testicular cancer. (Risk criteria for testicular cancer include history of undescended testes, single testicle).

- Sports injuries, other orthopedic problems.

Nutrition

Adolescence is the period of growth spurt, so nutrient requirements increase during this period to support the dramatic growth and development (Fig. 5.69). They need to eat three meals per day and breakfast is especially important. Eating meals with family on a regular basis is important to cope up demands of this period. Adolescents need orientation to choose healthy nutritious snacks daily that are rich in complex carbohydrates and to limit high-fat or low-nutrient foods and beverages such as candy, chips, or soft drinks. Information regarding choosing plenty of fruits and vegetables; breads, cereals, and other grain products; low-fat dairy products; lean meats; and foods prepared with little or no fat are necessary. Foods rich in calcium, iodine, vitamin A and D and iron, zinc in adolescents' diet are necessary for physical as well as intellectual development.

Multi-sectoral approach to ensure adequate food supply, equity in food distribution, improved knowledge about nutrition and gender issue are important aspects in improving nutritional need of adolescents. Help them to achieve and maintain a healthy weight and to manage weight through appropriate eating habits and regular exercise. Nutrition promotion should include healthy eating habits and lifestyles, availability of food, nutritional supplementation, prevention and management of nutritional risks, proper information by the media, magazines and internet.

Dental Health

Tooth eruption is completed during adolescence. Dental decay is one of the leading diseases in adolescence which is caused by improper diet and inadequate cleansing. Poor oral hygiene can result in gingivitis. They need to brush teeth twice a day with fluoridated toothpaste, and floss daily. Health professionals can meet up the queries adolescents have about how to handle dental emergencies, especially the loss or fracture of a tooth.

Accident Prevention

The teenage years mark the real beginning of a person's growing independence. It is when a child begins to flap their wings in the process of leaving home. Lifelong decisions are made and influenced during this time. It is a time of great learning but also a time of great danger.

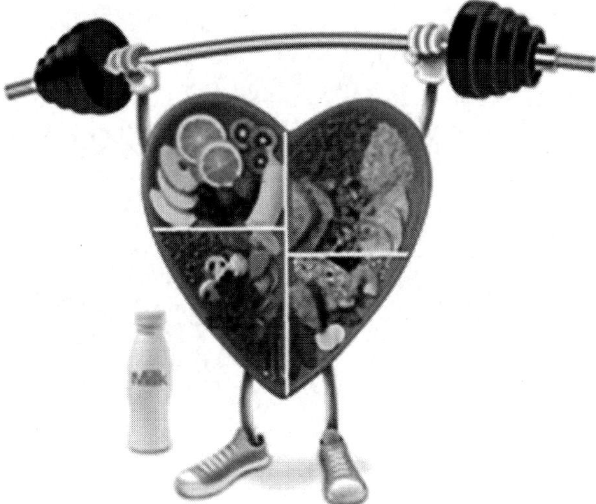

Fig. 5.69: Additional nutrition is necessary to support the dramatic growth and development during adolescence

Slightly more than 50% of all deaths among children between the ages of 1 to 14 years and almost 75% of deaths among youths aged between 15 and 24 years are not caused by disease. They are caused by injuries, which include unintentional injuries, suicides, and homicides. Data show clearly that child injuries take an unacceptably high toll on children's health and development and on society. Furthermore, if current trends continue, the global burden of injuries is expected to rise in the next 20 years. If the groundwork to prevent child injuries is not laid now, the processes that currently drive change in our world are likely to exacerbate the problem.

Adolescence is a developmental period characterized by behavior that involves taking risks, because 'invincible phenomenon' exists among them. Some of this behavior is associated with a misperception of the risks associated with certain activities (Figs 5.70A and B). Parents of teens have an important role to play in lessening the risk of road injuries in their children. They should try to provide vehicles for their children to drive that protect occupants well during crash, and restrict their teen's exposure to night driving, especially with other adolescent passengers.

Any parent who owns firearms should restrict their access by locking them in secured storage or placing them in a combination gun safe. It is recommended to avoid keyed devices because adolescents know where to find keys. If any member is a substance misuser or has a mental illness, firearms should be removed from that family.

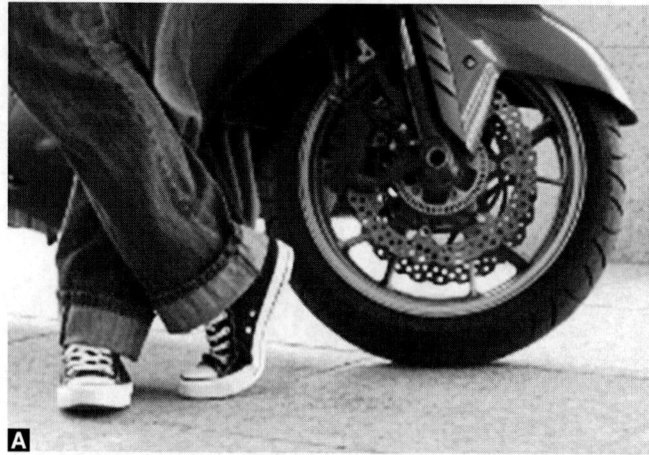

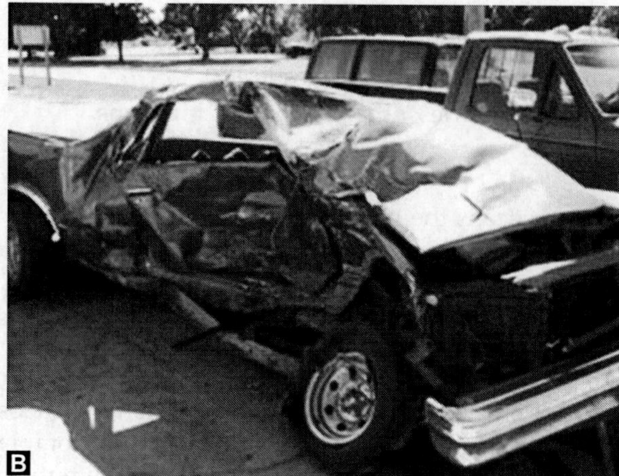

Figs 5.70A and B: Risky behavior and its consequences; **A.** Traffic accidents are the leading cause of death among adolescents between 17 and 21 years of age; **B.** Car crashes are the major cause of fatal head trauma among teens

Physicians can help by providing accurate information to both adolescents and their parents about the magnitude of risk reduction afforded by key measures designed to prevent injury.

Some processes such as globalization and urbanization may bring benefits that can bolster prevention efforts, e.g. increased resources, improvements in access to and quality of health services, knowledge transfer of effective injury prevention measures, and fostering a culture of safety. Without a concerted effort to harness these benefits in the implementation of child injury prevention measures, however, the negative effects of the processes will prevail.

Prevention of Risky Behavior

V–Identify–A problem adolescent
Self-concept
• **Behavior:** Agitation, restlessness, lack of concentration
• **Scholastic:** Drop in grades, adverse reports, abstinence
• **Addiction:** Tobacco, alcohol, drugs
• **Psychotic:** Hysterical, depression, suicidal thoughts
• **Organic:** Bed-wetting, stammering
• **Anti-social-Legal:** Fine, punishment, sexual crimes.

Taking risks is fairly common in adolescence. Risky behaviors precipitate serious, long-term, and—in some cases—life-threatening consequences. Preventing adolescent risky behaviors is important for several reasons. One is that engaging in a risky behavior can set the stage for engaging in other risky behaviors, thus increasing the likelihood of self-injury, victimization by others, and other negative consequences that result from these behaviors.

What makes an effective prevention intervention?

- Decreases risks factors, increases protective factors
- Address all forms of drug use
- Is tailored to the target population
- Establish norms and expectations
- Use cognitive-behavioral methods
- Emphasize development of social, communication and problem-solving skill
- Increase self-efficacy and drug resistance skills
- Take place at the level of school, family or community.

Some feasible strategies and relevant programs which can prevent risky behaviors are:

- Support and strengthen family functioning
- Increase connections between students and their schools
- Make communities safe and supportive for children and youth
- Promote involvement in high quality out-of-school-time programs
- Promote the development of sustained relationships with caring adults
- Provide children and youth opportunities to build social and emotional competence
- Provide children and youth with high quality education during early and middle childhood.

CHAPTER 6

Behavioral Pediatric and Pediatric Nursing

Chapter Outline

- Behavioral Pediatrics and Pediatric Nursing
- Common Behavioral Problems and Their Management
- Temper Tantrums
- Enuresis
- Toilet Training Difficulties
- Child Guidance Clinic
- Educational Guidance
- Role of a Pediatric Nurse in Child Guidance Clinic

BEHAVIORAL PEDIATRICS AND PEDIATRIC NURSING

According to 'Meeting Children's Needs' in *Principles of Parenting* by H. Wallace Goddard, a child development specialist, the way parents respond to their child's needs or demands teaches the child about the world he lives in and how to react to it. Children learn to feel safe, loved and emotionally supported from their parents. However, parents can identify their child's physical needs: nutritious food, warm clothes when it is cold, bedtime at a reasonable hour easily, but a child's mental and emotional needs may not be as obvious. Good mental health allows children to think clearly, develop socially and learn new skills. Children need the opportunity to explore and develop new skills and independence (Fig. 6.1). At the same time, children need to learn that certain behaviors are unacceptable and that they are responsible for the consequences of their actions. Additionally, good friends and encouraging words from adults are all important for helping children develop self-confidence, high self-esteem, and a healthy emotional outlook on life.

What is Behavioral Pediatrics?

Behavioral pediatrics is a stream of medicine which deals with developmental, learning, or behavioral problem of child. Developmental-Behavioral Pediatrics (DBP) is a unique area that focuses on a child's strengths and challenges within the context of the family using a biopsychosocial perspective. The experts possess training and experience to consider, in their assessments and treatments, the medical and psychosocial aspects of children's and adolescents' developmental and behavioral problems. They guide to early recognition and intervention in the significant problems increasingly affecting the emotional health of children and adolescents and thus to prevent mental illness.

Development and behavior of children happen first and foremost in the context of the family, so experts seek to understand the family's view of the problem and the effect of the child's problem on the family. Developmental-behavioral problems need to handle by working closely with schools, nursery, creche and other agencies involved with developmental care and education. Goddard, previously mentioned child development specialist adds that when parents/

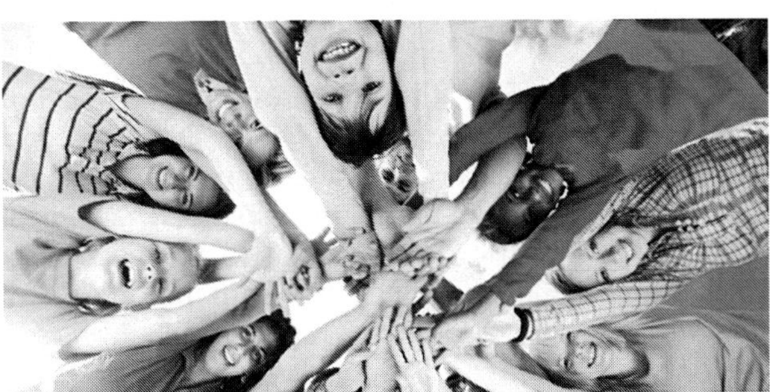

Fig. 6.1: Maximize physical and psychological potentialities of children

adults show concern and compassion in meeting their children's needs, they help them grow up to be stable, caring, healthy and independent adults. The lists of children's needs vary, but these five show up in each: physical needs, a sense of safety and security, affection, self-esteem and education and information.

Behavioral Pediatrics, the specialty within pediatrics focuses to:

- Understand the complex developmental processes of infants, children, adolescents, young adults and their families in the context of their families and communities
- Understand the biological, psychological, and social influences on development in the emotional, social, motor, language and cognitive domains
- On the mechanisms for primary and secondary prevention of disorders in behavior and development
- Identify and treat of disorders of behavior and development throughout childhood and adolescence.

Parent-Child Relationship

The parent-child relationship consists of a combination of behaviors, feelings, and expectations that are unique to a particular parent and a particular child (Figs 6.2A and B). The relationship between parent and the child is the most important relationship among the many different relationships people form over the course of the life span. Because the children who are loved, thrive better than those who are not. The relationship involves the full extent of a child's development.

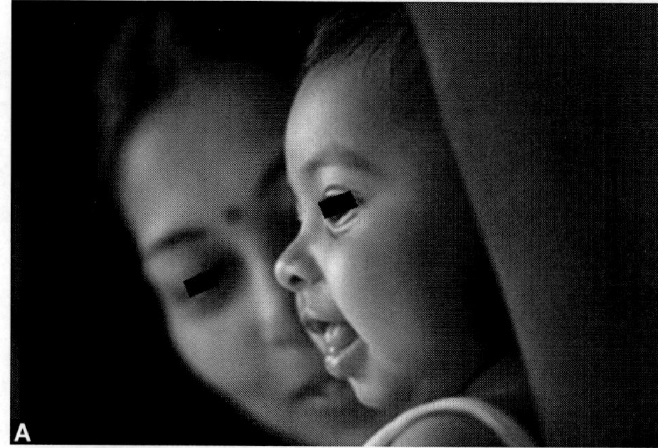

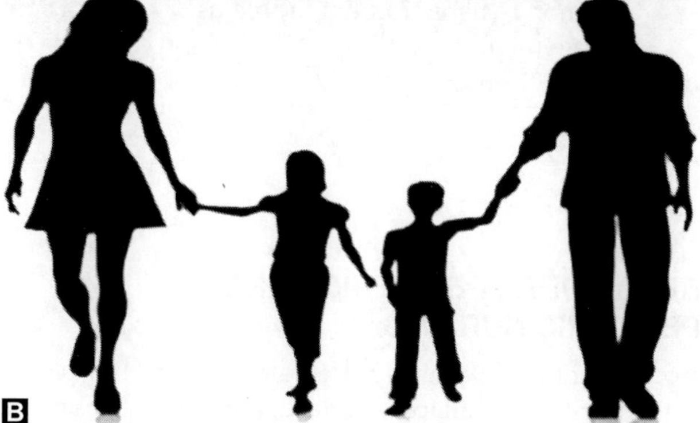

Figs 6.2A and B: A. The child is happy with the mother; **B.** Child needs both parents for love and security

Babies are cared for by their parents, and both parties develop understanding of the other. Gradually, babies start to expect that their parent will care for them when they cry. Gradually, parents respond to and even anticipate their babies' needs. This exchange and knowing each other (familiarity) create the basis for a developing relationship. Moreover, when parents can adapt to their babies, meet their needs, and provide nurturance, the attachment is secure. Psychosocial development can continue based on a strong foundation of attachment.

During toddlerhood, the parent-child relationship begins to change and goes beyond nurturing and predictability. In this period socialization is an important element in the parent-child relationship. It includes various child rearing practices, such as weaning, toilet training and discipline. Various parenting styles emerge during the preschool years. Preschoolers with authoritative parents are curious about new experiences, focused and skilled at play, self-reliant, self-controlled, and cheerful.

The natural broadening of psychosocial and cognitive abilities of child occurs in school age. The child's social world expands to include more people and settings beyond the home environment, but this is not a sign of disinterest in the parent-child relationship. The parents who are both responsive and demanding, their children continue to thrive psychologically and socially during middle childhood years. The biological, cognitive, and emotional changes of child transform the parent-child relationship during adolescence. Adolescents who have been reared authoritatively continue to show more success in school, better psychological development, and fewer behavioral problems.

Parenting Style

Parenting has four main style; authoritarian, authoritative, permissive and detached. Although parent does not use a single style in all situations, they do follow some general tendencies in their approach to child rearing. The parent-child relationship is described by the prevailing style of parenting.

Authoritarian parents: Authoritarian parents are rigid in their rules; they expect absolute obedience from the child without questioning. Children raised with this parenting style are often moody, unhappy, fearful, and irritable. They tend to be shy, withdrawn, and lack of self -confidence. If affection is withheld, the child commonly is rebellious and antisocial.

Authoritative: Authoritative parents show respect for the opinions of each of their children by allowing them to be different. Although there are some rules in the family, the children are allowed to discuss if they do not understand or agree with the rules. The authoritative parents have final authority, they are both responsive and demanding; they are firm, but they discipline with love and affection, rather than power, and they are allowing discussion and negotiation and are likely to explain rules and expectations to their children instead of simply asserting them. The children nurtured by this type of parenting style develop high self-esteem and are independent, inquisitive, happy, assertive and interactive.

Permissive parents: These parents are responsive but not demanding. Permissive (indulgent) parents have little or no control over the behavior of their children. Children follow the rules of the home inconsistently, there are empty threats of punishment without setting limits. Role reversal occurs; the children act more like the parents, and the parents behave like the children. Characteristics of the children of permissive parents may be disobedient, disrespectful, aggressive, irresponsible and defiant. They lack guidelines to direct their behavior and are insecure. Although low in both independence and social responsibility, they are more cheerful than the conflicted and irritable children of authoritarian parents.

Detached parents: Detached parents are neither responsive nor demanding. They may be careless or unaware or bother the needs of the child for affection and discipline. The children under this type of parenting style have higher numbers of psycho-social difficulties and behavior problems than other children.

Effective parenting also involves gaining knowledge and learning skills designed to improve a parent's ability to listen, understand and accept their child. For example, parents should know that love, security and acceptance should be at the heart of family life. Children need to feel that parents love does not depend on his or her accomplishments. Their mistakes and/or defeats should be expected and accepted. Confidence grows in a home that is full of unconditional love and affection. **Children's confidence and self-esteem need to be nurtured in the family, and parents' attention helps build children's self-confidence and self-esteem.** Effective parenting also includes learning some skills. The intent of these skills is to communicate that a child's emotions and thoughts are meaningful, understandable and authentic. Validating a child can decrease intense emotions and increase communication, which allows parents to identify the right problems to solve and propose strategies that fit their child's ability level and personality. Parental self-confidence is an important indicator of parental competence which is needed for validation own child. Moreover, validation does not mean that a parent agrees with the child or that their behavior was ok. It does communicate that the parent understands the child's behavior in the context of the child's life.

At the same time, parents need to know the strategies to respond to their child's behaviors with greater effectiveness. They may need training on mindfulness, interpersonal effectiveness, emotion regulation and distress tolerance. At this, they will learn how to guide the children to focus their attention on effective strategies for coping with interpersonal conflict, how to regulate painful emotions and skills to deal with the pain and distress, that is a part of life. They will able to teach the skills aimed specifically at improving their child's behaviors such as how to shape their child towards constructive activities, how to use punishment minimally though effectively and to use contracts and positive reinforcement to maintain limits and expectations.

The combination of information, specific skills and a non-judgmental approach appears to generate optimism. Ultimately the goal is to allow families to live meaningful and enjoyable lives. Although family life may differ from parent's initial vision, with this treatment many have described an increase of calm in their lives and a closer relationship with their children.

Basic Behavioral Pediatric Principles

A basic principle of behavior modification is that it is much easier to teach children what we want them to do in response to the triggers than to keep them from doing something that is inappropriate! As a result, teaching, modeling, and reinforcing good behavior is an active and often exhausting process. If children are responding to common events in a positive manner, these positive responses must be acknowledged, celebrated, and reinforced. If they are not, children will often adopt negative and often escalating behaviors to those events in the future.

Developmentally, it is expected that young children will have a difficult time controlling their emotions, particularly if tired, hungry or stressed. Toddlers and preschoolers often lack the self-control necessary to express anger and other unpleasant emotions peacefully. When this happens it is important for the child's caregiver to be able to provide him or her with the support to deal with these difficult and uncomfortable feelings. Children learn a lot through their parents' modeling of behaviors and this is the main reason for parents needing to be most in control when their children are feeling out of control.

Luckily for their parents, most children want to please their parents. Parents can therefore use this to their advantage when deciding how to change children's behavior and discipline them. When a parent shows joy for a behavior that is good, the child will be positively reinforced for doing this behavior. On the other hand if a parent shows disapproval for a behavior, the child is less likely to repeat this behavior given the basic principle that children want to please their parents.

Discipline is the system in which parents guide and teach their children. This word is often confused with the term punishment. The purpose of discipline is to teach children the difference between right and wrong behavior, to tolerate delayed gratification and to incorporate a sense of limits and appropriate behavior. Teaching discipline is a challenging task for parents and caregivers and not one that is taught overnight. Reinforcement is used to help increase the probability that a specific behavior will occur in the future by delivering a stimulus immediately after a response/ behavior is exhibited. Reinforcement for desired behaviors increases the likelihood events will occur.

Positive Reinforcement

Positive reinforcement can range from smiles to praise, edible treats, earned privileges (e.g. computer time), or even the opportunity to engage in a self-stimulating behavior for a specified period (e.g. twirling a favorite string). A variation on this is the star or sticker chart where a child earns a token or symbol for desired behaviors that can be traded at a future time for a reinforcer. Reinforcement varies with the developmental level and interests of each child. It takes many years for most children to be able to achieve self-control. Also, as children grow and develop, so do the types of things that they must be taught. The method of reinforcement must grow and change with the child. Caregivers need to be flexible because of changes in children and their environment as children mature and grow.

Negative Reinforcement

Negative reinforcement occurs when a certain stimulus (usually an aversive stimulus) is *removed* after a particular behavior is exhibited. The likelihood of the particular behavior occurring again in the future is increased because of removing/avoiding the negative consequence. For example a company has a policy that if an employee completes their assigned work by Friday, they can have Saturday off. Working Saturday is the negative reinforcer, the employee's productivity will be increased as they avoid experiencing the negative reinforcer.

Negative reinforcement should not be thought of as a punishment procedure. With negative reinforcement, behavior modifier is increasing a behavior, whereas with punishment, policy maker is decreasing a behavior.

Negative reinforcement is a term described by B. F. Skinner in his theory of operant conditioning. The basic definition is that a positive reinforcer *adds* a stimulus to increase or maintain frequency of a behavior while a negative reinforcer *removes* a stimulus to increase or maintain the frequency of the behavior. Positive and negative reinforcement are components of operant conditioning. In negative reinforcement, a response or behavior is strengthened by stopping, removing, or avoiding a negative outcome or aversive stimulus (*See* aggressive behavior management).

Functional Behavioral Assessment (FBA)

Functional behavioral assessment (FBA) is a comprehensive and individualized process to identify the purpose or function of a problem behavior. An FBA involves observation of the child in the setting(s) in which the behavior(s) occurs, analysis of data, and development of a plan to change the behavior.

When a child has disruptive behaviors (e.g. aggression in the classroom, self-injury, noncompliance), then the child's family can request an FBA from the school as per suggestion of clinician to generate a behavioral plan. Information from the FBA will identify the antecedent, label the behavior (what happened), and identify the consequence, or ABC data. It uses these data to figure out if the behavior is in response to things in the environment and if the consequence serves to reinforce it; in other words, what the function of the behavior is. The goal is to prevent further disruptive behavior and increase positive behaviors.

COMMON BEHAVIORAL PROBLEMS AND THEIR MANAGEMENT

Infancy and childhood are very much important in determining the future behavior and character of the children. Childhood is the period of dependency. Gradually child learns how to adjust in his/her environment. But when there is any complexity around them they cannot adjust with the circumstances. Then they become unable to behave in the socially acceptable way and behavioral problems develop with them.

Parents and family members are usually the first to notice if a child has problems with emotions or behavior. It can be difficult to assess whether the behavior of such children is normal or sufficiently problematical to require intervention. The observations of parents with those of teachers and other caregivers may lead to seek help for the child. Judgment will need to take into account the frequency, range and intensity of symptoms and the extent to which they cause impairment. If parents suspect a problem or have questions, consultation with pediatrician or a mental health professional is important.

The child's problems are often multifactorial such as parenting style which is inconsistent or contradictory, family or marital problems, child abuse or neglect, overindulgence, injury or chronic illness, separation or bereavement. The way in which children express their problems may be influenced by a range of factors including developmental stage, temperament, coping and adaptive abilities of family, and the nature and the duration of stress. In general, chronic stressors are more difficult to deal with than isolated stressful events.

Warning signs: There are signs which may indicate the need for professional assistance or evaluation. Those signs are:

- Poor grades in school result despite strong efforts
- Regular worry, restlessness or anxiety
- Repeated refusal to go to school or take part in normal children's activities
- Unable to share or take turns with other children
- Persistent nightmares
- Hyperactivity or fidgeting
- Persistent disobedience or aggression
- She has extreme fears that interfere with daily activities
- Frequent temper tantrums
- Depression, sadness or irritability
- Extremely 'rigid' about routines, and becomes extremely upset when things are changed and the child has extreme difficulty in separating from parent
- Too passive or fearful, and does not want to try things other children his age are doing, she/he has extreme fears that interfere with daily activities
- He is not interested in playing with other children.

All children will at some developmental stage display repetitive behaviors, but whether they may be considered as disorders depends on their frequency and persistence and the effect they have on physical, emotional and social functioning. These habit behaviors may arise originally from intentional movements which become repeated and then become incorporated into the child's customary behavior. Some habits arise in imitation of adult behavior. Other habits such as hair pulling or head banging develop as a means of providing a form of sensory input and comfort when the child is alone.

Causes of Behavioral Problem

Faulty parental attitude: Overprotection in the family, dominance, unrealistic expectations, over-criticism, unhealthy comparison, lack of discipline or imposition of rigid discipline, etc. are the responsible factors for development of behavioral problem.

Inadequate family environment: Poor economic status, cultural pattern, family habits, child rearing practices, superstitions, parents' mood and job satisfaction, parental illiteracy, inappropriate relationship among family members—these all have influence on child's behavior and may cause behavioral disorder.

Handicapped conditions: Child with sickness and disability may have behavioral problems. Chronic illness and prolong hospitalization can lead to this problem.

Influence of social relationship- Maladjustment at home and school, disturbed relationship with neighbours, school teachers, schoolmates, and playmates may predispose behavioral problems.

Influence of mass media: Television, radio, periodicals and high tech communication systems affects the school children and adolescents leading to conflict and tension which may cause behavioral disorder.

Influence of social change: Social unrest, violence, unemployment, change in value orientation, group interaction and hostility, frustration, economic insecurity etc. affect older children along with their parents and family members resulting abnormal behavior. The changing structure of the family, modernization, industrialization, globalization, and urbanization has impact on child's mental health.

India has the largest number of children (375 million) in the world, nearly 40% of its population.

The development of any country is dependent on positive mental development of its children. But often we see, the health of child and adolescent, who are

Table 6.1: Prevalence of children's behavioral and mental disorders in percentage

	5–10 years old		*11–16 years old*		*All 5–16 years old*
	Boys	*Girls*	*Boys*	*Girls*	
Emotional disorders	2.2	2.5	4.0	6.1	3.7
Conduct disorders	6.9	2.8	8.1	5.1	5.8
Hyperkinetic disorders	2.7	0.4	2.4	0.4	1.5
Less common disorders	2.2	0.4	1.6	1.1	1.3
Any disorder	10.2	5.1	12.6	10.3	9.6

future of a country, is given inadequate attention. Sixty nine percent of Indian children are victims of physical, emotional, or sex-abuse. Considering the size of the population involved and the nature and complexity of the problem, the total responsibility of welfare has to be borne cumulatively by the family, the regional community, and the State at different levels. The primary mission of the Child Guidance Clinic shall be to provide multi-disciplinary support services to children with special needs by providing preventative, consultative, diagnostic, and intervention services (Table 6.1).

Aggressive Behavior

Usually, aggressive behavior is common at one time or another and should subside as a child learns impulse control. Aggressive behavior is seen in toddlers as they lack the language to share their feelings or get their needs met. So, instead of being able to say 'Give that back' when his brother takes the ball out of his hand, he may hit or bite. The cause of aggressive behavior of school children may be the inability to regulate their emotions. When they are angry, they do not know how to calm down and may lash out. They too, may lack the ability to say, 'I'm really angry right now' and might show their anger with their behaviors. Sometimes kids behave aggressively because it actually works for them. For example, if a child bullies his brother, his brother may give him what he wants.

If the child is exhibiting frequent aggressive behaviors, it is important to develop a behavior management plan that can help parents determine how to respond to each aggressive behavior. It is important to provide an immediate consequence after each incident of aggressive behaviors.

Age appropriate discipline strategies are needed to handle childhood aggression. Young children up to about age 10 or 11, can benefit from a time out. Time out is a brief removal of the student from the setting (may be from the class) due to problem behavior. This can provide an immediate consequence and can also teach them how to calm themselves down. A time out alone is likely enough of a consequence for preschool children. Older children will likely require an additional consequence.

Loss of privileges is another great disciplinary strategy for aggression, which is called as 'response cost'. Response cost is the taking away of privileges or other valued elements in response to student misbehavior. Taking away the child's favorite activity for 24 hours can be very effective. For example, all electronics can be kept away from the child for one day.

Natural consequences work well when destruction of property is involved. For example, a teenager who kicks his foot through the wall will have to do chores to earn enough money to purchase the materials to fix the wall and then participate in repairing the damage.

Make sure that the consequence constitutes discipline and not punishment. *Shaming or embarrassing the child can backfire and may lead to increased acts of aggression.*

Positive discipline strategies can be effective in reducing aggression as well. For example, praise can motivate children to keep using their pro-social behaviors. Reward systems can also motivate children to 'keep their hands to themselves.'

Teaching New Skills

Attention is to given to find the skills the child may be lacking such as social skill. Sometimes kids who lack social skills may do things such as grab toys from other children which can eventually lead to aggressive behaviors. Teaching new skills should model to children what to do instead of behaving aggressively. For example, the child will learn to 'use their words,' or problem-solving with them when they have a problem.

A behavior conference is a brief meeting between teacher and students to discuss the student's problem behavior. It will typically include some elements like:

- Description of the problem behavior
- Open ended questions and student input to fully understand the factors are contributing to the problem behavior
- Teacher and student discuss solutions to the problem behavior and agree to plan and to carry out
- **Disciplinary reminders:** The teacher concludes the conference by informing the student of the disciplinary consequence that will occur if the problem behavior continues.

Defusing technique is another strategy where a teacher/adult take actions to calm a student/child or otherwise defuse a situation with the potential for confrontation or emotional escalation. The teacher/parent temporally removes academic work from the student who is reacting negatively to the assignment.

TEMPER TANTRUMS

A temper tantrum is an uncontrollable release of anger, lasting longer than a few minutes. Screaming, throwing, yelling, hitting, crying, biting, and head-banging are all hallmarks of tantrum behavior. They are equally common in boys and girls and usually occur between the ages of 1 to 3 years, some children may experience regular tantrums, whereas others have them rarely. Toddlers try to master their world as they have developed their motor skill but when they are not able to accomplish a task, they turn to one of the only tools at their disposal for venting frustration is called tantrum.

Causes and Types

Toddler develops the motor skills he needs to really explore his world and he can run and jump and climb. However, he does not yet have the knowledge he needs to keep himself safe. The frontal lobe of toddler's brain which controls logic, reasoning, planning, judgment, self-control, and emotional processing; is underdeveloped.

In his mind, scaling a 7 foot tall bookcase is *fun*. So, when his parent pulls him down to safety, he does not understand that parent is helping; all he knows is that parent has betrayed him by thwarting his climbing adventure or autonomy. The child feels frustrated and angry that he can not climb the bookcase, but he can't mentally process those feelings of reasoning, and safety. He lacks the self-control necessary to keep those emotions in check, and he certainly can not express his feelings verbally, the way an adult would. Therefore, he resorts to kicking and shrieking and throwing things, because those are skills he does have. He figures this out, and responds to anger and frustration, starts to assert his independence in a big way (Figs 6.3A to C).

Three types of toddler tantrums—frustration tantrums, exhaustion tantrums and temper tantrums. Toddlers' world is egocentric (narcissistic) and it is coupled with an incomplete and unbalanced development of expressive language skills; causes temper tantrum. Tantrums more often occur when toddlers are hungry, tired, bored or excessively tired.

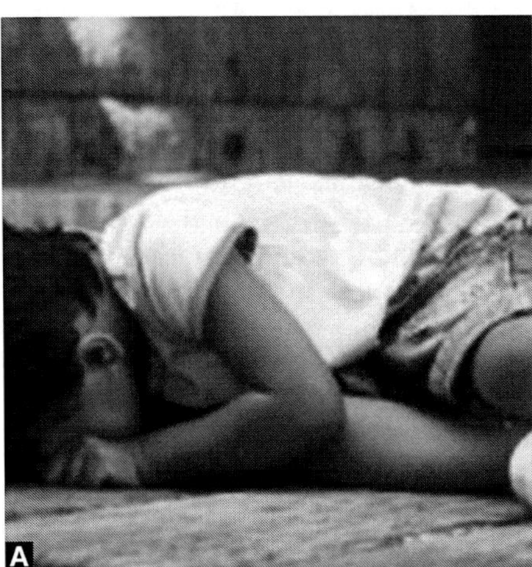

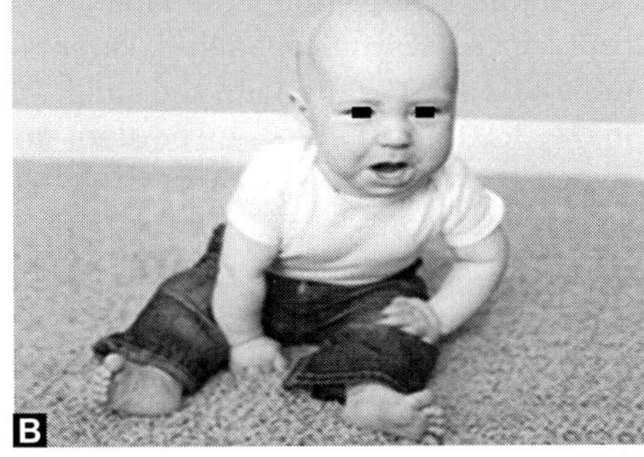

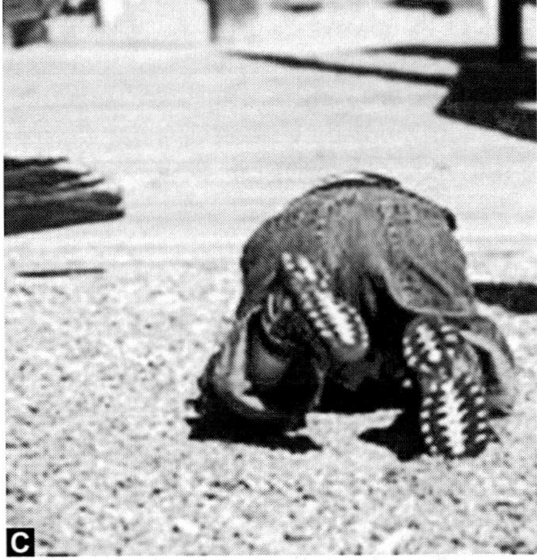

Figs 6.3A to C: For children, tantrums often stem from trying to communicate a need but not having the language skills to do it. For older toddlers, tantrums are more of a power struggle

Management

With sustained tantrums, it is important to take a thorough history which includes: time, location, duration and frequency of the tantrums. It is also need to inquire about precipitating factors, parties involved, and how the tantrums are managed. Children with severe temper tantrums (three or more tantrums per day those last more than 15 minutes) may be associated with behavior/emotional problems.

Parents can be guided to identify strategies to decrease the frequency of tantrums. Parents can anticipate periods of fatigue, they can have the child's food ready before the child gets too hungry and they can offer the toddler choices when possible; can minimize temper tantrums. Toddlers need appropriate and consistent limits. Children can be allowed to control over little things whenever possible by giving choices. A little bit of power given to the child can stave off the big power struggles later. 'Which do you want to do first, brush your teeth or put on your pajamas?' Children can be distracted by redirection to another activity when they tantrum over something they should not do or cannot have. They may be told, 'Let us see the album together.'

Safe isolation and to ignore the child is probably the most effective method to handle tantrums. They must learn that nothing is gained from tantrums, not even attention. Giving in to the child's demands or scolding the child only increases the behavior. Parents should remain calm and do not argue with the child, yelling at the child makes the tantrum worse. Toddlers stop using tantrums when they do not achieve their goals and as their verbal skills increase.

The child needs to learn how to try a more successful way of interacting with a peer or sibling, how to express his or her feelings with words and recognize the feelings of others without hitting and screaming. No reward is to be given to the child after a tantrum for calming down. Some children will learn that a temper tantrum is a good way to get a treat later. The temper tantrum should not interfere with otherwise positive parent child relationship, but they need assistance to gain self-control and to express anger constructively.

Pica (Geophagia)

Pica is an eating disorder that includes the ingestion, and sometimes mouthing of poisonous or inedible substances. Pica is characterized by an appetite for substances that are largely non-nutritive, such as paper, clay, metal, chalk, soil, glass, or sand. Pica usually begins in childhood and typically lasts for just a few months. It is more commonly seen in women and children, and in areas of low socioeconomic status. According to DSM-IV criteria, for these actions to be considered pica, they must persist for more than one month at an age where eating such objects is considered developmentally inappropriate, not part of culturally sanctioned practice and sufficiently severe to warrant clinical attention. However, it is likely to be more difficult to manage in children who are developmentally disabled.

Pica has been linked to mental disorders and they often have psychotic comorbidity. Stressors such as maternal deprivation, family issues, parental neglect, poverty, and a disorganized family structure are strongly linked to pica. There is no specific way to prevent pica. However, careful attention to eating habits and close supervision of children known to put things in their mouths may help catch the disorder before complications can occur.

If pica is suspected, a medical evaluation is important to assess for possible anemia, intestinal blockages, or potential toxicity from ingested substances. If symptoms are present, an evaluation begins by performing a complete medical history and physical exam. Certain tests such as X-rays and blood tests are done to check for anemia and look for toxins and other substances in the blood, and to check for blockages in the intestinal tract. Other tests are conducted for possible infections caused by eating items contaminated with bacteria or other organisms. A review of the child's eating habits also may be conducted.

Before making a diagnosis of pica, the presence of other disorders such as mental retardation, developmental disabilities, or obsessive-compulsive disorder—as the cause of the odd eating behavior are to be evaluated. This pattern of behavior must last at least one month for a diagnosis of pica to be made.

Treatment for pica may vary by patient and suspected cause and may emphasize psychosocial, environmental and family-guidance approaches. Dietary changes may be done to correct iron deficiency. An initial approach often involves screening for and, if necessary, treating any mineral deficiencies or other co-morbid conditions. If, pica that appears to be of psychotic etiology, close collaboration with a mental health team skilled in treating pica is ideal for optimal treatment of these complex cases. Therapy and medication such as SSRIs have been used successfully. However, previous reports have cautioned against the use of medication until all non-psychotic etiologies have been ruled out. Behavior-based treatment options can be useful for developmentally disabled and mentally ill individuals with pica. These may involve using positive reinforcement normal behavior. Many use aversion therapy, where the patient learns through positive reinforcement which foods are good and which ones they should not eat.

There are many potential complications of pica, such as:

- Lead to poisoning, increases the child's risk of complications including learning disabilities and brain damage. This is the most concerning and potentially lethal side effect of pica.
- Eating non-food objects can interfere with eating healthy food, which can lead to nutritional deficiencies.
- Eating objects that cannot be digested, such as stones, can cause constipation or blockages in the digestive tract, including the intestines and bowels. Also, hard or sharp objects (such as paperclips or metal scraps) can cause surgical emergency as it tears in the lining of the intestines.
- Bacteria or parasites from dirt or other objects can cause serious infections. Some infections can damage the kidneys or liver.
- Co-existing developmental disabilities can make treatment difficult.

Nail Biting (Onychophagia)

Biting fingernails (onychophagia) is an oral compulsive habit that often starts in childhood. Child may bite his nails for different reasons like curiosity, boredom, stress relief, habit, or imitation. Nail-biting is the most common of the so-called 'nervous habits,' which include thumb-sucking, teeth grinding, nose picking, hair twisting or tugging.

Growing up can make children anxious, and many of these tensions and pressures are invisible to parents. Onychophagia is an unwanted behavior which can make a person nervous in social situations. It might be a sign of anxiety and might serve as an anxiety-reducing function. Studies show 60% of children and 45% of teenagers bite their nails. Nail biting becomes less common after age 18, but it can continue into adulthood. Many adults and children are often unaware they are biting their nails because doing so has become a habit.

The problem can range from a mild, occasional habit to an ongoing and more serious problem.

If child bites moderately and does not injure himself or does it unconsciously while watching television, or if he tends to bite in response to specific situations (such as performances or tests), it is just his way of coping with minor stress and parents need not to worry about. But many adults and children are often unaware they are biting their nails because doing so has become a habit.

Severe nail-biting signals excessive anxiety. The child makes his fingertips sore or bloody, he does other worrisome behaviors (such as picking at his skin or pulling out his eyelashes or hair), or he does not sleep well. Nail biting presents in a significant proportion of referrals to a mental healthcare clinic setting. Its detection can then be followed by looking for other more subtle stereotypic or self-mutilating behaviors. Biting fingernails can also be a symptom of a psychological condition, such as OCD (obsessive-compulsive disorder). Patient with OCD may also bite their nails as part of the same spectrum of behaviors. Many children who are nail biters also have other psychiatric disorders, such as attention deficit hyperactivity disorder (ADHD), oppositional defiant disorder (ODD), separation anxiety disorder, or bed-wetting.

Onychophagia is reported to be a difficult behavior to modify. Research has shown that drugs are not effective for treatment of nail biting. It is essential to deal with the underlying causes of the behavior and to think about whether there is stress in child's life that can be addressed by parents. The most common treatment, which is cheap and widely available, is to apply a clear, bitter-tasting nail polish (denatonium benzoate, the most bitter chemical compound) to the nails, which discourages the nail biting. Other behavioral techniques that have been investigated with preliminary positive results are self-help techniques are trimming short the nails, the use of wristbands as non-removable reminders. Mental health professional is to be contacted if fingernail biting persists along with anxiety and stress. It could be a sign of a more serious psychological problem, including OCD, which can be treated with counseling, or medications.

ENURESIS

The word enuresis is derived from a Greek word (*enourein*) that means 'to void urine.' It can occur either during the day or at night and commonly known as 'bedwetting'. Enuresis can be divided into primary and secondary forms.

The cause of nighttime incontinence is not clearly known. Young children who experience bedwetting tend to be physically and emotionally normal. Most cases probably result from a mix of factors including slower physical development, an overproduction of urine at night, a lack of ability to recognize bladder filling when asleep, and, in some cases, anxiety. For many, there is a strong family history of bedwetting, suggesting an inherited factor.

The most important reason for treating enuresis is to minimize the embarrassment and anxiety of the child and the frustration experienced by the parents. Preliminary management focusing on behavioral modification and positive reinforcement is often helpful. Bladder training exercises are not recommended. The only therapies proved to be effective are alarm therapy and treatment with desmopressin acetate or imipramine. Enuresis is not a surgically treated condition.

Encopresis—Discussed in G. I chapter.

TOILET TRAINING DIFFICULTIES

Toilet training can be defined as delayed if the child is over 3 years of age, has normal development, and is not toilet trained after three or more months of training. Although the Diagnostic and Statistical Manual for Primary Care *Child and Adolescent Version* uses 4 years of age as a cut-off for abnormal toilet training delays, it makes sense to evaluate delays at 3 years of age to prevent ongoing harmful approaches by parents. **A toddler is not able to 'hold on' to a stool that is ready to come out. Children are often busy with what they are doing, so they do not always notice that their stool or urine is coming until it starts to come out, or it is too late to run to the toilet. They will have lots of 'accidents' while they are still learning.**

In order for a toddler to be successfully potty trained, she needs to be able to sense the urge to go, be able to understand what the feeling means, and then be able to verbalize that she needs parent's help to make it to the toilet and actually go. Waiting until the child is truly ready will make the experience much faster and more pleasant for everyone involved.

Toilet training delays have several causes, both behavioral and organic. The cause is most often behavioral. Organic causes are rare. The most common organic cause of isolated daytime wetting is a urinary tract infection. Other causes to consider are urethritis, giggle incontinence, urgency incontinence, or an ectopic ureter. Questions about neurologic causes arise often, but if the child can postpone urinating or defecating or hide to do it, neurologic input is clearly intact.

Moreover, most children who are resistant to toilet training are enmeshed in a power struggle with their parents. The cause of the power struggle is usually reminder resistance—an oppositional response to excessive reminders to sit on the toilet. If the parents are mishandling toilet training problems, it is a mistake to allow them to continue to do so for an additional year before intervening. If, for example, parents are punishing the child for noncompliance or forcibly holding the child on the toilet, these negative interactions will be much harder to undo and repair with time. Calling delays abnormal can wait until 4 years of age, but evaluation and intervention should begin sooner.

Parents need guidance to handle the toilet training resistance. They need to **transfer all responsibility to the child.** The child is to be explained that it is her body, and the stool and urine belong to her. She does not need anybody to help her any more, that it is up to her.

Reminders and practice runs are what keep the power struggle going on, so that to be stopped. Children older than 3 years never need reminders to help them become toilet trained. Make the child think that using the toilet is her idea. Once the power struggle has been dismantled, parents need to come up with the right incentive to achieve a breakthrough.

CHILD GUIDANCE CLINIC

For the all-round development of a child the child's physical and physiological functioning and the environment to which he is exposed at home and school, should be taken care off. All this is possible through interaction with and counseling of the child and his family by a health care team. Child guidance Clinic was established for those children who were not fully adjusted to their environment. They are guided and prevented from becoming psychotic and neurotics in later life. It was first started in Chicago in 1909 to deal with problems of juvenile delinquency.

Later, CGCs have come up with the purpose of understanding, preventing, and relieving psychologically-based distress and to promote subjective well-being and personal development in children. Child Guidance Clinic is specialized in diagnosing mental distress, psychological testing and psychotherapy within four primary theoretical orientations—psychodynamic, humanistic, behavior therapy/cognitive behavioral, and systems or family therapy. The first CGC was started in India in 1939 at the Tata Institute Mumbai. The CGC in Delhi was started in 1955 at RAK College of Nursing, simultaneously with Madras.

Definition

Child guidance clinic are specialized clinics that deal with children of normal and abnormal intelligence, exhibiting a range of behaviors and psychological problems which are summed up as maladjustments. A child guidance clinic is one of the medico-social amenities for the organized and scientific study and treatment of maladjustment in children.

Purpose

The philosophy CGC is, if sound mental health can develop in childhood the same will continue into adulthood.

The development of any country is dependent on positive mental health of its children. India has the largest number of children (375 million) in the world, nearly 40% of its population. But the health of child and adolescent, who are future of our country, is given inadequate attention. Sixty nine percent of Indian children are victims of physical, emotional, or sex-abuse and they suffer with other problems too. Considering the size of the population involved and the nature and complexity of the problem, the total responsibility of welfare has to be borne cumulatively by the family, the regional community, and the State at different levels. The concept of child guidance clinic has emerged in this context. The primary mission of the child guidance clinic is to provide multidisciplinary support services to children. Provision of preventative, consultative, diagnostic, and intervention services can increase positive functioning of the children across the multiple setting home, community and school.

Objectives of child guidance clinic:

- To ensure all round development of children and to maximize their potential to learn and grow
- To provide counseling, guidance and information to parents regarding care and upbringing of children
- To train parents to facilitate development and to prepare the children for placement in the appropriate educational setup
- To organize remedial help for school children facing achievement problems
- To work out behavior modification schedules for children presenting behavior problems
- To motivate parents for increased involvement for psychosocial adjustments
- To start early intervention of developmentally delayed children.

Team

The care of the child is carried out in a CGC by a team of workers. The team of staff members is constituted of a clinical psychologist, educational psychologist, a psychiatrist, a pediatrician, a PHN, and speech therapist, a psychiatric social worker, and playroom workers; who treat a child as a whole. As the personality has many aspects, *viz.* physical, intellectual, educational, emotional, social and economic, etc. Each of these aspects is studied by the respective staff member who has specialized in that particular field.

Services

Usually CGCs deal with psychological, emotional, and perception changes that occur in children through motor skills and psycho-physiological processes. Cognitive development involves areas such as problem-solving, moral understanding, and conceptual understanding; language acquisition; social, personality, and emotional development; and self-concept and identity formation.

Problems/deficiencies seen in children attending CGCs are:

- Poor school performance and learning disorders
- Academic skill deficits in reading, writing, spelling, math, etc.
- Speech and language disorders: Stuttering, aphasias, etc
- Motor skill deficits; poor handwriting, clumsiness, etc.
- Attention deficit hyperactivity disorders (ADD/ADHD)
- Behavioral problem like pica, bed-wetting, sleep walking
- Children with mental retardation
- Defiant/Oppositional behavior, conduct disorders
- Addiction to TV/Internet, disorganized routines
- Tics/Tourette Disorder, 'silent' epilepsy
- Obsessive behavior/disorders; obsessive slowness/procrastination
- Anxiety, school phobia, exam phobia and various Fears in the child
- Depression, social withdrawal, loss of interest
- Developmental neurological disorders
- 'Functional' symptoms like headache, breathlessness, stomach ache, frequent sickness, absenteeism from school, etc.

Some special features/rules maintained in the CGCs are:

- No medicines without physician's/psychiatrist's advice
- No labelling of the child/client
- Strict confidentiality is maintained in keeping client's data
- Child friendly approach is adopted
- Overall child development is the goal of CGC
- Team approach with collaboration with family, school and other community centers.

EDUCATIONAL GUIDANCE

Educational guidance primarily concerned with the students' success in his/her educational career. It is a process concerned with bringing about an individual with his distinctive characteristics on his own hand. In case of differently-abled children guidance given after some standardized test like intelligence quotient, aptitude test etc. After test students are placed/handled accordingly.

Principles of educational guidance:

- Development of self realization
- Development of human relationship
- All round personality development
- Develop individual potentialities to the fullest.

Educational Guidance Help the Students

To orient themselves to new purpose of philosophy and education; to make appraisal of own abilities and interests; to develop study habits appropriate to the study; to make own choices on course; to adjust with the learning environment; to understand own strength and weakness; to increase the accuracy of self-perception; identify learning difficulties and remedial measures to overcome.

Personal Guidance

Personal guidance is the assistance offered to the individual to solve his emotional, social, ethical moral and health problems.

Principles of Personal Guidance

- Focus on problems of life.
- Concerned with social and civic activities.
- Concerned with health and physical activities.
- Deals with healthy use of leisure time and character building.

Personal Guidance Helps Individual

Pre-primary stage: The child is helped in achieving emotional control and developing desirable social relationships.

Elementary stage: To develop self-discipline

Junior high-school: To help preadolescents to become adjusted in their new environment.

They learn to develop a feeling of belongingness and to function in a group with team spirit.

Guidance given to develop a positive attitude to seek counseling, it is needed in life.

To stimulate their desire to develop qualities needed for healthful living.

High-school stage: Efforts should be made to offer personal guidance for adjustment. Information pertaining to sex life may be provided. Discussion regarding cultural framework of the society, and healthy recreational activities can be done. A sense of social responsibilities and community services in children can be developed.

Nutritional guidance: It is the most important guidance to the parents and as well as for children, with the goal of achieving optimum nutrition throughout the years of growth and development. The nutritional status of the children is of vital importance in their growth and development, in the promotion and maintenance of health and prevention of diseases and restoration of health following illness and injury.

During infancy: Mother is the significant person who is responsible for maintenance of nutrition and promotion of health during this period. Mother needs guidance for breastfeeding so information regarding positioning, feeding schedule, timing and technique should be given.

In the latter half of infancy, guidance should concern about different aspects of weaning. Weaning is an important transitional period in relation to child's nutrition. Information should provide regarding importance of calm quite and relaxed approach during weaning. Selection of food with high nutrient content and cultural preferences is important. Forced feeding should be avoided.

For toddler: It is the period of autonomy and self-awareness which may cause refusal of food and assistance in feeding by which the toddler asserts himself or herself. In this period child may have decreased appetite due to slower growth rate and may be ritualistic in food preference.

Parents need guidance regarding balanced diet and independence of the child during feeding but to provide assistance whenever necessary.

For preschooler: A preschooler usually develops to have complete independence at meal time with increased imitation. Nutritional habits are developed in this period that become part of child's lifetime practice.

For school-age: Guidance is useful for the school age to help them to select food items wisely and to begin to plan and prepare for meal.

For adolescents: special emphasis should given on nutritional need related to the growth, selection of iron rich food items and preparing favourite adolescent food for physical fitness.

ROLE OF A PEDIATRIC NURSE IN CHILD GUIDANCE CLINIC

In CGC, a pediatric nurse acts as resource person. She is expected to apply expert knowledge and skills to a particular situation to achieve positive outcomes.

Education: Role of nurse is not only encouraging, but educating the public. She provides information and helps the client to learn or acquire new knowledge and technical skills. She encourages in compliance of prescribed therapy, promotes healthy lifestyle.

Identification of children with adjustment problems: Community health nurses identify the risk cases in the community through home visiting, school health program, and conducting clinics.

Lobbying for child rights: Involves concern for and actions in behalf of the client to bring about a change. Pediatric nurse promotes what is best for the client, ensuring that the client's needs are met and protecting the client's right and provides explanation in clients language and support clients decisions. She lobbies for established laws on child health as well as for rights of children.

Provide holistic nursing care: A pediatric nurse possesses professional skills and a developmental orientation that is naturally suited to the child care environment. When functioning as a child care health consultant (CCHC), a nurse has the opportunity to practice true holistic nursing.

Research: Nurse plays an important role in the child guidance clinic, she also undertakes research studies herself. She can participate in identifying significant researchable problems, participates in scientific investigation and must be a consumer of research findings, and must be aware of the research process, language of research, a sensitive to issues related to protecting the rights of human subjects.

Role model: Nurse helps in establishing good child parent bond; as well as good teacher parent-child bond. Be an exemplary role model and by guiding them.

Facilitation: As a facilitator, pediatric nurse can influence not only the immediate environment, but also has the potential to positively affect the total well-being of the children and family members through questioning, insights, and other counseling techniques, to discover the answers and solutions on his/her own. One of the most powerful goal as a facilitator is to impart a sense of self-efficacy and empowerment in clients.

Counselling: She helps client to recognize and cope with stressful psychologic or social problems; to develop an improved interpersonal relationships and to promote personal growth. She tries to:

- Provide emotional, intellectual and psychologic support
- Focus on helping a client to develop new attitudes, feelings and behaviors rather than promoting intellectual growth.
- Encourage the client to look at alternative behaviors; recognize the choices and develop a sense of control.

CHAPTER 7

Assessment of Pediatric Patient

Chapter Outline

- Importance of Assessment in Pediatric Patients
- Skills Used for Assessment
- Assessment of Pediatric Patient
- Admission Assessment
- Developmental Assessment
- Assessment of Nutritional Status
- Purposes of Nutritional Assessment
- Various Techniques with Different Approaches

'When I think about all the patients and their loved ones that I have worked with over the years, I know most of them don't remember me nor I them. But I do know that I gave a little piece of myself to each of them and they to me and those threads make up the beautiful tapestry in my mind that is my career in nursing.'

—Donna Wilk Cardillo

Assessing the pediatric patient can be one of the most challenging and stressful tasks for nurses (Fig. 7.1). Assessment is a key component of nursing practice, required for planning and provision of patient and family-centerd care through nursing process. Assessment is an important part of the nursing process. According to the Nursing and Midwifery Board of Australia (NMBA) in the national competency standard for registered nurses, 'The registered nurse assesses, plans, implements and evaluates nursing care in collaboration with individuals and the multidisciplinary health care team so as to achieve goals and health outcomes.' This nursing process is accepted by professional nurses as the foundation for their practice and it provides the framework for the care of the pediatric patients.

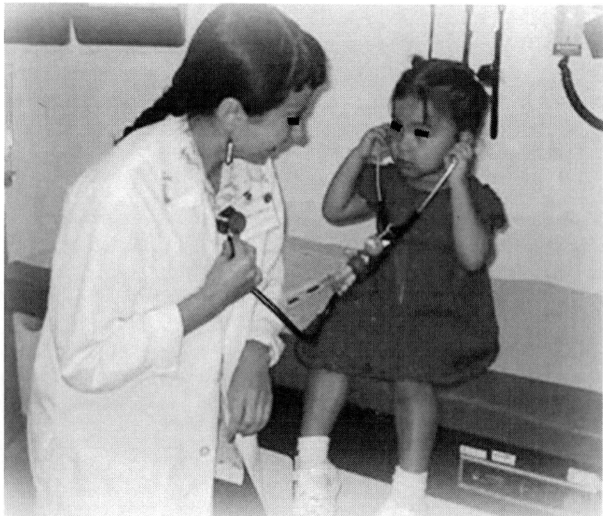

Fig. 7.1: Complete physical assessment of pediatric patients is a challenging task for nurses

The first step in the nursing process is **assessing**. Nurses use a systematic, dynamic way to collect and analyze data about a patient, the initial step in delivering nursing care. In this phase, data is gathered about the patient, family or community that the nurse is working with. Objective data can be collected through examination, is measurable. This includes things like vital signs, oxygenation level or observable patient behaviors. Nursing assessments provide the starting point for determining nursing diagnoses. For accurate determination of nursing diagnoses, a useful, evidence-based assessment framework is best practice.

Assessment includes not only physiological data, but also psychological, sociocultural, spiritual, economic, and life-style factors as well (Fig. 7.2). For example, a nurse's assessment of a hospitalized patient in pain includes not only the physical causes and manifestations of pain, but the patient's response—an inability to get out of bed, refusal to eat, withdrawal

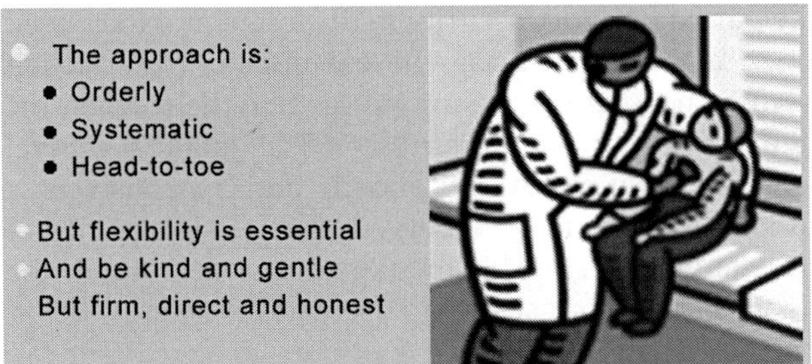

Fig. 7.2: Systematic physical assessment of child

from family members, anger directed at hospital staff, fear, or request for more pain medication.

IMPORTANCE OF ASSESSMENT IN PEDIATRIC PATIENTS

Anatomical, physiological, and psychological differences between children and adults have important implications for the initial assessment and management of pediatric patient (sickness/trauma). Children and infants are not only smaller than adults, but also significantly different physiologically. Knowledge of pediatric anatomic and physiologic differences will aid in recognizing normal variations found during the physical examination. It also assists with understanding the different physiologic responses children have to illness and injury. Importance of assessment in pediatric patients can be explained in following way:

Patients' perspective: Children are rate-dependent for respiratory and cardiovascular function. Unable to significantly increase cardiovascular stroke volume or respiratory tidal volume, they compensate by increasing heart and respiratory rate. This is the reason tachycardia is better tolerated than bradycardia specific to the pediatric patient.

Children have a different physiological response to major trauma compared to adults, in that they maintain a near-normal blood pressure even in the face of 25% to 30% of blood volume loss. In these situations, subtle changes in the heart rate and extremity perfusion may signal impending cardiorespiratory failure, and should not be overlooked.

Their larger body surface area to body mass ratio predisposes children to larger heat and insensible fluid loss than adults, resulting in higher fluid and caloric requirements. So, quick and proper assessment is imperative.

Children may not cope well emotionally in the aftermath of an illness/accident. They need to be managed in a calm, child-friendly environment. The presence of a parent or guardian in the resuscitation/treatment room may help the treatment team by minimizing the sick/injured child's fear and anxieties.

Nurses' perspective: Assessment guides nurses to take steps to identify patient's problems to set realistic goals and to intervene individualized care.

Assessment encourages for identification and utilization of child's strength. It enhances communication and interpersonal relationship with patients, families and team members.

Definition of Terms

Admission assessment: Comprehensive nursing assessment including patient history, general appearance, physical examination and vital signs completed at the time of admission.

Shift assessment: Concise nursing assessment completed at the commencement of each shift or if patient condition changes at any other time during your shift.

Focused assessment: It is detailed nursing assessment of specific body system(s) relating to the presenting problem or current concern(s) of the patient. This may involve one or more body system.

SKILLS USED FOR ASSESSMENT

Assessment of patient means collection of data. Types of data include, subjective data, i.e. facts expressed by the patients or relatives which are not observable and measurable and objective data are the facts observable and measurable by health personnel. Courteousness, calm and open mindedness, undivided attention and listening are important for effective communication. Overreaction and judgmental/critical comment are to be avoided for better assessment of the child.

The followings are the skills used for assessment of subjective data of pediatric clients:

- Skill for appropriate introduction
- Skill for maintaining privacy and confidentiality
- Skill for communicating with parents
- *Skills for communicating with children:* Allow children time to feel comfortable and avoid sudden or rapid advances, be aware about nonverbal cues such as extended eye contact, or other gestures that may be seen as threatening, talk to parent if child is initially shy, communicate through transition objects such as dolls, puppets, and stuffed animals before questioning a young child directly, give older children opportunity to talk in the parents' absence, assume a

position that is at eye level with the child, speak in a quiet, unhurried and confident voice, speak clearly, be specific and use simple words and short sentences, state directions and suggestions positively, offer a choice only when one exists, be honest with children, allow them to express their concerns and fears, use a variety of communication techniques.

- *Skill for communicating with adolescents:* Build a foundation.

Spend time together, encourage expression of ideas and feelings, respect their views, tolerate differences, praise good points, respect their privacy, set a good example.

Skills for Collecting Objective Data

Following are the specific examination techniques in assessment of patient
• *Inspection:* Purposeful observation of the child's physical features and behaviors. Physical feature characteristics include size, shape, color, movement, position, and location. Detection of odors is also a part of inspection.
• *Ipation:* Use of touch to identify characteristics of the skin, internal organs, and masses. Characteristics include texture, moistness, tenderness, temperature, position, shape, consistency, and mobility of masses and organs. The palmar surface of the fingers and finger pads helps determine position, size, consistency, and masses. The ulnar surface of the hand is best to detect vibrations.
• *Auscultation:* Listening to sounds produced by the airway, lungs, stomach, heart, and blood vessels to identify their characteristics. Auscultation is usually performed with a stethoscope to enhance the sounds heard.
• *Percussion:* Striking the surface of the body, either directly or indirectly, to set up vibrations that reveal the density of underlying tissues and borders of internal organs.

DEVELOPMENTAL APPROACH TO THE EXAMINATION

The sequence and approach to the examination varies by age (Table 7.1). A comfortable atmosphere for the examination is needed with privacy so that modesty is respected. Explaining the procedures is to be done before to begin to perform them. In young children, a foot-to-head sequence is often used so that the least distressing parts of the examination are completed first. In older cooperative children, the head-to-toe approach is generally used.

Infants Below 6 Months

Infants are among the easiest children to examine, as they do not resist the examination procedure. Presence of the parent provides security to the infant and they need physical comfort during the examination. Distraction such as rocking or clicking noises may help when the infant begins to get distressed. The infant's general level of activity, overall mood, and responsiveness to handling are to be observed. Keep the sequence of the examination flexible to take advantage of times the infant is quiet or asleep to auscultate the lungs, heart, and abdomen. If the infant continues to be quiet or can be quieted with a pacifier, palpate the abdomen while the muscles are relaxed. Portions of the examination that will disturb the infant, such as the examination of the hips, should be performed at the end.

Infants Above 6 Months

Because of developing separation and stranger anxiety, the nurses need to be careful to approach the baby. Smile and talk soothingly to the infant during handling him/her and avoid rapid advances. Because the infant may be fearful of being touched by a stranger, begin with the feet and hands before moving to the trunk. However, take advantage of opportunities presented when the infant is sleeping or quiet to auscultate the heart and lungs. The infant will not object to having clothing removed, but make sure the room is warm for the infant's comfort. Observe the infant's general level of activity, mood, and responsiveness to handling by the parent. A pacifier or toys can be used to distract the older infant. The infant and toddler can be examined on the parent's lap and then held against the parent's chest for some steps, such as the ear examination.

Toddlers

Developmentally the toddlers may be active, curious, shy, cautious, or slow to warm up. Because of stranger anxiety, keep toddlers with their parents, often examining them on the parent's lap. Much of the neurologic and musculoskeletal assessment can be conducted by observing the child play and walk around in the examining room. The child is to be told what nurse will do at each step of the examination, using a confident voice that expects cooperation rather than asking. When a choice is possible, let the child have some control. For example, let the toddler choose which ear to examine first or to stand or sit for a certain part of the examination.

To overcome fear and anxiety, let the child hold a security object if it helps. Attempt to reduce the child's anxiety by demonstrating the use of instruments on the parent or doll (security object). Begin the examination

Table 7.1: Age-specific approaches to physical examination during childhood

Position	*Sequence*	*Preparation*
Infant • Before able to sit alone: supine or prone, preferable in parent's lap; before 4–6 mo, can place on examining table • After able to sit alone; sitting in parent's lap • Whenever possible; if on table, place with parent in full view	• If child is quiet, auscultate heart, lungs, abdomen • Record heart and respiratory rates • Palpate and percuss same areas • Proceed in usual head-to-toe direction • Perform traumatic procedures last (eyes, ears, mouth [while crying]) • Elicit reflex as body part is examined • Elicit Moro reflex last	• Completely undress if room temperature permits. • Leave diaper on male infant. • Gain cooperation with distraction, bright objects, rattles, talking. • Smile at infant; use soft, gentle voice. • Pacify with bottle of sugar water or feeding. • Enlist parent's aid for restraining to examine ears, mouth. • Avoid abrupt, jerky movements.
Toddler • Sitting or standing on or by parent • Prone or supine in parents lap	• Inspect body area through play: count fingers', 'tickle toes' • Use minimum physical contact initially. • Introduce equipment slowly • Auscultate, percuss, palpate whenever quiet • Perform traumatic procedures last (same as for infant)	• Have parent remove outer clothing • Remove underwear as body part is examined • Allow to inspect equipment; demonstrating use of equipment is usually ineffective • If uncooperative, perform procedures quickly • Use restraint when appropriate; request parent's assistance • Talk about examination if cooperative; use short phrases. • Praise for cooperative behavior
Preschool Child • Prefer standing or sitting • Usually cooperative prone or supine • Prefer parent's closeness	• If cooperative, proceed in head-to-toe direction • If uncooperative, proceed as with toddler	• Request self-undressing • Allow to wear underpants if shy • Offer equipment for inspection; briefly demonstrate use • Make up story about procedure (e.g. 'I am seeing how strong your muscles are' (blood pressure) • Use paper-doll technique • Give choices when possible • Expect cooperation; use positive statements (e.g. 'open your mouth')
School-Age Child • Prefer sitting • Cooperative in most positions • Younger child prefers parent's presence • Older child may prefer privacy	• Proceed in head-to-toe direction • May examine genitalia last in older child	• Respect need for privacy • Request self-undressing • Allow to wear underpants • Give gown to wear • Explain purpose of equipment and significances of procedure, such as otoscope to see eardrum, which is necessary for hearing • Teach about body function and care.
Adolescent Same as for school-age child Offer option of parent's presence	• Same as older school-age child • May examine genitalia last	• Allow to undress in private • Give gown • Expose only area to be examined • Respect need for privacy • Explain findings during examination: 'your muscle are firm and strong' • Matter-of-factly comment about sexual development: 'your breasts are developing as they should be' • Emphasize normalcy of development • Examine genitalia as any other body part; may leave to end

by touching the feet and then moving gradually toward the body and head. Instruments to examine the ears, eyes, and mouth are usually viewed as the most fearful and should be used at the end of the examination.

Preschoolers

Most children in this age group are cooperative during the physical examination. Allow the child to touch and play with the equipment. Give simple explanations about the assessment procedures, and offer choice where there is one during the examination. Younger children will often prefer to be examined on the parent's lap, while older children will be comfortable on the examining table. Most children are willing to undress, but leave the underpants on until conducting the genital examination. Some children will prefer to have the head, eyes, ears, and mouth examined first while others will prefer to postpone them to the end. Use distraction to gain the child's cooperation during the examination, such as asking the child to count, name colors, or talk about a favorite activity. Give positive feedback when the child cooperates.

School-age Children

School-age children willingly cooperate during the examination and sit on the examining table. Anticipate the development of modesty in school-age children and offer a patient gown to cover the underwear. Let the older school-age child determine if the examination will be conducted in privacy or with the parent or siblings present. A head-to-toe sequence can be used in this age group. Demonstrate how the instruments are used and let the child handle them if they wish. During the examination, tell the child what you are doing and why. Offer as many choices as possible to help the child feel empowered. The examination is a good opportunity to teach the child about how the body works, such as letting the child listen to heart and breathe sounds.

Adolescents

Protect the adolescent's modesty by providing a private place to undress and put on the patient gown, and then during the examination by covering the parts of the body not being assessed. Use the head-to-toe sequence and the same procedures used for adults. Perform the examination in private without parent or siblings unless the adolescent specifically requests the parent's presence. Provide a chaperone when the parent or accompanying adult is not present during the examination. Adolescents often have a lot of concerns regarding their developing bodies. When appropriate, provide reassurance about the normal progression of secondary sexual characteristic development and what further changes to expect.

ASSESSMENT OF PEDIATRIC PATIENT

It includes gathering of subjective and objective data is done by collection of data through:

- History taking
- Family assessment
- Developmental assessment
- Physical assessment
- Nutritional assessment
- Review of investigation's report and record analysis.

Pediatric assessment triangle (PAT)

- General appearance
- Work of breathing
- Circulation to skin.

ADMISSION ASSESSMENT

An admission assessment should be completed by the nurse with a parent or caregiver, ideally upon arrival to the ward or preadmission, but must be completed within 24 hours of admission. Admission assessment is to be documented on the nursing admission form. Privacy of the patient needs to be considered all times.

Pediatric History Taking and Family Assessment

History collection is the part of health assessment. History of current illness/injury (i.e. reason for current admission), relevant past history, allergies and reactions, medications, immunization status and family and social history are to be taken.

A pediatric history and family assessment help the nurse to gain a comprehensive view of the child and the family. It is an important aspect to evaluate the child's condition. It helps in diagnosis and planning care. For neonates and infants consider maternal history, antenatal history, delivery type and complications if any, APGAR score, resuscitation required at delivery and newborn screening tests, etc. History regarding the child's illness is to be collected from the parent or significant others, and even from the child himself. Strategies are to be adopted for gaining cooperation during history taking. Purposes of history taking are:

- To aid in diagnosis and treatment of the child
- To collect subjective data to initiate nursing process
- To establish relationship with the child and his/her family members
- To assess the understanding of the family members about their child's health
- To give information to the family members regarding the child's health condition.

The format used for history taking may be:

- **Direct,** where the health care provider asks for information via direct interview with the informant or

- **Indirect,** where the informant supplies information by completion type of questionnaire.

History taking of a pediatric patient and his/her family assessment includes:

- Identifying information or identification data
- *Chief complaints:* It may be viewed as the theme, with the present illness viewed as the description of the problem
- *Present history of illness:* The details of onset, the present status, the reason for seeking help now
- *Past history of illness, injuries and operations:*
  - Family history and family medical and surgical history
  - Birth history
  - History of growth and development
  - Immunizations
  - Dietary history
  - Rest and sleep
  - Habits
  - Play and activities
  - Toilet training
  - Allergy history
  - Current medications
  - Personal hygiene and elimination
  - School history
  - Sociocultural history
  - Sexual history, in case of older children
  - Medical and surgical history (present and past).

General Appearance

Assessment of the patient's overall physical, emotional and behavioral state is explored and general appearance is observed. Considerations for all patients include: Looks well or unwell, pale or flushed, lethargic or active, agitated or calm, compliant or combative, posture and movement.

- Neonate and infant
  - Parent-infant, infant-parent interaction
  - Body symmetry, spontaneous position and movement
  - Symmetry and positioning of facial features
  - Strong cry.

Young Child

- Parent-child, child-parent interaction
- Mood and affect
- Gross and fine motor skills
- Developmental milestones
- Appropriate speech.

Adolescent

- Mood and affect
- Personal hygiene
- Communication.

Vital Signs

Baseline observations are recorded as part of an admission assessment and documented on the patients observation chart.

- *Temperature:* Tympanic temperatures for children older than 6 months. Less than 6 months use digital per axilla.
- *Respiratory rate:* Count the child's breaths for one full minute. Assess any respiratory distress.
- *Heart rate:* Palpate brachial pulse (preferred in neonates) or femoral pulse in infant and radial pulse in older children. To ensure accuracy, count pulse for a full minute.
- *Blood pressure:* Baseline measurement should be obtained for every patient. Selection of the cuff size is an important consideration. A rough guide to appropriate cuff size is to ensure it fits a 2/3 width of upper arm. For neonates without previous hospital admissions do a blood pressure on all 4 limbs.
- *Oxygen saturation:* As clinically indicated.
- *Pain:* FLACC, faces, numeric scale, neonatal pain assessment tool.
- Current pain relief medications/practices.

Additional Measurements

- *Weight:* On admission and/or weekly/daily as clinically indicated.
- *Height:* As clinically indicated.
- *Head circumference:* As clinically indicated.
- *Blood sugar level (BSL):* As clinically indicated.

Physical Assessment

A structured physical examination allows the nurse to obtain a complete assessment of the patient. Observation, inspection, palpation, percussion and auscultation are techniques used to gather information. The purposes of physical assessments are:

- To aid diagnosis, to plan and provide best treatment
- To safeguard the child and to prevent various complications
- To teach the family to correct health habits and to practice healthful living
- To provide preventive care to the children by early detection of deviation of deviations from the normal health.
- To provide follow-up care.

Table 7.2: Physical assessment: Review of the systems

Body systems	Examples of problems to identify
General	General growth pattern, overall health status, ability to keep up with other children or tires easily with feeding or activity, fever, sleep patterns, allergies, type of reaction (hives, rash, respiratory difficulty, swelling, nausea), seasonal or with each exposure
Skin and lymph	Rashes, dry skin, itching, changes in skin color or texture, tendency for bruising, swollen or tender lymph glands
Hair and nails	Hair loss, changes in color or texture, use of dye or chemicals on hair abnormalities of nail growth or color
Eyes	Vision problems, squinting, crossed eyes, lazy eye, wears glasses, eye infections, redness, tearing, burning, rubbing, swelling eyelids
Ears	Ear infections, frequent discharge from ears, or tubes in ears, no response to loud noises
Nose	Nosebleeds, nasal congestion, colds with runny nose, sinus pain or infections, nasal obstruction, difficult breathing
Mouth and throat	Mouth breathing, difficulty swallowing, sore throats, strep infections, mouth odor, tooth eruption, cavities, braces; voice change, hoarseness, speech problems
Heart and hematologic	Heart murmur, anemia, hypertension, cyanosis, edema, rheumatic fever, chest pain
Respiratory	Trouble breathing, choking episodes, cough, wheezing, cyanosis, exposure to tuberculosis, other infections
Gastrointestinal	Bowel movements, frequency, color, regularity, consistency, discomfort, constipation or diarrhea, abdominal pain, bleeding from rectum, flatulence, nausea or vomiting, appetite
Renal	Frequency, urgency, dysuria, dribbling, strength of urinary stream: Toilet trained—age when day and night dryness attained, enuresis
Musculoskeletal	Weakness, clumsiness, poor coordination, balance, tremors, abnormal gait, painful muscles or joints, swelling or redness of joints, fractures
Neurological	Brain or head injuries; seizures, fainting spells, dizziness, numbness; learning problems, attention span, hyperactivity, memory problems
Reproductive	For pubescent children
Female	Menses onset, amount, duration, frequency, discomfort, problems; vaginal discharge, breast development
Male	Puberty onset, emissions, erections, pain or discharge from penis, swelling or pain in testicles
Both	Sexual activity, use of contraception, sexually transmitted diseases

The review of systems is a specific review of each body system, following an order similar to that of the physical examination (Table 7.2). Clinical judgment should be used to decide on the extent of assessment required. Assessment information includes, but is not limited to:

- *Airway:* Noises, secretions, cough, artificial airway
- *Breathing:* Bilateral air entry and movement, breath sounds (normal and adventitious), respiratory rate, rhythm, work of breathing: Spontaneous/labored/supported/ventilator dependent, any oxygen requirement and delivery mode.
- *Circulation:* Pulses (location, rate, rhythm and strength); peripheral temperature, skin color and moisture, skin turgor, capillary refill time; lip, oral mucosa and nail bed color.
- *Disability:* Use assessment tools such as, alert voice pain unresponsive score (AVPU), gross motor function classification system (GMFCS). Identify any aids required such as mobility aids, transfer needs, glasses, hearing aids, prosthetics, orthotics etc. Any abnormal movement or gait.
- *Focused assessment:* Detailed nursing assessment of specific body system(s) relating to the presenting problem or current concern(s) of the patient. This may involve one or more body systems. For example, cardiovascular, respiratory, neurological (Table 7.2).
- *Skin:* Color, turgor, lesions, bruising, wounds, pressure injuries and other skin conditions (Table 7.3).
- *Input/Nutrition:* Appetite, appropriate weight for age, food intolerance, nausea or vomiting, dietary requirements, breastfed, formula, oral, NG, Gastrostomy, Jejunal, IV Fluids, hydration state.
- *Output/Elimination:* Bowel and bladder routine(s), incontinence management, drains and other losses.

Table 7.3: Examination of skin conditions
Cyanosis: Bluish tone through skin; reduced (deoxygenated) hemoglobin
Pallor: Paleness; may be sign of anemia, chronic disease, edema, or shock
Erythematic: Redness; may be result of increased blood flow from climatic conditions, local inflammation, infection, skin irritation, allergy, or other dermatomes or may be caused by increased numbers of red blood cells as compensatory response to chronic hypoxia
Ecchymosis: Large, diffuse areas, usually black and blue, caused by hemorrhage of blood into skin; typically result of injuries
Petechiae: Same as ecchymosed except for size: small, distinct, pinpoint hemorrhages 2 mm or less in size; can denote some type of blood disorder, such as leukemia
Jaundice: Yellow staining of skin usually caused by bile pigments

Social/Cultural

Parents/carers/guardian, living arrangements, siblings, visiting plans, transport, specific cultural requirements.

General Appearance

The child's general appearance is a cumulative, subjective impression of the child's physical appearance, state of nutrition, behavior, activity level, reaction to stress, request, frustration, degree of alzzertness, speech development, motor skills, coordination and recent area of achievement, (e.g., an 18-month-old child: 'motor development advanced for age; climbs runs, jumps, manipulates small objects with ease, excellent coordination and balance, beginning to name many objects, uses two word phrases, and enjoys talking to self and others), personality, interaction with the parents and others, overall state of health, fatigue, posture, position, general alertness, activity, movement of limbs, crying, response to stimulus, sleeping pattern, recent or unexplained weight gain or loss (period of time for either), contributing factors (change of diet, illness, altered appetite), fevers (time of day), chills, night sweets (unrelated to climatic conditions), frequent infections, general ability to carry out activities of daily living.

Measurements

Measurement of physical growth in childzren is a key element in evaluating their health status (Table 7.1). Physical growth parameters include weight, height (length), skin fold thickness, arm circumference, and head circumference. Values for these growth parameters are plotted on percentile charts. This chart is known as growth chart. Growth chart will be discussed later on, in nutritional assessment.

- *Length and height:* The term length refers to measurements taken when children are supine (also referred to as recumbent length). Recumbent length is measured up to 2 years of age (or 36 months if using the chart for birth to 36 months). Crown to heel length is taken by using a measuring board or infantometer, place the head firmly at the top of the board and heels of the feet firmly against the footboard. At first fully extend the body by holding the head in midline, secondly grasp the knees together gently, and thirdly, push down on the knees until the legs are fully extended and flat against the table.
  The term height (or stature) refers to the measurement taken when children are standing upright. Increase in height indicates skeletal growth. The measurement of height is taken (by using a wall-mounted unit or stadiometer) when children are standing upright.
  - At birth, average length of a healthy Indian newborn baby is 50 cm
  - 3 months: 60 cm
  - 9 months: 70 cm
  - 1 year: 75 cm (50 + 25 cm)
  - 2 year: 87 cm (12 cm increase)
  - 3 years: 96 cm (9 cm increase)
  - 4 years: 103 cm (7 cm increase)
  - 5 years: 109 cm (6 cm increase)

  So the child doubles the birth length by 4 to 4.5 years of age. Afterwards there is about 5 cm increase in every year till onset of puberty. Gradual slow increase in length is usually found up to the period of post-pubescence.
- *Weight:* Weight is the best criteria for assessment of growth and a good indicator of health and nutritional status of child. Among the Indian children, weight of the full term neonate at birth is approximately 2.5 kg to 3.8 kg. There is about 10% loss of weight during first week of life, which regains by 10 days of age. Then, weight gain is about 25 to 30 gm per day for first 3 months and 400 gm per month till one year of age.
  - The infants doubled their birth weight by 5 months of age.
  - Triple by 1 year
  - 4 times by 2 years
  - 5 times by 3 years

- 6 times by 5 years
- 7 times by 7 years
- 10 times by 10 years

- *Head circumference:* Average head circumference measures about 35 cm at birth.
  - At 3 months: 40 cm
  - At 6 months: 43 cm
  - At 1 year: 45 cm
  - At 2 years: 48 cm
  - At 7 years: 50 cm
  - At 12 years: 52 cm (almost same as adult)
  - Head and chest circumference are equal at the age of 6–12 months.

  Measure the head at its greatest circumference, usually slightly above the eyebrows and around the occipital prominence at the back of skull.
- *Fontanelle:* At birth, anterior and posterior fontanelle are usually present. Posterior fontanelle closes at birth or early within few weeks (6–8 weeks) of age. The anterior fontanelle normally closes by 12–18 months of age.
- *Chest circumference:* At birth it is 2–3 cm less than head circumference. At 6–12 months of age both become equal. After 1st year of age, chest circumference is greater than head circumference by 2.5 cm and by the age of 5 years, it is about 5 cm larger than head circumference.

  At birth chest is round in shape with nearly equal transverse and anteroposterior diameter. Thereafter, the width of chest becomes greater than depth due to rapid increase in transverse diameter.
- *Arm circumference:* Arm circumference is an indirect measure of muscle mass. Place the tape vertically along the posterior aspect of the upper arm to the acromial process and to the olecranon process; half the measured length is the midpoint. The average mid-upper arm circumference at birth is 11–12 cm at 1year of age it is 12–16 cm, at 1–5 years 16–17 cm, at 12 years it is 17–18 cm, and at 15 years it is 20–21 cm.
- *Physiologic measurements:* Physiologic measurements, key elements in evaluating physical status of vital functions, include temperature, pulse, respiration and blood pressure. For best result in taking vital sign of infants, count respiration first (before the infant is disturbed), take pulse next, and measurement temperature last. (*See* annexure for age-wise normal value)
- *Temperature:* Temperature is the measure of heat content within an individual's body. The 'core' temperature most closely reflects the temperature of the blood flow through the carotid arteries to the hypothalamus. For neonates, a core body temperature between 36.5 °C is a desirable range.

  Rectal—36.6–38 °C
  Oral—35.5–37.5 °C
  Axillary—34.7–37.3 °C
  Ear—35.8–38 °C.

Skin: Skin is assessed for color, texture, temperature, moisture, and turgor (Table 7.3). Examination of the skin and its accessory organs primarily involves inspection and palpation. Touch allows the health care provider to assess the texture, turgor and temperature of the skin. Normal color in the light skinned children varies from a milky white and rose to a deeply hued pink. Dark skinned children have inherited various brown, red, yellow, olive green and bluish tones in their skin. Normally the skin texture of young children is smooth, slightly dry and not oily or clammy.

Determine the tissue turgor or elasticity in the skin, by grasping the skin on the abdomen between the thumb and index finger, pulling it taut and quickly releasing it. Elastic tissue immediately assumes its normal position without residual marks or creases.

Lymph nodes: Lymph nodes are usually assessed when the part of the body in which they are located is examined. The body's lymphatic drainage system is extensive.

Palpate nodes using the distal portion of the fingers and gently but firmly pressing in a circular motion along the regions where nodes are normally present. During assessment of the nodes in the head and neck, tilt the child's head upward slightly but without tensing the sternocleidomastoid or trapeziums muscles. This position facilitates palpation of the submental, submandibular, tonsillar, and cervical nodes. Palpate the axillary nodes with the arms relaxed at the sides but slightly abducted. Assess the inguinal nodes with the child in the supine position.

Head and neck: Observe the head for general shape and symmetry. Palpate the skull for patent sutures, fontanels, fractures, and swellings. Normally the posterior fontanel closes by the second month of life, and the anterior fontanel fuses between 12 and 18 months of age (Table 7.2).

While examining the head, observe the face for symmetry, movement and general appearance. Note any unusual facial proportion, such as an unusually high or low forehead; wide or close-set eyes; or a small, receding chin. Inspect the neck for size and palpate its associated structures. The neck is normally short, with skinfolds between the head and shoulders during infancy; however, it lengthens during the next 3–4 years.

Face: Should be observed for symmetry, paralysis, shape, swelling and abnormal movements.

Eyes: Should be checked for edema, conjunctivitis or discharge, subconjunctival hemorrhage (due to traumatic delivery), color of sclera (blue color is indicative ontogenesis imperfect and yellow discoloration of the sclera indicates jaundice).

- Brash field's spots in the iris (Down syndrome Trisomy-21)
- Abnormal placement of the days (chromosomal anomalies)
- Abnormal distance between two eyes.

Nose: Observe in overall size and in diameters of the nares, any deviation of nasal bridge, alae nasi for any sign of flaring.

Mouth and throat: Observe the lips, oral cavity, gums, teeth, tongue, palate uvula, tonsils for color, white patches ulceration, bleeding, sensitivity, and moisture.

Ears: Assess the pinna firmness. Measure the height alignment of the pinna by drawing an imaginary line from the outer orbit of the eye to the occiput, or most prominent protuberance of the skull. Top of the pinna should meet or cross this line. Inspect the skin surface around the ear for small openings, extra tags of skin, or sinuses. Also assess the ear for hygiene. Look into the external canal to note the presence of cerumen. Look for any discharge, its color and odor are noted.

Chest: Inspect the chest for size, shape, symmetry, movement, breast development, and the bony landmarks formed by the ribs and sternum, or breast bone, located in the middle of the trunk. During infancy the chest's shape is almost circular.

Movement of the chest wall should be symmetric bilaterally and coordinate bilaterally and coordinated with breathing during inspiration the chest rises and expands, the diaphragm descends, and the costal angle increases. During expiration the chest falls and decreases in size, the diaphragm rises, and costal angle narrows. In children younger than 6 or 7 years of age, respiratory movement is principally abdominal or diaphragmatic. In older children, particularly girls, respirations are chiefly thoracic.

While inspecting the skin surface of the chest, observe the position of the nipples, as well as any evidence of breast development. Normally the nipples are located slightly lateral to the mid-clavicular line between the fourth and fifth ribs. Note symmetry of nipple placement and normal configuration of a darker pigmented areola surrounding a flat nipple in the pre-pubertal child.

Pubertal breast development usually begins in girls between 10 and 14 years of age. Early or delayed breast development is to be recorded, as well as evidence of any other secondary sexual characteristics. In males breast enlargement may be caused by hormonal or systematic disorders, but more commonly it is a result of adipose tissue from obesity or a transitory body change during early puberty. In either situation investigate the child's feelings regarding breast enlargement.

In adolescent girls who have achieved sexual maturity, palpate the breasts for evidence of any masses of hard nodules. Use this opportunity to discuss the importance of routine breast self-examination. Emphasize that most palpable masses are benign to decrease any fear or concern that results when a mass is felt.

Lungs: Inspection of the lungs primarily involves observation of respiratory movements. Evaluate respirations for rate (number per minute), rhythm (regular, irregular, or periodic), depth (deep or shallow), and quality (effortless automatic, difficult, or labored). Note the character of breath sounds, such as noisy, grunting, snoring, or heavy.

Evaluate respiratory movements by placing each hand flat against the back or chest with the thumbs in midline along the lower costal margin of the lungs. The child should be sitting during this procedure and, if cooperative, should take several deep breaths.

- *Auscultation:* Auscultation involves using the stethoscope to evaluate breath sounds. Breath sounds are best heard if the child inspires deeply. In the lungs breath sounds are classified as vesicular, bronchovesicular, or bronchial.

  Absent or diminished breath sounds are always an abnormal finding warranting investigation. Fluid, air or solid masses in the pleural space all interfere with the conduction of breath sounds.

  These sounds occur in addition into two main groups: crackles, which result from the passage of air through fluid or moisture, and wheezes, which are produced as air passes through narrowed passageways, regardless of the cause, such as exudates, inflammation, spasm, or tumor. Considerable practice with an experience tutor is necessary to differentiate the various types of lung sounds.

Heart: The heart is situated in the thoracic cavity between the lungs in the mediastinum and above the diaphragm. The heart is positioned in the thorax like a trapezoid.

Inspection is best done with the child sitting in a semi-Fowler position. Look at the anterior chest wall from an angle, comparing both sides of the rib cage with each other. Normally they should be symmetric. In children with thin chest walls, a pulsation may be visible.

Use palpation to determine the location of the apical impulse (AI), the most lateral cardiac impulse that may correspond to the apex.

Auscultation

Origin of heart sounds: The opening and closing of the valves and the vibration of blood against the walls of the heart and vessels. Normally two sounds— S1 and S2—are heard, which correspond, respectively, to the familiar 'lub dub' often used to describe the sounds.

- S1 is caused by closure of the tricuspid and mitral valves (sometimes called the atrioventricular valves). S1 is louder at the apex of the heart in the mitral and tricuspid area.
- S2 is the result of closure of the pulmonic and aortic valves (sometimes called semi lunar valves). S2 is louder near the base of the heart in the pulmonic and aortic area.
  Normally the split of the two sounds in S2 is distinguishable and widens during inspiration.
  Two other heart sounds S3 and S4 may be produced.
- S3 is normally heard in some children.
- S4 is rarely heard as a normal heart sound.
  Another important category of heart sounds is murmurs, which are produced by vibrations within the heart chambers or in the major arteries from the back-and-forth flow of blood. The description and classification of murmurs are skills that require considerable practice and training.

Abdomen: Examination of the abdomen involves inspection, followed by auscultation and then palpation.

Inspection: Inspect the contour of the abdomen with the child erect and supine. Normally the abdomen of infants and young children is cylindric. In the supine position the abdomen appears flat. The skin covering the abdomen should be uniformly taut, without wrinkles or crease.

Observe movement of the abdomen. Normally chest and abdominal movements are synchronous. In infants and thin children peristaltic waves may be visible through the abdominal wall; they are best observed by standing at eye level to and across from the abdomen.

Examine the umbilicus for size, hygiene, and evidence of any abnormalities, such as hernias. The umbilicus should be flat or only slightly protruding. If a herniation is present, palpate the sac for abdominal contents and estimate the approximate size of the opening.

A femoral hernia, which occurs more frequently in girls, is felt or seen as a small mass on the anterior surface of the thigh just below the inguinal ligament in the femoral canal (a potential space medial to the femoral artery). Feel for a hernia by placing the index finger of your right hand on the child's right femoral pulse (left hand for left pulse) and the middle finger flat against the skin toward the midline. The ring finger lies over the femoral canal, where the herniation occurs.

Auscultation: The most important finding to listen for is peristalsis, or bowel sounds, which sound like short metallic clicks and gurgles. Bowel sounds may be stimulated by stroking the abdominal surface with a fingernail.

Palpation: `Two types of palpation are performed: superficial and deep. For superficial palpation, lightly place hand against the skin and feel each quadrant, noting any areas of tenderness, muscle tone, and superficial lesions such as cysts.

Deep palpation is used for palpating organs and large blood vessels and for detecting masses and tenderness that were not discovered during superficial palpation. Palpation usually begins in the lower quadrants and proceeds upward to avoid missing the edge of an enlarged liver or spleen.

Palpate the femoral pulses by placing the tips of two or three finger (index, middle, or ring) along the inguinal ligament about midway between the iliac crest and symphysis pubis.

- ***Back and Extremities:***
  - *Spine:* The general curvature of the spine is noted. Normally the back of a newborn is rounded or C-shaped from the thoracic and pelvic curves. The development of the cervical and lumbar curves approximates development of various motor skills, such as cervical curvature with head control, and gives the older child the typical double S curve.
    A slight limp, a crooked hemline, or complaints of a sore back are other and symptoms of scoliosis. Inspect the back especially along the spine, for any tufts of hair, dimples, or discoloration. Mobility of the vertebral column is easily assessed in most children because of their propensity for constant motion during the examination. Movement of the cervical spine is an important diagnosis sign of neurologic problems, such as meningitis.
  - *Extremities:* Inspect each extremity (Hands and legs) for symmetry of length and size; refer

any deviation for orthopedic evaluation. Count the fingers and toes to be certain of the normal number. This is so often taken for granted that an extra digit (polydactyly) or fusion of digits may go unnoticed. Inspect the arms and legs for temperature and color.

Assess the shape of bones. Several variations of bone shape may be observed in children. Bowleg, or genu varum, is lateral bowing of the tibia. Toddlers are usually bowlegged after beginning to walk until all their lower back and leg muscles are well developed. Unilateral or asymmetric bowlegs that are present beyond the age of 2 to 3 years.

Knock-knee, or genu valgum, appears as the opposite of bowleg, in that the knees are close together but the feet are spread apart. Measuring the distance between the malleoli, which normally should be less than 7, 5 cm (3 inches). Knock-knee is normally present in children from about 2 to 7 years of age. Knock-knee that is excessive, asymmetric, accompanied by short stature, or evident in a child nearing puberty requires further evaluation.

- *Joints:* Evaluate the joints for range of motion. Normally this requires no specific testing if the nurse has observed the child's movements during the examination.
- *Muscles:* Note symmetry and quality of muscle development, tone, and strength. Observe development by looking at the shape and contour of the body in both a relaxed and a tensed state. Estimate tone by grasping the muscle and feeling its firmness when it is relaxed and contracted. A common site for testing tone is the biceps muscle of the arm. Children are usually willing to 'make a muscle' by clenching their fist.

Estimate strength by having the child use an extremity to push or pull against resistance, as in the following examples.

- *Arm strength:* Child holds the arms outstretched in front of the body and tries to raise the arms while downward pressure is applied.
- *Hand strength:* Child shakes hands with nurse and squeezes one or two fingers of the nurse's hand.
- *Leg strength:* Child sits on a table or chair with the legs dangling and tries to raise the while downward pressure is applied.

Genitalia: Examination of genitalia conveniently follows assessment of the abdomen while the child is still supine. In adolescents inspection of the genitalia may be left to the end of the examination. The best approach is to examine the genitalia matter-of-factly, placing no more emphasis on this part of the assessment than on any other segment.

If it is necessary to ask questions, such as about discharge or difficulty urinating, respect the child's privacy by covering the lower abdomen with the gown or underpants. To prevent embarrassing interruptions, keep the door or curtain closed and post a 'do not disturb' sign.

The genital examination is an excellent time for eliciting questions of concern about body function or sexual activity. Also use this opportunity to increase or reinforce the child's knowledge of reproductive anatomy.

- *Male genitalia:* Note the external appearance of the glans and shaft of the penis, the prepuce, the urethral meatus, and the scrotum.

  Examine the glans (head of the penis) and shaft (portion between the perineum and prepuce) for signs of swelling, skin lesions, inflammation, or other irregularities. The urethral meatus is carefully inspected for location and evidence of discharge.
  - Hair distribution is also noted.
  - The location and size of the scrotum are noted.
  - Palpation of the scrotum includes identification of the testes, epididymis, and, if present, inguinal hernias.
- *Female genitalia:* The examination of female genitalia is limited to inspection and palpation of external structures. A convenient position for examination of the genitalia involves placing the young child supine on the examining table or in a semireclining position on the parent's lap with the feet supported on your knees as you sit facing the child. Divert the child's attention from the examination by instructing her to try to keep the soles of her feet pressed against each other. Separate the labia majora with the thumb and index finger and retract outward to expose the labia minora, urethral meatus, and vaginal orifice.
  - Examine the female genitalia for size and location of the structures of the vulva, or pudendum. The appearance of soft, downy hair along the labia majora is an early sign if sexual maturation.

  The urethral meatus is located posterior to the clitoris and is surrounded by Skene glands and ducts. Although not a prominent structure, the meatus appears as a small v-shaped slit. The vaginal orifice is located posterior to the urethral meatus.

Anus: After examination of the genitalia, the anal area is examined, although the child should be placed on the abdomen. Note the general firmness of the buttocks and symmetry of the gluteal folds. Assess the tone of the anal sphincter by eliciting the anal reflex. An obvious quick contraction of the external anal sphincter results in gentle scratching of the anal areas.

Neurological assessment: The assessment of the nervous system is the broadest and most diverse part of the examining process. Much of the neurologic examination has already been discussed, such as assessment of behavior, sensory testing, and motor function. Reflexes are also important neurological assessment (Table 7.4).

- *Cerebellar function:* The cerebellum controls balance and coordination is included in observing the child's gross motor skills.
- *Finger-to-nose test:* With child's arm extended, ask child to touch the nose with the index finger with eyes open and then closed.
- *Heel-to-shin test:* Have child stand and run the heel of one foot down the shin or anterior aspect of the tibia of the other leg, both with eyes opened and then closed.

Table 7.4: Assessment of cranial nerve functioning

Description and Function	*Tests*
I—Olfactory nerve: Olfactory mucosa of nasal cavity Smell	With eyes closed, have child identify odors such as coffee, alcohol from a swab, or other smells; test each nostril separately.
II—Optic nerve: Rods and cones of retina, optic nerve Vision	Check for perception of light, visual acuity, peripheral vision, color vision, and normal optic disc.
III—Oculomotor nerve: Extraocular muscle of eye: Superior rectus(SR)—moves eyeball up and in Inferior rectus(IR)—moves eyeball down and in Medial rectus(MR)—moves eyeball nasally Inferior oblique(IO)—moves eyeball up and out Pupil constriction and accommodation Eyelid closing	Have child follow an object (toy) or light in 6 cardinal positions of gaze Perform PERRLA (stands for 'pupils equal, round to light, and accommodation') Check for proper placement of lid.
IV—Trochlear nerve: Superior oblique muscle (SO)—moves eye down and out	Have child look down and in
V—Trigeminal nerve: Muscle of mastication Sensory: Face, scalp, nasal and buccal mucosa	Have child bite down hard and open jaw; test symmetry and strength. With child's eyes closed, see if child can detect light touch in mandibular and maxillary regions. Test corneal and blink reflex by touching cornea lightly (approach from side so that child does not blink before cornea is touched).
VI—Abducent nerve: Lateral rectus (LR) muscle—moves eye temporally	Have child look toward temporal side
VII—Facial nerve: Muscle for facial expression Anterior 2/3 of tongue (sensory)	Have child smile, make funny face, or show teeth to see symmetry of expression. Have child identify sweet or salty solution; place each taste on anterior section and sides of protruding tongue; if child retracts tongue, solution will dissolve toward posterior part of tongue.
VIII—Auditory, acoustic, or vestibulocochlear nerve: Internal ear Hearing and balance	Test hearing; note any loss of equilibrium or presence of vertigo.

Contd...

Contd...

IX—Glossopharyngeal nerve: Pharynx, tongue Posterior 1/3 of tongue (sensory)	Stimulate posterior pharynx with a tongue blade; child should gag. Test sense of sour or bitter taste on posterior segment of tongue.
X—Vagus nerve: Muscle of larynx, pharynx, some organs of gastrointestinal system, sensory fibers of root of tongue, heart, and lung	Note hoarseness of voice, gag reflex, and ability to swallow. Check that uvula is in midline; when stimulated with tongue blade; it should deviate upward and to stimulated side.
XI—Accessory nerve: Sternocleidomastoid and trapezius muscle of shoulder	Have child shrug shoulders while applying mild pressure; with examiner's hands placed on shoulders, have child turn head against opposing pressure on either side; note symmetry and strength.
XII—Hypoglossal nerve: Muscle of tongue	Have child move tongue in all directions; have child protrude tongue as far as possible; note any midline deviation. Test strength by placing tongue blade on one side of tongue and having child move it away.

- *Romberg test:* Have child stand with eyes closed and heels together; falling or learning to one side is abnormal and is called Romberg sign.

DEVELOPMENTAL ASSESSMENT

Developmental assessment of development is essential to detect abnormal developmental delays. The most widely used screening for detecting developmental delays in infancy and preschool years is known as Denver Developmental Screening Test (DDST). It is a worldwide popular test developed in 1967 for the assessment of four areas, i.e, gross motor, fine motor, language and personal social behavior. DDST was modified in 1992 in the form of Denver II, with 125 items.

Other developmental tests include Borada DST, Trivandrum DST etc. In India Baroda Screening test was developed by Dr Pramila Pathak with 25 test items primarily for psychological aspects. The test is relevant for age 0 to 3 months. Gross motor, fine motor and cognitive aspects are evaluated in 10 minutes.

Trivandrum Development Screening test is the simplified version of Baroda DST that can be used by the health workers, nurse and pediatricians/physicians. It has 17 test items relevant for 0 to 2 years of age. The children are evaluated in three domains, i.e. gross motor, fine motor and cognitive for five minutes only.

See growth and development of children chapter for detail developmental assessment.

ASSESSMENT OF NUTRITIONAL STATUS

Knowledge of the child's dietary intake is an essential component of a nutritional assessment. The nutritional status of an individual is influence by the adequacy of food intake both in terms of quantity and quality and also by the physical health of the individual. Dietary evaluation is an important component of the child's assessment.

The dietary reference intakes are a set of nutrient-based reference values that provide quantitative estimates of nutrient intake for use in assessing and planning dietary intake. The specific DRIs include:

- Estimated average requirement (EAR): Nutrient intake estimated to meet the requirement of half the healthy individuals (50%) for a specific age and gender group.
- *Recommended dietary allowance (RDA):* Average daily dietary intake sufficient to meet the nutrient requirement of nearly all (97 to 98%) healthy individuals for a specific age and gender group.
- *Adequate intake (AI):* Recommended intake level based on estimates of nutrient intake by healthy groups of individuals.
- *Tolerable upper intake level (UL):* Highest average daily nutrient intake level likely to pose no risk of adverse health effects. As intake increases above the UL, risk of adverse effects increases.

PURPOSES OF NUTRITIONAL ASSESSMENT

- To detect nutritional problems
- To develop the plan to meet the nutritional needs.

VARIOUS TECHNIQUES WITH DIFFERENT APPROACHES (TABLE 7.5)

The assessment of nutritional status involves various techniques with different approaches. The assessment method includes:

- Dietary history
- Clinical examination

Table 7.5: Nutritional assessment of children

Assessment on	*Evidence of assessment nutrition*	*Evidence of deficient or excess nutrition*	*Deficiency or excess*
General growth	• Within 5th and 9th percentiles for height, weight and head circumference • Steady gain with expected growth spurts during infancy and adolescence • Sexual development appropriate for age	• Below 5th or above 95th percentile for growth • Absence of or delayed growth spurts; poor weight gain • Delayed sexual development	• Protein, calories, fats, and other essential nutrients, especially, Vitamin-A, pyridoxine, niacin, calcium, iodine, manganese, zinc • Excess vitamins A, D
Skin	• Smooth, slightly, dry to touch • Elastic and firm • Absence of lesions • Color appropriate to genetic background	• Hardening and scaling • Seborrheic dermatitis • Dry, rough, petechiae • Delayed wound healing • Scaly dermatitis on exposed surfaces • Wrinkled, flabby • Crusted lesions around orifices, especially nares • Pruritus • Poor turgor • Edema • Yellow tinge (jaundice) • Depigmentation • Pallor (anemia) • Paresthesia	• Vitamin A • Excess niacin • Riboflavin • Vitamin C • Riboflavin, vitamin C, zinc • Niacin • Protein, calories, zinc • Excess vitamin A, riboflavin, niacin • Water, sodium • Protein, thiamine • Excess sodium • Vitamin B_{12} • Excess vitamin A, niacin • Protein, calories • Pyridoxine, folic acid, vitamins B_{12}, C, E (in premature infants), iron • Excess vitamin C, zinc • Excess riboflavin
Hair	Lustrous, silky, strong, elastic	• Stringy, friable, dull, dry, thin • Alopecia • Depigmentation • Raised areas around hair follicles	• Protein, calories • Protein, calories, zinc • Protein, calories, copper • Vitamin C
Head	• Even molding, occipital prominence, symmetric facial features • Fused sutures after 18 months	• Softening of cranial bones, prominence of frontal bones, skull flat and depressed toward middle • Delayed fusion of sutures • Hard, tender lumps in occiput • Headache	• Vitamin D • Vitamin D • Excess vitamin A • Excess thiamine
Neck	Thyroid not visible, palpable in midline	Thyroid enlarged; may be grossly visible	Iodine
Eyes	• Clear, bright • Good night vision • Conjunctiva—pink, glossy	• Hardening and scaling of cornea and conjunctiva • Night blindness • Burning, itching, photophobia, cataracts, corneal vascularization	• Vitamin A • Vitamin A • Riboflavin
Ears	Tympanic membrane pliable	Calcified (hearing loss)	Excess vitamin D
Nose	Smooth, intact nasal angle	Irritation and cracks at nasal angle	Riboflavin Excess vitamin A

Contd...

Contd...

Assessment on	*Evidence of assessment nutrition*	*Evidence of deficient or excess nutrition*	*Deficiency or excess*
Mouth	Lips—smooth, moist, darker color than skin Gums—firm. coral pink color, stippled Mucous membranes—bright pink, smooth, moist Tongue—rough texture, no lesions, taste sensation Teeth—uniform white color, smooth, intact	Fissures and inflammation at corners Spongy, friable, swollen, bluish red or black color bleed easily • Stomatitis • Glossitis • Diminished taste sensation • Brown mottling, pits, fissures • Defective enamel • Caries	• Riboflavin • Excess vitamin A • Vitamin C • Niacin • Niacin, riboflavin, folic acid • Zinc excess fluoride • Vitamins A, C, D, calcium, phosphorus • Excess carbohydrates
Chest	In infants, shape almost circular In children, lateral diameter increased in proportion to anteroposterior diameter Smooth costochondral junctions Breast development—normal for age	Depressed lower portion of rib cage Sharp protrusion of sternum Enlarged costochondral junctions Delayed development	Vitamin D Vitamin D Vitamins C, D See under general growth; especially zinc
Cardiovascular system	Pulse and blood pressure (BP) within normal limits	Palpitation Rapid pulse Arrhythmias Increased BP Decreased BP	Thiamine Potassium Excess thiamine Magnesium, potassium Excess niacin, potassium Excess sodium Thiamine; excess niacin
Abdomen	In young children, cylindric and prominent In older children, flat Normal bowel habits	Distended, flabby, poor musculature Prominent, large Potbelly, constipation Diarrhea Constipation	Protein, calories Excess calories Vitamin D Niacin Excess vitamin C Excess calcium, potassium
Musculoskeletal system	Muscles—firm, well-developed, equal strength bilaterally Spine—cervical and lumber curves (double S curve) Extremities—symmetric; legs straight with minimum bowing Joints—flexible, full range of motion, no pain or stiffness	Flabby, weak generalized wasting Weakness, pain, cramps Muscle twitching, tremors Muscular paralysis Kyphosis, lordosis, scoliosis Bowing of extremities, knock-knees Epiphyseal enlargement Bleeding into joints and muscles, joint swelling, pain Thickening of cortex of long bones with pain and fragility, hard tender lumps in extremities Osteoporosis of long bones	Protein, calories Thiamine, sodium, chloride, potassium, phosphorus, magnesium Excess thiamine Magnesium Excess potassium Vitamin D Vitamin D, calcium, phosphorus Vitamin A, D Vitamin C Excess vitamin A Calcium Excess vitamin D

Contd...

Contd...

Assessment on	*Evidence of assessment nutrition*	*Evidence of deficient or excess nutrition*	*Deficiency or excess*
Neurologic system	Behavior—alert, responsive, emotionally stable	Listless, irritable, lethargic, apathetic (sometimes apprehensive, anxious, drowsy, mentally slow, confused)	Thiamine, niacin, pyridoxine, vitamin C, potassium, magnesium, iron, protein, calories
			Excess vitamins A, D, thiamine, folic, folic acid, calcium
		Mask like facial expression, blurred speech, involuntary laughing	Excess manganese
	Absence of, convulsions	Convulsions	Thiamine, pyridoxine, vitamin D, calcium, magnesium
			Excess phosphorus (in relation to calcium)
		Peripheral nervous system toxicity (unsteady gait, numb feet and hands, fine motor clumsiness)	Excess pyridoxine
	Intact peripheral nervous system		
	Intact reflexes	Diminished or absent tendon reflexes	Thiamine, vitamin E

- Anthropometrical measurement
- Biochemical evaluation and laboratory tests
- Functional assessment
- Radiology.

CHAPTER 8

Preventive Pediatrics

Chapter Outline

- Aim
- Preventive Pediatrics: Few Related Concepts
- Milestones in the History of MCH Care in India
- Child Health
- ICDS
- IMNCI
- Handicapped Child Care
- Adolescent Health
- School Health
- Center for International Child Health are WHO, UNICEF, FAO, CARE, USAID
- National Organizations
- Nurses Role in Preventive Pediatrics

Children are vulnerable to malnutrition and infectious diseases many of which can be effectively, prevented or treated.

INTRODUCTION

Despite health improvements over the last thirty years, lives continue to be lost to early childhood diseases, inadequate newborn care and childbirth-related causes. More than two million children die every year from preventable infections. Preventive care for children and adolescents is a corner stone of public health and well-being for the population. Through the use of screening, education and proper preventive medicine, many serious and devastating illnesses can be avoided (Fig. 8.1). Prevention is one of the hallmarks of pediatrics and pediatric nursing which includes diverse activities as physical screening, immunization, nutrition, growth monitoring, accident prevention, psychological assessment, love and support, work with child's family, school and so on so forth.

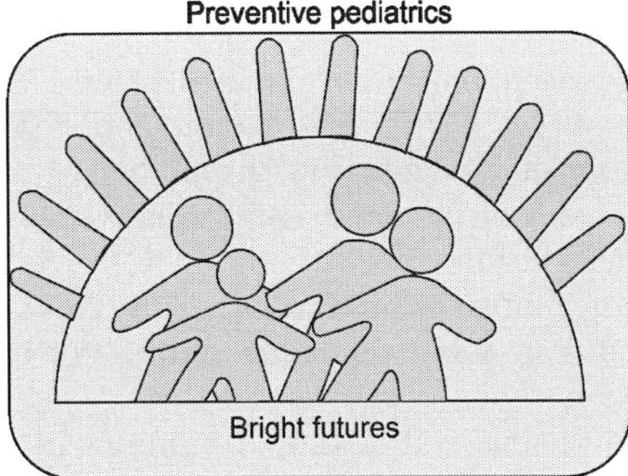

Fig. 8.1: Preventive pediatrics aims to enhance the health and well-being of children of the country

Preventive pediatrics aims to enhance the health and well-being of the children of the country. Early childhood care and development is a critical foundation not only of children but of society on the whole. This branch of science commits to all children of the country, through advocacy, health promotion, and community outreach through outreach programs to promote prevention of illness and early identification of life-threatening diseases. To provide early, accessible, preventive and interventional health services to improve the health status of children and adolescents in India by early identification of risk factors that affect their health through the implementation of clinical, educational and research programs.

DEFINITION

Preventive pediatrics is defined as the prevention of diseases and promotion of physical, mental and social welfare of children with the aim of attaining a positive health.

Preventive pediatric is a branch of medicine that deals with the care and management of children from conception to adolescence in health and disease state.

AIM

The aims of preventive pediatrics are similar to that of preventive medicine, i.e. prevention of disease and promotion of physical, mental, and social well-being of children so that each child may achieve the genetic potential with which he/she is born. To achieve these aims, hospitals for children have adopted the strategy of 'primary health care' to improve activities like growth monitoring, oral rehydration, nutritional surveillance, promotion of breastfeeding, immunization, community feeding, regular health check-ups, etc. Primary health care with its potential for vast increased coverage through an integrated system of service delivery is increasingly looked upon as the best solution to reach to millions of children, especially those who are in most need of preventive and curative services.

Preventive care aims to avoid or delay the occurrence of diseases, to timely detect a disease, to avoid or delay complications when the condition is already present, to avoid premature deaths and to improve efficiency. Prevention is a cornerstone of primary health care. When it is provided comprehensively, it increases the access and uptake of preventive services, which in turn results in better health and improved quality of care. So preventive pediatric aims:

- At the prevention of disease in children rather than focusing on cure of disease
- At the prevention of disease, means the child can attain their genetic potential
- To ensure adequate physical, mental and social growth of children
- At timely detection of disease of child to avoid or delay complications.

PREVENTIVE PEDIATRICS: FEW RELATED CONCEPTS

Child Health Protection

Child health protection refers to measure taken, at the population level to protect children from illness, injuries, and specific risks to their development. Child health protection is a form of primary prevention that in contrast with child health promotion, gives individuals a passive role. Protective measures are numerous and stretch from legislation to immunization and involve healthy public policy across all sectors of government not just health departments. Of particular note are legislation to protect children from abuse, neglect, and corporal punishment, social protection for children and families through taxation policy to redistribute societal wealth and reduce child and family material disadvantage, and education policy ensuring affordable childcare and schooling for all children.

Child Health Promotion

Health promotion is the process of enabling children and families to increase control over, and to improve, their health. It includes measures taken at the population and individual level to promote the health of children through personal skills development, building healthy public policy, and creating supportive environments. Child health promotion focuses on health rather than disease prevention and requires the active participation of individuals or families. Health promoting measures seek to ensure that children and their parents have the opportunity to adopt healthy lifestyles through the provision of education and information and health supportive environments (for example, with legislation). Therefore, health promotion is not just the responsibility of the health sector, but goes beyond health lifestyles to well-being.

School Health

Term refers to both the delivery of health services within school settings and the study of the effects of health on educational attainment and the effects of school on health. Although mainly concerned with health surveillance and identification of children with physical, psychological, learning and adaptive problems.

Classification

As this branch of medical science deals with the care of child from conception to adolescence, preventive pediatric can be broadly divided into two areas—antenatal preventive pediatric (APP), postnatal preventive pediatric (PPP).

APP focuses on mothers, for healthy child and safe delivery, and emphasize are being given on their health, environment and family. It includes birth preparedness and maternity services. APP is important for following reasons.

- Since conception, the development of fetus (40 weeks) takes place in mother's womb and receives all nutrition and oxygen from the mother
- The health of the child is intricately linked to the mother's health
- Healthy mother brings forth a healthy child. Healthy mother can avoid premature birth, still birth and abortion
- Certain habits and diseases conditions of expected mother will affect the child health, i.e taking drugs, syphilis, German measles, etc.

PPP is the extended arena of child health which targets prevention of diseases and overall development of child. It comprises efforts to avert rather than cure diseases and disabilities through newborn care and treatment; immunization, including polio; maternal and young child nutrition; treatment of child illnesses; and household-level improvement of water, sanitation, and environment. PPP should be highlighted for following reasons.

- After birth, the child is completely dependent on the mother, for various reasons at least for one year; separation hinders the growth and development (psychosocial, etc.)
- Child learns so many self-care tasks from mother
- The mental and social development of the child is also dependent on the mother. The mother is the earlier teacher of child
- The physical and mental development of child depends on knowledge, attitude and health practices of mother.

Maternal health is an important determinant in child health outcomes, and can affect fetal and child cognitive and behavioral development; risk of impairments and disabilities; and risk of developing chronic health conditions. Maternal health may be affected by a range of factors, such as:

- Access to prenatal and postnatal health and information services.
- Access to community support services such as breastfeeding or sleep clinics.
- The level of support provided within the family and the level of contact with other family members.
- The level of support provided at work, before and after childbirth (such as time off to avail antenatal services/medical appointments; maternity benefits; breastfeeding breaks, etc.).

Mother and child health (MCH): MCH is an integral part of the health care delivery system organized in India in 1921. MCH refers to the promotive, preventive, curative, and rehabilitative health care for mother and child. Presently the objectives of MCH are reduction in the maternal, perinatal, infant and child mortality and morbidity, promotion of reproductive health, promotion of physical and psychological development of child and adolescent within the family.

Maternal health: In many developing countries, complications of pregnancy and childbirth are the leading causes of death among women of reproductive age. A woman dies from complications from childbirth approximately every minute. According to the WHO, poor maternal conditions account for the fourth leading cause of death for women worldwide, after HIV/AIDS, malaria, and tuberculosis. Maternal health refers the health of women before pregnancy (prenatal care), during pregnancy (antenatal care), childbirth, and the postpartum period. It encompasses the health care dimensions of family planning, preconception, prenatal, and postnatal care in order to reduce maternal morbidity and mortality.

Preconception care: Preconception care can include education, health promotion, screening and other interventions among women of reproductive age to reduce risk factors that might affect future pregnancies. The goal of prenatal care is to detect any potential complication of pregnancy early, to prevent them if possible, and to direct the woman to appropriate specialist medical services as appropriate.

Antenatal health: Antenatal care services are the first steps towards ensuring the health of mothers and the newborn. This is the key component for achieving Millennium Development Goals by 2015. But India's performance continues to be poor in providing antenatal care services to its huge population, particularly in the rural areas. Antenatal care (ANC) consists of few care like registration and physical check up of pregnant woman, adequate nutrition and other care, prevention of communicable diseases, preparation for delivery, breastfeeding and mother crafts.

Antenatal care refers to the regular medical and nursing care recommended for women during pregnancy. It is a type of preventive care consists of prenatal checkup, physical examination and testing of mother, nutritional supplementation (iron and folic acid), tetanus toxoid, etc. with the goal of providing care to prevent potential health problems throughout the course of the pregnancy while promoting healthy lifestyles that benefit both mother and child. During checkups, women receive medical information over maternal physiological changes in pregnancy, biological changes, and prenatal nutrition including prenatal vitamins. Recommendations on management and healthy lifestyle changes are also made during regular checkups. The availability of routine prenatal care has played a part in reducing maternal death rates and miscarriages as well as birth defects, low birth weight, and other preventable health problems.

Good care during pregnancy is important for the health of the mother and the development of the unborn baby. Pregnancy is a crucial time to promote healthy behaviors and parenting skills. Good ANC links the woman and her family with the formal health system, increases the chance of using a skilled attendant at birth and contributes to good health through the life cycle. Inadequate care during this time breaks a critical link in the continuum of care, and affects both women and babies.

Postnatal health: Postnatal period is a very critical time for the mother and her newborn baby. The time when effective postnatal care can make the most difference to the health and life chances of mothers and newborns is in the early neonatal period, the time just after the delivery and through the first 7 days of life. However, the whole of the neonatal period, from birth to the 28th day after the birth, is a time of increased risk. Deaths during the first 28 days of babies who were born alive is reported by all countries in the world as the neonatal mortality rate (the number of babies who die in the first 28 days) per 1,000 live births. Similarly, reports of maternal mortality include deaths of women from complications associated with postnatal problems, not just problems arising during the birth. Both these rates are important indicators of the effectiveness of postnatal care. Postnatal care issues include recovery from childbirth, concerns about newborn care, nutrition, breastfeeding, and family planning.

Post natal health care consists of basic care for all newborns. It should include promoting and supporting early and exclusive breastfeeding, keeping the baby warm, increasing handwashing and providing hygienic umbilical cord and skin care, identifying conditions requiring additional care and counseling on when to take a newborn to a health facility. Newborns and their mothers should be examined for danger signs at home visits. At the same time, families should be counseled on identification of these danger signs and the need for prompt care seeking if one or more of them are present. Newborns with who have preterm birth or low birth weight, who are sick or are born to HIV-infected mothers need special care.

Women are offered information to enable them to promote their own and their baby's health and well-being and to recognize and respond to problems. At the first postnatal contact, women are advised of the signs and symptoms, and appropriate action for potentially life-threatening conditions. Breastfeeding is encouraged by maternity care providers. Usually at each postnatal contact, women are asked about their emotional well-being, what family and social support they have and their usual coping strategies for dealing with day-to-day matters. Women and their families/partners are encouraged to tell their health care professional about any changes in mood, emotional state and behavior that are outside of the woman's normal pattern. At each postnatal contact, health education is offered to enable them to:

- Assess their baby's general condition
- Identify signs and symptoms of common health problems seen in babies
- Contact a health care professional or emergency service if required.

WHO and UNICEF suggest that newborns born in health facilities should not be sent home in the crucial first 24 hours of life, and postnatal visits should be scheduled. Ideally, postnatal care is best delivered in a health facility. However, due to many socioeconomic and cultural reasons, such as the distance to travel and the cost of attending, most rural mothers give birth at home. For all home births a visit to a health facility for postnatal care as soon as possible after birth is recommended. In high mortality settings and where access to facility-based care is limited, WHO and UNICEF recommend at least two home visits for all home births: The first visit should occur within 24 hours from birth and the second visit on day 3. If possible, a third visit should be made before the end of the first week of life (WHO-UNICEF Joint Statement on Home Visits for Newborn Care).

> According to WHO up to two-thirds of the 3.1 million newborn deaths that occurred in 2010 can be prevented if mothers and newborns receive known, effective interventions. A strategy that promotes universal access to antenatal care, skilled birth attendance and early postnatal care will contribute to sustained reduction in maternal and neonatal mortality. A little less than half of all mothers and newborns in developing countries do not receive skilled care during birth, and over 70% of all babies born outside the hospital do not receive any postnatal care.

Family planning: India suffers from the problem of overpopulation. India launched a nationwide family planning program in 1952, which was later, expanded to cover maternal and child health, family welfare and nutrition. Commonly practiced family planning methods include birth control pills, condoms, sterilization and IUD (Intrauterine device).

Everyday, women who have access to family planning (FP) services are empowered to make lifesaving choices such as delaying motherhood, spacing their pregnancies and avoiding unintended pregnancies and abortions. Each year, women who make these choices and plan their families prevent as many as one in every three maternal deaths and more than two million infant and child deaths.

Yet, many more lives could be saved. By integrating FP with a variety of reproductive health (RH) services, it can be brought closer to the women who need them. Postpartum women need to know the advantages of timing and spacing their next pregnancy for their own and their baby's health, and that it is possible to become pregnant before the return of menses. If they are not breastfeeding, their fertility may return by 6 weeks after childbirth. So immediate postpartum visits that included FP counseling and services are most important, providers can help women avoid the dangerous cycle of unwanted pregnancy.

Women who seek HIV counseling and testing (HCT) services and clients who seek FP services are often the same people, and they are often women. Clients, providers and programs can all benefit from the synergies of these two types of services. For example, by averting unintended and high-risk pregnancies among HIV-positive women, FP reduces mother-to-child transmission of HIV. Women who do not seek postnatal care for themselves can be reached during well-child visits. By providing an integrated package of care during well-child visits—adding information about FP options and breastfeeding—we can reach women who might otherwise miss this opportunity to avoid unplanned pregnancies. FP services consists of condom distribution, oral contraceptives, counseling on IUD, IUD and sterilization services, medical termination of pregnancy (MTP) services.

The integration of FP and MCH programs and services provides multiple opportunities to streamline and improve care at favorable and critical times for maximizing women's RH and the health of their children. The benefits associated with combining FP and MCH services are directly related to achieving Millennium Development Goals reduce child mortality and improve maternal health.

Through collaboration with a number of international partners, the USAID ACCESS-FP program has been working to expand the integration of FP with MCH programs in these priority areas: (1) policies and strategies to include FP in national maternal and newborn essential care packages; (2) postpartum (PP) information on return to fertility, pregnancy spacing and FP methods in curricula, standards, and guidelines for training and service delivery; (3) behavior change communication strategies promoting pregnancy spacing and FP; and (4) facility and community-based approaches for integrating ANC, safe delivery, essential newborn care, and PP care for mothers and newborns (USAID, 2008a). ACCESS-FP is integrating women's needs for RH care and postpartum family planning (PPFP) with newborn and child health services, including prevention of mother-to-child transmission of HIV, during the extended PP period (i.e. through the first year after delivery).

FP use during the first year PP has the potential to significantly reduce the number of unplanned pregnancies and research has shown a large unmet need among women in the extended PP period. Meeting these needs could substantially increase contraceptive prevalence, reduce the percentage of birth intervals that are dangerously close, and reduce maternal and child mortality (Cleland et al., 2006). In 2005, a WHO technical consultation recommended the minimum interval of 24 months after a live birth before attempting the next pregnancy in order to reduce risk of adverse maternal, perinatal, and infant outcomes (WHO 2006). Greater FP use during the extended PP period, fully breastfeeding, and slower return to sexual activity can combine to lengthen birth intervals. From a programmatic standpoint, women who use maternal health services are more likely to use FP services during the extended postpartum period. Increasing contraceptive usage and family planning also improves maternal health through reduction in numbers of higher risk pregnancies.

MILESTONES IN THE HISTORY OF MCH CARE IN INDIA

Establishment of training of dais in Amritsar in 1880 to reproductive and child health care (RCH II) 2005.

Reproductive and Child Health (RCH) Program

Introduction

In order to effectively improve the health status of women and children and fulfill the unmet need for family welfare services in the country, especially the poor and under served by reducing infant child and maternal mortality and morbidity, Government of India during 1997–98 launched the RCH program for implementation during the 9th plan period by integrating child survival and safe motherhood (CSSM) program with other RCH services. In addition, a new component for management of reproductive tract infection (RTI) and sexually transmitted infection (STI) has also been incorporated. The RCH program is partly funded by World Bank, UNICEF, UNFPA and European Commission, etc. RCH program was launched by Government of India in Oct 1997, as per recommendations of the conference of International Council of Population Development (ICPD) at Cairo 1994.

Women in the reproductive age group

Under the reproductive and child health (RCH) program, care provider must ensure the following.

Counseling on:
- Care of girl child
- Optimal timing and spacing of birth
- Small family norms
- Use and choice of contraceptives
- Prevention of RTI/STIs

Definition of RCH

RCH has been defined as a state in which 'people have the ability to reproduce and regulate their fertility; women are able to go through pregnancy and childbirth safely, the outcome of pregnancy is successful in terms of maternal and infant survival and well-being; and couples are able to have sexual relations free of the fear of pregnancy and contract diseases'.

This means that every couple should be able to have child when they want, that the pregnancy is uneventful, that safe delivery services are available, that at the end of the pregnancy the mother and the child are safe, well and that contraceptives by choice are available to prevent pregnancy and of contracting diseases.

Components

RCH is a program for mother and child. First phase RCH-I launched in the year 1998 and second phase of RCH-II commenced from 1st April 2005. Main objective of the program is to bring about the change mainly in the three critical health indicators:

1. Reduce total fertility rate
2. Infant mortality rate
3. Maternal mortality ratio.

With a view to realizing the outcome envisioned in the Millennium Development goal, National Population policy, and National health policy, vision 2020 India.

In RCH program, the contour was broadened with major emphasis on Integrated delivery of services for fertility regulation, maternal health, child health, safe abortions, nutrition, communication for behavior changes, RTIs/STIs, adolescent health.

The essential elements of reproductive and child health services will help to understand how the reproductive and child health services have been going on at the community level. The different services for mothers provided under RCH program are tetanus toxoid immunization, prevention and treatment of anemia, antenatal care and early identification of maternal complications, deliveries by trained personnel, promotion of institutional deliveries, management of obstetric emergencies, birth spacing. Child health services under RCH are essential newborn care, exclusive breastfeeding and weaning, immunization, appropriate management of diarrhea, appropriate management of ARI, vitamin A prophylaxis, treatment of anemia. Services for eligible couple are prevention of pregnancy, safe abortion. Special emphasis has been given on adolescents' health. Special features under RCH are involvement of male persons, importance of care of girl child, optimal timing and spacing of birth, emphasis on small family norms, use and choice of contraceptives, prevention and treatment of RTI/STI.

The package of RCH services is being implemented in the community level, sub-center level, primary health center level, first referral unit (FRUs) and district level.

The new approach under the RCH program places special emphasis on client-centered, demand driven, participatory, bottom up, high quality, integrated services based on the need of the community, evolved through decentralized participatory planning

Remember:

Pre-eclampsia should be detected and managed early. Thus, one can prevent 9% all deaths which occur due to eclampsia.

CHILD HEALTH

There is a famous saying healthy children contribute to healthy nation. Prevention is the best measure to maintain health, an old saying, 'a stich in time saves nine' supports this. Child survival strategies are extremely important to tackle current problems of malnutrition, infections, diarrheal diseases and poor maternal health. Government of India has accepted the approach of low cost interventions acceptable to the people. Primary health care activities for prevention of diseases such as growth monitoring, promotion of breastfeeding and weaning, oral rehydration, community feeding, immunization, nutritional surveillance, regular health checkups and aware generation on health habits and hygiene are being implemented in different health care settings.

Major Milestones in Mother and Child Health Programs in India

For the welfare of children and development of human resources, integrated child development services (ICDS) was started in India in the year 1975. ICDS scheme is working at village level in rural areas and also in urban and tribal areas. It is designed to offer a package of services for prevention of diseases and promotion of health of children.

Till 1977 the major health activity was family planning which was changed into family welfare program with maternal and child health becoming an integral part of family planning program with the vision that reduction in birth rate has a direct relationship with reduction in infant and child mortality.

Under Five Clinic

National health policy 1983 envisioned significant reduction in IMR, NMR and CMR by 2000. All the child health programs are directed towards achieving these goals.

The diarrheal disease control program was started in the country in 1978. The main objective of the program was to prevent death due to dehydration caused by diarrheal diseases among children under 5 years of age due to dehydration. Health education aimed at rapid recognition and appropriate management of diarrhea has been a major component of the CSSM, 1992. Under the CSSM program, a massive expansion of MCH services has occurred at the sub-district and the district levels.

Under the RCH program 1997, ORS is supplied in the kits to all sub-centers in the country every year.

Universal immunization program (UIP) against six preventable diseases, namely, diphtheria, pertussis, childhood tuberculosis, poliomyelitis, measles and neonatal tetanus was introduced in the country in a phased manner in 1985, which covered the whole of India by 1990. Significant progress was made under the program in the initial period when more than 90% coverage for all the six antigens was achieved. The UIP was taken up in 1986 as National Technology Mission and became operational in all districts in the country during 1989–90. UIP become a part of the intensified pulse polio campaign and pulse polio immunization.

School Health Program

CSSM program was launched in 1992 and RCH program in 1997. Universal immunization against 6 vaccine preventable diseases (VPD) by 2000 was one of the goals set in the National Health Policy (1983).

To boost up the breastfeeding practices and to oppose the trends of bottle feeding, the baby friendly hospital initiative was launched in the year 1992 in India.

Different Nutritional Programs for children were started

- Nutritional blindness prevention program
- Anemia prevention by distribution of iron and folifer tablet
- Mid-day meal program.

The ARI control program was started in India in 1990. It sought to introduce scientific protocols for case management of pneumonia with cotrimoxazole. Initially 14 pilot districts were selected and later on new districts were included. A review of the health facility done in 1992 revealed that although 87% of personnel were trained and the drug supply was regular yet there were problems in correct case classification and treatment. Since 1992 the program was implemented as part of CSSM and later with RCH. Cotrimoxazole tablets are supplied as part of drug kit for use by different category of workers for managing cases of pneumonia. Under RCH-II, activities are proposed to be implemented in an integrated way with other child health interventions.

The child survival and safe motherhood program jointly funded by World Bank and UNICEF was started in 1992–93 for implementation up to 1997–98. The child survival and safe motherhood program was implemented in a phased manner covering all the districts of the country by the year 1996–97. The objectives of the programs were to improve the health status of infants, child and maternal morbidity and mortality. The programs seek to sustain high coverage levels achieved under the universal immunization program (UIP) in good performance areas and strengthen the immunization services of poor performing areas. The program also provides for augmenting various activities under the oral rehydration therapy (ORT) program, universalizing prophylaxis schemes for control of anemia in pregnant women and control of blindness in children and initiating a program for control of acute respiratory infection (ARI) in children.

Reproductive Child Health (RCH) Program

Reproductive and child health program is in its operation and is currently operational in entire country. The program follows a differential strategy with inputs under the program linked to the needs of the area coupled with the capacity for implementation. Efforts were made to strengthen the routine immunization as well as PPI by launching a project for immunization strengthening with the World Bank assistance.

Integrated Management of Neonatal and Childhood Illnesses (IMNCI)

It offers a comprehensive package for the management of the most common causes of childhood illnesses, i.e. sepsis, measles, malaria, diarrhea, pneumonia and malnutrition. It is supported by appropriate strengthening of the health care system and promotion of positive health care practices of the community.

Currently the initiatives that are being implemented by the Department of Family Welfare for reduction of IMR, NMR, CMR are:

- Reproductive and Child Health program
- Universal Immunization Program
- Pulse Polio Immunization (intensified campaign)
- Integrated Child Development Services
- Control of deaths due to acute respiratory infection
- Control of deaths due to diarrheal diseases
- UIP and intensified Pulse Polio Immunization
- Provision of essential newborn care
- Vitamin A supplementation for children between the ages of 6 months to 3 years
- Iron Folic Acid supplementation to children under 5 years of age
- Implementation of exclusive breastfeeding up to the age of 6 months and appropriate practices related to complementary feeding
- Integrated Management of Neonatal and Childhood Illnesses (IMNCI).
- National Rural Health Mission and all national programs to prevent and control of communicable and non-communicable diseases.

Other Initiatives in Child Health

Under Five Clinic

Child under 5 years of age need a special health care program because they constitute a large sector of the total population. They are vulnerable group: As they undergo physical and mental development, which call for preventive care. There is high morbidity, children suffer from infectious, nutritional and parasitic diseases. In developing countries, 50% of total deaths occur among under five compared to < 5% in the developed countries. The important causes of morbidity and mortality of this group are mainly neonatal and perinatal diseases, ARI, diarrheal diseases, infections and accidents, which are mostly preventable with care and support. Under five clinic serves that purpose of prevention and most morbidity and mortality of children are prevented by the primary level of prevention, e.g. immunization, sound nutrition, health education and environmental sanitation (Fig. 8.2). Prevention of certain adulthood health problems could be initiated in childhood period, e.g. early treatment of streptococcal infection prevents rheumatic heart disease. Moreover, obesity, hypertension, cardiovascular diseases may be initiated in early life. The services provided by the clinic are set out in the symbol, which was proposed for under-five clinic in India.

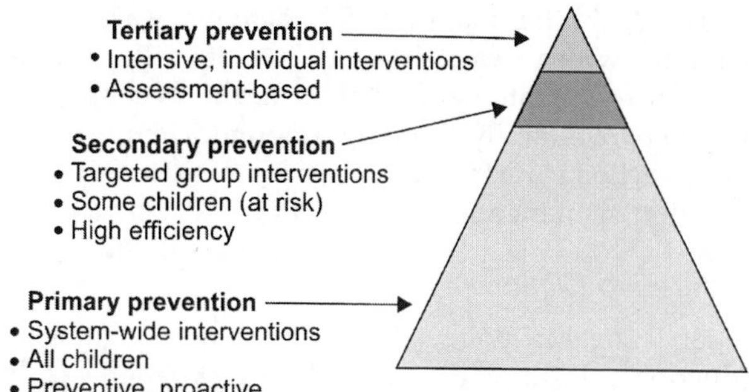

Fig. 8.2: Different levels of preventive and curative activities to protect child health

The symbol of under five clinic is triangular in shape. The apex of the large triangle represents care in illness, the left and right triangle consecutively indicates nutrition and immunization. The central triangle represents family planning. The outer border of the large triangle indicates health education to the parent.

- Care in illness under this clinic includes
  - Diagnosis and treatment of acute illness, e.g. oral rehydration therapy
  - Diagnosis and treatment of chronic diseases like physical, mental, congenital and acquired abnormalities
  - Treatment of growth and developmental disorders
  - X-ray and laboratory services
  - Referral services.
- *Criteria for identifying at risk children:* Birth weight < 2500 grams, twins, birth order > 5th, artificial feeding, weight below 60% of the expected weight for age, failure to gain weight for three successive months, child having protein energy malnutrition (PEM), children having frequent diarrhea or ARI, infants of working mothers.
- *Adequate nutrition:* Growth and development of children depends on adequate nutrition, so health care providers should give importance on breastfeeding, weaning, and balanced diet of the under five children. In this age group, nutritional disorders like PEM, anemia, nutritional blindness, rickets are common. Early detection and control of these conditions can be done through growth monitoring periodically. Monthly weighing of children up to one year of age then bimonthly checkup till second year, and every 3 months thereafter up to the age of 5 to 6 years. The child's weight is plotted on 'road to health card' and 'growth

curve' which helps in detecting early onset of growth failure (*see* chapter 4 of this edition). Health checkup are done every 3–6 months by physical examination and laboratory tests. The child's 'health card' is maintained which assists to identify 'at risk' children who are being registered for special care and referral for better treatment. Health education on nutrition is an important component of under five clinic. At present supplementary feeding of children (under 6 years) are carried out by ICDS projects.

- *Immunization:* The right triangle of under 5 clinic symbol represents the immunization, which indicates coverage of at least six killer diseases like diphtheria, tetanus, pertussis, tuberculosis, poliomyelitis and measles. The national immunization schedule must be known by all health care providers for maximum coverage of immunization thus to prevent morbidity, mortality and disability condition due to these six killer diseases.
- *Family planning:* FP services include counseling and checkup of the mothers and free distribution of devices.
- Health education is most important component of this clinic. Awareness on child care and child rearing practices are conducted among mothers. They receive information about prevention and control of malnutrition and infections.

The under five clinic is usually located in low socioeconomic areas like village, slum and labor colony and conducted by staff trained in child health and nutrition. She makes home visit to educate the mothers on prevention and promotion of child health and to make sure that they care to bring their children in the clinic for regular checkup, immunization, etc.

ICDS

Full form of ICDS is Integrated Child Development Scheme. The ICDS services is India's response to the challenge of meeting the holistic need of the child (Fig. 8.3). The ICDS is one of the world's largest and most unique outreach program for early childhood care and development. It symbolizes India's commitment to its children. ICDS was evolved to make a coordinated effort for an integrated program to deliver a package of services (Figs 8.4A to C) comprising supplementary

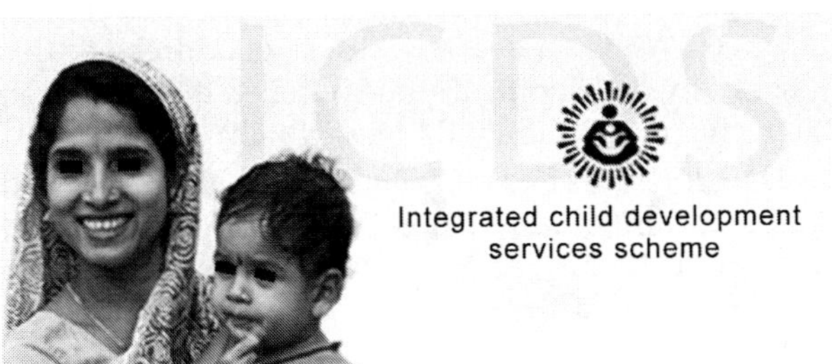

Fig. 8.3: Popular logo of integrated child development scheme

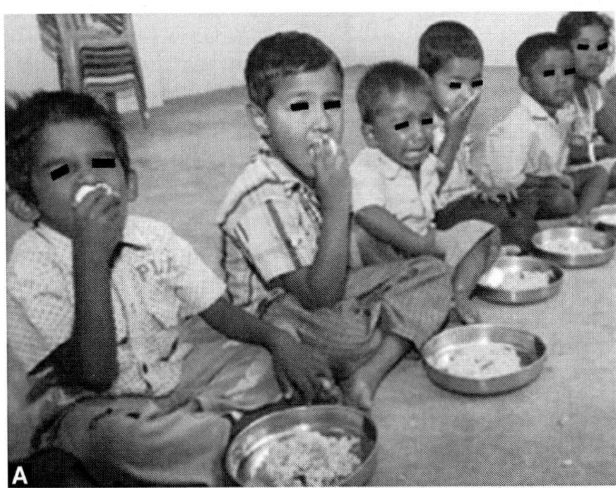

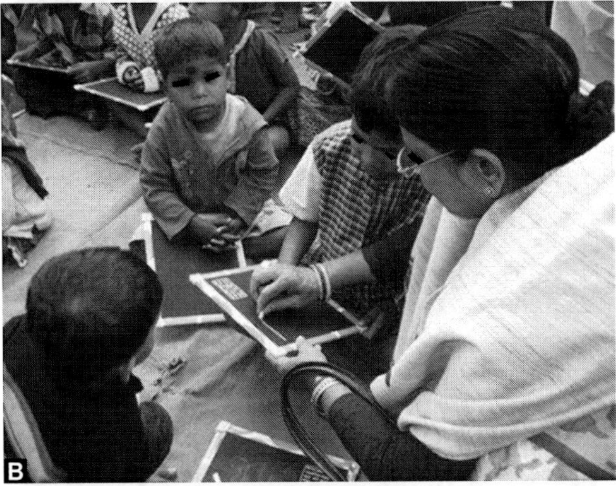

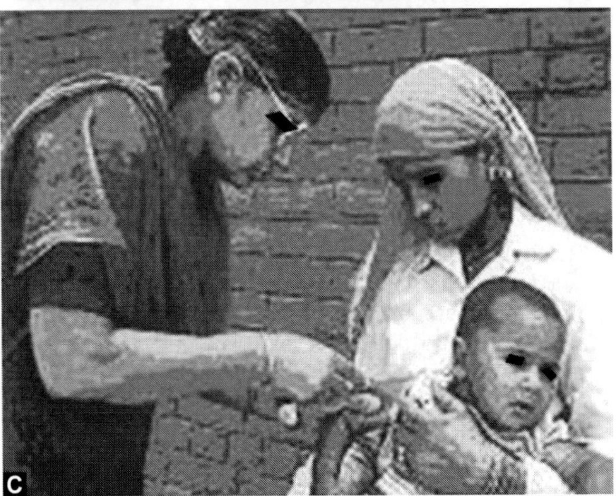

Figs 8.4A to C: Different activities in ICDS center

nutrition, immunization, health checkup, referral services to children below six years of age and expectant and nursing mothers. Non-formal preschool education is imparted to children of the age group 3–6 years and health and nutrition education to women in the age group 15–45 years. High priority is accorded to the needs of the most vulnerable younger children under 3 years of age in the program through capacity building of caregivers to provide stimulation and quality early childhood. The blueprint for the scheme was drawn by the Ministry of Social Welfare, Government of India in 1975. The scheme called for coordinated and collective effort by different Ministries, Departments and Voluntary Organizations. Considering the magnitude of the task, it was decided to set up 33 projects on an experimental basis in the year 1975–76. The scheme was formally launched in India with 33 project in all over the country on 2nd October, 1975, ICDS project Jama Masjid was the milestone project for the state of Delhi. Today, the ICDS has a network of more than 5000 projects covering the rural and urban slum pockets of the country.

Objectives of ICDS

- Improve the nutritional and health status of children below the age of six years.
- Lay the foundation for the proper psychological, physical and social.
- Reduce the incidence of mortality, morbidity malnutrition and school dropouts.
- Achieve effective coordinates of policy and implementation among various departments to promote child development.
- Enhance the capability of the mother to look after the normal health and nutritional needs of child, through proper health and nutrition education.

Services Provided Under the ICDS Program

- **Supplementary Nutrition**—to provide cooked food to children and lactating mothers
- Health check-up
- Immunization–with the help of auxiliary nursing midwives (ANM)
- Referral services–hospitals and health centers
- Nutrition and health education
- Nonformal preschool education for the 0–6 children
- **Health checkup**, again, has four direct interventions:
  - Antenatal and postnatal checkup of mothers
  - Detection of anemia and other diseases
  - Prevention of disabilities
  - Child growth monitoring through regular weighing and height measurement
- **Prenursery education**

National prophylaxis program for prevention of blindness caused by deficiency of vitamin A, and control of nutritional anemia among mothers and children are two direct nutrition interventions integrated in ICDS. For dietary promotion the food rich in vitamin A, iron, folic acid and vitamin C is an important part of nutrition and health education. At 9 months of age, 100,000 IU of vitamin A solution is administered to infants along with immunization against measles. Children in the age group of 1–5 years receive 200,000 IU of vitamin A solution every 6 months, with priority given to children under 3 years of age. Tablets of iron and folic acid are administered to expectant mothers for prophylaxis and treatment and to anemic children. The usage of only iodized salt is promoted, especially in the food supplement provided towards preventing iodine deficiency disorders.

Administrative setup of ICDS in India

Government of India Department of Women and Child Development

State level:	Department of social welfare/Rural Development/ Community Development/Tribal welfare/Women and Child Development Department
District level:	**District** Welfare Officer/District ICDS cell
Block level:	**BDO**—Child Development Project Officer—Medical Officer
Sector level:	**Mukhya** Sevika—Supervisor—Health Assistant (female)
Village level:	**Auxilliary** Nurse Midwives
	Anganwadi workers, Trained Birth Attendants
	Village Health Guides

IMNCI

Everyday, millions of parents seek health care for their sick children, taking them to hospitals, health centers, doctors and traditional healers. Health professionals often rely on history and signs and symptoms to determine a course of management that makes the best use of the available resources. These factors make providing quality care to sick children a serious challenge. WHO and UNICEF have addressed this challenge by developing a strategy called the Integrated Management of Childhood Illness (IMCI).

The Integrated Management of Neonatal and Childhood Illness (IMNCI) is the Indian adaptation of the WHO-UNICEF generic IMCI strategy and is the centerpiece of newborn and child health strategy under RCH-II and National Rural Health Mission.

The strategy provides an integrated approach for standard management of major causes of childhood morbidity and mortality like pneumonia, diarrhea, malnutrition, neonatal problems, measles, malaria in the outpatient settings. With the implementation of IMNCI strategy in the country, more and more newborns and children are being referred to health facilities for inpatient care.

Government of India recognizes the need to strengthen child health activities in the country too. In order to do so and introduce IMCI in the country, a core group was constituted which included representatives from Indian Academy of Pediatrics (IAP), National Neonatology Forum of India (NNF), National Anti Malaria Program (NAMP), Department of Women and Child Development (DWCD), Child-in-Need Institute (CINI), WHO, UNICEF, eminent Pediatricians and Neonatologists, and the representatives from Ministry of Health and Family Welfare Government of India. The adaptation group developed Indian version of IMCI guidelines and renamed it as Integrated Management of Neonatal and Childhood Illness (IMNCI).

What is IMCI?

IMCI is an integrated approach to child health that focuses on the well-being of the whole child. IMCI aims to reduce death, illness and disability, and to promote improved growth and development among children under 5 years of age. IMNCI includes both preventive and curative elements that are implemented by families and communities as well as by health facilities.

The major components of this strategy are:

- Strengthening the case management skills of the health care workers
- Strengthening the health care infrastructure (health system)
- Involvement of the community. Improving family and community health practices.

The first two components are the facility based IMNCI and the third is the commnity based IMNCI. The major highlights of Indian adaptation are:

- Incorporation of neonatal care as it now constitutes two thirds of infant mortality
- Inclusion of 0–7 days
- Incorporating National guidelines on malaria, anemia, vitamin A supplementation and Immunization schedule
- Training schedule reduced from 11 to 8 days
- Training begins with sick young infant up to 2 months.

The Government has initiated implementation of the IMNCI strategy in different districts in selected states of India.

The complete IMCI case management process involves the following elements.

- *Assess* a child with history taking and examination for danger signs and other health problems, checking nutrition and immunization status
- Classify a child's illness using a color coded triangle system. Each illness is classified as:
  - Urgent pre-referral treatment or referral
  - Specific medical treatment and advice
  - Simple advice on home management
- *Identify:* After classifying the child the specific treatment is identified. Treatment must be given before urgent referral. First dose of drug and immunization (if the child is not immunized) are to be given in the clinic, before sending the child for home treatment.
- *Treatment:* Practical treatment instructions are to be given to the care givers. Counseling regarding child's condition, signs needed immediate attention, importance of follow-up are to be done for the parents.
- *Counseling* of mothers about breastfeeding/feeding, immunization or other queries are to be made. Counsel the mother about her health.
- *Give follow-up care* when a child is brought back to the clinic, if necessary, reassess the child for new problems.

Comprehensive integrated strategies such as IMNCI are feasible to deliver and can significantly affect infant mortality; neonatal mortality is substantially improved among those born at home. The major challenges before IMNCI are the feasibility of provision of health care using IMNCI at sub-center and village level by ANMs and Anganwadi workers (AWWs) considering the irregular supply of drugs and logistics, lack of proper supervision, sustaining what is initiated through indicator-based monitoring, making home-based care of young infants operational by ANMs and AWWs and a high staff turnover. Thus, IMNCI offers a strategy for improving the state of health of children in India. This approach could help the country in achieving the Millennium Development Goals of reducing the under-five mortality.

FACTS ON CHILD HEALTH—World Scenario

From 1 month to 5 years of age, the main causes of death are pneumonia, diarrhea, malaria and measles. *Malnutrition is estimated to contribute to more than one third of all child deaths.*

- **Pneumonia** is the prime cause of death in children under 5 years of age. Addressing the major risk factors —including malnutrition and indoor air pollution—is essential to preventing pneumonia, as are vaccination and breastfeeding. Antibiotics and oxygen are vital tools for effectively managing the illness.
- **Diarrheal diseases** are a leading cause of sickness and death among children in developing countries. Breastfeeding helps prevent diarrhea among young children. Treatment for sick children with Oral Rehydration Salts (ORS) combined with zinc supplements is safe, cost-effective, and saves lives.
- One child dies every minute from malaria. Insecticide-treated nets prevent transmission and increase child survival.
- Over 90% of **children with HIV** are infected through mother-to-child transmission; this can be prevented with antiretrovirals, as well as safer delivery and feeding practices.
- Worldwide, about 20% of deaths among children under-five could be avoided if feeding guidelines are followed. WHO recommends exclusive breastfeeding for 6 months, introducing age-appropriate and safe complementary foods at 6 months, and continuing breastfeeding for up to 2 years or beyond.

WHO update—September 2013

HANDICAPPED CHILD CARE

The convention of the rights of people with disabilities adopted in the year 2006, defines a disability as: 'persons with disabilities include those who have long-term physical, mental, intellectual or sensory impairments which in interaction with various barriers may hinder their full and effective participation in society on an equal basis with others (Fig. 8.5).'

It is considered that around 150 million children in the world live with a disability; 80% of them live in developing countries. Most often, these children do not receive necessary treatment and most of them are discriminated. State parties of the convention of the Rights of Children (CRC) recognized that a mentally or physically disabled child should enjoy a full and a decent life, in conditions which ensure dignity, promote self-reliance and facilitate the child's active participation in the community.

The second paragraph of article no. 23 CRC, dedicated to children with disabilities guarantees their right to get special care and to request the granting of state assistance, adapted to the child's country and to the financial standing of his parents or his guardian.

It is obvious that children with disabilities are entitled to special treatment, but in practice, most of

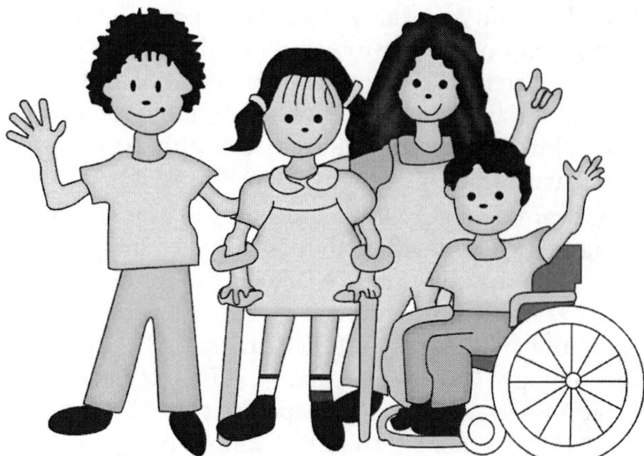

Fig. 8.5: Differently abled children

these children are entirely deprived of even proper medical treatment. Their chance of recovering or in the least of living with less suffering are thus reduced to zero.

ADOLESCENT HEALTH

The 11 to 19 year old age is called adolescence. This is the period of rapid change and maturation when the child grows into the adult. This is one of the most enjoyable stages of one's life and it has to be experienced with joy and friendship paving the way for building a healthy society with good social relationships. In India, it represents almost one-third of the total country's population. The National Population Policy 2000 identified adolescents as an under-served group for which health needs and within this reproductive and sexual health interventions are to be designed. The National Youth Policy 2003 recognizes 13 to 19 years as a distinct age group which had to be covered by special programs in all sectors including health.

A large number of adolescents of our country are out of school, get married early, work in vulnerable situations, are sexually active, and are exposed to peer pressure. These factors have serious social, economic and public health implications. Adolescents are not a homogenous group. Their situation varies by age, sex, marital status, class, region and cultural context. This calls for interventions that are flexible and responsive to their disparate needs. Adolescents have a number of unmet health needs in different areas, among which we mention violence, reproductive health and nutritional problems such as anorexia, overweight and obesity. Some of the public health challenges for adolescents include unplanned pregnancy, excess risk of maternal and infant mortality, sexually transmitted infections and reproductive tract infections in adolescence, and the rapidly rising incidence of HIV in this age group. Preventive services are essential to tackle the above-mentioned problems. To be effective, services should be easily accessible, high quality and comprehensive.

Adolescent Reproductive and Sexual Health (ARSH) is a key objective of RCH-II program and National Rural Health Mission. The goals of the Government of India RCH-II program are reduction in IMR, MMR and TFR. In order to achieve these goals, RCH-II has four technical strategies. One of these is Adolescent Health. Strategy for ARSH has been approved as part of the RCH-II National Program Implementation Plan (PIP). This strategy focuses on reorganizing the existing public health system in order to meet the service needs of adolescents. Steps are to be taken to ensure improved service delivery for adolescents during routine sub-center clinics and ensure service availability on fixed days and timings at the PHC and CHC levels. This is to be in tune with outreach activities. A core package of services includes preventive, promotive, curative and counseling services.

Some of the specific strategies undertaken by various governments are Kishori Balika scheme under ICDS by Department of Women and Child Development. Weekly once 100 mg iron Folic Acid supplementation of all adolescent girls through schools and anganwadi centers are distributed in Andhra Pradesh. 'Annesa' special clinic on adolescents' health is being carried out in the state of West Bengal. Services rendered on adolescents' special needs, special emphasis on counseling on family life and reproductive health are given in these clinics.

Although adolescents are apparently healthy, they are practicing unhealthy behaviors that will ultimately result in much death and disability. This is an immense public health issue. Therefore, focusing attention both on diseases experienced during adolescence and on risk factors with their roots in adolescence makes sense. Adolescent health efforts should emphasize prevention because so much of the disease burden is preventable and because prevention is a particularly cost-effective strategy in relation to adolescents, given the long duration over which benefits will be reaped and adolescents' greater openness to change than adults.

Different studies highlighted the need of a more positive approach to promote higher retention of girls at schools. This would also encourage their participation in the workforce. It is important to bring social pressure on errant families and specific communities by women's groups and organizations. Promotion of healthy lifestyles through sports competition or a cultural program for youth can also bring positive change. Some activities can provide opportunities for youth to take part together. A health component that has behavior change communication, counseling and service delivery aspects could be built into these.

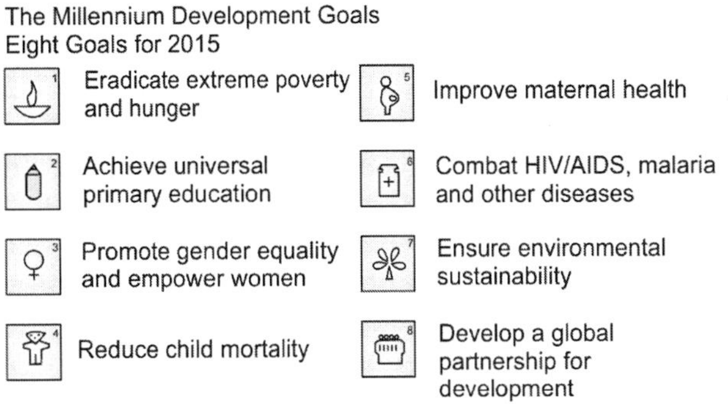

The Millennium Development Goals
Eight Goals for 2015

1 Eradicate extreme poverty and hunger
2 Achieve universal primary education
3 Promote gender equality and empower women
4 Reduce child mortality
5 Improve maternal health
6 Combat HIV/AIDS, malaria and other diseases
7 Ensure environmental sustainability
8 Develop a global partnership for development

Fig. 8.6: The millennium development goals

The Road Ahead

India is a signatory to the Millennium Development Goals (MDGs) (Fig. 8.6). The fourth millennium development goal is reduction of child mortality and the target for this is to reduce by two thirds, between 1990 and 2015 the mortality rate of children under five. This is reflected in the tenth five year plan (2002–2007), which states that Infant mortality rate is to be reduced to 45/1000 by 2007 and 28/1000 live births by 2012.

SCHOOL HEALTH

After the child's home, school represents the second most influential environment in a child's life. In India a school health committee was formed to examine the health and nutritional status of the school children in 1960. As per recommendations of the said committee, school health program was started in India in the year 1962.

School health services include preventive and screening services, health education and assistance with decision-making about health, nutrition and immunization against preventable diseases. Moreover there are provisions for treatment of communicable diseases, acute and chronic illnesses, injuries and emergencies (through referral system to the institution). Necessary interventions are being made on common problems like malnutrition, nutritional anemia, vitamin A deficiency, skin diseases, worm infestation, dental caries, diseases of eye, ear and nose. If problems like obesity, substance use and abuse, mental problems, adolescent pregnancy, vision difficulty detected, the student is referred for specific investigations and treatment. At present reproductive health care has been considered under the ongoing program of reproductive and child health.

Objectives of the school health services are as follows:

- The promotion of positive health
- The prevention of diseases
- Early diagnosis, treatment and follow-up of defects
- Awakening health consciousness of children
- The provision of healthful environment.

School Health Program—Appraisal

Appraisal aspects: These are organized activities carried out to assess the physical, mental and social status of the school children through periodic medical examination and daily observation/inspection by the school teacher. It should cover not only the students but also the teachers and other school personnel (Fig. 8.7).

Components of Appraisal

History taking, observation, screening test, examination, laboratory test are the primary components of school health program appraisals.

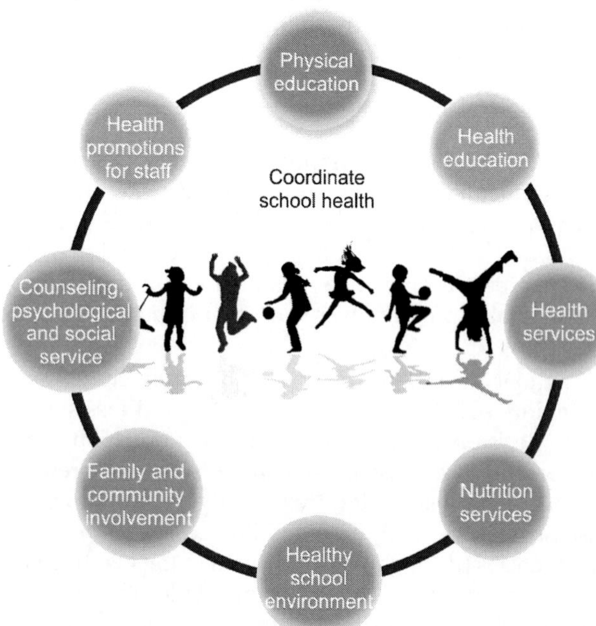

Fig. 8.7: The components of school health program

Preventive Aspects

- Prevention and control of communicable diseases.
- Early detection and treatment of non-communicable diseases.
- Early identification and education of children with special needs.
- Emergency services and first aid services.

Curative Services

Children showing signs and symptoms should be referred to the school medical officers, of health care institutions for appropriate treatment and follow-up.

Nutritional Services

Few nutritional programs are being carried out in India to overcome the nutritional problems among children like PEM, vitamins, iron and minerals deficiencies, etc.

Nutritional Programs

- Mid-day school meal
- Applied nutrition program
- Specific nutrients.

Health Education

It is part of the education given in the school by the school.

Methods of school health education:

- Formal health education
- Inter-related health education
- Incidental health education.

Healthful School Environment

- Psychosocial and emotional environment include school schedule. Duration and timing of school day, amount and timing of home work
- Healthful environment through teacher-student, student-student relationship.

Physical Environment

- Safe sanitary facilities lighting, furniture, play facility, garbage
- School health administration—there is no uniform pattern of it. In India, school health and committees services are administered by different department mainly health and education. It is important function of PHC.
- The school health committee (1961), in India recommended the formation of school health committee from village to national level. These committees should mobilize community Resources

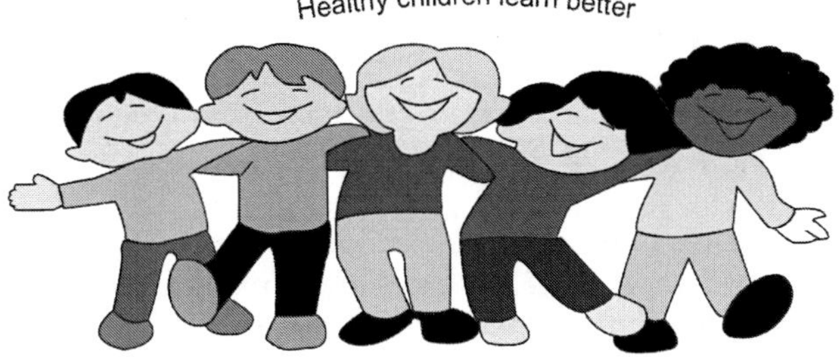

Fig. 8.8: School nurse is the key person in school health program

and make the school health program continuous and self-supporting.

Role of school health nurse: School health nurses facilitate positive student responses to normal development (Fig. 8.8); promote health and safety; intervene with actual and potential health problems; provide case management services; and actively collaborate with others to build student and family capacity for adaptation, self-management, self-advocacy, and learning. The school nurse has a unique role in provision of school health services for children with learning disability, behavioral and other mental health problems, special health needs, including children with chronic illnesses and disabilities of various degrees of severity.

More school-based health centers are needed in rural and urban communities where poverty levels are higher and medical care harder to come by. With parents' consent, nurses can diagnose illness, give minor ailments medications and render preventive care. A growing number can be provided dental care.

School nurses are well-positioned to take the lead for the school system in partnering with physicians, other health professionals, ongoing national and public health programs, community physicians, and community organizations.

Child guidance clinic (CGC): Concept of child guidance clinic was emerged for the all-round development of a child, the child's physical and physiological functioning and the environment to which he is exposed at home and school, should be taken care off. All this is possible through interaction with and counseling of the child and his family by a health care team. Child guidance clinic were started in 1922, as part of program sponsored by a private organization 'Commonwealth Fund's Program' for the prevention of juvenile delinquency. The first CGC was started in India in 1939 at the TATA institute Mumbai. The CGC in Delhi was started in 1955 at RAK con, simultaneously with Chennai (*See* the behavioral pediatric chapter 6).

International and National Welfare Organizations

A large number of organizations of various sizes provide international health aid. Besides financial aid, the international health organizations are a major source of expert technical advice and training for local health professionals. International health organizations are usually divided into three groups: Multilateral organizations, bilateral organizations, and non-governmental organizations (NGOs).

The term multilateral means that funding comes from multiple governments (as well as from non-governmental sources) and is distributed to many different countries. The major multilateral organizations are all part of the United Nations. Other premier international health organizations are WHO, World Bank, UNICEF, etc.

Bilateral agencies are governmental agencies in a single country which provide aid to developing countries. The largest of these is the United States Agency for International Development (USAID).

Non-governmental organizations (NGOs), also known as private voluntary organizations (PVOs), provide approximately 20% of all external health aid to developing countries. Most of these organizations are quite small; many are church-affiliated. In the very poorest countries, hospitals and clinics run by missionary societies are especially important. The largest NGO devoted to international health in the United States is Project Hope, with an annual budget exceeding $100 million. Worldwide, the most important NGO in long-term international health is probably Oxfam International.

CENTER FOR INTERNATIONAL CHILD HEALTH ARE WHO, UNICEF, FAO, CARE, USAID

World Health Organization

The World Health Organization (WHO) is the premier international health organization. Technically, it is an 'intergovernmental agency related to the United Nations.' WHO and other such intergovernmental agencies are 'separate, autonomous organizations which, by special agreements, work with the UN and each other through the coordinating machinery of the Economic and Social Council.' According to its constitution (1948) its principal goal is 'the attainment by all peoples of the highest possible level of health.'

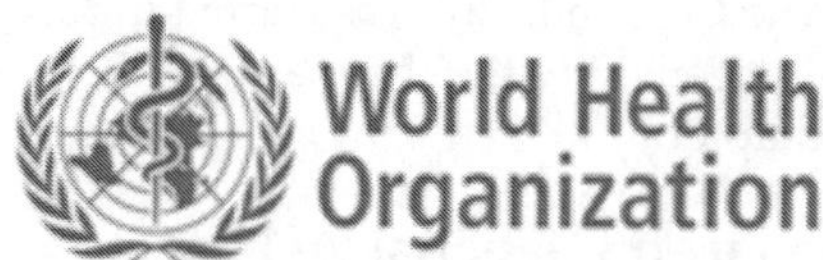

Fig. 8.9: Logo of world health organization

The principal work of WHO is directing and coordinating international health activities and supplying technical assistance to countries. It develops norms and standards, disseminates health information, promotes research, provides training in international health, collects and analyzes epidemiologic data, and develops systems for monitoring and evaluating health programs.

The WHO organized in 1948 is one of the specialized agencies of the United Nations. Through this organization the public health and medical professions of more than 100 countries exchange their knowledge and experience and work together in an effort to achieve the highest possible level of health throughout the world (Fig. 8.9). The organization is not concerned with problems that individual countries or territories can solve with their own resources. Instead, it focuses on those problems that can be satisfactorily solved only through the cooperation of all or certain groups of countries. For example, the eradication of malaria and the control of cholera, plague, yellow fever, and smallpox are international problems.

WHO is the directing and coordinating authority for health within the United Nations system. It is responsible for providing leadership on global health matters, shaping the health research agenda, setting norms and standards, articulating evidence-based policy options, providing technical support to countries and monitoring and assessing health trends. Structurally, World Health Assembly is the supreme governing body of WHO, consists of members from each member state. The next tier of administration is Executive Board, which is composed of 31 technically competent members. The head office of WHO Secretariat is in Geneva, which has different divisions. WHO has established six regions, India is a member of South East Asia region; whose head quarter is located at New Delhi.

UNICEF

United Nations International Children's Emergency Fund (UNICEF) is another most important agency of United Nations, established in 1946 (Fig. 8.10).

UNICEF spends the majority of its program (non-administrative) budget on health care. UNICEF makes the world's most vulnerable children its top priority, so it devotes most of its resources to the poorest countries and to children younger than 5 years. UNICEF runs many of the child health programs in cooperation with WHO. It also works with UNDP, FAO, and UNESCO.

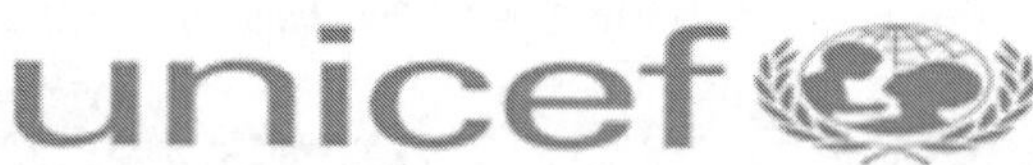

Fig. 8.10: Logo of UNICEF

At present the greater attention of UNICEF is 'Whole Child'. They render help not only for health and nutrition but for overall development of children, and to the development of country in which they live. This approach is known as 'country health promotion'. In India, UNICEF has provided substantial aid for safe water supply, production of vaccines and sera, supported BCG vaccination program from its inception. This organization has assisted in establishing DDT plant (Pune), for manufacturing penicillin, triple vaccine and iodized salt. The purpose is not only to reduce child illness and death but to improve the quality of life in the villages.

UNICEF supported supplementary feeding program in India through low cost nutrimix packet. With collaboration with FAO, UNICEF started to help in 'Applied Nutrition' program. They stimulate the rural population to grow and eat the foods it required for better child nutrition. Specific aid has been given to fight anemia, goiter, xerophthalmia. More recently, much emphasize has been given by FAO, UNICEF, WHO to develop food and nutrition policy of the countries to ensure child nutrition.

FAO

The Food and Agriculture Organization of the United Nations (FAO) is an agency of the United Nations that leads international efforts to defeat hunger (Fig. 8.11). It was established in 1945, with head quarter at Rome. Serving both developed and developing countries, FAO acts as a neutral forum where all nations meet as equals to negotiate agreements and debate policy. FAO is also a source of knowledge and information, and

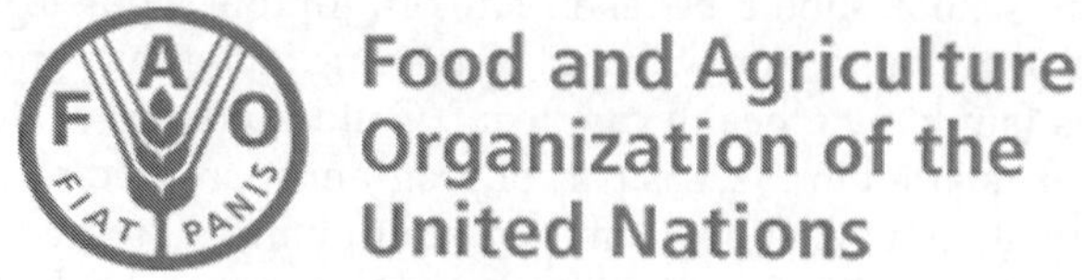

Fig. 8.11: Logo of FAO

helps developing countries and countries in transition, modernize and improve agriculture, forestry and fisheries practices, ensuring good nutrition and food security for all. The most important aspect of FAO's work is towards increased production of food to keep pace with the ever growing world population. Joining with WHO, FAO participates in applied nutrition program, nutritional surveys training programs, etc. The most important priority area FAO has outlined in its fight against hunger for the coming biennium, 2014–2015 is given below:

- Help eliminate hunger, food insecurity and malnutrition
- Contribute to the eradication of hunger by facilitating policies and political commitments to support food security and by making sure that up-to-date information about hunger and nutrition challenges and solutions is available and accessible.

CARE

CARE (Cooperative for Assistance and Relief Everywhere) is a major international humanitarian agency delivering broad-spectrum emergency relief and long-term international development projects. Founded in 1945, CARE's programs in the developing world address a broad range of topics including emergency response, food security, water and sanitation, economic development, climate change, agriculture, education, and health (Fig. 8.12). CARE also advocates at the local, national, and international levels for policy change and the rights of poor people. Within each of these areas, CARE focuses particularly on empowering and meeting the needs of women and on promoting gender equality. CARE provides emergency food aid and supports the prevention of malnutrition through demonstrating proper breastfeeding, providing education focusing on the cultivation and preparation of nutritious food, and improving infrastructure.

care®

Defending dignity.
Fighting poverty.

Fig. 8.12: Logo of CARE

USAID

The United States Agency for International Development (USAID) is the United States federal government agency primarily responsible for administering civilian foreign aid. USAID seeks to 'extend a helping hand to those people overseas struggling to make a better life, recover from a disaster or striving to live in a free and democratic country (Fig. 8.13).'

USAID's commitment to improving global health includes confronting global health challenges through improving the quality, availability, and use of essential health services. USAID's objective is to improve global health, including child, maternal, and reproductive health, and reduce abortion and disease, especially HIV/AIDS, malaria, and tuberculosis.

Newborn deaths are a large contributor to child deaths and USAID's leadership is helping to increase access to essential newborn care and addressing one of the three big killers of newborns—birth asphyxia, through resuscitation. USAID assistance is also instrumental in improving child and maternal health in other ways, such as increasing access to family planning and reducing the burden of HIV/AIDS and other infectious diseases.

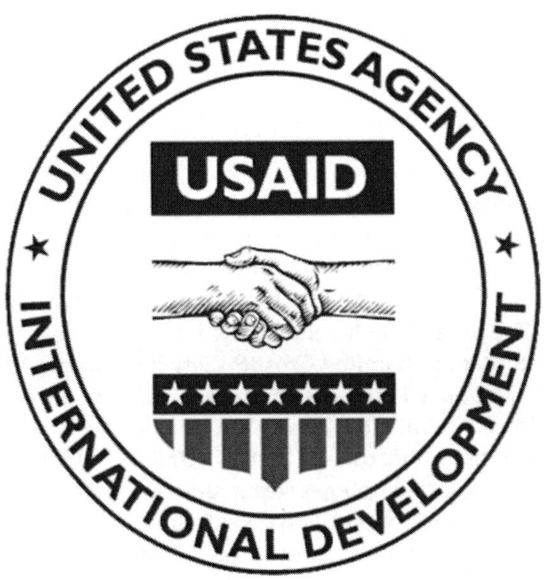

Fig. 8.13: Logo of USAID

NATIONAL ORGANIZATIONS

Indian Council for Child Welfare (ICCW)

ICCW was established in 1952 and affiliated with international union of child welfare. Its state and district councils have been working for India's children, those opportunities and facilities by law and other means which are necessary to enable them all round health. ICCW mobilizes its members to initiate, innovate and accelerate change to fulfill our paramount obligations to deliver to our children the support, protection and services that are their birth right.

Central Social Welfare Board

The central social welfare board came into being in early fifties, in an era when welfare services for the disadvantaged sections of society were not systematized and the welfare infrastructure was not yet a format construct.

A total of 33 State Social Welfare Board are functioning in each state capital and union territory of the country with an object to implement various schemes for the welfare and development of women and children through registered voluntary organizations. The state board is headed by a non-official chair person who is renowned woman social worker of the state. The Central Welfare Board provides support to voluntary organizations under a variety of programs in order to facilitate and strengthen their role in empowering women through education and training, through collective mobilization and awareness creation, through income generating facilities and by the provision of support services.

Red Cross

The Indian Red Cross Society is a voluntary humanitarian organization having a network of over 700 branches throughout India, providing relief in times of disasters/emergencies and promoting health and care of the vulnerable people and communities (Fig. 8.14).

On June 7, 1920, Indian Red Cross Society was constituted. Indian Red Cross Society has a partnership with National Red Cross and Red Crescent Societies, St. John Ambulance. It also coordinates with Indian Government and other agencies (UNDP, WHO, etc.). Red Cross society follows seven fundamental principles like Humanity, Impartiality, Neutrality, Independence, Voluntary services, Unity and Universality in its functioning.

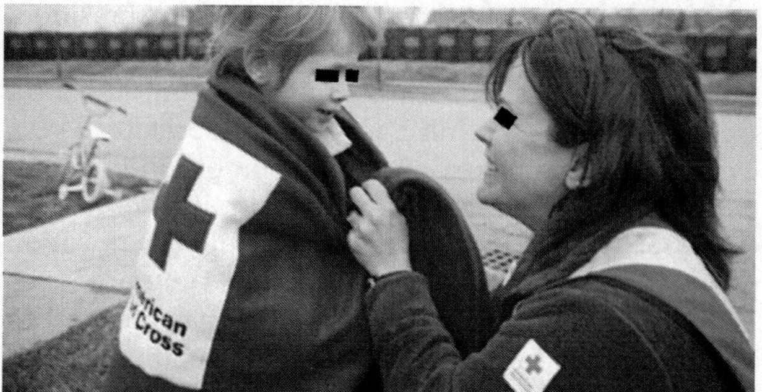

Fig. 8.14: Logo of Red Cross

Ongoing Child Welfare Programs in India

Social welfare programs aim at enabling the deprived sections of the population to overcome their social, economic or physical handicaps and improve their quality of life. They supplement the developmental programs in general in dealing with the problems of poverty and unemployment and are meant in particular, to assist the most disadvantaged groups below the poverty line, especially children from poor families, women, the handicapped and the infirm. The program of services for children in need of care and protection needs suitable, modified and cheaper models with better standards of services.

NURSES' ROLE IN PREVENTIVE PEDIATRICS

Nurses provide preventive services comprehensively than other health care professionals because they carry out in-hospital and outreach activities and are trained to address the family and the community. In a real sense, nurses are seen as active members of the community, and they value 'Health Promotion' that is focused on community participation.

Government and other health agencies have been undertaken different initiatives for progress in child survival and disease control (Table 8.1). A few million children under 5 are being saved each year as nurses carry out the interventions, such as newborn resuscitation for birth asphyxia, oral rehydration therapy (ORT), zinc supplementation to treat diarrhea, basic immunizations for common ailments, micronutrient supplementation to treat malnutrition and many more tasks.

Preventive care evolves continuously to keep the pace of the epidemiology of the population. Thus, nurses must acquire new competencies that, in turn, imply their involvement to identify and tackle emergent problems in addition to the existing ones.

Table 8.1: Different initiatives undertaken by government and other health agencies for progress in child survival and disease control

S.No.	*Child welfare programs*	*Year of beginning*	*Objectives/Description*
1.	Integrated Child Development Services (ICDS)	1975	It is aimed at enhancing the health, nutrition and learning opportunities of infants, young children (0–6 years) and their mothers.
2.	Creche scheme for the children of working mothers	2006	Overall development of children, childhood protection, complete immunization, awareness generation among parents on malnutrition, health and education.
3.	Reproductive and child health program	1951	To provide quality integrated and sustainable primary health care services to the women in the reproductive age group and young children and special focus on family planning and immunization.
4.	Pulse polio immunization program	1995	To eradicate poliomyelitis (polio) in India by vaccinating all children under the age of 5 years against polio virus.
5.	Sarva Shiksha Abhiyan	2001	All children in school, Education Guarantee Center, Alternate School, 'Back-to-School' camp by 2003; all children complete 5 years of primary schooling by 2007; all children complete 8 years of elementary schooling by 2010; focus on elementary education of satisfactory quality with emphasis on education for life; bridge all gender and social category gaps at primary stage by 2007 and at elementary education level by 2010; universal retention by 2010.
6.	Kasturba Gandhi Balika Vidyalaya	2004	To ensure access and quality education to the girls of disadvantaged groups of society by setting up residential schools with boarding facilities at elementary level.
7.	Mid-day meal scheme	1995	Improving the nutritional status of children in classes I–VIII in Government, Local Body and Government aided schools, and EGS and AIE centers. Encouraging poor children, belonging to disadvantaged sections, to attend school more regularly and help them concentrate on classroom activities. Providing nutritional support to children of primary stage in drought-affected areas during summer vacation.
8.	Integrated program for street children	1993	Provisions for shelter, nutrition, health care, sanitation and hygiene, safe drinking water, education and recreational facilities and protection against abuse and exploitation to destitute and neglected street children.
9.	The national rural health mission	2005	Reduction in child and maternal mortality, universal access to public services for food and nutrition, sanitation and hygiene and universal access to public health care services with emphasis on services addressing women's and children's health universal immunization, etc.

An appropriate example is ICDS program. The natural activity of this program is the provision of preventive services. It allows identifying prevalent diseases, monitoring child growth and development and provision of health education to the child and parents. This means that nurses need to be updated with the clinical information about the vaccines and spend more time with parents explaining the benefits and potential secondary effects of the newly introduced vaccines. Also, because they are the 'front line' of preventive services, nurses should be trained to identify the side effects of the vaccines and contribute in generating the pharmacoepidemiological information.

Among children overweight and obesity, diabetes are on the rise. Currently, preventive care for these children is mostly focused on screening of these conditions. This is a limited perspective. Further training and involvement of nurses to care for this problem are needed. Nurses need to be updated about the nutritional aspects of overweight and obesity, diabetes and learn motivational techniques for parent and children counseling. In addition, they should be actively included in the coordination with other health providers for treating children experiencing these conditions.

CONCLUSION

Nearly 6.9 million children under the age of five died in 2011—nearly 800 every hour, 6.6 million children under the age of five died in 2012—more than 750 every hour. Most of these children could survive and thrive with access to simple, affordable interventions. The loss of a child is a tragedy—families suffer and human potential is wasted. Preventive pediatrics has an important role in disease prevention, health policy/advocacy and health promotion efforts by addressing the health needs of children and adolescents. This vision will be driven by ongoing monitoring, assessment leading to policy-making oriented towards the prevention of diseases and related risk factors, therefore improving morbidity and mortality rates is to promote and advance the field of health promotion and disease prevention through research, education, service, and policy advocacy.

Progress in child survival and disease control has long been steady, and remains among the countries' major accomplishments. Worldwide, few million children under 5 are saved each year through basic interventions, such as:

- Newborn resuscitation for birth asphyxia
- Oral rehydration therapy (ORT)
- Zinc supplementation to treat diarrhea
- Basic immunizations for common ailments
- Micronutrient supplementation to treat malnutrition.

Preventive pediatrics and pediatric nursing aim in improving child and maternal health in other ways too, such as increasing access to family planning and reducing the burden of HIV/AIDS and other infectious diseases.

CHAPTER 9

Hospitalized Child

Chapter Outline

- Meaning of Hospitalization
- Need for Hospitalization
- Modern Concepts of Hospitalization
- Effects of Hospitalization on Child and Family
- I. Manifestation of Separation Anxiety in Young Children
- II. Manifestation of Loss of Control
- III. Manifestation of Bodily Injury and Pain
- Preparation of the Child for Hospitalization
- Nursing Care of the Child Who is Hospitalized
- Nursing Management of a Child in the Hospital
- Summarization

Disease and hospitalization can be the first crisis that a child encounters. Children's way of reacting to this crisis depends on the age at which the previous experience of disease and isolation took place, hospitalization, compatibility skills, gravity of the illness, and support systems present. Research has shown that previous experience and familiarity with medical procedures do not reduce fear in children. In fact, a previous experience may be a cause of substituting a known or unknown fear. The state of the illness can cause an experience of invasive and traumatic procedures. These factors can cause adverse emotional effects on children resulting from hospitalization. The recent trends of shortened hospital stays, increased use of outpatient care and ambulatory surgery, and managed care have had a direct impact on the practice of pediatric nursing (Fig. 9.1). The challenge for nurses is to adapt practices by supporting the physical, emotional, and developmental needs of the child and family while reducing costs without negatively influencing the quality of care provided.

MEANING OF HOSPITALIZATION

Hospitalization is admittance to the hospital as a patient. Patients are admitted to the hospital for a variety of reasons, including scheduled tests, procedures, or surgery; emergency medical treatment; administration of medication; or to stabilize or monitor an existing condition.

Pediatric hospitalization means the confinement of a child or infant in a hospital for diagnostic testing or therapeutic treatment. Regardless of age or the degree of illness or injury, hospitalization constitutes a major crisis in the life of a child, and the emotional trauma may elicit various behavioral reactions that the nurse must recognize and be prepared to cope with to facilitate recovery.

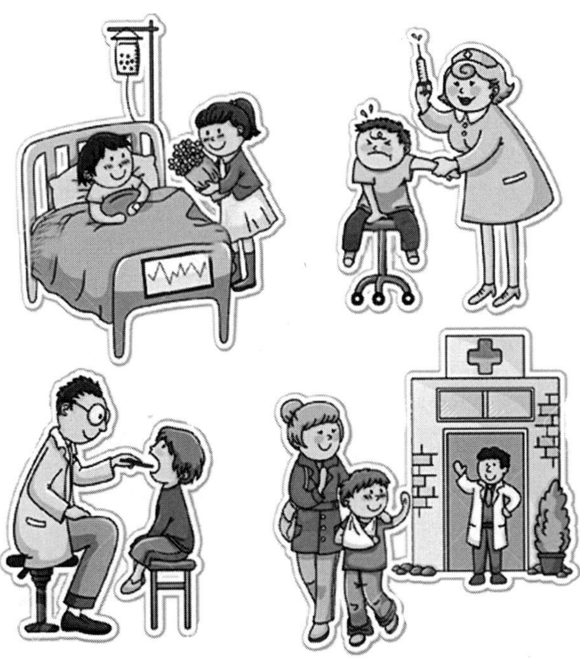

Fig. 9.1: Children in different situations related to health care

NEED FOR HOSPITALIZATION

In spite of best preventive health care and promotive care, some children become sick and need hospitalization. Still there are so many factors which seek hospitalization for the child. So hospitalization is needed:

- To reduce infant mortality rate.
- To cure the child from acute and chronic diseases.
- To early diagnosis and treatment of diseases.
- To provide advance technical treatment method to save the life of the child.
- To meet the intensive care of the child.
- To reduce the severity of the diseases.
- To provide periodical special care like blood transfusion to a thalassemic child, radiotherapy and chemotherapy to a leukemic child, etc.

MODERN CONCEPTS OF HOSPITALIZATION

Children may react to the stresses of hospitalization before admission, during hospitalization and after discharge. So, there are some modern concept to minimizes the stresses of hospitalization.

Visiting

Many years ago, when parents were permitted to visit their hospitalized child for only 1 hour once a month, but today many hospitals permit visiting from 2–8 pm or early in the morning to bedtime. Some institutions encourage flexible unlimited visiting at any time during the day or night. Some hospitals permit visiting by siblings between 2 and 12 years of age during certain hours of the day though siblings of ill child are not permitted to visit the child. Some hospitals have a closed-circuit television or telephone video that allows two-way visits between the child and visitors of all ages.

Rooming in

Some hospital provides comfortable lounge or waiting room for the parents where they can relax. In some institution, meals can be served to the parents in the child's room so they can eat with their child or they may eat in the hospital cafeteria or coffee shop. Food may be brought from home for the child if there are no dietary restriction and if the policy of the institution permits this to be done. Usually mothers of seriously ill children may be allowed to stay in the hospital if they desire to do so and if facilities are available for their comfort.

Care by Parent Unit

Some hospitals have care by parent or family participation units where parents actually live in the hospital with the child. This method of care has its roots in the orient, where the whole family become involved with the care of the sick. In this unit, parents are prepared naturally and effectively for the care their child will need at home. In some care by units, the parents are totally responsible for their child's care. In care by unit, older children may care for themselves, providing self-care under the direction of the nurse or the parents or both.

Parent Support Group

Many support groups for parents meet outside the hospital. Recent support group also have been started within the hospital for parents of hospitalized children. Such groups may be conducted by nurses, by play therapists, or by child life program staff, who act as facilitators to develop a support system among the parents. In this group, a nonthreatening atmosphere prevails, where parents may feel comfortable enough and ventilate their feelings and concerns to relieve their anxiety and stress.

Self-care

Within the self-care framework, nurses have the responsibility of assessing the abilities of the hospitalized child and then helping the child to learn self-care skills. The time and methods used in teaching these skills depend on the child's cognitive abilities, emotional state, and readiness to learn.

EFFECTS OF HOSPITALIZATION ON CHILD AND FAMILY

During the early years, children are particularly vulnerable to the crises of illness and hospitalization. The dominant factors influencing stress, which vary according to the child's developmental age, his or her previous experience with illness, and the seriousness of the condition, include separation from the parents and familiar environment, disruption of routine patterns of daily life, loss of independence, and worry about bodily injury or painful experiences.

Major stressors and Children's Response to Hospitalization/Illness

- Fear of the unknown
- Separation anxiety
- Fear of bodily injury resulting in discomfort, pain or mutilation
- Loss of control
- Anger
- Guilt
- Regression.

Infants: Birth to 18 Months

Hospital Stressors

- Disruption of routine, sleep and feeding patterns
- Loud noises, sudden movements and bright lights
- Separation from parents.

Common Reactions

Observed behaviors during later infancy cries, screams, searches for parent with eyes, clings to parents, avoids and rejects contact with stranger (Figs 9.2A and B). Additional behaviors observed during toddler are verbal attacks to strangers (e.g. 'go away'), physical attacks to strangers (e.g. Kicks, bites, hits, pinches), attempts to escape to find parent. These behaviors possibly last from hours to days. Protest, such as crying, often continues, ceasing only with physical exhaustion.

Increased Protest Precipitates by Approach of Strangers

Phase of despair of hospitalized child is characterized as inactive, withdrawn from other, depressed, sad, uninterested in environment, uncommunicative. He/she shows regression to earlier behavior (e.g. thumb sucking, bed-wetting, use of pacifier, and use of bottle). These behaviors last for variable length of time. The child's physical condition deteriorates from refusal to eat, drinks, or move.

Child shows phase of detachment as his interest in surroundings increases. He interacts with strangers or familiar caregivers, forms new but superficial relationships, appears happy. Detachment of child occurs usually after prolonged separation from parent, rarely seen in hospitalized children.

How Parents can Help

- Spend time with, hold and talk to the baby as much as possible
- Decrease noise level and bright lights
- Swaddle in blanket when not holding
- Provide calming music.

Toddlers and Preschoolers: 18 Months to 5 Years

Hospital Stressors

- Fear of separation from parents
- Stranger anxiety, fear of medical staff
- Unfamiliar environment
- Loss of control, independence and mobility.

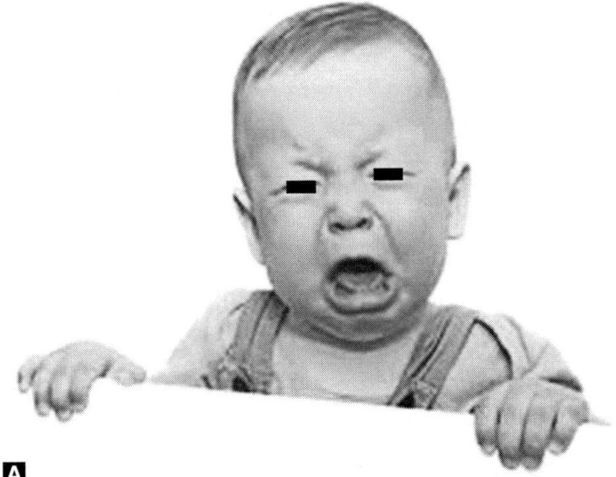

A

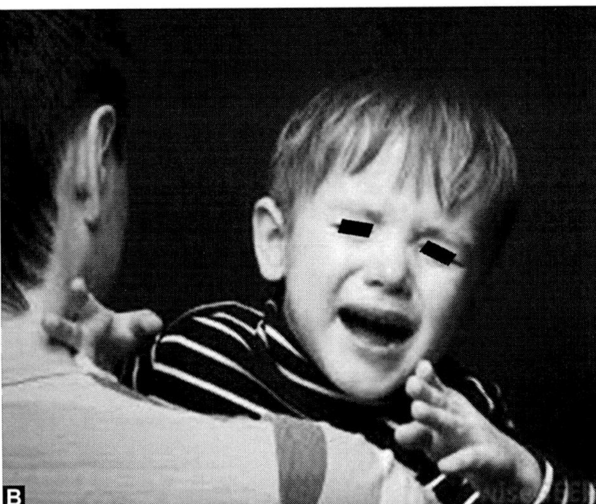

B

Figs 9.2A and B: A. Incessant cry of toddler lasts for variable length of time in separation anxiety; **B.** In the protest phase of separation anxiety, children cry loudly and are inconsolable in their grief for the parent

Common Reactions

- Clinging to parents
- Irritability and crying
- Regression of recently learned developmental skills
- Uncooperative and resistant behavior.

How Parents can Help

- Provide physical and emotional support with hugs and encouraging words
- Allow your child to make appropriate choices to feel more 'in control'
- Let your child play: Bring favorite toys or stuffed animals

- Normalize the environment by hanging up pictures of family and friends.

School-age: 6 to 12 Years

Hospital Stressors

- Misconceptions about hospitalization
- Loss of control, independence and mobility
- Fear of pain.

Common Reactions

- Regression
- Acting out
- Withdrawn.

How Parents can Help

- Encourage play and expression of emotions
- Allow child participation in care
- Be honest and use child-friendly language to help them understand their illness and treatment
- Treat as normally as possible.

Adolescents: 13 to 18 Years

Hospital Stressors

- Separation from friends, school and extracurricular activities
- Loss of independence and privacy
- Fear of bodily harm/deformity and death.

Common Reactions

- Anger and frustration
- Withdrawn.

How Parents can Help

- Allow peer contact and visitation
- Respect privacy
- Involve adolescent in medical care and decisions
- Communicate honestly
- Continue education/schooling.

Care of Hospitalized Child

- Prepare for hospitalization
- Prevent/minimize separation
- Minimize loss of control
- Prevent minimize bodily injury
- Allow for regression
- Provide pain management (= Atraumatic care)
- Provide for developmentally appropriate play activities
- Provide opportunities for play/expressive activities
- Maximize potential benefit of hospitalization

Focus on development age rather than chronological age

I. MANIFESTATION OF SEPARATION ANXIETY IN YOUNG CHILDREN

Phase of Protest

Observed behaviors during later infancy are cries, screams, searches for parent with eyes, clings to parent, avoids and rejects contact with stranger.

Additional behaviors observed during toddler

- Verbally attacks strangers (e.g. 'go away').
- Physically attacks strangers (e.g. kicks, bites, hits, pinches).
- Attempts to escape to find parent.
- Attempts to physically force parent to days.
- Behaviors possibly lasting from hours to days.
- Protest, such as crying, often continuous, ceasing only with physical exhaustion.
- Increased protest precipitated by approach of strangers.

Phase of Despair

- Inactive
- Withdrawn from other
- Depressed, sad
- Uninterested in environment
- Uncommunicative
- Regress to earlier behavior (e.g. thumb sucking, bed-wetting, use of pacifier, and use of bottle)
- Behaviors lasting for variable length of time
- Child's physical condition deteriorating from refusal to eat, drinks, or move.

Phase of Detachment

- Shows increased interest in surroundings.
- Interacts with strangers or familiar caregivers.
- Forms new but superficial relationships.
- Appears happy.
- Detachment occurring usually after prolonged separation from parent, rarely seen in hospitalized children.
- Behaviors representative of a superficial adjustment to loss.

Behavior Observed in Older Children

- Emotional coldness followed by demanding dependence on parents.
- Anger toward parents.
- Jealousy toward others.

II. MANIFESTATION OF LOSS OF CONTROL

One of the factors influencing the amount of stress imposed by the hospitalization is the amount of control that children perceive themselves as already have. Lack of control increase the perception of threat and can affect children's coping skills. Sometimes the additional hospital sight, sound, and smell may be overwhelming for the child.

In infant—crying or smiling.

In toddler—negativism, temper tantrum, etc.

In preschoolers—become shameful, feel guilt and fear.

In school age—hostility, depression and frustration.

In adolescent—rejection, uncooperativeness, withdrawal, self-assertion, anger or frustration.

III. MANIFESTATION OF BODILY INJURY AND PAIN

Fears of bodily injury and pain are prevalent among children. The consequences of these fears can be far reaching; adult who experience more medical fear in childhood are more fearful of medical pain as adult.

In infant: Cry loudly with body jerking in a different position like squirming, writhing, flailing and refuse to lie still, attempt to push the person away or try to escape.

In toddlers: Behavior indicate pain including grimacing, clenching the teeth or lips, opening the eyes wide, rocking, rubbing, aggressiveness such as biting, kicking, hitting, or running away, etc.

In preschoolers: They response more favorably to preparatory interventions, such as explanation and distraction, than younger children. Physical and verbal aggression is more specific and goal directed. Instead of showing total body resistance, preschoolers may push the offending person away, try to secure the equipment, or attempt to lock themselves in a safe place.

In school age: They express their discomfort in a way such as holding rigidly still, clenching their fists or teeth or trying to act brave. They display signs of over resistance, such as biting, kicking, pulling away, trying to escape, crying, or plea bargaining, etc.

In adolescent: They express their feeling by asking numerous questions, withdrawing, rejecting others, or questioning the adequacy of care. Sometimes they show overconfidence to overcome body image change. They are able to describe the intensity of pain and to use the pain assessment tools developed for adults.

Effects on nutritional status of the hospitalized child: An understanding of the nutritional status of hospitalized children is of fundamental importance to establishing a strategy for maintaining and/or recovering nutritional status during their hospital stay. Dietary care is of fundamental importance in the context of clinical treatment, irrespective of the disease responsible for admission, particularly in regions with high rates of child malnutrition. Weight loss during hospitalization had a significant relationship with prolonged hospital stays and with the disease responsible for hospitalization. The fact that the nutritional status of children who had been admitted in a well-nourished state deteriorated while they were in hospital must lead us reflect on the need for a culture that values the nutritional condition of hospitalized patients, in particular children, because of their increased nutritional vulnerability.

Risk factors that increases children's vulnerability to the stresses of hospitalization:

- 'Difficult' temperament.
- Lack of fit between child and parent.
- Age especially between (6 months to 5 years).
- Male gender.
- Below-average intelligence.
- Multiple and continuing stresses. (e.g. frequent hospitalization).

Different reactions among different age group of child due to hospitalization:

Hospitalization and prolonged illness can retard growth and development and cause adverse reactions in the child based on stage of development.

- *Reactions of neonates:* Effects of hospitalization and prolonged illness interrupt in the early stages of development of a healthy mother-child relationship and family integration. Impairment of bonding and trusting relationship, inability of the baby to respond to parents and family members are the common reactions.
- *Reactions of infants:* Separation anxiety and disturbance of development of basic trust are the main reactions here as the infant is separated from mother and illness interferes to meet the need of the infants. Emotional withdrawal and depression (4–8 months) are found along with the delayed growth and development. They have limited tolerance due to separation anxiety which is found as fear of strangers, excessive crying, clinging and overdependence on mother.
- *Reactions of toddlers:* There reactions are found as protest, despair, denial and regression. They protest by frequent crying, shaking crib, rejecting nurses' attention, urgent desire to find mother and showing signs of distrust with anger and tears, mostly when with mother. In despair, the toddler becomes

hopeless, apathetic, anorectic, listless, looks sad, cry continuously or intermittently and use comfort measures by thumbsucking, fingering lip and tightly clutching a toy. In denial, child accepts care without protest and shows more attachment with nurses than mother. They represses all feelings.

- *Reactions of preschool child:* They adopt various mental mechanisms (defense mechanism) to adjust with the stressful experiences. They react by exhibiting regression, repression, projection, displacement, identification, aggression, denial, withdrawal and fantasy. They may simply show similar behaviors of the toddlers also.
- *Reactions of school-aged child:* They are concerned with fear, worry, mutilation, fantasies, modesty and privacy. They react with defence mechanism like regression, phobia, unrealistic fear, suppression or denial of symptoms and conscious attempts of mature behavior.
- *Reactions of adolescents:* They are concerned with lack of privacy, separation from peers or family and school, interference with body image or independence or self-concept and sexuality. They react with anxiety related to loss of control and insecurity in strange environment. They may show anger and demanding behavior or increased dependency on parents or staff. They may adopt mental mechanism like intellectualization about disease, rejection of treatment, depression, denial or withdrawal.

Children's developmental concepts of illness and pain: Piaget (1969) has been called the father of child psychology. His work concerning cognitive development in children is based on the premise that human intelligence is an extension of biological adaptation, or one's ability to adapt psychologically to the environment. From his extensive studies he discovered four major stages:

1. *From birth to 2 years of age:* The child in this stage develops sensorimotor perception and sense of self with increased mobility develops from the external environment. The concepts of object permanence emerge's as the ability to form mental images evolves.
2. *From 2–7 years of age:* Development of understanding of symbolic gestures, can express self with language and achieve object permanence. They perceive illness as an external cause and relates pain as a punishment for wrong doing. This is the stage of preoperational stage.
3. *From 7–12 years of age:* Development of understanding of reversibility and spatially, logical thinking socialization, differentiation, classification and application of rules develops in this stage. They perceive illness as an external cause but located inside the body and relate pain physically and able to perceive psychologic pain. This is the stage of concrete operational stage.
4. *From 12–15+ years of age:* Here the child learn's to logical thinking and abstract reasoning, making and testing hypotheses and cognitive maturity achieved. The children can explain illness in sequence of events and mature understanding about pain are present here. This is the formal operational stage.

Effects of hospitalization on the family of the child: Parents whose children have been admitted to the hospital feel not only separation from their children but also they may have feeling of inadequacy as others (nurses, doctors) provide care for their children. They feel anxiety, anger, fear, disappointment, self-blame and possible guilt feeling due to lack of confidence and competence for caring the child in illness and wellness.

Factors affecting parents' reactions to their child's illness

- Seriousness of the threat to the child.
- Previous experience with illness or hospitalization.
- Medical procedures involved in diagnosis and treatment.
- Available support systems.
- Personal ego strengths.
- Previous coping abilities.
- Additional stresses on the family system.
- Cultural and religious beliefs.
- Communication patterns among family members.

Other than that there are so many factors which may increase the parental anxiety. The anxious parent can be recognized by the trembling, coarse or waver voice, restlessness, irritability, withdrawal or erratic body movements. Hostile and aggressive behavior may be evident towards those caring for the child. The reaction of the family members can be influenced by cultural and spiritual beliefs. They think that illness is due to any fault in child rearing and considered as punish by god.

Siblings reactions: siblings may experiences loneliness, fears and worry for their ill siblings. The following factor are related to increase the effects on the siblings:

- Being younger and experiences many changes.
- Being cared for outside the home by care providers who are not relatives.
- Receiving little information about their ill brother or sister.

- Perceiving their parents as treating them differently compared with before their sibling's hospitalization.

However, the perception of stress varied significantly in relation to the type of sibling relationship and frequency of sibling visitation.

Altered family roles: In addition to the effects of separation on family roles, loss of the parent and sibling roles may affect each family member differently. Without an understanding of the interpersonal dynamics between siblings and parents are likely to blame the well child for antisocial behavior. Rivalry tends to be greatest with the siblings who are nearest the ill child's age. Illness may also result in a child's loss of status within either the family or peer group.

PREPARATION OF THE CHILD FOR HOSPITALIZATION

Preparation for hospitalization is important to prevent psychologic or emotional trauma of hospitalization. Both planned and emergency admission require special preparation for the child by the parents, health team members and nurses, to promote coping with the traumatic event. The following concepts help to minimize the emotional trauma to the children and their parents for better adjustment during hospital stay:

- Family integrity and child's relationship should be maintained to follow the child's behavior and reaction.
- The sick child should be supported and guided to learn to handle new experiences and feelings by family participation to provide love and security during illness and hospital.
- Needs of each child are different based on individual differences, family background, level of growth and development and degree of illness.
- The pediatric nurse seeks to promote, maintain and restore health in both children and their parents by health counseling and teaching about the needs.
- Hospitalized child should be cared by the professional nurses following scientific principles of disease process and nursing process with appropriate therapeutic and nursing interventions.
- Family participation for planning, implementation and evaluating plan of care is essential for optimal outcome by continuity of care.
- Sick child needs expert physical care, emotional support, expression of feelings (through play) and continuation of school education to promote continued growth both in acute and chronic illness.
- A trusting relationship is needed between parents and health care team and parents should have permission for expression of feelings and emotions in the hospital environment.
- Parents and family members of terminally ill or dying child must be supported so that the child can die with dignity and with a feeling of being loved.
- As hospitalization is the break in the unity of the family so, the emotional effects should be considered first, because it is often mistakenly accorded less importance than physical care given to the sick child.

NURSING CARE OF THE CHILD WHO IS HOSPITALIZED

Children and their families require competent and sensitive care to minimize the potential negative effects of hospitalization and also to promote benefits from the experience. Interventions should focus on (1) eliminating or minimizing the stressors of separation, loss of control, and bodily injury and pain for children and (2) providing specific supportive strategies for family members, such as fostering family relationships and providing information.

Adaptation in nursing care of the sick child: Even with the best preparation some children and their parents may still feel severe stress during illness and admission to hospital. The sources of stress included the five following categories:

1. *Psychological stress* due to separation from home, parents, other family members and friends, change in role, anxiety, fear and pain.
2. *Physiological stress* due to loss of sleep, diagnostic and treatment procedures, trauma, burns, surgery, immobilization and physical restraint.
3. *Environmental stress* due to loss of daily routine, unfamiliar noise, strange odor and stimuli and various gadgets especially in intensive care unit.
4. *Biological stress* due to pathological organisms and cross infections.
5. *Chemical stress* due to drugs, toxic substances, reactions to blood transfusions, anesthesia, etc. Stress is the nonspecific response to stressors or demands made on the body. Coping is the way an individual deals with a situation and adapts to it. The nurse can assist the child and parents in coping efforts in regard to hospitalization by using reality oriented and task oriented coping strategies.

The strategies for adaptation in nursing care:

- Welcome the child and parents heartily during each nursing interventions.

- Call by name and touch the child gently with love.
- Explain the interventions in simple sentence according to the level of understanding and tell about the event, what will exactly happen.
- Ask for cooperation and its benefit.
- Encourage to express the feelings, allow verbalizing and answering question.
- Demonstrate the interest and empathy to the child and family members.
- Explain and reason out any unpleasant experience of the past which will reduce anxiety level and help to obtain cooperation.
- Discuss about cultural and religious belief of the family, never condemned those beliefs.
- Allow parent or significant other during any treatment.
- Maintain privacy; minimize exposure and gentle handling of the child.
- Provide physical comfort by appropriate positioning, warmth, bladder evacuation, etc. before and during the intervention.
- Take opinion of the parents and the child during any decision making regarding any treatment plan and intervention.
- Maintain eye level contact during conversation.
- Divert the child's attention by toys or telling story or simply taking with him/her.
- Restraints should be used only if there is no alternative.
- Skillful and confident approach to be practiced throughout the procedures.
- Protect the child from physical injury and infections.
- Assure about the confidentiality of the information for older children.
- Patience, tenderness and emotional strength are essential during nursing care to the children.
- Never tell lie and negative statement to the child, honest explanation is important for positive approach.
- Praise the child for cooperation, never threat or blame the child for non-cooperation.
- Establishment of rapport and friendly approach are the key points to gain cooperation.

NURSING MANAGEMENT OF A CHILD IN THE HOSPITAL

Focused Assessment

Assessment is done for any problems related to the hospital admission by identifying pertinent historical data on the admission data sheet and analyzing the results of the physical examination. Important assessment areas that can cause problems for hospitalized children include:

Nutrition

- Assessment is performed for the child's calorie intake, and comparison is taken with the requirements for age and weight.
- Notification is to be performed to identify the abnormalities if any after plotting and recording height and weight percentiles.
- Child's favorite foods and customary rituals around mealtime in addition to cultural or religious dietary practices that may restrict a child's food choices is to be determine.

Elimination

- Any regression the child may be having in bowel or bladder control is to be assess.
- Enquiry is to be carried out for specific terms, the child uses for elimination and it is useful to verbalize those terms to provide comfort and assistance to the child.

Sleep

- Understanding and communicating the child's usual sleep patterns and routines to others will assist in planning care.
- Determination of child's usual bedtime, hygiene practices used before sleep and bedtime rituals like rocking, prayers, stories, snacks, etc. are to be carried out.
- Notification of any alterations in the number of hours the child is sleeping, and compare with the norm for the child's age are to be performed.

Self-care

The child's usual self-care activities (eating, bathing, dressing, brushing teeth) must be assessed and note. Alteration may indicate increasing anxiety or loss of control.

Emotional/social Status

- Signs of anxiety (crying, temper tantrums, withdrawal, decreased communication) or fear related to the hospital setting must be assessed.
- Assess the child's ability to keep in touch with peers.
- Note whether the child readily participate in unit activities or not.

Nursing Diagnosis

Imbalanced nutrition less than body requirements related to unfamiliar foods, separation from caregiver, strange environment or disease process.

Expected outcomes: The child will:

- Eat the appropriate number of calories and variety of nutrients according to age.
- Maintain prehospital weight.

Intervention

- The cause of the child's decreased intake is to be identified.
- Parents are to be encouraged to bring foods from home and to be with the child during meals.
- The child is to be allowed to select food from the menu.
- Communicate to the other staff with the types of foods the child particularly likes.
- Small portion, small dishes, cups and glasses are to be offered to the child.
- If parents cannot be available during meals, the child is to be allowed to eat with other children.
- A dietary consultation is to be arranged for the child.

Evaluation

- Is the child's nutritional intake appropriate for age?
- Did the child maintain baseline body weight during hospitalization?

Nursing Diagnosis

Delayed growth and development, regression in toilet training or self-care skills, related to separation and hospitalization.

Expected outcomes: The child will maintain usual self-care activities of feeding, toileting, dressing and bathing and any regression reverses quickly after discharge.

Intervention

- Home routines of elimination is to be followed.
- The incontinent child must not be scolded.
- Explanation should be given to parents that some regression in all self-care activities is normal in hospitalized children and that most children resume their normal routines soon after discharge.
- Parents are to be discouraged from beginning toilet training during hospitalization.
- The child is to be encouraged to participate in self-care according to developmental abilities.
- The child is to be assisted when the ability to perform self-care is limited, because of fatigue, discomfort or other factors related to the disease process.
- The child is to be provided the necessary equipment for self-care and place if within easy reach.
- The child is to be offered choices and allowed to make decisions when appropriate.

Evaluation

- Is the child able to feed, toilet, dress and bathe at the same level as before the illness?
- Does the child readily participate in self-care activities?

Nursing Diagnosis

Disturbed sleep pattern related to unfamiliar environment, anxiety or discomfort.

Expected outcomes: The child will sleep the appropriate number of hours for age.

Intervention

- Prior planning for care should be prepared to allow time for periods of sleep.
- Care can be organized so that vital signs can be measured and other procedures performed when medication is given.
- A sign on the door is to be posted when the child is asleep to prevent other staff and visitors from awaking the child and phone must be unplugged, television must be turn off, etc.
- A night light must be provided.
- If the parents are not with the child, then explanation must be given to the child that the parents will be nearby and will check during the night.

Evaluation

Does the child take naps and sleep an appropriate amount of time on the basis of age requirements?

Nursing Diagnosis

Anxiety related to fear of the unknown and separation from significant others and familiar surroundings.

Expected outcomes: The child will:

- Decrease indication of distress (e.g. crying, withdrawal, irritability).
- Verbalize feelings of anxiety.
- Play appropriately and maintain contact with peers.

Intervention

- The child and parent to the hospital and the routines of the unit must be oriented.
- The child and parents are to be prepared for all procedures in an age appropriate way.
- Parents are to be encouraged to stay with the child when possible and to be involved in the child's care.
- The infant or young adult is to be hold, cuddle or rock.
- If the parents cannot stay with the child, a consistent caregiver should be provided.
- Home routine and rituals can be followed if possible.
- Parents are to be encouraged to be honest with the child when they leave and to inform the nurse where they can be reached and when they will return.
- The parents are to be encouraged to call while they are away, and older children can talk on the phone with their parents.
- The parents is to be encouraged to bring transitional objects (e.g. blanket, teddy bear) and to provide reminders of themselves if they cannot be with the child.
- The child is to be taken to the playroom and introduce to other children when appropriate or plan play activities (reading, board games, drawing) for a child unable to leave the room.
- For the older child, peer contact through visits, phone calls and letters are to be arrange.
- The child is to be offered choices and allowed to make decisions when appropriate.
- The older child is to be encouraged to wear street clothes and to decorate the room.
- Opportunities must be provided for the older child to express feelings about the illness and hospitalization; communicate with the child life specialist about the child's identified needs (e.g. anxiety, anger, boredom, lack of information).
- Information must be provided to the parents about diagnosis, treatment and prognosis and the child's need for sleep and nutrition.

Evaluation

- Is the child playing and communicating with other children and staff and showing decreased signs of distress?
- Is the child able to express feelings of anxiety either verbally or through play?

Nursing management of the family of the hospitalized child:

Focused assessment:

- Assessment for the factors that affect a family's adjustment to illness and hospitalization is to be done.
- Special attention should also be given to any information obtained in the admission interview.
- Try to determine whether the parents and siblings are experiencing stress and how they are coping with hospitalization.
- Compare assessment with concerns expressed on the child's admission history like:
  - Was the admission an emergency?
  - Were there previous admissions?
  - How did the parents perceive those hospitalization?
  - How serious is the illness or trauma?
  - Are some factors unknown such as the cause of the disease or the child's prognosis?

Nursing Diagnosis

Interrupted family processes related to the child's hospitalization and illness.

Expected outcomes: The parents will:

- Participate in the child's care.
- Meet the needs of other family members.
- Use appropriate support systems.
- Identify ways to cope.
- Assist the child to move from a sick role to a well role.

Intervention

- The parents is to be oriented to the hospital and to provide information related to their physical needs (e.g. food, sleep, bathing).
- Family members (parents, siblings) are to be encouraged to express their feelings and to ask questions about the child's illness.
- Information about the child's condition, treatment and support systems must be provided to the family and begin to prepare them for the child's discharge.
- Family coping strategy should be identified and their parenting skill must be supported.
- The family is to be refered to other professionals (e.g. social worker, clinical psychologist, clinical specialist, psychiatrist, clergy) when their problems are not within scope of nursing.

Evaluation

- Are the parents able to participate in their child's care while meeting the needs of other family members?
- Do family members support each other and seek other resources when necessary?
- Are family members able to describe and use positive coping skills?

- Are the parents able to assist the child to move from a sick to a well role?

Information for discharge:

After assessing the family's knowledge, the information should be provided to the families need to know to help the child's transition from hospital to home:

- Information about the illness or trauma and expected outcome is to be told to the parents when they consult to the physician or nurse.
- Medications or treatments are to be given at home and information about time, route, side effects and any special care to be taken when giving the medication and written information is valuable.
- Information about any special nutritional needs should be given.
- Specific activities the child may, may not and sometimes should participate in like :
  - The date when the child may return to school.
  - The date to bring the child back to the hospital, clinic or office for follow-up care must be informed.
- Information about any referral agency needed for the child or family.
- The unit phone number should be provided.
- Return demonstration about any procedures that will be performed in the home should be taken from the parents or family member.

SUMMARIZATION

So, we discussed today about the definition of hospitalization, philosophy of pediatric care in hospital, need for hospitalization, modern concepts of hospitalization, children's developmental concepts about illness and pain, preparation of the child for hospitalization, effects of hospitalization on the child, risk factors that increase the vulnerability to stressors on hospitalized child and reaction formation among different age group child, effects of hospitalization on the family of the child, nursing care of the hospitalized child and nursing care of the family of the hospitalized child.

CONCLUSION

Although hospitalization can and usually is stressful for children, it can also be beneficial. The most obvious benefit is the recovery from illness, but hospitalization also can present an opportunity for children to master stress and feel competent in their coping abilities. The hospital environment can provide children with new socialization experiences that can broaden their interpersonal relationship.

CHAPTER 10

Integrated Management of Neonatal and Childhood Illness (IMNCI)

Chapter Outline

- The IMNCI Package
- Principles of IMNCI Integrated Care

'Close to 50 percent of newborn deaths in India occur during the first seven days of birth'.

IMCI is an integrated approach to child health that focuses on the well-being of the whole child. IMCI aims to reduce death, illness and disability, and to promote improved growth and development among children under five years of age. It focuses primarily on the most common causes of child mortality, i.e. diarrhea, pneumonia, measles, malaria, malnutrition, illness affecting children aged one week to two months, two months to five years (Fig. 10.1). IMCI includes both preventive and curative elements that are implemented by families and communities as well as by health facilities.

Annually, over 10 million children in low and middle income countries including India die before they reach their fifth birthday and 7 out of 10 of these deaths are due to some common treatable or preventable conditions such as diarrheal dehydration, acute respiratory infections, measles, malaria, and malnutrition. Delay in seeking treatment and lack of quality care in health facilities are important cause of death in such conditions, as parents fail to recognize warning signs and sick children not being taken to health facilities on time. Moreover, according to the world bank report 1993, in situations where laboratory support and clinical resources are limited, a syndromic approach with comprehensive health care strategies is more realistic and cost-effective. It also has the potential to make the greatest impact on the global burden of disease. Considering this situation, during the year 1992, WHO, in collaboration with UNICEF and some other agencies, institutions and individuals, responded to the challenge by adopting a strategy known as integrated management of childhood illness (IMCI).

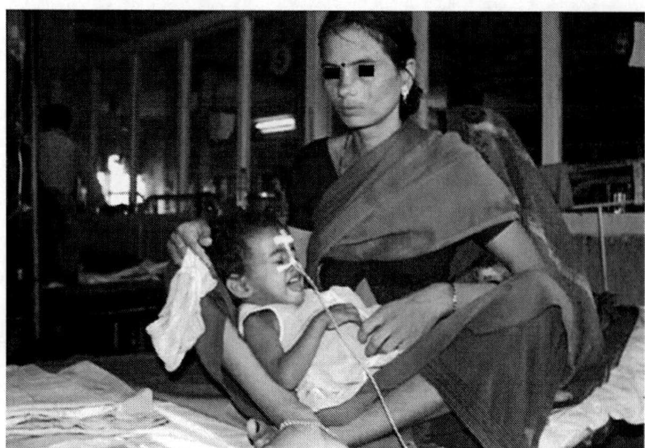

Fig. 10.1: IMNCI emphasizes on integrated approach for treating the sick children

The Government of India along with other experts also recognized the need for a strategy like IMCI. Moreover, close to 50 percent of newborn deaths in India occur during the first seven days of birth. In Indian scenario, neonatal mortality constitutes a substantial (64%) proportion of 'under 5 mortality,' all neonates starting from the day of birth were included in the strategy. Thus for Indian version, IMCI was adapted as integrated management of neonatal and childhood illness (IMNCI). It focuses on strengthening home-based care and provides special care for under-nourished newborns. During home visits by health workers the mother is taught how to recognize diseases early and when to seek medical help. She is also educated on the benefits of exclusive breastfeeding. So beneficiaries of IMNCI care of young infants for newborns (under 2 months), young children (2 months–5 years).

DEFINITION

IMNCI is an integrated approach to child health that focuses on the *well-being of the whole child.* It focussed primarily on the most common causes of child mortality-diarrhea, pneumonia, measles, malaria, malnutrition, illness affecting children aged 1 week to 2 months, 2 months to 5 years including both preventive and curative elements to be implemented by families.

The objectives of the IMNCI strategy are:

- To reduce mortality and morbidity associated with the major causes of disease in children less than five years of age
- To reduce the frequency and severity of illness and disability
- To contribute to the healthy growth and development of children.
- To ensure that the relevant needs of the child are looked at and attended during the contact of the child with the health care personnel.

Operationalization of these objectives need to determine baseline mortality among children under 5 years of age (NMR, IMR, USMR) to determine prevalence of fever, loose stools, cough and any other illness (morbidity density) in two weeks prior to day of field survey among children under 5 years of age to assess effective program coverage for specific disease condition (loose stool with dehydration) occurring in two weeks prior to day of field survey.

Why Integrated Approach?

WHO/UNICEF have developed a new approach to tackling the major diseases of early childhood called the integrated management of childhood illnesses (IMCI). Studies show that children presenting with any illness often suffer from more than one disease. For instance, a child presenting with diarrhea may also be malnourished and may not have received the immunization as per the National Immunization schedule. The integrated approach ensures that all relevant needs of the child are looked at and attended to during the contact of the child with the health workers.

- Integrated approach is child centered.
- *Five conditions:* Pneumonia, diarrhea, measles, malaria and malnutrition are major cause of death.
- Three out of four children seeking health care in developing countries suffers from one of these conditions.
- Children likely to be suffering from more than one condition.
- Often combination of these conditions leads to fatal result.
- Making a single diagnosis may be difficult.
- Such children often need combined therapy for successful treatment.

When correctly applied, IMNCI has the following advantages:

- Promotes the accurate identification of childhood illnesses in out-patient settings, hence prompt referral.
- Speeds up the urgent treatment and treatment seeking practices. Ensures appropriate combined treatment of all major childhood illnesses.
- Aims to improve the quality of care of sick children at the referral level.
- Strengthens the counselling of mothers or caregivers, involves parents in effective care of baby at home.
- Strengthens the provision of preventive services.
- Involves prevention of diseases by active immunization, improved nutrition and exclusive breastfeeding practices (community IMNCI).
- Highly cost-effective.
- It avoids wastages of resources by using most appropriate medicines and treatment.
- It reduces duplication of effort.
- Partial success of individual disease control program.

THE IMNCI PACKAGE

The health care experts including the child health researchers, academicians the indian academy of pediatrics (IAP) and the national neonatology forum (NNF) has developed IMNCI package to adapt it for the specific requirements of children in India. Since newborn care is an important issue for bringing down the infant mortality rate in India, this aspect has been included in the package adapted by India. Depending on the child's age, various clinical signs and symptoms differ in their degrees of reliability, and diagnostic value and importance. For this reason , the children are broadly categorized as two groups; (1) young infants up to 2 months, (2) children aged 2 months to 5 years. IMNCI package includes three important components:

I. Integrated management of childhood illness.

- IMCI strategy are most effective when all three components are implemented simultaneously.
- Care of newborns and young infants (infants under 2 months):
  - Keeping the child warm.
  - Initiation of breastfeeding immediately after birth and counselling for exclusive breastfeeding and non-use of prelacteal feeds.
  - Cord, skin and eye care.

- Recognition of illness in newborn , management and/or referral.
- Immunization.
- Home visits in the postnatal period.

Home visits are an integral part of this intervention. Home visits by health workers help mothers and families to understand and provide essential newborn care at home and detect and manage newborns with special needs due to low birth weight or sickness.

- Home visits by health workers (ANMs, AWWs, ASHAs).
- 3 home visits are to be provided to every newborn:
    - First visit on the day of birth (day 1)
    - Next two visit on day 3 and day 7
- For low birth weight babies, 3 more visits—on day 14, 21 and 28
- Care of mothers during the postpartum period.

- Care of infants (2 months to 5 years)
    - Management of diarrhea, acute respiratory infections (pneumonia), malaria, measles, acute ear infection, malnutrition and anemia.
    - Recognition of illness and at risk conditions and management/referral.
    - Prevention and management of iron and vitamin A deficiency.
    - Feeding counselling for all children below 2 years
    - Feeding counselling for malnourished children between 2–5 years.
    - Immunization (Fig. 10.2).
- Who will provide IMNCI services?
    - The health workers in the community (ANM, AWW, ASHA) or
    - Providers at the facility (PHC/CHC/FRU).

After neonatal period, IMNCI package is accessed by the family for their newborns and other children from the health workers in the community. In addition the opportunity of home visit is to be used for the care of mothers during the postpartum period. This will help mothers and families on how to recognize and manage minor conditions and will ensure timely referral of severe cases.

II. Improvements to the health system. The essential elements include:
- Ensuring availability of the essential drugs with workers and at facilities covered under IMNCI.
- Improve referral to identified referral facility.
- Referral mechanism to ensure that an identified sick infant or child can be quickly transferred to a higher level of care when needed. Every health worker must be aware of where to refer a sick child and the staff at appropriate health facilities must be in position to identify and acknowledge the referral slips and give priority care to the sick children.
- Functioning referral centres, especially where healthcare systems are weak, referral institutions need to be reinforced or private/public partnerships established
- Ensuring availability of health workers/providers at all levels
- Ensuring supervision and monitoring through follow up visits by trained supervisors as well as on the job supportive supervision

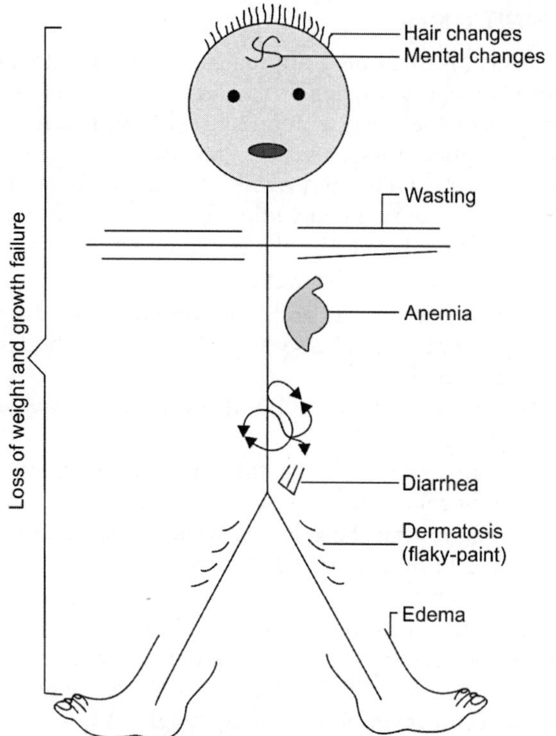

Fig. 10.2: Disorders of malnutrition

III. Community IMCI or promotion of key family and community practices
- Improvement of family and community practices counseling of families and creating awareness among communities on their role is an important component of IMNCI. This includes:

IIIrd Promoting healthy behaviors such as breast feeding, illness recognition, early case seeking, etc.

IEC campaigns for awareness generation.

Counseling of care givers and families, as part of management of the sick child when they are brought to the health worker/health facility.

During home visits: Home visits provide an opportunity for identification of sickness and focused BCC for improving newborn and child care practices.

Collaboration/coordination with other departments, panchayati raj institution (PRIs), self help groups, mahila swasthya sangha (MSS), etc. Implementation of IMNCI in an effective way in any district would be possible only with the total involvement of ANM and *anganwadi* workers of ICDS, and grassroot functionaries of other sectors. Community ownerships and participation is of paramount importance. Therefore active involvement of PRI, self-help groups and women's groups is a must. Special effort will thus be required on the part of the district CMOs to involve the concerned departments.

- IMNCI is a skill based training. The training is based on a participatory approach combining classroom sessions with hands-on clinical sessions in both facility and community settings.

  Broadly, two categories of training are included, one for medical officers and a second for front-line functionaries including ANM's and *anganwadi workers* (AWW's).

  For accredited social health activist (ASHA) and link volunteers if any, a separate package consistent with IMNCI focusing on the home care of newborn and children is in preparation keeping in mind their educational status. The essential purposes of training are:
- Ensuring availability of health workers/providers at all levels.
- Ensuring availability of the essential drugs.
- Improve referral to identified referral facility.
- Referral mechanism to ensure hassle free transfer to higher level of care when needed.
- Awareness of health worker for when and where to refer a sick child.
- The staff at appropriate health facilities must identify and acknowledge the referral slips and give priority care to the sick children.
- Functioning referral centers, especially where health care systems are weak need to be reinforced or private/public partnerships established.
- Ensuring supervision and monitoring through follow-up visits by trained supervisors.
- On the job supportive supervision.

PRINCIPLES OF IMNCI INTEGRATED CARE

- All, under five years of age sick children must be examined for conditions which need immediate hospitalization or referral.
- Routine assessment of all children for major symptoms, nutritional and immunization status, feeding problems and other potential problems.
- Only a few carefully selected clinical signs are used based on evidence of their sensitivity and specificity to detect disease.
- The child is placed in a classification (color coded) based on the presence of selected clinical signs. Classifications are not specific diagnoses but categories that are used to determine the treatment.
- IMNCI guidelines address most common, but not all pediatric problems.
- Only essential drugs, few in number are used.
- Caregivers are actively involved in the treatment of children.
- Orientation and counselling about home care and when to return to health care facility.

Color coded case management strategy:

- *Light gray classification*: Child needs inpatient care
- *Dark gray classification*: Child needs specific treatment, provide it at home (e.g. antibiotics, antimalarial, ORT)
- *Extra dark gray classification*: Child needs no medicine, advise home care (original color code used in government protocol is as follows: light gray–pink; dark gray–yellow; extra dark gray–green).

Six steps of IMNCI case management process (Flowchart 10.1 and 10.2)

1. Assess the young infant/child
2. Classify illness
3. Identify treatment
4. Treat the young infant/child
5. Counsel the mother/caregiver
6. Provide follow-up care

Step 1–3: Assess, Classify, Identify Treatment

The above mentioned classification chart describes the steps of IMNCI case management process. In the classification table, a child receives classification in one color only. If the child shows signs from more than one row, select the most severe classification.

Table 10.1: Classification table for dehydration and preferred treatment of children

	Signs	*Classify as*	*Identify treatment (urgent prereferral treatments are in bold print)*
A.	Two of the following signs: • Lethargic or unconscious • Sunken eyes • Not able to drink or drinking poorly • Skin pinch goes back very slowly	Severe dehydration	**If child has no other severe classification:** • Give fluid for severe dehydration (plan C) Or **If child also has another severe classification:** • **Refer urgently to hospital with mother giving frequent sips of ORS on the way** • **Advise the mother to continue breastfeeding** • **If child is 2 years or older and there is choldra in your area, give antibiotic for choldra.**
B.	Two of the following signs: • Restless, irritable • Sunken eyes • Drinks eagerly, thirsty • Skin pinch goes back slowly	Some dehydration	Give fluid and food for some dehydration (plan B) **If child also has a severe classification:** • **Refer urgently to hospital with mother giving frequent sips of ORS on the way** **Advise the mother to continue breastfeeding** • Advise mother when to return immediately. • Follow-up in 5 days if not improving.
C.	Not enough signs to classify as some or severe dehydration	No dehydration	Give fluid and food to treat diarrhea at home (plan A) Advise mother when to return immediately. Follow-up in 5 days if not improving.

A. Light gray B. Dark gray C. Extra dark gray

Classification of IMNCI starts with the light gray rows. If the child does not have the severe classifications, look at the dark gray rows. If the child does not have any of the signs in the light gray or dark gray rows, the classification is set in the extra dark gray rows.

Potential problem of the child (very low weight, anemia) are assessed and information in this regard is collected from mother. The children should be routinely assessed for symptoms of diarrhea and for feeding problems. Health education on feeding, immunization, potential health problems are to be given after identifying problems.

The 'identify treatment' column of annexure shows all the treatments required for the sick child. If a sick child has more than one classification, treatment required for all the classifications must be identified. All sick children should be assessed for possible bacterial infection, jaundice or hypothermia. The child is classified based on severity rather than the diagnosis.

Based on the classifications and 'treatment identified', an infant is managed with prereferral treatment for severe classification, OPD treatment and management at home.

Step 4: IMNCI Process

Treat the Young Infant/Child

Children with severe classification (light gray) are referred to a hospital after assessment and administration of prereferral treatment. In case of the signs and symptoms of bacterial infection the prereferral treatment includes administration of first dose of antibiotic (a single dose of ceftriaxone 100 mg/kg or cefotaxime 50 mg/kg), treating hypoglycemia, providing warmth to prevent hypothermia (in case of LBW /preterm baby).

In case of diarrhea, assessment of level of dehydration, administration of fluid is urgently needed. If infection is present, the child is to be referred to the hospital quickly. ORS is to be given during transportation.

If the child is convulsing, give diazepam 0.2/kg (0.05 mL/kg) IV or rectally. If convulsions continue after 10 minutes, give a second dose of diazepam. Injection phenobarbital (20 mg/kg) is also used in case of infants less than 2 weeks of age.

Outpatient treatment: Children with nonreferral classification (dark gray and extra dark gray) are catered in outpatient treatment. The treatment usually starts with a first line of drug (essential drug). Next line of drug is used if the illness of the child does not respond in the first line drug. The health worker needs to teach the mother or other caregivers regarding administration of drug.

Step 5: IMNCI Process

Counselling a mother or caregiver (Community IMNCI)

- Counselling of families and creating awareness among communities.
  This includes:

Flowchart 10.1: Six steps of IMNCI case management process is shown in this algorithm

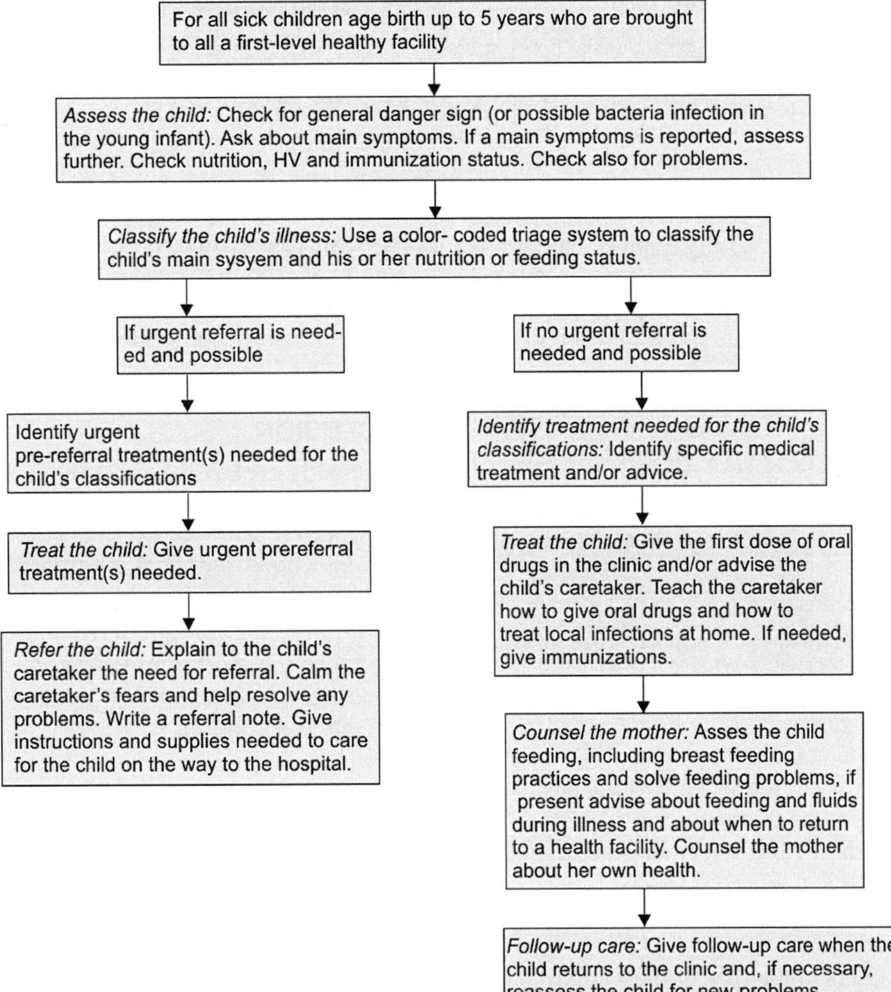

- Promoting healthy behaviors such as breastfeeding, illness recognition, early care seeking, etc.
- IEC campaigns for awareness generation.
- Counselling of caregivers and families as part of management of the sick child when they are brought to the health worker/health facility.
- *During home visits:* Identification of sickness and focused BCC for improving newborn and child care practices.

16 key family practices identified under four broad heading:

- *The promotion of growth and development of the child:*
  - Exclusive breastfeeding for six months. Good quality complementary foods after six months. Continue breastfeeding for two years or longer.
  - Ensure enough micronutrients—such as vitamin A, iron and zinc—in diet or through supplements.
  - Promote mental and social development by responding to a child's needs for care and by playing, talking and providing a stimulating environment.
- *Disease prevention:*
  - Dispose of all feces safely, wash hands after defecation, before preparing meals and before feeding children.
  - Protect children in malaria endemic areas, by ensuring that they sleep under insecticide—treated bed nets.
  - Provide appropriate care for HIV/AIDS affected people, especially orphans, and take action to prevent further HIV infections.

Flowchart 10.2: Six steps of IMNCI case management process is shown in this algorithm

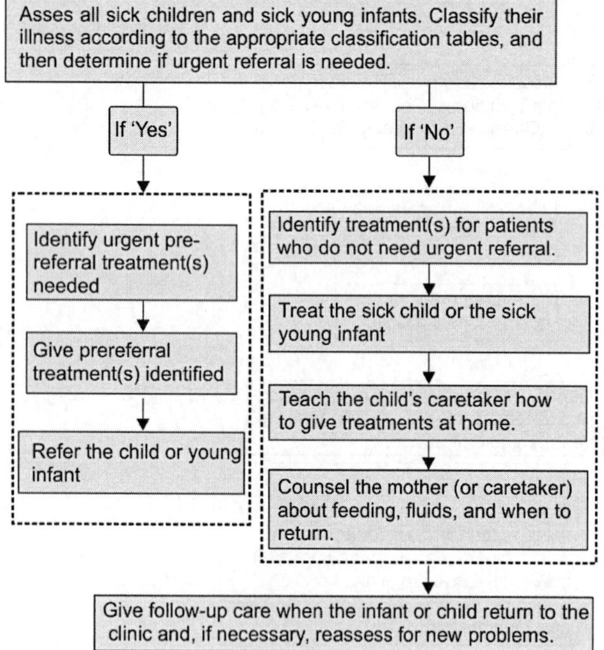

- *Appropriate care at home:*
  - Continue to feed and offer more fluids, including breast milk to children when they are sick.
  - Appropriate home treatment for infections.
  - Protect children from injury and accident and provide treatment when necessary.
  - Prevent child abuse and neglect, and take action when it does occur.
  - Involve fathers in the care of their children and in the reproductive health of the family.
- *Care-seeking outside the home:*
  - Recognize when sick children need treatment outside the home and seek care from appropriate providers.
  - Complete a full course of immunization before first birthday.
  - Follow the health provider's advice on treatment, follow-up and referral.
  - Ensure that every pregnant woman has adequate antenatal care, and seeks care at the time of delivery and afterwards.

Step 6: IMNCI Process

Follow-up Care

At a follow-up visit, the child is assessed whether he/she is improving on the drug or other treatment that was prescribed. Some children need change of antibiotic or antimalarial , and may need to try a second line of drug. The child is referred to the hospital if condition worsens. If the child has a new problem, the IMNCI protocol is used afresh.

CONCLUSION

IMCI, already in place in almost all countries and IMNCI in India, provides a unique opportunity to rapidly scale up newborn health interventions, especially care of serious infections. India has set goals of IMNCI as:

- Standardized case management of (evidence based syndromic approach) sick newborns and children
- Focus on the most common causes of mortality
- Nutrition assessment and counselling for all sick infants and children
- Home care for newborns to (1) promote exclusive breastfeeding; (2) prevent hypothermia; (3) improve illness recognition and timely care seeking.

Strengthening the newborn component of IMCI implemented at the community, first level health facility, and referral levels is likely to contribute to improved newborn survival especially in the difficult and underserved areas of the country. There are several challenges in implementing IMNCI in an effective way to improve newborn survival. In most situations, IMCI has been implemented to include infants and children in health facilities, but is not proactive in reaching children in the community, which is especially detrimental to newborn health. Complementary strategies such as home visits by facility based or community-based health workers to provide routine post natal care may be necessary.

CHAPTER 11

The Child: A Fluid and Electrolyte Alteration

Chapter Outline

- Review of Fluid and Electrolytes in Children
- Overview of Dyselectrolytemias
- Disturbances in Acid-base Status
- Fluid Imbalance
- Maintenance of Fluid and Electrolyte Balance: Nursing Responsibilities

REVIEW OF FLUID AND ELECTROLYTES IN CHILDREN

Body Fluid and Its Composition

Total body weight (TBW) constitutes approximately 75% of the body weight at birth and declines to about 60% from the age of 2 years onwards. TBW is compartmentalized into intracellular fluid (ICF) and extracellular fluid (ECF) (Fig. 11.1).

The extracellular fluid found outside the cell comprises of (i) plasma, (ii) interstitial fluid, (iii) transcellular fluid. The proportion of extracellular water to body weight is about 40% at birth, 25% at 2 years of age and 20% after the age of 7 years.

- *Interstitial fluid:* Fluid surrounding the cell, including lymph fluid.
- *Intravascular fluid:* Fluid contained with the blood vessel (e.g. plasma).
- *Transcellular space:* Cerebral fluid, pericardial, pleural, synovial, sweat, digestive secretions.

ECF is lost first when fluid loss occurs (illness, fever, trauma).

ICF: Intracellular fluid found within the cells, comprising approximately two thirds of the body's fluid in older children and about half of the fluid in the infants.

The distribution of body fluid is determined by the composition of electrolytes and proteins in different fluid compartments.

Electrolytes: In chemistry, an **electrolyte** is any substance containing free ions that make the substance electrically conductive. Electrolytes exist as ions namely cations and anions. The cations are positively charged, i.e. Na^+, K^+, etc. and anions are negatively charged, i.e. Cl^-, hydrogen carbonate HCO_3^- etc. The number of cations in body is equal to the number of anions. Electrolytes commonly exist as solutions of acids, bases or salts.

Electrolytes are minerals in blood and other body fluids that carry an electric charge. Common electrolytes

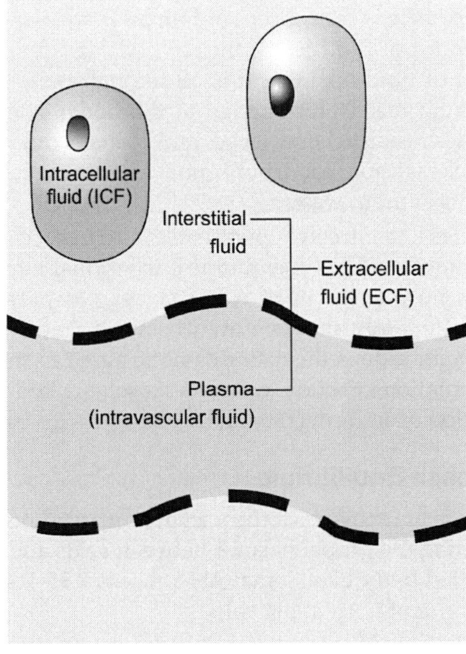

Fig. 11.1: Intracellular and extracellular fluid

include calcium, chloride, magnesium, phosphorus, potassium, sodium.

ECF: ECF has a high concentrations of sodium, chloride and bicarbonate.

ICF: Potassium, magnesium, and phosphate are predominantly intracellular ions.

The concentrations of electrolytes are generally expressed as milliequivalent per liter (mEq/L). Electrolytes affect the amount of water in body, the acidity of blood (pH), muscle function, and other important processes. Man loses electrolytes when he/she sweats. They must replace them by drinking fluids.

Molality and Molarity

Molarity (M) and molality (m) are both measures of concentration of solutions. Molality is the ratio of moles of solute to volume of the solution (number of moles in a kg of solvent) and the other is the ratio of moles of solute to the mass of the solution (number of moles in liter of solution). The osmolality (expressed by mols per kg) of solutions determines the movement of water across an intervening semi-permeable membrane.

It is important to know that despite the differences in compositions each compartment in itself is electroneutral and all compartments have the same osmolality (290 mOsm/kg).

Regulation of Body Water and Electrolytes

Fluid balance is the concept of human homeostasis that the amount of fluid lost from the body is equal to the amount of fluid taken in. It is all the more essential as there is no real water storage in the body: The water man loses needs to be replaced, and humans can survive 4–6 weeks without food, but cannot survive more than a few days without water.

Water is freely permeable across capillary membranes and cell membranes. In normal situations there is no movement of water across compartments, since water only moves down osmotic gradients. As sodium chloride is the major osmotic agent in the ECF, the regulation of body water is closely linked to the regulation of sodium (Flowchart 11.1).

Acid-base Equilibrium

Acid-base homeostasis is the part of human homeostasis concerning the proper balance between acids and bases, also called body pH. Nomal pH value is 7.35–7.45. The importance of normal pH value:

- Maintenance of cellular function (affect cellular metabolism)

Flowchart 11.1: Regulation of water and sodium balance in the body

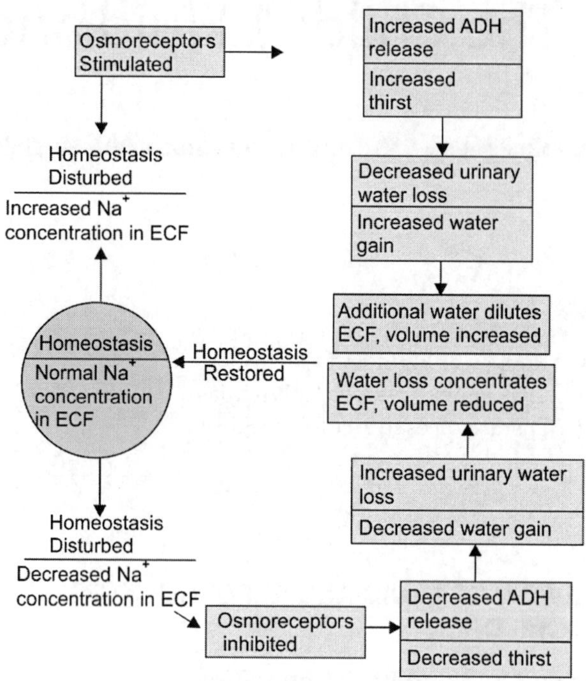

- Enzymatic process-enzymatic activity
- Keep stable neuromuscular membrance potential.

Acidosis: Anormal accumulation of acid or loss of bases from the body, pH value: ≤ 7.35.

Alkalosis: Abnormal accumulation of bicarbonate or loss of acid in the body, pH value: ≤ 7.45.

Buffer System

The body's acid-base balance is normally tightly regulated by buffering agents, the respiratory system, and the renal system, keeping the arterial blood pH between 7.38 and 7.42. Buffer system resist marked changes in [H^+], provided moderate amount of acid or base are added to them.

Compensatory changes by lungs: Remove CO_2 from the blood and to decrease carbonic acid, and thus to raise blood pH.

Acidosis: Respiratory rate and depth will increase, removing CO_2 and raising blood pH.

Alkalosis: Respiratory rate and depth will decrease, thus lowering blood pH.

Compensatory changes by kidneys : Renal compensatory process work more slowly than respiratory mechanism, usually within 1–2 days. It regulates bicarbonate and removes hydrogen ions from the blood.

- *Alkalosis:* Kidney conserve hydrogen ions, thus lower blood pH
- *Acidosis:* Kidneys excrete hydrogen ions and conserve bicarbonate, raising blood pH.

Fluid and Electrolyte Balance: Pediatric Differences (Table 11.1)

In caring for children, especially infants and young children, it is important to be aware that there are some significant differences in their ability to maintain fluid and electrolyte balance. Infants and young children are at greater risk than adults for disturbance in fluid and electrolyte balance due to difference in body position, higher metabolic rate, and immaturity for physiologic regulation systems. Look at the following chart to see what those differences are and their clinical implications.

OVERVIEW OF DYSELECTROLYTEMIAS

Hyponatremia

Hyponatremia, defined as a serum sodium (Na) concentration of less than 135 mEq/L, can lead to hyponatremic encephalopathy, particularly in prepubescent pediatric patients. Classification is traditionally according to volume status:

- Hypovolemic hyponatremia (sodium depletion in excess of water depletion)
- Euvolemic hyponatremia (normal body sodium with increase in total body water)
- Hypervolemic hyponatremia (increase in total body sodium with greater increase in total body water)
- Hyponatremia must also be evaluated with regard to changes in body fluid tonicity (effective osmolality).
- At any volume status, hyponatremia must be further subclassified into the following:
  - Hypotonic hyponatremia, [Na < 135 (130) meg/L]
  - Isotonic hyponatremia [Na (135–145 meg/L)]
  - Hypertonic hyponatremia [Na >145 (150 meg/L)]

Only hypotonic hyponatremia is of clinical significance regarding necessity for treatment and its urgency.

Etiology

Primary sodium deficit with sodium depletion occurs in renal sodium losses in prematurity, fever, malnutrition, decreased sodium intake, burns and wounds, diarrhea, vomiting, nasogastric suction, cystic fibrosis, diabetic ketoacidosis, SIADH **(syndrome of inappropriate antidiuretic hormone secretion,** abnormal water and sodium retention occur in nephritic syndrome, renal failure, cirrhosis of liver, congestive heart failure (CHF).

Table 11.1: Fluid and Electrolyte Balance: Pediatric Differences

Pediatric differences	*Clinical implications*
Immature kidneys—infants and young children are unable to concentrate or dilute urine as well as adults and also unable to conserve or excrete sodium as well.	Infants are more likely to become dehydrated more quickly. In gastroenteritis, their bodies do not conserve fluid well and the loss of intake and increased output produce exaggerated effects. On the other hand, children, who are given an overload of fluid are also unable to compensate well and can easily get into cardiac overload.
Surface area—an infant has a greater surface area to body mass than an adult, therefore insensible loss can be greater. Metabolism is also greater because of the larger mass of active tissue.	Infants with fevers will have greater fluid loss from sweating than older children. During a fever the infant's metabolism will also climb which will increase the fluid loss through the respiratory system. Children are prone to illnesses that involve fluid losses and fevers. Given an already high metabolism, the addition of illness (fever, infection) causes to produce increased wastes via metabolism. The immature kidneys may have difficulty filtering large amounts of wastes.
Total body water—proportionately, infants and small children have greater percentages of body water which is replaced by fat and muscle in the older child/adult. Until about the age of 2, one half of the total body water (TBW) is extracellular.	Infants and children are prone to illnesses that increase water losses.
Intake and output—children take in and excrete a larger amount of fluid proportionately than an older child. Because the daily exchange of ECF is high in the infant, there is little fluid reserve.	Dehydration during vomiting or diarrhea happens quickly because there is a smaller reserve of fluid in the infant.

Signs and Symptoms

Usually do not show signs until sodium reaches 125 mEq/L. Early signs of hyponatremia include the central nervous system (CNS) findings like anorexia, headache, nausea, emesis, restlessness.

Advanced signs include impaired response to verbal stimuli, impaired response to painful stimuli, bizarre behavior, hallucinations, obtundation, incontinence, respiratory insufficiency, seizure activity (Fig. 11.2).

Far-advanced signs include decorticate or decerebrate posturing.

- Altered temperature regulation
- Dilated pupils
- Seizure activity
- Respiratory arrest
- Coma.

Cardiovascular and musculoskeletal findings

- *Cardiovascular:* Hypotension and tachycardia
- *Musculoskeletal:* Weakness and muscular cramps.

Management

Acute severe hyponatremia (i.e. less than 125 mmol/L) usually is associated with neurologic symptoms such as seizures and should be treated urgently because of the high-risk of cerebral edema and hyponatremic encephalopathy. The initial correction rate with hypertonic saline should not exceed 1 to 2 mmol/L per hour. To correct the sodium deficit the fluid needs to administer as 10 mL/kg body weight, at the rate of 1 mL per minute intravenously. Thereafter, calculated extra sodium should be administered slowly in 24 to 48 hours.

In most cases of chronic asymptomatic hyponatremia, removing the underlying cause of the hyponatremia suffices. Otherwise, fluid restriction (less than 1 to 1.5 L per day) is the mainstay of treatment and the preferred mode of treatment for mild to moderate SIADH and to safeguard against pulmonary edema and CHF. The combination of loop diuretics with a high-sodium diet may be required to achieve an adequate response in patients with chronic SIADH.

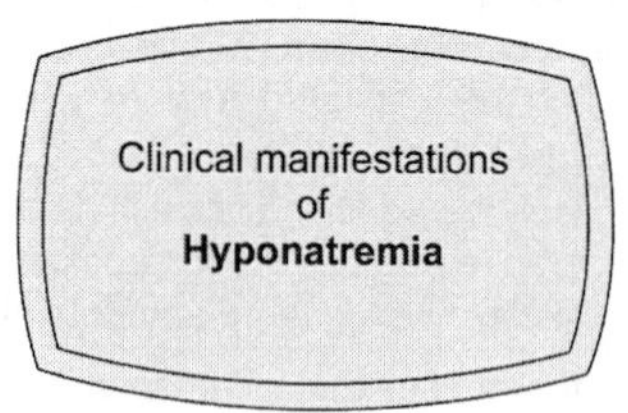

Fig. 11.2: Progressive signs of hyponatremia

Rapid correction of sodium deficit is not suggested in both symptomatic and asymptomatic hyponatremia as it may cause pontine myelinolysis.

Central pontine myelinolysis (CPM) is a neurological disorder that most frequently occurs after too rapid medical correction of sodium deficiency (hyponatremia). The rapid rise in sodium concentration is accompanied by the movement of small molecules and pulls water from brain cells. Through a mechanism that is only partly understood, the shift in water and brain molecules leads to the destruction of myelin, a substance that surrounds and protects nerve fibers. Nerve cells (neurons) can also be damaged. Certain areas of the brain are particularly susceptible to myelinolysis, especially the part of the brainstem called the *pons.*

Hypernatremia

Hypernatremia is defined as a serum sodium concentration of more than 150 mEq/L. It is characterized by a deficit of TBW relative to total body sodium levels due to either loss of free water, or infrequently, the administration of hypertonic sodium. There is hypertonicity of all body fluids, manifested by elevated sodium concentration in the plasma and ECF, and by increased intracellular potassium concentration. Sodium concentrations greater than 155 mEq/L may be life-threatening.

- Wide range of causes, but commonly related to net water loss relative to body sodium content, due to inadequate water intake in the presence of continuing renal or extrarenal free water losses, i.e. renal disease, diuresis, diarrhea, vomiting, burns or excessive sodium intake, diabetes insipidus.
- Symptoms include intense thirst, anorexia, restlessness, nausea, and vomiting, dry and sticky mucus membrane, flushed skin, oliguria followed by progressive alteration in mental status, from initial lethargy or irritability to stupor or coma. Physical findings may underestimate the degree of dehydration. It can be associated with hydration, i.e. normal hydration, dehydration and over hydration status (Figs 11.3A and B).

Diagnosis: The diagnosis is established by measuring serum sodium.

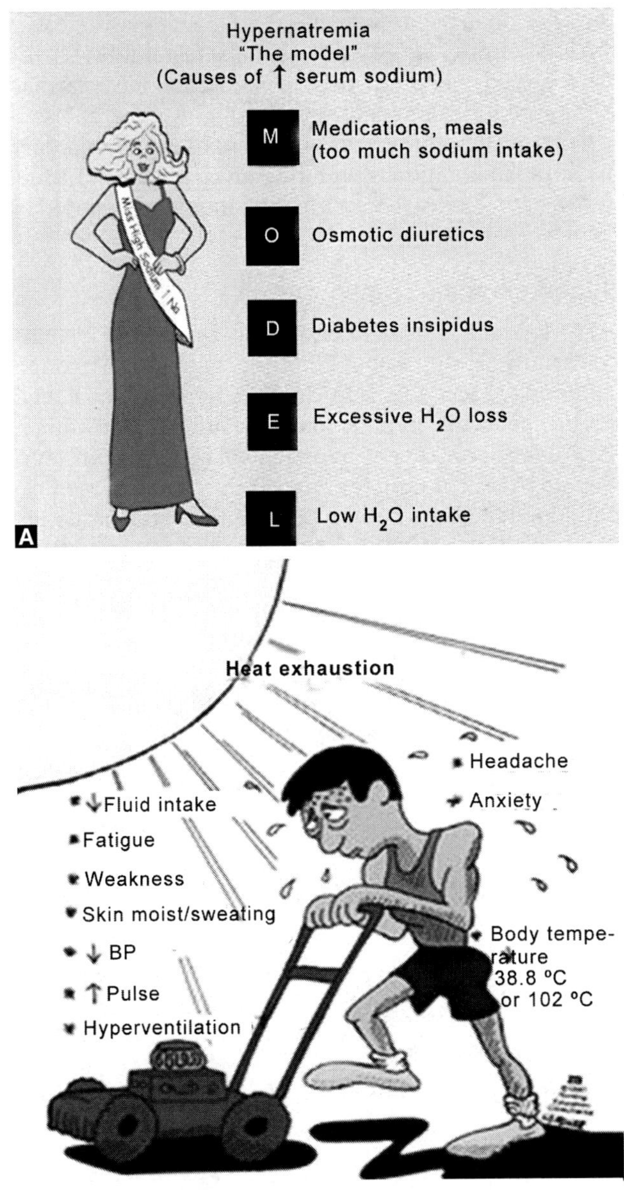

Figs 11.3A and B: **A.** Hypernatremia: etiology; **B.** Hypernatremia: manifestations

Management

The patient is stabilized by correcting volume deficits with isotonic or hypotonic saline. Patients with an increase in total body sodium may require 5% dextrose, with or without furosemide. Those with hypothalamic diabetes insipidus may require desmopressin.

In correcting hypernatremia, do not rapidly decrease the sodium level because a rapid decline in the serum sodium concentration can cause cerebral edema. The recommended rate of sodium correction is 0.5 mEq/h or as much as 10–12 mEq/L in 24 hours. Dehydration should be corrected over 48–72 hours. If the serum sodium concentration is more than 200 mEq/L, peritoneal dialysis should be performed using a high-glucose, low-sodium dialysate.

The selection of intravenous fluid is based on the following:

- If the patient is hypotensive, normal saline (lactated ringer solution, or 5% albumin solution) should be used regardless of a high serum sodium concentration.
- In hypernatremic dehydration, 0.45% or 0.2% NaCl should be used as a replacement fluid to prevent excessive delivery of free water and a too rapid decrease in the serum sodium concentration.
- In cases of hypernatremia caused by sodium overload, sodium-free intravenous fluid (e.g. 5% dextrose in water) may be used, and a loop diuretic may be added.
- The serum sodium concentration should be monitored frequently to avoid too rapid correction of hypernatremia.
- In cases of associated hyperglycemia, 2.5% dextrose solution may be given. Insulin treatment is not recommended because the acute decrease in glucose, which lowers plasma osmolality, may precipitate cerebral edema.
- Once the child is urinating, add 40 mEq/L KCl to fluids to aid water absorption into cells.
- Calcium may be added if the patient has an associated low serum calcium level.
- Serum sodium levels should be monitored every 4 hours.

Hypokalemia

Hypokalemia refers to the condition in which the concentration of potassium (K^+) in the blood is less than 3.5 mEq/L. Normal plasma potassium levels are between 3.5 to 5.0 mEq/L, about 98% of the body's potassium is found inside cells, with the remainder in the extracellular fluid including the blood.

Causes of hypokalemia may be one or more like inadequate potassium intake, gastrointestinal or integument potassium loss (diarrhea, vomiting, perspiration, nasogastric tube), stress, starvation, malabsorption. Hypokalemia may occur due to administration of IV fluid without added potassium, diuretic drugs (especially furosemide, ethacrynic acid, thiazide), corticosteroids, etc.

Clinical Presentation

Mild hypokalemia is often without symptoms, although it may cause a small elevation of blood pressure, and can occasionally provoke cardiac arrhythmias. Besides that muscle weakness, paralysis, leg cramp, decreased bowel sound, ileus, weak and irregular pulse, tachycardia, bradycardia, cardiac arrhythmias, hypotension, irritability, fatigue may occur due to low potassium level in the body (Fig. 11.4). Hypokalemia affects the bioelectric processes including nerve conduction, myocardial pacing, and muscle contraction.

Management

- The most important treatment in severe hypokalemia is addressing the cause, such as improving the diet, treating diarrhea or stopping an offending medication, as treatment of hypokalemia carries with it a significant risk of iatrogenic hyperkalemia.
- Transient, asymptomatic, or mild hypokalemia may spontaneously resolve or may be treated with enteral potassium supplements.
- Symptomatic or severe hypokalemia should be corrected with a solution of intravenous potassium.
- Patients without a significant source of potassium loss and who show no symptoms of hypokalemia may not require treatment.
- Mild hypokalemia (>3.0 mEq/L) may be treated with oral potassium chloride supplements. As this is often part of a poor nutritional intake, potassium-containing foods may be recommended, such as leafy green vegetables, tomatoes, coconut water, citrus fruits, oranges or bananas. Both dietary and pharmaceutical supplements are used for people taking diuretic medications.
- Severe hypokalemia (<3.0 mEq/L) may require intravenous (IV) supplementation. Typically, a saline solution is used, with 20–40 mEq KCl per liter over 3–4 hours. Giving IV potassium at faster rates (20–25 mEq/hr) may predispose to ventricular tachycardias and requires intensive monitoring. A generally safe rate is 10 mEq/hr. Even in severe hypokalemia, oral supplementation is preferred given its safety profile. Sustained release formulations should be avoided in acute settings.

Hyperkalemia

Hyperkalemia is usually defined as a serum or plasma potassium greater than 5.5 mEq/L (mmol/L). Although children are less likely to develop hyperkalemia than adults, pediatric hyperkalemia is not an uncommon occurrence, and severe hyperkalemia (potassium level greater than 7 mEq/L [mmol/L]) is a serious medical problem that needs immediate attention. Hyperkalemia is classified as mild (K 5.5–6.0), moderate (K 6.1–6.9) or severe (K >7.0).

Releasing too much potassium from cells to ECF can result from hemolysis, rhabdomyolysis (break down of muscle tissue), burns, trauma, other tissue injury, uncontrolled diabetes, acidosis, hemorrhage.

It may be precipitated due to increased intake of potassium (i.e. salt substitutes), decreased urine output, kidney failure, severe dehydration, too rapid IV administration of potassium.

Clinical Presentation

Symptoms of hyperkalemia can include irritability, anxiety, twitching, hyper-reflexia, abnormal heart rhythm—arrhythmia (that can be life-threatening), slow heart rate, weakness, flaccid paralysis bradycardia, apnea, respiratory arrest (Fig. 11.5).

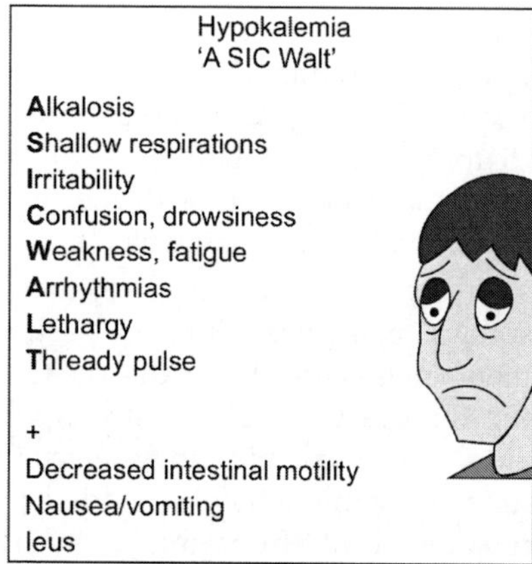

Fig. 11.4: Hypokalemia

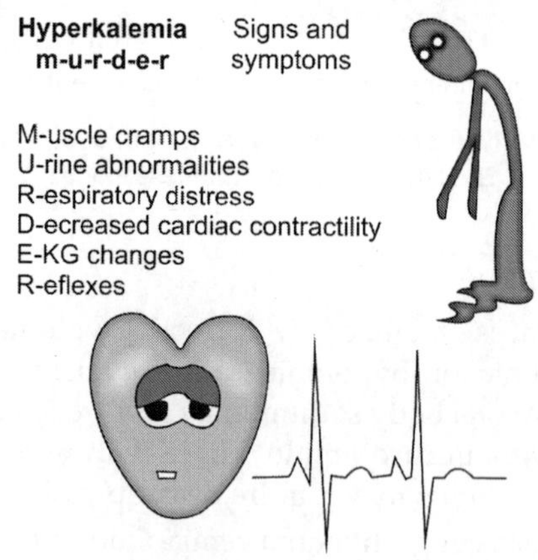

Fig. 11.5: Hyperkalemia

Potassium and homeostasis

The body needs a delicate balance of **Potassium** for the normal functioning of the muscles, heart, and nerves. It plays an important role in controlling activity of smooth muscle (such as the muscle found in the digestive tract) and skeletal muscle (muscles of the extremities and torso), as well as the muscles of the heart. It is also important for normal transmission of electrical signals throughout the nervous system within the body to help the heart and other muscles work properly. The potassium gradient is critically important for many physiological processes, including maintenance of cellular membrane potential, homeostasis of cell volume, and transmission of action potentials in nerve cells, etc. But too much potassium in blood can lead to dangerous and possibly deadly changes in heart rhythm.

Normal blood levels of potassium are critical for maintaining normal heart electrical rhythm. Both low blood potassium levels (hypokalemia) and high blood potassium levels (hyperkalemia) can lead to abnormal heart rhythms. The most important clinical effect of hyperkalemia is related to electrical rhythm of the heart. While mild hyperkalemia probably has a limited effect on the heart, moderate hyperkalemia can produce ECG changes, and severe hyperkalemia can cause suppression of electrical activity of the heart and can cause the heart to stop beating.

Hyperkalemia is diagnosed by laboratory testing of blood. If hyperkalemia is suspected, an electrocardiogram is often performed, since the ECG may show changes typical for hyperkalemia in moderate to severe cases. The ECG will also be able to identify cardiac arrhythmias that result from hyperkalemia. Generally, blood tests for renal function (creatinine, blood urea nitrogen), glucose and occasionally creatine kinase and cortisol are done. Calculating the transtubular potassium gradient can sometimes help in distinguishing the cause of the hyperkalemia.

Management

The definitive management of severe hyperkalemia is hemodialysis which are the most rapid methods of removing potassium from the body. These are typically used if the underlying cause cannot be corrected swiftly while temporizing measures are instituted or there is no response to these measures. Dialysis recommended, particularly if other measures have failed or if renal failure is present.

Several medical treatments shift potassium ions from the bloodstream into the cellular compartment, thereby reducing the risk of complications. The effect of these measures tends to be short-lived, but may temporize the problem until potassium can be removed from the body.

Treatment of hyperkalemia may include any of the following measures, either singly or in combination:

- A diet low in potassium (for mild cases).
- Discontinue medications that increase blood potassium levels.
- Intravenous administration of glucose and insulin, which promotes movement of potassium from the extracellular space back into the cells. Insulin (e.g. intravenous injection of 10–15 units of regular insulin along with 50 mL of 50% dextrose to prevent hypoglycemia) will lead to a shift of potassium ions into cells. Its effects last a few hours, so it sometimes needs to be repeated while other measures are taken to suppress potassium levels more permanently. The insulin is usually given with an appropriate amount of glucose in order to prevent hypoglycemia following the insulin administration.
- Salbutamol (albuterol, ventolin), a β_2-selective catecholamine, is administered by nebulizer (e.g. 10–20 mg). This drug also lowers blood levels of K^+ by promoting its movement into cells.
- Though previously recommended, IV bicarbonate as a method to shift potassium into cells is no longer recommended. Not only has it been effective in controlled trials but it lowers ionized calcium levels, theoretically increasing the risk of cardiac arrhythmia.
- Intravenous calcium to temporarily protect the heart and muscles from the effects of hyperkalemia.
- Diuretic administration to decrease the total potassium stores through increasing potassium excretion in the urine. It is important to note that most diuretics increase kidney excretion of potassium. Only the potassium-sparing diuretics mentioned above to decrease kidney excretion of potassium.
- Medications known as cation-exchange resins, which bind potassium and lead to its excretion via the gastrointestinal tract.

Treatment of hyperkalemia naturally also includes treatment of any underlying causes (for example, kidney disease, adrenal disease, tissue destruction) of hyperkalemia.

Hypocalcemia

Calcium in the blood exists in three primary states: Bound to proteins (mainly albumin), bound to anions such as phosphate and citrate, and as free (unbound) ionized calcium. Only the ionized calcium is physiologically active. Normal blood calcium level is between 8.5 to 10.5 mg/dL (2.12 to 2.62 mmol/L) and that of ionized calcium is 4.65 to 5.25 mg/dL (1.16 to 1.31 mmol/L). Calcium is necessary to keep bones strong and to help them grow or heal.

Hypocalcemia is the term for an abnormally low level of calcium in the body (calcium <8.5 mg/dL, ionized <4.5 mg/dL). Hypocalcemia may be the result of low calcium production or insufficient calcium circulation in the body. A deficiency of magnesium or vitamin D is linked to most cases of hypocalcemia.

Common causes of hypocalcemia include inadequate intake of calcium, hypoparathyroidism, vitamin D deficiency, and chronic kidney disease, calcium losses, i.e. infection and burns, alkalosis, administration of diuretics, inadequate exposure to sun.

Symptoms of hypocalcemia include neuromuscular irritability (including muscles cramp, tetany as manifested by Chvostek's sign or Trousseau's sign, bronchospasm, laryngospasm), electrocardiographic changes, seizures, hypotension and cardiac arrest.

Management

Treatment is dependent upon the cause, but most commonly includes supplementation of calcium and some form of vitamin D or its analogues.

Intravenous calcium gluconate 10% can be administered, or if the hypocalcemia is severe, calcium chloride is given instead. This is only appropriate if the hypocalcemia is acute and has occurred over a relatively short time frame. But if the hypocalcemia has been severe and chronic, then this regimen can be fatal, because there is a degree of acclimatization that occurs. The neuromuscular excitability, cardiac electrical instability, and associated symptoms are then not cured or relieved by prompt administration of corrective doses of calcium, but rather exacerbated. Such rapid administration of calcium would result in effective over correction—symptoms of hypercalcemia would follow.

Primary Prevention

- Child's diet should be sufficient in fat-soluble vitamins (including D) and dietary calcium
- Child should get a moderate amount of sun exposure to maintain appropriate vitamin D hydroxylation in the skin.

Hypercalcemia

Calcium is a mineral that is important in the regulation and processes of many body functions including bone formation, hormone release, muscle contraction, and nerve and brain function. Hypercalcemia is the term that refers to elevated levels of calcium in the bloodstream (calcium >11.0 mg/dL, ionized calcium 5.5 mg/dL).

Causes: One of the most common causes of hypercalcemia is hyperparathyroidism. Other causes may be transient neonatal hyperparathyroidism, vitamin D excess, William's syndrome, thyrotoxicosis, prolonged immobilization, hypoproteinemia, acidosis, milk-alkali syndrome, renal disease, etc.

The signs and symptoms of hypercalcemia can be remembered by the phrase 'moans, stones, groans, and bones.'

- Stones (renal or biliary)
- Bones (bone pain), bony changes especially in parathyroid disorder
- Groans (abdominal pain, nausea and vomiting)
- Thrones (polyuria)
- Psychiatric overtones (Depression 30–40%, anxiety, cognitive dysfunction, insomnia, coma). It is extremely rare (calcium >15 mg/dL)
- Other symptoms can include fatigue, anorexia, thirst, itching and pancreatitis.

Management

Treatment depends on the underlying cause of hypercalcemia as well as the degree of severity and prognosis depends on the underlying cause of hypercalcemia. The initial therapy is fluids and diuretics.

- Hydration, increasing salt intake, and forced diuresis.
- Hydration is needed because many patients are dehydrated due to vomiting or renal defects in concentrating urine.
- Increased salt intake also can increase body fluid volume as well as increasing urine sodium excretion which further increases urinary calcium excretion (In other words, calcium and sodium (salt) are handled in a similar way by the kidney.
- Large volume intravenous salt and water replacement while minimizing the risk of blood volume overload and pulmonary edema. In addition, loop diuretics tend to depress renal calcium reabsorption thereby helping to lower blood calcium levels.
- Can usually decrease serum calcium by 1–3 mg/dL within 24 hour.
- Caution must be taken to prevent potassium or magnesium depletion.

DISTURBANCES IN ACID-BASE STATUS

When body fluids contain too much acid, this is known as acidosis. Acidosis occurs when kidneys and lungs cannot keep body's pH in balance.

There are two types of acidosis—metabolic and respiratory. Metabolic acidosis occurs when kidneys cannot get rid of acid buildup or when body gets rid of too much base. Bases neutralize acids, and vice versa.

Respiratory acidosis occurs when lungs do not properly eliminate the carbon dioxide (CO_2). When CO_2 builds up in blood, it becomes more acidic (Table 11.2).

Respiratory Acidosis

Respiratory acidosis (low pH of body fluid) is characterized when too much CO_2 builds up in the body. Normally the lungs remove CO_2 while man breathes. However, sometimes body cannot get rid of enough CO_2. This may happen because of:

- Pulmonary diseases with alveolar hypoventilation, like asthma, pneumothorax
- Injury to the chest, deformed chest structure
- Obesity, which can make breathing difficult
- Muscle weakness in the chest
- Problems with the nervous system.

Clinical Manifestation

The manifestations of hypercapnia are not always obvious, unless it is severe. Clinical manifestations include increasing heart rate, arrhythmias with hypotension, increasing rate and depth of respiration and forceful use of accessory muscles with retraction and cyanosis, flushed skin, muscular tremor, etc. The child usually presents with headache, irritability, restlessness, depression due to rise of intracranial pressure.

Management

Respiratory acidosis is best treated by correction of underlying disease and correction of ventilation problem by the use of oxygen, intubation, mechanical ventilation. Tight fitting oxygen mask and head box may precipitate dangerous elevation of pCO_2.

Metabolic Acidosis

Metabolic acidosis is defined as an arterial blood pH <7.35 with plasma bicarbonate <22 mmol/L.

It starts in the kidneys instead of the lungs. Metabolic acidosis may result from increased production of metabolic acids or disturbances in the ability to excrete acid via the kidneys. Renal acidosis is associated with an accumulation of urea and creatinine as well as metabolic acid residues of protein catabolism.

Mild metabolic acidosis is characterized by nausea, vomiting, headache and abdominal pain. The clinical features of chronic acidosis are anorexia, lethargy and fatigue. Patients with acute metabolic acidosis (pH is below 7.2) have deep and rapid breathing (Kussmaul breathing). Severe acidosis may cause confusion, drowsiness, muscles weakness and flaccidity, myocardial depression and shock.

There are three major forms of metabolic acidosis:

- Diabetic acidosis occurs in people with poorly managed diabetes. Ketones build up in the body and acidify the blood.
- Hyperchloremic acidosis results from a loss of sodium bicarbonate. This base helps to keep the blood neutral. Both diarrhea and vomiting can cause this type of acidosis.
- Lactic acidosis as seen in hypoperfusion, hypoxia, septicemia. Even prolonged exercise can lead to lactic acid build-up.

Other factors that can contribute to risk of metabolic acidosis include:

- Eating a high-fat, low-carbohydrate diet
- Kidney failure
- Dehydration
- Aspirin or methanol poisoning.

Diagnosis

Early diagnosis can make a big difference in recovery of acidosis.

An arterial blood gas analysis gives the picture of oxygen and carbon dioxide level in blood. It also reveals blood pH. A series of blood tests give the status of kidney functioning and pH balance and it also measures calcium, protein, blood sugar, and electrolyte levels. Taken together, these tests can identify the different types of acidosis.

If it is diagnosed with respiratory acidosis, this may involve a chest X-ray or a pulmonary function test.

Urine testing is important if metabolic acidosis is suspected. To check the pH and kidney functioning (properly eliminating acids and bases or not) is important. Additional tests may be needed to determine the cause of acidosis.

Management

Patients with metabolic acidosis are often very ill and prone to rapid deterioration. Quick history taking of the child and assessment (physical and laboratory) are important. In mild and moderate cases, correction of acidosis is usually not recommended. Treatment of underlying condition improves acidosis. Severe acidosis requires urgent measures like:

- Shifting the patient in the resuscitation area, or to transfer to a high-dependency area as soon as feasible and to place him on an ECG monitor, SaO_2 monitor and BP/HR monitor.
- In patients who are clinically unwell and have deteriorating SaO_2 levels or conscious levels, intubation and assisted ventilation is to be considered.
- A central venous line may be needed for aggressive rehydration.
- Consider catheterization to monitor urine output and obtain urine for analysis.
- If there is any possibility of drug or toxin ingestion, initial therapies should be started such as activated charcoal/chelating agents/emetics, dependent on the specific compound ingested and latest local guidelines for poisoning.
- Liaise with local or national toxicology/poisoning services if there has been ingestion of a potentially dangerous substance.

Correction of Acidosis

Treatment of the underlying cause is the aim. Empirical therapy with bicarbonate is not recommended as it can lead to a fatal outcome. Bicarbonate therapy has a role only when the pH is less than 7.25 because pH in this range causes myocardial depression and hypotension. The therapy consists of $NaHCO_3$, K^+ replacement and mechanical ventilation as indicated. Half of the calculated sodium bicarbonate with proper dilution (with at least equal volume of distil water may be administered immediately and other half is given in next 12 to 24 hours in slow drip.

THAM (trihydroxymethyl aminomethadone), the alkalinizing agent may be used to correct acidosis where use of sodium bicarbonate is considered hazardous. This drug rapidly increases pH of body fluids and tissues including CNS and transiently lower pCO_2.

Respiratory Alkalosis

High pH is characterized by a decreased pCO_2, primarily due to hyperventilation in case of assisted ventilation and hyperventilation from CNS stimulation such as emotions, fear, pain, hysteria, salicylate poisoning. Compensatory renal responses lead to increased excretion and decreased serum bicarbonate level.

Respiratory alkalosis may be caused due to decreased lung compliance and hypoxemia from conditions such as pulmonary edema, CHF, pneumonia, asthma, pulmonary emboli.

Clinical manifestations of the condition include light headedness, dizziness, paresthesias and diaphoresis. In severe cases numbness, tetany, convulsions and arrhythmias (changes in ST-T wave) may be present.

Management should be directed at the underlying disorder. Mild to moderate respiratory alkalosis usually does not require specific treatment. If condition is severe, mechanical ventilation may be started.

Metabolic Alkalosis

Metabolic alkalosis is a metabolic condition in which the pH of tissue is elevated beyond the normal range (7.35–7.45). This is the result of decreased hydrogen ion concentration, leading to increased bicarbonate, or alternatively a direct result of increased bicarbonate concentrations.

Mild metabolic alkalosis has no signs and symptoms. Severe type causes decreased respiratory rate and depth, increased heart rate, arrhythmias, muscles weakness, change in level of consciousness from apathy and confusion to stupor. Metabolic alkalosis is further classified into two variants; chloride responsive and chloride resistant. Chloride responsive alkalosis is associated with volume depletion related conditions such as vomiting, pyloric stenosis, gastric drainage and diuretics.

Management

Along with the treatment of underlying disease, chloride correction is given with NaCl and KCl in fluid. Along with isotonic saline solution, an H_2 receptor antagonist to decrease gastric hydrochloric acid, acidifying agents, and potassium sparing diuretics may be used.

In chloride resistant type, mild cases respond to sodium chloride restriction, spirolactone therapy and potassium supplements. Very rarely, in severe refractory cases of metabolic alkalosis ($pH > 7.5$), does one need to infuse dilute hydrochloric acid or ammonium chloride.

FLUID IMBALANCE

Dehydration is the excessive loss of body water which accompany disruption of metabolic processes. Dehydration occurs when water loss in the body exceeds the water intake. Most people can tolerate less than three percent decrease in body water without difficulty. A 5 to 8% decrease can cause fatigue and dizziness. Over 10% can cause physical and mental deterioration, accompanied by severe thirst. A decrease more than 15 to 25% of the body water is invariably fatal. Dehydration of skin and mucous membranes can be called medical dryness.

Table 11.2: Laboratory values: Acid-base disturbances

Test	*Respiratory acidosis*	*Metabolic acidosis*	*Respiratory alkalosis*	*Metabolic alkalosis*
ABG; pH	< 7.35	< 7.35	> 7.45	> 7.45
$PaCO_2$ (mm Hg)	> 45	< 40	< 35	> 45
PaO_2 (mm Hg)	Decreased	WNL or slightly decreased	Decreased	Decreased
HCO_3 (mEq/L)	WNL or slightly increased	< 22	Decreased	>26
K^+ (mEq/L)	WNL	< 4.0	Slightly decreased	Decreased
Na^+ (mEq/L)	WNL	Varies according to condition	do -	do -
Cl^- (mEq/L)	WNL	Usually increased	do -	do -

Abbreviations: ABG = arterial blood gas; WNL = within normal limit; PaO_2 = partial pressure of oxygen in arterial blood; $PaCO_2$ = partial pressure of carbon dioxide in arterial blood

Estimated percentage dehydration	*Physical examination findings*
< 5	History of fluid loss but no findings on physical examination
5	Dry oral mucous membranes but no panting or pathological tachycardia
7	Mild to moderate decreased skin turgor, dry oral mucous membranes, slight tachycardia, and normal pulse pressure.
10	Moderate to marked degree of decreased skin turgor, dry oral mucous membranes, tachycardia, and decreased pulse pressure.
12	Marked loss of skin turgor, dry oral mucous membranes, and significant signs of shock.

Water goes out of the body in many ways, and they can be categorized into either 'sensible' water loss or 'insensible' water loss. Human body loses water in following ways (Table 11.3):

- Through the respiratory tract (by breathing)
- Through the gastrointestinal tract (feces)
- Through the skin (perspiration and sweating)
- Through the kidneys (urine excretion).

Dehydration produces both fluid and electrolyte deficiencies. It is one of the most common causes of hospitalization in infants and children. According to the status of serum sodium concentration dehydration is classified as isonatremic, hyponatremic and hypernatremic.

Table 11.3: Average water loss from human body	
Kidneys	1.5 L
Respiratory tract	0.4 L
Gastrointestinal tract	0.2 L
Skin	0.5 L
Total	**2.6 L**

Pathophysiology of Dehydration

The decrease in total body water causes reductions in both the intracellular and extracellular fluid volumes. All types of lost fluid contain electrolytes in varying concentrations, so fluid loss is always accompanied by some degree of electrolyte loss. The exact amount and type of electrolyte loss varies depending on the cause (e.g. significant amounts of HCO_3^- may be lost with diarrhea but not with vomiting). However, fluid lost always contains a lower concentration of Na than the plasma. Thus, in the absence of any fluid replacement, serum Na rises (hypernatremia). Hypernatremia causes water to shift from the intracellular and interstitial space into the intravascular space, helping, at least temporarily, to maintain vascular volume. With hypotonic fluid replacement (e.g. with plain water), serum Na may normalize but can also decrease (hyponatremia). Hyponatremia results in some fluid shifting out of the intravascular space into the interstitial space at the expense of vascular volume.

Young children are more susceptible to dehydration due to larger body water content, renal immaturity, and inability to meet their own needs independently. Older children show signs of dehydration sooner than infants due to lower levels of extracellular fluid (ECF). Clinical manifestations of dehydration are most closely related to intravascular volume depletion. As dehydration progresses, hypovolemic shock ultimately ensues, resulting in end organ failure and death.

Causes of Dehydration

- *Diarrhea and vomiting:* Diarrhea is the most common reason for a person to lose excess amounts of water. A significant amount of water can be lost with each bowel movement. Worldwide, more than four million children die each year because of dehydration from diarrhea. Severe, acute diarrhea—that is, diarrhea that comes on suddenly and violently—can cause a tremendous loss of water and electrolytes in a short amount of time. Vomiting along with diarrhea means more fluids and minerals loss. Children and infants are especially at risk. Diarrhea may be caused by a bacterial or viral infection, food sensitivity, a reaction to medications or a bowel disorder.

Table 11.4: Types of dehydration

Isotonic dehydration Na (135–145 meg/L)	*Hyponatremic dehydration* Na < 135 (130) meg/L	*Hypernatremic dehydration* Na >145 (150 meg/L)
Etiology—diarrhea, vomiting, low fluid intake with increased exercises	*Etiology*—diuretics, hyperglycemia, nephritis, adrenal insufficiency and other losses like vomiting, diarrhea, burns, SIADH, CHF	*Etiology*—diuretics, diabetes incipidus, adrenal insufficiency and other losses like vomiting, diarrhea
Clinical manifestations	*Clinical manifestations*	*Clinical manifestations*
Skin Color—gray Temperature—cold Turgor—poor, feel dry Mucous membranes—dry Tearing and salivation—absent Eyeball—sunken Fontanel—sunken Body temperature—subnormal elevated Pulse—rapid Respirations—rapid Behavior—irritable to lethargic	Skin Color—gray Temperature—cold Turgor—very poor Feel—clammy Mucous membrane—slightly moist Tearing and salivation—absent Eyeball—sunken Fontanel—sunken Temperature—subnormal or elevated Pulse—very rapid Respirations—rapid Behavior—lethargic, comatose, convulsions	Skin Color—gray Temperature—cold or hot Turgor—fair, feel thickened Mucous membranes—parched Tearing and salivation—absent Eyeball—sunken Fontanel—sunken Body temperature—sub-normal or elevated Pulse—moderately rapid Respirations—rapid Behavior—marked lethargy

- *Vomiting:* Vomiting can also be a cause of fluid loss. Not only can an individual lose fluid in the vomitus, but it may be difficult to replace water by drinking because of that same nausea and vomiting.
- *Fever:* In general, higher the fever, the more dehydration may occur. If the child has a fever in addition to diarrhea and vomiting, he/she may lose even more fluids.
- *Excessive sweating:* Sweating causes loss of water. If somebody does vigorous activity and does not replace fluids as he goes along, he can become dehydrated. Hot, humid weather increases the amount of sweat and the amount of fluid losses. Man can also become dehydrated in winter if he does not replace lost fluids. Preteens and teens who participate in sports may be especially susceptible, both because of their body weight, which is generally lower than that of adults, and because they may not be experienced enough to know the warning signs of dehydration.

  The body can lose significant amounts of water in the form of sweat when it tries to cool itself. Whether the body temperature is increased because of working or exercising in a hot environment or because a fever is present due to an infection; the body uses water in the form of sweat to cool itself.
- *Inability to drink fluids:* The inability to drink adequately is the other potential cause of dehydration. Whether it is the lack of availability of water, intense nausea with or without vomiting, or the lack of strength to drink, this, coupled with routine or extraordinary water losses can compound the degree of dehydration.

'Dehydration', is a term that has loosely been used to mean loss of water, regardless of whether it is as water and solutes (mainly sodium) or free water. In children, the most commonly seen type of dehydration by far is isotonic (isonatremic) dehydration (sodium level 138–145 mEq/L), but this effectively refers to hypovolemia. In hyponatremic dehydration, the electrolyte loss is greater than water loss (serum level is less than 135 mEq/L). In hypernatremic dehydration, the water loss is greater than the electrolyte (serum sodium concentration is more than 150 mEq/L) (Table 11.4).

Those who refer to hypotonic dehydration therefore refer to solute loss and thus loss of intravascular volume but in the presence of exaggerated intravascular volume depletion for a given amount of total body water gain. It is true that neurological complications can occur in hypotonic and hypertonic states. The former can lead to seizures, while the latter can lead to osmotic cerebral edema upon rapid rehydration. It is thus important to distinguish 'dehydration' from 'hypovolemia' and maybe limit the term 'dehydration' to states of 'hypernatremia' and call all other usage 'hypovolemia' as that would greatly facilitate management.

Dehydration in Children

Millions of children die worldwide each year because of dehydration, often because of diarrhea. As well, the temperature regulation and sweat mechanism of infants are not well developed, and this increases their risk of heat related illness. Dehydration occurs because there is too much water lost, not enough water taken in, or most commonly, a combination of the two. It is important to remember that infants and children are dependent upon others to provide them with water and nutrition. Infants cannot tell their parents or care providers when they are thirsty. Moreover, dehydration in sick children is often a combination of refusing to eat or drink anything and losing fluid from the body. Enough fluid needs to be provided so that the dehydration can be prevented. This is especially true if increased water loss occurs because of fever, vomiting or diarrhea. Infants and children are more likely to become dehydrated than adults because they weigh less and their bodies turn over water and electrolytes more quickly.

Therapeutic Management of Dehydration

Fluid and Electrolyte Therapy

Oral Rehydration Therapy (ORT) for mild or moderate dehydration:

- Mild or moderate dehydration can usually be treated very effectively with ORT.
- Vomiting is generally not a contraindication to ORT. If evidence of bowel obstruction, ileus, or acute abdomen is noted, then intravenous rehydration is indicated.
- Dehydration correction starts with calculation of fluid deficit. Physical findings consistent with mild dehydration suggest a fluid deficit of 5% of body weight in infants and 3% in children. Moderate dehydration occurs with a fluid deficit of 5–10% in infants and 3–6% in children. The fluid deficit should be replaced over 4 hours.
- The oral rehydration solution should be administered in small volumes very frequently to minimize gastric distention and reflex vomiting. Generally, 5 mL of oral rehydration solution every minute is well tolerated. Hourly intake and output should be recorded by the caregiver. As the child becomes rehydrated, vomiting often decreases and larger fluid volumes may be used.
- If vomiting persists, infusion of oral rehydration solution via a nasogastric tube may be temporarily used to achieve rehydration. Intravenous fluid administration (20–30 mL/kg of isotonic sodium chloride 0.9% solution over 1–2 hour) may also be used until oral rehydration is tolerated.
- Replace ongoing losses from stools and emesis (estimate volume and replace) in addition to replacing the calculated fluid deficit.

An age appropriate diet may be started as soon as the child is able to tolerate oral intake.

Severe Dehydration

Laboratory evaluation and intravenous rehydration are required in severe dehydration. The underlying cause of the dehydration must be determined and appropriately treated. Primary focus of IV fluid replacement therapy is to provide for a child's maintenance and deficit fluid needs. Fluid and electrolyte therapy is divided in three phases.

Maintenance fluid needs—it is met by replacing fluids and electrolytes lost through normal body processes (for example, metabolism and respiration).

Deficit fluid needs—it is met by replacing fluids and electrolytes lost before therapy started.

Correction of ongoing losses—additional fluid may be needed to replace abnormal losses that continue during therapy (persistent vomiting, diarrhea, on nasogastric tube drainage). Severe dehydration by clinical examination suggests a fluid deficit of 10–15% of body weight in infants and 6–9% of body weight in older children. The daily maintenance fluid is added to the fluid deficit. In general, the recommended administration is one half of this volume administered over 8 hours and administration of the remainder over the following 16 hours. Continued losses (e.g. emesis, diarrhea) must be promptly replaced.

Application: Daily fluid maintenance formula is used in calculating 24 hours fluid requirement of sick child. Then determine the amount of fluid (in milliliter) each child needs per hour.

(i) Piu, age 10 years, kilogram weight = 32.7 kg
Fluid maintenance needed per 24 hours ______.
Fluid maintenance needed per hour ______.

(ii) Sona, age 2 years, kilogram weight = 11.8 kg
Fluid maintenance needed per 24 hours ______.
Fluid maintenance needed per hour ______.

(iii) Sama, age 4 weeks, kilogram weight = 3.6 kg
Fluid maintenance needed per 24 hours ______.
Fluid maintenance needed per hour ______.

(iv) Sabnam, age 7 years, kilogram weight = 22 kg
Fluid maintenance needed per 24 hours ______.
Fluid maintenance needed per hour ______.

Table 11.5: Scale: Fluid maintenance requirements

Body weight	*Fluid and Electrolyte needs/24 hours*	*By body surface area per 24 hours*
New born (0–72 hours)	60–100 mL/kg	
0–10 kg	100 mL/kg	150 mL/m² (range 1200–1800 mL)
11–20 kg	1000 mL + 50 mL/kg > 10 kg	
> 20 kg	1500 mL + 20 mL/kg > 20 kg	
Sodium	3–4 mEq/kg/day	40–60 mEq/m²
Potassium	2–3 mEq/kg/day	30–40 mEq/m²
Chloride	3-4 mEq/kg/day	

Application Answers

All answers below are based on the (Table 11.5: Scale: Daily maintenance fluid needs)

(i) 1500 mL + (20 mL/kg × 12.7 kg) = 1754 mL per 24 hours. 1754 mL/24 hours = 73 mL per hour.

(ii) 1000 mL + (50 mL/kg × 1.8 kg) = 1090 mL per 24 hours. 1090 mL/24 hours = 45 mL per hour.

(iii) 100 mL/kg = 100 × 3.6 kg = 360 mL per 24 hours. 360 mL/24 hours = 15 mL per hour.

(iv) 1500 mL + (20 mL/kg × 2 kg) = 1540 mL per 24 hours. 1540 mL/24 hours = 64 mL per hour.

The 4:2:1 Rule

The 4:2:1 rule simplify and speeds up calculations. IV fluid rates are written per hour rather than per day. The 4:2:1 rule closely approximates the long route. Consider that 100 mL/kg/day/24 hours = 4.2 mL/kg/hour (close to 4), 50 mL/kg/day/24 hours = 2.1 mL/kg/hour (close to 2), 20 mL/kg/day/24 hours = 0.8 mL/kg/hour (close to 1).

Example: Sabnam, age 7 years, kilogram weight = 22 kg. Fluid maintenance needed per hour = 4 × 10 + 2 × 10 + 2 × 1 = 62 mL/hour (approx).

Health education

When to seek medical attention in dehydration?

- The child does not urinate for > 6 hours.
- Crying without tears or dry mucous membranes
- Sunken fontanel
- Blood in the diarrhea or diarrhea become severe
- Frequency of diarrhea >1/hr, > 10 times/day
- Severe abdominal cramps occur
- Dizzy with standing
- Very sick, the child starts acting
- Fever > 37.8 °C for more than 72 hours
- Mild diarrhea > 7 days
- The child's behavior and mental status changes

MAINTENANCE OF FLUID AND ELECTROLYTE BALANCE: NURSING RESPONSIBILITIES

Fluid balance assessment is a fundamental aspect of caring for the ill children with hypovolemia. Early recognition and treatment is paramount to prevent potentially life-threatening hypovolemic shock. The management of fluid balance requires the nurse to have a mixture of different skills, including an understanding of the principles of fluid balance in the body and of the different intravenous fluids. The nurse must also have an understanding of the pathophysiologic responses of body to fluid depletion and be able to recognise those signs and respond appropriately. It is necessary as dehydration can develop very quickly in infants and young children; especially in the conditions such as diarrhea, fever, vomiting, burns, trauma, diabetes; moreover the condition of the child can change rapidly when body lacks its homeostasis, i.e fluid and electrolyte imbalance.

Nursing Diagnosis and Planning

Deficient fluid volume related to gastric or intestinal infection or inflammation, hemorrhage, burns, or failure of fluid regulatory mechanisms.

Expected Outcome

The child will display adequate fluid volume and electrolyte balance as evidenced by age appropriate urine output and urine specific gravity, BP and heart rate, gain of weight, and normal skin turgor and moist mucous membrane; serum pH and electrolyte levels within normal limits.

Interventions

One of the major preventive activities of community health nurse is to aware families to prevent dehydration. They should be taught to give additional fluid to the child during summer, avoid over dressing and to encourage frequent rest periods during high energy play and exercises. Parents should give additional fluid during minor ailments like fever, diarrhea, dysentery, vomiting to avoid complications. They should learn about early signs and symptoms of dehydration and replacement of fluids, oral rehydration, nutrition and other management (discussed above). Nursing interventions for the hospitalized child with fluid and electrolyte imbalance include:

- Obtain patient history to ascertain the probable cause of the fluid disturbance, which can help to guide interventions.

- Assess for signs and symptoms of dehydration, type and level of dehydration (see above)
- Monitor weight daily and consistently, with same scale, and preferably at the same time of day which facilitate accurate measurement and follow trends.
- Evaluate fluid status/dehydration level in relation to dietary intake. Determine if patient has been on a fluid restriction or suffering from minor ailments.
- Encourage patient to drink prescribed fluid amounts or administer parenteral fluids as ordered. Anticipate the need for an IV fluid challenge with immediate infusion of fluids for patients with abnormal vital signs.
- Monitor vital signs. Hypotension is evident in hypovolemia. Sinus tachycardia may occur with hypovolemia to maintain an effective cardiac output. Usually the weak and may be irregular pulse occur if electrolyte imbalance also develops.
- Monitor serum electrolytes and urine osmolality and report abnormal values. Fluid deficit is identified by elevated hemoglobin and elevated blood urea nitrogen (BUN), increased urine specific gravity.
- Dehydration can alter mental status. Document baseline mental status and record during each nursing shift.
- During treatment, monitor closely for signs of circulatory overload (headache, flushed skin, tachycardia, venous distention, elevated central venous pressure (CVP), shortness of breath, increased BP, tachypnea, cough).
- Explain importance of maintaining proper nutrition and hydration.
- Parents need to understand the importance of drinking extra fluid during bouts of diarrhea, fever, and other conditions causing fluid deficits. Teach interventions to prevent future episodes of inadequate intake.

Evaluation

- The child is alert
- The child will maintain fluid balance within normal limits
- Age-appropriate urine output
- Serum pH and electrolyte levels within normal limits
- Capillary refilling time < 2 seconds
- Elastic skin turgor
- Moist mucous membranes
- Maintenance of pre-illness weight.

CHAPTER 12

The Child with a Gastrointestinal Disorder

Chapter Outline

- Review of the Gastrointestinal (GI) System
- Pediatric Differences in the GI System
- Endoscopy
- Colonoscopy
- Disorders of Prenatal Development
- Motility Disorders
- Inflammatory and Infectious Disorders
- Obstructive Disorders
- Malabsorption Disorders
- Hepatic Disorders
- Hepatitis

INTRODUCTION

The gastrointestinal system of human is also called the GI system, GI tract, or digestive system. It is one of the most fascinating systems in the human body. Not only the GI system is responsible for the entry and exit of food, water, and nutrients, but it also plays a key role in a number of body functions. These include energy production, blood flow, nerve signaling (the body's nerve communication system), hormone control, metabolic reactions, and detoxification. In addition, the GI system is one of the largest disease battling, or immune systems in the body.

REVIEW OF THE GASTROINTESTINAL (GI) SYSTEM

The GI tract is a series of hollow organs joined in a long, twisting tube from the mouth to the anus (Fig. 12.1). The movement of muscles in the GI tract, along with the release of hormones and enzymes, starts the digestion to convert food into energy and basic nutrients to feed the entire body. The upper GI tract includes the mouth, esophagus, stomach, small intestine, and duodenum, which is the first part of the small intestine. The lower GI consists of jejunum and ileum (part of small intestine), large intestine, rectum, anal canal. In addition to the alimentary canal, there are several important accessory organs that help body to digest food but do not have food pass through them. Accessory organs of the digestive system include the teeth, tongue, salivary glands, liver, gallbladder, and pancreas. To achieve the goal of providing energy and nutrients to the body, six major functions take place in the digestive system:

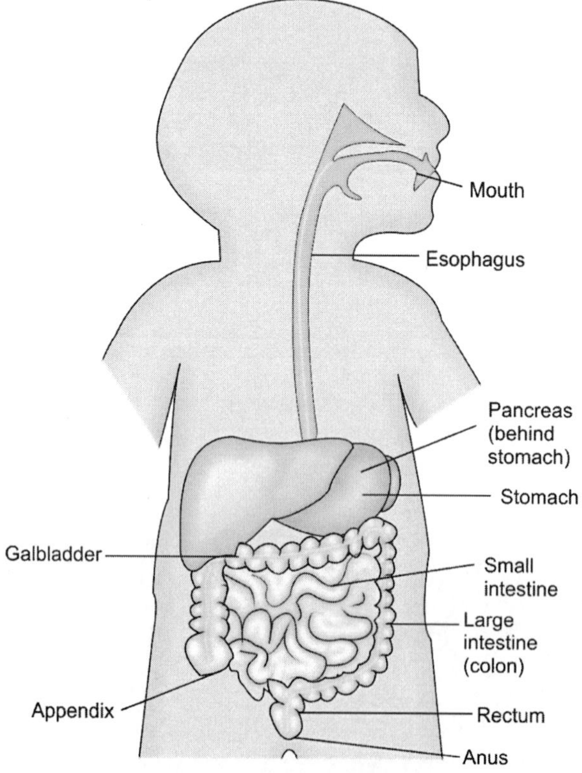

Fig. 12.1: Gastrointestinal system

1. Ingestion
2. Secretion
3. Mixing and movement
4. Digestion
5. Absorption
6. Excretion.

What is peristalsis?

Beginning in the esophagus, food moves smoothly through entire digestive tract by a process called peristalsis, a coordinated, rhythmic wave of muscular contraction that travels in a single direction. Peristalsis works independently of gravity. This means if man eats while standing on his head, the food would still move properly from esophagus to stomach through digestive system.

PEDIATRIC DIFFERENCES IN THE GI SYSTEM

Infants have minimal saliva. Swallowing is not under voluntary control until 6 weeks. Smaller stomach capacity.

Age	*Capacity of stomach (mL)*
New born	10–20
1 week	30–90
2–3 weeks	80–100
4 weeks	90–150
12 weeks	150–200
1 year	210–360
1–6 years	500
10 years	750–900
12–21 years	1000–1500
Adults	2000–3000

Reverse peristaltic waves in infancy causes regurgitation and vomiting. Food remains in the stomach in shorter duration due to faster peristalsis. Hydrochloric acid concentration is low until school age, and pepsinogen approximates adults level by 3 months.

- The liver is proportionately larger than adults and is immature until 1 year. Immature neonatal liver not yet efficient in ability to detoxify, results in less vitamins and mineral breakdown than in older children.
- Fever increases the rate of propulsion in children.
- Neonate's GI tract is immature.
- Large intestine relatively short, with less epithelial lining to absorb water. Peristalsis matures by 8 months, causing stools to be more formed.
- The large surface area and prolonged exposure time increase risk of toxin-mediated damage, and increased permeability in early infancy may augment this further.
- GI malfunction can impact normal growth and development.

Major Digestive Enzymes and Hormones

Digestive enzymes are enzymes that breakdown polymeric macromolecules into their smaller building blocks, in order to facilitate their absorption by the body. Digestive enzymes are diverse and are found in the oral cavity, the stomach, and the small intestine. Digestive enzymes are secreted by different exocrine glands including salivary glands, secretory cells in the stomach, secretory cells in the pancreas, secretory glands in the small intestine.

Digestive enzymes are classified based on their target substrates:

- Proteases and peptidases split proteins into small peptides and amino acids.
- Lipases split fat into three fatty acids and a glycerol molecule.
- Carbohydrases split carbohydrates such as starch and sugars into simple sugars such as glucose.
- Nucleases split nucleic acids into nucleotides.

Small amounts of starch placed in the mouth are digested by the amylase present in saliva. The chief cells of stomach synthesize and secrete pepsinogen, the precursor to the proteolytic enzyme pepsin. It breaks long polypeptide chains into shorter lengths. Pancreatic amylase hydrolyzes starch into a mixture of maltose and glucose. Pancreatic lipase. The enzyme hydrolyzes ingested fats into a mixture of fatty acids and monoglycerides. Its action is enhanced by the detergent effect of bile. Three protein-digesting enzymes secreted by the pancreas are serine proteases, named as chymotrypsin, trypsin, elastase. Further digestion occurs by enzymes which are incorporated in the plasma membrane of the microvilli in the small intestine. Aminopeptidases attack on peptides producing amino acids, disaccharidases convert disaccharides into their monosaccharide subunits, maltase hydrolyzes maltose into glucose, sucrase hydrolyzes sucrose (common table sugar) into glucose and fructose, lactase hydrolyzes lactose (milk sugar) into glucose and galactose.

There are at least **five hormones** that aid and regulate the digestive system in mammals. There are variations across the vertebrates, as for instance in birds. Arrangements are complex and additional details are regularly discovered. For instance, more connections to metabolic control (largely the glucose-insulin system) have been uncovered in recent years.

- *Gastrin:* It is in the stomach and stimulates the gastric glands to secrete pepsinogen (an inactive form of the enzyme pepsin) and hydrochloric acid. Secretion of gastrin is stimulated by food arriving in stomach. The secretion is inhibited by low pH.
- *Secretin:* Secretin is in the duodenum and signals the secretion of sodium bicarbonate in the pancreas and it stimulates the bile secretion in the liver. This hormone responds to the acidity of the chyme.
- *Cholecystokinin (CCK):* It is in the duodenum and stimulates the release of digestive enzymes in the pancreas and stimulates the emptying of bile in the gall bladder. This hormone is secreted in response to fat in chyme.
- *Gastric inhibitory peptide (GIP):* It is in the duodenum and decreases the stomach churning in turn slowing the emptying in the stomach. Another function is to induce insulin secretion.
- *Motilin:* It is in the duodenum and increases the migrating myoelectric complex component of GI motility and stimulates the production of pepsin.

Significance of pH in Digestion

Digestion is a complex process controlled by several factors. pH plays a crucial role in a normally functioning digestive tract. In the mouth, pharynx, and esophagus, pH is typically about 6.8, very weakly acidic. Saliva controls pH in this region of the digestive tract. Salivary amylase is contained in saliva and starts the breakdown of carbohydrates into monosaccharides. Most digestive enzymes are sensitive to pH and will denature in a high or low pH environment.

The stomach's high acidity inhibits the breakdown of carbohydrates within it. This acidity confers two benefits: it denatures proteins for further digestion in the small intestines, and provides non-specific immunity, damaging or eliminating various pathogens.

In the small intestines, the duodenum provides critical pH balancing to activate digestive enzymes. The liver secretes bile into the duodenum to neutralize the acidic conditions from the stomach, and the pancreatic duct empties into the duodenum, adding bicarbonate to neutralize the acidic chyme, thus creating a neutral environment. The mucosal tissue of the small intestines is alkaline with a pH of about 8.5.

Common Symptoms and Signs of GI Disorders

Failure to thrive (FTT): It is a term used in child health to indicate insufficient weight gain or inappropriate weight loss. It is usually defined in terms of weight, and can be evaluated either by a low weight for the child's age, or by a low rate of increase in the weight. The weight of the child consistently remains below the 3rd percentile or body mass index (BMI) below the 5th percentile.

FTT covers poor physical growth of any cause and does not imply abnormal intellectual, social, or emotional development, although of course it can subsequently be a cause of such pathologies. Traditionally, causes of FTT have been divided into endogenous and exogenous causes. Initial investigation should consider physical causes, calorie intake and psychosocial assessment.

Problems with the GI system such as gas and acid reflux are painful conditions which may make the child unwilling to take in sufficient nutrition. FTT is caused due to malabsorption syndromes like cystic fibrosis, diarrhea, liver disease, and celiac disease. Weight gain of child is hampered by physical deformities such as cleft palate and tongue tie. Milk allergies can cause endogenous FTT. Also the metabolism may be raised by parasites, asthma, urinary tract infections, and other fever-inducing infections, or heart disease so that it becomes difficult to get in sufficient calories to meet the higher caloric demands.

Exogenous causes of FTT of children come from caregiver's actions, like physical inability to produce enough breastmilk, inability to procure formula when needed, purposely limiting total caloric intake, and not offering sufficient age-appropriate solid foods for babies and toddlers over the age of 6 months.

Regurgitation or spitting up: It occurs when stomach contents flow back up into the esophagus—the muscular tube that carries food and liquids from the mouth to the stomach. It is also called *acid reflux* or *acid regurgitation* because the stomach digestive juices contain acid. Infants spit up liquid mostly made of saliva and stomach acids. It is common in infants under 2 years of age. About half of all infants spit up, or regurgitate, many times a day in the first 3 months of life. Most healthy infants experience few to no symptoms and stop spitting up between the ages of 12 and 14 months.

If an infant's regurgitation progresses to GERD, additional symptoms—such as vomiting and poor feeding—occur and can adversely affect the child's overall health and temperament. Infants with severe symptoms or with regurgitation that lasts beyond 12–14 months may actually have GERD and should seek medical attention.

Nausea and vomiting: Unpleasant sensation vaguely referred to the throat or abdomen with an inclination to vomiting is called nausea. Forceful ejection of gastric content is known as vomiting. Vomiting involves a complex process under central nervous system (CNS) control that causes salivation, sweating, pallor and tachycardia. Vomiting occurs when nerves in the body or brain sense a trigger, such as food poisoning, certain infections or medicines, or motion. Nausea sometimes, but not always, occurs before vomiting. Younger children may not be able to describe nausea, although they may complain of a stomach ache or have other general complaints. There are dozens of conditions that can lead to vomiting or nausea, but a few more common causes are gastroenteritis, food allergies and irritations, anxiety and stress, the flu and other illness, eating too much, food poisoning.

Projectile vomiting: This is a form of vomiting where the stomach contents are forcibly pushed out of the body through vigorous vomiting. Projectile vomiting can strain the esophagus and stomach. While projectile vomiting can be a short-lived event in many children, it can also be an indication of serious health issues like food poisoning, pyloric stenosis, intestinal obstruction, hepatitis, flu. Dehydration is a significant risk, particularly if the vomiting continues over a period of several days or longer and is accompanied with fever and diarrhea.

Abdominal pain: There are many causes of abdominal pain (Fig. 12.2). Some common causes are functional abdominal pain, gastroesophageal reflux (heartburn), excess sugar intake, constipation, inflammation, kidney or liver or pancreas problems, and pain associated with anxiety. This pain may be sudden onset or episodic severe pain; localised or diffuse, acute or chronic; often caused by obstruction, haemorrhage. The child seems unwell, is doing less than usual, or lying down, not wanting to move or wriggling around trying to find a position that makes the pain feel better.

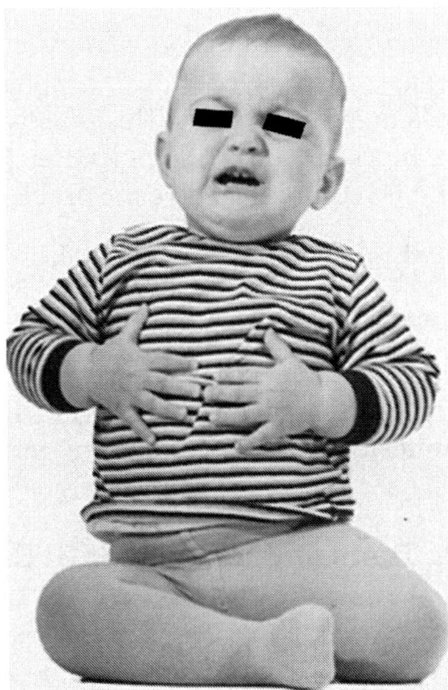

Fig. 12.2: Pain abdomen is a common symptom of gastrointestinal disorders

Abdominal distension: Abdominal distension in children is bloating or enlargement of child's abdomen. Abdominal distension occurs when substances, such as air or fluid, accumulate in the abdomen causing its outward expansion beyond the normal girth of the stomach and waist. A major cause of abnormal bloating is excessive eating and sleep swallowing, known as aerophagia. Other causes of bloating include inflammatory bowel diseases such as Crohn's disease and ulcerative colitis, irritable bowel syndrome, functional dyspepsia or transient constipation. In rare cases, bloating may occur in individuals who have milk intolerance (lactose intolerance), parasite infections like giardia, food poisoning (bacteria), celiac disease, severe peptic ulcer disease, bowel obstruction or after certain types of abdominal surgery.

Dehydration: It is a condition that can occur with excess loss of water and other body fluids. Dehydration is significant depletion of body water and, to varying degrees, electrolytes. Symptoms and signs include thirst, lethargy, dry mucosa, decreased urine output, and, as the degree of dehydration progresses, tachycardia, hypotension, and shock. Children are particularly susceptible to dehydration with acute gastroenteritis or other illnesses that cause vomiting, diarrhea and fever.

Clinical signs of dehydration

- Decrease in skin turgor
- Dry mucous membranes
- Decreased production of tears and urine
- Increased pulse
- Decreased blood pressure
- Sunken eyes
- Delayed capillary refill

Diarrhea: It is defined by the World Health Organization (WHO) as having three or more loose or liquid stools per day, or as having more stools than is normal for that person. Diarrhea is the frequent stool with an increased water content as a result of alterations of water and electrolyte transport by the GI tract; it may be acute or chronic.

Constipation: It is a condition of the digestive system in which there is difficulty in emptying the bowels. It is usually associated with hardened feces and is present for two or more weeks. In most cases, this occurs because the colon has absorbed too much of the water from the food that is in the colon. The slower the food moves through digestive tract, the more water the colon will absorb from food. Consequently, the feces become dry and hard. It may include blood streaked stools and abdominal discomfort. Defecation (emptying the bowels) can become very painful, and in some serious cases there may be symptoms of bowel obstruction. When the constipation is very severe; when the constipation prevents the passage of feces and gas, it is called obstipation.

Encopresis: Many children with constipation will ultimately pass either an overly large and/or hard stool resulting in a painful experience. The rational step (from the child's perspective) is to avoid stooling and thus avoid further pain. Consequently stool accumulates in the rectum and becomes desiccated and thus more difficult and more painful to pass. This recurrent cycle reinforces the child's behavior to avoid stooling at all costs. Children who develop encopresis may develop abnormal stretching and enlargement of the rectal area that reduces the reflex urge to stool. This cycle can result in so deeply conditioning the holding response that the rectal anal inhibitory response (RAIR) or anismus results. As a consequence, the impacted stool mass may allow 'upstream' semisolid stool to leak around the 'downstream' stool obstruction, causing soiling in clothes as well as occasional chunks of stool to also be passed without the child's knowledge or desire.

Hypoactive, hyperactive or absent bowel movement: Abdominal sounds are the noises made by the intestines. Abdominal sounds (bowel sounds) are made by the movement of the intestines as they push food through. Since the intestines are hollow, bowel sounds can echo through the abdomen much like the sounds heard from water pipes. Evidence of intestinal motility problems may be caused by inflammation or obstruction.

Reduced (hypoactive) bowel sounds include a reduction in the loudness, tone, or regularity of the sounds. They are a sign that intestinal activity has slowed. Hypoactive bowel sounds are normal during sleep, and also occur normally for a short time after the use of certain medications and after abdominal surgery. Decreased or absent bowel sounds often indicate constipation.

Hyperactive bowel sounds mean there is an increase in intestinal activity. This can sometimes occur with diarrhea and after eating.

No bowel sounds after a period of hyperactive bowel sounds can mean there is a rupture of the intestines, or strangulation of the bowel and death (necrosis) of the bowel tissue. Very high-pitched bowel sounds may be a sign of early bowel obstruction.

Gastrointestinal bleeding: Gastrointestinal bleeding or gastrointestinal hemorrhage describes every form of hemorrhage in the GI tract, from the pharynx to the rectum and can be defined as acute or chronic bleeding. An upper source is characterized by hematemesis (vomiting up blood) and melena (tarry stool containing altered blood). About half of cases are due to peptic ulcer disease esophagitis and erosive disease is the next most common causes. In those with liver cirrhosis 50–60% of bleeding is due to esophageal varices. Passage of bright red blood per rectum, usually indicating lower GI tract bleeding is hematochezia.

Jaundice: Yellowing of the skin or whites of the eyes, arising from excess of the pigment bilirubin and typically caused by obstruction of the bile duct, by liver disease, body fluids may also be yellow. The color of the skin and sclerae varies depending on levels of bilirubin; mildly elevated levels display yellow skin and sclerae, while highly elevated levels display brown.

Dysphagia: Dysphagia means swallowing difficulties, and usually caused by neuromuscular problems. Dysphagia may occur due to gastroesophageal reflux disease (GERD), neuromuscular problems in pharynx, upper esophageal sphincter.

- Oropharyngeal dysphagia (high dysphagia). The problem is in the mouth and/or throat. This is usually caused by a neurological problem—there is something wrong with the nerves (and muscles).
- Esophageal dysphagia (low dysphagia). The problem is in the esophagus. This is usually because of some blockage or irritation. Often, a surgical procedure is required to solve the problem.

Dysfunctional swallowing: Impaired swallowing defects caused by CNS defects or structural defects of the oral cavity, or esophagus, can cause feeding problems or aspirations.

Fever: Common diseases in children with GI disorders; usually manifested with dehydration, inflammation, infection.

Laboratory Tests and Images for GI Disorders

Stool

A stool (feces) sample can provide valuable information about what is going on when a child has a problem in the stomach, intestines, or other part of the GI system.

Ova and parasites: Stool is examined microscopically for presence of parasites and their eggs in case of diarrhea and abdominal pain. Microscopy is particularly useful in diarrhea, may show protozoa like giardia, ova, cyst and other infective agents. No special patient preparation is necessary but sample should be free from urine and water. One to three samples are collected and delivered to the laboratory either fresh or in preservatives.

Culture and sensitivity: The stool culture might be ordered if the child has diarrhea for several days or has bloody diarrhea, especially if there has been an outbreak of food borne illness in community. It identifies infective organisms and determine their antibiotic sensitivity. Organism from a small sample of stool are grown in culture media. A stool culture is performed to look for illness-causing bacteria such as *Shigella, Salmonella, Yersinia, Campylobacter, Escherichia coli* (*E. coli*). On occasion some other illness-causing bacteria may be noted.

No special preparation is required, but the lab will need a fresh or refrigerated sample of stool without contamination. The stool should be collected into clean, dry plastic jars with screw-cap lids or any clean, sealable container could do the job. For best results, the stool should then be brought to the laboratory immediately. Barium, antacids, mineral oil, and antibiotics may interfere with the results. The best samples are of loose, fresh stool; well-formed stool is rarely positive for disease-causing bacteria. Sometimes swabs from a child's rectum also can be tested for viruses. Although this is not done routinely, it can sometimes give clues about certain illnesses, especially in newborns or very ill children. Viral cultures can take a week or longer to grow, depending on the virus.

Occult blood (guaiac, hematest): Testing for blood in the stool is done in certain kinds of infectious diarrhea, bleeding within the GI tract, and other inflammatory conditions, bowel necrosis. However, most of the time, blood streaking in the stool of an infant or toddler is from a slight rectal tear, called a fissure, which is caused by straining against a hard stool (this is fairly common in infants and kids with ongoing constipation).

Testing for blood in the stool is often performed with a quick test. First, stool is smeared on a card, then a few drops of a developing solution are placed on the card. An instant color change shows that blood is present in the stool. Sometimes, stool is sent to a laboratory to test for blood, and the result will be reported within hours.

Urine

Laboratory or dip stick analysis is done to determine bile by products in urine.

Urobilinogen level is determined in hepatic dysfunction and obstruction cases. No special preparation is needed for this test.

Blood

- Routine blood tests may reveal anemia, high CRP or low albumin; which shows a high correlation for the presence of an organic disease. In this setting, microcytic anemia usually implies iron deficiency and macrocytosis can be caused by impaired folic acid or vitamin B_{12} absorption or both. Low cholesterol or triglyceride may give a clue toward fat malabsorption. Low calcium and phosphate may give a clue toward osteomalacia from low vitamin D.
- Specific vitamins like vitamin D or micronutrient like zinc levels can be checked. Fat soluble vitamins (A, D, E and K) are affected in fat malabsorption. Prolonged prothrombin time can be caused by vitamin K deficiency.
  - Serological studies. Specific tests are carried out to determine the underlying cause.
  - IgA Anti-transglutaminase antibodies or IgA anti-endomysial antibodies for coeliac disease (gluten sensitive enteropathy).
- Liver function test: Serum levels are measured to give an indication of liver function.

X-ray Exams of the Digestive Tract

Flat Plate of Abdomen

It includes anterior and posterior radiographs of abdomen.

Radiographs shows the patency of GI tract and stool and gas pattern. It is used in cases of abdominal pain, appendicitis, imperforate anus, intussusceptions.

Usually no preparation is needed, except to allay the anxiety of child and family.

Radiographs with Barium

There are X-ray tests that allow to examine the digestive tract from the esophagus to the rectum. These tests utilize barium or an iodine-containing agent that allows visualization of the digestive tract and a form of X-ray machine called fluoroscopy. Fluoroscopy allows part of the body to be studied in motion and recorded on a video monitor.

Upper GI tests use X-rays to examine the esophagus, stomach, and first part of the small intestine (the duodenum). For these tests, patients need to drink barium. As the barium passes through the digestive tract, it fills and coats the esophagus, stomach, and first part of the small intestine making them more visible with X-ray. Then a fluroscopy machine is held over the part of the body being examined and transmits continuous images to a video monitor. This upper GI test is used to diagnose, hiatal hernias, ulcers, tumors, esophageal varices, obstruction or narrowing of the upper GI tract.

It may also be used to determine the cause of swallowing problems, reflux symptoms (dyspepsia or heartburn), abdominal pain, diarrhea, unexplained vomiting, weight loss, or bleeding. Preparation for upper GI or lower GI testing usually includes making dietary changes (such as following a low-fiber diet for two to three days before the test), not smoking for 12–24 hours before the test, not taking any medications for up to 24 hours before the test and not eating anything for 12 hours before the test.

Lower GI Tests

Lower GI tests or barium enemas are used to examine the large intestine and the rectum. For this test, barium or an iodine-containing liquid is introduced gradually into the colon through a tube inserted into the rectum. As the barium passes through the lower intestines, it fills the colon, allowing the radiologist to see growths or polyps and areas that are narrowed. The fluoroscope is held over the part of the body being examined and transmits continuous images to the video monitor.

This lower GI testing is used to detect colon polyps, tumors, diverticular disease, gastroenteritis, strictures or sites of narrowing and obstruction, ulcerative colitis or Crohn's disease. Other causes of abdominal pain or blood, mucus, or pus in the stool.

There are several types of tests used to view the lower GI, including:

- *Air contrast barium enema (double contrast barium enema):* This is an X-ray examination of the large intestine (colon). Barium and air are introduced gradually into the colon by a rectal tube. Approximate time: 1 hour.
- *Barium enema:* This is an X-ray examination of the large intestine (colon). Barium is introduced gradually into the colon by a rectal tube. Approximate time: 1 hour.

With the barium or contrast enema, the colon is filled with a contrast material containing barium or iodine-containing contrast (a liquid that lights up on X-ray) by running it through a tube inserted into the rectum. The barium blocks X-rays; therefore the colon, when filled with the agent, shows up clearly on the X-ray picture.

The air contrast study is slightly different. The colon is first filled with some barium, and then the colon is filled with air. This technique provides a more detailed picture of the lining of the colon, improving the procedure›s ability to detect small polyps or inflammation.

Preparation before the Upper or Lower GI Studies

Preparation for upper GI or lower GI testing usually includes making dietary changes (such as following a low-fiber diet for two to three days before the test), not smoking for 12–24 hours before the test, not taking any medications for up to 24 hours before the test and not eating anything for 12 hours before the test. Additional preparation for the lower GI test usually includes taking oral laxatives and an enema the night before the test.

What Happens During the GI Tests?

- Patients will be positioned on a tilting X-ray table by the technologist. For an upper GI test, the table usually starts in a vertical position, with the person standing. For a lower GI test, the table usually starts in a horizontal position, with the person lying on his or her back or stomach. The table will be tilted at various angles during the test to help spread the barium solution throughout the body so that different views can be seen on the fluoroscope. During the test, the radiologist may put pressure on your abdomen to get a clearer image on the fluoroscope.
- Although the barium solution given in an upper GI test is unpleasant tasting, there is no pain and little discomfort during the procedure. The lower GI test may cause some discomfort, including cramps and a strong urge to have a bowel movement.
- After the barium enema is administered in a lower GI test and a few X-rays are taken, you will be helped to the bathroom (or given a bedpan) and asked to move your bowels to expel as much of the barium as possible. Then you will go back to the X-ray examination room where more X-rays will be taken of the barium solution that remains on the lining of the intestine. In some cases, air will be injected slowly into the colon (air contrast barium enema) to provide further contrast on the X-rays to detect abnormalities.

What Happens after the GI Tests?

Generally patient can resume usual activities and normal diet immediately after GI tests. But, drinking plenty of fluids (unless fluid is restricted for another medical condition), especially if the test is an upper GI and/or small bowel series. The barium tends to constipate people. Drinking 8–10 glasses of water or juice per day for three days will help you to eliminate the barium from your colon.

It is normal that stool to have a white or light color for up to three days after the test.

The barium enema given during the lower GI test may cause you to feel week or dizzy.

Are these GI Tests Safe?

There is virtually no risk with the upper and lower GI tests, unless they are repeated several times within a few months' time, when radiation exposure can become a risk. Although radiation exposure is minimal, it is greater than for standard still X-rays. Steps will be taken during the test to minimize radiation exposure.

Other risks include infection (very low risk with both the upper and lower GI tests), tearing the intestinal wall during a lower GI test. Should this occur, surgery may be necessary. This is a very rare complication.

Who Should Not Receive GI Tests?

If there is existing blockage or tear in the intestinal wall, the upper and lower GI tests should not be performed.

When to need medical attention after GI tests

After the GI tests, medical attention is needed if the patient is having:

- A temperature of 101 °F or higher. This could be a sign of infection and should be treated right away.
- A marked change in bowel habits (such as no bowel movement in two or three days after the test). Remember, it is normal for your stool to have a white or light color for up to three days after the test.
- Worsening of pain
- Any unusual rectal drainage.

ENDOSCOPY

There are times when a child has symptoms, such as vomiting, diarrhea, constipation or pain and the reason for these symptoms is not easily explained by physical examination and other laboratory tests or X-rays. When this happens, examine the inside of the child's stomach or intestines (colon) is done by using an endoscope, a small flexible tube with a camera on the end of it. The tube of the endoscope is passed through the mouth or through the rectum, depending on the area of the body that needs to be examined. The image from inside the body is projected onto a monitor for examination. Advances in endoscopy and anesthesia have enabled GI endoscopy for children since 1960.

The procedure allows direct viewing of the lining of the esophagus, stomach and proximal duodenum. Materials for biopsies and cultures are collected by this method. It is used to rule out various upper GI tract disorders.

Preparation for GI endoscopy in children should respect the special physiology as well as the psychosocial and emotional needs of pediatric patients and their parents. Informed consent of the parents or guardians has to be obtained. Parents and children should be provided with sufficient information about potential risks and benefits of the procedure using an age-appropriate language. The important elements of this discussion should be acknowledged in writing and signed to provide legal documentation.

Preprocedure assessment includes a systematic review and physical examination with a special focus on the airway system. Examination and documentation of loose teeth, oral piercings and enlarged tonsils is very important. Loose teeth can be accidentally dislodged and may cause complications when entering the airways. Enlarged tonsils can provoke breathing difficulties and obstructive apnea in sedated patients and should be evaluated by the physician before sedation. Laboratory tests may include coagulation and liver function tests. To reduce anxiety in the younger patients, the presence of parents for preprocedural preparation is usually essential. Premedication with benzodiazepines has been shown to reduce anxiety and fear prior to endoscopy. Oral or nasal application is possible.

Contraindications: Absolute contraindications include unstable airway, cardiovascular collapse, intestinal perforation and peritonitis. Relative contraindications are bowel obstruction, severe thrombocytopenia, coagulopathy, recent GI surgery, respiratory infections and recent food intake. The procedure should be delayed or cancelled in the absence of signed consent.

Patient monitoring: In most hospitals an interdisciplinary team of pediatric gastroenterologists, anesthetists and specialized nurses is involved in the endoscopy procedures. All patients should be monitored regarding the cardiovascular system including oxygen-saturation. Monitoring should be continued for 15–30 minutes after the procedure. Afterwards the patient should stay on the ward for at least two hours. Intake of clear fluid is possible one hour after sedation. Discharge is possible if sufficient cardiovascular function and airway patency is confirmed, the patient is fully oriented and protective reflexes are intact.

COLONOSCOPY

Colonoscopy is done in the detection of lower GI tract pathology in children. The indications for diagnostic colonoscopy in children are basically similar to the ones in adults. The colon is viewed directly by a fiberoptic scope and camera inserted rectally. As shown, the main causes leading to colonoscopy in children are hematochezia, abdominal pain and diarrhea. The most common endoscopic diagnoses are IBD (diagnosis or review), juvenile polyps, polyposis syndromes (diagnosis or review), allergic colitis and miscellaneous (vascular anomaly, infective colitis, tumors.

Preprocedural preparation should be individualized according to the child's age, cooperation of the child. In infants, adequate preparation can usually be obtained with the use of small-volume enemas and by substituting clear liquids for milk 12–24 hours prior to the procedure.

Absolute contraindications to colonoscopy in pediatric patients are suspected bowel perforation and acute peritonitis.

CT Abdominal Scans in Children

A CT abdominal scan is a type of medical exam that uses X-ray equipment and a computer to make many cross-sectional images of the abdomen. These images can be studied on a computer, printed, or put on a CD. A CT scan of the abdomen is an important test to diagnose abdominal problems in newborns, infants, and children. It is called a noninvasive medical test because it does not involve an incision or procedure that goes inside child's body. An abdominal CT scan allows to get a better picture of what is going on inside the abdomen than a plain X-ray. Some childhood diseases that an abdominal CT scan can help diagnose include appendicitis, inflammatory bowel disease, abdominal tumors, and birth defects. Important organs that can be evaluated include the stomach, liver, kidney, and spleen. The preparations for the procedure needed are:

- Doctor should be informed regarding allergies child has, medication he takes, suffers from any medical condition (heart disease, asthma, thyroid).
- Child needs to stop eating and drinking several hours before the exam. Children who are having general anesthesia usually must stop all food and drink 8 hours in advance.
- Leave all metal objects, such as jewelry and hair barrettes, at home since metal can affect CT imaging.
- Dress the child in comfortable clothes on the day of the exam.

The CT scanner is a large machine with a tunnel that an examination table passes through. The steps followed here are:

- Child will be positioned on the exam table.
- If child is having anesthesia or sedation, an IV line will be placed in your child's hand or arm.
- If contrast material is given through an IV, child may feel a warm sensation when it is injected and may have a metallic taste for a short time. Contrast material may be given as a drink, possibly mixed with juice or soda to mask the taste.
- The scan itself is painless and lasts between 5 and 20 seconds. Child may hear clicking, whirring, and buzzing sounds as the scanner rotates around the exam table.
- Child may be asked to hold his or her breath during the scan if possible.
- After the scan, child will probably need to wait while the images are checked to make sure they are acceptable.
- Most often, child will be able to get back to his or her usual schedule right away. If child had sedation or anesthesia, he or she may be observed for a while in a recovery area. In this case or if child was given contrast material, may be given some instructions for care at home, depending on child's particular situation.

Others

Ultrasound

Abdominal ultrasonography is a form of medical ultrasonography to visualize abdominal anatomical structures. It uses transmission and reflection of ultrasound waves to visualize internal organs through the abdominal wall (with the help of gel which helps transmission of the sound waves). The sound waves cannot be heard by the human ear and cannot be felt by the child having the ultrasound study.

Abdominal ultrasound studies are most commonly performed to investigate the causes of abdominal pain or whether there is a mass of tissue or 'lump'. This type of study is particularly useful in examining the liver, pancreas, spleen, kidney but can provide very useful information about other organs.

Hydrogen Breath Test (HBT)

Hydrogen breath testing is simple noninvasive test is used to evaluate several different GI problems including intolerance of various sugars (such as lactose intolerance) and overgrowth of bacteria in the small intestine. Bacteria in the intestinal tract can produce hydrogen when they are exposed to unabsorbed sugars. This hydrogen gets into the bloodstream, is taken to the lungs, and then removed from the body in the breath. To do this test, the child prepares by fasting for 4–5 hours and asked to blow into a bag (to get a baseline reading). Then they are given a measured amount of a specific sugar to drink. At intervals after this, the child blows into a bag. The hydrogen in their breath will be measured. The test takes about 4 hours. So, HBT is performed to diagnose maldigestion or malabsorption syndromes.

DISORDERS OF PRENATAL DEVELOPMENT

Cleft Lip and Palate

Cleft lip (cheiloschisis) and palate (palatoschisis) are facial and oral malformations that may occur individually together. A cleft is a birth defect that occurs when the tissues of the lip and/or palate of the fetus do not fuse very early in pregnancy. Babies born with cleft lips will have an opening involving the upper lip. The length of the opening ranges from a small notch, to a cleft that extends into the base of the nostril. Cleft lips may involve one or both sides of the lip (Figs 12.3A to C). It is one of the most common congenital abnormalities with a worldwide incidence as high as 1 in 700. The incidence of cleft palate alone is about 1 in 2,000.

Babies born with cleft palates have openings in the palate, which is the roof of the mouth. The size and position of the opening varies. The cleft may be only in the hard palate, the bony portion of the roof of the mouth, opening into the floor of the nose. It may be only in the soft palate, the soft portion of the roof of the mouth. The cleft palate may involve both the hard and soft palate and may occur on both sides of the center of the palate. Cleft palate is found mostly in girls and cleft lip alone or together with cleft palate is found mostly in boys These are separate anomalies but are closely related to etiology, pathophysiology and nursing care.

Pathophysiology

Cleft lip and palate refer to facial malformations that evolve during embryonic development, resulting in nonunion of the bones and tissues of the lip and palate.

During the first six to eight weeks of pregnancy, the shape of the embryo's head is formed. The development of the face is coordinated by complex morphogenetic events and rapid proliferative expansion, and is thus

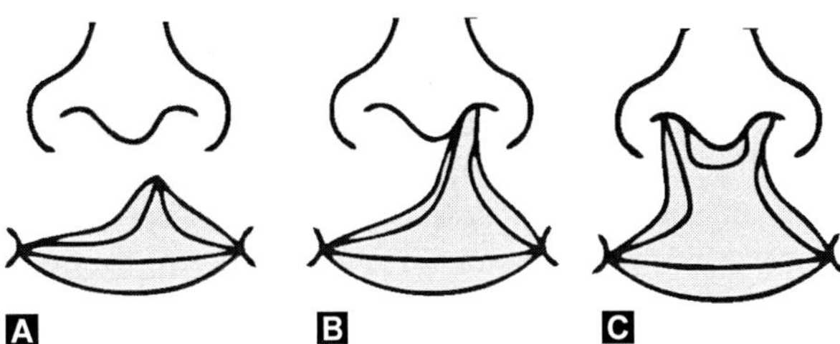

Figs 12.3A to C: Types of cleft lip. **A.** Unilateral incomplete; **B.** Unilateral complete; **C.** Bilateral complete

highly susceptible to environmental and genetic factors, rationalising the high incidence of facial malformations. Cleft lip occurs when the medial nasal and maxillary processes fail to form. Cleft palate occurs when the bone and tissue of the primary palatial shelves or processes fail to fuse at about 7–12 weeks of gestation, causing a communication between the mouth and nose.

Cleft lip and palate can occur on one or both sides of the mouth. Because the lip and the palate develop separately, it is possible to have a cleft lip without a cleft palate, a cleft palate without a cleft lip, or both a cleft lip and cleft palate together.

Cleft lips and palates not associated with a syndrome are caused by a combination of genetic and environmental factors. Inheritance caused by such a combination is called multifactorial. The risk of a baby being born with a cleft lip or palate increases with the number of affected relatives and the number of relatives that have more severe clefts. The embryo inherits genes that increase the risk for cleft lip and/or palate. When an embryo with such genes is exposed to certain environmental factors the embryo develops a cleft. Environmental factors that increase the risk of cleft lip and palate include cigarette and alcohol use during pregnancy. Some drugs, such as phenytoin, sodium valproate, and methotrexate, also increase the incidence of clefting. The pregnant mother's nutrition may affect the incidence of clefting as well. Cleft lip and palate may also occur as a result of exposure to viruses or chemicals while the fetus is developing in the womb.

What Problems are Associated with Cleft Lip and/or Cleft Palate?

- *Eating problems:* With a separation or opening in the palate, food and liquids can pass from the mouth back through the nose. Fortunately, specially designed baby bottles and nipples that help keep fluids flowing downward toward the stomach are

available. Children with a cleft palate may need to wear a man-made palate to help them eat properly and ensure that they are receiving adequate nutrition until surgical treatment is provided.
- *Ear infections/hearing loss:* Children with cleft palate are at increased risk of ear infections since they are more prone to fluid build-up in the middle ear. If left untreated, ear infections can cause hearing loss. To prevent this from happening, children with cleft palate usually need special tubes placed in the eardrums to aid fluid drainage, and their hearing needs to be checked once a year.
- *Speech problem:* Children with cleft lip or cleft palate may also have trouble speaking. Because of the gap, air leaks into the nasal cavity resulting in a hypernasal voice resonance and nasal emissions while talking. Secondary effects include speech articulation errors (e.g., distortions, substitutions, and omissions) and compensatory misarticulations and mispronunciations. Possible treatment options include speech therapy, prosthetics, augmentation of the posterior pharyngeal wall, lengthening of the palate, and surgical procedures. These children's voices do not carry well, the voice may take on a nasal sound called 'glottal' sound, and the speech may be difficult to understand. Not all children have these problems and surgery may fix these problems entirely for some.
- *Dental problems:* Children with clefts are more prone to a larger than average number of cavities and often have missing, extra, malformed, or displaced teeth requiring dental and orthodontic treatments. In addition, children with cleft palate often have an alveolar ridge defect. The alveolus is the bony upper gum that contains teeth. A defect in the alveolus can (1) displace, tip, or rotate permanent teeth, (2) prevent permanent teeth from appearing, and (3) prevent the alveolar ridge from forming. These problems can usually be repaired through oral surgery.
- *Psychosocial problem:* Most children who have their clefts repaired early enough are able to have a happy youth and social life. Adolescents with cleft palate or lip are at an elevated risk for developing psychosocial problems especially those relating to self-concept, peer relationships and appearance. Adolescents may face psychosocial challenges but can find professional help if problems arise. A cleft palate or lip may impact an individual's self-esteem, social skills and behavior. There is research dedicated to the psychosocial development of individuals with cleft palate. Self-concept may be adversely affected by the presence of a cleft lip and or cleft palate, particularly among girls.

Treatment

Due to the number of oral health and medical problems associated with a cleft lip or palate, a team of health professionals and other specialists is usually involved in the care of these children. Members of a cleft lip and palate team typically include.
- Plastic surgeon to evaluate and perform necessary surgeries on the lip or palate
- An otolaryngologist (an ear, nose, and throat doctor) to evaluate hearing problems and consider treatment options for hearing problems
- An oral surgeon to reposition segments of the upper jaw when needed, to improve function and appearance and to repair the cleft of the gum
- An orthodontist to straighten and reposition teeth
- A dentist to perform routine dental care
- A prosthodontist to make artificial teeth and dental appliances to improve the appearance and to meet functional requirements for eating and speaking
- A speech pathologist to assess speech and feeding problems
- A speech therapist to work with the child to improve speech
- An audiologist (a specialist in communication disorders stemming from a hearing impairment); to assess and monitor hearing
- A nurse coordinator to provide ongoing supervision of the child's health
- A social worker/psychologist to support the family and assess any adjustment problems
- A geneticist to help parents and adult patients understand the chances of having more children with these conditions.

The health care team works together to develop a plan of care to meet the individual needs of each patient. Treatment usually begins in infancy and often continues through early adulthood.

MOTILITY DISORDERS

Gastroesophageal Reflux

Gastroesophageal reflux (GER) is regurgitation of stomach contents back into the esophagus and sometimes into or out of the mouth. Usually, infants with the condition are otherwise healthy; all adults and infants periodically experience reflux, especially after meals. Refluxed stomach acid that touches the lining of the esophagus can cause heartburn. Also called acid indigestion, heartburn is an uncomfortable, burning feeling in the midchest, behind the breastbone, or in the upper part of the abdomen.

In older children, the causes of GER are also different than what is seen in infants and adults; and does not always mean they have GER disease. Children and adolescents may be able to control GER by:

- Avoiding foods and beverages that contribute to heartburn, such as chocolate, coffee, peppermint, greasy or spicy foods, tomato products, and alcoholic beverages
- Avoiding overeating
- Quitting smoking
- Losing weight if they are overweight
- Not eating 2–3 hours before sleep
- Taking over-the-counter medications

Gastroesophageal Reflux Disease

Gastroesophageal reflux disease (GERD) is a more serious, chronic—or long lasting—form of GER. GER that occurs more than twice a week for a few weeks could be GERD, which over time can lead to more serious health problems.

Etiology

Anything that causes the muscular valve between the stomach and esophagus (the lower esophageal sphincter or LES) to relax, or anything that increases the pressure below the LES, can cause GERD. Such things include obesity, overeating, constipation, and certain foods, beverages, and medications.

GERD is a more serious, chronic—or long lasting—form of GER. GER that occurs more than twice a week for a few weeks could be GERD, which over time can lead to more serious health problems.

Babies with cerebral palsy, Down's syndrome, head injury; have other problems affecting their nerves, brain, or muscles, and may affect the transmission of neural signals to the LES (lower esophageal sphincter). Hiatal hernias, partial or incomplete swallowing dysfunctions also promote GERD.

Increased intra-abdominal pressure while incurred by crying, coughing, straining tends to promote increased episodes of GER. According to the National Digestive Disease Information Clearing house, a child's immature digestive system (short abdominal LES) is usually to blame. They add that most infants grow out of GERD by the time they are 1-year-old.

Pathophysiology of GERD

At the lower end of the esophagus, where it joins the stomach, there is a circular ring of muscle called the lower esophageal sphincter (LES). Stomach content is kept in the stomach by this valve. When food reaches the LES, it relaxes so that food enters the stomach. The muscle then squeezes shut to prevent food and acid from backing up into the esophagus.

The LES is innervated by vagal nerves and receives signals from various organs. Problems with this nerve make the valve open or close. A defect in the neural control may result in a dysfunctional LES with periods of transitory spontaneous relaxation. This period of relaxation allow gastric contents to back into the esophagus (Fig. 12.4).

Moreover, the anatomical position of esophagus is between the thoracic and abdominal cavities, with the LES positioned strategically between the two. Usually LES remains in the abdominally. The greater the length of the intra-abdominal esophagus, the more competent this valve becomes. The reflux of gastric contents seen more where the abdominal segment of LES is shorter due to any reason.

Manifestations and Diagnostic Evaluation

Common GERD symptoms include vomiting after meal, hiccupping, and recurring otitis media due to pooled secretions in the nasopharynx. Besides that a dry, chronic cough; wheezing; asthma or recurrent pneumonia; nausea; vomiting; a sore throat, hoarseness, or laryngitis—swelling and irritation of the voice box; difficulty swallowing or painful swallowing; pain in the chest or the upper part of the abdomen; dental erosion and bad breath.

Immediate medical attention is needed if the child:

- Vomits large amounts or has persistent projectile, or forceful, vomiting
- Vomits fluid that is green or yellow, looks like coffee grounds, or contains blood
- Has difficulty breathing after vomiting

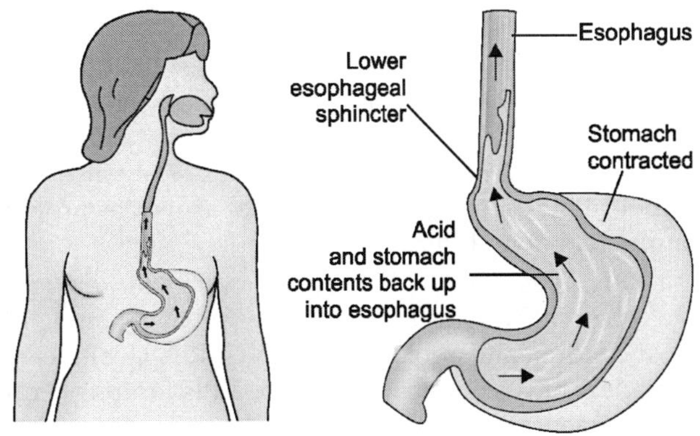

Fig. 12.4: Gastric regurgitation

- Has pain related to eating
- Has difficulty swallowing or painful swallowing
- Refuses food repeatedly, resulting in weight loss or poor weight gain
- Shows signs of dehydration, such as no tears when crying.

Diagnostic tests include barium swallow examination, upper GI series study, endoscopy, esophageal manometry, pH study, ultrasound, gastroesophageal scintigraphy, CT scan of chest.

Management

Treatment for GERD for children may involve one or more of the following, depending on the severity of symptoms: lifestyle changes, medications, or surgery.

Lifestyle Changes

Some children and adolescents can reduce GERD symptoms by:

- Losing weight, if needed
- Small frequent feeding, thickened feeding
- Caffeine and fatty foods lowers LES pressure and should be eliminated
- Wearing loose-fitting clothes around the stomach area, as tight clothing can constrict the area and increase reflux
- Remaining upright for 3 hours after meals
- Raising the head of the bed 6–8 inches by securing wood blocks under the bedposts—just using extra pillows will not help
- Keep the child away from smoking.

Medications

Antacids, which, are a first-line approach most health care providers usually recommend to relieve heartburn and other mild GERD symptoms. Antacids, however, can have side effects, including diarrhea and constipation.

H2 blockers, H2 blockers provide short-term or on-demand relief and are effective for many children and adolescents with GERD symptoms. They also can help heal the esophagus, although not as well as proton pump inhibitors (PPIs).

PPIs: PPIs are more effective than H2 blockers and can relieve symptoms and heal the esophageal lining in most children and adolescents with GERD. Health care providers most commonly prescribe PPIs for long-term management of GERD. However, studies show they are more likely to cause hip, wrist, and spinal fractures when taken long-term or in high doses. Children and adolescents should take these medications on an empty stomach in order for stomach acid to activate them.

Prokinetics help make the stomach empty faster. Prokinetics can interact with other medications, so caregivers should tell the health care provider about all medications the child or adolescent takes.

Antibiotics, including one called erythromycin, have been shown to improve gastric emptying.

Surgery

Surgery recommended when children and adolescents cannot manage severe GERD symptoms through medication or lifestyle changes. Surgery is also needed where GERD symptoms lead to severe respiratory problems. Fundoplication is the standard surgical treatment for GERD and leads to long-term reflux control in most cases. A pediatric gastroenterologist or surgeon may also use endoscopic techniques to treat GERD. Adolescents and children are more likely to develop complications from surgery than from medications; however, anti-reflux surgery is more successful in children and adolescents than in adults.

Fundoplication is an operation to sew the top of the stomach around the esophagus to add pressure to the lower end of the esophagus and reduce reflux. A pediatric surgeon performs fundoplication using a laparoscope, a thin tube with a tiny video camera attached used to look inside the body. Endoscopic techniques, such as endoscopic sewing and radiofrequency, help control GERD in a small number of children and adolescents. Endoscopic sewing uses small stitches to tighten the sphincter muscle. Radiofrequency creates heat lesions that help tighten the sphincter muscle. Surgery for both techniques requires an endoscope.

Constipation and Encopresis

Constipation and encopresis (fecal soiling) are common childhood disorders that may lead to significant functional impairment. The etiology and course of constipation and encopresis are increasingly conceptualized from a broad biopsychosocial perspective, and therefore a holistic approach to assessment and treatment is indicated. Successful treatment of constipation and encopresis requires a combination of patient and parent education, medical therapy, nutritional intervention, behavioral modification, and long-term monitoring of compliance.

Constipation basically refers to bowel movements that are hard, infrequent or difficult to pass or the sensation of incomplete bowel evacuation. Constipation is a common cause of painful defecation and/or occur less often than every 3 days, and can even escalate to menacing heights if not taken seriously. Constipation is a symptom, not a diagnosis, that has multiple etiologies and multiple alternative treatments.

Irritable Bowel Syndrome

Irritable bowel syndrome (IBS) is defined as chronic or recurrent abdominal pain, altered bowel habits, and bloating, with the absence of structural or biochemical abnormalities to explain these symptoms. IBS is not a disease; it is a group of symptoms that occur together. The most common symptoms of IBS are diffuse abdominal pain or discomfort not related to food and activity, often reported as cramping, along with diarrhea, constipation, or both.

Etiology and Incidence

The causes of IBS are not well understood. The possible causes of IBS in children include brain-gut signal problems, GI motor problems, hypersensitivity, mental health problems, bacterial gastroenteritis, small intestinal bacterial overgrowth, and genetics. In infants it is not associated with psychopathology but it may be related to lactase deficiency. Sometimes it is called nonspecific diarrhea which may occur in toddlers and adolescents.

- Limited information is available about the number of children with IBS. Thirty-three percent of adults who have irritable bowel syndrome can trace their symptoms back to childhood.
- Girls are affected by the disorder slightly more often than boys.
- There is no known gene that causes irritable bowel syndrome, but the disorder does seem to occur more often in families where either a child or a parent has the disorder.

The causes of IBS are not well understood. Researchers believe a combination of physical and mental health problems can lead to IBS. The possible causes of IBS in children include the following:

- *Brain-gut signal problems:* Signals between the brain and nerves of the small and large intestines, also called the gut, control how the intestines work. Problems with brain-gut signals may cause IBS symptoms, such as changes in bowel habits and pain or discomfort.
- *GI motor problems:* Normal motility, or movement, may not be present in the colon of a child who has IBS. Slow motility can lead to constipation and fast motility can lead to diarrhea. Spasms, or sudden strong muscle contractions that come and go, can cause abdominal pain. Some children with IBS also experience hyperreactivity, which is an excessive increase in contractions of the bowel in response to stress or eating.
- *Hypersensitivity:* Children with IBS have greater sensitivity to abdominal pain than children without IBS. Affected children have been found to have different rectal tone and rectal motor response after eating a meal.
- *Mental health problems:* IBS has been linked to mental health, or psychological, problems such as anxiety and depression in children.
- *Bacterial gastroenteritis:* Some children who have bacterial gastroenteritis—an infection or irritation of the stomach and intestines caused by bacteria—develop IBS. Research has shown a connection between gastroenteritis and IBS in adults but not in children. But researchers believe postinfectious IBS does occur in children. Researchers do not know why gastroenteritis leads to IBS in some people and not others.
- *Small intestinal bacterial overgrowth (SIBO):* Normally, few bacteria live in the small intestine. SIBO is an increase in the number of bacteria or a change in the type of bacteria in the small intestine. These bacteria can produce excess gas and may also cause diarrhea and weight loss. Some researchers believe that SIBO may lead to IBS, and some studies have shown antibiotics to be effective in treating IBS. However, the studies were weak and more research is needed to show a link between SIBO and IBS.
- *Genetics:* Whether IBS has a genetic cause, meaning it runs in families, is unclear. Studies have shown that IBS is more common in people with family members who have a history of GI problems. However, the cause could be environmental or the result of heightened awareness of GI symptoms.

Pathophysiology: Irritable bowel syndrome

Normally large intestine (colon) absorbs water and nutrients from the partially digested food that enters the colon from the small intestine. Anything that is not absorbed is slowly moved on a pathway out of your body. These undigested and unabsorbed food particles are also known as stool, a bowel movement.

In IBS, intestine gets 'irritable', but cause is unknown. The condition results in two distinct problems. To have a bowel movement, the muscles in the colon and the rest of the body have to work together. If this process is somehow interrupted, the contents of the colon can not move along very smoothly. It sorts of stops and starts, doesn't move, or sometimes moves too fast. This disorganization causes alternately diarrhea and constipation with abdominal pain. This can hurt and make a kid feel awful. The second component is excess production of mucus in the lumen of bowel. This produces mal-digestion and the passage of incompletely digested food and nutrients.

Manifestations and Diagnostic Evaluation

The abdominal pain or discomfort associates with bowel movements that occur more or less often than usual, start with stool that appears looser and more watery or harder and more lumpy than usual, improve with a bowel movement.

Other symptoms of IBS may include diarrhea—having loose, watery stools three or more times a day and feeling urgency to have a bowel movement, constipation—having hard, dry stools; two or fewer bowel movements in a week; or straining to have a bowel movement; feeling that a bowel movement is incomplete; passing mucus, a clear liquid made by the intestines that coats and protects tissues in the GI tract; abdominal bloating.

IBS is diagnosed when a child who is growing as expected has abdominal pain or discomfort once per week for at least 2 months without other disease or injury that could explain the pain. The medical history will include questions about the child's symptoms, family members with GI disorders, recent infections, medications, and stressful events related to the onset of symptoms. IBS is diagnosed when major GI pathologic conditions (Crohn's disease, lactose intolerance, giardiasis) are excluded and the physical exam does not show any cause for the child's symptoms and the child meets all of the following criteria:

- has had symptoms at least once per week for at least 2 months
- is growing as expected
- is not showing any signs that suggest another cause for the symptoms

Investigations often used to diagnose IBS are stool for ova and parasites and culture, ultrasound, radiologic examinations of abdomen, and age appropriate gynecologic examination.

Therapeutic and Nursing Management

Though there is no cure for IBS, the management targets to identify and reduce the triggers and reducing the bowel spasms. The primary nursing intervention is to give mental support and explanation regarding this self-limiting problem. The symptoms can be treated with a combination of the changes in eating, diet, and nutrition, medications, probiotics, therapies for mental health problems.

Nutrition

Large meals can cause cramping and diarrhea, so eating smaller meals more often, or eating smaller portions, may help IBS symptoms. Eating meals that are low in fat and high in carbohydrates, such as pasta, rice, whole-grain breads and cereals, fruits, and vegetables may help.

Certain foods and drinks may cause IBS symptoms in some children, such as:

- Foods high in fat
- Milk products
- Drinks with caffeine
- Drinks with large amounts of artificial sweeteners, which are substances used in place of sugar
- Foods that may cause gas, such as beans and cabbage

Dietary fiber may lessen constipation in children with IBS, but it may not help with lowering pain. Fiber helps keep stool soft so it moves smoothly through the colon. The Academy of Nutrition and Dietetics recommends children consume 'age plus 5' grams of fiber daily. A 7-year-old child, for example, should get '7 plus 5,' or 12 grams, of fiber a day. Fiber may cause gas and trigger symptoms in some children with IBS. Increasing fiber intake by 2–3 grams per day may help reduce the risk of increased gas and bloating.

Medications

The health care provider will select medications based on the child's symptoms. Caregivers should not give children any medications unless told to do so by a health care provider.

- *Fiber supplements:* Fiber supplements may be recommended to relieve constipation when increasing dietary fiber is ineffective.
- *Laxatives:* Constipation can be treated with laxative medications. Laxatives work in different ways, and a health care provider can provide information about which type is best. Caregivers should not give children laxatives unless told to do so by a health care provider.
- *Antidiarrheals:* Loperamide has been found to reduce diarrhea in children with IBS, though it does not reduce pain, bloating, or other symptoms. Loperamide reduces stool frequency and improves stool consistency by slowing the movement of stool through the colon. Medications to treat diarrhea in adults can be dangerous for infants and children and should only be given if told to do so by a health care provider.
- *Antispasmodics:* Antispasmodics, such as hyoscine, cimetropium, and pinaverium, help to control colon muscle spasms and reduce abdominal pain.

- *Antidepressants:* Tricyclic antidepressants and selective serotonin reuptake inhibitors in low doses can help relieve IBS symptoms including abdominal pain. These medications are thought to reduce the perception of pain, improve mood and sleep patterns, and adjust the activity of the GI tract.

Probiotics

Probiotics are live microorganisms, usually bacteria, that are similar to microorganisms normally found in the GI tract. Studies have found that probiotics, specifically *Bifidobacteria* and certain probiotic combinations, improve symptoms of IBS when taken in large enough amounts. But more research is needed. Probiotics can be found in dietary supplements, such as capsules, tablets, and powders, and in some foods, such as yogurt. A health care provider can give information about the right kind and right amount of probiotics to take to improve IBS symptoms. More information about probiotics can be found in the National Center for Complementary and Alternative Medicine fact sheet—An Introduction to Probiotics.

Therapies for Mental Health Problems

The following therapies can help improve IBS symptoms due to mental health problems:

- *Talk therapy:* Talking with a therapist may reduce stress and improve IBS symptoms. Two types of talk therapy used to treat IBS are cognitive behavioral therapy and psychodynamic, or interpersonal, therapy. Cognitive behavioral therapy focuses on the child's thoughts and actions. Psychodynamic therapy focuses on how emotions affect IBS symptoms. This type of therapy often involves relaxation and stress management techniques.
- *Hypnotherapy:* In hypnotherapy, the therapist uses hypnosis to help the child relax into a trancelike state. This type of therapy may help the child relax the muscles in the colon.

Most children with irritable bowel syndrome continue to grow and develop normally. However, some children may eat less to avoid the pain that can accompany digestion, and therefore, lose weight. They do not feel well, may be embarrassed and avoid socialization with friends. Its greatest morbidity resides in the fact that it affects normal daily activity of the child, affecting school or peer relations. Environmental modification is important to identify the stresses surrounding the child and reverse them. Parents and school teachers must support the child rather than concentrating on the pain. Try to help the child focus on something fun or pleasant during a painful episode.

INFLAMMATORY AND INFECTIOUS DISORDERS

Peptic Ulcer Disease

Peptic ulcer disease (PUD) in children is reported worldwide, although it is relatively rare as compared with adults. **Peptic ulcers** are ulcers that form in the stomach or the upper part of the small intestine, called the duodenum. An ulcer in the stomach is called a **gastric ulcer** and an ulcer in the duodenum is called a **duodenal ulcer**. Most primary ulcers occur in the absence of predisposing factor and tend to be chronic, occurring more frequently in the duodenum. Stress ulcer is occurred due to stress of a severe underlying disease or injury (sepsis, burn, severe trauma, multi-organ failure), which are frequently acute and gastric. Primary ulcers are common in older children (more than 6 years), stress ulcers are common in infants younger than 6 months.

Etiology

The etiology of peptic ulcer disease remains unclear. Besides genetic factors, infectious and environmental factors appear to play an important role. The mucous—bicarbonate barrier in children is altered due to several reasons like.

Helicobacter pylori (HP), gram negative spiral bacterium infection is a common cause of PUD in the pediatric age. It may cause ulcers by weakening the gastric mucosal barrier and allowing acid to damage the mucosa (Figs 12.5A and B). *H. pylori* infection also induces an inflammatory reaction that reduces bicarbonate secretion by duodenal epithelial cells. Thus, the capacity of the duodenal mucosa to buffer the caustic effects of gastric acid is reduced.

Excessive acid secretion, and multiple ulcers are occurred in Zollinger-Ellison syndrome, hyperthyroidism, etc.

Prostaglandins augment both the mucous gel lining and bicarbonate secretion. Impairment of the mucous—bicarbonate barrier of stomach is caused due to deficiency of mucosal secretion of prostaglandins.

Other risk factors include the use of nonsteroidal anti-inflammatory agents (NSAIDs), steroids, immunosuppressive drugs, and stressful events.

Emotional factors also seem to be important. Children with peptic ulcer disease tend to be of above-average intelligence, are often overachievers who have trouble dealing with frustration, and tend to internalize their feelings.

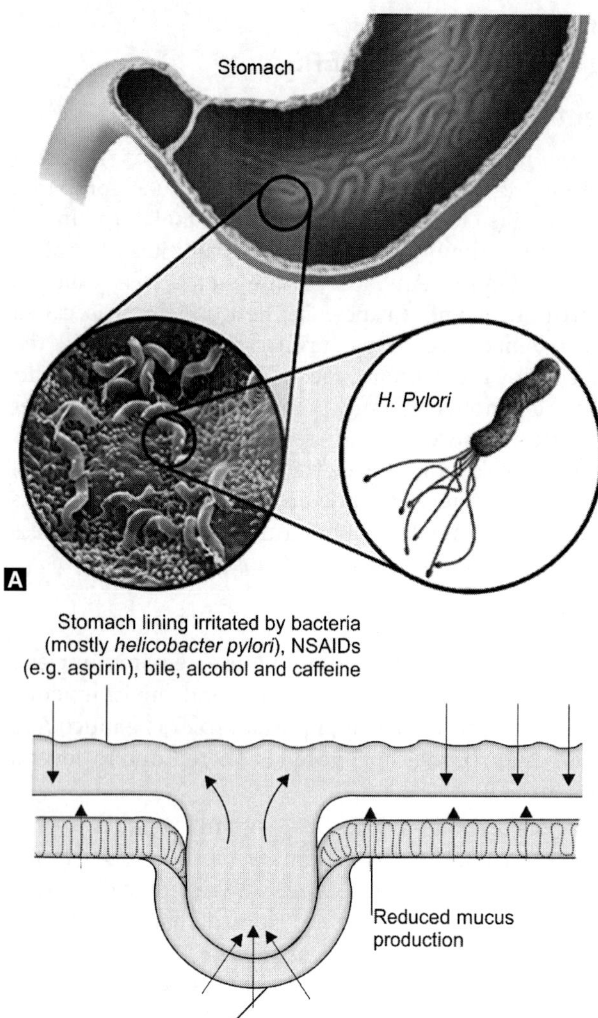

Figs 12.5A and B: Stomach ulcer due to *H. Pylori* infection

Recently, local factors such as gastric mucus, alkaline secretion by the gastric mucosal cells, gastric blood flow, and prostaglandins have been shown to be important in local tissue resistance to acid and to digestive enzymes.

> **Pathophysiology**
>
> **Peptic ulcer disease (PUD)** is a distinct breach in the mucosa of the stomach as a result of caustic effects of acid and pepsin in the lumen. Histologically, peptic ulcer is identified as necrosis of the mucosa which produces lesions equal to or greater than 0.5 cm (1/5").
>
> The stomach and duodenum is lined by thick mucus layer (mucus-bicarbonate layer) which acts as buffer zone for acid neutralization. Surface epithelial cells liberate bicarbonate

Contd...

Contd...

> ions and diffuse stomach acids slowly. The establishment of a neutral pH at the gastric epithelial surface provides protection from the combined effects of acid and pepsin. The disruption of equilibrium between aggressive and protective factors of gastric secretion precipitates ulcers in the stomach and duodenum. Due to some factors (HP infection, inflammation) peptic ulcers tend to occur within the section of the GI tract that is in contact of gastric juice containing acid and pepsin.

Diagnostic Evaluation

The diagnosis of peptic ulcer includes taking of history, physical examination and diagnostic testing. Although gnawing pain, burning discomfort, and tenderness in the epigastric area are the symptoms and signs most commonly associated with PUD, focus to be given on oral regurgitation, nocturnal pain, hematemesis, heartburn. Nausea and vomiting may also occur in conjunction with the pain. The finding of occult blood in the stool definitely warrants a diagnostic evaluation.

The timing of the symptoms in relation to the meal may differentiate between gastric and duodenal ulcers: A gastric ulcer would give epigastric pain during the meal, as gastric acid production is increased as food enters the stomach. Symptoms of duodenal ulcers would initially be relieved by a meal, as the pyloric sphincter closes to concentrate the stomach contents, therefore acid is not reaching the duodenum. Duodenal ulcer pain would manifest mostly 2–3 hours after the meal, when the stomach begins to release digested food and acid into the duodenum.

Laboratory Studies may Include

An upper GI tract radiographic series with small bowel follow-through should be done first. If this is nondiagnostic in a child with persistent pain or in a child with blood in the stool, upper GI tract endoscopy is indicated. This procedure can usually be done under local sedation with minimal discomfort, either psychologic or physical, to the patient; to visualize the lining of esophagus, stomach and proximal end of duodenum and to collect biopsy or culture material. Ultrasound may be done to rule out gallstones, tumours and any other obstruction. The fecal occult blood test may be done to check for GI bleeding.

So, the diagnostic tests include endoscopy and upper GI barium X-ray, analysis of stool specimens for occult blood, gastric secretory studies, and biopsy and histology with culture to detect *H. pylori* (serologic testing, stool antigen tests, or a breath test may also detect *H. pylori*).

Therapeutic Management

The goal of ulcer treatment is to relieve pain, heal the ulcer, and prevent complications.

Hydrochloric acid has traditionally been implicated in the pathogenesis of peptic ulcer and most therapies are directed at either 'neutralizing' acid or blocking its secretion. Antacids neutralize existing acid in the stomach. However, the neutralizing action of these agents is short-lived, and frequent dosing is required. Magnesium containing antacids, can cause diarrhea, while aluminum containing agents can cause constipation. Ulcers frequently return when antacids are discontinued.

H2 receptor antagonists and proton pump inhibitor drugs are prescribed for suppression of acid secretion in the stomach. PPIs are the drugs of choice for managing patients with peptic ulcers, regardless of the cause. They suppress the production of stomach acid by blocking the gastric acid pump–the molecule in the stomach glands that is responsible for acid secretion.

PPIs can be used either as part of a multidrug regimen for *H. pylori*, or alone for preventing and healing NSAID-caused ulcers. They are also useful for treating ulcers caused by Zollinger-Ellison syndrome. They are considered to be more effective than H2 blockers.

Drugs used to strengthen gastric mucous lining are misoprostol (cytotec), sucralfate (carafe), etc.

When the underlying cause of PUD is addressed, the prognosis is excellent. Antibiotics combined with proton pump inhibitors and bismuth salts to suppress *H. Pylori* (HP). Standard triple therapy, bismuth-based quadruple therapy, and the sequential therapy represent the current recommended treatments for *Helicobacter pylori* related ulcers. Eradication of the bacteria *H. pylori* not only heals ulcers but also prevents the recurrence of ulcer disease.

NSAIDs related ulcers are treated by stopping the causative medications and by administration of proton-pump inhibitors or anti-secretory drugs.

Diet—There is no conclusive evidence that dietary restrictions and bland diets play a role in ulcer healing. Usually a diet for PUD is designed to accomplish the following:

- Restrict or avoid those foods that may cause irritation to the digestive system
- Reduce excessive acid production
- Prevent unpleasant side effects, such as heartburn.

Large amounts of food should be avoided, as it stretches the stomach and can result in pain. Four to five small meals a day are suggested instead of 3 larger meals. Small frequent feeding with milk is not recommended as protein and calcium of milk stimulate more acid secretions.

Diet rich in fiber, especially from fruits and vegetables, poly unsaturated oils are prescribed.

It is important to take rest and relax a few minutes before and after each meal, as well as remaining relaxed during meals.

A regular diet low in caffeine is generally recommended because caffeine is a potent stimulant of acid secretion and exacerbates GERD.

Surgery

With the advent of H2 receptor antagonists, surgical intervention is less common.

- If recommended, surgery is usually for intractable ulcers (particularly with Zollinger–Ellison syndrome), life threatening hemorrhage, perforation, or obstruction. Surgical procedures include vagotomy, vagotomy with pyloroplasty, or Billroth I or II.
- Patients with ulcer bleeding may report passage of black tarry stools (melena), weakness, a sense of passing out upon standing (orthostatic syncope), and vomiting blood (hematemesis). Initial treatment involves rapid replacement of lost blood intravenously, usually with fluids. Patients with persistent or severe bleeding may require blood transfusions. An endoscopy is performed to establish the site of bleeding and to stop active ulcer bleeding with the aid of specialized endoscopic instruments.

Nursing Considerations

The major focus of nursing care is teaching, which includes review of pathophysiology of peptic ulcer, medication administration, diet and early assessment of complications.

Nursing assessment includes pain assessment and methods used to relieve it; a thorough history, food habits, medication use (NSAIDs), and level of tension or nervousness, family history of ulcer disease.

Assess vital signs for indicators of anemia (tachycardia, hypotension), hematemesis present or not.

Assess for blood in the stools with an occult blood test. Palpate abdomen for localized tenderness.

The major goals of the patient may include relief of pain, reduced anxiety, maintenance of nutritional requirements, knowledge about the management and prevention of ulcer recurrence, and absence of complications.

Nursing interventions include:

- Administration of prescribed medications.
- Avoid aspirin, which is an anticoagulant, and foods and beverages that contain acid enhancing caffeine (colas, tea, chocolate), along with decaffeinated coffee.
- Regularly spaced feeding of the child is to be done in a relaxed atmosphere; obtain regular weights.

Health Education

- Assist the patient in understanding the condition and factors that help or aggravate it.
- Orient the patient and caregivers about personal hygiene, food hygiene
- Teach patient about prescribed medications, including name, dosage, frequency, and possible side effects. Also identify medications such as aspirin that patient should avoid.

Parent Teaching

- Instruct parent about particular foods that will upset the gastric mucosa, such as coffee, tea, colas which have acid producing potential.
- Encourage parent to feed child regular meals in a relaxed setting and to avoid overeating.
- Teach stress reduction activities
- Do not administer antacids within one hour of other antiulcer medicines
- Do not use over the counter medications without consulting physician.
- Alert parent to signs and symptoms of complications to be reported. These complications include hemorrhage (cool skin, confusion, increased heart rate, labored breathing, and blood in the stool), penetration and perforation (severe abdominal pain, rigid and tender abdomen, vomiting, elevated temperature, and increased heart rate), and pyloric obstruction (nausea, vomiting, distended abdomen, and abdominal pain). To identify obstruction, insert and monitor nasogastric tube; more than 400 mL residual suggests obstruction.

CONCLUSION

PUD still represents a major concern in the pediatric age. A careful differential diagnosis and an adequate treatment constitute an excellent prognosis. PUD may persists into adult life if adequate treatment not provided to the child.

Infectious Gastroenteritis

Gastroenteritis is a bowel infection which causes diarrhea (runny, watery stool) and sometimes vomiting. Infective gastroenteritis in young children is characterised by the sudden onset of diarrhea, with or without vomiting. Most cases are due to a viral infection but some are caused by bacterial or protozoal infections (Table 12.1). The illness usually resolves without treatment within days but severe diarrhea can rapidly cause dehydration, which may be life-threatening. Acute gastroenteritis accounts for millions of deaths each year in young children, mostly in developing communities.

Gastroenteritis literally means inflammation of the GI tract, involves both the **stomach** (*'gastro'*-) and the small intestine (*'entero'*), resulting in some combination of **diarrhea**, **vomiting**, and **abdominal** pain and cramping. Viral gastroenteritis is also called 'stomach flu.' The severity can range from a mild tummy upset for a day or two with some mild diarrhea, to severe diarrhea and vomiting for several days or longer. It is extremely common, especially in children, and is highly contagious. Many viruses, bacteria and other microbes (germs) can cause gastroenteritis and may result in massive fluid and electrolyte loss, sepsis, and death.

Etiology and Incidence

Acute gastroenteritis accounts for millions of deaths each year in young children, mostly in developing communities. Worldwide, 3–5 billion cases of acute gastroenteritis and nearly 2 million deaths occur each year in children under 5 years. Children with poor nutrition are at increased risk of complications. In the developing countries children are brought for admission with gastroenteritis, malnutrition, comorbidity, and electrolyte disturbance (especially hypokalemia) and stay a longer period in the hospital for treatment.

A virus is the most common cause of gastroenteritis. Rotavirus, norovirus, and astrovirus are known to cause viral gastroenteritis. Rotavirus is the most common virus causing gastroenteritis in children below 5 years, and produces similar incidence rates in both developed and developing world. Viruses cause about 70% of episodes of infectious diarrhea in the pediatric age group. Rotavirus is less common in adults due to acquired immunity. Adenoviruse are another common group of viruses that cause gastroenteritis in children under 2 years of age. Adenovirus and rotavirus infection are more common in infants and younger children than in teenagers. Like the adenovirus, astrovirus can infect people of all ages but is most likely to affect infants and

Table 12.1: Infectious gastroenteritis: Difference in characteristics

Infectious Agent	*Charateristics*	*Clinical manifestations*	*Diagnostic findings*	*Treatment*
Rotavirus	Incubation 1–3 days	Symptoms usually last for 2-6 days. H/O Preceding or concurrent resp. illness	Virus in stool detected by enzyme Immunoassay test	No drug treatment. Contact precautions
Giardia lamblia	Common cause of parasitic diarrhea Water borne infection	No fever, abdominal distension, flatulence, Variable diarrhea	Ova and parasites fond in stool, no blood Or PMNs Parasites found on duodenal biopsy	Metronidazole for 7 days Contact precautions Safe drinking water (with chlorine/iodine)
Shigella (entero invasive with cytotoxin)	Incubation period 1–7 days. Most common in summer Fecal – oral spread Remains communicable For 1–3 weeks	Symptoms last for 5–10 days Watery stool in the beginning, then small stool with blood and mucus Severe abdominal pain, High fever Neurologic symptoms (headache, nuchal rigidity, convulsions)	Blood, mucus, WBCs in stool. Low platelet count, poor kidney function, low blood cell count	Bactrim 8–10 mg/kg/day × 5 days OR Ampicillin 50–100 mg/kg/day × 5 days Contact precautions Identify source if possible
Salmonella (enteroinvasive)	Incubation 6 hr to 3 days Usually food borne infection Common in summer	Secretory diarrhea, abdominal pain, nausea and vomiting for 2–5 days	Blood and PMNs in stool	For infants younger than 12 weeks, same as for shigella. Contact precautions Source identification if possible
Escherichia coli (enteroinvasive with cytotoxin)	Variable incubation Most common in Summer. Food borne most common	Green and watery stool, fever, secretory diarrhea.	Blood and PMNs in stool Low platelet count, poor kidney function, low blood cell count	Same as *Shigella*. Contact precautions
Compylobacter	Incubation 2–5 days. Raw and undercooked poultry, unpasteurized milk, contaminated water	It is characterized by inflammatory, sometimes bloody diarrhea or dysentery syndrome, mostly including cramps, fever, and pain		The infection is usually self-limiting and in most cases, symptomatic treatment by liquid and electrolyte replacement is enough in human infections. The use of antibiotics, though, is controversial.Symptoms typically last five to seven days.

young children. It is most common in winter, although it can occur at any time of year.

From the feces, viruses find their way into food or water or onto insects or people who later touch and contaminate food (fecal-oral transmission). Unfortunately, these viruses are tough enough to beat modern sanitation practices. Viruses cause disease by infecting or irritating cells within the wall of the small intestine. This causes fluids, minerals, and salts to flush into the intestines, leaving the body as diarrhea.

Food poisoning results when a person eats food that has grown bacteria that can cause gastroenteritis. The symptoms of food poisoning are caused either by the bacteria themselves or by the byproducts (toxins) they produce. Symptoms of food poisoning can begin within a few hours or a few days after eating the contaminated food, depending on whether the bacteria or the toxin causes the problem.

Manifestations

- The main symptom is diarrhea, often with vomiting as well. Diarrhea means loose or watery stools (faeces), usually at least three times in 24 hours. Blood or mucus can appear in the stools with some infections.

- Crampy pains in the abdomen (tummy) are common. Pains may ease for a while each time some diarrhea is passed.
- A high temperature (fever), headache and aching limbs sometimes occur.
- A child with a significant degree of dehydration may have a prolonged capillary refill, poor skin turgor, and abnormal breathing. It occurs if the water and salts that are lost in child's stools, or when they vomit, are not replaced by them drinking enough fluids.

Diagnostic Evaluation

- Gastroenteritis should be suspected if there is a sudden change in stool consistency to loose or watery stools, and/or a sudden onset of vomiting.
- Children are often febrile with any type of infective gastroenteritis. Check temperature, blood pressure, pulse rate and and respiratory rate.
- Bloody diarrhea should arouse suspicion of bacterial infection. Bloody diarrhea in children, when due to acute enteric infection, is usually caused by either *Campylobacter* , and *E. coli* infections.
- Most children do not become significantly dehydrated but always assess for the presence and degree of dehydration. Assess for features of dehydration:
  - *Mild dehydration:* lassitude, anorexia, nausea, light-headedness, postural hypotension.
  - *Moderate dehydration:* Apathy, tiredness, dizziness, muscle cramps, dry tongue, sunken eyes, reduced skin elasticity, postural hypotension (systolic blood pressure >90 mmHg), tachycardia, oliguria.
  - *Severe dehydration:* Profound apathy, weakness, confusion (leading to coma), shock, tachycardia, marked peripheral vasoconstriction, systolic blood pressure <90 mmHg, oliguria or anuria.
- Abdominal examination (including any areas of tenderness, any masses, distension and bowel sounds) is to be done. Record findings, even if negative. Always repeat a thorough examination if the situation changes or does not settle as expected.
- *Stool investigations:* Microscopy (include ova, cysts and parasites), culture and sensitivity.

A stool sample should be sent for microbiological investigation if there is blood and/or mucus in the stool.

Other potential causes of signs and symptoms that mimic those seen in gastroenteritis that need to be ruled out include appendicitis, volvulus, inflammatory bowel disease, urinary tract infections and diabetes mellitus.

Dehydration

Severity clinical signs of dehydration (Fig. 12.6)			
	Mild	*Moderate*	*Severe*
Water loss	< 5%	50~100 mL/kg	10~120 mL/kg
By weight spirit	< 5% Slightly dispirited Slightly agitated	5%~10% Dispirited Agitated	> 10% Extremely dispirited apathy, hypnody, coma
Skin Mocous	Slightly dry Slightly dry	Dry pale Very dry	Gray mottled Parched
Anterior fontanel and eye ball	Slightly depressed	Depressed	Depressed greatly
Tear Urine output Peripheral circulation	Normal Slightly reduced Normal	Reduced Little or No Little cool	No No urine output Cool, weak pulse, shock

Therapeutic Management and Nursing Considerations

Gastroenteritis is usually an acute and self-limiting disease that does not require medication. Diarrhea is the manifestation of secretion/absorption disturbance and disordered motility: a symptom of damage already done in the infected gut. Antidiarrheal medication is not advised. Antidiarrheal formulations aim to reduce intestinal motility, reduce secretion of water and electrolytes, and adsorb fluid and toxins, thereby reducing the number of stools seen in the diaper; however, none treat the cause of diarrhea or actual pathology, and their use may be associated with more

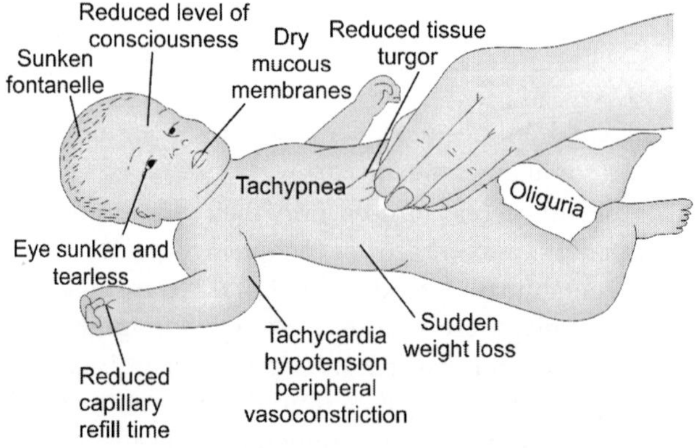

Fig. 12.6: Signs and symptoms of dehydration

side-effects in young children than in adults. The preferred treatment in those with mild to moderate dehydration is oral rehydration therapy (ORT).

Rehydration Therapy

Dehydration is classified into three types on the basis of osmolality and depends on the sodium level in the blood: (1) isotonic, (2) hypotonic, (3) hypertonic. When dehydration does not affect the concentration of sodium in the extracellular fluid, it is called isonatremic dehydration or isotonic or iso-osmolar dehydration.

When dehydration results in an increased sodium concentration of the extracellular fluid, it is called hypernatremic dehydration or hypertonic or hyperosmolar dehydration.

When dehydration results in a decreased sodium concentration of the extracellular fluids, it is called hyponatremic or hypotonic or hypoosmolar dehydration.

Dehydration, electrolyte disturbance and metabolic acidosis in gastroenteritis can be prevented and treated by fluid therapy. Optimal management with oral or intravenous fluids minimises the risk of dehydration and its adverse outcomes.

Most children with mild-moderate dehydration can be treated with oral or enteral rehydration using low osmolality oral rehydration solutions. Maintenance therapy includes providing anticipated water and electrolyte needs for the next 24 hours in the child who is now euvolemic with expected normal urine output. Severely dehydrated or shocked children usually need IV fluids and institutional care. Intravenous fluids are administered whenever the child is unable to ingest sufficient amount of fluid and electrolytes. This fluid replacement therapy aims to (1) meet ongoing daily physiologic losses, (2) replace previous deficits, and (3) replace ongoing abnormal losses.

Oral rehydration solutions usually come in sachets and are available without a prescription, over the counter. Dissolve them in water helps in replace of salt, glucose and other important minerals that are lost through dehydration. If child vomits after drinking an oral rehydration solution, 5–10 minutes time to be given before giving them some more. However, drink to be given slowly; may be a spoonful every few minutes.

It is usually recommended that child drinks an oral rehydration solution each time they pass a large amount of watery stools. The exact amount that they should drink will depend on their size and weight. A home-made salt-and-sugar solution (SSS) (half a teaspoon of salt plus 8 teaspoons of sugar per litre of water) is useful, but of unpredictably variable concentration may aggravate dehydration. However, glucose-linked sodium absorption with secondary water uptake is maintained even in secretory states like cholera. This is the basis of oral rehydration therapy (ORT). Hypotonic fluids with a sodium content of 45–65 mmol/l (e.g. rehidrat, sorol) allow more rapid rehydration than fluids with a higher sodium content,but hypertonic sugar-based drinks with little sodium (e.g. cola and sports drinks) may result in osmotic aggravation.

Daily fluid requirement of child	*Model for rehydration in child's diarrhea*
Calculate body weight of child in kg	Rehydration solution should contain 75–90 mEq of sodium (Na+)/Liter Administer 40 to 50 mL/kg of rehydration solution.
Allow 100 mL fluid/kg for first 10 kg	Replacement and maintenance solution should contain 40–60 mEq of Na^+ per Liter.
Allow 50 mL fluid/kg for second 10 kg	Re-evaluate the child's need for further rehydration; initiate maintenance therapy using maintenance formulations; and daily volume should not exceed 150 mL/kg/day
Allow 20 mL/kg for reminder of weight in kg	If additional fluids are required, low salt fluids such as breast milk or water to be given
Hourly fluid requirement of child	
Calculate body weight of child in kg Allow 4 mL fluid/kg for first 10 kg Allow 2 mL fluid/kg for second 10 kg Allow 1 mL/kg for reminder of weight in kg	

The primary treatment of gastroenteritis in both children and adults is rehydration. This is preferably achieved by oral rehydration therapy, although intravenous delivery may be required if a there is a decreased level of consciousness or if dehydration is severe. Oral replacement therapy products made with complex carbohydrates (i.e. those made from wheat or rice) may be superior to those based on simple sugars. Drinks especially high in simple sugars, such as soft drinks and fruit juices, are not recommended in children under 5 years of age as they may increase diarrhea. Plain water may be used if more specific and effective ORT preparations are unavailable or are not palatable. A nasogastric tube can be used in young children to administer fluids if warranted.

Dietary Interventions

It is recommended that breastfed infants continue to be nursed in the usual fashion, and that formula-fed infants continue their formula immediately after rehydration with ORT. Lactose-free or lactose-reduced formulas usually are not necessary. Children should continue their usual diet during episodes of diarrhea with the exception that foods high in simple sugars should be avoided. The BRATT (bananas, rice, applesauce, toast and tea) is no longer recommended, as it contains insufficient nutrients (low in energy and protein), low in electrolytes and has no benefit over normal feeding.

Consumption of solid food should be guided by appetite. Small, light meals are to be given and avoidance of fatty, spicy, or heavy food is needed. There is little evidence on any benefit of fasting or dieting for the treatment of acute diarrhea. Starchy simple foods are best try and offer foods such as bread or toast, porridge, rice, potatoes, plain biscuits, yoghurt, milk pudding.

Some probiotics have been shown to be beneficial in reducing both the duration of illness and the frequency of stools. They may also be useful in preventing and treating antibiotic associated diarrhea. Fermented milk products (such as yogurt) are similarly beneficial.

Zinc supplementation appears to be effective in both treating and preventing diarrhea among children in the developing world.

Foods and drinks should not be given to the child with diarrhea are:

- Fluid/juice contains too much sugar and can make child's diarrhea worse
- Coffee and tea—these can make child become dehydrated
- Fatty or sugary foods such as chippies, sweets, cakes, chocolate, ice cream, cream, coconut cream
- Chicken or meat broth is not given as it contains excessive sodium and inadequate carbohydrate.

Treatment

Diarrhea is the manifestation of secretion/absorption disturbance and disordered motility, a symptom of damage already done in the infected gut. Drugs are usually unnecessary and may do harm. The body clears out the virus on its own without treatment. Prevention is the key to controlling gastroenteritis, and recently licensed, highly effective rotavirus vaccines will have a major effect on public health.

Antidiarrheal medication is not advised. Antidiarrheal formulations aim to reduce intestinal motility, reduce secretion of water and electrolytes, and adsorb fluid and toxins, thereby reducing the number of stools seen in the diaper; however, none treat the cause of diarrhea or actual pathology, and their use may be associated with more side-effects in young children than in adults. Furthermore, adsorbents (e.g. kaolin) hide the true extent of water loss, risking underestimation of the amount of fluid required for hydration in severe diarrhea.

Drugs are usually unnecessary and may do harm. Routine use of antibiotics, antidiarrheal agents, and antiemetics is not recommended in gastroenteritis as it may cause harm. Viral gastro cannot be treated with antibiotics. The body clears out the virus on its own without treatment. Prevention is the key to controlling gastroenteritis, and recently licensed, highly effective rotavirus vaccines will have a major effect on public health.

Antibiotics

Major cause of infective gastroenteritis of children is viral origin and viral gastro cannot be treated with antibiotics. The body clears out the virus on its own without treatment. Antibiotics are not recommended with acute diarrhea of unknown pathology but may be appropriate when gastroenteritis is due to a known bacterial or protozoal cause.

In bacterial infection, antibiotic therapy generally does not shorten the length of diarrhea, except when administered early in the case of dysentery (ciprofloxacin for 3 days is recommended). Rather, antibiotics are required to prevent or limit the spread of infection to others (e.g. early in cholera), and should be prescribed for evident parenteral infection (e.g. urinary tract infection or otitis media). In those with *Giardia* species or *Entamoeba histolytica*, tinidazole treatment is recommended and superior to metronidazole. The WHO recommends the use of antibiotics in young children who have both bloody diarrhea and fever.

Antiemetics

Vomiting is largely attributed to local factors and poor gastric emptying, and should not be treated with antiemetic drugs. Cyclizine and prochlorperazine have not proven useful and may carry a higher risk of toxic side-effects in young infants, and in the presence of dehydration. Ondansetron is moderately effective, but the cost and quantity required for a clinically significant effect negates general recommendation.

In early gastroenteritis, solids or foods with a high protein, fat or fibre content slow down gastric emptying and may aggravate vomiting. Substitution with a clear, hypotonic fluid may result in earlier cessation of vomiting.

Abdominal Pain

Abdominal pain is usually spasmodic due to disordered motility, or is associated with colitis in dysentery. Metoclopramide should be considered in severe pain, at a dose of 0.1 mg/kg of body mass to a maximum of 10 mg; a total daily dose of 0.5 mg/kg should not be exceeded. The extrapyramidal side-effects of metoclopramide in young infants should warrant caution. Frequent small oral sips of a clear hypotonic glucose-containing fluid correct ketosis and prevent gastric overdistension, in addition to contributing to rehydration.

Antimotility Agents

Antimotility drugs should be avoided if there is blood and/or mucus in the stools, or high fever.

Loperamide, an opioid analogue, is commonly used for the symptomatic treatment of diarrhea. Loperamide is not recommended in children, however, as it may cross the immature blood–brain barrier and cause toxicity.

Micronutrient

Zinc acetate for 2 weeks reduces duration and recurrence risks.

Care of Buttock

Diarrheal stools are highly irritating to the skin and care is needed to protect the skin from excoriation. Diarrhea can cause a rash; after each bowel motion wash and dry child's buttock well and then apply a protective cream or ointment (such as zinc and castor oil cream or vaseline).

Gastroenteritis: Antibiotics

Routine use of antibiotics, antidiarrheal agents, and antiemetics is not recommended and may cause harm. Prevention is the key to controlling gastroenteritis, and diarrheal diseases.

Antibiotics are not routinely used to treat gastroenteritis in children because:

- Most cases of gastroenteritis in children are caused by viruses (the rotavirus).
- Even if gastroenteritis is caused by bacteria, research shows that antibiotics are often no more effective than waiting for the symptoms to pass, and they can cause unpleasant side effects.
- Every time antibiotics are used to treat mild conditions, their effectiveness for treating more serious conditions is reduced.

Preventing gastroenteritis

As gastroenteritis is highly infectious. Routine use of antibiotics, antidiarrheal agents, and antiemetics is not recommended and may cause harm. Prevention is the key to controlling gastroenteritis. It is important to take steps to prevent it from spreading to other people. These include:

- Full and exclusive breastfeeding on demand: this protects against intestinal infections prevents exposure to environmental contamination. Breastfed babies under 6 months of age do not require water supplements, even in hot weather.
- Washing hands thoroughly after going to the toilet and before eating or preparing food, especially after going to the toilet, after nappy changing and before handling food; encourage your child to wash and dry their hands after using the toilet.
- Provision of safe water for drinking and food preparation. Avoiding sharing food and drink.
- Full immunisation including rotavirus vaccines: the new rotavirus vaccines are safe and reduce the severity of infection and prevent deaths, but they do not prevent all cases of rotavirus diarrhea.
- Safe disposal of human and other waste.
- Child should be kept away from friends and other children until vomiting and diarrhea have stopped; children with diarrhea must stay away from daycare, kindergarten and school until the diarrhea has stopped.

Complications

- Dehydration and electrolyte imbalance is a common complication of gastroenteritis. Hypernatremia, hyponatremia, and hypoglycemia occasionally complicate dehydration. Serum electrolyte levels should be measured in children with severe dehydration and in those with moderate dehydration that presents in atypical ways.
- **Repeat infections** are typically seen in areas with poor sanitation, and malnutrition, stunted growth, and long-term cognitive delays can result.
- **Reactive complications.** Rarely, other parts of the body can react to an infection that occurs in the gut. This can cause symptoms such as arthritis (joint inflammation), skin inflammation and eye inflammation (either conjunctivitis or uveitis). Reactive complications are uncommon if it is a virus causing gastroenteritis.
- **Spread of infection** to other parts of your child's body such as their bones, joints, or the meninges that surround their brain and spinal cord. This is rare. If it does occur, it is more likely if gastroenteritis is caused by *Salmonella* spp. infection.
- **Irritable bowel syndrome** is sometimes triggered by a bout of gastroenteritis.
- **Lactose intolerance** can sometimes occur for a while after gastroenteritis. It is known as secondary or

acquired lactose intolerance. Your child's gut lining can be damaged by the episode of gastroenteritis. This leads to lack of an enzyme (chemical) called lactase that is needed to help the body digest a sugar called lactose that is in milk. Lactose intolerance leads to bloating, abdominal pain, wind and watery stools after drinking milk. The condition gets better when the infection is over and the gut lining heals.

- **Hemolytic uremic syndrome** is a rare complication. It is usually associated with gastroenteritis caused by a certain type of *E. coli* infection–*E. coli O157*. It is a serious condition where there is anemia, a low platelet count in the blood and kidney failure. If recognized and treated, most children recover well.
- **Malnutrition** may follow some gut infections. This is mainly a risk for children in developing countries.
- Repeat infections are typically seen in areas with poor sanitation, and malnutrition, stunted growth, and long-term cognitive delays can result.
- Risk of infection is higher in children due to their lack of immunity and relatively poor hygiene. Risk is greatest at the extremes of life and those with immunocompromise (PLHIV).

Dysentery

Dysentery is a type of gastroenteritis. Dysentery is an inflammatory disorder of the intestine, especially of the colon, marked by frequent watery stools, often with blood and mucus. It is clinically characterized by abdominal pain, tenesmus, fever, and dehydration.

> **Pathophysiology : Dysentery**
>
> Each specific pathogen has its own mechanism or pathogenesis, but in general the result is damage to the intestinal lining, leading to the inflammatory immune response. They penetrate the lining of the intestine, causing swelling, ulcerations, and severe diarrhea containing blood and pus. This can cause elevated temperature, painful spasms of the intestinal muscles (cramping), swelling due to water leaking from capillaries of the intestine (edema), and further tissue damage by the body's immune cells and the chemicals, called cytokines, they release to fight the infection. The result can be impaired nutrient absorption, excessive water and mineral loss through the stools due to breakdown of the control mechanisms in the intestinal tissue that normally remove water from the stools, and in severe cases the entry of pathogenic organisms into the bloodstream.
>
> **Some microorganisms**—for example, bacteria of the genus *Shigella*, secrete substances known as cytotoxins, which kill and damage intestinal tissue on contact. Viruses directly attack the intestinal cells, taking over their metabolic machinery to make copies of themselves, which leads to cell death.

Types

Dysentery results from viral infections, bacterial infections, or parasitic infestations. These pathogens typically reach the large intestine after entering orally, through ingestion of contaminated food or water, oral contact with contaminated objects or hands, and so on.

Bacillary dysentery Bacillary dysentery, is caused by invasive bacteria. Bacterial infections are by far the most common causes of dysentery. These infections include *Shigella, Campylobacter, E. coli,* and *Salmonella* species of bacteria. The frequency of each pathogen varies considerably in different regions of the world. For example, shigellosis is most common in Latin America while *Campylobacter* is the dominant bacteria in Southeast Asia.

Dysentery caused by *Shigella* is also known as bacillary dysentery. There are four different species of *Shigella: Shigella dysenteriae, Shigella flexneri, Shigella boydii* and *Shigella sonnei.*

If someone is infected with shigella, the bacteria can pass out in their stools (feces). Infection may be passed on to others if drinking water is contaminated with infected faeces or if food is washed in contaminated water and then eaten. Because shigella infection can be passed on by drinking contaminated water or eating contaminated food, shigella can be a cause of food poisoning.

Signs and symptoms of bacillary dysentery tend to appear from one to three days after the person has been infected. Most typically, there is just mild stomach-ache and diarrhea, and no blood or mucus in the feces. For many, symptoms are so mild that they do not need medical attention, and the problem resolves in a few days. Initially, the infected person goes to the toilet frequently with diarrhea. Although much less common, some people with bacillary dysentery may have blood or mucus in their feces, abdominal pain may be intense, there may be an elevated body temperature (fever), nausea and vomiting.

Amoebic dysentery (amoebiasis)—*Amoebic dysentery* or *intestinal amoebiasis,* is caused by a single-celled, microscopic parasite living in the large bowel. *Entamoeba histolytica,* a type of amoeba, is a protozoan (single-celled) organism that constantly changes shape. These species are able to burrow through the intestinal wall and spread through the bloodstream to infect other organs, such as the liver, lungs and brain. The amoeba group together and form a **cysts**, the cysts come out of the body in human feces. In areas of poor sanitation, these cysts (which can survive for a long time), can contaminate food and water, and infect other humans. The cysts can also linger in infected people's hands after going to the toilet. Good hygiene practice reduces the risk of infecting other people. It is more common in tropics.

Symptoms of amoebic dysentery include abdominal pain, fever and chills, nausea and vomiting, watery diarrhea, which can contain blood, mucus or **pus**, painful passing of stools, fatigue, intermittent constipation.

Prevention

To reduce the risk of contracting dysentery the following are suggested:

- Washing one's hands after using the toilet, after contact with an infected person, and regularly throughout the day
- Washing one's hands before handling, cooking and eating food, handling babies, and feeding young or elderly people
- Keeping contact with someone known to have dysentery to a minimum
- Washing laundry on the hottest setting possible
- Avoiding sharing items such as towels and face cloths.

Treatment

The treatment of dysentery should aim at removing the offending and toxic matter from the intestines and for alleviating painful symptoms, stopping the virulence of the bacteria and promoting healing of the ulcer.

Rehydration therapy: Initially this is done using oral rehydration; the patient is encouraged to drink plenty of liquids. Diarrhea, as well as vomiting results in loss of fluids that have to be replaced to prevent dehydration. If this treatment cannot be adequately maintained due to vomiting or the profuseness of diarrhea, hospital admission may be required for intravenous fluid replacement. If symptoms are not severe and it is Bacillary dysentery *(Shigella)*, the patient most likely will receive no medication, in the vast majority of cases the illness will resolve within a week. Oral rehydration is important.

Antibiotics and amoebicidal drugs: In ideal situations, no antimicrobial therapy should be administered until microbiological microscopy and culture studies determine whether the illness is being caused by bacterium or amoeba. When laboratory services are not available, it may be necessary to administer a combination of drugs, including an amoebicidal drug, to kill the parasite and an antibiotic to treat any associated bacterial infection.

Antibiotics are used to treat shigella infection in children. This is one of the few times that antibiotics are used to treat infections of the bowels (intestines), called gastroenteritis. It may help to reduce the chance that child passes on shigella infection to someone else and also may help to reduce the number of days that the child suffers from their symptoms. The usual antibiotic used is ciprofloxacin. However, the antibiotic may vary depending on laboratory report of stool sample. The exact antibiotic that is recommended is likely to depend on the organism's pattern of resistance to some antibiotics. Antibiotic resistance is where the medicines are no longer able to kill the bacteria that they are meant to fight.

Antibiotics are not prescribed for mild cases of dysentery. This is because generally, overusing antibiotics to treat minor ailments can make them less effective in treating more serious or life-threatening conditions.

Nursing Interventions

Assess level of dehydration—*See* management of diarrhea.

The child should be kept on complete bed rest as movement induces pain and aggravates distressing symptoms. Hot water bag may be applied over the abdomen.

The child-patient should be kept on liquid diet for the first 24 hours. The use of butter milk will be especially beneficial as it combats offending bacteria and helps establishment of helpful micro-organisms in the intestines.

After acute symptoms are over, the child may be allowed rice, curd, fresh ripe fruits, especially bael, banana and pomegranate and skimmed milk. Solid foods should be introduced very careful and gradually according to the pace of recovery. Fresh fruits and vegetable salads which have a detoxifying and cleansing effect upon the intestine.

OBSTRUCTIVE DISORDERS

- Hypertrophic pyloric stenosis
- Intussusception
- Volvulus
- Hirschsprung disease.

MALABSORPTION DISORDERS

Lactose Intolerance

Lactose intolerance means the body cannot easily digest lactose, a type of natural sugar found in milk and dairy products. Lactose cannot be absorbed directly by the body but must be hydrolysed into its monosaccharide components of glucose and galactose. This process is assisted in the body by the enzyme lactase (beta-galactosidase) which is situated in the brush border cells in the microvilli in the small intestine. Once absorbed, these simple sugars enter the bloodstream and act as nutrients. Lactose intolerant individuals have insufficient levels of lactase, an enzyme that catalyzes hydrolysis of lactose into glucose and galactose, in their digestive system. The exact reason of this deficiency is unknown.

Lactase deficiency: Causes and classification:

- Primary lactase deficiency is genetic, only affects adults and is caused by the absence of lactase persistence allele.
- Secondary, acquired, or transient lactase deficiency is a more common type. It is caused by an injury to the small intestine, usually during infancy, from acute gastroenteritis, diarrhea, chemotherapy, intestinal parasites or other environmental causes.
- Congenital lactase deficiency is a very rare, autosomal recessive genetic disorder that prevents lactase expression from birth.

Lactose intolerance is not an allergy because it is not an immune response, but rather a problem with digestion caused by lactase deficiency. Milk allergy is a separate condition, with distinct symptoms that occur when the presence of milk proteins trigger an immune reaction.

Pathophysiology : Lactose intolerance

Lactose intolerance occurs when the lactase enzyme is absent (alactasia) or deficient (hypolactasia), leading to reduced activity in the normal functioning of the small intestine. The undigested sugars are unable to participate in the normal absorption process and remain in the intestinal lumens and draw fluid into the intestine by a process of osmosis. In addition, the bacteria in the colon act on the undigested sugars, causing hydrogen gas and lactic acid to be produced. The outcome of this fermentation process initiates the main signs and symptoms associated with lactose intolerance.

Manifestations and Diagnostic Evaluation

Symptoms of lactose intolerance can be mild to severe, depending on how much lactase body makes. Symptoms usually begin 30 minutes to 2 hours after child eats or drink milk products.

- *Diarrheal stools*: Frequent, explosive, acidic and watery (may be green or yellow in colour depending on severity)
- A persistently unsettled, crying infant
- Pain and distension of the abdomen
- *Excess gas/flatus*: 'A windy baby' with loud bowel sounds
- Vomiting
- Possible dehydration and weight loss
- Acidic breath.

For diagnosis of lactose intolerance usually blood test, stool acidity test and lactose hydrogen breath tests, stool pH are performed. Lactose intolerance manifestations include diarrhea that is frothy but not fatty, abdominal distension and excessive flatus. If the infant is acutely unwell, an acid stool test may be a preferred choice of investigation. This test measures the amount of acid in the infant's stools. If lactose is undigested in the bowel, the fermentation process creates actic acid, which can then be measured. A stool pH of 5.5 can be an indication of lactose intolerance and can be a useful aid to diagnosis, especially in infants and young children.

Treatment

Cutting down or removing milk products from child's diet usually eases symptoms. In most cases total elimination of milk is unnecessary. Most children with low lactase levels can drink less amount of milk at one time without having symptoms. Larger servings may cause problems for children with lactase deficiency.

Milk products may be easier to digest include:

- Buttermilk and cheeses (have less lactose than milk)
- Fermented milk products, such as yogurt
- Goat's milk
- Ice cream, milkshakes, and hard cheeses
- Lactose-free milk and milk products
- Lactase-treated cow's milk for older children and adults
- Soy formulas for infants younger than 2 years
- Soy or rice milk for toddlers.

Lactose also appears to enhance the absorption of several minerals, including calcium, magnesium, and zinc. Not having milk in diet can lead to a shortage of calcium, vitamin D, riboflavin, and protein. Child needs 800–1,500 mg of calcium each day depending on age and body weight. Besides supplementation, calcium containing foods such as leafy greens, oysters, sardines, canned salmon, shrimp, and broccoli, orange can be given to the child.

Nursing Considerations

Assessment: An accurate history of the infant and family is essential, together with a detailed picture of feeding patterns and bowel habits.

A thorough physical examination is required to determine the infant's overall condition, and should include hydration and nutrition status.

Baseline observations of temperature, pulse, respirations and blood pressure are required, together with growth and development measurements in relation to weight, height and head circumference.

Interventions

If the infant is acutely unwell and is admitted to hospital, initial treatment will focus on rehydration and control of electrolyte imbalance. This will depend on the degree of intolerance and the severity and duration of the symptoms.

In the case of secondary lactose intolerance, when these acute symptoms have been alleviated management should continue in a supportive way. Milk, whether breast or formula, should be reintroduced to the infant, but the response of the child should be observed and the feeding regime manipulated in a controlled way.

If child can tolerate small amount of milk, food and lactase preparations simultaneously with milk may be offered to the child.

Dietary management and supplementation of micro nutrients are needed as discussed above.

Reassurance should be given that symptoms can often be minimised through nutritional support, with dietary control preventing further complications for the infant.

Evaluation

- Is the child happy and out of symptoms?
- Do the parents follow the diet schedule? Do they able to say what foods are essential to avoid?
- Are the stools of the child are soft and formed?
- Do the parents know about intake of micronutrients supplementation?

> WHO (1997) infers that lactose intolerance is rare when breast milk is the only source of lactose entering the infant's body. This is interesting, as breast milk contains a higher proportion of lactose than some formula milks (approximately 7 g per 100 mL), but it tends to be well tolerated - possibly because the amount of lactose reaching the intestine at any one time is low. This is not to say that breastfed infants never become lactose intolerant; by suggesting simple changes in breastfeeding patterns the effects of lactose intolerance can be eliminated. Infants should be encouraged to nurse fully on one breast before being offered the second.

Celiac Disease

Celiac disease is an immune-mediated enteropathy caused by a permanent sensitivity to the gliadin protein fraction of gluten found in cereal grains including wheat, rye, and barley.

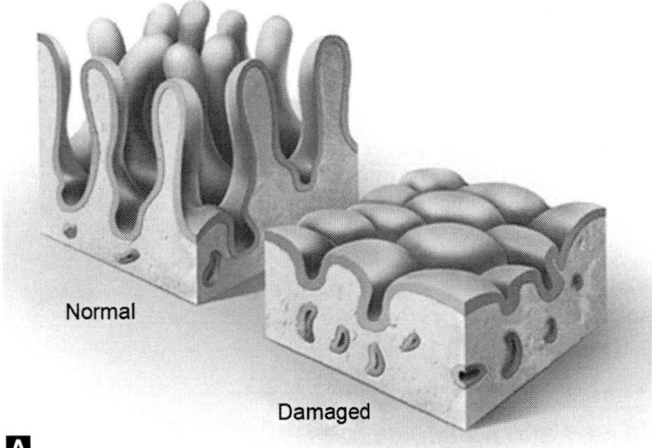

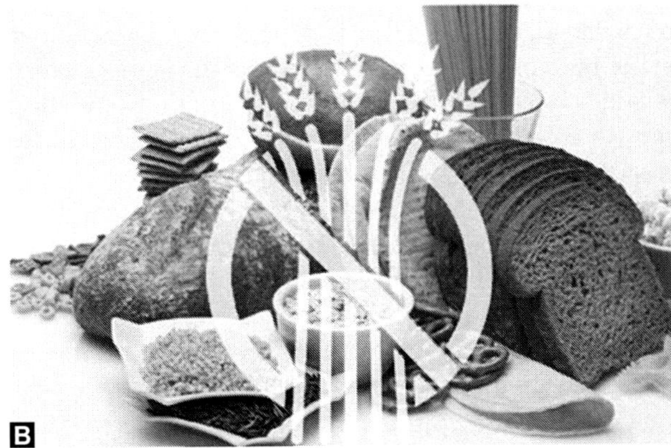

Figs 12.7A and B: A. Intestinal villus atrophy seen in celiac disease; **B.** Caution about these food stuff in celiac disease

It is a disease of the proximal small intestine characterized by abnormal mucosa and intolerance to gluten. It is an condition where the immune system reacts abnormally to the protein gluten.

Celiac disease occurs in genetically susceptible individuals who ingest gluten, a protein found in certain grains (Figs 12.7A and B). In these individuals, gluten causes an abnormal T cell–mediated immune response and inflammatory injury to the mucosa of the small intestine, resulting in malabsorption of nutrients.

> **Pathophysiology**
>
> Celiac disease is an autoimmune disease caused by the ingestion of gluten. Gliadin is a glycoprotein extract from gluten that is felt to be directly toxic to the enterocytes of individuals with celiac disease. When the body's immune system overreacts to gluten in food, the immune reaction damages the

Contd...

Contd...

tiny, hair-like projections (villi) that line the small intestine and which normally absorb vitamins, minerals, and nutrients from the ingested food. Susceptible individuals are unable to digest the gliadin component of gluten, resulting in an accumulation of a toxic substance that is damaging to the mucosal cells. The damage resulting from celiac disease makes the inner surface of the small intestine inflamed and flattened and it appear more like a tile floor. This is referred to as villous atrophy. Villous atrophy reduces the surface area of the bowel available for nutrient absorption. As a result body is unable to absorb nutrients necessary for health and growth (fat, calorie, carbohydrates,vitamin deficiency). Celiac crisis is manifested through diarrhea and severe dehydration.

Causes and Manifestations

The most important genes associated with susceptibility to coeliac disease are HLA DQ2 and HLA DQ8. Either one or both of these genes are present in virtually every person with coeliac disease. While 30% of the population carry one or both of these genes, only 1 in 30 of these people (approximately) will get coeliac disease.

A first degree relative (parent, sibling, child) of someone with coeliac disease has about a 10% chance of also having the disease. If one identical twin has coeliac disease there is an approximate 70% chance that the other twin will also have coeliac disease (but may not necessarily be diagnosed at the same time).

Gene changes (mutations) appear to increase the risk of developing the disease. But having those gene mutations doesn't mean the child will get celiac disease, meaning other factors must be involved.

Sometimes celiac disease is triggered, or becomes active for the first time, after surgery, viral infection or severe emotional stress.

In celiac disease, eating gluten triggers an immune response in small intestine. Over time, this reaction produces inflammation that damages the small intestine's lining and prevents absorption of some nutrients (malabsorption).

The intestinal damage can cause weight loss, bloating and sometimes diarrhea. Eventually, brain, nervous system, bones, liver and other organs can be deprived of vital nourishment.

In children, malabsorption can affect growth and development. The intestinal irritation can cause stomach pain, especially after eating.

Investigation

The first step in diagnosing celiac disease is through blood tests to check for the presence of certain antibodies. If a patient tests positive for celiac disease, an intestinal biopsy is necessary to confirm the diagnosis.

- *Blood tests:* The test for total serum IgA is suggested because there is a high prevalence of IgA deficiency in patients with celiac disease.
- *Endoscopy:* Sometimes endoscopy is done to view small intestine and to take a small tissue sample (biopsy) to analyze for damage to the villi.
- *Capsule endoscopy:* Capsule endoscopy uses a tiny wireless camera to take pictures of your entire small intestine.

Management

Diet

Gluten free diet: Although the diet is called 'gluten' free, but it is impossible to exclude every source of this protein. Corn and rice become main source of substitute of grain source for celiac disease child.

Vitamin and mineral supplementation: In severe nutritional deficiencies vitamin and mineral supplements like calcium, folate, iron, vitamin B_{12}, Vitamin D, Vitamin K, Zinc, may be needed.

Vitamin supplements are usually taken in pill form. If digestive tract has trouble absorbing vitamins, it may be given them by injection.

Drugs

If small intestine is severely damaged, steroids may be recommended to control inflammation. Steroids can ease severe signs and symptoms of celiac disease while the intestine heals.

If skin problem like itchy, blistering skin rash that sometimes accompanies celiac disease, a skin medication (dapsone) along with the gluten-free diet may be ordered.

Complications

Untreated, celiac disease can cause:

- *Malnutrition:* The damage to your small intestine means it cannot absorb enough nutrients. Malnutrition can lead to anemia and weight loss. In children, malnutrition can cause stunted growth and delayed development.
- *Loss of calcium and bone density:* Malabsorption of calcium and vitamin D may lead to a softening of the bone (osteomalacia or rickets) in children and a loss of bone density (osteoporosis) in adults.
- Damage of small intestine may cause to abdominal pain and diarrhea after eating lactose-containing

dairy products, even though they do not contain gluten. Once intestine has healed, child may be able to tolerate dairy products again. However, some children continue to experience lactose intolerance despite successful management of celiac disease.

Nursing Considerations

Nursing diagnosis: Altered nutrition: Less than body requirements related to decreased maldigestion and malabsorption.

Outcomes: Nutritional status: food and fluid intake; nutrient intake; biochemical measures; body mass; energy; Endurance.

Interventions: Nutrition management; Nutrition therapy; Nutritional counseling and monitoring; Fluid/ electrolyte management.

When someone with celiac disease eats gluten-containing foods, the immune system overreacts and attacks healthy intestinal tissue. This damages the intestinal villi and increases the risk for malabsorption of nutrients. Nurses should conduct thorough assessments on those who display the signs of celiac disease, as an early diagnosis can prevent substantial intestinal damage. For patients hospitalized with a celiac crisis, appropriate nursing interventions can relieve discomfort and prevent additional intestinal inflammation.

Nursing Assessment

In patients 3–9 months of age, this condition causes severe diarrhea and vomiting, irritability and an increased risk of failure to thrive. Patients 9–18 months old may experience weight loss, abdominal distension, muscle wasting in the buttocks and extremities, abnormal stools, mood changes, dermatitis, hypotonia and vomiting that usually occurs in the evening.

In older children and adults, signs and symptoms are often related to the vitamin, mineral and protein deficiencies that occur as a result of damage to the intestinal villi. These deficiencies include anemia, calcium deficiency, hypoproteinemia and a lack of prothrombin. Older children and adults with celiac disease also experience abdominal pain, constipation, flatulence, weight loss, fatigue and fatty stools.

Diagnostic Criteria

Laboratory testing may show elevated prothrombin time, decreased total protein and albumin levels, elevated immunoglobulin. A endomysium antibodies and reduced hemoglobin, vitamin K and folic acid levels. A small bowel biopsy will reveal the presence of abnormal mucosa.

Interventions

One of the most helpful therapeutic interventions for patients with celiac disease is modification of the diet. Those with celiac disease should follow a gluten-free diet that excludes all foods containing wheat, barley and rye. In some cases, the patient also needs to avoid foods made with oats. Due to decreased disaccharide activity, some celiac patients also follow a low-lactose, low-sucrose diet for 6–8 weeks. Nursing interventions for this condition help alleviate pain and discomfort, prevent additional intestinal damage and prevent complications associated with celiac disease.

Nurses should monitor intake and output, hydration status, dietary intake, patient weight and electrolyte levels. Monitoring dietary intake involves a careful balance between making sure the diet is free of gluten and ensuring that the patient receives essential nutrients.

Because celiac disease causes loose or fatty stools in some patients, nurses should pay close attention to the condition of the skin around the anus. Lubricating the skin and keeping it clean prevents skin breakdown and other complications.

Parent Teaching

For pediatric cases of celiac disease, educating parents about the disease and the need for a gluten-free diet is critical.

HEPATIC DISORDERS

Liver Disease: Common Signs and Symptoms

Jaundice: Occurs when serum bilirubin rises above 50–100 μmol/L. High concentrations lead to deposits in the skin and eyes, with the patient's color going from a pale yellow to green if very severe. This is often accompanied by dark urine and pale stools. A complication of unconjugated hyperbilirubinemia is severe brain damage (kernicterus). Treatment includes drugs and phototherapy for some unconjugated disorders.

- *Pruritus:* It is intense itching caused by the irritation of the cutaneous sensory nerves, probably by retained bile salts. Treatments include pharmacological and complementary therapies, but these have minimal effect. Severe pruritus can reduce quality of life significantly and can be an indication for liver transplantation.
- *Hepato/splenomegaly:* A fibrotic liver is enlarged and hard. The spleen enlarges because of the hyperplasia of the reticuloendothelial tissue and congestion. Hepato/splenomegaly is often associated with portal hypertension.

Portal hypertension (PHT) is an increase in portal venous pressure above 5–10 mmHg and the formation of portosystemic collaterals, which divert blood to the systemic circulation, bypassing the liver. PHT can be intrahepatic or extrahepatic. In extrahepatic PHT, the liver works normally. The main complication is ruptured varices. The commonest presentation is malena or hematemesis. Once collaterals are formed, resistance to portal blood flow is higher than normal, so they do not provide total decompression. Varices develop from the collateral circulation and, where they extend toward a superficial surface, such as the rectum, they may rupture, which can be life threatening. Ruptured varices are treated endoscopically with sclerotherapy, or the varix will be banded. Many patients will be given intravenous octreotide acetate. Propranolol is often used, although the efficacy of this in children has not been established.

Ascites is a protein-rich fluid, which accumulates in the peritoneal cavity. It is associated with portal hypertension, hepatocellular damage and a drop in serum albumin. Ascites is thought to develop due to a combination of factors and can compromise the patient's health in a number of ways:

- Pressure on the abdomen causes diaphragmatic splinting and can result in respiratory distress
- Increased pressure in the abdomen reduces stomach capacity, causing nausea, vomiting, poor weight gain in children and abdominal compartment syndrome
- Poor mobility and resulting impeded development.

Treatments of ascites include ascitic tap or intravenous low-sodium albumin infusions to increase oncotic pressure.

Coagulopathy: The liver plays a central role in the clotting process, coagulation disorders occur in acute and chronic liver diseases due to multiple causes: decreased synthesis of clotting and inhibitor factors, decreased clearance of activated factors, quantitative and qualitative platelet defects, hyperfibrinolysis, and accelerated intravascular coagulation. Patients with liver disease show the bleeding tendency and account for increased risk of morbidity and mortality who undergo diagnostic or therapeutic invasive procedures. Caution is needed with invasive procedures and coagulation factors and blood products may be needed.

Encephalopathy is usually observed in adults and some children with acute liver failure. Hepatic encephalopathy is the occurrence of confusion, altered level of consciousness, and coma as a result of liver failure. In the advanced stages it is called hepatic coma and may ultimately lead to death. It is caused by accumulation in the bloodstream of toxic substances that are normally removed by the liver.

Malnutrition and failure to thrive: Malnutrition is prevalent in all forms of liver diseases. As the liver is responsible for metabolism; malnutrition in adults and children and failure to thrive in infants is commonly observed. Although the pathogenesis of PCM is multifactorial, alterations in protein metabolism plays an important role. Malnutrition is prevalent in liver cirrhosis due to the presence of ascites, nausea, vomiting, insufficient food intake, malabsorption and metabolic disorders, poor dietary intake, malabsorption, increased intestinal protein losses, low protein synthesis, and hyper metabolism. Nutritional management is essential to promote recovery from disease, optimise preparation for liver transplantation and aid recovery after transplantation.

Xanthomas are caused by high serum cholesterol concentrations. Small, yellow nodules of fat, they accumulate under the skin, particularly around joints. They cannot be treated but are harmless and reabsorbed after transplantation.

Spider nevi are superficial arterioles developing into a series of fine, radiating branches on the face, neck, forearms and backs of hands. The presence of 10 or more suggests chronic liver disease.

Palmar erythema: The loss of capillary dilatation in severe liver disease results in the palms of the hands becoming mottled, bright red and warm. This is not life threatening.

Hepatorenal syndrome may occur in patients with chronic liver disease and PHT. Patients present with impaired renal function but normal tubular function. It may be difficult to distinguish hepatic from renal failure. Survival depends upon the reversibility of the liver disease.

Hepatopulmonary syndrome: About one-third of adult patients and some children with decompensated cirrhosis are cyanotic. Hypoxemia is common in patients with chronic liver disease. This may be due to intrapulmonary shunting through arteriovenous fistulae. Pulmonary symptoms are common in patients with liver disease. Dyspnea can be an early sign of pleural effusion, hepatopulmonary syndrome, or portopulmonary hypertension.

HEPATITIS

Hepatitis is a general term that simply means inflammation of the liver. There are many different causes of hepatitis like infection by different viruses, some toxins or disease state. Hepatitis may be sudden onset (acute) or chronic (long standing). Hepatitis is most commonly caused by a viral infection and there are five main hepatitis viruses, referred to as types A, B, C, D and E. Hepatitis A and E are typically caused by ingestion of contaminate food or water. Hepatitis B, C and D usually occur as a result of parenteral contact with infected body fluids (e.g. from blood transfusions or invasive medical procedures using contaminated equipment).

Hepatitis may be mild and self-limiting and resolve with no treatment, or it may become chronic and lead to liver failure requiring liver transplant. If the cause of the hepatitis can be treated quickly, the liver is likely to recover fully. There is a wide range of clinical finding with hepatitis depending on the severity of the inflammation. Although each type of hepatitis is unique, assessment findings and treatment have many similarities.

Viral Hepatitis

Hepatitis A

One of the more common causes of acute hepatitis is hepatitis A virus (HAV), which was isolated by Purcell in 1973. Humans appear to be the only reservoir for this virus. Hepatitis A (also called infectious hepatitis) is a common form of hepatitis in children. It is caused by the hepatitis A virus (HAV), which is primarily spread when an uninfected (and unvaccinated) person ingests food or water that is contaminated with the feces of an infected person. The infected stool might be found in small amounts in food and on household objects (such as doorknobs and diapers). Hepatitis A can remain in the stool for several months after the initial illness, especially in younger babies and children. The disease is closely associated with a lack of safe water, inadequate sanitation and poor personal hygiene.

HAV is a single-stranded, linear RNA enterovirus. In humans, viral replication depends on hepatocyte uptake and synthesis, and assembly occurs exclusively in liver cells. Acquisition results almost exclusively from ingestion (e.g. fecal-oral transmission), although isolated cases of parenteral transmission have been reported.

Unlike hepatitis B and C, hepatitis A infection does not cause chronic liver disease and is rarely fatal, but it can cause debilitating symptoms and fulminant hepatitis (acute liver failure), which is associated with high mortality.

Hepatitis B

Hepatitis B is a potentially life-threatening liver infection caused by the hepatitis B virus. Hepatitis B is a type that can move from one person to another through blood and other body fluids. People can also get it through having sex or from needles—like needles shared by drug or steroid users who have the virus, or tattoo needles that have not been properly sterilized. And a pregnant woman can pass hepatitis B to her unborn baby. The hepatitis B virus can survive outside the body for at least seven days. During this time, the virus can still cause infection if it enters the body of a person who is not protected by the vaccine.

Pathophysiology of viral hepatitis

Necrosis and Inflammation of hepatic cells, low liver function, circulating immune complexes and complement system activation, impaired bilirubin metabolism and obstruction of bile flow, acholic stool, urobilinogen in urine jaundice.

Hepatitis viruses cause necrosis of the parenchymal cells of the liver cells. Along with the development of inflammation in the liver, the normal pattern in the hepatic impaired. Disruption of the normal blood supply to the cells causes hepatic necrosis and damage to liver cells. Inflammation of the liver due to viral invasion would lead to an increase in body temperature and stretching the liver capsule which lead to feelings of discomfort in the upper right abdominal quadrant. This is manifested by the presence of nausea and pain in the gut. Onset of jaundice because the liver parenchymal cell damage. Although the number billirubin that has not undergone conjugationinto the liver remained normal, but due to liver cell damage and intra-hepatic bile ductuli, then there is the difficulty of transporting bilirubin in the liver. There was also a difficulty in terms of conjugation. As a result, billirubin imperfect through the ductus hepaticus issued, due to retention (due to cell damage excretion) and regurgitation in the ductuli, bile has not undergone conjugation (indirectbilirubin), or already experiencing the conjugation of bilirubin (direct bilirubin). So here jaundice arising mainly due to difficulties in transport, conjugation and excretion of bilirubin. Feces contain little stercobilin therefore pale stools (abolis). Because water-soluble conjugated bilirubin, the bilirubin can be excreted into the urine, causing urinarybilirubin and dark colored urine. Elevated levels of bilirubin can be accompanied by an increase in the conjugated bile salts in the blood which will cause itching in jaundice.

After passing the time, the liver cells become damaged eliminated from the body by the immune system response and replaced by new cells of a healthy liver. Therefore, most clients who have hepatitis recovered with normal liver function.

Manifestations

The symptoms of hepatitis are similar regardless of the cause of inflammation.

It includes jaundice, dark urine, extreme fatigue, nausea, vomiting and abdominal pain. Initially the child may have nonspecific flu-like symptoms including fever, fatigue, muscle aches, vomiting, diarrhea and rash. Abdominal pain (right upper quadrant), yellowing of the skin and eyes (jaundice), and dark urine may occur. Enlargement of the liver may be found on exam.

As hepatitis becomes chronic, the liver may actually become smaller as inflammation is replaced by scarring (fibrosis) of the liver. Extensive scarring of the liver can lead to cirrhosis.

The liver may be unable to produce the proteins needed for normal body functions. This can lead to swelling of the abdomen with fluid (ascites), fluid accumulation of the legs, enlargement of the spleen, or easy bleeding and bruising.

Varices may develop. These are enlarged veins in the esophagus, stomach, intestine, and other organs that may produce life-threatening bleeding. Severe hepatitis may lead to problems with other organ systems such as lung, kidney, and CNS as well.

Hepatitis A is rarely severe disease, and fulminant hepatitis is caused primarily by hepatitis B and hepatitis C.

Diagnostic Evaluation

It is important to seek medical attention if yellow coloration of eyes and skin of child is seen. Laboratory tests are done to identify the extent of liver involvement as well as measure the function of the liver. Physical examination and serologic markers (antibodies and antigens) indicate the presence of active infection with hepatitis A, B, and C or previous infection (Table 12.2). Liver function tests like aspartate transaminase (AST), alanine transaminase (ALT), bilirubin test and sedimentation tests are done for detection of liver damage by hepatitis. Serum bilirubin levels peak 5–10 days after jaundice appears.

Hepatitis is diagnosed by identification of the antigens like HbsAg, HBeAg, HBcAg responsible for the disease, antibodies (anti-HAV, anti-HBcAg, anti-HCV), or polymerase chain reaction (i.e. HCV RNA). In hepatitis A, immunoglobulins M (IgM) and HAV antibodies are present. Radiology studies of the liver (ultrasound, MRI, etc.) may also be done. An abdominal ultrasound provides measurement of the liver size, detection of cystic lesions, and stones, and imaging of gallbladder.

At times, a biopsy of the liver is most informative. This is a procedure where a piece of liver tissue is obtained to be evaluated under a microscope. It is done to evaluate the chronic active forms of the disease and to determine the extent of damage in advanced fulminant cases.

Incidence

Hepatitis A occurs sporadically and in epidemics worldwide, with a tendency for cyclic recurrences. Every year there are an estimated 1.4 million cases of hepatitis A worldwide. The hepatitis A virus is one of the most frequent causes of food borne infection.

Epidemics related to contaminated food or water can erupt explosively, such as the epidemic in Shanghai in 1988 that affected about 300000 people. Hepatitis A viruses persist in the environment and can resist food-production processes routinely used to inactivate and/or control bacterial pathogens.

Hepatitis B is a major global health problem. More than 240 million people have chronic (long-term) liver infections. About 600000 people die every year due to the acute or chronic consequences of hepatitis B.

A vaccine against hepatitis B has been available since 1982. Hepatitis B vaccine is 95% effective in preventing

Table 12.2: Differential diagnosis of viral hepatitis

Type	*Transmission incubation*	*Incubation period*	*Clinical manifestations*	*Recovery prognosis*
Hepatitis A	Fecal–oral Water and food contaminated with HAV.	15–45 days (average 30 days)	No jaundice and mostly asymptomatic in children. In general and in adolescents flu like features, i.e. fever, malaise, anorexia, nausea, jaundice.	Prognosis good. Life –long immunity
Hepatitis B	Blood, blood products, body fluids, prenatally, perinatally, breast milk.	45–180 days (average 90 days)	Same as HAV. Anicteric/asymptomatic most common in children. Disease ranges from asymptomatic to fulminating infection	Usually full recovery, except in chronic carriers
Hepatitis C	Blood, blood products, IDUs, perinatally, unsterile tattoos/body piercing.	14–115 days (average–45 days)	Same as HAV	More than 50% progress to chronic hep.
Hepatitis D	Blood, blood products, body fluids, IDUs.	30–60 days	Children have chronic hepatitis	More likely to develop fulminant hepatitis than other strains.
Hepatitis E	Fecal–oral	Unknown	Same as HAV	Children usually asymptomatic. Dangerous to pregnant women.

infection and its chronic consequences, and was the first vaccine against a major human cancer.

Hepatitis B prevalence is highest in sub-Saharan Africa and East Asia. Most people in these regions become infected with the hepatitis B virus during childhood and between 5–10% of the adult population is chronically infected. High rates of chronic infections are also found in the Amazon and the southern parts of eastern and central Europe. In the Middle East and the Indian subcontinent, an estimated 2–5% of the general population is chronically infected. Less than 1% of the population in Western Europe and North America is chronically infected.

Treatment

Treatment for hepatitis involves largely supportive therapy. Medications may be used to correct any abnormalities associated with liver dysfunction. Treatment is aimed at maintaining comfort and adequate nutritional balance. Sometimes child may be admitted to the hospital for observation or treatment. Nonessential drugs are not to be given during infection.

Severe cases of hepatitis can cause significant dysfunction and be life threatening. These patients are critically ill and require careful monitoring in the intensive care unit. Patient needs to provide hemostasis, nutritional and fluid support, neurological assessment and management. They may be placed on a ventilator to support breathing. They may require dialysis to support kidney function.

Medications and other techniques may be needed to maintain neurologic status. Significant bleeding is a risk with severe hepatitis and may require a procedure or surgery to stabilize.

If the underlying cause of hepatitis can be found, therapy may be direct toward that as well. In severe cases, liver transplant may be an option.

Prognosis

Prognosis for hepatitis is extremely variable. Some cases are transient mild elevation of liver enzymes that resolve with no intervention. These patients will typically have no further episodes of hepatitis and no future liver problems.

Other cases of hepatitis can lead to chronic hepatitis. These patients need to be followed by a pediatric gastroenterologist or pediatric hepatologist and their liver function followed closely. They may need medications to maintain liver function, but otherwise can be fairly healthy and active. Liver fibrosis increases with the duration of HCV infection. They may be at risk for liver cancers later in life. Severe cases may lead to liver failure.

Cirrhosis of Liver

Cirrhosis is an abnormal liver condition in which there is irreversible scarring of the liver. It is a chronic disease characterized by replacement of normal liver tissue with diffuse fibrosis that disrupts the structure and function of the liver. The fibrosis alters liver structure and vasculature, impairing blood and lymph flow and resulting in hepatic insufficiency and hypertension in the portal vein. After years of liver inflammation, it will gradually lose its ability to function well, which can lead to a serious problem in other parts of the body. According to Medilexicon's medical dictionary:

Cirrhosis is *'A chronic liver disease of highly various etiology characterized by inflammation, degeneration, and regeneration in differing proportions; pathologic hallmark is formation of microscopic or macroscopic nodules separated by bands of fibrous tissue; impairment of hepatocellular function and obstruction to portal circulation often lead to jaundice, ascites, and hepatic failure.'*

Causes

Viral or autoimmune hepatitis: This disease appears to be caused by the immune system and inflammatory responses by attacking the liver and causing damage, and eventually scarring of the liver tissues.

Bile ducts obstruction: The duct that carry the bile out of the liver blocked, bile backs up and damages liver tissue.

Drugs and toxin: Prolonged exposure to drugs and environmental toxins can lead to hepatic cell damage.

Genetic or inherited disorder: It also can result from inherited diseases like cystic fibrosis, hemophilia, Wilson disease, etc. Cirrhosis is a progressive disease, developing slowly over many years, until eventually it can stop liver function (liver failure).

Pathophysiology

Cirrhosis

The liver carries out several essential functions, including the synthesis of proteins (for example, albumin, clotting factors and complement), detoxification, and storage (e.g. vitamin A), it also purifies the blood and manufactures vital nutrients. In addition, it participates in the metabolism of lipids and carbohydrates.

The pathological hallmark of cirrhosis is the development of scar tissue that replaces normal parenchyma. This scar tissue blocks the portal flow of blood through the organ therefore disturbing normal function. Recent research shows the pivotal role of the stellate cell, a cell type that normally stores vitamin A,

Contd...

Contd...

in the development of cirrhosis. Damage to the hepatic parenchyma (due to inflammation) leads to activation of the stellate cell, which increases fibrosis and obstructs blood flow in the circulation.

The fibrous tissue bands (septa) separate hepatocyte nodules, which eventually replace the entire liver architecture, leading to decreased blood flow throughout. Liver cirrhosis increases resistance to blood flow and higher pressure in the portal venous system, resulting in portal hypertension. Effects of portal hypertension include Splenomegaly (increase in size of the spleen) is found in 35–50% of patients. Esophageal varices result from collateral portal blood flow through vessels in the stomach and esophagus (a process called Portacaval anastomosis). When these blood vessels become enlarged, they are called varices and are more likely to burst. The spleen becomes congested, which leads to hypersplenism and increased sequestration of platelets. Portal hypertension is responsible for most severe complications of cirrhosis. Due to decreased functioning/dying of liver cells, liver cannot produce necessary proteins and bile and as a result malabsorption and malnutrition developed. This scar tissue causes blood flow to be blocked and waste products to build-up in the body.

Manifestations

If cirrhosis is mild the liver can make repairs and continue functioning properly. If the cirrhosis is advanced and more and more scar (fibrous) tissue forms in the liver, the damage is irreparable. Children exhibit jaundice, poor growth, anorexia, itchy skin, loss of appetite, loss of body weight, nausea, muscle weakness and lethargy. Impaired intra-hepatic blood flow may cause abdominal pain, ascites, edeme, GI bleeding, anemia. Pulmonary function may be impaired due to pressure against the diaphragm from hepatospleenomegaly and ascites. Hypoxemia may develop due to development of intrapulmonary arteriovenous shunts. Spider angiomas and prominent blood vessels (blood capillaries) are often visible on the upper abdomen.

Diagnosis

- Following tests are performed to confirm or rule out the diagnosis of cirrhosis. Tests may include (but are not limited to):
  - *CT scan or ultrasound, MRI:* Show shrinkage or abnormal appearance of the liver.
  - *Laboratory studies:* Bilirubin, albumin, alanine transaminase (ALT), aspartate transaminase (AST), prothrombin time, and serum ammonia—to check for elevated values, which indicate hepatic cell destruction.
  - *Laparoscopy and liver biopsy:* Direct visualization of the liver, analyzing a sample of liver tissue removed via a thin needle inserted into the liver.
  - *Paracentesis:* To examine ascetic fluid for cell, protein and bacterial counts.
  - *Esophagoscopy:* To determine the presence of esophageal varices.

Therapeutic Management

In general, cirrhosis cannot be cured or reversed, treatment aims to:

- Control the cause of the liver damage
- Prevent additional damage
- Treat symptoms and complications
- Treat underlying medical conditions.

Drugs are administered to treat the underlying cause of the liver disease. Other medications may be used to control symptoms or fight infections. Some medications are prescribed to get rid of excess fluid in the body or reduce the risk of a blood vessel breaking. Others help child's body cut down on its absorption of harmful waste products or toxins.

If the complications of cirrhosis can no longer be controlled, or if the liver is in danger of no longer functioning, a liver transplant is often the best option.

Many of the liver disorders that cause childhood cirrhosis are not preventable, but there are precautions parent can take. Completion of immunizations including influenza and hepatitis vaccines at the times it is recommended, prevention of hepatitis B, C infection, awareness about medicines that may damage liver are important to prevent cirrhosis in children.

Balanced nutritional intake is important for patients who already have cirrhosis of the liver can prevent or slow further liver damage. Child may need extra calories to grow properly and to maintain adequate overall strength. If the cirrhosis is more advanced and compromises the liver's ability to process protein properly, limiting protein may be recommended. Limiting salt in child's diet is necessary, because salt tends to make the body retain water. They may also advise avoiding raw seafood. Make sure child takes any vitamin supplements prescribed. Due to increased risk of infections, vaccines against flu, pneumonia, and hepatitis for people with cirrhosis may be recommended.

One of the dangerous complications that can arise in an individual with cirrhosis is variceal hemorrhage. This occurs when an enlarged blood vessel in the esophagus and/or stomach breaks open and causes bleeding. Typically if this occurs one may vomit blood (which could be bright red or black like coffee grounds). Alternatively, blood might be noted in the stools—it could be bright red or black and tarry. This occurrence is a medical emergency so immediate medical attention should be sought for.

Nursing Management

Assessment: Monitor vital signs, intake and output and electrolyte levels to determine fluid volume status. Monitoring the child's weight on daily and weekly basis and recording intake and output can provide critical information about edema and growth. To assess fluid retention, measure and record abdominal girth every shift. Weight the patient daily and document his weight.

Observe and document for bleeding gums, ecchymoses, epistaxis, petechiae and degree of sclerae, skin jaundice. Remain with the patient during the hemorrhagic episodes.

Inspect stools for amount, color and consistency. Test stools and vomitus for occult blood as ordered.

Watch for signs of anxiety, epigastric fullness, restlessness and weakness.

Psychological support: Observe closely for signs of behavioral changes. Report increasing stupor, lethargy, hallucinations or neuromuscular dysfunction. Arouse the patient periodically to determine level of consciousness. Offer psychological support and encouragement, when appropriate.

Watch for asterixis, a sign of developing encephalopathy. Asterixis (also called the flapping tremor, or liver flap) is a tremor of the hand when the wrist is extended, sometimes said to resemble a bird flapping its wings. This motor disorder is characterized by an inability to actively maintain a position, which is demonstrated by jerking movements of the outstretched hands when bent upward at the wrist.

Stabilize patient and secure airway, with critical care intervention if necessary. Assess for precipitating factor(s) with appropriate treatment as indicated; in particular look for gastrointestinal bleeding and sepsis.

Nutritional support: As the liver is responsible for metabolism, malnutrition in children and failure to thrive in infants is commonly observed. Nutritional management is essential to promote recovery from disease, optimise preparation for liver transplantation. The diet needs to be high carbohydrates, normal protein, high calorie and low fat. As anorexia remains a problem, tube feeding or TPN may be needed. Restrict sodium and fluid intake as prescribed.

Vitamin support: In children with cholestasis, fat soluble vitamin absorption is severely affected. Even with vigilant monitoring of levels and extensive supplementation, diseases of vitamin deficiency can occur specially if the child has chronic liver disease.

Some of the common deficiencies seen in children with cholestasis are vitamin A—night blindness and the skin becoming dry and pimply vitamin A deficiency hemorrhages, loose teeth and gingivitis due to vitamin C deficiency, rickets or osteoporosis with brittle bones due to vitamin D deficiency, Vitamin E deficiency causes red blood cell hemolysis and if severe; impairment of muscle power and peripheral nerve function in feet. Vitamin K deficiency causes clotting abnormalities. All children with jaundice will require fat soluble vitamin supplementation and the dosing is likely to be significantly higher than what is generally recommended.

Skin care: Pruritus is intense itching caused by the irritation of the cutaneous sensory nerves, probably by retained bile salts. Treatments include pharmacological and complementary therapies, like colloidal oatmeal baths and calamine lotion are used for temporary relief. Drugs are not usually used as impaired liver function affects metabolism of drugs. Keeping nails trimmed short and use of cotton gloves during sleep can minimize damage to the skin from scratching. Caring the bruising can prevent further complication.

Prevention of Complications

- *Ascites:* Monitoring intake-output and weight, maintaining fluid balance, monitoring abdominal girth and distension are nursing concerns. Monitoring of edema, giving low sodium diet and administration of diuretics are usual interventions done for management of ascites.
  Moreover treatments of ascites include ascitic tap or intravenous low-sodium albumin infusions to increase oncotic pressure. Monitoring of intra-abdominal pressure may guide further management. Administer diuretics, potassium and protein supplements as directed. Restrict sodium and fluid intake as prescribed. Maintain some periods of rest with legs elevated to mobilize edema and ascites. Child with edema needs alternate rest periods with ambulation.
- *Coagulopathy:* Vitamin K deficiency causes coagulopathy, putting infants and children at risk of intracranial bleeds. Many children will require regular IV vitamin K (usually weekly) in addition to daily oral administration to assist in the maintenance of safe clotting levels. Identify bleeding as soon as possible and protect the child from injury. Nursing care in the hospital includes transfusing blood and blood products safety, maintaining fluid balance, monitoring vital signs, administering oxygen therapy, assisting in advanced medical interventions like endoscopic sclerotherapy, placement of a Sengstaken-Blakemore tube for compression of bleeding esophageal varices.

- *Encephalopathy:* May develop in some children with acute liver failure. This results from a buildup of ammonia in the blood from the incomplete breakdown of protein. Nursing responsibilities includes limiting protein in diet, giving lactulose as prescribed to decrease the GI bacteria that produce ammonia, administering antibiotics, and monitoring behavior changes and changes in level of consciousness.

Patient Teaching for Home Care

- To minimize the risk for bleeding, warn the parents against giving nonsteroidal anti-inflammatory drugs, preventing child from straining to defecate and blowing his nose or sneezing to vigorously, and use of a soft toothbrush.
- Advise the patient that rest and good nutrition conserve energy and decrease metabolic demands on the liver. Urge mothers to provide frequent small meals. Teach child to alternate periods of rest and activity to reduce oxygen demand and prevent fatigue.
- Providing developmental stimulation on a daily basis is essential, and parents need education and support services to achieve this.

Acute Abdomen

Acute abdomen is the medical term used for pain in the abdomen that usually comes on suddenly due to numerous disorders and is so severe that one may have to go to the hospital. Among children the most common medical cause is gastroenteritis, and the most common surgical cause is appendicitis. In the acute surgical abdomen, pain generally precedes vomiting, while the reverse is true in medical conditions. The challenge for the clinician is to identify those patients with abdominal pain who have either serious, potentially life-threatening conditions, such as appendicitis or bowel obstruction (as can occur from volvulus, intussusception, or adhesions), or infections that require specific treatment (i.e. streptococcal pharyngitis or pneumonia). The likely diagnosis is often suggested by the child's age and clinical features (i.e. associated symptoms, past medical history and physical examination).

Etiology

Infantile Colic

Ten to twenty percent of infants suffer from abdominal colic during the first three to four weeks of life. Typically, infants with colic scream, draw their knees up against their abdomen, and appear to be in severe pain.

Gastroenteritis

Gastroenteritis is the most common cause of abdominal pain in children. Viruses such as rotavirus, enterovirus, Norwalk virus, and adenovirus are the most frequent causes. The most common bacterial agents include *Escherichia coli, Campylobacter, Salmonella,* and *Shigella.*

Appendicitis

Appendicitis is the most common surgical condition in children who present with abdominal pain. Lymphoid tissue or a fecalith obstructs the appendiceal lumen, the appendix becomes distended, and ischemia and necrosis may develop. Patients with appendicitis classically present with visceral, vague, poorly localized, periumbilical pain. Within 6 to 48 hours, the pain becomes parietal as the overlying peritoneum becomes inflamed; the pain then becomes well localized and constant in the right iliac fossa.

Mesenteric Lymphadenitis

The condition mimics appendicitis, except the pain is more diffuse, signs of peritonitis often are absent, and generalized lymphadenopathy may be present. Mesenteric lymphadenitis often is associated with adenoviral infection.

Constipation

Constipation may be acute and chronic in nature. Acute constipation usually has an organic cause (e.g. gastroenteritis, appendicitis), while chronic constipation usually has a functional cause (e.g. low-residue diet). Abdominal pain resulting from constipation is most often left-sided or suprapubic.

Abdominal Trauma

Abdominal trauma may occur in children due to accident. Blunt abdominal trauma is more common than penetrating injury. Abdominal trauma may cause musculocutaneous injury, bowel perforation, intramural hematoma, laceration or hematoma of the liver or spleen, and avulsion of intra-abdominal organs or vascular pedicles.

Intestinal Obstruction

Causes of intestinal obstruction include volvulus, intussusception, incarcerated hernia, and postoperative adhesions. Intestinal obstruction produces a characteristic cramping.

Pathophysiology

Clinically, abdominal pain falls into three categories: visceral (splanchnic) pain, parietal (somatic) pain, and referred pain. Visceral receptors respond to mechanical and chemical stimuli whereas mucosal receptors respond primarily to chemical stimuli.

Visceral pain occurs when noxious stimuli affect a viscus, such as the stomach or intestines. Tension, stretching, and ischemia stimulate visceral pain fibers. Tissue congestion and inflammation tend to sensitize nerve endings and lower the threshold for stimuli. Because visceral pain fibers are bilateral and unmyelinated and enter the spinal cord at multiple levels, visceral pain usually is dull, poorly localized, and felt in the midline. Pain from foregut structures (e.g. lower esophagus, stomach) generally is felt in the epigastrium. Midgut structures (e.g. small intestine) cause periumbilical pain, and hindgut structures (e.g. large intestine) cause lower abdominal pain.

Parietal pain arises from noxious stimulation of the parietal peritoneum. Pain resulting from ischemia, inflammation, or stretching of the parietal peritoneum is transmitted through myelinated afferent fibers to specific dorsal root ganglia on the same side and at the same dermatomal level as the origin of the pain. Parietal pain usually is sharp, intense, discrete, and localized, and coughing or movement can aggravate it.

Referred pain has many of the characteristics of parietal pain but is felt in remote areas supplied by the same dermatome as the diseased organ. It results from shared central pathways for afferent neurons from different sites. A classic example is a patient with pneumonia who presents with abdominal pain because the T9 dermatome distribution is shared by the lung and the abdomen.

Management

Acute abdomen can be defined as a medical emergency in which there is sudden and severe pain in abdomen with accompanying signs and symptoms that focus on an abdominal involvement. Treatment should be directed at the underlying cause. In a sick patient the initial steps include rapid IV access and normal saline 20 mL/kg (in the presence of shock/hypovolemia), adequate analgesia, nothing per oral/IV fluids, Ryle's tube aspiration and surgical consultation. Traditionally, the use of analgesics is discouraged in patients with abdominal pain for fear of interfering with accurate evaluation and diagnosis. However, several prospective, randomized studies have shown that judicious use of analgesics actually may enhance diagnostic accuracy by permitting detailed examination of a more cooperative patient.

An ultrasound abdomen is the first investigation in almost all cases with moderate and severe pain with localizing abdominal findings. In patients with significant abdominal trauma or features of pancreatitis, a contrast enhanced computerized tomography (CECT) abdomen will be a better initial modality. Continuous monitoring and repeated physical examinations should be done in all cases. Specific management varies according to the specific etiology.

If amoebic dysentery is diagnosed the patient will probably start with a 10 days course of an antimicrobial medication, such as Flagyl (metronidazole). Diloxanide furoate, paromomycin (Humatin), or iodoquinol (Yodoxin) may also be prescribed to make sure the amoeba does not survive inside the body after symptoms have gone.

CHAPTER 13

A Child with Respiratory Disorders

Chapter Outline

- Disorders of Upper Respiratory Tract
- Foreign Body Aspiration
- Cystic Fibrosis
- Pleural Effusion
- Lung Abscess

RESPIRATORY SYSTEM

Prenatal Respiratory Development

The placenta performs oxygenation in utero, but many physiologic adaptations take place for the survival of humans at birth, among those, cardiorespiratory adaptation is by far the most crucial. The respiratory and circulatory systems must be developed sufficiently in utero for the newborn infant to withstand drastic changes at birth, from the fetal circulatory pattern with liquid-filled lungs to air breathing with transitional circulatory adaptation in a matter of a few minutes.

Postnatal Respiratory Changes

At birth the newborn infant must exercise an effective neuronal drive and respiratory muscles to displace the liquid filling the airway system. During vaginal delivery, compression of the thorax forces out some fetal lung fluid. Hypoxemia, hypercarbia, cold, tactile stimulation; and possible decrease in the concentration of prostaglandin E2 stimulate respiration. It introduces sufficient air against the surface force in order to establish sufficient alveolar surface for gas exchange. At the same time, pulmonary blood vessels must dilate rapidly to increase pulmonary blood flow and to establish alveolar ventilation/pulmonary perfusion for sufficient pulmonary gas exchange. Closures of the foramen ovale and the ductus arteriosus establish the pulmonary and circulatory systems. The neonatal adaptation of lung mechanics and respiratory control takes several weeks to complete.

Beyond this immediate neonatal period, the infant's lungs continue to mature at a rapid pace, and postnatal development of the lungs and the thorax surrounding the lungs continue well beyond the first year of life.

The respiratory system consists of the respiratory center in the brainstem; the central and peripheral chemoreceptors; the phrenic, intercostal, hypoglossal (efferent), and vagal (afferent) nerves; the thorax (including the thoracic cage; the muscles of the chest, abdomen, and diaphragm); the upper airway (extrathoracic) and lower (intrathoracic) airway; the lungs (Fig. 13.1); and the pulmonary vascular system. The upper airway consists of nose, mouth, nasal cavity, sinuses, pharynx. The lower respiratory tract includes the voice box (larynx), trachea, lungs, bronchi and bronchioles, alveoli (Fig. 13.2).

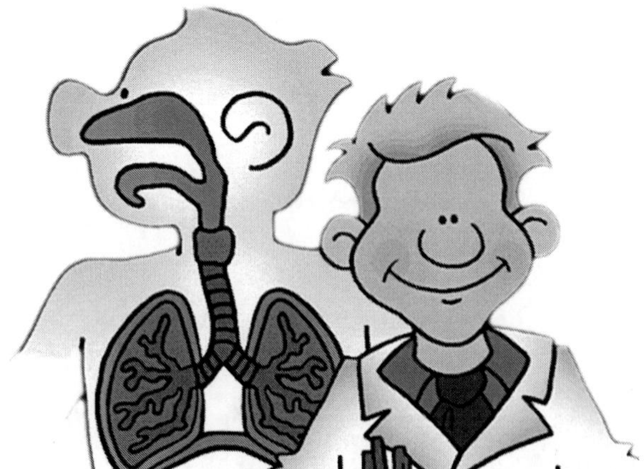

Fig. 13.1: Graphical representation of respiratory system of a child

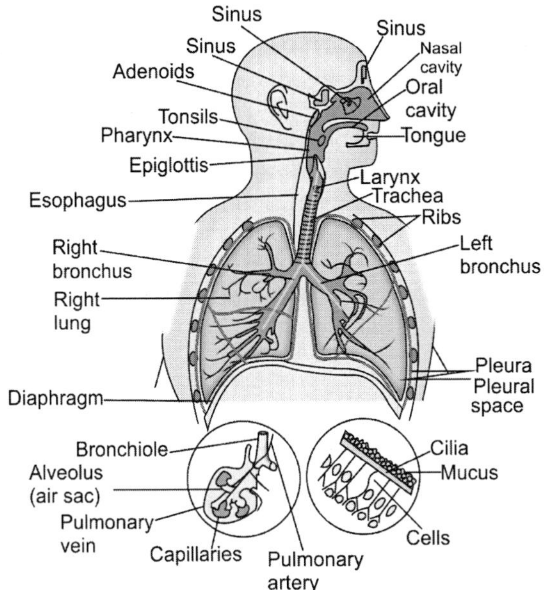

Fig. 13.2: The respiratory system

The principal function of the respiratory system is to maintain the oxygen and carbon dioxide (CO_2) equilibrium in the body. Respiration is the set of events that results in the exchange of oxygen from the environment and carbon dioxide from the body's cells (Fig. 13.3). The process of taking air into the lungs is inspiration, or inhalation, and the process of breathing it out is expiration, or exhalation. Four steps of respiration in human are:

1. *Breathing:* This involves inspiration of air into the lungs.
2. *External respiration:* This is the diffusion of oxygen, and carbon dioxide between air and blood in the alveoli.
3. *Internal respiration:* When the blood gives oxygen to the cells, and receives carbon dioxide to be carried away.
4. *Cellular respiration:* The mitochondria in cells use oxygen to breakdown sugar, to produce water.

The lungs also make an important contribution to the regulation of acid-base (pH) balance. The maintenance of body temperature (via loss of water through the lungs) is an additional but secondary function of the lungs. The lungs are also an important organ of metabolism.

Common Respiratory Symptoms

- *Wheezing:* Wheezing is a high-pitched whistling sound heard when a person breathes out. The child's wheezing may come and go before he is 3 years old. Then it may go away altogether. The child may wheeze only when he has a virus, such as a cold. He may wheeze even when he does not have a cold. He may wheeze when he is around things such as pet hair. His wheezing may decrease as he gets older.
- *Trouble breathing:* The child may tell that his chest feels tight. His nostrils may flare out as he tries to breathe. His stomach muscle or the skin over his ribs may move in deeply while he tries to breathe. He may also take shorter, faster breaths than usual.

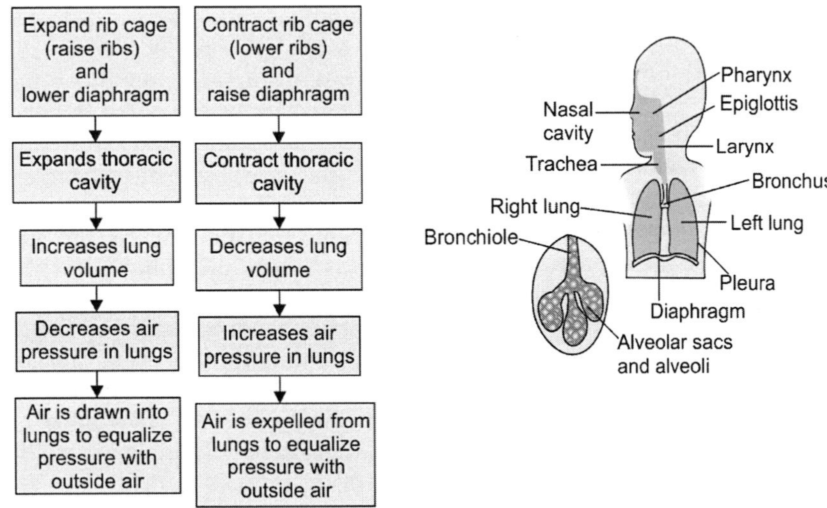

Fig. 13.3: Mechanism of respiration and respiratory system

- *Cough:* The child may have a cough that does not go away. Crackle sound may be heard when the child breathes or coughs.
- *Fast heartbeat:* When the child cannot breathe as well, his heart may beat faster than usual.
- *Runny nose:* The child may have a runny nose along with other signs and symptoms of reactive airway disease (RAD).

Respiratory Noises

Breath sounds are the noises produced by the structures of the lungs during breathing. The lung sounds are best heard with a stethoscope. This is called auscultation. Normal lung sounds occur in all parts of the chest area, including above the collarbones and at the bottom of the rib cage. Normal breathing sounds, decreased or absent breath sounds, and abnormal breath sounds may be heard by stethoscope. Absent or decreased sounds can mean:

- Air or fluid in or around the lungs (pneumonia, heart failure, and pleural effusion)
- Increased thickness of the chest wall
- Over-inflation of a part of the lungs (emphysema can cause this)
- Reduced airflow to part of the lungs

There are several types of abnormal breath sounds. The four most common are:

1. *Rales:* Small clicking, bubbling, or rattling sounds in the lungs. They are heard when a person breathes in (inhales). They are believed to occur when air opens closed air spaces. Rales can be further described as moist, dry, fine, and course.
2. *Rhonchi:* Sounds that resemble snoring. They occur when air is blocked or air flow becomes rough through the large airways.
3. *Stridor:* Wheeze-like sound heard when a person breathes. Usually it is due to a blockage of airflow in the trachea or in the back of the throat.
4. *Wheezing:* High-pitched sounds produced by narrowed airways. They are most often heard in when a person breathes out (exhales). Wheezing and other abnormal sounds can sometimes be heard without a stethoscope.

Investigations

Investigating respiratory illness in children is tricky because in young children respiratory illness does not necessarily have a respiratory presentation, the approach to investigation is incomplete, clinical syndromes overlap, pathogens hunt together.

Chest radiographs: X-rays are made by using low levels of external radiation to produce images of the body, the organs, and other internal structures for diagnostic purposes. Chest X-rays may be used to assess heart status (either directly or indirectly) by looking at the heart itself, as well as the lungs. Changes in the normal structure of the heart, lungs, and/or lung vessels may indicate disease or other conditions.

An abnormal chest X-ray may require further testing, including a chest computed tomography (CT) scan. If an abnormal growth is seen, a biopsy may be ordered.

Blood gas analysis: An arterial blood gas (ABG) is a **blood test** that is performed using **blood** from an **artery** (such as radial, femoral). ABG gives information regarding patient's oxygenation and acid base status. Arterial blood gas analysis reveals oxygenation status, adequacy of ventilation and acid-base balance. It plays a significant role in documenting and monitoring respiratory failure, especially during ventilator and oxygen therapy.

Cellular function is ultimately dependent on regular supply of glucose, oxygen and water. Consequently, volatile acids like carbonic acid (from tissue oxidation) and fixed acids like sulfuric acid, phosphoric acid, lactic acid, ketoacid (products of intermediary metabolism) are constantly poured into the general circulation. Respiratory system plays an important role in eliminating volatile acids while renal mechanisms eliminate fixed acids in the form of hydrogen ions. In pathological states, this homeostasis gets disturbed causing accumulation of the above acids and resulting in acid-base disturbance. Though renal and respiratory system take the brunt to mitigate the acid-base disturbance, the other important mechanism for immediate rescue is the buffer base system which includes intracellular and extracellular buffers.

If the acid base disturbances are mild, the pH variation is also within adjustable limits (7.3–7.5) and the clinical manifestations are not overt. In severe acidosis when pH falls below 7.20, grave features like poor myocardial performance, arrhythmias, hypotension, pulmonary edema and hyperkalemia occur. Similarly in severe alkalosis when the pH exceeds 7.5 features like mental confusion, muscular irritability, seizures, arrhythmias, generalized tissue hypoxia and hypokalemia occur. Identification of these clinical features is difficult in a sick child presenting predominantly with the features of primary disease.

An ABG is a test that measures the **arterial oxygen tension** (PaO_2), **carbon dioxide tension** ($PaCO_2$), and acidity (pH). In addition, arterial oxyhemoglobin saturation (SaO_2) can be determined. Such information is vital when caring for patients with critical illness or respiratory disease.

Pulse oximetry: It checks the oxygen content of the blood. The device used to perform the test is a **pulse oximeter**, which consists of a sensor that emits light in different wavelengths to measure how much oxygen is in the blood. A sticker or bandage is used to temporarily attach a sensor to the baby's finger, earlobe, or foot.

The sensor monitors how much oxygen is in the baby's blood in both arms and both feet. A newborn baby should have an oxygen saturation of greater than 95% and a difference of no more than 3% in the saturation in the arms and feet. The test is performed three times, an hour apart, ideally when the baby is 24 to 48 hours old.

Pulmonary function tests (PFT): PFT is a breathing test designed to give information about the actual objective measurements of the patient's respiratory physiology (Fig. 13.4A). It includes a series of breathing maneuvers that measure the amount of air in the lungs, and how well the lungs function in moving air in and out. They are painless, non-invasive, and most children age five or older are able to perform these tests by following some simple directions.

Bronchoscopy: Bronchoscopy is a procedure which can help to diagnose and treat some conditions of the airways (bronchi) and lungs (Fig. 13.4B). The bronchoscope is passed through the nose or mouth, down the back of the throat, into the trachea, and down into the bronchi. The fiber-optics allow light to shine around bends in the bronchoscope and so the doctor can see clearly inside your airways.

A rigid bronchoscope is like a thin, straight telescope. It may be needed for some procedures, and in children. It requires a general anesthetic whereas fiber-optic bronchoscopy only requires sedation. Both types of bronchoscope have a side channel down which thin instruments can pass. For example, a thin grabbing instrument can pass down to take a small sample from the inside lining of a bronchus, or from structures next to a bronchus.

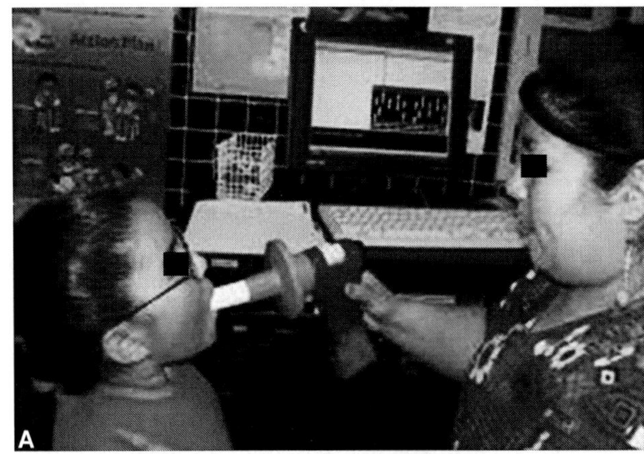

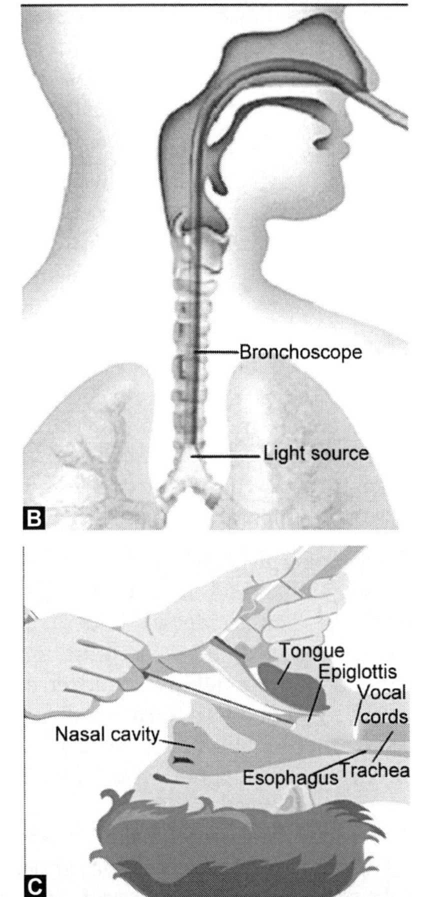

Figs 13.4A to C: A. Pulmonary function test; **B.** Broncoscopy; **C.** Laryngoscopy

Laryngoscopy: Laryngoscopy is a visual examination below the back of the throat, where the voice box (larynx) containing the vocal cords is located (Fig. 13.4C). It is an effective procedure for discovering the causes of voice and breathing problems, throat or ear pain, difficulty in swallowing, narrowing of the throat (strictures or stenosis), and airway blockages. The three kinds of laryngoscopy are indirect laryngoscopy, fiber-optic (flexible) laryngoscopy, direct laryngoscopy.

- Indirect laryngoscopy uses a small mirror held at the back of throat and doctor shines a light on the mirror to view the throat area. This is a simple procedure where medicine to numb the back of throat may be used.

- Fiber-optic laryngoscopy uses a small flexible telescope. The scope is passed through nose and into throat. This is the most common way that the voice box is examined. Patient remains awake for the procedure. Numbing medicine will be sprayed in nose. This procedure typically takes less than 1 minute.
- Laryngoscopy using strobe light can also be done. Use of strobe light can give the performer more information about problems with voice box.
- Direct laryngoscopy uses a tube called a laryngoscope. The instrument is placed in the back of throat. The tube may be flexible or stiff. This procedure allows the doctor to see deeper in the throat and to remove a foreign object or sample tissue for a biopsy. It is done under general anesthesia.

Transcutaneous (TC) monitoring: TC is an innovative and highly-accurate technology which provides quantitative information about cutaneous oxygenation and perfusion. Its power and appeal derive from a simple principle. Through a non-invasive sensor applied to the body, blood gases diffusing through the skin can be detected and estimated. For example, any changes in oxygen uptake, carbon dioxide washout, transport and release are reflected by $tcpO_2$ and $tcpCO_2$ values. Thus, it is ideal for neonatal intensive care units to monitor preterm babies or in sleep laboratories to track and diagnose sleep disorders. It is also extremely well suited for respiratory care, intensive care units.

Computed tomography: Computed tomography remains the imaging method of choice for investigating trauma (including non-accidental injury) and when hemorrhage is suspected, these account for a considerable portion of neuroimaging in children and young adults. The speed of modern computed tomography scanners is such that sedation or general anesthesia are rarely required, whereas magnetic resonance imaging in children may require anesthesia because it takes much longer to carry out. The small risks associated with anesthesia are comparable to, or sometimes greater than, the risks of exposure to radiation from computed tomography.

CT scanning, also called computed tomography, is a test using X-rays and powerful computers for diagnosis. X-rays are taken from a series of different angles around the body. CT detectors report the results of these X-rays to a powerful computer that uses the data to compute cross-sectional views of organs in the body.

CT can be utilized to evaluate abdomen—evaluation for neoplasm, inflammatory conditions, traumatic injury, chest, cardiovascular—heart and large blood vessel, musculoskeletal—bone and joints, neuroradiology—spine, neck, head.

Acute Respiratory Infections

Acute respiratory infections (ARIs) are the most common causes of both illness and mortality in children under five, who average three to six episodes of ARIs annually. ARIs are classified as upper respiratory tract infections (URIs) or lower respiratory tract infections (LRIs). ARIs are not confined to the respiratory tract and have systemic effects because of possible extension of infection or microbial toxins, inflammation, and reduced lung function. Diphtheria, pertussis, and measles are vaccine-preventable diseases that may have a respiratory tract component they also affect other systems of the body (*See* Chapter 20).

However, the proportion of mild to severe disease varies between high- and low-income countries, and because of differences in specific etiology and risk factors, the severity of LRIs in children under five is worse in developing countries, resulting in a higher case-fatality rate. Although medical care can mitigate both severity and fatality to some extent, many severe LRIs do not respond to therapy, largely because of the lack of highly effective antiviral drugs. Some 10.8 million children die each year. *The World Health Organization (WHO) estimates that 2 million children under five die of pneumonia each year.*

Disorders of Upper Respiratory Tract

The upper respiratory tract consists of the airways from the nostrils to the vocal cords in the larynx, including the paranasal sinuses and the middle ear. These structures direct the air that man breathes from the outside to the trachea and eventually to the lungs for respiration to take place.

An upper respiratory tract infection, or upper respiratory infection, is an infectious process of any of the components of the upper airway. Infection of the specific areas of the upper respiratory tract can be named specifically. Vast majority of upper respiratory infections are caused by viruses and are self-limited.

Common Cold

An upper respiratory infection (URI), also known as the common cold, is one of the most common illnesses, leading to more hospital/clinic visits and absences from school and work than any other illness every year. The common cold (viral upper respiratory tract infection, acute viral rhinopharyngitis, acute coryza or cold) is a contagious, viral infectious disease of upper respiratory system. Caused by a virus that inflames the membranes in the lining of the nose and throat, colds can be the result of more than 200 different viruses. However, among all of the cold viruses, the rhinoviruses cause the majority of colds. Other viruses include the corona virus, parainfluenza virus, adenovirus, enterovirus, and respiratory syncytial virus.

Pathophysiology

After the virus enters the child's body, it causes a reaction—the body's immune system begins to react to the foreign virus. This, in turn, causes an increase in mucus production (a runny nose). Congestion occurs due to swelling of the lining of the nose, and it makes it hard to breath. Sneezing may start from the irritation in the nose and cough from the increased mucus dripping down the throat.

Etiology and Incidence

What is referred to as 'a cold' can be caused by different viruses. These viruses spread easily from person to person both through the air and by touching germ-laden surfaces then touching nose, mouth or eyes. A cold is easy for children to spread because they touch their nose, mouth, and eyes often and then touch other people or objects and can spread the virus. It is important to know that viruses can be spread through objects, such as toys, that have been previously touched by someone with a cold. That is why handwashing for child and caregiver is so important.

Manifestations

Infants: Unable to sleep, fussiness, congestion in the nose, sometimes vomiting and diarrhea, fever.

Older children: Stuffy, runny nose, watery eyes, scratchy, tickly throat, sneezing (Fig. 13.5), mild hacking cough, congestion, sore throat, fever, achy muscles and joints, watery discharge from the nose that thickens and turns yellow or green.

Treatment for the Common Cold

It is important to remember that there is no cure for the common cold and that antibiotics will not help treat a common cold. Medications are used to help relieve the symptoms, but will not make the cold go away any faster. Therefore, treatment is based on helping the symptoms and supportive care.

Increased fluid intake helps to keep the lining of the nose and throat moist and help to prevent dehydration.

Avoidance of secondhand smoke—child should be kept away from passive (secondhand) smoke, as this will increase the irritation in the nose and throat.

To help relieve the congestion and obstruction in the nose for younger children, following applications may be considered:

- Saline nose drops may be used.
- Use a bulb syringe to help remove the mucus.
- Cool mist humidifier in the room help in easy respiration.
- Analgesics, such as acetaminophen, are sometimes helpful in decreasing the discomfort of colds.

Aspirin is contraindicated to a child who has fever. Aspirin, when given as treatment for viral illnesses in children, has been associated with Reye syndrome, a potentially serious or deadly disorder in children. So aspirin (or any medication that contains aspirin) not be used to treat any viral illnesses (such as colds, flu, and chickenpox) in children.

There are other medications for congestion, cough, or runny noses but over-the-counter cough and cold medicines for children are not recommended.

Complications

The possible complications from having a cold are ear infections, sinus infections, pneumonia and throat infections.

Prevention

Taking proper preventive measures can reduce the risk of child developing a cold. Preventive measures may include:

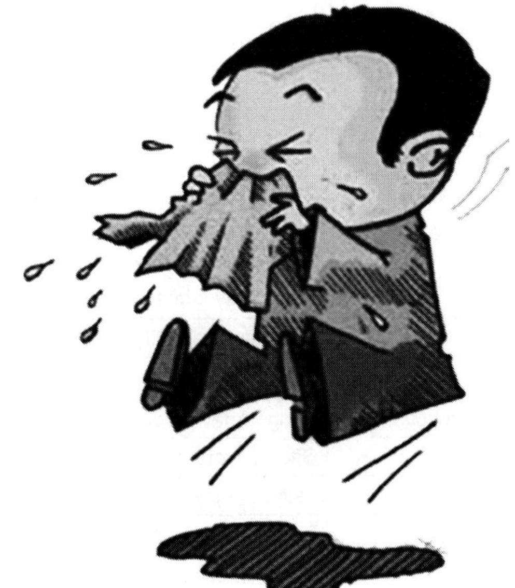

Fig. 13.5: Common cold

- Keep child away from a person with a cold.
- Encourage child to wash his or her hands frequently and not to touch his or her mouth, eyes, or nose until their hands are washed.
- Make sure toys and play areas are properly cleaned, especially if multiple children are playing together.

Influenza (Flu)

Like a cold, influenza affects the upper respiratory system. Unlike a cold, though, it often causes severe illness and complications. Flu is highly contagious disease and can seasonal epidemics manifesting as an acute febrile illness with variable degrees of severity, ranging from mild fatigue to respiratory failure and death. It is caused by one of three types of influenza viruses. Types A and B are responsible for the yearly flu epidemics, and type C flu virus causes sporadic mild illness. Type A flu virus is further divided into different subtypes based on the chemical structure of the virus.

Flu is spread among children when a child either inhales infected droplets in the air (coughed up or sneezed by an infected person) or when the child comes in direct contact with an infected person's secretions. A person can be contagious one day before onset of symptoms and 5–7 days after being sick. This can happen, for example, when they share pencils at school or play computer games and share the remotes or share utensils such as spoons and forks. Hand to hand contact is also important to consider when thinking about how flu can spread.

Manifestations

The symptoms of flu in children are more severe than symptoms of a childhood cold. Symptoms of flu in children start abruptly and usually cause kids to feel the worse during the first two or three days of onset. A clear picture of symptoms of flu and cold is given below:

Cold symptoms	*Flu symptoms*
Low or no fever	High fever up to 104 °F. Chills and shakes with the fever
Sometimes a headache	Commonly a headache
Stuffy, runny nose	Sometimes a stuffy nose
Sneezing	Sometimes sneezing
Mild, hacking cough	Cough, may progress
Slight aches and pains	Often severe aches and pains
Mild fatigue	Fatigue, may persist
Sore throat	Sometimes a sore throat
Normal energy level	Exhaustion

Management

Supportive care for pediatric influenza can include the following:

- Acetaminophen for fever
- Steam inhalation
- Oral or intravenous fluids if dehydration occurs
- Antiviral therapy for selected patients.

Avian Influenza

World Health Organization (WHO) recommendations for the management of avian influenza are as follows:

- Patients with confirmed or suspected H5N1 infection should be treated with oseltamivir as soon as possible
- Zanamivir may be considered as an alternative if the patient is capable of using an inhaler
- If neuraminidase inhibitors are available, amantadine and rimantadine should not be used as first-line therapies, because of potential resistance
- If neuraminidase inhibitors are available and if the virus is susceptible, a combination of neuraminidase inhibitors and M2 inhibitors can be used in confirmed cases of H5N1 infection
- If neuraminidase inhibitors are not available, amantadine can be used as a first-line therapy, provided the virus is susceptible
- If neuraminidase inhibitors are not available, rimantadine can be used if the virus is known to be susceptible, because it has fewer side effects than amantadine
- For prophylaxis in high-risk and moderate-risk exposures, give oseltamivir for 7–10 days from the day of exposure
- Prophylaxis is not recommended for low-risk groups.

Vaccination in the Pediatric Population

Influenza vaccination in targeted high-risk populations is the best means of preventing severe disease caused by influenza virus. Vaccines made using inactivated influenza virus provide 60–90% protection against influenza when the vaccine matches the epidemic strain. Monovalent 2009 H1N1 influenza vaccine and seasonal trivalent inactivated influenza vaccine are well tolerated among children.

Live Attenuated Vaccine

Influenza vaccine is also available as a nasal spray (Flu Mist Quadrivalent) for healthy children aged 2 years or older, adolescents, and adults. Children who take aspirin, have asthma, or have had a wheezing episode in the preceding 12 months should not receive the intranasal vaccine. Several studies have demonstrated superior efficacy of the live attenuated vaccine in children.

General Influenza Prevention

Handwashing with soap and water is the most appropriate way to prevent infection by an influenza virus. Other preventive measures are to avoid touching of eyes or nose before washing hands, and to avoid sharing personal items with another person during an influenza outbreak.

Patients with influenza who are clinically stable and are able to convalesce at home are instructed to stay at home to avoid spread in the community.

Sinusitis

Sinusitis is an infection of the sinuses near the nose. These infections usually occur after a cold or after an allergic inflammation.

Child's sinuses are not fully developed until late in the teen years. Although small, the maxillary and ethmoid sinuses are present at birth. Unlike in adults, pediatric sinusitis is difficult to diagnose because symptoms of sinusitis can be caused by other problems, such as viral illness and allergy.

Etiology

Sometimes, a sinus infection happens after an upper respiratory infection (URI) or common cold. The URI causes inflammation of the nasal passages that can block the opening of the paranasal sinuses, and result in a sinus infection. Allergies can also lead to sinusitis because of the swelling of the nasal tissue and increased production of mucus. There are other possible conditions that can block the normal flow of secretions out of the sinuses and can lead to sinusitis including the following:

- Abnormalities in the structure of the nose
- Enlarged adenoids
- Diving and swimming
- Infections from a tooth
- Trauma to the nose
- Foreign objects stuck in the nose
- Cleft palate
- Gastroesophageal reflux disease (GERD)
- Secondhand smoke.

When the flow of secretions from the sinuses is blocked, bacteria may begin to grow. This leads to a sinus infection, or sinusitis. The most common bacteria that cause sinusitis include the following:

- *Streptococcus pneumoniae*
- *Haemophilus influenzae*
- *Moraxella catarrhalis.*

Pathophysiology

Viral infections and allergies affect sinuses the same way they affect the nasal passages, causing swelling and producing extra mucus. This makes it difficult for the sinuses to drain properly and as mucus accumulates, the sinuses become a safe haven for germs to grow. The resulting infection can cause sinus pressure and pain.

Manifestations

The symptoms of sinusitis depend greatly on the age of the child. The following are the most common symptoms of sinusitis. However, each child may experience symptoms differently. Symptoms may include:

- Younger children show symptoms such as runny nose, lasts longer than 7 to 10 days, discharge is usually thick green or yellow, but can be clear, night-time cough, occasional daytime cough, swelling around the eyes, usually no headaches younger than 5 years of age.
- Older children and adults show symptoms like runny nose or cold symptoms lasting longer than 7 to 10 days, drip in the throat from the nose, headache, usually in children age six or older, facial discomfort, bad breath, cough, fever, sore throat, swelling around the eye, often worse in the morning, irritability or fatigue.

Young children are more prone to infections of the nose, sinus, and ears, especially in the first several years of life. These are most frequently caused by viral infections, and they may be aggravated by allergies. However, if child remains ill beyond the usual week to ten days, a sinus infection may be the cause.

Sinus infections can be reduced for child by reducing exposure to known environmental allergies and pollutants such as tobacco smoke, reducing his/her time at day care, and treating stomach acid reflux disease.

Diagnosis

A thorough history and examination usually leads to the correct diagnosis. Occasionally, special instruments will be used to look into the nose. An X-ray called a CT scan may help to determine how completely the child's sinuses are developed, where any blockage has occurred, and confirm the diagnosis of sinusitis.

- **Sinus X-rays:** Diagnostic test which uses invisible electromagnetic energy beams to produce images of internal tissues, bones, and organs onto film. (X-rays are not typically used, but may help assist in the diagnosis).
- **Computed tomography (CT or CAT scan):** A diagnostic imaging procedure that uses a combination of X-rays and computer technology to produce horizontal or axial images (often called slices) of the body. A CT scan shows detailed images of any part of the body, including the bones, muscles, fat, and organs. CT scans are more detailed than general X-rays.
- **Cultures from the sinuses:** Laboratory tests that involve the growing of bacteria or other microorganisms to aid in diagnosis.

Treatment

The goal in treating these children is to combine antibiotic therapy with treatment of associated conditions for a time sufficient to allow resolution of symptoms with return of normal sinus physiology and mucociliary clearance.

Acute sinusitis: Most children respond very well to antibiotic therapy. Nasal decongestant sprays or saline nasal sprays may also be prescribed for short-term relief of stuffiness. Nasal saline drops or gentle spray can be helpful in thinning secretions and improving mucous membrane function. Over-the-counter decongestants and antihistamines are not general effective for viral upper respiratory infections in children, and the role of such medications for treatment of sinusitis is not well-defined. Such medications should not be given to children younger than 2 years old.

Symptoms of a child with acute sinusitis, should improve within the first few days of treatment. Even if child improves dramatically within the first week of treatment, it is important that to complete the antibiotic therapy. To treat child with additional medicines if he/she has allergies or other conditions make the sinus infection worse.

Chronic sinusitis*:* If child suffers from one or more symptoms of sinusitis for at least 12 weeks, he or she may have chronic sinusitis. Chronic sinusitis or recurrent episodes of acute sinusitis numbering more than four to six per year, are indications that parents should seek consultation with an otolaryngologist. The ear, nose and throat (ENT) may recommend medical or surgical treatment of the sinuses.

Surgery is considered for the small percentage of children with severe or persistent sinusitis symptoms despite medical therapy. Using an instrument called an endoscope, the ENT surgeon opens the natural drainage pathways of child's sinuses and makes the narrow passages wider. This also allows for culturing so that antibiotics can be directed specifically against child's sinus infection. Opening up the sinuses and allowing air to circulate usually results in a reduction in the number and severity of sinus infections. Surgical removal of adenoid tissue from behind the nose may be a part of the treatment for sinusitis. Although the adenoid tissue does not directly block the sinuses, infection of the adenoid tissue, called adenoiditis (obstruction of the back of the nose), can cause many symptoms that are similar to sinusitis, namely, runny nose, stuffy nose, post-nasal drip, bad breath, cough, and headache.

Otitis Media

Acute ear infection occurs with up to 30 percent of URIs. In developing countries with inadequate medical care, it may lead to perforated eardrums and chronic ear discharge in later childhood and ultimately to hearing impairment or deafness. Chronic ear infection following repeated episodes of acute ear infection is common in developing countries, affecting 2 to 6 percent of school-age children. The associated hearing loss may be disabling and may affect learning. Repeated ear infections may lead to mastoiditis, which in turn may spread infection to the meninges. Mastoiditis and other complications of URIs account for nearly 5 percent of all ARI deaths worldwide.

Pharyngitis and Tonsillitis

Pharyngitis and tonsillitis are infections in the throat that cause inflammation. Examination of patients who present with sore throat may reveal tonsillitis, tonsillopharyngitis, or nasopharyngitis.

Pharyngitis is inflammation of the structures of pharynx and lymphoid tissues. It is also called sore throat. It is relatively minor and self-limiting disease but bacteria like Group A beta-hemolytic streptococci (GABHS), can have serious complications like rheumatic fever and glomerular nephritis.

The term tonsillitis is commonly used to describe inflammation and infection of the two palatine tonsils. Adenoiditis is the inflammation of the adenoids (pharyngeal tonsils), which are located above palatine tonsils on the posterior wall of the nasopharynx. When the tonsils become infected they isolate the infection and stop it spreading further into the body.

As a child's immune system develops and gets stronger, the tonsils become less important and usually shrink. In most people, the body is able to fight infection without the tonsils, but sometimes the tonsils become a site for infection.

A child might even have inflammation and infection of both the tonsils and the throat. This would be called pharyngotonsillitis.

Etiology and Incidence

Pharyngitis is uncommon in children below 1 year of age but its incidence is peak around 5–6 years when most children's schooling starts. Tonsillitis most commonly affects children between preschool ages and the mid-teenage years.

There are many causes of infections in the throat. Viruses are the most common cause and do not require antibiotics. Treating viral pharyngitis and tonsillitis is a common reason for the inappropriate use of antibiotics, which should be used only for bacterial infections. Causes of throat infections include viruses like Adenovirus, Influenza virus, Rhinovirus, Coxsackie virus, Epstein-Barr virus (mononucleosis), Herpes simplex virus and bacteria like GABHS, *Neisseria gonorrhoeae, Haemophilus influenzae* type b, *Mycoplasma, Chlamydia pneumoniae* and fungal and parasitic infection.

The primary concern for pharyngitis and tonsilitis in children aged 2 years or older is that untreated GABHS pharyngitis may subsequently cause rheumatic fever. The absence of pharyngeal inflammation or the presence of rhinorrhea is much more likely to be associated with viral infection. However, no physical findings clearly separate GABHS from viral, other bacterial, or noninfectious causes.

Pathophysiology

Acute pharyngitis is defined as an infection of the pharynx and/or tonsils. It is a very common pathology among children and adolescents. Pharyngitis often associates with common cold and clinical manifestations include sore throat and fever with sudden onset, red pharynx, enlarged tonsils covered with a yellow, blood-tinged exudate. Inflamed palatine tonsils may meet in the midline and cause difficulty in swallowing and breathing. The Eustachian tubes may be obstructed due to enlargement of adenoids and it may cause otitis media and hearing impairment. Hypertrophied adenoids can block the passageway between the nose and throat, and may precipitate mouth breathing or obstructive sleep apnea.

Manifestations

Common signs and symptoms of pharyngitis are pain during swallowing, hoarseness, cough, runny or stuffy nose, itchy or watery eyes, a rash on the body, fever and headache. Usually low-grade fever in viral infection and high-grade fever in bacterial infection is observed. Erythema and inflammation of the pharynx and tonsils, cervical lymph nodes may be enlarged and tender, nausea, vomiting, diarrhea, or stomach pain.

Common signs and symptoms of tonsillitis include red, swollen tonsils, white or yellow coating or patches on the tonsils, sore throat, difficult or painful swallowing, fever, enlarged, tender glands (lymph nodes) in the neck, a scratchy, muffled or throaty voice, bad breath, stomachache, particularly in younger children, stiff neck, headache.

In young children who are unable to describe how they feel, signs of tonsillitis may include drooling due to difficult or painful swallowing, refusal to eat and unusual fussiness.

Diagnosis

In some cases, it is hard to distinguish between a viral sore throat and a strep throat based on physical examination. As a result, some children, when they have the above symptoms, will receive a strep test and possibly a throat culture to determine if it is an infection caused by GABHS. This usually involves a throat swab test in the clinic.

A throat swab is collected for throat culture. A cotton swab is rubbed against the back of the child's throat. This test may show if bacteria are causing the child's sore throat and the type of bacteria that are causing it.

Quick tests, called rapid strep tests, may be performed. Rapid antigen detection assays for GABHS are diagnostic if positive because the specificity of such tests is 98–99% (1–2% false-positive results); however, their sensitivity is only 70% (30% false-negative results), necessitating follow-up cultures for negative results.

This may immediately show as positive for GABHS and antibiotics will be started. If it is negative, part of the throat swab will usually be kept for a throat culture. This will further identify, in 2 to 3 days, if GABHS is present. The treatment plan is determined based on the findings.

Treatment

In acute phase of pharyngitis and tonsillitis, treatment is symptomatic. If bacteria are not the cause of the infection, then the treatment is focused on the comfort of the child. Antibiotics will not help treat viral sore throats. Treatment may include:

- Acetaminophen or ibuprofen for pain relief and anti-inflammatory effect.

- Rest—encourage the child to get plenty of sleep and to rest his or her voice.
- Increased fluid intake
- Throat lozenges (for children old enough to handle hard candies)
- Antibiotics (if the cause of the infection is bacterial, not viral)—the drug of choice for treatment of GABHS remains penicillin V, which is given two to three times daily for 10 days. Although many experts recommend shorter courses of antibiotics like amoxicillin, cephalosporins, azithromycin because of its efficacy like penicillin, superior compliance and adherence, lower incidence of side effects, improved parent satisfaction and lower drug costs.
- Surgical removal of tonsils/adenoids—surgery to remove the tonsils (a tonsillectomy) is usually only recommended in cases where there have been several severe episodes of tonsillitis over a long period of time, or if repeated episodes disrupt normal activities.

A tonsillectomy may also be performed if tonsillitis results in difficult-to-manage complications, such as obstructive sleep apnea, breathing difficulty, swallowing difficulty, an abscess that does not improve with antibiotic treatment.

Electrosurgical tonsillectomy is a newer method that uses electromagnetic radiation to generate heat within tissue for cutting and coagulation. The risk for bleeding may be lessen by this technique and produce less patient's discomfort than traditional surgical method. Generally, tonsillectomy is not done in children under 3 years of age as of the tendency for remaining tonsillar tissues to hypertrophy. Tonsillectomy is also contraindicated in active infection and cleft palate. Adenoidectomy is also done in case of repeated otitis media caused by obstruction of eustachian tube and or for persistent nasal and airway obstruction.

LOWER RESPIRATORY TRACT DISORDERS

The lower respiratory tract covers the continuation of the airways from the trachea and bronchi to the bronchioles and the alveoli.

Acute Tracheolaryngobronchitis/Infectious Croup

The common early childhood ailment is known as (tracheolaryngobronchitis) involves inflammation of the trachea, the larynx and the bronchioles. Croup is a syndrome and recognized by a distinctive 'barking cough' and varying degree of respiratory distress that usually starts suddenly and at night. Children ages 3 months to 3 years are most susceptible to croup. The major types of croup include acute laryngotracheitis, spasmodic croup, bacterial tracheitis, laryngotracheobronchitis, and epiglottitis.

Etiology and Incidence

Croup is usually deemed to be due to a viral infection and also due to bacterial infection. Viral croup or acute laryngotracheitis is caused by parainfluenza virus, primarily types 1 and 2, in 75% of cases. Other viral causes include influenza, measles, adenovirus and respiratory syncytial virus (RSV). Spasmodic croup is caused by the same group of viruses as acute laryngotracheitis, but lacks the usual signs of infection (such as fever, sore throat, and increased white blood cell count).

Bacterial tracheitis is less common than laryngotracheobronchitis and acute spasmodic croup. Laryngeal diphtheria is due to *Corynebacterium diphtheriae* while bacterial tracheitis, laryngotracheobronchitis, and laryngotracheobronchopneumonitis are usually due to a primary viral infection.

Children are most likely to get croup between 3 months and 5 years of age. As they get older, it is not as common because the windpipe is larger and swelling is less likely to get in the way of breathing. Croup can occur at any time of the year, but it is more common in the pre-winter and winter months. It has a slightly higher frequency in boys than in girls. Bacterial croup is an infection of the same structures that are affected during a viral process.

Pathophysiology

Croup is the infection of upper airway, often caused by viruses, with parainfluenza virus as the most common. In all forms of croup the entire upper airway is involved to some extent and it is named according to the anatomic area most severely involved. In spasmodic croup the larynx is the area of most severe inflammation. Other types are laryngotracheitis croup, laryngotracheobronchitis, and laryngotracheobronchopneumonitis.

The viral infection that causes croup leads to swelling of the larynx, trachea, and large bronchi due to infiltration of **white blood cells**. The swelling causes the airway below the vocal cords to become narrow and produces airway obstruction which, when significant, leads to dramatically increased work of breathing and the characteristic turbulent, noisy airflow known as stridor. In all forms of croup, the airway becomes narrow due to inflammation and edema. The narrowing of airway is dangerous to children because of their small airway diameter, and flexible larynx, which is more susceptible to spasm.

Mucosal inflammation and sudden onset of symptoms: Respiratory distress—sternal retraction, edema, narrow airway, croup, pallor, cyanosis, increased HR, hypoxia.

Types and Manifestations

Viral croup

This is the most common type of croup. It is caused by a viral infection of the voice box and windpipe. It often starts out just like a cold, but then slowly turns into a barky cough. The child's voice will become hoarse and her breathing will get noisier. She may make a coarse musical sound each time she breathes in called stridor. Most children with viral croup have a low fever, but some have temperatures up to 104 °F (40 °C).

Spasmodic Croup

This type of croup is thought to be caused by an allergy or by reflux from the stomach. It can be scary because it comes on suddenly, often in the middle of the night. The child may go to bed well and wake up in a few hours, gasping for breath. She will be hoarse and have stridor when she breathes in. She also may have a barky cough. Most children with spasmodic croup do not have a fever. This type of croup can recur. It is similar to asthma and often responds to allergy or reflux medicines.

Stridor

Stridor is common with mild croup, especially when a child is crying or active. But if a child has stridor while resting, it can be a sign of more severe croup. As child's effort to breathe increases, she may stop eating and drinking. She also may become too tired to cough, and parent may hear the stridor more with each breath.

The danger of croup with stridor is that sometimes the airway may swell so much child may barely be able to breathe (Fig. 13.6). In the most severe cases, child will not be getting enough oxygen into her blood. If this happens, she needs to go to the hospital. Luckily, these most severe cases of croup do not occur very often.

The severity of symptoms is proportional to the amount of relative narrowing of the airway. The more severe the vocal cord narrowing the more effort is required to inhale. A severely sick child will refuse to lie down, demanding to remain in an upright position. They will show retractions of the skin above the collarbone and between the ribs with inspiration and may develop facial cyanosis. Apparent exhaustion and decreased respiratory effort are an indication of impending respiratory failure and are cause for immediate paramedic evaluation and transport to the emergency department of the closest hospital.

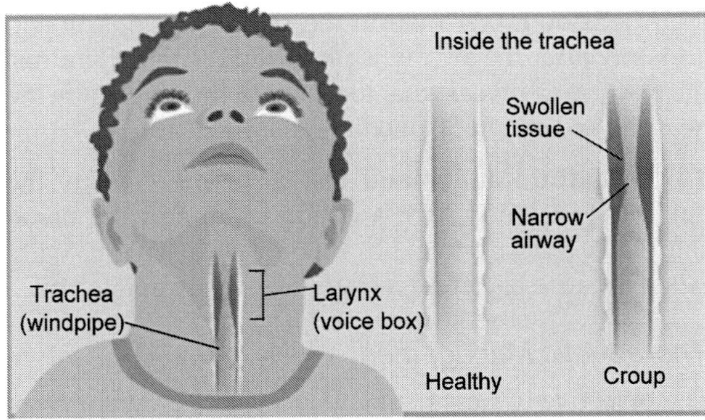

Fig. 13.6: A child with tracheolaryngobronchitis

Diagnostic Evaluation

Croup is diagnosed based on child's clinical symptoms and a physical examination. Pulse oximeter may be used to make sure that enough oxygen is reaching the blood or not. Differentiation between viral croup and bacterial epiglottitis is very important as treatment differs. Arterial blood gas values may be monitored to detect decreased PaO_2 levels.

Therapeutic Management

Croup can be frightening for both children and parents. Therefore, comforting and reassuring the child is the first step. Breathing difficulties can develop and worsen rapidly. Close monitoring of the child is important during the early phases of the illness. The goal of treatment is to maintain patent airway.

Urgent care or emergency department treatment of croup depends on the degree of respiratory distress. In mild croup, a child may present with only a croupy cough and may require nothing more than parental reassurance, given alertness, baseline minimal respiratory distress, proper oxygenation, and stable fluid status (oral fluid) may be increased if the child is not in respiratory distress. The caregivers may only need education regarding the course of the disease and supportive homecare guidelines.

Oral or parenteral corticosteroid therapy may be administered in this disease to reduce inflammatory edema and to destruction of ciliated epithelium. Nebulization with budesonide may also be continued. In case of bacterial infection, antibiotic is administered. Intravenous fluid is given until respiratory distress subsides. Sedatives are contraindicated as they depress respiratory center and could mask restlessness, an early sign of hypoxia.

To help the child breathe more comfortably, a cool or warm mist vaporizer can be placed near the child. The humidified air promotes reduction of vocal cord swelling and thus lessens symptoms. To avoid scalds burns, cool mist humidifiers are recommended. When cough or stridor worsens at night, 10 or 15 minutes sitting or driving in the cool night air can also help the child breathe.

However, any infant/child who presents with significant respiratory distress/complaints with stridor at rest must have a thorough clinical evaluation to ensure the patency of the airway and maintenance of effective oxygenation and ventilation. Keep young children as comfortable as possible, allowing him or her to remain in a parent's arms and avoiding unnecessary painful interventions that may cause agitation, respiratory distress, and lead to increased oxygen requirements. Persistent crying increases oxygen demands, and respiratory muscle fatigue can worsen the obstruction.

Epiglottitis

Epiglottitis is an inflammation of the epiglottis and/or the supraglottic tissues surrounding the epiglottis. This includes the aryepiglottic folds, arytenoid soft tissue, and occasionally, the uvula. Due to its place in the airway, swelling of this structure can interfere with breathing, and constitutes a life-threatening emergency. Infection can cause the epiglottis to obstruct or completely close off the airway.

Etiology

Epiglottitis is usually an infectious process of bacterial etiology, but it can be caused by caustic ingestion, thermal injury, or direct trauma. Epiglottitis, most often is caused by *Haemophilus influenzae* type B, other organisms such as *Streptococcus pneumoniae, Streptococcus agalactiae, Staphylococcus aureus, Streptococcus pyogenes, Haemophilus influenzae,* and Group A beta hemolytic streptococcus, may also cause the infection (less frequently).

Epiglottitis is more common in children ages 3 to 7 years. With the advent of the Hib vaccine, the incidence of epiglottitis has decreased, but the condition has not been eliminated.

Pathophysiology
Epiglottitis, also termed supraglottitis is an inflammation of structures above the insertion of the glottis and is most often caused by bacterial infection. Affected structures include the epiglottis, aryepiglottic folds, arytenoid soft tissue, and occasionally, the uvula. Epiglottis becomes edematous and cherry red color with high fever. The edema is severe and painful. The epiglottis is the most common site of swelling, which obstruct the airway. Secretions pool in the hypopharynx and larynx and the child is unable to swallow and begins to drool. Acute epiglottitis and associated upper airway obstruction has significant morbidity (stridor, cough, hypoxia, acidosis) and mortality and may cause respiratory arrest and death.

Manifestations

Epiglottitis commonly affects children, and it is associated with fever, difficulty in swallowing, drooling, hoarseness of voice, and typically stridor. Stridor is a sign of upper airways obstruction and is a surgical emergency. The child often appears acutely ill, anxious, and has very quiet shallow breathing with the head held forward, insisting on sitting up in bed. The early symptoms are insidious but rapidly progressive, and swelling of the throat may lead to cyanosis and asphyxiation.

Cardinal signs and symptoms of epiglottitis	
Drooling *Dysphagia* *Dysphonia* *Distress in respiratory effort*	[In case of suspected epiglottitis, examination or obtain material for culture is contraindicated, as any stimulation with tongue depressor or culture swab could trigger complete airway obstruction. The child should not leave alone]

Diagnosis

Blood oxygen level: Measures an estimation of the saturation of oxygen in blood is done by pulse oxymeter.

Examination of epiglottis: An edematous, cherry red epiglottis is the most reliable diagnostic sign of epiglottitis. Laryngoscopy is the best way to confirm the diagnosis of epiglottitis, but this **should not be** done outside the operating room or where an immediate airway can be obtained. Simply depressing the child's tongue with a tongue blade may help in visualizing the epiglottitis but it is contraindicated. Some concern exists regarding the safety of such procedures, which can provoke anxiety and increased respiratory effort or laryngospasm during examination, leading to airway obstruction.

Chest or neck X-ray: Because of the danger of sudden breathing problems, children may have X-rays taken at their bedside rather than in the radiology department, and only after the airway is protected. With epiglottitis, the X-ray may reveal what looks like a thumbprint in the neck, an indication of an enlarged epiglottis.

Throat culture and blood tests: For the culture, the epiglottis is wiped with a cotton swab and the tissue sample is checked for Hib. Blood cultures are usually taken because bacteremia may accompany epiglottitis.

Therapeutic Management

The objective of treatment is to achieve a patent airway as quickly as possible.

If the child has adequate oxygenation, urgent transport to the health care setting is required. Everything should be done to keep the child calm, often in the arms of a parent.

The conscious and stable child should be allowed to assume a position of comfort. Oxygen may be administered if it does not disturb the child. Obtaining vital signs or any other diagnostic procedures are secondary to assuring an adequate airway.

If the child has a respiratory arrest, first attempt ventilation with a bag-valve mask. Long, slow ventilations are best. Orotracheal intubation should be attempted if emergency service personnel are unable to ventilate the child. Orotracheal intubation or needle cricothyroidotomy (also known as percutaneous transtracheal ventilation or translaryngeal ventilation) may be necessary in emergent situations.

Oxygen may be administered if it does not disturb the child. Once airway is secured the child is transferred to intensive care unit and following steps are to be taken:

- Intravenous fluids for nutrition and hydration until the child is able to swallow again
- Antibiotics to get rid of a bacterial infection. Antibiotic therapy is necessary but should be initiated after securing the airway. Empiric antimicrobial therapy must cover all likely pathogens in the context of the clinical setting.
- Anti-inflammatory medication, such as corticosteroids, to reduce the swelling of the throat
- A minor surgical procedure requiring a needle insertion into the trachea tissue, also known as a tracheotomy (in very severe cases) to allow exchange of oxygen and to prevent respiratory failure. This procedure allows air into the child's lungs while bypassing the larynx.

Bronchiolitis

Bronchiolitis is an acute viral infection of the lower respiratory tract affecting infants below two years and is characterized by respiratory distress, wheezing, and crackles. It is usually caused by a virus which causes inflammation of the tiny airways called the bronchioles that lead to the lungs. As these airways become inflamed, they swell and fill with mucus, making breathing difficult (Fig. 13.7). The inflammation partially or completely blocks the airways, which causes wheezing. This means that less oxygen enters the lungs, potentially causing a decrease in the blood level of oxygen.

Etiology and Incidence

More than 50% of bronchiolitis or inflammation of bronchioles are usually caused by Respiratory Syncytial Virus (RSV). Children who are older than two years typically do not develop bronchiolitis, but can be infected with RSV. RSV infection is common in children older than 2 years. RSV is transmitted through droplets that contain viral particles; these are exhaled into the air by breathing, coughing, or sneezing. These droplets can be carried on the hands, where they survive and can spread infection for several hours. If someone with RSV on his or her hands touches a child's eye, nose, or mouth, the virus can infect the child. It causes symptoms similar to those of the common cold or mild wheezing and infants usually acquire the disease from an older child or adult.

Although it is not airborne, it is highly communicable and needs thorough handwashing. Other causative organisms of bronchiolitis are *Mycoplasma*, parainfluenza virus, and some adenovirus.

Bronchiolitis is a common cause of illness and is the leading cause of hospitalization in infants and young children. Typically, the peak time for bronchiolitis is during the winter months. It can cause serious illness in some children. Infants who are very young, born early, have pulmonary or heart disease, or have difficulty fighting infections or handling oral secretions are more likely to have severe disease with bronchiolitis. The incidence peaks at age of six months. Nearly 100% children will have had RSV by age of 2 years. Immunity does not occur, but the incidence and severity decrease with age.

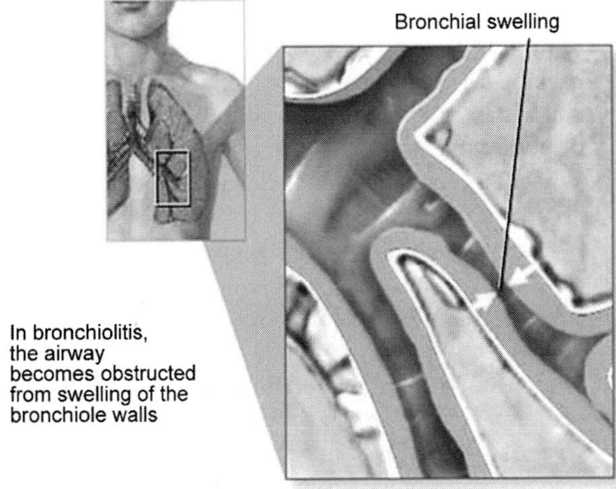

Fig. 13.7: Obstructed airways in bronchiolitis

Pathophysiology

In bronchiolitis, the obstruction of the bronchioles is caused by edema and accumulation of mucus and cellular debris. The virus spreads from the upper respiratory tract to the medium and small bronchi and bronchioles, causing epithelial necrosis and initiating an inflammatory response. Infants' bronchioles are very small and can become obstructed quickly. The developing edema and exudate result in partial obstruction, which is most pronounced on expiration and leads to alveolar air trapping. Complete obstruction and absorption of the trapped air may lead to multiple areas of atelectasis, which can be exacerbated by breathing high inspired O_2 concentrations. The child with bronchiolitis is most acutely ill during initial 24–48 hours after the onset of the disease. Improvement of this condition is usually occurs in a few days.

- URI usually by RSV (Respiratory Syncytial Virus)
- Epithelial necrosis and initiation of inflammatory response obstruct bronchioles
- Bronchioles constrict during breathing out, causing hyperinflation of lungs
- Atelectasis occurs due to complete obstruction and absorption of trapped air
- Normal exchange of gases impaired
- Hypoxemia
- Metabolic acidosis and mild respiratory alkalosis

Manifestations

Bronchiolitis usually develops from mild upper respiratory tract infection (common cold symptoms) like nasal congestion and discharge, a mild cough, fever (temperature higher than 100.4 °F or 38 °C), decreased appetite.

As the infection progresses and the lower airways are affected, other symptoms may develop, including the following:

- Breathing rapidly (60 to 80 times per minute) or with mild to severe difficulty. The effort required to breathe faster and harder is tiring. In severe cases, a child may not be able to continue to breathe on his or her own.
- Wheezing, crackles, rhonchi which usually lasts about 7 days.
- Persistent coughing, which may last for 14 or more days.
- Intercostal and subcostal retractions with or without nasal flaring.
- Difficulty feeding related to nasal congestion and rapid breathing, which can result in dehydration.
- Cyanosis—cyanosis may first be noticed in the finger and toenails; ear lobes; tip of the nose, lips, or tongue; and inside of the cheek.
- Apnea (a pause in breathing for more than 15 or 20 seconds) can be the first sign of bronchiolitis in an infant. This occurs more commonly in infants born prematurely and infants who are younger than 2 months.
- Grunting—a child who is grunting, appears to be tiring, stops breathing, or has cyanosis needs urgent medical attention.

Diagnosis

- Clinical presentation
- Pulse oximetry
- Chest X-ray as needed
- RSV antigen test on a nasal swab or washing for seriously ill children.

Diagnosis is suspected by history, examination, and occurrence of the illness as part of an epidemic. Symptoms similar to bronchiolitis can result from an asthma exacerbation, which is often precipitated by a respiratory viral infection and is more likely in a child > 18 month of age, especially if previous episodes of wheezing and a family history of asthma have been documented. Gastric reflux with aspiration of gastric contents also may cause the clinical picture of bronchiolitis; multiple episodes in an infant may be clues to this diagnosis. Foreign body aspiration occasionally causes wheezing and should be considered if the onset is sudden and not associated with manifestations of URI. Heart failure associated with a left-to-right shunt manifesting at age 2 to 3 month also can be confused with bronchiolitis.

Patients suspected of having bronchiolitis should undergo pulse oximetry to evaluate oxygenation. No further testing is required for mild cases with normal O_2 levels, but in cases of hypoxemia and severe respiratory distress, a chest X-ray supports the diagnosis and typically shows hyperinflated lungs, depressed diaphragm, and prominent hilar markings. Infiltrates may be present resulting from atelectasis and/or RSV pneumonia; RSV pneumonia is relatively common among infants with RSV bronchiolitis. RSV rapid antigen testing done on a nasal swab or washing is diagnostic but not generally necessary; it may be reserved for patients with illness severe enough to require hospitalization. Other laboratory testing is nonspecific; about two thirds of the children have WBC counts of 10,000 to 15,000/μL. Most have 50 to 75% lymphocytes.

The diagnosis of bronchiolitis is based upon a history and physical examination. Blood tests and X-rays are not usually necessary.

Treatment

- Supportive therapy
- O_2 supplementation as needed
- IV hydration as needed.

Treatment includes measures to ensure that the child consumes adequate fluids and is able to breathe without significant difficulty. Most children begin to improve 2 to 5 days after first developing breathing difficulties, but wheezing can last for a week or longer.

Emergent care: Parents should seek medical attention if the child seems to be worsening. A child who is grunting, appears to be tiring, stops breathing, or has blue-colored skin (cyanosis) needs urgent medical attention. Emergency medical services should be called, available in most areas of the United States by dialing 911.

Severe bronchiolitis should be evaluated in an emergency department or clinic capable of handling urgent respiratory illnesses. This is a life-threatening illness and treatment should not be delayed for any reason.

Symptomatic care: There is no cure for bronchiolitis, so treatment is aimed at the symptoms (e.g. difficulty breathing, fever). Treatment at home usually includes making sure the child drinks enough and saline nose drops (with bulb suctioning for infants).

Monitoring: Monitoring at home involves observing the child periodically for signs or symptoms of worsening. Specifically, this includes monitoring for an increased rate of breathing, worsening chest retractions, nasal flaring, cyanosis, a decreased ability to feed or decreased urine output. Parents should contact their child's health care provider to determine if and when an office visit is needed, or if there are any other questions or concerns.

Fever control: Parents may give acetaminophen (sample brand names: Tempra, Tylenol) to treat fever if the child is uncomfortable. Ibuprofen (sample brand names: Advil, Motrin) can be given to children greater than six months of age. Aspirin should not be given to any child under age 18 years. Parents should speak with their child's health care provider about when and how to treat fever.

Nose drops or spray: Saline nose drops or spray might help with congestion and runny nose. For infants, parents can try saline nose drops to thin the mucus, followed by bulb suction to temporarily remove nasal secretions. An older child may try using a saline nose spray before blowing the nose.

Encourage fluids: Parents should encourage their child to drink an adequate amount of fluids; it is not necessary to drink extra fluids. Children often have a reduced appetite, and may eat less than usual. If an infant or child completely refuses to eat or drink for a prolonged period, urinates less often, or has vomiting episodes with cough, the parent should contact their child's health care provider.

Other therapies: Other therapies, such as antibiotics, cough medicines, decongestants, and sedatives, are not recommended. Cough medicines and decongestants have not been proven to be helpful, and sedatives can mask symptoms of low blood oxygen and difficulty breathing.

Coughing is one way for the body to clear the lungs, and normally does not need to be treated. As the lungs heal, the coughing caused by the virus resolves. Smoking in the home or around the child should be avoided because it can worsen a child's cough.

Antibiotics are not effective in treating bronchiolitis because it is usually caused by a virus. However, antibiotics may be necessary if the bronchiolitis is complicated by a bacterial infection, like an ear infection or bacterial pneumonia (very uncommon).

Sometimes, keeping the child's head elevated can reduce the work of breathing. A child may be propped up in bed with an extra pillow. Pillows should not be used with infants younger than 12 months of age.

Hospital care: Approximately 3% of children with bronchiolitis will require monitoring and treatment in a hospital. Most children receive monitoring of vital signs and supportive care, including supplemental oxygen and intravenous fluids, if necessary. Other treatments are individualized, based upon the child's needs and response to therapy.

Isolation precautions: Because the viruses that cause bronchiolitis are contagious, precautions must be taken to prevent spreading the virus to other patients and/or children. Parents may visit (and stay with the child) but siblings and friends should not. Toys, books, games, and other activities can be brought to the child's room. All visitors (nurses, doctors, parents) must wash their hands before and after leaving the room.

Feeding: Most infants and children can continue to eat, breastfeed, or drink normally while in the hospital. If the child is unable or unwilling to eat or drink adequately, the respiratory rate is too fast, or the child is having significant difficulty breathing or stops breathing, fluids and nutrition should be given into a vein (intravenously).

Treatments: In some cases, an inhaled medication is given to open the child's airways (a bronchodilator). If the medication is helpful, it may be given every 4 to 6 hours as needed to ease breathing.

Supplemental oxygen may be needed for children who are unable to get enough oxygen from room air; this is usually given by placing a tube (called a nasal cannula) under a child's nose or by placing a face mask over the nose and mouth. For infants, an oxygen head box (a clear plastic box) may be used. The child is tested periodically to determine the blood oxygen level when oxygen is turned off. The goal is to slowly reduce and then discontinue supplemental oxygen when the child is ready.

If a child is severely ill and unable to breathe adequately on his or her own, or if the child stops breathing, a breathing tube (endotracheal tube) may be inserted into the mouth and throat. This is connected to a machine (called a ventilator) that breathes for the child at a regular rate. The use of an endotracheal tube and ventilator is a temporary measure that is discontinued when the child improves.

Discharge to home: Most children who require hospitalization are well enough to return home within 3 to 4 days. Children who require a machine to help them breathe usually need to stay in the hospital for four to eight days or longer before they are ready to go home.

Recovery: Most children with bronchiolitis who are otherwise healthy begin to improve within 2 to 5 days. However, wheezing persists in some infants for a week or longer, and it may take as long as 4 weeks for the child to return to his or her 'normal' self. Recovery may take longer in younger infants and those with underlying medical problems (e.g. prematurity, other lung diseases). The child should be kept out of daycare and/or school until the fever and runny nose have resolved (i.e. the time during which they are most contagious).

Bronchitis

Acute bronchitis is a clinical syndrome produced by swelling and irritation in air passages. This irritation may cause the child to cough or have other breathing problems. Acute bronchitis often starts because of another illnesses of the upper and lower respiratory tracts. Symptoms of acute bronchitis usually include productive cough and sometimes retrosternal pain during deep breathing or coughing. The illness spreads from the child's nose and throat to his windpipe and airways. Bronchitis is often called a chest cold. It can be confused with asthma. Generally, the clinical course of acute bronchitis is self-limited, with complete healing and full return to function typically seen within 10–14 days following symptom onset.

Etiology and Incidence

Acute bronchitis is generally caused by respiratory infections; approximately 90% are viral in origin, and 10% are bacterial. Chronic bronchitis may be caused by repeated attacks of acute bronchitis, which can weaken and irritate bronchial airways over time, eventually resulting in chronic bronchitis. Rhinoviruses are the most common causative organisms. Other viruses which cause bronchitis are adenovirus, influenza, parainfluenza, respiratory syncytial virus.

Secondary bacterial infection as part of an acute upper respiratory tract infection or some other airway problems may occur. Air pollutants, such as those that occur with smoking and from second-hand smoke, also cause incident bronchiolitis.

Bronchitis, both acute and chronic, is prevalent throughout the world and is one of the top 5 reasons for childhood physician visits in countries that track such data. The incidence of bronchitis in British schoolchildren is reported to be 20.7%, among German schoolchildren 28%, etc.

Pathophysiology

Acute bronchitis leads to the hacking cough and phlegm production that often follows upper respiratory tract infection. A child with bronchitis have more mucus than normal because of either increased production or decreased clearance. Coughing is the mechanism by which excess secretion is cleared. Cough may be associated with wheezing or crackles on auscultation. Because of nonspecific leukocytic migration purulent secretions can occur even in the absence of a bacterial infection.

In children, chronic bronchitis follows either an endogenous response (e.g. excessive viral-induced inflammation) to acute airway injury or continuous exposure to certain noxious environmental agents (e.g. allergens or irritants). Normally 3 functional compartments of the mucociliary apparatus [the cilia, a protective mucus layer, and an airway surface liquid (ASL) layer], work together to remove inhaled particles from the lung. An airway when undergoes such an insult (by irritant exposures of airborne particulates) responds quickly with bronchospasm and cough, followed by inflammation, edema, and mucus production. Elements of these descriptors are present in the working definitions of asthma, as well.

Acute bronchitis is a self-limiting disease. Chronic bronchitis is recurring inflammation and degeneration of the bronchial tubes that may be associated with active infection. In case of children, chronic bronchitis may indicate an underlying chronic respiratory dysfunction.

Manifestations

Acute bronchitis begins as a respiratory tract infection that manifests as the common cold. Symptoms often include coryza, malaise, chills, slight fever, sore throat, and back and muscle pain.

The cough in these children is usually accompanied by a nasal discharge. The discharge is watery at first, then after several days becomes thicker and colored or opaque. It then becomes clear again and has a mucoid

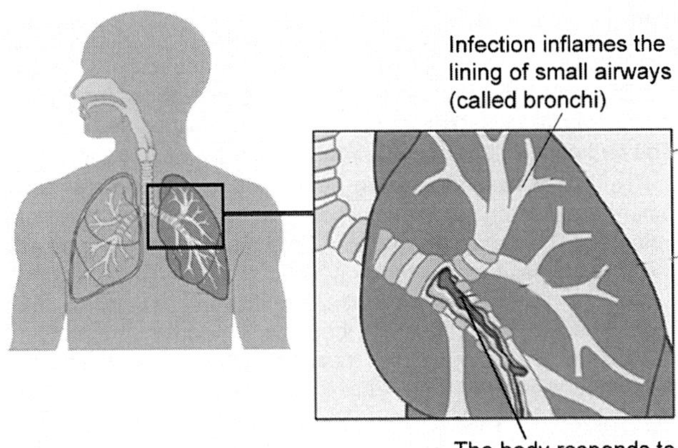

Fig. 13.8: Bronchial tree and internal structure of bronchus during inflammation

watery consistency before it spontaneously resolves within 7–10 days. Purulent nasal discharge is common with viral respiratory pathogens and, by itself, does not imply bacterial infection. The child may show short of breath and wheezes (makes a high-pitched noise) when he breathes. The child is more tired than usual.

Diagnostic Evaluation

The diagnosis of bronchitis is usually done on the basis of clinical picture (Fig. 13.8). Chest X-rays are usually normal.

The following conditions are to be considered in the diagnosis of bronchitis in pediatric patients:

- Retained foreign body
- Bronchopulmonary allergy
- Immunosuppression.

Chronic bronchitis is often part of an underlying disease process, such as asthma, cystic fibrosis, dyskinetic cilia syndrome, foreign body aspiration, or exposure to an airway irritant. Recurrent tracheobronchitis may also be seen in patients with tracheostomy or with certain forms of immunodeficiency. In all of these patient groups, chronic bronchitis should not be the primary diagnosis, because it does not describe the pathology of the underlying disorder.

Therapeutic Management

Treatment is mainly symptomatic. In pediatric patients, treatment includes rest, use of antipyretics, adequate hydration, and avoidance of smoke.

Analgesics and antipyretics target the symptoms of pediatric bronchitis. Antihistamines should be avoided because of their drying effect on secretions. Antibiotics should be considered only after establishing the diagnosis of bacterial infection through culture or if the clinical picture supports the diagnosis. In chronic cases, bronchodilator therapy should be considered. Oral corticosteroids should be added if cough continues and the history and physical examination findings suggest a wheezy form of bronchitis.

Pneumonia

Pneumonia is a form of acute respiratory infection that affects the lung parenchyma. Pneumonia is an inflammatory condition of the lung affecting primarily the microscopic air sacs known as alveoli. Normally, these alveoli fill with air when a healthy person breathes in. When a child has pneumonia, the alveoli are filled with pus and fluid, which makes breathing painful and limits oxygen intake (Figs 13.9A and B).

It is usually caused by infection with viruses or bacteria and less commonly other microorganisms, certain drugs and other conditions such as autoimmune diseases. The viruses and bacteria that are commonly found in a child's nose or throat, can infect the lungs if they are inhaled. They may also spread via airborne droplets from a cough or sneeze. In addition, pneumonia may spread through blood, especially during and shortly after birth.

Etiology and Incidence

Pneumonia is caused by a number of infectious agents, including viruses, bacteria and fungi. The most common are:

- *Streptococcus pneumoniae* and *staphylococous aureus* are the most common cause of bacterial pneumonia in children;
- *Haemophilus influenzae* type b (Hib)—the second most common cause of bacterial pneumonia;
- RSV—respiratory syncytial virus is the most common viral cause of pneumonia; pneumonia is also caused by adenoviruses, influenza viruses, cytomegalo virus (mainly in neonates). About 80–85% of all childhood pneumonias are caused by viruses.
- In infants infected with HIV, *Pneumocystis jiroveci* is one of the commonest causes of pneumonia, responsible for at least one quarter of all pneumonia deaths in HIV-infected infants.

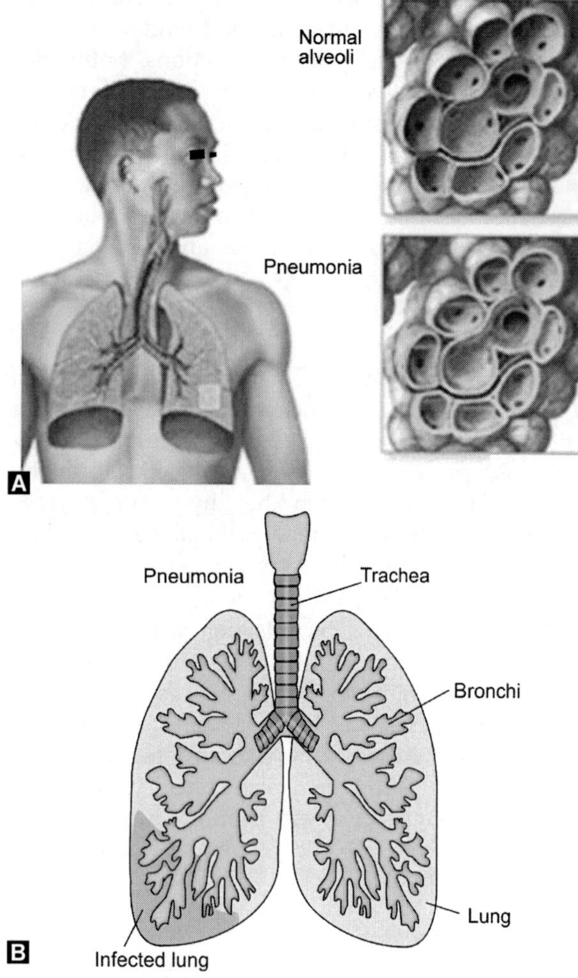

Figs 13.9A and B: Normal respiratory alveoli and collection in alveoli during pneumonia

Global mortality in children younger than 5 years has fallen substantially in the past two decades from more than 12 million in 1990, to 6·9 million in 2011, still pneumonia and diarrhea are the two leading causes of death in this age group and have overlapping risk factors. The United Nations Children's Fund (UNICEF) estimates that pediatric pneumonia kills 3 million children worldwide each year. These deaths occur almost exclusively in children with underlying conditions, such as chronic lung disease of prematurity, congenital heart disease, and immunosuppression.

Pathophysiology

Pneumonia is an infection of lungs in which the lung tissue of an infected child is filled with fluid or pus. People suffering from

Contd...

Contd...

this condition tend to experience some symptoms and these include rapid breathing, fever, chills, chest and abdominal pain, presence of brown, yellow or green colored mucous and cough. The pathophysiology of such a condition is :

Pneumonia may be caused by viruses, bacteria, fungi and other parasites and in this infection afflicting the lungs may get inflamed. The organism invading the immune system causes the symptoms in this condition as it provokes the immune system to respond. As a result of the invading organisms the blood vessels within the lungs leak and this causes the protein rich fluid to seep into alveoli. Mucous further decreases the gas exchange within the lung. Fluid continues to fill in the alveoli and the debris resulting from the white blood cells fighting the infection also fill the alveoli.

Cell destruction with sloughing of cellular debris into lumen of terminal airways and alveoli causes patchy infiltrate that affects multiple lobes. This results in less area for exchange of oxygen and carbon dioxide. As the patient is deprived of oxygen the breathing becomes faster so as to bring more oxygen and release the carbon dioxide. Vital capacity and lung compliance decrease as consolidation increases.

Alveoli are actually air spaces that are hollow however these tend to become solid because of the debris and fluid collection. This is called consolidation and is a classical feature seen in bacterial pneumonia cases (Fig. 13.10). In mycoplasma pneumonia cases along with viral pneumonia, the alveoli walls are infected and consolidation does not occur in these cases.

Manifestations

The presenting features of viral and bacterial pneumonia are similar. However, the symptoms of viral pneumonia may be more numerous than the symptoms of bacterial pneumonia. Cough is the most common symptom of pneumonia in infants, along with tachypnea, retractions, and hypoxemia. These may be accompanied by congestion, fever, rapid breathing, irritability, decreased activity and poor eating, a grunting sound

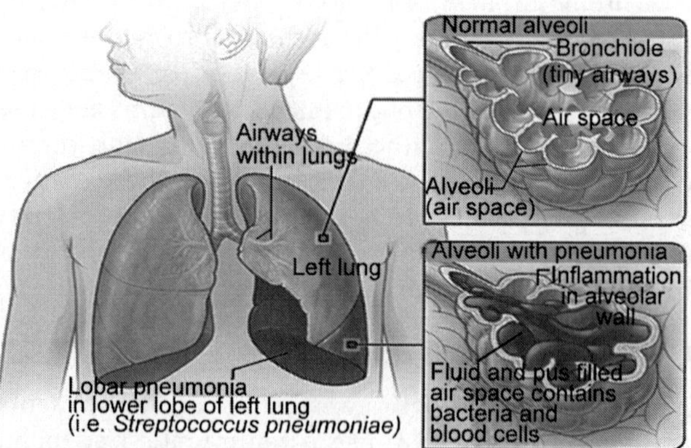

Fig. 13.10: Alveoli are actually air spaces that are hollow. But in pneumonia, alveoli tend to become solid because of the debris and fluid collection, called consolidation

when the child exhales, in drawing of muscles, and skin around neck and chest with each breath.

In children under 5 years of age, who have cough and/or difficult breathing, with or without fever, pneumonia is diagnosed by the presence of either fast breathing or lower chest wall indrawing. Wheezing is more common in viral infections. Feeding difficulty may occur in very severely ill infants and may also experience unconsciousness, hypothermia and convulsions.

Diagnostic Evaluation

The signs and symptoms of pneumonia are often nonspecific and widely vary based on the patient's age and the infectious organisms involved.

The signs and symptoms of pneumonia are often nonspecific and widely vary based on the patient's age and the infectious organisms involved.

Observing the child's respiratory effort during a physical exam is an important first step in diagnosing pneumonia. The World Health Organization (WHO) respiratory rate thresholds for identifying children with pneumonia are as follows:

- Children younger than 2 months: Greater than or equal to 60 breaths/min
- Children aged 2–11 months: Greater than or equal to 50 breaths/min
- Children aged 12–59 months: Greater than or equal to 40 breaths/min.

Hypoxemia, a frequent complication of pneumonia, is a risk factor for death. Such an association between hypoxemia and pneumonia suggests that its early detection and treatment are important aspects in the management of children with pneumonia. Assessment of oxygen saturation by pulse oximetry should be performed early in the evaluation when respiratory symptoms are present. Cyanosis may be present in severe cases. Capnography may be useful in the evaluation of children with potential respiratory compromise.

Other diagnostic tests may include the following:

- Auscultation by stethoscope
- Cultures
- Serology
- Complete blood cell count (CBC)
- Chest radiography—X-ray presentations of pneumonia may be classified as lobar pneumonia, bronchopneumonia (also known as lobular pneumonia), and interstitial pneumonia. Aspiration pneumonia may present with bilateral opacities primarily in the bases of the lungs and on the right side. Radiographs of viral pneumonia may appear normal, appear hyper-inflated, have bilateral patchy areas, or present similar to bacterial pneumonia with lobar consolidation.
- Ultrasonography (USG)—lung ultrasound is a simple and reliable tool that can be used in the case of suspected pneumonia. Lung USG is a simple and reliable imaging technique that is nearly as reliable as chest X-ray in identifying the lung lesions that are diagnostic for community acquired pneumonia, and also show that it is even more effective than chest X-ray in diagnosing pleural effusion. New data show that point-of-care ultrasonography accurately diagnoses most cases of pneumonia in children and young adults.

Therapeutic Management

Oral antibiotics, rest, simple analgesics, and fluids usually suffice for complete resolution.

Initial priorities in children with pneumonia include the identification and treatment of respiratory distress, hypoxemia, and hypercarbia. Grunting, flaring, severe tachypnea, and retractions should prompt immediate respiratory support. Children who are in severe respiratory distress should undergo tracheal intubation if they are unable to maintain oxygenation or have decreasing levels of consciousness. Increased respiratory support requirements such as increased inhaled oxygen concentration, positive pressure ventilation, or CPAP are commonly required before recovery begins.

Antibiotics

The majority of children diagnosed with pneumonia in the outpatient setting are treated with oral antibiotics. High-dose amoxicillin is used as a first-line agent for children with uncomplicated community-acquired pneumonia. Second- or third-generation cephalosporins and macrolide antibiotics such as azithromycin are acceptable alternatives. Combination therapy (ampicillin and either gentamicin or cefotaxime) is typically used in the initial treatment of newborns and young infants.

Hospitalized patients can also usually be treated with a narrow-spectrum penicillin such as ampicillin. The choice of agent and dosing may vary based on local resistance rates (high rates of intermediate or resistant pneumococcus may require higher dosing of ampicillin to surmount the altered penicillin-binding protein that is the cause of resistant pneumococcus). In areas where resistance is very high (>25% of strains being nonsusceptible), a third-generation cephalosporin might be indicated instead. Older children, in addition, may receive a macrolide to cover for atypical infections.

Although the fluoroquinolones would cover all the common respiratory pathogens of childhood, they are

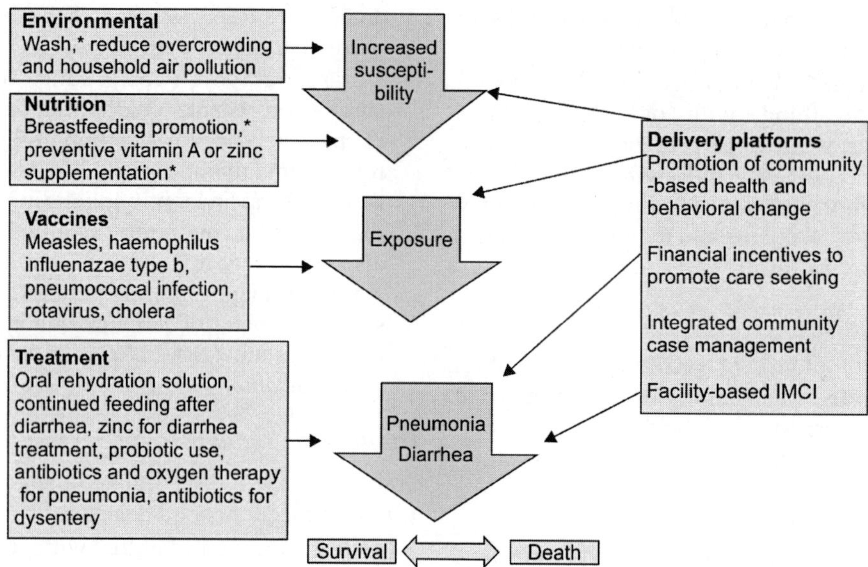

Fig. 13.11: Graphical representation of preventive and curative management of pneumonia and diarrheal diseases within community settings

not approved for this indication and have significant potential adverse effects, including short-term tendon damage and long-term impact on antibiotic resistance. They should be reserved for cases in which other therapies have failed and ideally should be used after consultation with an infectious disease specialist with whom other options, or alternative diagnoses, can be considered.

Children who are toxic appearing should receive antibiotic therapy that includes vancomycin (particularly in areas where penicillin-resistant pneumococci and methicillin-resistant *S aureus* [MRSA] are prevalent) along with a second- or third-generation cephalosporin.

Vaccines

Aside from avoiding infectious contacts (difficult for many families who use daycare facilities), vaccination is the primary mode of prevention. Influenza vaccine is recommended for children aged 6 months and older. The pneumococcal conjugate vaccine (PCV13) is recommended for all children younger than 59 months old. The 23-valent pneumococcal polysaccharide vaccine (PPVSV) is recommended for children 24 months or older who are at high-risk of pneumococcal disease.

WHO Response

The United Nations Children's Fund (UNICEF) estimates that pediatric pneumonia kills 3 million children worldwide each year. These deaths occur almost exclusively in children with underlying conditions, such as chronic lung disease of prematurity, congenital heart disease, and immunosuppression.

The WHO and UNICEF integrated Global action plan for pneumonia and diarrhea (GAPPD) aims to accelerate pneumonia control with a combination of interventions (Fig. 13.11) to protect, prevent, and treat pneumonia in children with actions to:

- Protect children from pneumonia including promoting exclusive breastfeeding and adequate complementary feeding
- Prevent pneumonia with vaccinations, handwashing with soap, reducing household air pollution, HIV prevention and cotrimoxazole prophylaxis for HIV-infected and exposed children
- Treat pneumonia focusing on making sure that every sick child has access to the right kind of care—either from a community-based health worker, or in a health facility if the disease is severe—and can get the antibiotics and oxygen they need to get well.

Nursing Interventions

Nursing Diagnosis

Ineffective airway clearance related to edema, and accumulation of secretions.

Expected Outcome

Child can breathe effectively, lung ventilation is adequate and there is no buildup of secretions.

Interventions and Rationale

- Monitor respiratory status every 2 hours, review the respiratory status, abnormal breath sounds and color of skin. Monitor blood gas analysis to assess respiratory status. Provide cool mist. Ensure that that the airway is patent. Perform percussion, vibration and postural drainage every 4–6 hours. It helps in loosening the secretions and reduces bronchial edema.
- Give the comfortable position that allows the patient to breathe. Do chest physiotherapy and postural drainage. Provide steam inhalation. It drains out secretion.
- Continue oxygen therapy as indicated, Help cough up secretions/suction mucus if needed. Adequate hydration, preferably warm fluids. It can help in mobilization and expectoration of secretions.
- Create a comfortable environment, plan daily care activities without disturbing his/her rest, so that patients can sleep calmly. Rest and sleep minimizes extra respiratory efforts as well anxiety and confusion.
- Provide sputum for culture/sensitivity test. Administer antibiotics as prescribed to control infection.

Nursing Diagnosis

Impaired gas exchange related to changes in alveolar capillary membrane due to infection of lung parenchyma.

Expected Outcome

Child will show improvement in ventilation, as it will be evidenced in normal respiratory rate and absence of cyanosis.

Nursing Intervention with Rationale

- Elevate head end of the bed (Fowler position semi-Fowler), which lowers diaphragm and promotes chest expansion.
- Observation of the level of consciousness, respiratory status, cyanosis signs every 2 hours. Give oxygen, monitor blood gas analysis and observe SaO_2 level. Monitoring and observing these areas help to understand the patient's respiratory status and to take necessary measure.
- Create an environment of calm and comfort patients and prevent the occurrence of fatigue in patients.

Nursing Diagnosis

Fluid volume deficit related to inadequate oral intake, fever, tachypnea.

Expected outcome: Patient will maintain normal body fluids.

Nursing Interventions

- Encourage the child to take fluids orally. Parent should avoid the cold or thick milk/drink as it may induce cough.
- Monitor fluid balance in the mucous membranes, skin turgor, rapid pulse, decreased consciousness, vital signs.
- Keep drip infusion accuracy according to the program. Record intake and output of fluids.
- Perform oral hygiene.

Nursing Diagnosis

Hyperthermia related to the infection process

Expected Outcomes

Maintains normal body temperature is 36.5 to 37.5 °C.

- Nursing interventions and rationale monitor the temperature every 2 hours and monitor vital signs and signs of dehydration. Effect of temperature increase is a change in pulse, respiration and blood pressure, and body loses water through the skin and evaporation.
- So anti-pyrexia drug is administered to reduce body temperature of the patient.
- Child is encouraged to drink about 2000 mL/day, cold compress/bath given. Hydrotherapy reduces body temperature, decreases metabolic demands and oxygen consumption. Monitor signs of seizures, as high body temperature risks for a seizure.

Nursing Diagnosis

Activity intolerance related to decreased blood oxygen levels.

Expected Outcome

Patients can do activities based on conditions.

Interventions

- Assess the patient's physical tolerance.
- Assist patients in activities of daily activities.
- Provide age-appropriate games that patients with activities that do not spend a lot of energy, match the activity with the condition.
- Give oxygenation as prescribed or child complaints respiratory difficulty during play/ADL.

Foreign Body Aspiration

Foreign body aspiration can be a life-threatening emergency, which is seen most frequently in children ages 6 months to 5 years. An aspirated solid or semisolid object may lodge in the larynx or trachea. If the object is large enough to cause nearly complete obstruction of the airway is caused with large object, asphyxia may rapidly cause death. Certain items have an increased incidence of aspiration in children. Lesser degrees of obstruction or passage of the obstructive object beyond the carina can result in less severe signs and symptoms.

Etiology and Incidence

Children are at risk for putting small toys, candies, or nuts into their mouths. Children aged 1–3 years chew incompletely with incisors before their molars erupt, and objects or fragments may be propelled posteriorly, triggering a reflex inhalation. The male-to-female ratio is 2:1, depending on the study. Few aspects of developmental characteristics like children's curiosity, oral needs, exploration of his/her immediate world, contribute to the occurrence of foreign body aspiration. Occasionally lack of supervision, food given to the infants and smaller children for which they are not developmentally prepared to ingest (hard candy, peanuts, popcorn), precipitate this hazard. Childhood aspiration can occur at any age but the children of 1 to 3 years of age is most vulnerable group as it occurs most frequently in this period of life.

Pathophysiology

Most foreign body aspiration occurs in the bronchi, and right bronchus is a more common site than the left bronchus because of its anatomic development. Near-total obstruction of the larynx or trachea can cause immediate asphyxia and death. The location of the aspiration would depend on the child's age and physical position at the time of the aspiration. Because the angles made by the main stem bronchi with the trachea are identical until age 15 years, foreign bodies are found on either side with equal frequency in persons in this age group. With normal growth and development, the adult right and left main stem bronchi diverge from the trachea with very different angles, with the right main stem bronchus being more acute and therefore making a relatively straight path from larynx to bronchus. Objects that descend beyond the trachea are more often found in the right endobronchial tree than in the left. Obstruction in bronchus causes edema and inflammation and manifests as obstructive emphysema, pneumonia and atelectasis. The likelihood of complications increases after 24–48 hours, making expeditious removal of the foreign body is imperative.

Organic foreign bodies such as oily nuts induce inflammation and edema. Local inflammation, edema, cellular infiltration, ulceration, and granulation tissue formation may contribute to airway obstruction while making bronchoscopic identification and removal of the object more difficult. Mediastinitis or tracheoesophageal fistulas might result. Distal to the obstruction, air trapping might lead to local emphysema,

Contd...

Contd...

atelectasis, hypoxic vasoconstriction, suppurative pneumonia, or bronchiectasis. Bronchoscopically, the object may appear as a tumor, and scar carcinoma may develop over time. Even if the object is removed, the inflammatory changes may not be completely reversible.

Manifestations

Immediate sign and symptoms of complete obstruction include sudden violent coughing, respiratory distress, aphonia, cyanosis, loss of consciousness, and death occur in quick succession unless the object is dislodged. When the degree of obstruction is less severe or when the aspirated object descends beyond the carina, the presentation is less dramatic. Signs and symptoms of laryngeal and tracheal obstruction include choking, dysphagia, croupy cough, stridor, hoarseness of voice, and possibly dyspnea and cyanosis.

Local inflammation, edema, cellular infiltration, ulceration, and granulation tissue formation may contribute to airway obstruction while making bronchoscopic identification and removal of the object more difficult. The airway becomes more likely to bleed with manipulation; the object is more likely to be obscured and becomes more difficult to dislodge. Mediastinitis or tracheoesophageal fistulas may result. Distal to the obstruction, air trapping may occur, leading to local emphysema, atelectasis, hypoxic vasoconstriction, postobstructive pneumonia, and the possibility of volume loss, necrotizing pneumonia or abscess, suppurative pneumonia, or bronchiectasis.

A history of a choking episode is not always obtained or may have initially been ignored or misdiagnosed. Most patients or parents can identify a specific episode of choking; however, presentation is often delayed by more than a week. The latency period prior to the onset of symptoms may last months or years if the foreign body is inert bone or inorganic material. Presenting symptoms (other than cough) include fever, hemoptysis, dyspnea, and chest pain.

Diagnostic Evaluation

Most foreign bodies are radiolucent. Less than 20% of aspirated foreign bodies are radiopaque. The diagnosis is based on a correct history and clinical manifestations. Fluoroscopy and X-ray chest are used to reveal the presence of a foreign object in the respiratory tract. Standard posteroanterior inspiratory chest radiography is performed to look for unilateral hyperinflation, lobar or segmental atelectasis, mediastinal shift, or pneumomediastinum.

Bronchoscopy (both rigid and flexible) can be used diagnostically and therapeutically. Most aspirated foreign bodies are radiolucent. Radiologic procedures do not have extreme diagnostic accuracy, and aspiration events are not always detected. Other medical conditions are possible. Rigid bronchoscopy confirms the diagnosis and provides an avenue for removing the object.

Arterial blood gas analysis is useful for judging the adequacy of ventilation and identifying the evolution of acute ventilatory failure. This test is done in conjunction with an assessment of appearance, voice, speech, vital signs, physical examination, and pulse oximetry.

CT scanning of the chest may show the object or may identify localized air trapping. The presence of a foreign body and its condition, anatomic location (i.e. larynx, trachea, main, lobar or segmental bronchus), shape, composition, position, size (i.e. number of fragments), and extent of entrapment by edema or granulation tissue must be identified prior to attempts at extraction.

Fluoroscopy of the chest can be performed to observe diaphragmatic and mediastinal shifting of air trapping while the patient is breathing if the diagnosis is in doubt or if the patient cannot cooperate.

Therapeutic Management

Acute choking, with respiratory failure associated with tracheal or laryngeal foreign body obstruction, may be successfully treated at the scene with the Heimlich maneuver, back blows, and abdominal thrusts. Even in nonemergency situations, expeditious removal of tracheobronchial foreign bodies is recommended.

Rigid bronchoscopy is the procedure of choice for removing foreign bodies in children and in most adults. Success rates for extracting foreign bodies are reportedly more than 98%. Large solid and semisolid objects are best managed emergently in the operating room with a rigid bronchoscope and appropriate grasping instruments.

Flexible bronchoscopy can be performed to confirm, localize, and visualize the foreign body in the tracheobronchial tree. The flexible bronchoscope can provide access to subsegmental bronchi beyond that provided by the rigid bronchoscope. If gas exchange is already compromised or if insertion of the flexible bronchoscope would result in significant impairment of gas exchange, flexible bronchoscopy is contraindicated. Diagnostic flexible bronchoscopy prior to rigid bronchoscopy has even been advocated for nonasphyxiating children in whom the diagnosis of foreign body aspiration cannot be confirmed.

Almost all aspirated foreign bodies can be extracted bronchoscopically. If rigid bronchoscopy is unsuccessful, surgical bronchotomy or segmental resection may be necessary. Chronic bronchial obstruction with bronchiectasis and destruction of lung parenchyma may require segmental or lobar resection.

Observing patients for 1–2 days postextraction may be appropriate, in case complications from impaction or extraction arise. Noncardiogenic re-expansion pulmonary edema, airway inflammation, hemoptysis, pneumothorax, tracheoesophageal fistula, pneumonia, atelectasis, fever, or ventilatory failure may require continued hospitalization, including ICU monitoring, intubation, mechanical ventilation, repeated bronchoscopic procedures (e.g. directed suctioning of inspissated pus, laser therapy of bleeding, obstructing granulation tissue or polyps), antibiotics, corticosteroids, bronchodilators, or chest physical therapy.

Cystic Fibrosis

Cystic fibrosis (CF) is an autosomal recessive genetic disorder that affects multisystem mostly the lungs but also the pancreas, liver, and intestine. CF is an inherited disease of the mucus and sweat glands. It affects mostly your lungs, pancreas, liver, intestines, sinuses and sex organs. CF causes your mucus to be thick and sticky. The mucus clogs the lungs, causing shortness of breath problems and making it easy for bacteria to grow. This can lead to problems such as repeated lung infections and lung damage. Other symptoms include sinus infections, poor growth, and infertility, affect other parts of the body.

The name *cystic fibrosis* refers to the characteristic scarring (fibrosis) and cyst formation within the pancreas, first recognized in the 1930s.

Pathophysiology

An inherited condition, cystic fibrosis affects the cells that produce mucus, sweat and digestive juices. Normally, mucus is a thin, slippery, watery substance. It keeps the linings of certain organs moist and prevents them from drying out or getting infected. But in cystic fibrosis, a defective gene causes the secretions to become thick and sticky. Instead of acting as a lubricant, the secretions plug up tubes, ducts and passageways, especially in the lungs and pancreas.

It is caused by one of many different mutations in the gene for the protein cystic fibrosis transmembrane conductance regulator (CFTR). This protein is required to regulate the components of sweat, digestive fluids, and mucus. Healthy people have two working copies of the CFTR gene. People with CF have no working copy. Carriers have one working copy. Therefore CF has autosomal recessive inheritance and precipitates abnormal transport of chloride and sodium across the epithelium. This leads to thick, viscous secretions, which builds up in lungs and blocks airways. The buildup of mucus makes it easy for bacteria to grow. This leads to repeated, serious lung infections. Over time, these infections can severely damage child's lungs.

Clinical Manifestations

Cystic fibrosis signs and symptoms vary, depending on the severity of the disease. In some children, symptoms begin during infancy. Other people may not experience symptoms until adolescence or adulthood.

The thick and sticky mucus associated with cystic fibrosis clogs the tubes that carry air in and out of your lungs. This can cause a persistent cough that produces thick sputum and mucus, wheezing, breathlessness, a decreased ability to exercise, repeated lung infections, inflamed nasal passages or a stuffy nose. Pneumothorax, hemoptysis, clubbing of fingers and toes are clinically seen.

The thick, sticky mucus also can block tubes, or ducts of pancreas. As a result, the digestive enzymes that pancreas makes cannot reach small intestine and absorption of fats and proteins will be decreased. This can cause vitamin deficiency and malnutrition because nutrients pass through the body without being used. The child may have bulky stools, intestinal gas, a swollen belly from severe constipation, and pain or discomfort.

CF also causes sweat to become very salty, and large amounts of salt will be lost from the body. This can upset the balance of minerals in blood and cause many health problems. Examples of these problems include dehydration, increased heart rate, fatigue, weakness, decreased blood pressure, heat stroke, and rarely, death. Other complications associated to CF are:

- *Bronchiectasis:* Cystic fibrosis is one of the leading causes of bronchiectasis, the condition which damages the airways, making it harder to move air in and out of the lungs.
- *Chronic infections:* Bacteria and fungi easily breed in thick mucus in the lungs and sinuses. Child with cystic fibrosis may have frequent bouts of sinusitis, bronchitis or pneumonia.
- *Nasal polyps:* Polyps can be developed as the lining inside the nose is inflamed and swollen. Nasal polyps can obstruct breathing during sleep.
- *Cough up blood:* Over time, cystic fibrosis can cause thinning of the airway walls, which may result in hemoptysis.
- *Pneumothorax:* This condition, in which air collects in the space that separates the lungs from the chest wall, is also more common in older people with cystic fibrosis. Pneumothorax can cause chest pain and breathlessness.
- Pancreatitis
- *Collapsed lung:* Repeated lung infections damage the lungs, making it more likely for the lung to collapse.
- *Respiratory failure:* Over time, cystic fibrosis can damage lung tissue so badly that it no longer works. Lung function typically worsens gradually, and it eventually can become life-threatening.

Diagnostic Evaluation

Sweat test: A sweat-producing chemical is applied to a small area of skin (on the forearm or on the thigh) and electrodes are attached. With a mild electric current the skin is stimulated to sweat, which does not cause pain or harm to the child. The collected sweat is then tested to see if it is saltier than normal, may suggest CF.

Genetic testing: DNA samples from blood or saliva can be checked for mutations in the CFTR gene, the specific defects on the gene responsible for cystic fibrosis.

Chest X-ray: The changes in lungs are detected by:

Pulmonary Function Test (PFT)

Imaging tests: Damage to lungs or intestines can be monitored with X-rays, CT scans and MRI.

Lung function test: These tests measure the size of your lungs, how much air you can breathe in and out, how fast you can breathe in and out, and how well your lungs deliver oxygen to your blood.

Sputum culture: Sputum is analyzed for bacteria.

Organ function tests: Blood tests can measure the health of your pancreas and liver. Children with cystic fibrosis should be regularly tested for diabetes after age 10.

Therapeutic Management

There is no cure for cystic fibrosis, but several treatment methods may be adopted to manage CF. The cornerstones of management include proactive treatment of airway infection, and encouragement of good nutrition and an active lifestyle. Because of the wide variation in disease symptoms, treatment should be done at specialist multidisciplinary centers. Different treatment modalities aim at maximizing organ function, to ease severity of symptoms and therefore quality of life.

Treatment of airway obstruction: The most consistent aspect of therapy in cystic fibrosis is limiting and treating the lung damage caused by thick mucus and infection, with the goal of maintaining quality of life. Intravenous, inhaled, and oral antibiotics are used to treat chronic and acute infections. Mechanical devices and inhalation medications are used to alter and clear the thickened mucus. These therapies, while effective, can be extremely time-consuming. Several mechanical techniques such as chest physiotherapy, exercises are used to dislodge sputum and encourage its expectoration.

Pleural Effusion

Pleural effusion, which in pediatric patients most commonly results from an infection, is an abnormal collection of fluid in the pleural space (Fig. 13.12). Pleural effusion develops because of excessive filtration or defective absorption of accumulated fluid.

Parapneumonic effusion is defined as fluid in the pleural space in the presence of pneumonia, lung abscess, or bronchiectasis. Nontuberculous bacterial pneumonia constitutes the most frequent origin of pleural effusion in children.

Etiology

Pleural effusion in children is usually a manifestation of an underlying disorder, and its prevalence mirrors that of the underlying disease. Pleural effusions in children most commonly are infectious (50% to 70% parapneumonic effusion); congestive heart failure is a less frequent cause (5% to 15%), and malignancy is a rare cause. Pleural effusions caused by nonbacterial infectious agents are more common than those caused by bacterial organisms. Viral effusions are usually asymptomatic and resolve without therapy. Parapneumonic effusion and empyema are serious complications of bacterial pneumonia. Pleural effusion occurs in a large number of cases of pulmonary tuberculosis in children. Tuberculous pleural effusions can be either primary or the result of reactivation disease. Tuberculous pleural effusion commonly occurs in adolescents and is uncommon in the preschool-aged child.

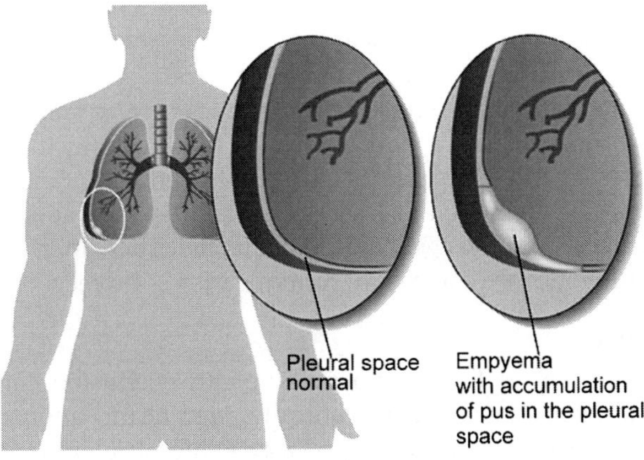

Fig. 13.12: Pleural effusion

Congestive heart disease is a less-common cause of pleural effusion in children than it is in adults, where effusions are usually bilateral and transudative. Lymphoma is the most common of all childhood malignancies that is associated with pleural effusion.

Parapneumonic effusions and empyema are more common in boys than girls. In addition, parapneumonic effusions and empyema are more commonly encountered in infants and young children than in older children.

Pathophysiology

Parapneumonic effusion is defined as pleural effusion associated with lung infection (i.e. pneumonia). These effusions result from the spread of inflammation and infection to the pleura. Much less commonly, infections in other adjacent areas, such as the retropharyngeal, vertebral, abdominal, and retroperitoneal spaces may spread to the pleura resulting in the development of effusion.

Early in the course of parapneumonic effusion, the pleura becomes inflamed; subsequent leakage of proteins, fluid, and leukocytes into the pleural space forms the effusion. At the time of formation, the pleural effusion is usually sterile with a low leukocyte count. With time, bacteria invade the fluid, resulting in empyema, which is defined as the presence of grossly purulent fluid in the pleural cavity. The development of pleural empyema is determined by a balance between host resistance, bacterial virulence, and timing of presentation for medical treatment.

The etiologic mechanisms involved in the formation of most pleural effusions include pleural space infection (empyema), abnormal capillary permeability (exudates), increased hydrostatic or decreased oncotic pressure in the setting of normal capillaries (transudates), abnormal lymphatic clearance (exudates), and blood in the pleural space (hemothorax).

Clinical Manifestations

Children with pleural effusions may come from different disease backgrounds. These children usually present with the following symptoms:

Symptoms Related to the Size and Location of Effusion

An accumulation of a small amount of fluid may be asymptomatic. A large collection of fluid leads to dyspnea, respiratory distress, dull pain, and coughing. These symptoms may vary with an alteration in body position. Subpulmonic fluid collection can be associated with vomiting, abdominal pain, and abdominal distention caused by partial paralytic ileus.

Chest pain: Chest pain is pleuritic in origin. Patients with an exudative effusion are more likely to have pain than are patients with a transudative effusion. The pain can be localized or referred to the shoulder and

Children with complication of pneumonia often have a history of recent URTI, bronchitis, or pneumonia.	*Children with tuberculous pleural effusions may present with the following symptoms*	*Malignant effusions*	*Transudative effusions*
Persistent fever Cough Anorexia Malaise Tachypnea Dyspnea Chest pain	Cough Pleuritic chest pain Dyspnea Night sweats Fever Hemoptysis Weight loss	Causes no symptoms or only cough and low-grade fever. Pleural effusion due to a malignant lymphoma may present with respiratory distress, because of the size of the effusion, the mediastinal mass, or both.	Effusions in congestive heart failure, nephrotic syndrome, the underlying disease usually determines the presenting symptoms. Occasionally the child may be asymptomatic until the accumulation becomes large enough to cause symptoms

abdomen. It is typically described as sharp or stabbing and worsens with inspiration. The pain intensity lessens as the effusion increases in size; as the effusion increases, it separates the pleural membranes, and the pain becomes dull or disappears.

Diagnostic Evaluation

Blood test: A complete blood count (CBC) with differential, blood cultures, and C-reactive protein (CRP) may help to establish the presence of infection. The white blood cell (WBC) count and CRP may be useful in monitoring treatment progress in infectious effusions. A positive blood culture finding may facilitate the selection of antibiotics in sterile empyema. (Approximately 10–22%) of children with complicated parapneumonic effusions have a positive blood culture result.

Analysis of pleural fluid: Analysis of the pleural fluid is the single best method to determine the cause of a pleural effusion. Pleural fluid analysis involves inserting a needle into the pleural space to remove fluid and then sending it to a lab for testing. Simple observation of the gross appearance of the fluid may provide a clue as to the cause of the pleural effusion, as follows:

- Grossly purulent fluid indicates an empyema
- A putrid odor suggests an anaerobic empyema
- Clear, pale yellow fluid suggests a transudate
- Milky fluid is consistent with a chylothorax
- Bloody pleural fluid is seen with trauma, malignancy, tuberculosis, uremia, and empyema due to group A *Streptococcus.*

X-ray chest: A chest radiograph, is the simplest and least expensive method of identifying a pleural effusion. X-rays in different positions to check whether fluid is free-flowing, which would indicate that infection is not present. A chest radiograph may also reveal underlying pneumonia before pleural fluid starts accumulating.

USG of chest and CT scan: Pleural ultrasonography permits easy characterization of pleural effusion. Ultrasonography may also facilitate the identification of the best site for thoracocentesis or insertion of a thoracotomy tube. Ultrasound or CT scan to view the amount and nature of fluid.

Treatment

Noninflammatory pleural effusions (such as transudates) are managed by treating the underlying cause and by supportive care of any functional disturbances. Treatment of tuberculous pleural effusion (TPE) is similar to that of pulmonary tuberculosis.

Currently available treatment options for pediatric parapneumonic effusion and empyema include antibiotics alone or in combination with thoracocentesis, chest tube drainage with or without instillation of fibrinolytic agents, and surgery.

If a causative organism is identified, antibiotic choice should be guided by the sensitivity pattern of the organism. Some groups of antibiotics such as penicillins, cephalosporins, aztreonam, clindamycin, and ciprofloxacin exhibit more satisfactory pleural fluid penetration than others (e.g. aminoglycosides).

In a hospitalized patient with complicated parapneumonic effusion, antibiotics are commonly administered intravenously while a thoracostomy tube is present and the patient is febrile. Intravenous antibiotics may be continued at least 48 hours after the patient is afebrile and the chest drain is removed. Thereafter, oral antibiotics are commonly continued for 2–4 weeks.

Diet

Children with complicated pleural effusion and empyema may have clinically significant anorexia and increased needs. High-calorie, high-protein foods that appeal to the child should be provided early, and nasogastric feeds should be considered early, particularly in young children. Chylothorax may respond to a diet with fat supplied as medium-chain triglycerides (MCTs), with a resolution of the chylous effusion at the end of 2 weeks.

Activity

Pain and chest-tube placement may limit the patient's motility. Analgesia can facilitate cough and clearance of the airway, especially in the presence of an underlying pneumonic process.

Chest Drainage

Effusions that are enlarging or compromising respiratory function in a febrile, unwell child require drainage (Fig. 13.13). A small-bore tubes (e.g. pigtail catheters) are commonly used for free-flowing fluid and large-bore tubes are commonly employed for thick pus. When combined with fibrinolytic therapy (use of streptokinase, urokinase and alteplase), the use of small chest tubes found to have some advantages over large tubes.

The timing of elective removal of the drain depends on numerous factors, including the amount of fluid draining, the child's overall clinical condition, the presence of fever, and the radiographic and ultrasonographic appearance of the chest, as well as a fall in acute phase reactants. In most cases, the chest tube may be removed when the pleural drainage becomes minimal (< 10–15 mL/24 hr) and the fluid is clear or yellow.

As the effusion becomes fibrinopurulent and subsequently organizes, chest tubes often become ineffective because fibrinous strands and loculations divide the pleural space into compartments. Fibrinolytics instilled into the pleural cavity may facilitate drainage by lysing fibrinous strands and clearing lymphatic pores.

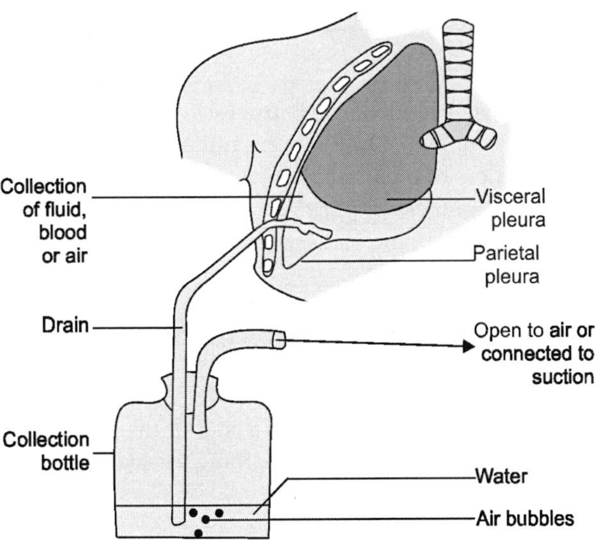

Fig. 13.13: Chest drainage

Surgery

Indications for surgery include persistent sepsis in association with a persistent pleural collection (despite antibiotics, chest tube drainage, and fibrinolytics), complex empyema with significant lung pathology (e.g. delayed presentation with a significant peel and trapped lung), and bronchopleural fistula with pyopneumothorax.

Three surgical options are noted for management of children with parapneumonic effusion and empyema:

- VATS
- Minithoracotomy
- Open thoracotomy with decortication.

ALLERGIC DISORDERS

Bronchial Asthma (Reactive Airway Diseases)

Reactive airways disease (RAD) is a term used to describe breathing problems in children up to 5 years old. It is common for infants and children to cough and wheeze when they have a cold. It may be difficult to know if a child has asthma, bronchiolitis, or airway hyper-responsiveness. Airway hyper-responsiveness is quick narrowing of child's airways, making it hard for him to breathe. Child may also have pneumonia, or simply a cold. Child's symptoms may go away as he gets older, or he may have asthma, or another breathing disorder, later in life.

Asthma is one of the most common chronic diseases in childhood, with increasing prevalence in the past 3 decades. Pediatric asthma is a chronic, multifactorial, lower airway disease that affects 5–15% of children. Asthma is characterized by bouts of dyspnea as a result of temporary narrowing of bronchi due to bronchial spasm, mucosal edema and thick secretions. Children with asthma have sensitive, easily irritated airways in their lungs. When these airways exposed to triggers like viruses, allergens, secondhand smoke, chemical irritants, pollution or cold air; the airways become more inflamed, produce more increased mucus, mucosal swelling and muscle contraction. This results in airway obstruction, chest tightness, shortness of breath, coughing and wheezing (Fig. 13.14). Asthma is a chronic condition affecting children as well as adults. It cannot be cured, only controlled. Asthma is one of the most common causes of hospital admission and visits to

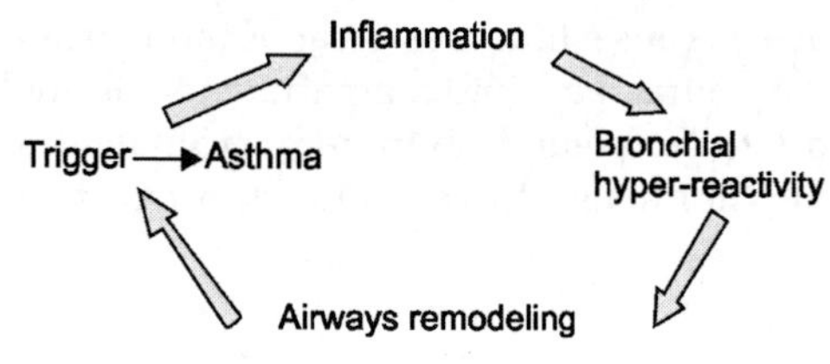

Fig. 13.14: Asthma cycle

health clinic of children. Most common chronic disease of childhood; primary cause of school absences.

Etiology and Incidence

It is not clear why some people get asthma and others do not, but it is probably due to a combination of environmental and genetic factors.

Not all children who wheeze have asthma. Most children younger than 3 years who wheeze are not predisposed to asthma. Only 30% of infants who wheeze go on to develop asthma. To establish the diagnosis of asthma, certain criteria should be met, i.e. at least 5 years of age, episodic symptoms of airflow obstruction or airway hyper-responsiveness, reversible airflow obstruction of predicted forced expiratory volume in one second (FEV1) after use of short-acting β_2 agonist of at least 10% cases, alternative diagnoses have been excluded.

Asthma prevalence appears to be increasing worldwide. Air pollutants may play a role in the prevalence increase. Higher prevalence occurs in poverty stricken urban areas where children are less likely to have routine doctor visits and access to the availability of medications.

A correlation may exist between high levels of exposure to cockroach allergen and the frequency of asthma-related health problems in inner-city children. Homes in poverty areas were more likely to have high cockroach allergen levels. Asthma may develop in children from early exposure to cockroach allergen. An association may exist between obesity and childhood asthma. Increased resistin, an adipokine produced by adipose tissue, may play a negative predictive role in asthma. The peak prevalence of asthma is in those aged 6–11 years, the male-to-female ratio is 1.5:1. So asthma symptoms flare up in certain situations:

- Exercise-induced asthma, which may be worse when the air is cold and dry, smoke, fumes
- Occupational asthma, triggered by workplace irritants such as chemical fumes, gases or dust
- Allergy-induced asthma, triggered by particular allergens, such as pet dander, cockroaches or pollen
- Medications, including beta blockers, aspirin, ibuprofen and naproxen (Aleve)
- He/she had a lung infection caused by a virus, such as respiratory syncytial virus (RSV)
- Parental/familial history.

Pathophysiology

Numerous environmental stimuli induce an allergen-antibody interaction, causing a release of mediators that create airway inflammation. Airway inflammation is the primary factor responsible for smooth muscle hyper-responsiveness, edema, and increased mucous production. A complex interaction occurs between inflammatory cells and airway epithelium. Mast cells, eosinophils and lymphocytes secrete mediators include histamine, tryptase, heparin, leukotrienes, platelet-activating factor, cytokines, interleukins, and tumor necrosis factor and create an environment toxic to respiratory epithelial cells by causing edema, mucous secretion. Next, small muscles around the airways go into spasm. As they become active, they shorten and tighten around the tubes in the lung. This narrows the airways and reduces airflow, much like wrapping somebody's hand around a soft garden hose and squeezing to reduce the flow of water. During an asthma attack, both inflammation and resulting airway spasm cut the air flow. This causes bronchospasm, shortness of breath, coughing, increased work of breathing and often wheezing through the narrowed airway tubes (Fig. 13.15).

The immature anatomy of infants and small children put them more distress on them. A child's airways are small and narrow, which easily fill and get blocked with mucus and decreased elastic lung recoil make them more prone to airway obstruction. The child's flexible rib cage and underdeveloped chest muscles and diaphragm lead to exhaustion when respiratory effort increases. As the children get older, the severity of asthma attacks decreases because of increased airway size, matured diaphragmatic support and better clearing of mucus.

Manifestations

Asthma is reversible obstructive airway disease characterized by the following symptoms :

- Shortness of breath
- Chest tightness or pain
- Trouble sleeping caused by shortness of breath, coughing or wheezing
- Wheezing on expiration. It is a whistling sound when exhaling (wheezing is a common sign of asthma in children)
- Coughing or wheezing attacks that are worsened by a respiratory virus, such as a cold or the flu
- Increasing difficulty in breathing, measurable with a peak flow meter
- Rapid heart rate
- Restlessness, apprehension, diaphoresis. Difficulty

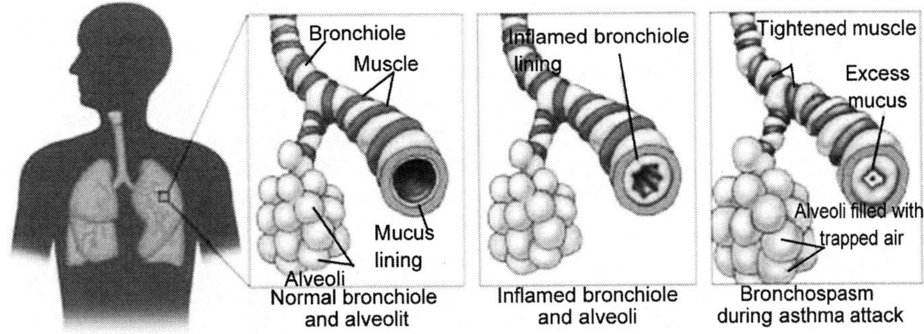

Fig. 13.15: Normal bronchioles and alveoli and Inflammation and Bronchospasm

in performing simple tasks (eating, talking, walking), because of shortness of breath

- Allergic shiner (dark semicircles of skin under the eyes)
- Transverse nasal skin fold from repeatedly rubbing the nose
- Flaring of nasal alae.

Diagnosis

A complete blood count (CBC) may be indicated for a suspected viral infection (lymphocytosis, leukopenia), parasitic infection (eosinophilia), or hemosiderosis.

Chest X-ray shows patchy atelectasis and generalized emphysema.

An arterial blood gas (ABG) determination should be performed for any patient in status asthmaticus to check for hypoxia, hypercarbia, or acidosis; alternatively, a venous blood gas measurement can be used to assess for hypercarbia and acidosis and combined with pulse oximetry monitoring.

An assessment of electrolyte levels may reveal hypokalemia in patients who are using albuterol.

Pulmonary function test—these tests show a decreased forced expiratory volume in 1 second, increased residual volume from air trapping, and decreased vital capacity (the maximum amount of air exhaled after a maximum inhalation).

Peak expiratory flow (PEF) is the most common form of pulmonary function test monitoring. Record the best of 3 attempts. Possible life-threatening asthma exacerbation with PEF predicted of less than 30%; severe exacerbation, with less than 50%; and moderate exacerbation, with less than 80%.

Therapeutic Management

Pharmacologic management includes the use of control agents such as inhaled corticosteroids, inhaled cromolyn or nedocromil, long-acting bronchodilators, theophylline, leukotriene modifiers, and more recent strategies such as the use of anti-immunoglobulin E (IgE) antibodies (omalizumab). Relief medications include short-acting bronchodilators, systemic corticosteroids, and ipratropium.

β-Agonists—this long-acting preparation of a β_2 agonist is used primarily to treat nocturnal or exercise-induced symptoms. β-Agonists are sympathomimetic agents that cause bronchodilatation due to bronchial smooth muscle relaxation by activating β_2-adrenergic receptors, which increase intracellular cyclic adenosine monophosphate (cAMP) concentrations within smooth muscles. It has no anti-inflammatory action and is not indicated in the treatment of acute bronchospastic episodes. It may be used as an adjunct to inhaled corticosteroids to reduce the potential adverse effects of the steroids.

Inhaled Steroids

Steroids are the most potent anti-inflammatory agents. Inhaled forms are topically active, poorly absorbed, and least likely to cause adverse effects. They are used for long-term control of symptoms and for the suppression, control, and reversal of inflammation. Inhaled forms reduce the need for systemic corticosteroids.

Inhaled steroids block late asthmatic response to allergens; reduce airway hyper-responsiveness; inhibit cytokine production, adhesion protein activation, and inflammatory cell migration and activation; *and reverse β_2-receptor downregulation and subsensitivity (in acute asthmatic episodes with LABA use).*

Systemic Steroids

These agents are used for short courses (3–10 days) to gain prompt control of inadequately controlled acute asthmatic episodes. They are also used for long-term prevention of symptoms in severe persistent asthma as well as for suppression, control, and reversal of inflammation. Frequent and repetitive use of β_2 agonists has been associated with β_2-receptor subsensitivity and downregulation; these processes are reversed with corticosteroids.

Corticosteroids are the first line of treatment for severe acute asthma, because of the inflammatory process. Steroids control airway inflammation through a number of mechanisms, such as reducing the number and activation of lymphocytes, eosinophils, mast cells, and macrophages; suppressing the production of cytokines, tumor necrosis factor-α, granulocyte-macrophage colony-stimulating factor, adhesion molecules, and inducible enzymes, including nitric oxide synthase and cyclooxygenase.

Higher-dose corticosteroids have no advantage in severe asthma exacerbations, and IV administration has no advantage over oral therapy, provided that GI transit time or absorption is not impaired. The usual regimen is to continue frequent multiple daily dosing until the FEV_1 or peak expiratory flow (PEF) is 50% of the predicted or personal best values; then, the dose is changed to twice daily. This usually occurs within 48 hours.

Omalizumab

Omalizumab is a recombinant, DNA-derived, humanized IgG monoclonal antibody that binds selectively to human IgE on surface of mast cells and basophils. It reduces mediator release, which promotes allergic response. It is indicated for moderate-to-severe persistent asthma in patients who react to perennial allergens in whom symptoms are not controlled by inhaled corticosteroids.

Methylxanthines (such as Theophylline) is available in short-acting and long-acting formulations. Because of the need to monitor serum concentrations, this agent is used infrequently. The dose and frequency depend on the particular product selected.

Ipratropium (Atrovent)

Chemically related to atropine, protropium has antisecretory properties and, when applied locally, inhibits secretions from serous and seromucous glands lining the nasal mucosa. The MDI delivers 17 mcg/actuation. Solution for inhalation contains 500 mcg/2.5 mL (0.02% solution for nebulization).

Magnesium Sulfate

Magnesium is a calcium antagonist that causes smooth muscle relaxation as a result of the inhibition of calcium uptake. It is used in severe acute asthma attacks, along with other treatments. With respect to asthmatic patients, mechanisms such as the inhibitory action on smooth muscle contraction, histamine release from mast cells, acetylcholine release from nerve terminals, and sedative action may contribute to its therapeutic effects.

Helium-Oxygen Mixture (Heliox)

Helium is a low-density gas that, when used in a mixture with oxygen, reduces turbulent airflow, enhancing laminar flow and in consequence reducing airflow resistance. It may also be considered in unresponsive cases.

Asthma in children varies by age group, and infants, toddlers and 4-year-olds are diagnosed and treated differently than teens and adults. The way asthma affects a child also varies from person to person, and symptoms may get better or worse at certain times. In some children, asthma symptoms get better as the child grows. While asthma cannot be cured, symptoms can be managed by the treatment plan developed on child's respiratory status.

Give oxygen through a nasal or face mask or cannula
The flow of 1–6 liters/minute oxygen concentration produces 24–44%
The flow of 5–8 liters/minute oxygen concentration produces 40–60%
The flow of 8–12 liters/min oxygen concentration produces 60–80%
The flow of 8–12 liters/min oxygen concentration producing 90%

Severe acute asthma is currently the most common medical emergency in children. Different terms have been described for severe acute asthma exacerbation, which include *status asthmaticus, near-fatal asthma, sudden asphyxic asthma,* and *acute fatal asthma.* Status asthmaticus refers to an acute asthma exacerbation in which bronchial obstruction is severe and continues to worsen or not improve despite the institution of adequate standard therapy, leading to respiratory failure. Near-fatal asthma was described as an asthma exacerbation of sudden onset that rapidly progresses to hypercapnia and hypoxemia, leading to respiratory arrest. The near-fatal attribute of the exacerbation was due to the severe asphyxia rather than cardiac arrhythmias. Sudden asphyxic asthma was characterized in a group of young patients presenting with rapid decompensation in less than 3 hours after onset of symptoms, severe.

Acute Asthma Management

Treatment goals for acute severe asthmatic episodes are as follows:

- Correction of significant hypoxemia with supplemental oxygen; in acute stages, alveolar hypoventilation requires mechanically assisted ventilation
- Rapid reversal of airflow obstruction with repeated or continuous administration of an inhaled β_2-agonist; early administration of systemic corticosteroids (e.g. oral prednisone or intravenous methylprednisolone) is suggested in asthmatic children that fails to respond promptly and completely to inhaled β_2-agonists (Fig. 13.16).
- Reduction in the likelihood of recurrence of severe airflow obstruction by intensifying therapy: Often, a short course of systemic corticosteroids is helpful.

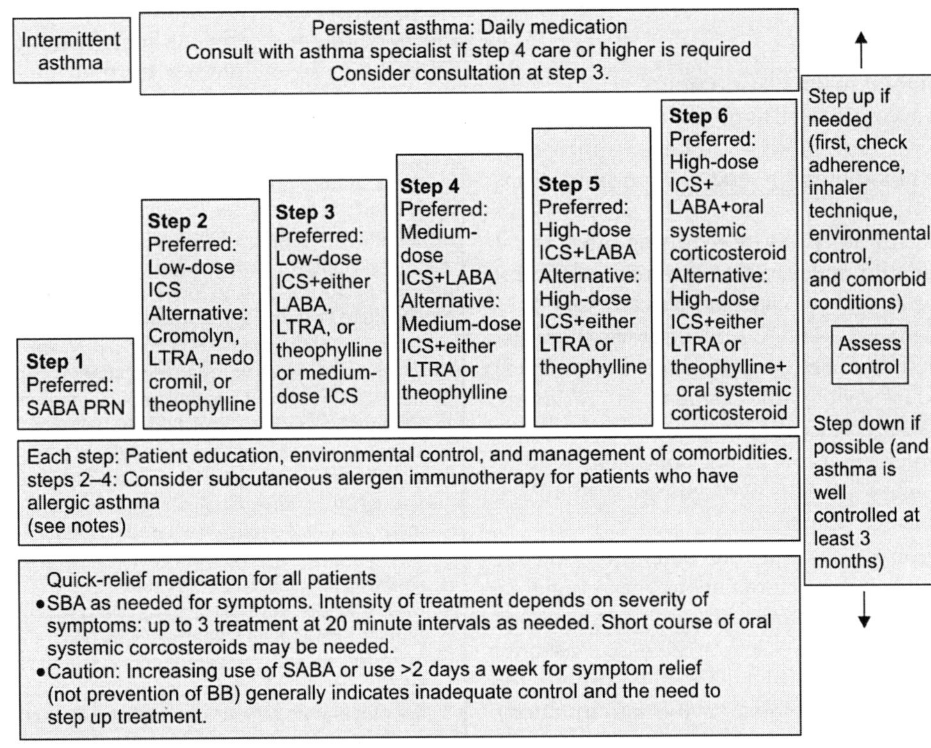

Key: Alphabetical order is used when more than one treatment option is listed within either preferred or alternative therapy. ICS, inhaled corticosteroid; LABA, inhaled long-acting beta 2-agonist, LTRA, leukotriene receptor antagonist; SABA, inhaled short-acting beta 2-agonist.

Notes:
- The stepwise approach is meant to assist, not replace, the clinical decision- making required to meet individual patient needs.
- If alternative treatment is used and response is inadequate, discontinue it and use the preferred treatment before stepping up.
- Theophylline is a less desirable alternative due to the need to monitor serum concentration levels.
- Step 1 and step 2 medications are based on evidence a. Step 3 ICS + adjunctive therapy and ICS are based on evidence b for efficacy of each treatment and extrapolation from comparator trials in older children and adults—comparator trials are not available for this age group; steps 4–6 are based on expert opinion and extrapolation from studies in older children and adults.
- Immunotherapy for steps 2–4 is based on evidence b for house-dust mites, animal danders, and pollens; evidence is weak or lacking for molds and cockroaches. Evidence is strongest for immunotherapy with single allergens. The role of allergy in asthma is greater in children than in adults. Clinicians who administer immunotherapy should be prepared and equipped to identify and treat anaphylaxis that may occur.

Fig. 13.16: Stepwise approach for managing asthma in children 5–11 years of age

The use of the peak flow rate or FEV_1 values, patient's history, current symptoms, and physical findings to guide treatment decisions is helpful in achieving the aforementioned goals. When using the peak expiratory flow (PEF) expressed as a percentage of the patient's best value, the effect of irreversible airflow obstruction should be considered. For example, in a patient whose best peak flow rate is 160 L/min, a decrease of 40% represents severe and potentially life-threatening obstruction.

Patients admitted to the PICU require:

- Intravenous access, as well as continuous monitoring of their cardiorespiratory status, including noninvasive blood pressure and oxygen saturations (SpO_2).
- Those with respiratory failure requiring mechanical ventilation should undergo the placement of central venous, arterial, and urinary bladder catheters.
- During patient assessment a respiratory therapist will document the Pediatric Asthma Score (PAS) every 2 hours while the patient is receiving continuous albuterol treatment.
- Advancement in therapy to the next level will be performed when there is worsening of the PAS, using the stepwise approach.
- Administration of short acting beta-adrenoceptor agonists (SABA) by powdered nebulizer or metered dose inhaler. If symptoms do not improve or if the child's PEFR is less than 70% of baseline. Corticosteroids are the first line of treatment for severe acute asthma, because of the inflammatory process. Mucous production is decreased, and inflammatory cell infiltration and activation are reduced. In children with severe acute asthma, systemic corticosteroids are indicated and in the intensive care unit setting the intravenous route is preferred. Antibiotics may also be administered to treat concurrent infection.
- *Oxygen:* Children with severe acute asthma possibly will have ventilation/perfusion mismatch as an effect of mucus plugging and atelectasis, causing hypoxemia. Treatment with β-agonists may aggravate hypoxemia by increasing cardiac output and eliminating the compensatory hypoxic pulmonary vasoconstriction. Oxygen should be used as carrier gas for intermittent or continuous nebulization and to keep oxygen saturation above 92%.
- *Fluids:* Children with severe acute asthma are often dehydrated because of poor oral intake and increased insensible fluid losses. Appropriate fluid resuscitation and maintenance fluids are indicated. The key is to avoid over hydration because of the increased risk of transpulmonary edema in children with severe asthma associated with large fluctuations in intrathoracic pressures. The use of half normal saline or isotonic solution in dextrose is preferred in the pediatric population.

Long-term asthma management: Long-term asthma management aims to minimize symptoms, avoid side effects of therapy, prevent acute asthma episodes and helps the child maintain a normal life. Children with asthma and their parents need to know the Asthma Action Plan discussed below:

Asthma action plan: The child and/or parent will work with their health-care provider to develop tailored guidelines (also called an action plan) to follow when symptoms increase.

Asthma symptoms are divided into three zones, which are assigned colors similar to those of a traffic light. These zones can be used to make decisions about the need for treatment:

- **Green:** Green signals that the lungs are functioning well. When asthma symptoms are not present or are well controlled, patients should continue their regular medicines and activities.
- **Yellow:** Yellow is a sign that the airways in the lungs are somewhat narrowed, making it difficult to move air in and out; this occurs when there is an increase in asthma symptom frequency or severity. A short-term change or increase in medication is generally required. Patients should change or increase their asthma medication according to the plan that was discussed with their provider.
- **Red:** Red is a sign that the airways are severely narrowed and requires immediate treatment; this occurs with a significant increase in asthma symptoms. The quick-acting reliever inhaler should be used according to the plan discussed with the provider and the child should be evaluated by a medical professional.
- **Emergency care plan:** Parents should work with their child's healthcare provider to formulate an emergency care plan that explains specifically what to do if asthma symptoms worsen. This may include more frequent use of a reliever medication. However, if asthma symptoms worsen or do not improve after use of a quick-acting reliever medication, the parent should immediately be shifted to health care setting. Severe asthma attacks can be fatal if not treated promptly.

Nursing Management and Interventions

The immediate nursing care of patients with asthma depends on the severity of symptoms. The patient and family are often frightened and anxious because of the patient's dyspnea which is caused due to airway spasm, secretion retention, amount of mucus. Therefore, a calm approach is an important aspect of care.

Assess the patient's respiratory status by monitoring the severity of symptoms, breath sounds, peak flow, pulse oximetry, and vital signs. It is necessary to determine therapy based on oxygen saturation.

Free the airway (suction if needed), monitor the chest wall retraction, assess the rate and type of respiration and use of accessory muscles. Observe the cerebral function. Maintain oxygen saturation above 90%. Provide mist inhalation. Encourage the child to bring out sputum.

Listen to lung sounds, encourage the patient to drink warm, monitor oxygen delivery, evaluation of lung sounds after suction. Monitor Vital signs; respiration, pulse, blood pressure, temperature. Position the patient in semi-Fowler position with back support. Provide chest table with extra pillows if child prefers leaning forward.

Effective gas exchange is to be established by correcting impaired gas exchange and related to bronchospasms and damage to the alveoli. Airway management is to be done by positioning the patient in upright position, auscultation of breath sounds of patients, patient's fluid balance, monitor respiration rate and effort.

Identify medications the patient is currently taking. Teach the child/parent to use an inhaler, to relax smooth muscle and dilate the airway. Administer medications as prescribed and monitor the patient's responses to those medications; medications may include an antibiotic if the patient has an underlying respiratory infection.

Acid-base management: Monitor blood gas analysis, monitor electrolyte levels, monitor oxygen saturation, administration of medication to maintain the acid-base balance (sodium bicarbonate), monitor hemodynamic status:

- Administer fluids if the patient is dehydrated.
- Assist with intubation procedure, if required.
- Monitor for deteriorating respiratory status and note sputum characteristics.
- Administer IV medications to control asthma as bolus on admission. It quickly relieves symptom, exacerbations, and reverse airflow obstruction.

Bronchiectasis

Bronchiectasis is a lung condition that causes bronchi to permanently widen. Bronchiectasis is a lung disease that usually results from an infection or other condition that injures the walls of the airways in lungs. This injury is the beginning of a cycle in which airways slowly lose their ability to clear out mucus, resulting in mucus buildup and an environment in which bacteria can grow. Normally lungs make mucus to trap and remove germs and irritants that man breathes. In bronchiectasis, child's lungs cannot clear mucus as it loses the ability to do so. This leads to repeated serious lung infections that cause more damage to airways. Over time, the airways become stretched out, flabby, and scarred, and unable to move air in and out. Bronchiectasis usually begins in childhood, but symptoms may not appear until months or even years after the child started having repeated lung infections.

Etiology of Bronchiectasis

- *Chemical damage:* Gastroesophageal reflux (GER) from child's stomach or breathing in harmful fumes may damage child's airways.
- *Immune system problems:* These include conditions such as allergies, rheumatoid arthritis (RA), inflammatory bowel disease (IBS), or HIV infection. These may increase the risk of infection or cause damage to child's airways.
- *Genetic diseases:* Child with some health condition, such as cystic fibrosis, makes it difficult to clear mucus.
- *Obstructions:* Food may accidentally get stuck in child's airways while he/she eats. Tumors in child's chest may grow large and block his airway. This may lead to inflammation or infection.
- *Past lung infections:* Lung infections, such as measles, whooping cough, pneumonia and tuberculosis, can damage child's airways.

Pathophysiology

The bronchi of lungs are lined with cilia, which work to sweep mucus upwards within the lungs, allowing it to be easily coughed out. In bronchiectasis, some of the bronchi become scarred and permanently enlarged. In this disease process the cilia are damaged so that they are unable to effectively sweep away the mucus. So mucus accumulates in parts of the lung that are affected and the risk of developing lung infections is increased. Recurrent infections can then cause further scanning and bronchial enlargement thereby precipitating the condition.

Signs and Symptoms

- A productive cough (over months and years)
- Foul-smelling sputum
- Repeated lung infection
- Weakness and fatigue
- Shortness of breath, wheezing or trouble breathing
- Loss of appetite or weight loss
- Clubbing of your child's fingers or toes
- Chest pain
- Coughing up blood or bloody mucus
- Weight loss
- Fatigue
- Sinus drainage.

Bronchiectasis can also lead to other serious health conditions, including collapsed lung, heart failure and brain abscess.

Diagnosis

- Chest X-ray of the heart and lungs to detect any signs of infection and scarring of the airway walls.
- Computed tomography (CT) scan to provide a computer generated image of the airways and other tissue in the lungs.
- Blood tests to detect a disease or condition that can lead to bronchiectasis. They can also reveal an infection or low levels of certain infection-fighting blood cells.
- Sputum culture to detect bacteria, fungi, or tuberculosis.
- Lung function tests to measure how well the lungs move air in and out.
- Sweat test or other tests for cystic fibrosis.
- *Pulmonary function tests:* Pulmonary function tests (PFTs) help to learn how well child's body uses oxygen. How much air he breathes in and out over a certain amount of time.

Treatment

The mainstays of treatment for bronchiectasis is to clear mucus from the chest, reduce frequency of acute pulmonary exacerbations, preserve lung function, and maintain a good quality of life. Medications—especially antibiotics, bronchodilators, steroid inhalers, expectorants.

Antibiotic selection for acute infective episodes is based on results of lower airway culture, clinical severity and patient tolerance. Hospitalization for more intensive treatments including intravenous antibiotics is necessary, when patients whose condition does not respond promptly or adequately to oral antibiotics.

- Oxygen therapy through mask.
- *Chest physical therapy (CPT)*: Chest physiotherapy and regular exercise should be encouraged.
- *Surgery*: The part of the lung causing symptoms may need to be removed.

Lung Abscess

Lung abscess was a dreaded disease in the earlier part of the last century. At present lung abscess is infrequently encountered in the pediatric population after the introduction of modern antibiotics.

Lung abscess is a severe, localized, suppurative infection in the substance of the lung, associated with necrotic cavity formation. The process is usually surrounded by a fibrous reaction, forming the abscess wall. Multiple small abscess formation may occur and is sometimes referred to as 'necrotizing pneumonia'.

Etiology and Other Risk Factors

Lung abscess in pediatric patients is believed to develop secondary to bacterial pneumonia. Immunodeficiency or immunosuppressant states caused by viral infections are the other predisposing causes. Other less common causes of lung abscess are cystic fibrosis, alpha-1 antitrypsin deficiency, anesthesia and dental surgery. Mechanisms precipitating abscess formation include:

- Inhalation of foreign body.
- Bacteremia seeding in the lungs.
- Tricuspid endocarditis leading to septic pulmonary embolus.
- Extension of hepatic abscess.
- Associated with lung cancer.
- Proximal to bronchial obstruction.
- Complication of severe or incompletely treated pneumonia (particularly staphylococci or klebsiella).
- Penetrating pulmonary trauma, e.g. a stab wound.
- Choking/aspiration/near drowning
- Severe periodontal disease.

Causative Organisms

Common pathogens causing lung abscess include anaerobes, *Staphylococcus aureus* and enteric Gram-negative rods like *Klebsiella pneumoniae.* Common anaerobes responsible for lung abscess are *Peptostreptococcus, Bacteroides, Fusobacterium,* Microaerophilic streptococci.

Common aerobes responsible for lung abscess are *S. Aureus, Streptococcus pyogenes, Haemophilus influenza, Pseudomonas aeruginosa, K. pneumoniae*—becoming more prevalent, *Streptococcus pneumonia, Proteus mirabilis, Pasteurella multocida*—zoonotic infection from cats/dogs/cattle.

Other organisms may cause lung abscess such as Mycobacterial infections—predominantly tuberculosis (TB), Fungal lung infections such as *Aspergillus, Cryptococcus, Histoplasma, Blastomyces, Coccidioides* species, Parasites such as *Entamoeba histolytica, Paragonimus* (seen in immunocompromised child).

Types

Primary lung abscesses are the ones developing in a previously healthy child, whereas secondary lung abscesses are those developing in a child with some other disease or in a child with predisposing factors like aspiration, pneumonia, cystic fibrosis, gastroesophageal reflux or immunodeficiency. The side and the lobar involvement is greatly influenced by the etiology, e.g. primary lung abscess is predominantly a right-sided disease and if aspiration is the cause then the upper lobes of either side are commonly involved.

Clinical Manifestations

- Onset of symptoms is often insidious (more acute if following pneumonia)
- Spiking temperature with rigors and night sweats
- Tachypnea, tachycardia
- Cough ± phlegm production (frequently foul-tasting and foul-smelling and often blood-stained)
- Pleuritic chest pain
- Breathlessness present
- Localized dullness on percussion (if consolidation or effusion is present)
- Crepitations (if consolidation)
- Dehydration.

Diagnostic Evaluation

Following tests are done to diagnose lung abscess:

- *Blood test:* CBC, ESR/CRP. ESR/CRP usually elevated.
- Renal function.
- Liver function tests.
- Blood cultures and sputum cultures (including AAFB).
- *CXR:* shows walled cavity, usually with a fluid level; may also be presence of an empyema or effusion.
- Tapping or draining of fluid or empyema with microbiology and cytology of samples.
- CT scan of the thorax—may detect multiple small abscesses.
- Fiber-optic bronchoscopy can exclude obstruction and provide samples for culture.
- Trans-thoracic biopsy/aspiration (usually with ultrasound guidance) or trans-tracheal biopsy.

Management

Management of lung abscess predominantly is based on administration of parenteral antibiotics with anaerobic and staphylococcal coverage, replacing the older methods like pneumonostomy, catheter drainage and resectional surgery. Additional computerized tomography (CT)-guided percutaneous drainage or other surgical interventions may become mandatory occasionally, if there is an incomplete or inadequate response to parenteral antibiotics alone. Transtracheal aspiration and drainage are very recently introduced techniques. Complications like pleural hemorrhage, empyema, bronchopleural fistula, or pneumothorax may occur with all these procedures. A thoracotomy may be done in case of a lung abscess for which tube drainage may be done.

Complications

These include:

- Empyema
- Pneumatocele
- Bronchopleural fistula
- Bronchiectasis
- Brain tumor.

Prognosis

Children with a lung abscess, both primary and secondary, have a significantly better prognosis than adults with the same condition. There is an overall 90% cure rate with prolonged courses of antibiotic therapy. Prognosis is adversely affected by older age and multiple comorbidities. Other poor prognostic factors include pneumonia, reduced level of consciousness, anaemia and infection with *P. aeruginosa*, *S. aureus* and *K. pneumoniae*.

CHAPTER 14

Child with Genitourinary Disorders

Chapter Outline

- Review of Renal System
- Congenital Abnormalities
- Congenital Abnormalities Related to Bladder and Lower Urinary Tract
- Other Disorders of GU System of Children
- Dialysis

REVIEW OF RENAL SYSTEM

The kidneys are two bean-shaped organs, each about the size of a fist (in adolescent and adult), lie one on each side of spinal column. The upper portion of left kidney lies near the twelfth rib, it is located slightly more superior than the right kidney due to the larger size of the liver on the right side of the body. Unlike the other abdominal organs, the kidneys lie behind the peritoneum that lines the abdominal cavity and are thus considered to be retro-peritoneal organs.

The urinary system consists of:

- *The kidneys:* The majority of humans have two kidneys, one on either side of the abdomen. Kidneys clear toxins from blood. Urea is the most important part of the waste products that are taken out by the kidneys. The kidneys also regulate acid concentrations, as well as maintaining water balance in the body by excreting urine. Water is mixed with urea to produce urine.
- *The ureters:* Urine passes through the connecting tubes called *ureters* from the kidneys to the bladder. Each kidney has one ureter connecting it to the bladder. Most of us have two kidneys, and therefore two ureters. People with just one kidney have just one ureter.
- *The bladder:* A hollow organ (sac) in the lower abdomen that stores urine. Known as the urinary bladder.
- *The urethra:* A tube that carries urine from the bladder to outside the body. In males the urethra goes down the middle of the penis to an opening at the end. In males the urethra also carries semen to outside the body. In females the urethra goes from the bladder to above the vaginal opening. The urethra in females is shorter than in males.

A thin fibrous capsule encases the kidney. The outer region of the kidney is the cortex which contains the glomeruli and tubules, and the inner region medulla contains renal pyramid. The gross structures of kidney are:

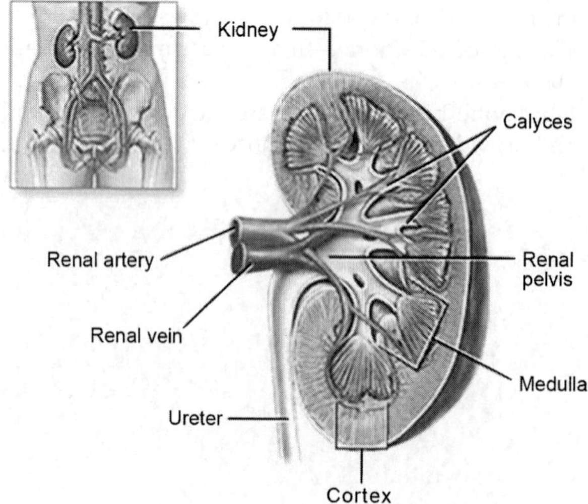

Fig. 14.1: Structure of a kidney

Gross Structures of Kidney (Fig. 14.1)

- *Outer cortex:* Glomeruli and convoluted tubules
- *Inner medulla:* Collecting ducts, Henle's loops and osmotic gradient
- *Collecting system:* Calices, pelvis and ureter
- Bladder and urethra.

Microscopic

- *Nephron:* Glomerulus and its tubule. Each kidney is made up of about a million filtering units called nephrons, which are the basic working units of the kidney (Fig. 14.2).
- *Glomerulus:* Compact tuft of capillary loops surrounded by Bowman's capsule.
- Cells and protein are held within blood while small solutes/water pass into tubules.
- *Tubule:* It is divided into segments—proximal, distal, loop of Henle. Proximal convoluted tubule controls absorption of glucose, sodium and other solutes. Absorption (water, sodium, glucose, etc.), secretion (K^+, H^+), formation of osmotic gradient (loop of Henle, distal tubule).
- *Collecting ducts:* Concentration of urine under control of ADH.

Each nephron filters a small amount of blood. The nephron includes a filter, called a glomerulus, and a tubule. The nephrons work through a two-step process. The glomerulus lets fluid and waste products pass through it; however, it prevents blood cells and large molecules mostly proteins, from passing. The filtered fluid then passes through the tubule, which changes the fluid by

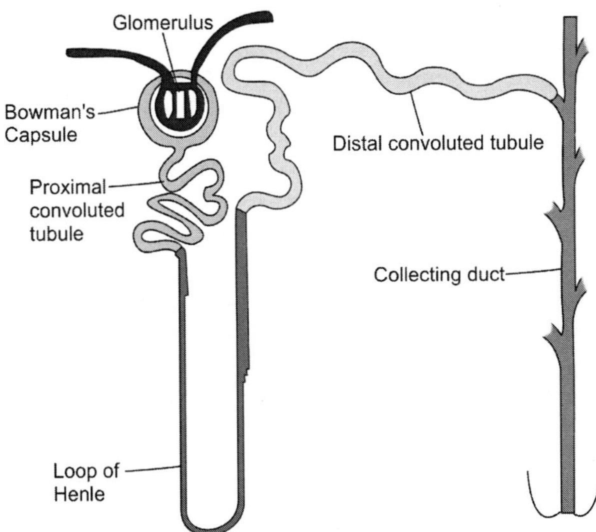

Fig. 14.2: Structure of a nephron

sending needed minerals back to the bloodstream (such as sodium, phosphorus, and potassium), and removing wastes. The final product becomes urine. Each day your kidneys process around 200 L of blood, with around 1 to 2 L of waste leaving the body as urine.

Blood Supply

- The kidneys are supplied by renal arteries which are branch of the abdominal aorta: 25% of cardiac output to glomerulus interlobar arteries → arcuate arteries → interlobular arteries → afferent arterioles → glomerulus → efferent artery → peritubular plexus (superficial and middle cortex) → vasa recta (juxtamedullary cortex).

The kidneys are master chemists of the body, excrete the end products of metabolism, intervene in many processes and balances in the body to keep the composition and volume of body fluids within normal range. The major roles of the kidneys are to act as filters for body to clean blood of wastes, yet retain essential elements needed by the body, to keep the proper balance of salts and acids, produce hormones and enzymes. Kidneys make three important hormones—erythropoietin, renin and active vitamin D. Erythropoietin stimulates the production of red blood cells, renin is involved in the control of blood pressure and active vitamin D controls calcium uptake and helps make strong bones. So functions of kidney are:

- Regulate total body water
- Control body's blood pressure (renin-angiotensin-aldosterone)
- Regulate acid base status
- Make red blood cells and help to maintain blood composition and pH levels
- Regulate electrolytes, calcium and phosphorus
- Maintain strong and healthy bones and help to keep mineral balance
- Remove nitrogenous wastes
- Drug metabolism and removal.

The kidneys work around the clock; a person does not control what they do. Ureters are the thin tubes of muscle—one on each side of the bladder that carry urine from each of the kidneys to the bladder. As the bladder fills with urine, it compresses the distal ureters, preventing urine reflux. The bladder capacity of infant/child is approximately equal to 10 mL/kg body weight. The bladder muscles (the detruser muscles) is capable of distending to accept urine without increasing the pressure inside. The urethra leads from the bladder, and it has two sphincters (internal and external) which control urination. The size of the urethra is longer in boys than girls.

Pediatric Differences in the Genitourinary System

Kidney begins to reach adult functioning about one year of age. Infants cannot concentrate urine as efficiently as older children and adults. Filtration capacity of the glomeruli is less and kidney; urine is voided frequently and has a low specific gravity; clear urine and lots of it. Kidneys operate at a functional level appropriate for body size of the child.

Fluid is large fraction of total body weight, kidneys less efficient to regulate electrolyte and acid-base balance and elimination drugs from body.

The neonate's bladder remains in the lower abdominal cavity and gradually sinks into the pelvis cavity during early childhood.

The capacity of bladder is around 20–50 mL at birth to 700–1000 mL at adult; stretch receptors at the age of 2 years and complete bladder control by the age of 4 to 5 years. Child has shorter urethra which contributes to frequent UTIs. The kidneys can get injured/trauma as much fat does not protect the organs.

Approach to the Child with Genitourinary Disorders

Clinical history and physical examination: The mode of onset gives information about the etiology of the ailment. The first component to any genitourinary (GU) evaluation is a medical history. The initial GU history taken for all children should encompass the mother's pregnancy and the child's birth history, including any anomalies, prematurity, and birth weight. It is also important to ask about any fevers of unknown origin, since this could have been an undiagnosed pyelonephritis. A voiding history of the child like dysuria, frequency of urination, urgency, hesitancy, quality of urinary stream, straining, pre- or postvoid leaking, day or nighttime wetting and quality and quantity of fluid intake, are to be explored. A detailed bowel history is important to evaluate for concurrent constipation, which is linked to both incontinence and UTI.

For male children, the circumcision status, retractability or ballooning of the prepuce with urination, any inguinal bulge or scrotal swelling, and whether or not the testicles are descended or not, are to be examined. Once a baseline has been established, future history taking can be tailored to the specific complaint.

Developmental history – It is necessary to identify whether the ailment has impact on development of the child or not.

Clinical Features

Abnormalities of Micturition: Micturition, the process of passing urine may change on several factors such as temperature, physical exertion and fluid intake. An increase in the quantity of urine can be caused by taking in a lot of fluids, specially diuretics like alcohol and tea. It can also be caused by certain medical conditions such as chronic nephritis, hypertension, diabetes mellitus and hyperparathyroidism.

A decrease in the quantity of urine is also caused by a number of factors which include taking in less fluid, losing a lot of fluids through other channels like perspiration, diarrhea, vomiting or fever. It can also be caused by medical conditions such as acute nephritis, lowered blood pressure, and severe gastroenteritis. Frequent or less frequent urination can also be considered an abnormality.

Moreover, persistent dribbling or a poor urinary stream in the presence of full bladder suggests abnormalities of micturition. Micturition reflex contraction cannot occur if the sensory nerve fibers from the bladder to the spinal cord are destroyed, thereby preventing transmission of stretch signals from the bladder and child loses bladder control.

Edema: Edema forms in patients with kidney disease for two reasons viz a heavy loss of protein in the urine, impaired kidney function. The heavy loss of protein in the urine (over 3.0 g/day) with its accompanying edema is termed the nephrotic syndrome. Nephrotic syndrome results in a reduction in the concentration of albumin in the blood (hypoalbuminemia). Since albumin helps to maintain blood volume in the blood vessels, a reduction of fluid in the blood vessels occurs. The kidneys then register that there is depletion of blood volume and, therefore, attempt to retain salt. Consequently, fluid moves into the interstitial spaces, thereby causing pitting edema. Besides salt restriction the loss of protein in the urine may be reduced by the use of ACE inhibitors and angiotensin receptor blockers (ARBs).

Salt and excess fluid can build up in the body if the glomeruli and kidneys are not working normally. Acute glomerulonephritis is characterized with facial puffiness and gross hematuria. Edema of GN is turgid and does not pit readily on pressure. The patients with kidney failure from whatever cause will develop edema if their intake of sodium exceeds the ability of their kidneys to excrete the sodium.

Hematuria: History of present illness includes duration of hematuria and any previous episodes. Urinary obstructive symptoms (e.g. incomplete emptying, nocturia, difficulty starting or stopping) and irritative symptoms (e.g. irritation, urgency, frequency, dysuria) should be noted. Patients should be asked about the presence of pain and its location and severity and whether they have vigorously exercised.

Presence of fever, night sweats, or weight loss should also be noted. Past medical history should include questions about any recent infections, particularly a sore throat that may indicate a group A β-hemolytic streptococcal infection which cause glomerular disorder. Also, conditions that predispose to a glomerular disorder, such as a connective tissue disorder (particularly SLE and RA), endocarditis, shunt infections, and abdominal abscesses, should be identified. Drug history should note use of anticoagulants, antiplatelet drugs, and heavy analgesic use.

Vital signs should be reviewed for fever and hypertension. The heart should be auscultated for murmurs (suggesting endocarditis). The abdomen should be palpated for masses; flanks should be percussed for tenderness over the kidneys. The face and extremities should be inspected for edema (suggesting a glomerular disorder), and the skin should be inspected for rashes (suggesting vasculitis, SLE).

A fresh specimen of urine is examined for red cells, red cell casts, and protein. In glomerular disease, urine shows smoky brown and cola-colored, dysmorphic red cells of different shapes (conical, bleb, folded-shaped), whereas in bleeding from renal pelvis or the lower urinary tract, the red cells maintain their normal morphology.

Oliguria: Oliguria is the low output of urine. In humans, it is clinically classified as an output more than 100 mL/day but less than 400 mL/day and commonly follows dehydration. Oliguria, in infant is defined as urine output less than 1 mL/kg/hour. It may occur due to prerenal cause, e.g. hypoperfusion of kidney (dehydration by poor oral intake, cardiogenic shock, diarrhea, G6PD, massive bleeding or sepsis); renal cause (kidney damage), postrenal cause (obstruction of the urine flow).

Dysuria, Renal colic, Flank pain: Dysuria is painful or uncomfortable urination, typically a sharp, burning sensation. It results from irritation of the bladder trigone or urethra. Dysuria is typically caused by urethral or bladder inflammation or stricture of the urethra which precipitates difficulty in starting urination and burning on urination. Some disorders cause a painful ache over the bladder or perineum. Dysuria is an extremely common symptom in women, but it can occur in men and can occur at any age.

Renal colic typically begins in the abdomen and often radiates to the hypochondrium or the groin. It is typically colicky due to ureteric peristalsis, but may be constant. During passage, calculi may irritate the ureter and may become lodged, obstructing urine flow and causing hydroureter and sometimes hydronephrosis. Large calculi can remain in the renal parenchyma or renal pelvis usually asymptomatically unless they cause obstruction and/or infection. Severe pain, often accompanied by nausea and vomiting, usually occurs when calculi pass into the ureter, cause obstruction, or both. Sometimes gross hematuria also occurs.

Flank pain is a common complaint with acute ureteral obstruction being the most common cause. The 'flank' describes the posterior portion of the body between the ribs and the ilium. Pain in this area arises from a myriad of locations ranging from the skin and superficial muscles to deeper abdominal structures. The distinction between nephrolithiasis and renal colic must be made clear. The simple presence of nephrolithiasis does not explain the presence of symptoms. It is only after passage of the stone out of the renal pelvis and into the collecting system that the muscular spasm felt as renal colic will occur. In fact, a large stone in the kidney is less likely to cause symptoms as it is unable to make such a passage.

Hypertension: The kidneys control blood pressure by regulating the amount of salt in the body and by making the enzyme renin that, along with other substances, controls the constriction of blood vessels. Symptomatic hypertension in children is most often secondary. High blood pressure is common in children with chronic kidney disease (CKD). Because of their young age when they develop CKD and high blood pressure, there is a high risk that these children may eventually have heart problems and a worsening of CKD. When the kidneys receive low blood flow, they act as if the low flow is due to dehydration. So they respond by releasing hormones that stimulate the body to retain sodium and water. Blood vessels fill with additional fluid, and blood pressure goes up.

Growth retardation: Growth retardation remains a major problem in patients with chronic kidney disease (CKD) and renal tubular disorders. Growth failure in the setting of kidney disease is multifactorial and is related to poor nutritional status as well as comorbidities, such as anemia, bone and mineral disorders, and alterations in hormonal responses, as well as to aspects of treatment such as steroid exposure. Moreover, progressive anorexia, decreased protein synthesis, and increased catabolism contribute to malnutrition in children with

CKD. Growth retardation in CKD probably reflects poorer nutritional status and increased catabolism, which is associated with increased rates of infections, hospitalizations, and other adverse effects.

Anemia: Normocytic normochromic anemia is a problem among children with chronic kidney disease (CKD). Lower levels of glomerular filtration rate (GFR) are associated with lower levels of hemoglobin. Diseased kidneys may not produce enough erythropoietin (EPO), a hormone that regulates red blood cell production. The liver is the primary source of EPO production in the fetus, but after birth, a group of peritubular interstitial cells in the kidney take over this function, becoming the major sites of EPO. In children, the relationship between GFR and anemia is less clear. Other factors that can contribute to anemia in patients with kidney disease include iron deficiency, some vitamin deficiencies, and the effects of poor nutrition or inflammation . However, treatment of anemia in both adults and children improve anemia dramatically.

Enuresis: When a child empties the urinary bladder at an inappropriate time and place it is called incontinence. When incontinence happens at night while asleep, it is called bedwetting. Most children with nocturnal enuresis have no evidence of renal disease. If enuresis persists in child after having achieved normal continence, urinalysis and culture are however recommended (discussed more in detail in behavioral pediatric chapter 6).

Abdominal pain: The abdominal pain can be dull and persistent ache or can be sharp, sudden and unbearable according to different renal pathologies. Major causes of abdominal pain include kidney stones, kidney cysts, kidney infection and polycystic ovary.

Moreover, infections in any part of the body can enter into the kidneys with blood circulation. In case of kidney infection, the pain is usually dull. Polycystic kidney disease or kidney cysts are common causes of abdominal pain. With continuous enlargement of the cysts, normal renal tissues get oppressed and replaced. In PKD, a numerous renal cysts are common in both kidneys.

Investigations of Renal Diseases

Urine examination: Presence of casts, protein, or dysmorphic RBCs (unusually-shaped, with spicules, folding, and blebs) indicates a glomerular disorder. WBCs or bacteria suggest an infectious etiology. However, because urinalysis shows predominantly RBCs in some patients with cystitis, urine culture is usually done. A positive culture result warrants treatment with antibiotics. If hematuria resolves after treatment and no other symptoms are present, no further evaluation is required for patients < 50 years, specially women.

Glomerular filtration rate: Glomeruli are the tiny filters in the kidneys that filter waste from the blood. Glomerular filtration rate (GFR) is a test used to check how well the kidneys are working. Specifically, it estimates how much blood passes through the glomeruli each minute.

Before the test antibiotics and stomach acid medicines needs to stop taking. According to the National Kidney Foundation, normal results range from 90—120 mL/min/1.73 m^2. Older people will have lower normal GFR levels, because GFR decreases with age. Levels below 60 mL/min/1.73 m^2 for 3 or more months are a sign of chronic kidney disease. GFR result lower than 15 mL/min/1.73 m^2 is a sign of kidney failure and requires immediate medical attention.

Creatinine clearance test: Creatinine is a breakdown product of creatine, which is an important part of muscle. The creatinine clearance test helps provide information about how well the kidneys are working. The test compares the creatinine level in urine with the creatinine level in blood. The creatinine clearance test is used to estimate GFR, as creatinine is removed from the body entirely by the kidneys. If kidney function is abnormal, creatinine level increases in the blood because less creatinine is released through the urine. Clearance is often measured as milliliters/minute (mL/min). Normal values are male: 97 to 137 mL/min; female: 88 to 128 mL/min.

Imaging of the urinary tract: It includes CT scan, voiding cystourethrogram, USG, IVP, radioactive imaging like dimercaptosuccinic acid (DMSA) renal scan, urodynamic studies for bladder function.

CONGENITAL ABNORMALITIES

Kidneys and Upper Urinary Tract

As a baby develops in the womb, part of the urinary tract can grow to an abnormal size or in an abnormal shape or position. Sometimes the kidneys do not develop properly and, as a result, do not function as they should. Often these problems are genetic and not due to anything a parent did or did not do.

Many of these problems can be diagnosed before a baby is born through routine prenatal testing and treated with medication or surgery while the child is still young. Other problems may appear later, with symptoms such as urinary tract infections (UTIs), growth problems, or hypertension.

Renal Agenesis, Hypoplasia

Renal agenesis is a medical condition in which one (unilateral) or both (bilateral) fetal kidneys fail to develop. It may be unilateral or bilateral. Renal agenesis is the name given to a congenital absence of one or both kidneys. The kidneys develop between the 5th and 12th week of fetal life, and by the 13th week they are normally producing urine. When the embryonic kidney cells fail to develop, the result is called renal agenesis. The presence of bilateral agenesis or hypoplasia is not compatible with life.

This absence of kidneys causes oligohydramnios, which can place extra pressure on the developing baby and cause further malformations (limb anomalies). Babies with BRA show wide-set eyes, prominent folds at the inner corner of each eye, sharp nose, and large low-set ears with lack of ear cartilage, and dry loose skin. They will typically have underdeveloped lungs, absent urinary bladder, anal atresia, esophageal atresia and unusual genitals. The lack of amniotic fluid causes some of the problems (undeveloped lungs, sharp nose, clubbed feet) and other problems occur because the kidneys and those affected structures are formed at the same time of fetal life (such as the ears, genitals, esophagus).

URA is common with intrauterine growth retardation and often results in premature birth. Babies may have low-set ears, so if ears are in this lower placement the baby should be examined for kidney problems. This is because the ears and kidneys are formed at the same time in fetal development. The ureters may also be abnormal and must be carefully examined early in life (by X-ray or ultrasound) so the kidney function of the one remaining kidney will be preserved. Unilateral renal agenesis is a relatively common congenital urinary malformation that is usually diagnosed during fetal ultrasonography. There are reports of hypertension and renal insufficiency (proteinuria, reduced GFR, edema, hematuria) in long-term studies of patients with a single kidney, and lifetime follow-up is recommended.

Certain genetic factors can create a higher risk for URA or BRA. The occurrence of renal agenesis has also been linked with several prenatal factors, such as diabetes mellitus, younger maternal age, and consumption of alcohol during pregnancy. Some drugs like retinoids, thalidomide, arsenates, and cocaine may contribute to defective renal development.

Treatment and Prognosis

BRA is not compatible with life outside the womb. The condition is typically fatal within the first few days of life. Newborns usually die from underdeveloped lungs shortly after birth.

Some newborns with BRA survive. They must have chronic peritoneal dialysis to replace their missing kidneys. Factors such as lung development, overall health, and family support determine the success of this treatment. The goal is to sustain these infants with *dialysis* until they grow strong enough to have a kidney transplant.

The prognosis for newborns with URA depends on the health of the solitary kidney and the presence of other abnormalities. Most individuals with URA do not experience any complications or limitations. Once diagnosed, children with one kidney (also called solitary kidney) will be encouraged to protect the remaining kidney from infection or injury. They will receive examinations of the kidney periodically and require prompt treatment of any urinary tract infection. They may be counseled to avoid contact sports where the kidney could be injured. Blood pressure monitoring will be essential throughout life since its elevation can cause kidney damage. Once diagnosed, children with URA need to have their blood pressure, urine, and blood tested annually to ensure the health of the remaining kidney. Blood pressure monitoring will be essential throughout life since its elevation can cause kidney damage. They will receive examinations of the kidney periodically and require prompt treatment of any urinary tract infection. They may be counseled to avoid contact sports where the kidney could be injured.

Renal Ectopia, Horse Shoe Kidney

Renal ectopy and fusion are common congenital anomalies of the kidney and urinary tract, and result from disruption of the normal embryologic migration of the kidneys. An ectopic kidney may lie in the pelvis or the iliac fossa. Horse shoe kidney, where the two kidneys are fused into one arched kidney that usually functions normally (Fig. 14.3A), but is more prone to develop problems later in life. It results as a consequence of abnormal renal ascent in embryogenesis with fusion of the kidneys within the pelvis. It is thought to occur in the first trimester, at around 4th to 8th week of fetal life.

Although children with these anomalies are generally asymptomatic, some children develop

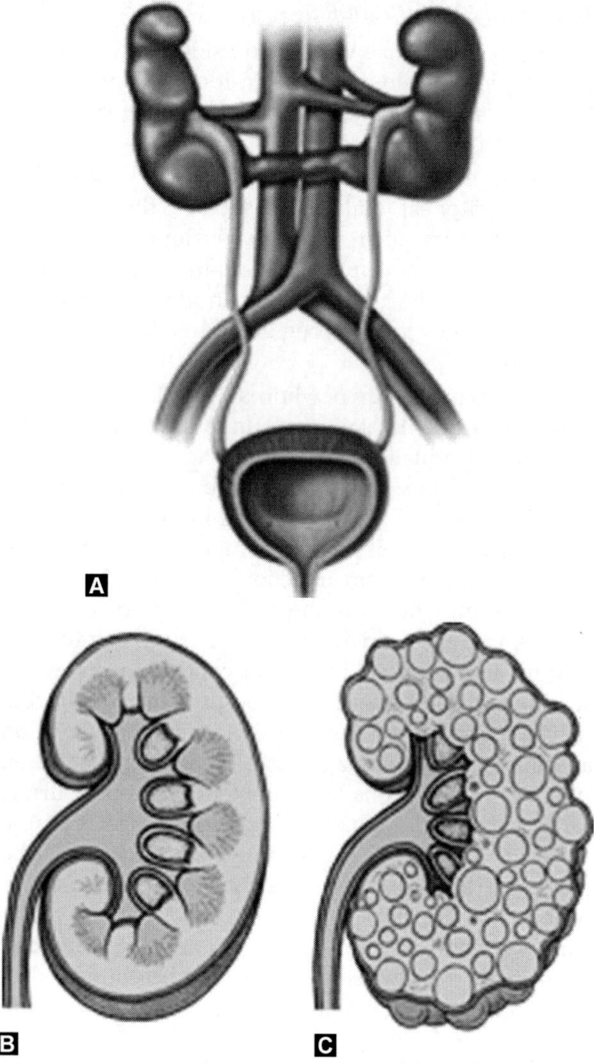

Figs 14.3A to C: A. Horse shoe kidney; B. Normal kidney; C. Polycystic kidney

symptoms due to complications, such as infection, renal calculi, and urinary obstruction.

The most common problem associated with an ectopic kidney is vesicoureteric reflux which occurs in up to 85% of children, pelviureteric junction obstruction is present in 33–52%. This is frequently due to a high insertion of the ureter on the renal pelvis, malrotation of the kidney or an anomalous blood supply which obstructs the collecting system. Renal calculi are also seen in this condition.

Crossed fused ectopia usually does not require any primary treatment (medical or surgical), but it does need to be checked regularly. However, understanding is essential before planning any surgical intervention in the renal region. The blood supply to cross-fused kidney is usually anomalous and angiography recommended before surgical intervention.

Complications of a crossed fused renal ectopic kidney are nephrolithiasis, infection, and hydronephrosis.

Renal Dysplasia, Multicystic Kidney

Renal dysplasia implies abnormal development of renal parenchyma. Multicystic dysplastic kidney (MCDK) is a congenital maldevelopment (nonfunctioning kidney) in which the renal cortex is replaced by numerous cysts of multiple sizes. A dysplastic parenchyma anchors the cysts, the arrangement of which resembles a bunch of grapes. The calyceal drainage system is absent. This is when large cysts develop in a kidney that has not developed properly, eventually causing it to stop working. While polycystic kidney disease (PKD) always affects both kidneys, MKD usually affects just one kidney.

Multicystic dysplastic kidney is the most common type of renal cystic disease, and it is one of the most common causes of an abdominal mass in infants. Fortunately, the unaffected kidney (Fig. 14.3B) takes over and most people with MKD will have normal kidney function. MKD usually is diagnosed by prenatal ultrasound before birth. Therapeutic management is done by monitoring blood pressure and screening for UTIs when needed. Very rarely, surgical removal of the kidney might be necessary.

The multicystic dysplastic kidney has an excellent long-term prognosis, and an affected patient will most likely have one normally functioning kidney for the remainder of their life.

There is no way to prevent multicystic dysplastic kidney from occurring early in a baby's development, and there is no known way to prevent it from happening.

Polycystic Kidney

Polycystic kidney disease (PKD) is a condition in which many fluid-filled cysts develop in both kidneys (Fig. 14.3C). Polycystic kidney disease is an inherited disease that affects both kidneys. Affected individuals are born with normal kidneys, and the cysts develop over time. Age of onset and severity are variable and depends on the genetic pattern of the disease in a given family. The cysts can multiply so much and grow so large that they lead to kidney failure. Most forms of PKD are inherited. The cysts are numerous and are fluid-filled, resulting in massive enlargement of the kidneys. The disease can also damage the liver, pancreas, and in some rare cases, the heart and brain.The two major forms of polycystic kidney disease are distinguished by their patterns of inheritance (autosomal dominant, autosomal recessive).

PKD can be diagnosed before or after the child is born. In some cases, there are no symptoms; in others, PKD can lead to UTIs, kidney stones, and high blood pressure. Treatment for PKD varies. The goal of PKD treatment is to manage symptoms. Controlling high blood pressure is the most important part of treatment. Treatment may include pain medication, blood pressure medication, antibiotics to treat UTI, diuretics, surgery (to drain cysts and help relieve discomfort). In some cases PKD can be managed with dietary changes; others require a kidney transplant or dialysis.

Duplication of the Ureters

Duplication of the ureters is a common anomaly which may be either complete or incomplete and is often accompanied by various complications (Figs 14.4A and B). The ureteric bud, the embryological origin of the ureter, splits (or arises twice), resulting in two ureters draining a single kidney. In most cases, the kidney is divided into two parts—an upper and lower lobe, with some overlap due to intermingling of collecting tubules. Ureteral duplication may be partial, i.e. the two ureters drain into the bladder via a single common ureter and complete, in which the two ureters drain separately. Complete ureteral duplication may result in one ureter opening normally into the bladder, and the other being ectopic, ending in the vagina, the urethra or the vulval vestibule, ejaculatory duct, seminal vesicles in male. These cases occur when the ureteric bud arises twice (rather than splitting).

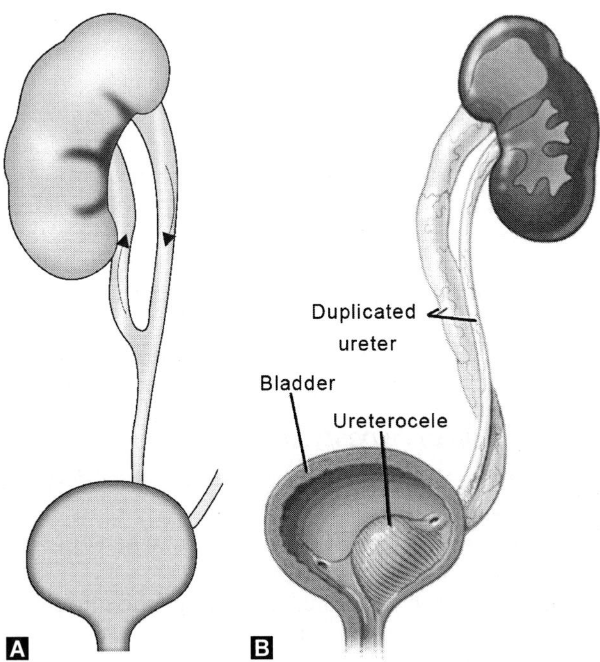

Figs 14.4A and B: A. Duplication of ureter (partial type); **B.** Duplication of ureter (complete type)

Ectopia or stenosis of one or both orifices, vesico-ureteral reflux into the lower ureter or both ureters, and ureterocele may occur. Surgery may be necessary if there is obstruction, vesicoureteral reflux, or urinary incontinence. Incomplete duplication is rarely of clinical significance. Duplication of the ureters can lead to urinary tract infections over time and can be treated with medication or, in some cases, with surgery.

CONGENITAL ABNORMALITIES RELATED TO BLADDER AND LOWER URINARY TRACT

Exstrophy of Bladder

Bladder exstrophy occurs when the bladder does not develop normally and is exposed through an opening on the abdominal wall. It is a rare congenital anomaly and known as *Ectopia Vesicae*. Urine produced by the kidneys drains into this open area and is not stored normally in the bladder. The disorder may occur in varying degrees from a mild to a severe defect that involves the genitalia and pelvis. Bladder exstrophy presents with:

- The bladder is turned inside out and exposed on the abdominal wall. The bladder neck has not developed properly and the bladder itself is usually small.
- *Presence of epispadias:* In males, the urethral opening is usually on the topside of the penis and not the tip. They may experience chordate. In girls, the urethral opening may be positioned further up between the divided clitoris and labia minora.
- *Widening of the pubic bones:* The pubic bones usually join to protect and support the bladder, urethra and abdominal muscles. In children with exstrophy, the pubic bones do not join, leaving a wide opening. This causes external rotation of the pelvis.
- *Vesicoureteral reflux (VUR):* Normally the kidneys make urine and drain down the ureters into the bladder. VUR is a condition where urine travels back up into the kidneys. This may develop after the bladder is reconstructed.
  - Abnormal development of genitalia with exstrophy of bladder
    - *Boys:* The size of the penis may develop shorter and curved in an upward direction.

The testicles may not be in a normal position in the scrotum and a hernia may be seen.
   - *Girls:* The clitoris and labia minora remain separated and spread apart; the vagina and urethra are shorter. The uterus, fallopian tubes and ovaries are generally normal.
- Displacement of the umbilicus and/or an umbilical hernia.

Diagnosis

Exstrophy of the bladder can usually be diagnosed by fetal ultrasound prenatally. Other tests are urine test (urine culture and urine analysis) to check for UTI and to test kidney function, blood tests (complete blood count, electrolytes, and BUN, record of urine output, X-ray of child's lower stomach and bones, ultrasound of child's kidneys.

Treatment

Treatment of exstropy of bladder comprises of surgical correction which may be complete repair of exstrophy, or two/three phased surgery. One time surgery includes bladder closure, bladder neck reconstruction, epispadias repair and pelvic osteotomy (closing the pelvic bones). Closing the bladder early allows the bladder to cycle (fill and empty urine) which optimizes bladder growth and development.

In by phased surgeries, the first surgery separates the exposed bladder from the abdomen wall and closes the bladder, the bladder neck and urethra are repaired. A suprapubic catheter is placed to drain urine from the bladder and a second catheter is left in the urethra to promote healing (for 3–4 weeks).

The second surgery, pelvic bone surgery is done along with the bladder repair. It may be delayed for weeks or months. After pelvic bone surgery, child will need to be in a lower body cast or sling for 4 to 6 weeks. This helps the bones to stabilize and hold anatomical position and thus to promote healing.

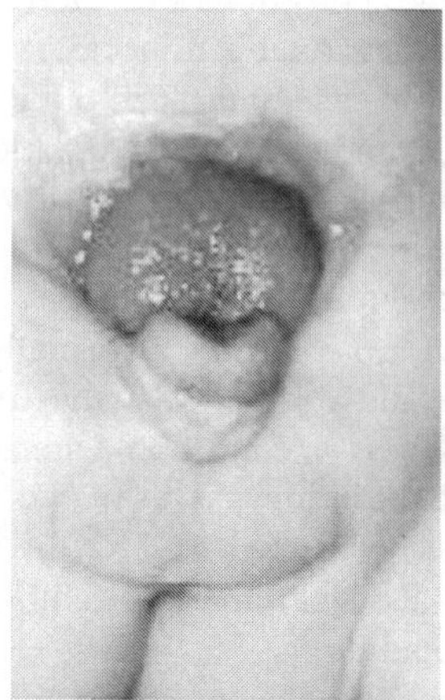

Fig. 14.5: Extrophy of bladder

Consecutive surgeries may be needed if there is a bowel defect, genital anomaly.

Wound care, pain management, and antibiotics are used as needed.

Urine samples will need to be checked to detect any infection from the procedure.

Long-term goals of surgery for children with exstrophy of bladder and other anomalies, are to :

- Allow the child to optimize continence (normal urinary control), volitional voiding and normal renal function.
- To have a cosmetically acceptable genitalia and avoid future problems with sexual function.
- Improve the child's physical appearance (genitals will look more normal).
- Prevent infection that could harm the kidneys.

Hypospadias and Epispadias

Hypospadias is a congenital anomaly of the male urethra and phallus. It is characterized by shortening of the urethra and ectopia of the external urethral opening. Instead of opening at the tip of the glans of the penis, a hypospadic urethra may open slightly ventral to the glance or as far back as penoscrotal junction. Hypospadias may accompany chordee, or downward curvature of the penile shaft. Associated anomalies, like undescended testes and inguinal hernia may be present with hypospadias.

Epispadias represents a congenital anomaly which is characterized by short phallus with marked upward curvature (dorsal chordee). The corresponding defect in females is a fissure in the upper wall of the urethra and is quite rare. The problem can also include like an abnormal clitorus and labia. The urethral opening is often between the clitoris and the labia, but it may be in the belly area. They may have trouble controlling urination (urinary incontinence).

Classification of Hypospadias

Classification of hypospadias is done by the position of the urethral meatus. The types are:

- Distal glandular, most common form when opening is found near the head of the penis.
- Midshaft, when opening is found in the middle to the lower shaft of the penis.
- Penoscrotal, when opening is on the scrotum.
- Perineal, when opening is behind the scrotal sac.

> **Pathophysiology**
> Hypospadias is the incomplete development of the anterior urethra and corpus spongiosum. The exact cause of the disorder is not known, but may have relation with genetic, environmental and maternal-fetal hormonal interactions. Usually the urinary continence is not interfered by the ectopic position of the urethral meatus. But stenosis of the urethral opening may give rise to partial obstruction of out flowing urine. If it is left uncorrected, this penile disorder has its social and sexual impact in child's future life.

Clinical Features

The signs and symptoms of hypospadias may include:

- Opening of the urethra at a location other than the tip of the penis (opens anywhere along the urethral groove).
- Chordee or congential curvature of the penis (downward curve of the penis).
- Hooded appearance of the penis because only the top half of the penis is covered by foreskin.
- Altered urinary stream, having to sit down to urinate.

Diagnosis

It is almost always diagnosed immediately at birth upon initial examination; if on initial examination the foreskin is incompletely developed or asymmetrical, the child should be evaluated for hypospadias. Imaging tests may be done to look for other congenital defects.

Management

Hypospadias needs surgical intervention which is usually done through one stage or more. Surgery is usually done before the child starts school. Today, most urologists recommend repair before the child is 18 months old (before toilet training). Surgery can be done as young as 4 months old. The goals of surgical correction are to allow the child to void while standing, to straighten the penis, and to provide a symmetrical appearance to the penis and prepuce. It means to make urinary and sexual function as normal as possible and to improve the cosmetic appearance of the penis. The surgical steps are to release the chordate, lengthen the urethra, position the meatus at the tip of the penis (opening is corrected using tissue grafts from the foreskin) and reconstruction of the penis. Indwelling catheter or urethral stents are commonly used. The child's movement is restricted and kept in bed for several days. Infants with hypospadias should not be circumcised. The foreskin should be kept for use in later surgical repair.

The choice of dressings, addition of prophylactic antibiotics and decisions about urinary diversion depends on surgeon's preference, influenced by the severity of the hypospadias and the type of surgical repair employed.

The primary goals of treatment of epispadias are to: lengthen and straighten the penis by correcting dorsal bend and chordee; and create functionality and cosmetically acceptable external genitalia with as few surgical procedures as possible. If the bladder and bladder neck are also involved, surgical treatment is required to establish urinary continence and preserve fertility.

The prognosis for epispadias depends on the extent of the defect. Most males with relatively minor epispadias lead normal lives, including fathering children. As the extent of the defect increases, surgical reconstruction generally is acceptable. However, many of these men are unable to conceive children. Most epispadias in females can be surgically repaired. The chances of residual disfigurement increase as the extent of the epispadias increases. Fertility in females is not generally affected by epispadias.

Follow-up care

An ideal protocol should include an early evaluation within 3 months of surgery, followed by a review at 1 or 2 years, and again at 4 or 5 years. Subjective evaluation of quality of micturition and if possible objective assessment is to be done with uroflowmetry and ultrasound evaluation. With the onset of rapid growth at puberty there is potential for new problems to arise so reassessment during puberty and mid teen is important. By this time genital maturation will be at, or near completion and the patient is able to comment about social and sexual aspects of his penile surgery.

Phimosis

Phimosis is defined as the inability to retract the foreskin or prepuce covering the glans of the penis (Fig. 14.6A). Phimosis may appear as a tight ring or 'rubber band' of foreskin around the tip of the penis, preventing full retraction. Phimosis is divided into two forms—physiologic and pathologic.

> **Pathophysiology**
> Physiologic phimosis occurs in newborn males. The prepuce is adhered to glans at birth and this separates naturally over time (usually around 5 to 7 years of age). Enthusiastic attempts to retract foreskin in physiological phimosis causes micro-tears, infection, and bleeding with secondary scarring and true phimosis (pathologic). Poor hygiene and recurrent balanitis (infection of glans penis), posthitis (inflammation of foreskin), or both could lead to difficulty in retraction of foreskin and consequent true phimosis.

Clinical Features

Physiologic phimosis involves only nonretractability of the foreskin. There may be some ballooning during urination. On gentle traction, the prepuce puckers and the overlying tissue are pink and healthy. In pathologic phimosis, there is usually pain, ballooning of the foreskin with urination resulting in forceful/difficult of urination, irritation, local infections, bleeding, dysuria, hematuria, painful erection,frequent episodes of urinary tract infections, preputial pain, and weak urinary stream. Occasionally, enuresis or urinary retention is noticed. The meatal opening is small and the tissue in front of the foreskin is white and fibrotic.

Based on state of the foreskin, phimosis is categorized as:

- Fully retractable prepuce but tight behind glance—Grade I.
- Partial retractability with partial exposure of the glans—Grade II.
- Partial retractability with meatus just visible—Grade III.
- Slight retraction but neither meatus nor glans visible—Grade IV.

Diagnosis

Diagnosis of phimosis is primarily clinical and no laboratory tests or imaging studies are required. These may be required for associated urinary tract infections or skin infections.

Management

Treatments for phimosis vary depending on the child and severity of phimosis. When a child is brought with history of inability to retract the foreskin, it is important to confirm whether it is physiologic or pathologic. Management depends on age of child, type of nonretraction, severity of phimosis, cause, and associated morbid conditions. Treatments may include: gentle daily manual retraction (Fig. 14.6B), topical corticosteroid ointment application or circumcision.

When it is certain that phimosis in the child is not pathologic, it is vital to reassure the parents on normalcy of the condition in that age group. They should be taught how to keep the foreskin and its undersurface clean and hygienic. Normal washing with lukewarm water and gentle retractions during bathing and urination makes the foreskin retractile over time. Mild soap can be used, but avoid strong soaps as it could lead to chemical irritant dermatitis and further phimosis. Reassurance and reinforcement of proper preputial hygiene may need to be repeated at periodic intervals.

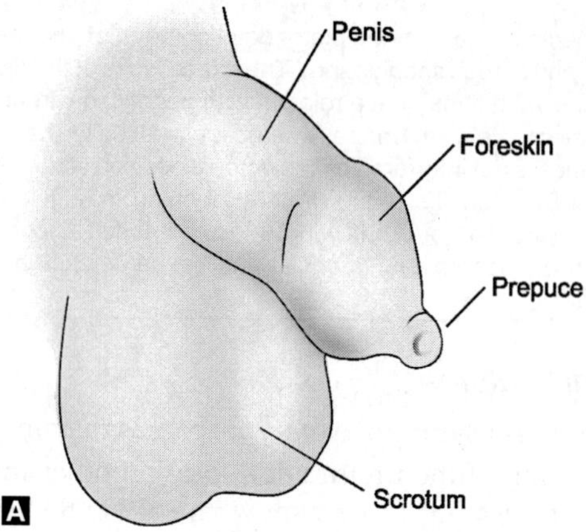

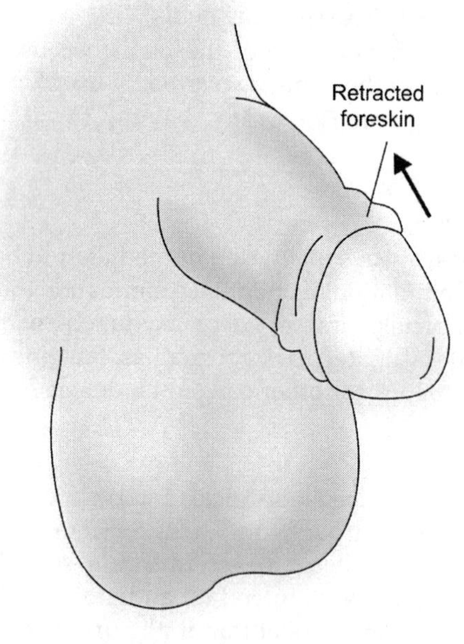

Figs 14.6A and B: A. Phimosis; **B.** Corrected Phimosis by retraction

Topical steroids have been tried in cases of phimosis since more than 2 decades. In recent years, topical application of steroids has provided an effective nonsurgical treatment for phimosis, and this treatment is, at present, the recommended management of phimosis. Overall, studies using topical creams for phimosis have yielded dramatic results. Mechanism of action of topical steroid therapy in phimosis is not exactly known. It is believed to act via its local anti-inflammatory and immunosuppressive action.

Surgery: In circumcision (the conventional intervention), phimotic foreskin is totally excised. Circumcision is one of the oldest elective operations known in humans which cures phimosis and prevents recurrence. It also prevents further episodes of balanoposthitis and lowers incidence of urinary tract infections.

If surgery is indeed needed, conservative plastic surgical techniques should be performed rather than the traditional circumcision. This would help the patients, their families, and the health care as well as the society at large.

Posterior Urethral Valve

Posterior urethral valves (PUV) are obstructing membranous folds within the lumen of the posterior urethra. Posterior urethral valves occur only in boys as a result of abnormal in utero development. It is one of the most common etiology of chronic kidney disease due to urinary tract obstruction in children. Diminished urinary output in utero usually results in oligohydramnios. This can also lead to pulmonary hypoplasia and respiratory distress syndrome.

Types

Each child who presents with PUV has a different amount of damage to the urinary system (bladder, ureters and kidneys) – some may have a mild problem whereas in others PUV may have caused severe damage in the womb.

Type I valves representing folds extending inferiorly from the veru to the membranous urethra.

Type II valves as leaflets radiating from the veru proximally to the bladder neck.

Type III valves as concentric diaphragms within the prostatic urethra, either above or below the veru.

By far the most common are Type I valves, and these are believed to result from failure of the posterolateral migration of the urethrovaginal folds, with fusion of the distal (or anterior) extension of these folds.

Pathophysiology

In true senses, the name PUV is a misnomer, since using the word valve implies that there exists a functional valve somewhere, which in this case is dysfunctional. The 'valve' in PUV is actually an overgrowth of urethral tissue that forms a membranous barrier to antegrade urine flow. A blockage to the urine flow through the urethra causes back pressure on the bladder which may enlarge considerably and/or develop a very thick muscle wall. This in turn can lead to further back pressure up the ureters and lead to excess fluid in the kidneys called hydronephrosis.

Clinical Manifestations

PUV may present with a broad array of symptoms or signs at any age during childhood and may vary from ascites in the neonate to renal failure in an infant or only minor voiding dysfunction in an older child. Urinary tract infection is common at all ages.

Inability to void is a common presentation. There may be dribbling or poor urine stream, infection or less commonly hematuria.

Diagnostic Investigations

The diagnosis is made radiologically with a voiding cystourethrogram (VCUG), where bladder thickening, urethral dilation and severe vesicoureteral reflux are seen PUV on voiding cystourethrogram is characterized by an abrupt tapering of urethral caliber near the verumontanum, with the specific level depending on the developmental variant. Vesicoureteral reflux is also seen in over 50% of cases.

This is usually done in conjunction with the renal ultrasound to evaluate the upper tracts. Ultrasound may show hydronephrosis and possibly increased renal echogenicity.

Diagnosis can also be made by cystoscopy, for direct visualization of the posteriorly positioned valve.

Renal function studies, in addition to serum studies, should determine the glomerular filtration by clearance values and some estimation made of urinary concentrating ability.

Management

Treatment is initially to drain the bladder, and after medical stabilization, valve ablation. The standard surgical intervention is primary (transurethral) ablation of the valves, where the valve is removed through the urethra without creation of stoma.There are specific endoscopic treatments of posterior urethral valves:

- *Vesicostomy followed by valve ablation:* A stoma is made in the urinary bladder, also known as *low diversion,* after which the valve is ablated and the stoma is closed.
- *Pyelostomy followed by valve ablation:* Stoma is made in the pelvis of the kidney as a slightly *high diversion,* after which the valve is ablated and the stoma is closed.

Following surgery, the follow-up in patients with posterior urethral valve syndrome is long term, and often requires a multidisciplinary effort between urologists, pulmonologists, neonatologists, radiologists, pediatric nurse and the family of the patient. Care must be taken to promote proper bladder compliance and renal function, as well as to monitor and treat the significant lung underdevelopment that can accompany the disorder.

Cryptorchidism and Inguinal Hernia

Different Surgical Procedures and Nursing Management of the Child with Urologic Surgery (*See* surgery Chapter 23).

OTHER DISORDERS OF GU SYSTEM OF CHILDREN

Urinary Tract Infection (UTI)

UTI is one of the most common pediatric infections characterized by the presence of bacteria to the urine along with systemic signs of infection. It distresses the child, concerns the parents, and may cause permanent kidney damage. Occurrences of a first-time symptomatic UTI are highest in boys and girls during the first year of life and markedly decrease after that.

An abnormality of the urinary tract: Structural abnormalities can cause retention of urine. The most common condition is called vesicoureteric reflux.

Etiology and Incidence

UTIs, except in newborn infants, can occur when bacteria like *E.coli* (most common bacteria), enterobacter species, *Klebsiella pneumoniae*, proteus species get into the bladder or the kidneys. These bacteria are common on the skin around the anus. They can also be present near the vagina.

Normally, there are no bacteria in the urinary tract. However, some things make it easier for bacteria to enter or stay in the urinary tract. These include:

Congenital or acquired anomalies/obstructions in the structure of the renal tract cause UTIs.

A problem in the urinary tract, called *vesicoureteral reflux*. This condition, which is most often present at birth, allows urine to flow back up into the ureters and kidneys. This is a problem at the junction where the ureter enters the bladder. In this condition, urine refluxes up the ureter from the bladder from time-to-time. This should not happen. The urine should only flow downwards out of the bladder when going to the toilet. This condition makes urine infections more likely. Infected urine that refluxes from the bladder back up to the kidneys may also cause hydronephrosis, kidney infection, scarring, and damage. In some cases this leads to severe kidney damage if urine infections recur frequently. Other rare problems that may be found include kidney stones, or congenital abnormalities of parts of the urinary tract.

- Brain or nervous system illnesses (such as myelomeningocele, spinal cord injury, hydrocephalus) that make it harder to empty the bladder.

Other conditions that increase the risk of a urine infection include:

- Patient is having diabetes, and a poorly functioning immune system. For example, children having chemotherapy.
- Not urinating often enough during the day.
- Wiping from back (near the anus) to front after going to the bathroom. In girls, this can bring bacteria to the opening where the urine comes out.

Nearly 1 in 20 boys, and more than 1 in 10 girls, have at least one urine infection by the time they are 16 years old. Children aged under 5 years are the most commonly affected.

Pathophysiology

Urinary Tract Infection

Most urine infections are due to bacteria that normally live in the bowel. They cause no harm in the bowel but can cause infection if they get into the urine. Fecal bacteria colonize around the perineal area or under the prepuce of uncircumcised infant boys. These bacteria can sometimes travel to the urethra and into the bladder. Some bacteria thrive in urine and multiply quickly to cause infection. The infection is commonly just in the bladder, is called cystitis, but may travel higher up to affect one or both renal parenchyma cause pyelonephritis. Pyelonephritis is more frequently seen in children with VUR (vesicoureteral reflux), but can occur in its absence. This condition, which is most often present at birth, allows urine to flow back up into the ureters and kidneys.

Recurrent urinary tract infections, which can predispose to scarring of the kidney. Scarring, may precipitate from inflammatory consequence of pyelonephritis, is more frequently seen in infants and is significant cause of hypertension during childhood. Arterial perfusion to the kidney is decreased due to scarring, which may results in volume depletion. This triggers the renin-angiotensin mechanism to increase aldosterone release and cause sodium and water retention. Hypertension is developed due to subsequent increase in circulating blood volume.

Clinical Manifestations

Children with UTIs may have a fever, poor appetite, vomiting, or no symptoms at all. Clinical manifestations of children with UTI vary widely due to underlying factors. Most urinary tract infections in children only involve the bladder. If the infection spreads to the kidneys (called pyelonephritis), it may be more serious.

Symptoms of a bladder infection in children include *blood in the urine*, cloudy urine, foul or strong urine odor, *frequent or urgent need to urinate,* malaise, dysuria, flank pain, wetting problems after the child has been toilet trained. Signs that the infection may have spread to the kidneys include chills with shaking, fever (104 °F), flushed, warm, or reddened skin, nausea, pain in the flank, severe pain in the abdomen and vomiting.

Diagnostic Evaluation

The physical examination of a child with suspected UTI should start with the vital signs. The presence of fever (specially over 102.2 °F or 39 °C) is highly correlated with the presence of a UTI. BP and assessment of height and weight provide helpful reassurance if normal or stable long-term renal function. Visual examination of the abdomen for enlargement related to potentially oversized kidney(s) or bladder is important. An abdominal mass can suggest hydronephrosis in an infant. Abdominal tenderness specially on the suprapubic region containing the bladder or the flank area is very helpful in establishing the diagnosis.

Examination of the genitalia is also very important to see if there is evidence of vaginal irritation (redness, discharge, evidence of trauma or foreign body). An *uncircumcised male* (specially with a foreskin which is difficult to retract) is more likely to experience a UTI.

A microscopic examination of urine may be indicative of a urinary tract infection. However, the urine culture is mandatory in confirming the diagnosis of a UTI. The culture provides both the exact bacterial cause as well as the antibiotic sensitivity profile to successfully treat the infection.

Certain children with UTIs may need more intensive evaluation for underlying structural abnormalities. Usually USG is done to detect kidney dilation resulting from obstruction, voiding cystourethrography or radionuclide cystography to detect vesicoureteral reflux (VUR).

Management

Antibiotic therapy for UTIs is based upon the sensitivity profile obtained from the urine-culture results. Cystitis should respond quickly to routine oral antibiotics. Pyelonephritis may need hospitalization for intravenous administration of antibiotics along with fluid therapy if the patient is experiencing associated vomiting and *dehydration*. Oral antibiotic therapy, however, may be appropriate if these complications are not present. Oral trimethoprim—sulfamethoxazole and cephalosporins are frequently used. A follow up urine culture evaluates treatment success.

The American Academy of Pediatrics has issued a position statement recommending follow-up studies for children who have experienced a urinary tract infection. Children who should be further evaluated include children 2 months to 2 years of age who sustain their first UTI, any male child who experiences a UTI, any child 3 years and older who has had more than one UTI, any child who has had pyelonephritis.

Some children may be treated with antibiotics for periods as long as 6 months to 2 years. This treatment is more likely when the child has had repeat infections or vesicoureteral reflux. Sometimes VUR is treated with the endoscopic injection of bulking material into the submucosa of the affected ureter. The material, Deflux injectable gel, builds a protective wall inside the ureter to prevent the backflow of urine.

Acute Glomerulonephritis (AGN)

AGN refers to an inflammation of the glomerulus, which is the unit involved in filtration in the kidney. The inflammatory process usually begins with an infection or injury (e.g. burn, trauma), then the protective immune system fights off the infection, scar tissue forms, and the process is complete. This damage interferes with the function of the glomeruli and it can interfere with the function of the kidneys as a whole. Salt and excess fluid can build up in the body if the kidneys are not working normally. This can lead to complications such as high blood pressure and, in some cases, AGN leads to acute renal failure (ARF).

Causes

- *Infections:* Bacterial infections (e.g. with streptococcus, staphylococcus, or pneumococcus), fungal and viral infections, parasitic infections (e.g. malaria), viral infections (e.g. hepatitis B and C or HIV infections). AGN that results from any of these infections is called postinfectious glomerulonephritis.
- *Vasculitis:* Cryoglobulinemia, eosinophilic granulomatosis with polyangiitis (formerly, Churg-Strauss syndrome), granulomatosis with polyangiitis (formerly, Wegener granulomatosis), microscopic polyangiitis.
- *Immune disorders:* AGN that develops into rapidly progressive glomerulonephritis most often results from conditions that involve an abnormal immune reaction (Goodpasture syndrome, systemic lupus erythematosus), immunoglobulin A nephropathy (IgA nephropathy, Berger's disease).
- *Other causes:* Hereditary nephritis, membranoproliferative nephritis (type of kidney inflammation), drugs (e.g. quinine, gemcitabine, or mitomycin).

Pathophysiology

Glomerulonephritis is the medical word used to describe swelling, redness and subsequent damage to the tiny filters, glomeruli in the kidneys. APGN commonly occurs as a result of an immunologic responses and one to two weeks after a sore throat or skin infection. APGN damages the kidney filters, which are responsible for the removal of waste and toxic products from the blood and out of the body via urine. After the strep. throat, or skin infection is gone, antibodies that help to fight the disease and antigen from the bacteria form an immune complex and travel through the circulation, and become trapped in the glomerulus. An inflammatory response is activated in the basement membrane of the glomerulus.

The bacteria do not infect the kidney filters; it is the immune complexes injure the filters. The renal injury occurs as a result of an immune-mediated process which involves the complement system. This leads to deposition of circulating immune complexes and/or their in situ formation in the kidney resulting in renal damage. Products of the inflammatory response stick to the kidney filters, cause swelling and reduction of the size of the capillary lumen and thus decrease GFR. Low GFR retains sodium and water in the body which leads to edema and hypertension. Permeability of the glomerular membrane increased due to injury and so that larger molecules and structures such as RBCs, casts, proteins can pass through it into urine. Treating the strep throat or skin infection with antibiotics does not prevent acute poststreptococcal glomerulonephritis.

Types

- *Primary glomerulonephritis:* It develops on its own and is not related to another pre-existing disease or condition in the body.
- *Secondary glomerulonephritis:* It develops because of another pre-existing disease or condition in the body such as systemic lupus erythematosus (SLE) and polyarteritis nodosa.

  The glomerulonephritis can be classified according to the changes that can be seen when the tissue sample is examined under a microscope. It can be classified as:
- *Focal and segmental glomerulosclerosis:* The glomeruli are sclerosed or scarred. Focal means that only some of the glomeruli are affected and segmental means that only parts of a glomerulus (and not the whole glomerulus) may be affected.
- *IgA and IgM glomerulonephritis:* These antibodies produced are deposited in the kidneys leading to inflammation, scarring and damage.
- *Membranoproliferative glomerulonephritis:* A glomerulus is made up of a membrane (the tiny blood vessels that filter the blood) and the mesangium which provides support to the glomerulus structure. In membranoproliferative glomerulonephritis, the membrane and the mesangium are both affected and damaged.
- *Membranous glomerulonephritis:* Just the membrane of the glomerulus is damaged and the mesangium is not affected in this type of glomerulonephritis.
- *Minimal change nephropathy:* Tissues look essentially normal under microscope, or there is minimal change—but symptoms of glomerulonephritis can still be present. This is a common type of glomerulonephritis in children.

Acute Poststreptococcal Glomerulonephritis (APSGN)

APSGN is a common form of glomerulonephritis in children. APSGN is active inflammation in the glomeruli. Infection with certain types of streptococcal bacteria (group A beta-hemolytic) is the most common infection that can trigger glomerulonephritis.

APSGN most often occurs as a complication of a throat or skin infection with streptococcus. Symptoms of glomerulonephritis typically develop between one and three weeks after the initial streptococcal pharyngitis and 3 to 6 weeks after streptococcus pyoderma. Glomerulonephritis that is triggered by an infection may occur at any age but it most commonly develops in children aged between 5 and 15 years and is uncommon before 3 years.

Clinical Features

In APSGN, a latent period (7–21 days) is seen between onset of the streptococcal infection and development of clinical glomerulonephritis. This latent period, more clearly defined after pharyngeal infections than after pyoderma, averages approximately 10 days. The most common feature in case of APSGN is edema and/or gross hematuria (classic description of smoky or tea- or cola-colored urine).

Hematuria or both hematuria and edema usually appear abruptly and may be associated with various degrees of malaise, lethargy, anorexia, fever, abdominal pain, joint pain and headache. Edema is the most frequent and sometimes the only clinical finding, usually appears abruptly and first involves the periorbital area and ankles but it may be generalized. The degree of edema widely varies and depends on a number of factors, including the severity of glomerular involvement, the fluid intake, and the degree of hypoalbuminemia. *The triad of edema, hematuria, and hypertension is classic for APSGN.* Three phases of the disease can be identified. These are—the latent phase, the acute phase, and the recovery phase.

Diagnosis

The diagnosis of APSGN is done on the basis of history, presenting symptoms and laboratory findings.

Patients with (AGN) have an active urinary sediment. This means that signs of active kidney inflammation can be detected when the urine is examined under the microscope. Such signs include red blood cells, white blood cells, proteinuria and 'casts' of cells that have leaked through the glomeruli and have reached the tubule, where they develop into cylindrical forms. Laboratory tests show variable amounts of protein and blood cells in the urine. Blood tests usually detect anemia. Electrolyte disturbances like high serum potassium and low serum bicarbonate levels can result from inadequate glomerular filtration.

Often kidney dysfunction is shown by a high concentration of urea and creatinine in the blood. The creatinine result can also be used to calculate the estimated glomerular filtration rate (eGFR). This gives a good measure of how well the kidneys are working.

Sometimes, a biopsy of a kidney is done to confirm the diagnosis, help determine the cause, and determine the amount of scarring and potential for reversibility. Kidney biopsy is done under ultrasound or computed tomography (CT) guidance to obtain a small amount of kidney tissue.

Additional tests are sometimes helpful for identifying the cause. For example, in the diagnosis of postinfectious glomerulonephritis, a throat culture may provide evidence of streptococcal infection. An antistreptolysin (ASO) titer, which indicates the presence of antibodies to streptococcal bacteria or a streptozyme test can be elevated. It is useful only if the infection is recent and the child has not taken antibiotic.

- *Chest X-ray:* This may be suggested if the child shows any breathing problems.
- *Ultrasound scan of the kidneys:* This can give information about the size of the kidneys, any blockages, etc.

Therapeutic Management

The goal of treatment is to stop the ongoing inflammation and lessen the degree of scarring that ensues.

Treatment of acute poststreptococcal glomerulonephritis (APSGN) is mainly supportive, because there is no specific therapy for renal disease. The goals of pharmacotherapy are to reduce morbidity, to prevent complications, and to eradicate the infection. Agents used include antibiotics, loop diuretics, vasodilators, and calcium channel blockers. The associated signs and symptoms are managed with supportive care and medical management.

- Treatment of any underlying cause of glomerulonephritis, e.g. treatment for an infection that may have triggered glomerulonephritis or for an underlying condition such as SLE. Usually a 10-day antibiotic course may be required.
- *Changes to diet and fluid intake:* The child may be kept on fluid restriction as well as the amount of salt and protein in diet.
- *Medicines to suppress immune system:* Because many cases of glomerulonephritis are thought to be caused by a problem with the immune system, steroid medicines, may be advised to help suppress immune system.
- *Angiotensin-converting enzyme (ACE) inhibitor medicines:* These may be advised to help reduce the amount of protein in urine. These medicines can also help to lower blood pressure if this is high.
- *Strict control of blood pressure:* It is accomplished by limiting sodium and water intake and by using antihypertensive or diuretic medicines.
- Treatment of anemia if present.
- *Plasma exchange:* This is a treatment similar to dialysis, which can be used to help suppress the immune system. Plasma is the fluid part of the blood containing antibodies. In plasma exchange, plasma is removed and replaced, either with other fluids or with plasma donated from other people that does not contain antibodies. Removing the antibodies may help to reduce the damage to the kidney tissues.
- Kidney dialysis and kidney transplant may be needed in severe cases.

Nursing Management

Assessment

- Obtain history focusing on immunologic issues like presence of SLE and infection of throat and skin (past and present), along with other history of illness.
- Complete physical examination, noting for presence of edema (on both foot, on both hands, periorbital area), hypertension and pulse rate, and hypervolemia as characterized by increased jugular venous pressure and engorged neck veins; assessment of skin condition.
- Assessment of fluid intake and calculation of urine output every 4 hourly.
- Assessment of pulmonary condition. Assessment for adventitious breath sounds.
- Monitor cardiac and serum laboratory values.

- Do routine laboratory workouts like urinalysis to assess for presence of blood and protein.

Nursing Diagnosis

- Excess fluid volume in the body due to decreased GFR, retention of sodium and fluid.
  Expected outcome: The child will maintain normal fluid status as evidenced by urine output (20 mL/per hour) and lesser edema (+) 1, normal BP, no increase in weight, no respiratory distress.
- Risk for impaired skin integrity due to edema and decreased activity.
  Expected outcome: The child will show intact skin with normal color and absence of tenderness.
- Altered nutrition, less than body requirement related to albuminuria and GI disturbances.
  Expected outcome: The child will have adequate nutrition as evidenced by maintenance of normal weight (preillness weight).
- Risk for activity intolerance due to fatigue and presence of edema.
  Expected outcome: The child will tolerate daily care and play activities.
- Anxiety related to knowledge deficit of disease process, care of child and hospitalization.
  Expected outcome: The child and family will show less anxiety. They will participate in care, child will show interest in age appropriate play. Parents will describe disease processes and its management and care.

Nursing Interventions

- Provide best rest during the acute phase and perform passive range of motion exercises for the patient on bed rest.
- Monitor intake and output and daily weight. Everyday there should be approximate loss of 0.5% body weight. Gain in weight indicates increased edema and fluid retention. Testing of urine at regular interval is to be done.
- Diuretic is to be administered as prescribed. After checking BP, antihypertensive is to be given.
- Consult the dietician about a diet high in calories and low in protein, sodium, potassium, and fluids.
- Provide skin care to maintain its integrity.
- Allow the patient to resume normal activities gradually as symptoms subside.
- Protect the debilitated patient against secondary infection by providing good nutrition and hygienic technique and preventing contact with infected people.
- Check the patient's vital signs and electrolyte values.
- Monitor intake and output and daily weight.
- Report peripheral edema (dependent) or the formation of ascites.
- Explain to the patient taking diuretics that he may experience orthostatic hypotension and dizziness when he changes positions quickly.
- Provide emotional support for the patient and his family.
- Provide developmentally appropriate play, when the child overcomes the acute phase.
- Orient the parents about continuation of care and follow-up.
- If the patient is scheduled for dialysis, explain the procedure fully.

Prognosis

Acute poststreptococcal glomerulonephritis resolves completely in most cases, specially in children. About 1% of children and 10% of adults develop chronic kidney disease.

Nephrotic Syndrome

Nephrotic syndrome is not a disease. It is a description of group of associated clinical features and laboratory abnormalities. Nephrotic syndrome is a collection of symptoms that indicate kidney damage. It is characterized by a number of signs like albuminuria, hyperlipidemia, edema (Fig. 14.7), hypoalbuminemia. The damage in renal bed causes increase in permeability of the capillary walls of the glomerulus leading to the presence of high levels of protein passing from the blood into the urine, low levels of protein in the blood.

Nephrotic syndrome in children can be caused by the following conditions:

- *Minimal change disease* is a condition characterized by damage to the glomeruli that can be seen only with an electron microscope. The cause of minimal change disease is unknown; some experts think it may occur after allergic reactions, vaccinations, and viral infections.
  Focal segmental glomerulosclerosis is scarring in scattered regions of the kidney, typically limited to a small number of glomeruli. *Membranoproliferative glomerulonephritis* is a group of autoimmune diseases that cause antibodies to build up on a membrane in the kidney.
  The prognosis of minimal change nephrotic syndrome is very good, chances of relapse with the age is usually less.

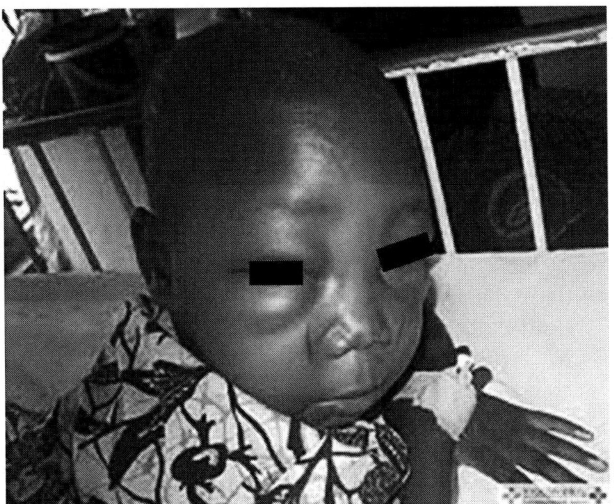

Fig. 14.7: A child with nephrotic syndrome

- *Systemic diseases:* Nephrotic syndrome in child may occur due to systemic diseases like SLE, hepatitis, heavy metal poisoning and cancer.

Pathophysiology

The basic cause of nephrotic syndrome (NS) is unknown, but it probably represents an antigenic response to a number of known and unknown stimuli in susceptible individuals. The syndrome may accompany many forms of renal and other pathology due to structural and functional changes in the glomerular capillary wall (GCW). Damage to the GCW causes increased permeability and loss of substances that would normally prevent negatively charged proteins from the capillary walls. As protein is lost in the urine, this leads to low levels of protein in the blood and the liver is unable to synthesize proteins to balance the loss.

Protein and other chemicals in the blood exert an osmotic pressure which tends to pull fluid into the blood vessels. If the concentration of protein in the blood reduces, the osmotic pressure reduces, and fluid comes out from the blood vessels into the tissues. This leads to edema which is the main symptom of nephrotic syndrome. This shift of fluid decreases renal blood flow which in turn initiates renin-angiotensin-aldosterone phenomenon (Fig. 14.8), and results in renal tubular reabsorption of sodium. The ultimate result of this phenomenon again is edema.

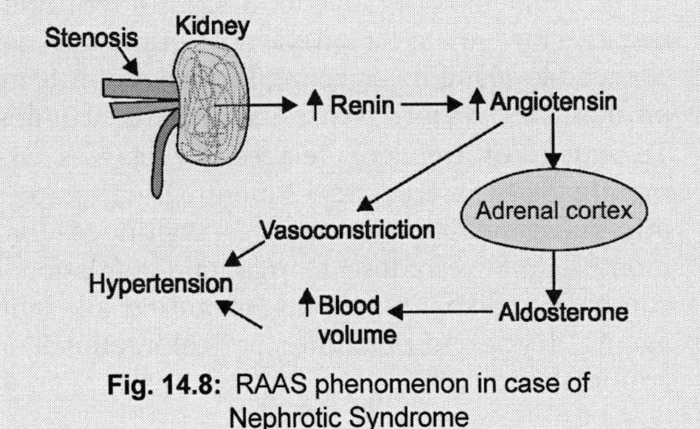

Fig. 14.8: RAAS phenomenon in case of Nephrotic Syndrome

Contd...

Contd...

Moreover, this progressive morphologic renal abnormalities elevates the serum values of cholesterol and triglycerides because proteinemia stimulates liver to produce more albumin to maintain normal oncotic pressure. At the same time, liver releases more cholesterol and triglycerides.

In NS, loss of immunoglobulins in urine is common. These children are prone to infection as the levels of immunoglobulin G are decreased in their body. They also suffer from hypercoagulability which may predispose them to venous thrombosis. Hypovolemia in NS leads to increased concentration of RBCs and platelets and slow circulation. The risk of thrombus formation is increased as a result of urinary loss of protein which usually inhibits coagulation.

Clinical Features

- *Proteinuria:* Damage to the glomeruli can also cause protein to leak into the urine. High levels of protein in the urine can make it frothy, it is considered to be in the nephrotic range when the urine protein is 3+/4+ on a dipstick test.
- Hypoalbuminemia (serum albumin <2.5 g/dL)
- Hyperlipidemia (serum cholesterol >200 mg/dL)
- *Edema:* Disease may be first noted with insidious edema around periorbital spaces. Edema develops due to the serum hypoalbuminemia. Lower serum oncotic pressure causes fluid to accumulate in the interstitial tissues. Sodium and water retention aggravates the edema. This may take several forms like puffiness around the eyes, characteristically in the morning, pitting edema over the legs, fluid in the lungs (pleural effusion, pulmonary edema) and ascites. This generalized edema is also known as anasarca or dropsy.
  Examination should also exclude other causes of gross edema, specially the cardiovascular and hepatic system.
- Usually child with NS remains normotensive. In some cases rise of blood pressure is observed.
- Anemia (iron resistant microcytic hypochromic type) may be present due to transferrin loss.
- Dyspnea may be present due to pleural effusion or due to diaphragmatic compression with ascites.
- Erythrocyte sedimentation rate is increased due to increased fibrinogen and other plasma contents.

Diagnostic Evaluation

In order to establish the presence of nephrotic syndrome, laboratory testing should include (*a*) Urinalysis; (*b*) complete blood count, blood levels of albumin, cholesterol, urea and creatinine; (*c*) blood levels of antistreptolysin O and C3 in patients with persistent microscopic or gross hematuria; (*d*) appropriate tests for underlying illness if clinically suspected (e.g. antinuclear antibodies for systemic lupus erythematosus); (*e*) urine culture, if urinary tract infection is suspected; (*f*) X-ray chest, Mantoux test; and (*g*) hepatitis B surface antigen.

Other tests like complete blood count, levels of serum electrolytes, calcium, phosphorus, and ionized calcium, as well as of blood urea nitrogen and creatinine, testing for hepatitis B and C, complement studies (C3, C4), antinuclear antibody are done to determine whether the nephrotic syndrome is idiopathic or secondary. Renal biopsy is indicated in case of atypical cases (presence of hematuria or hypertension), or the child who does not respond as expected to pharmacologic treatment.

The diagnosis of nephrotic syndrome is based on the presence of heavy proteinuria, hypoalbuminemia and edema. Once the diagnosis is made, a detailed evaluation of the patient is necessary before starting treatment with corticosteroids. The height, weight and blood pressure are recorded. A regular weight record, during a relapse, helps monitor the decrease of edema until dry weight is achieved.

Physical examination to detect infections is necessary, which if present should be treated promptly. The child is tested for exposure to tuberculosis and varicella because treatment of NS suppresses the immune system.

Patients should be examined for an underlying systemic disorder, e.g. systemic lupus erythematosus, amyloidosis and Henoch-Schonlein purpura.

Therapeutic Management

The objective of this treatment is to treat the imbalances brought about by the illness edema, hypoalbuminemia, hyperlipemia, hypercoagulability and infectious complications. Usually child is hospitalized for palliative care for edema, diagnostic evaluation, initiation of treatment and preparation of parent for necessary home care.

- *Edema:* A return to an unswollen state is the prime objective of this treatment of NS. It is carried out through the combination of a number of interventions.
- *Rest:* Depending on the seriousness of the edema and taking into account the risk of thrombosis caused by prolonged bed rest.
- Medical nutrition therapy is based on a diet with the correct energy intake and balance of proteins that will be used in synthesis processes and not as a source of calories. A total of 35 kcal/kg body weight/ day is normally recommended. This diet should also comply with two more requirements—the first is to not consume more than 1 g of protein/kg body weight/ day, as a greater amount could increase the degree of proteinuria and cause a negative nitrogen balance. It includes a moderate intake of foods rich in animal proteins.
- The second guideline requires that the amount of water ingested is not greater than the level of diuresis. Generally, for these whose illness condition and edema is very severe, they can drink water 500 mL more than their urine output the day before. In addition, if they found it is hard to not to drink water when they are extremely thirsty, they can daub their lips with wet swab, which will help them limit fluid intake strictly.

  In order to facilitate the fluid restriction, the consumption of salt must also be controlled, as this contributes to water retention. It is advisable to restrict the ingestion of sodium to 1 or 2 g/day, which means that salt cannot be used in cooking and salty foods should also be avoided.

  The pharmacological treatment of edema consists of diuretic drugs, specially loop diuretics. Loop diuretics, such as furosemide (starting at 1-2 mg/ kg/d), may improve edema. Metolazone may be beneficial in combination with furosemide for resistant edema.

  It may be necessary to give a patient potassium or require a change in dietary habits if the diuretic drug causes hypokalemia as a side effect.
- *Treatment by steroid (remission induction therapy):* Kidney damage is treated with corticosteroid therapy, and usually prednisolone at a dose of 2 mg/kg day (maximum 60 mg), divided into 2 to 3 doses are administered. This therapy is continued upto 4 to 6 weeks until the child is in remission (zero to trace albumin in urine for 5 to 7 consecutive days). After 4 to 6 weeks, the therapy is switched to 40 mg/ m^2 or 1.5 mg/kg (maximum 40 mg) on alternate days for 2 to 5 months with tapering, with a minimum total duration of treatment of 12 weeks.

  Treatment of infrequent relapse (1 relapse in 6 months or 1 to 3 relapses in 12 months): Steroid therapy will start at the dose (60 mg/m^2/day or 2 mg/kg/day) until urinary protein is negative for 3 days. After urine is negative for protein for 3 days, dose of prednisone is changed to 40 mg/m^2 or 1.5 mg/kg (maximum 40 mg) on alternate days for 4 weeks, then stop or taper dose.

  Treatment of frequent relapse (2 relapses in 6 months or ≥4 relapses in 12 months) – Therapy of infrequent relapse treatment is continued for 3 months at lowest dose to maintain remission or corticosteroid-sparing agents, including alkylating agents (cyclophosphamide or chlorambucil) is administered.

Antihypertensive Agents

Angiotensin-converting enzyme (ACE) inhibitors and angiotensin II receptor blockers (ARBs) can reduce hypertension and may also contribute to reducing proteinuria.

Infectious complications are treated with an appropriate course of antibacterial drugs according to the infectious agent.

In addition to these key imbalances, vitamin D and calcium are also taken orally in case the alteration of vitamin D causes a severe hypocalcemia, this treatment has the goal of restoring physiological levels of calcium in the patient.

Vaccination of child is to be completed except live vaccines (when the child is on steroid). In addition to killed virus vaccines, the child should receive pneumococcal and an influenza vaccine to prevent the exacerbations of those diseases.

Nursing Management

Assessment

Collection of subjective data through history taking. Recent known exposure to communicable diseases, immunization status.

- Monitoring vital signs for early signs of infection and hypovolemia.
- Careful documentation of child's fluid intake and urine output, taking daily weight.
- Assessment of edema in each shift, specifically in the periorbital areas, abdomen, genitalia, and lower extremities.

Lab Test—Urine for Protein

Nursing Diagnosis: Risk for impaired skin integrity due to edema and decreased circulation.

Expected outcome: The skin of the child will remain intact, as evidenced by the absence of redness, tenderness to touch, and ulceration.

Intervention with Rationale

Two hourly position changing is to be done. Elevation of edematous part with pillows, while the child is in bed or sitting in a chair. Position changing frequently decreases pressure on body parts and helps relieve edema in dependent parts.

Avoiding invasive procedure as possible. Good skin care, use of nonalcohol-based lotion for dry skin. Avoiding the contact of two edematous skin surfaces (thigh surfaces) to prevent friction. Daily change of linen. Frequent gentle massage and applying lotion helps in circulation. Change of linen gives comfort, otherwise body secretions and debris on linens can irritate the skin.

Promotion of physical activity as the child is able to tolerate by providing developmentally suitable play. Promotion of circulation is helped by increased activity.

Evaluation

Is the child's skin intact without redness and tenderness?

Nursing Diagnosis: Excess fluid volume related to decreased loss of sodium and fluid accumulation in tissue.

Expected outcome: No fluid overload as evidenced by stable body weight and normal respiratory pattern.

Intervention and Rationale

Record intake and output accurately in each shift. Report if child has output of less than 1 to 2 mL/kg/hour of urine. Daily evaluation is important for therapeutic efficacy and the basis for determining action.

Weigh weight each day in the same scale, same time, in a gown only. It estimates reduction in edema of the body. Concern regarding scale, time, and clothing is needed for accuracy of the readings.

Give fluids carefully sand low-salt diet. It prevents edema, gain weight.

Dietary protein 1 to 2 g/kg/day. High protein diet is necessary to compensate proteinuria.

Administer prescribed medicines (prednisolone, diuretics) orally. Ensure adequate potassium intake (fruit juice, banana). Elimination of excess fluid is done by diuretics. Diuretics can increase excretion of potassium.

Monitor pulmonary status by listening breath sounds for crackles, observing for signs of increased work of breathing and presence of cough. It is necessary as fluid overload can result in pulmonary edema.

Evaluation

Does the child maintain a stable weight?

Is there any incidence of respiratory distress of the child?

Nursing Diagnosed: Changes in nutrition from the space requirements associated with malnutrition secondary to protein loss and decreased appetite.

Expected outcome: The child will show better nutritional intake as evidenced by a good appetite, improved hypoproteinemia, and he/she is active and alert.

Intervention and Rationale

Encourage the child to take food. Record food intake and output accurately. Monitoring nutritional intake for the body.

Assess for anorexia, hypoproteinemia, diarrhea. Nutritional deficiencies can occur slowly and diarrhea occurs as intestinal edema reaction.

Make sure the child gets enough food diet, considering diet restrictions and likes and dislike of the child. Nutritional supplementation can be considered as needed. These steps prevent worse nutritional status.

Evaluation

Does the child show interest in eating? Does the child maintain a stable blood protein level? Does the child show interest in his environment?

Nursing Diagnosis: High risk of infection related to urinary loss of gammaglobulins decreased body immunity (immunosuppressive therapy).

Expected outcome: The child will not show an infection as evidenced by the criteria for signs of infection do not exist, vital signs within normal limits, and absence of cough and abdominal pain.

Intervention and Rationale

Protect children from people who are infected by restricting visitors. It minimizes the entry of organisms which may pose a serious threat to the child with immunosuppressive drugs.

Place the child in a room of noninfectious and wash hands before and after the action. It prevents the occurrence of nosocomial infections.

Monitor child for fever, sore throat, cough, or complaints of abdominal pain each shift. Monitor laboratory findings (TLC, DLC). Record vital signs. This nursing action ensures early detection of infectious processes. Abdominal pain can be a sign of peritonitis.

Administer antibiotics as prescribed, perform invasive aseptically. It is necessary to restrict the entry of bacteria into the body. Early detection can prevent sepsis infection.

Evaluation

Does the child maintain normal body temperature and show normal laboratory value? Is he/she free from any signs of infection?

Nursing Diagnosed: Child's fear and parental anxiety regarding treatment and associated with foreign environment (impact of hospitalization).

Expected outcome: The parents will demonstrate decreased anxiety as evidenced by participation in care, the child will communicate with others in his environment as show less fear.

Intervention and Rationale

To provide emotional support and validate feelings of fear or anxiety. Allowing parents in child care. Feelings are real and help patients to openly so that they can deal with it. Moreover, maintaining contact with parents, involving them in care and providing information regarding child's condition minimizes anxiety of family. Sometimes they may be allowed to express their frustration. Strengthening relationships with health care professionals increase the expression of feelings. Moreover, continuous support reduces the fear or anxiety faced by the parents.

Encourage parents to bring toys or family photos. Allowing play and self-care as tolerated by the child. They may be allowed to play with other children as it is not otherwise contraindicated. These actions minimize the impact of hospitalization separated from family members.

Evaluation

Does the child communicate and play with others? Do the parents involve in the child's care?

Acute Renal Failure (ARF)

ARF is characterized by the abrupt failure of the kidneys to regulate water and electrolyte homeostasis and filter waste products. ARFs in childhood due to dehydration, postinfectious acute glomerulonephritis, hemolytic-uremic syndrome; are reversible, but a small percentage may progress to chronic renal failure (CRF). ARF is an occasional but alarming complication of NS. ARF in childhood is associated with obstructive uropathy, congenital anomalies, and other causes.

ARF is divided into three forms—prerenal failure (most common), intrinsic renal failure, and postrenal failure. Treatment ranges from conservative medical management to dialysis or renal transplantation, depending on the severity of kidney disease and degree of renal function recovery. Worldwide, most cases of ARF in children are due to hemolytic-uremic syndrome or volume depletion.

Etiology and Incidence

ARF is a life-threatening, abrupt reduction of urinary output to less than 300 mL/m^2/day that is precipitated by prolonged renal ischemia in most cases.

- Prerenal failure (before the nephron)—Anything that originates in the circulatory blood supply of the nephron that impairs its function will be classed as prerenal acute renal failure. Prerenal failure occurs due to dehydration, perinatal asphyxia, hypotension, hemorrhagic shock and obstruction in the renal artery.
- *Intrinsic renal failure (within the nephron):* With intrarenal disorders, the problem arises from within the nephron tubules themselves, at some point from the proximal tubule to the collecting duct. Hemolytic -uremic syndrome (HUS), glomerulonephritis, pyelonephritis, nephrotoxic substances (drugs, pesticides, contrust dyes) cause intrinsic renal failure.
- *Postrenal failure (beyond the nephron and within urinary tract):* Postrenal disorders are those that originate in the urinary tract 'downstream' from the nephrons of the kidney. These disorders can involve the renal pelvis, the ureters or the bladder and urethra. Structural abnormalities like ureteropelvic obstruction, ureterovesical obstruction, PUV, neurogenic bladder, outlet obstruction by edema, stones and tumor cause postrenal failure.

Pathophysiology

ARF is not a single, uniform pathophysiological entity. Factors that can be singled out to contribute to the decrease in glomerular filtration rate (GFR) are a low renal perfusion pressure, a decreased filtration, high intratubular pressure, acute tubular necrosis (ATN), interstitial nephritis and interstitial oedema. This condition triggers oliguria, azotemia and other electrolyte imbalance. Tissue injury further magnifies the damage and the less perfusion.

In the case of overt hypotension, a prerenal cause can be suspected. The prerenal ARF is the result of decreased perfusion of the kidney as there is decreased blood flow and subsequent ischemia cause cellular swelling. This ischemia damages kidney tissue (intrarenal ARF). Obstruction of urine outflow increases pressure within the kidney, which decreases renal function (postrenal ARF).

- Reduced cardiac output and renal perfusion pressure
- Results in afferent arteriole constriction
- Avid sodium and water reabsorption
- Oliguria
- *Acute tubular necrosis* if prolonged hypoperfusion.

Clinical Manifestations

Symptoms of acute renal failure depend largely on the underlying cause. Nonspecific manifestations ARF include poor feeding, vomiting, lethargy, pallor, swelling of the tissues, seizure. Fluid and electrolyte imbalances, uncontrolled accumulation of nitrogenous waste products, i.e. BUN and serum creatinine, indicate established ARF.

Frequently this is led to massive fluid overload in the ARF patient with resultant pulmonary congestion, hypoxia, and premature need for mechanical ventilatory support and/or hemodialysis.

In children with HUS, gastrointestinal problems characterized by abdominal pain, fever, bloody diarrhea, vomiting may be present.

Diagnostic Evaluation

To find out the underlying cause of ARF is very important. The renal function usually returns to normal if the underlying cause can be reversed.

Physical examination: The child with ARF comes with edema resulting from decreased urine output and fluid overload. He/she may be hypertensive and may be in respiratory distress, due to fluid overload.

Medical history: The underlying cause ARF can be identified through medical history of the patient. History of fever, diarrhea, vomiting can give the clue of dehydration and prerenal ARF. History of recent throat infection and drug intake (recent and past) are important. It is important to find out any recent history of bloody diarrhea that might suggest HUS. Examination and history taking usually include—is there a prerenal cause? Could this be obstruction? Is intrinsic renal disease probable – what does urine analysis show?

Blood tests: The kidney function is assessed through serum creatinine, BUN and other electrolytes in the body. In ARF, the laboratory data may reflect as hyperkalemia, hyponatremia, hypocalcemia, metabolic acidosis or azotemia, disturbed coagulation factors. The child with HUS exhibits hemolytic anemia, thrombocytopenia.

Urine tests: The specific symptom of ARF is oliguria where urine output remains 0.5–1 mL/kg/hour. Urinalysis is done to explore proteinuria, hematuria, RBCs, casts, etc.

- *Chest X-ray:* It is done to see the pulmonary bed.
- *Bone scan:* A nuclear imaging method to evaluate any degenerative and/or arthritic changes in the joints; to detect bone diseases and tumors; to determine the cause of bone pain or inflammation.
- *Renal ultrasound and renal scan:* The test is used to determine the size and shape of the kidney, and to detect a mass, kidney stone, cyst, or other obstruction or abnormalities (cause of postrenal ARF). A renal scan can be helpful in assessing the cause of renal failure. The blood flow, function and obstruction of renal structure can be explored by renal scan.
- *Electrocardiogram (ECG or EKG):* This test records the electrical activity of the heart, shows abnormal

rhythms (arrhythmias or dysrhythmias), and detects heart muscle damage.

- *Renal biopsy:* Renal biopsy may be indicated when intrinsic renal disease is suspected, specially if serology is nondiagnostic.

Therapeutic Management

Treatment of acute renal failure depends on the underlying cause. Some children in ARF are managed without dialysis. Treatment may include:

- *Hospitalization:* Hospitalization is needed for treating any life-threatening features first like shock, respiratory failure, hyperkalemia, for meticulous monitoring of daily urine and other outputs and careful restoration of caloric, fluid, and electrolyte losses, and prevention of other complications.
- *Administration of intravenous (IV) fluids in large volumes (to replace depleted blood volume):* Fluid management should be guided by the principles of replacing the estimated insensible water loss (IWL) plus the loss from both volume and electrolytes from urinary or other outputs. *Fluid management depends on the patient's hemodynamic status and urinary output. The patient who presents with oliguria and hemodynamic instability should be given a fluid bolus of 20 mL/kg of an isotonic solution such as normal saline, packed red blood cells, or even albumin, although albumin's effectiveness is debated in the literature.* A daily weight loss of up to 1% of the body weight is expected during the management of the initial oliguric phase of ARF. Weight gain or hyponatremia during this period usually indicates fluid overload. In case of fluid overload and absence of urine output, fluid restriction is necessary.
- *Diuretic therapy or medications (to increase urine output):* Both mannitol and furosemide are used to increase urinary flow rate and decrease intratubular obstruction; both also may limit oxygen consumption in damaged cells. The patient's hemodynamic status should be assessed and intravascular volume to be restored carefully before furosemide or mannitol administration.

  Final fluid adjustments depend on daily weights and close monitoring of the patient's intake and output.
- *Close monitoring of important electrolytes such as potassium, sodium, and calcium:* Hyperkalemia (6.5 mEq/L [6.5 mmol/L]), with T-wave elevation on ECG examination is a medical emergency, which may precipitate cardiac arrhythmia. Treatment of this emergency comprises of, intravenous calcium gluconate solution (0.5 mL/kg of 10% calcium gluconate solution over 2 to 4 minutes), insulin therapy (1 unit of insulin in 5 g of dextrose to promote movement of potassium intracellularly through enhanced glucogenesis). Other measures like potassium restricted diet and IV fluids, nasogastric suction, administration of exchange resin (kayexalate) are undertaken to decrease the level of potassium in the blood.

  In ARF, sodium level may be elevated or decreased. Elevated sodium level is treated with fluid restriction.

Hyponatremia (sodium concentrations 130 mEq/L usually is associated with ARF. If the serum sodium concentration is greater than 120.0 mEq/L (120.0 mmol/L), fluid restriction or water removal with dialysis should be considered, and sodium should be corrected to at least 125 mEq/L by using the calculation: (125-plasma sodium) × (weight in kilograms) × (0.6) mEq Na. This amount of sodium should be delivered slowly over several hours.

Metabolic acidosis is another complication of ARF, as excretion of hydrogen ions and ammonia through the kidney is impaired (low serum bicarbonate). It requires judicious use of sodium bicarbonate therapy (when serum total bicarbonate falls below 10 mEq/L (10 mmol/L). Calculation for the amount of bicarbonate to administer to correct the acidosis is: mEq of bicarbonate = (desired-observed bicarbonate) × kg × 0.5.

The correction should be undertaken with care because this is only a temporizing measure, and overcorrecting the acidosis may cause hypocalcemia.

- *Medications (to control blood pressure):* Hypertension in ARF usually is due to volume overload or changes in vascular tone. If volume overload is present, diuresis with furosemide or dialysis should be initiated to return the patient to hemodynamic stability. If increased vascular tone is the cause of hypertension, intravenous antihypertensive treatment may be necessary. ARF with severe hypertension is treated with sodium nitroprusside. Sodium nitroprusside administration needs monitoring of thiocyanate concentrations because the kidney excretes this by product of metabolized nitroprusside.
- *Specific diet requirements:* The general principle of nutrition therapy in ARF is to give maximum calories and moderate restriction of protein. In critically ill child a minimum of 25% of the daily caloric requirement must be supplied to reduce the catabolism of ARF. This can be achieved by a 25% dextrose solution delivered via an indwelling cannula inserted into the superior vena cava to avoid peripheral venous thrombosis from such a hypertonic solution.

Intravenous infusion of essential amino acids has been advocated as therapy for patients who have ARF, based on the theory that accumulations of urea, creatinine, potassium, and phosphate are removed in the synthesis of nonessential amino acids from essential amino acids and the formation of new tissue.

The oliguric phase of ARF usually lasts from a few days to 2 weeks. A high-caloric supplement is needed when the child regains his or her appetite (toward the end of that period).

Chronic Renal Failure (CRF) and End Stage Renal Disease (ESRD)

Chronic Kidney Disease

Chronic renal failure means that kidney tissue has been destroyed gradually over a long period of time, and this is an irreversible loss of kidney function. Many people are unaware of the problem until more than 70% of kidney function has been lost. The aim of early detection of kidney disease and treatment (diet and medication) is to prevent or slow down progression of the disease. However, in some cases, the progression to end stage renal failure, when dialysis or transplantation is necessary, is not preventable.

The most common causes of end stage renal failure in are diabetes mellitus, glomerulonephritis, hypertension and polycystic kidney disease.

End Stage Kidney Disease

End stage renal failure occurs when the kidneys can no longer function adequately and survival depends on either dialysis or transplantation. Probably the child has reached, or are approaching this stage of kidney disease and his/her present treatment is aimed at easing the load on your damaged kidneys and minimizing the accumulation of waste products in child's body.

Nursing Management of Child with Renal Failure

Nursing Diagnosis

- Excess fluid volume and electrolyte shifts related to compromised regulatory mechanism.
- *Risk for decreased cardiac output (RF may include:* Fluid overload, fluid shifts, fluid deficit).
- *Risk for imbalanced nutrition:* Less than body requirements related to dietary restrictions and decreased appetite.
- Risk for infection
- Deficient knowledge about disease process, treatment and care
- Risk for impaired skin integrity related to edema and poor nutrition
- Disturbed family processes related to life-threatening disease of the child.

Nursing Intervention

Monitoring fluid and electrolyte balance:

- To prevent hyperkalemia; parenteral fluids, all oral intake, and all medications are to be screened for hidden sources of potassium. Cardiac function and musculoskeletal status are to be monitored for signs of hyperkalemia.
- Careful monitoring of fluid intake of patient (IV medications should be administered in the smallest volume possible), urine output, apparent edema, distention of the jugular veins, alterations in heart sounds and breath sounds, and increasing difficulty in breathing are important nursing interventions.
- Maintain daily weight and intake and output records.
- Fluid and electrolyte status monitoring, and immediate reporting of indicators of any deterioration regarding it is important. Prepare patient for dialysis as indicated to correct fluid and electrolyte imbalances.

Reducing Metabolic Rate

- Reduce exertion and metabolic rate with bed rest
- Prevent or treat fever and infection promptly.

Promoting Pulmonary Function

- Assist patient to change of position, cough and take deep breaths frequently
- Encourage and assist patient to move and turn
- Help the patient in chest physiotherapy.

Preventing Infection

- Practice asepsis when working with invasive lines and catheters.
- Use good hand hygiene technique and instruct the family members to do the same.
- Avoid indwelling catheters if possible.

Providing Skin Care

- Perform meticulous skin care to maintain skin integrity.
- Bath the patient with cool water, turn patient frequently, keep the skin clean and well-moisturized and fingernails trimmed for patient comfort and to prevent skin breakdown.

Discharge Goals

- Homeostasis is achieved.
- Complications regarding fluid and electrolytes are prevented or minimized.
- Dealing realistically with current condition of the child.
- Parents and family will be able to explain disease process, prognosis, and therapeutic regimen understood.
- Aware the family about referral, to meet needs after discharge.
- The child and family will achieve successful coping strategies and participate in care and access appropriate support.

DIALYSIS

Dialysis is a treatment that does some of the things done by healthy kidneys. It is the artificial process of eliminating waste (diffusion) and unwanted water (ultrafiltration) from the blood, where kidneys have failed or damaged and cannot carry out the function properly. The two types of dialysis are hemodialysis (HD) and peritoneal dialysis (PD). HD is more efficient and requires less time than PD.

Hemodialysis (HD)	*Peritoneal Dialysis (PD)*
Hemodialysis is a method where an artificial kidney (hemodialyzer) is used to achieve the extracorporeal removal of waste products such as creatinine and urea and free water from the blood when the kidneys are in a state of renal failure. HD occurs through a vascular access, such as double lumen central line or an arteriovenous fistula or shunt. Hemodialysis utilizes counter current flow, where the dialysate is flowing in the opposite direction to blood flow in the extracorporeal circuit. Ideally a patient with chronic kidney failure should have hemodialys is three times a week each session lasting from three and half to four hours. Side effects caused by removing too much fluid and/or removing fluid too rapidly include low blood pressure, fatigue, chest pains, leg-cramps, nausea and headaches, these symptoms collectively referred to as the dialysis hangover. The major complications of HD include access infection and access obstruction. HD is technically more difficult in case of infants and small children and fluid and electrolyte shifts are more pronounced.	PD is a treatment for patients with severe chronic kidney disease. The process uses the patient's peritoneum in the abdomen as a membrane across which fluids and dissolved substances are exchanged from the blood. Fluid is introduced through a permanent tube in the abdomen which remains in the cavity and flushed out either every night while the patient sleeps (automatic peritoneal dialysis) or via regular exchanges throughout the day (continuous ambulatory peritoneal dialysis). The total volume is referred to as a *dwell* while the fluid itself is referred to as dialysate. The dwell can be as much as 2.5 L, and medication can also be added to the fluid immediately before infusion. The dwell remains in the abdomen and waste products diffuse across the peritoneum from the underlying blood vessels. Usually, after 4–6 hours of dialysis, the fluid is removed and replaced with fresh fluid. The main complications of peritoneal dialysis are infections, weight gain, weakness of abdominal muscles.
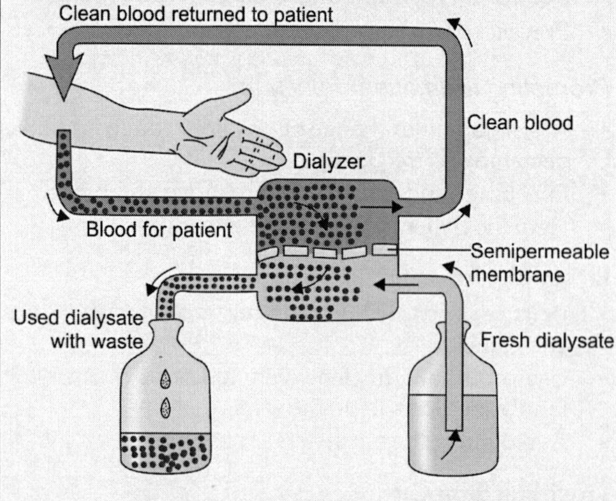 **Fig. 14.9:** Mechanism of hemodialysis	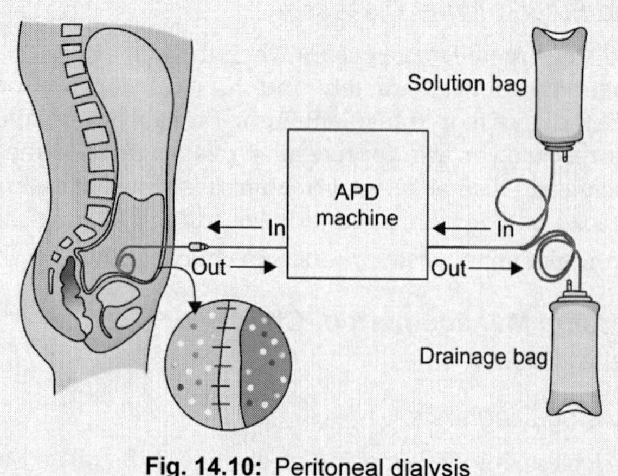 **Fig. 14.10:** Peritoneal dialysis

CHAPTER 15

The Child with a Hematologic Alteration

Chapter Outline

- Hematologic System
- Anemia

HEMATOLOGIC SYSTEM

The hematologic system is made up of the blood, the spleen, bone marrow, and the liver. The word 'heme' comes from the Greek for blood. Hematology is a branch of medicine concerning the study of blood, the blood-forming organs, and blood diseases. The hematopoietic system is not fully developed at birth, and the normal hematologic values of newborns and infants differ as compared to older children and adults. At birth and thereafter, the hematopoiesis is restricted to the bone marrow and continues to evolve in order to adapt to the new oxygen-rich environment and the needs of the growing organism. With age, the more membranous bones of the vertebra, sternum and ribs assume RBC production.

The principal component of the hematologic system is the blood (Fig. 15.1). Although blood appears to be red liquid it is actually composed of an yellowish liquid called plasma and billions of cells. The vast majority of these cells are red cells and these give blood its red color. Blood is made up of three main components—red blood cells, white blood cells, and plasma.

Plasma is a fluid made up of 90% of water, in which blood is suspended. Plasma allows blood cells to travel through vessels, in the water it contains. Plasma is also made up of minerals, nutrients, and electrolytes. It carries not only the blood cells but also nutrients such as sugars, amino acids, fats, salts, minerals, etc. waste products (CO_2, lactic acid, urea, etc.), antibodies, clotting proteins (called clotting factors), chemical messengers such as hormones, and proteins that help to maintain the body's fluid balance.

Hematopoietic stem cells (HSCs) reside in the medulla of the bone (bone marrow) and have the unique ability to give rise to all of the different mature blood cell types and tissues (Fig. 15.2). HSCs are self-renewing cells, when they proliferate, at least some of their daughter cells remain as HSCs, so the pool of stem cells does not become depleted. This phenomenon is called asymmetric division. The other daughters of HSCs (myeloid and lymphoid progenitor cells), however can commit to any of the alternative differentiation pathways that lead to the production of one or more specific types of blood cells, but cannot self-renew. The pool of progenitors is heterogeneous and can be divided into two—red blood cells and erythrocytes, are the most common blood cells. They appear as disks with an indent in the surface, and they lack a nucleus. Erythrocytes are

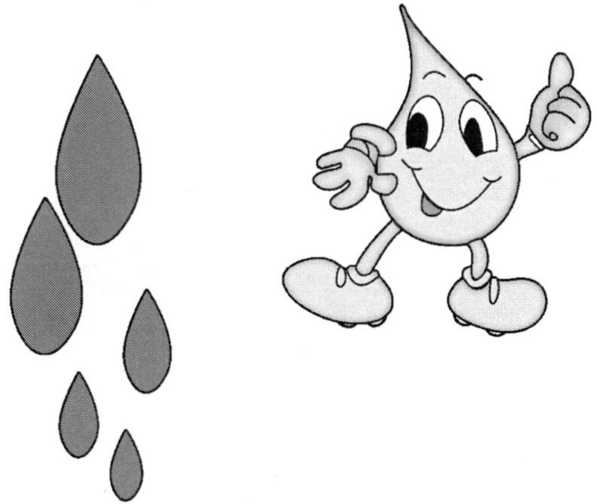

Fig. 15.1: Hematologic system

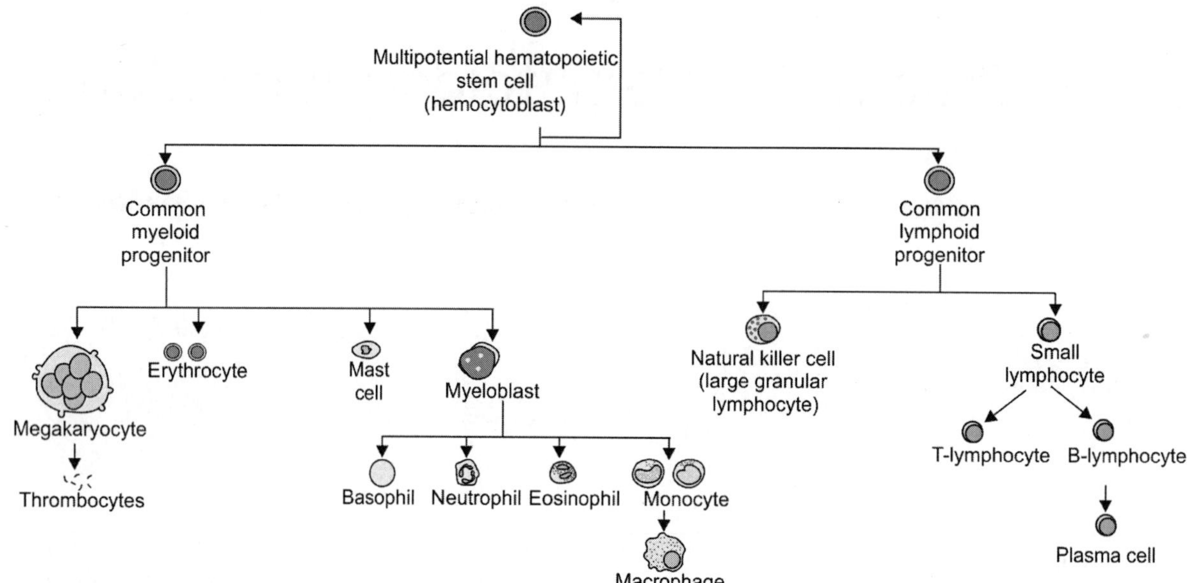

Fig. 15.2: Hemopoietic system

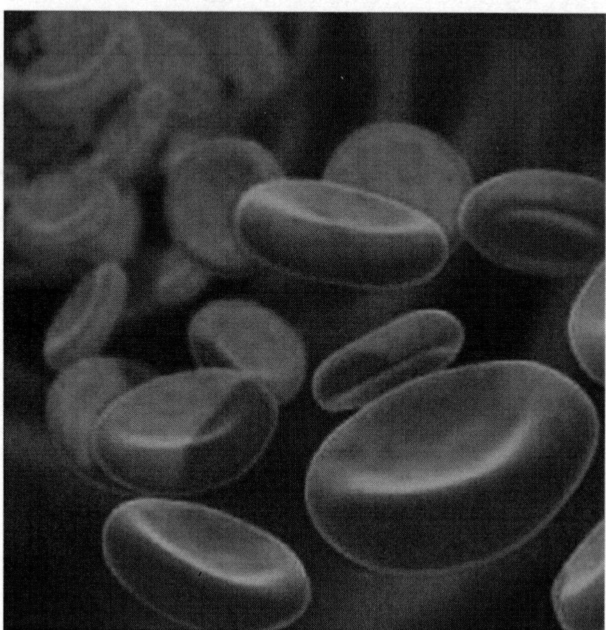

Fig. 15.3: Structure of RBCs

generally 6 to 8 micrometers in diameter (Fig. 15.3), and most adults have 20 to 30 trillion erythrocytes in their body at any given point. Their lifespan is about 100 to 120 days. Respiratory system gives oxygen and takes carbon dioxide to the erythrocytes, then the erythrocytes carry blood to all tissues, and supply what they carry, and carry away wastes. It takes about 20 seconds for an erythrocyte to make a complete loop from the heart, to tissue, back to the heart. While traveling, RBCs may take damage bouncing off of blood vessel walls. Without a nucleus, they have no means to repair themselves. The spleen is an important organ. It acts as a reservoir for blood, and it filters out erythrocytes that can no longer carry out their functions.

White blood cells: White blood cells or leukocytes, are one of the body's defenses. Besides the red cells, the blood also contains several types of infection-fighting white cells and tiny cell fragments called platelets which are essential for clotting. WBCs are formed in the bone marrow and in the lymphatic tissue. There are two types—granulocytes and agranulocytes. There are seven types of leukocytes. Neutrophils fight bacteria and fungi. Eosinophils fight larger parasites and modulate the inflammatory response with allergies. Basophils release histamine to induce an inflammatory response. There are three types of lymphocytes—B-cells, T-cells, and natural killer cells. B-cells release antibodies and assist T-cell activation. T-cells can be regulatory, which cause the body to return to normal after an inflammatory response, they can activate and regulate B- and T-cells, or they can attack virus infected or cancer cells. Natural killer cells attack virus infected and tumor cells as well. Monocytes move to tissues and then differentiate into macrophages. Macrophages are phagocytic cells, and they eat cellular waste, debris, and pathogens. They also stimulate lymphocytes. WBCs fight foreign bodies (bacteria, virus, parasites, etc.) through the process of phagocytosis and antibody production.

Platelets: Platelets are fragments of a much larger cell, the megakaryocyte, that stays in the bone marrow after it differentiates and matures from the stem cell.

The platelets leave the bone marrow and circulate throughout the body. It promotes homeostasis— the prevention of blood loss from the body. When stimulated by substances from damaged tissue, the platelets release substances necessary to help blood clot. This helps initiate the clotting sequence and protect the integrity of the vasculature. It can circulate in the blood for about 10 days before they die; however disease, fever and infection can shorten a platelet's lifetime. Platelets disorder may occur when bone marrow cannot meet the production demand of the body.

Diagnostic Tests

Hematology relies on blood tests as a primary diagnostic tool. Tests performed to diagnose illnesses include:

- *Blood count (CBC):* It helps in diagnosing anemia and certain blood cancers. A CBC also helps to monitor infection and blood loss.
- *Platelet count:* It helps for diagnosing diseases and monitoring bleeding and clotting diseases.
- *Erythrocyte sedimentation rate (ESR):* It measures the rate at which red blood cells fall to help diagnose sickle cell anemia, polycythemia, and congestive heart failure.
- *Prothrombin time (PT):* Evaluates bleeding and clotting diseases and can help monitor anticlotting therapies.
- *Bone marrow biopsies:* To test for abnormal red or white blood cell counts shown in cancerous diseases (leukemia or Hodgkin's disease) or anemia.
- *Antiglobulin or Coombs test:* It measures for antibodies that destroy red blood cells that may cause anemia, jaundice, mono syphilis, lymphoproliferative disorder, or blood transfusion reactions.
- *Diascopy:* A simple test to see how skin blanches under pressure to diagnose various conditions. It is a special technique for examination of erythematous skin lesions. If a clear glass slide, pressed over the lesion, causes color to fade, there is vascular engorgement; if it does not fade, it is hemorrhage in the skin.

Classification of Hematology

Hematology is classified into four major groups. These are:

1. **Hemoglobinopathy:** Studies abnormality in the globin chains of the hemoglobin molecule. Diseases such as thalassemia (or erythropoiesis) and sickle-cell anemia fall under the umbrella of hemoglobinopathy, which are more common in the ethnic African population.
2. **Hematological malignancies:** Diagnosis and treatment of cancers that affect bone marrow, blood, and lymph nodes. Leukemia, lymphomas, and myeloma fall into this category.
3. **Anemia:** Involves the loss of hemoglobin from the blood leading to low organ oxygenation.
4. **Coagulopathy:** Deals with diseases that encompass improper blood clotting and excessive bleeding.

ANEMIA

Anemia is a condition in which reduced hematocrit or hemoglobin levels lead to diminished oxygen-carrying capacity that does not optimally meet the metabolic demands of the body. Anemia is not a specific disease entity but is a condition caused by various underlying pathologic processes.

Iron Deficiency Anemia

Anemia caused by a low iron level is the most common form of anemia which is caused by insufficient dietary intake and absorption of iron, and/or iron loss from bleeding. Iron deficiency causes approximately half of all anemia cases worldwide. It is the most common cause of anemia during infancy, childhood and adolescence.

Etiology and Incidence

Normally the body gets iron through certain foods. It also reuses iron from old red blood cells. Because of the presence of maternal iron stores, this anemia is rare before age of 4 to 6 months; it occurs most often in children age 9 to 24 months as iron stores are depleted. A diet that does not have enough iron is the most common cause. Toddlers who drink too much cow's milk may also become anemic if they are not eating other healthy foods that have iron. During periods of rapid growth during puberty, even more iron is needed.

The most significant cause of iron-deficiency anemia in developing world children is—parasitic worms, hookworms, whipworms, and roundworms. Worms cause intestinal bleeding, which is not always noticeable in feces, and is specially damaging to growing children.

Other causes may be:

- The body is not able to absorb iron well, even though the child is eating enough iron.
- Slow blood loss over a long period, often due to menstrual periods or bleeding in the digestive tract.

- Iron deficiency in children can also be related to lead poisoning.

Classification

Anemia is usually classified based on the size of RBCs (microcytic, normocytic, or macrocytic), as measured by the mean corpuscular volume (MCV). Anemia can be microcytic (MCV typically less than 80 µm^3 [80 fL]), normocytic (80–100 µm^3 [80–100 fL]), or macrocytic (greater than 100 µm^3 [100 fL]). The RBC distribution width is a measure of the size variance of RBCs. A low RBC distribution width suggests uniform cell size, whereas an elevated width (greater than 14%) indicates RBCs of multiple sizes. Normocytic anemia may be caused by chronic disease, hemolysis, or bone marrow disorders. Workup of normocytic anemia is based on bone marrow function as determined by the reticulocyte count. If the reticulocyte count is elevated, the patient should be evaluated for blood loss or hemolysis. A low reticulocyte count suggests aplasia or a bone marrow disorder.

Common tests used in the evaluation of macrocytic anemias include vitamin B_{12} and folate levels, and thyroid function testing. A peripheral smear can provide additional information in patients with anemia of any morphology.

Manifestations

Most children with anemia are asymptomatic, and the condition is detected on screening laboratory evaluation. Mild anemia may have no symptoms. As the iron level and blood counts becomes lower, child may act irritable, become short of breath, eat less food, crave unusual foods, feel tired or weak all the time, have a sore tongue, have headaches or dizziness.

With more severe anemia, child may have extreme pallor with porcelain like skin, pale mucous membrane and conjunctiva, brittle nails.

Diagnostic Evaluation

Complete history taking to assess the nutritional intake. Physical examination of the child to identify the degree of anemia. Blood tests that measure iron level in the body include:

- *Complete blood count:* Child with IDA will show microcytic, hypochromic RBCs, with decreased mean cell volume. The reticulocyte count is usually normal or slightly elevated.
- *Hematocrit:* It will show low hemoglobin levels, 6 to 11 g/dL.
- *Serum ferritin.*
- *Serum iron:* A measurement called iron saturation (serum iron/TIBC) often can show whether the child has enough iron in the body.
- *Total iron binding capacity (TIBC):* Iron binding capacity is usually increased as a result of decreased serum iron levels.
- *Hemoglobin electrophoresis:* It may be done to rule out causes other than IDA.

Therapeutic Management

Since children only absorb a small amount of the iron they eat, most children need to have 8 to 10 mg of iron per day. Dietary intake and iron supplementation are needed to treat IDA. Eating healthy foods is the most important way to prevent and treat iron deficiency. Good sources of iron include chicken, fish, and other meats, dried beans, lentils, and soybeans, eggs, liver, green leafy vegetables, molasses, dates, raisins, etc.

Mild microcytic anemia may be treated presumptively with oral iron therapy in children 6 to 36 months of age who have risk factors for iron deficiency anemia. Follow up monitoring includes a CBC and reticulocyte count. An increased hemoglobin level can be expected in 4 to 30 days. If the anemia is severe or is unresponsive to iron therapy, the patient should be evaluated for gastrointestinal blood loss. Other tests used in the evaluation of microcytic anemia include serum iron studies, lead levels, and hemoglobin electrophoresis. Correction of anemia by blood transfusion is rarely indicated. RBC transfusions are reserved for severe anemia and cardiovascular compromise.

Complications

Acute and severe anemia can result in cardiovascular compromise. Acute anemia needs treatment immediately and appropriately, otherwise, the resulting hypoxemia and hypovolemia can lead to brain damage, multiorgan failure, and death. Long-standing anemia can result in failure to thrive.

Many studies have shown the deleterious effects of iron deficiency anemia or iron deficiency without anemia on the neurocognitive and behavioral development in children. Other complications can include congestive heart failure, hypoxia, hypovolemia, shock, seizure, and acute silent cerebral ischemic event.

Aplastic Anemia

Aplastic anemia is a syndrome of bone marrow failure characterized by peripheral pancytopenia and marrow hypoplasia. In case of aplastic anemia, the body does not make enough red blood cells, white blood cells, and platelets. This is because the bone marrow's stem cells are damaged. Aplastic anemia also is called bone marrow failure. The outcome is a deficiency of all three blood cell types (pancytopenia); red blood cells (anemia),white blood cells (leukopenia), and platelets (thrombocytopenia). Aplastic refers to inability of the stem cells to generate the mature blood cells.

A reduced number of red blood cells causes the red cell number and hemoglobin to drop. A reduced number of white blood cells causes the patient to be susceptible to infection. A reduced number of platelets can cause the blood not to clot the way it should.

Etiology and Incidence

Aplastic anemia in children has multiple causes. Some of these causes are idiopathic, other causes are secondary, resulting from a previous illness or disorder. Very often there is an immunological dysfunction or malignant (cancerous) change in the cells. Many childhood cases of aplastic anemia occur sporadically for no known reason. Acquired causes, however, may include history of specific infectious diseases, such as hepatitis, Epstein-Barr virus, cytomegalovirus, parvovirus, HIV. History of taking certain medications, exposure to certain toxins, such as heavy metals, exposure to radiation, history of an autoimmune disease, such as lupus, a developing acute lymphocytic leukemia.

Many diseases, conditions, and factors can damage the stem cells. These conditions can be acquired or inherited. Some disorders that are known to predispose a child to aplastic anemia include Fanconi anemia, reticular dysgenesis, familial aplastic anemias.

Aplastic anemia is thought to be more common in Asia than in the West. This increased incidence may be related to environmental factors, such as increased exposure to toxic chemicals, rather than to genetic factors (4 per million population approx). The male-to-female ratio for acquired aplastic anemia is approximately 1:1. Although aplastic anemia occurs in all age groups, a small peak in the incidence is observed in childhood because of the inclusion of inherited marrow-failure syndromes.

Manifestations

The following are the most common symptoms of aplastic anemia. However, each child may experience symptoms differently. Symptoms may include anemia with malaise, pallor and associated symptoms such as palpitations and fatigue, headache, dizziness, nausea, shortness of breath and swelling of foot. Thrombocytopenia, leading to increased risk of hemorrhage, bruising and petechiae. Leukopenia, leading to increased risk of infection, recurrent infections, mouth and pharyngeal ulcerations. Reticulocytopenia (low counts of reticulocytes, that is, immature red blood cells) is seen. Abnormal paleness or lack of color of the skin and mucous membrane, enlarged liver or spleen, are seen in aplastic anemia.

Diagnostic Evaluation

Aplastic anemia is diagnosed with blood and bone marrow studies.

CBC: A paucity of platelets, red blood cells (RBCs), granulocytes, monocytes, and reticulocytes is found in patients with aplastic anemia. Mild macrocytosis is occasionally observed. The degree of cytopenia is useful in assessing the severity of aplastic anemia.

Bone marrow biopsy: The definitive diagnosis is by bone marrow biopsy; normal bone marrow has 30 to 70% blood stem cells, but in aplastic anemia, these cells are mostly gone and replaced by fat. There may have relatively increased nonhematopoietic elements, such as mast cells.

Therapeutic Management

Aplastic anemia is a serious illness and treatment usually depends on the underlying cause. For certain causes, recovery can be expected after treatment; however, relapses can occur. To treat the low blood counts, initial treatment is usually supportive, meaning that it is necessary to treat the symptoms but not possible to cure the disease. Supportive therapy may include:

- Blood transfusion (both red blood cells and platelets)
- Preventative antibiotic therapy
- Meticulous handwashing
- Special care to food preparation (such as only eating well-cooked foods).

Pharmacotherapy

- *Immunosuppressive therapy:* The treatment of immune-mediated aplastic anemia involves suppression of the immune system which consists of immunosuppressive drugs, typically either anti-lymphocyte globulin or antithymocyte globulin, combined with corticosteroids and cyclosporine.
- Hormones or medications (to stimulate the bone marrow to produce cells)
- In addition, iron chelation may be required in chronically transfused patients who develop elevated serum ferritin levels above 1000 μg/L.

Sickle Cell Anemia

Sickle cell anemia is an inherited form of anemia, a condition in which there are not enough healthy red blood cells to carry adequate oxygen throughout the body. It is an inherited genetically determined autosomal recessive disorder.

Etiology

Sickle cell anemia is an autosomal recessive inheritance caused by hemoglobin beta gene (HBB) that affects the oxygen carrying pigment in red blood cells, hemoglobin. Changes in the hemoglobin-A chains of the red blood cells causes an alteration of the normal biconcave disk shape into the characteristic sickle cell shape. The molecular alteration of the hemoglobin-A chains that are characteristic of sickle cell anemia are renamed hemoglobin-S chains. Sickle cell anemia is believed to be the result of a natural adaptation that evolved to protect people from malaria.

> **Pathophysiology**
>
> Normally, red blood cells are flexible and round, moving easily through blood vessels. Sickle cell disease is a group of diseases characterized by an abnormal hemoglobin chain (normal hemoglobin HbA is partially or completely replaced by HbS, i.e. sickle cell hemoglobin or HbC) that results in a structural alteration of the red blood cells. The most common form of sickle cell disease is sickle cell anemia.
>
> In sickle cell anemia, the red blood cells become rigid and sticky and are shaped like sickles or crescent moons. These irregularly shaped cells can get stuck in small blood vessels, which can slow or block blood flow and oxygen to parts of the body.
>
> It is considered to be a chronic hemolytic anemia. Sickling occurs when normal hemoglobin molecules are replaced by hemoglobin S molecules. With each sickling episode, red blood cell membranes are progressively weakened, leading to hemolysis over time and impairing organ function (possibly causing hemosiderosis, or stored iron in the organs). Symptoms of sickle cell anemia are most likely to occur when the patient is under severe emotional or physical stress or dehydrated.

Manifestations

Patient may have a steady state of sickness or a period of sickle cell crises.

- *Episodes of severe pain:* Most likely to occur during times of physical or emotional stress.
- Severe and reoccurring infections
- Jaundice from hemolysis
- Chronic hemolytic anemia
- *Signs of poor oxygenation:* Pallor, hypotension or hypertension, shortness of breath, changes in level of consciousness, irritability, dizziness, lightheadedness, and increased capillary refill.
- Generalized weakness
- Dyspnea on exertion
- Pain and edema in the lower extremities
- Hypertension.

Sickle Cell Crisis

- *Sequestration crises:* Sickled red blood cells occlude vessels and become trapped in the spleen and liver.
- Pallor and cardiovascular collapse may occur from lack of circulation.
- *Diagnostic markers:* Severe anemia 2—3 g/100 mL, with a high reticulocyte count.
- An emergency blood transfusion is usually indicated.
- A splenectomy is curative is generally performed after two episodes.
- *Priapism:* Prolonged penile erection (more common in children than adults).

Diagnosis

- *Blood studies:* The presence of abnormal hemoglobin or gene.
- Confirmatory testing is performed by electrophoresis or other methods. Hemoglobin electrophoresis confirms SS hemoglobinopathy and distinguishes between those with sickle cell trait and those with sickle cell disease.
- Isoelectric focusing
- High performance liquid chromatography (HPLC)
- Hematological findings will reveal decreased hemoglobin, hematocrit, and platelets with high reticulocyte counts (due to hemolysis). In aplastic crises, the reticulocyte counts are elevated.

Management

While there is currently no known cure for SCA, early detection and management of symptoms is crucial in preventing progression of the disease. Treatment is focused on preventing and treating dehydration to replenish electrolytes, treating associated pain, antibiotics for secondary infections, and transfusions to delivers more oxygen to peripheral tissues. In rare cases, a bone marrow transplant is indicated.

Nursing Care of Children with Anemia

Nursing diagnosis: Ineffective tissue perfusion related to reduced oxygen carrying capacity of the blood.

Expected outcome: Maintaining adequate oxygenation and tissue perfusion.

Nursing Interventions with Rationale

- Monitor vital signs, capillary refill, skin color, mucous membranes. Monitor laboratory tests such as Hb level, CBC, MCV, peripheral smear as indicated; it helps to detect the severity of anemia.
- Elevate head of bed as tolerated. Assist the child to change position slowly, monitor for dizziness.
- Provide oxygen as needed. It improves respiration and tissue oxygenation. Higher concentration of oxygen promotes diffusion across the alveoli (oxygen therapy is concentrated whereas room air is only 22% oxygen).
- Provide rest and age appropriate nonstrenuous play. Stress and activities increase the need for administer or assist blood transfusions as prescribed, this promotes circulation and delivery of oxygen to tissues. Observe for any adverse reactions throughout the transfusion, for prevention of complications.

Nursing diagnosis: Activity intolerance due to decreased level of hemoglobin.

Expected outcome: Child can tolerate activity better, decrease in physiological signs of intolerance, such as pulse, respiration, and blood pressure is still within the normal range.

Nursing Interventions with Rationale

Assess the capability of child in doing the activity. Monitor vital signs during and after activity, and note his/her physiological response to activity (increased heart rate, increased blood pressure, or rapid breathing). Avoid any type of stress in the child and provide information to the patient or family to stop doing such activities. It is necessary to reduce oxygen demand of the body. Provide support to perform their daily activities according to the ability of the child. Create a schedule of activities involving other health team, to minimize strain and thus to provide rest and sleep.

Correct anemia by taking appropriate steps. Observe and record client's food intake, weigh periodically, give small, frequent meals and/or between meal nourishment. Bland diet with low in roughage and salt and spices is indicated.

Provide a high calorie, high protein, and iron containing diet; which minimizes risk of infection by maintaining optimal nutritional status. Give iron supplementation, treat the cause of anemia, administer blood transfusions as prescribed, etc.

Record and report occurrence of nausea or vomiting, flatus, and other related symptoms such as irritability or impaired memory. Encourage or assist with good oral hygiene.

Nursing diagnosis: High risk of infection related to an inadequate secondary defenses, (inflammatory response depressed).

Expected outcome: No sign of infection is present and hemoglobin level increased and no leukopenia.

Nursing Interventions with Rationale

- Good handwashing practice (patient and caregiver).
- Minimize exposure to infectious agents; it minimizes risk of infection by decreasing exposure.
- Monitor above mentioned laboratory tests, record vital signs and record and report signs and symptoms of infection promptly. Note the chills and tachycardia with or without fever. The process of inflammation or infection requires evaluation or treatment. Administer antibiotics as prescribed in case of any infection.
- Maintain strict aseptic technique in the procedure or treatment of injuries. Provide meticulous skin, oral, and perianal care. Encourage frequent position changes or ambulation, coughing, and deep-breathing exercises. Promote adequate fluid intake. These are necessary for reducing the risk of colonization or infection of bacteria.
- Observe erythema or wound fluid, which may be indicators of local infection. Note the formation of pus may not exist when granulocytes depressed.
- Take specimens for culture or sensitivity may be done to differentiate an infection, to identify the specific pathogen and administer appropriate antibiotic.

Nursing diagnosis: Deficient knowledge of the child and family regarding condition, prognosis, treatment, self-care, and discharge needs.

Expected outcome: The child and family will be able to talk about the disease process, diagnostic procedures, treatment and potential complications. They will initiate talk related to necessary behaviors or lifestyle change.

Nursing Interventions with Rationale

Provide information about specific anemia and therapy which depends on the type and severity of the anemia. Discuss effects of anemias on preexisting conditions, it can aggravate heart, lung, and cerebrovascular disease. It helps in informed decision and also allay anxiety. Anxiety or fear of the unknown increases stress level, which in turn increases the cardiac workload and more demand of oxygen.

Review required diet alterations to meet specific dietary needs. They must know good source of iron, folic acid and vitamin C (vitamin C enhances absorption of iron). Discuss foods to avoid (e.g. coffee, tea, egg yolks, milk, fiber, and soy protein) at the time when the child is eating high-iron foods. These foods block absorption of iron and should be taken at a different meal. For example, red meat and milk taken at the same time can block absorption of the iron from the meat.

Instruct and demonstrate parents for administration of oral iron preparations, i.e. administer the drug with meals or immediately after meals; tell them to dilute liquid preparations (preferably with orange juice) and administer through a straw; to avoid stain on teeth. Discuss importance of taking only prescribed dosages; and duration of therapy (usually 3–6 months).

Review good oral hygiene, necessity for regular dental care. Instruct to avoid use of aspirin products to avoid bleeding.

Refer to appropriate community resources when indicated; free supply of iron and folic acid supplementation, and other nutritional program in the community.

Thalassemia

Thalassemia is a problem with red blood cells synthesis that is passed down genetically from parents-to-children. It is a group of blood disorders that affect the way the body makes hemoglobin, a protein found in RBCs that is responsible for carrying oxygen throughout the body. This is a group of genetic disorders characterized by an abnormality in synthesis of hemoglobin that results from a reduction in or absence of one of the chains (alpha or beta chains) found in normal hemoglobin. Children with thalassemia do not create enough hemoglobin. It means that the body does not make enough red blood cells to begin with; the RBCs breakdown faster than normal; the red blood cells are smaller than normal; children with thalassemia have less hemoglobin in their red blood cells than normal. According to the site of aberrant globin synthesis, these disorders are categorized as alpha thalassemia, and beta thalassemia. The most severe form of this condition, beta thalassemia is called Cooley anemia, also known as thalassemia major.

Etiology

Thalassemias are inherited conditions—they are carried in the genes and passed on from parents-to-children. People who are *carriers* of a thalassemia gene show no thalassemia symptoms and might not know they are carriers. If both parents are carriers, they can pass the disease to their children (Fig. 15.4).

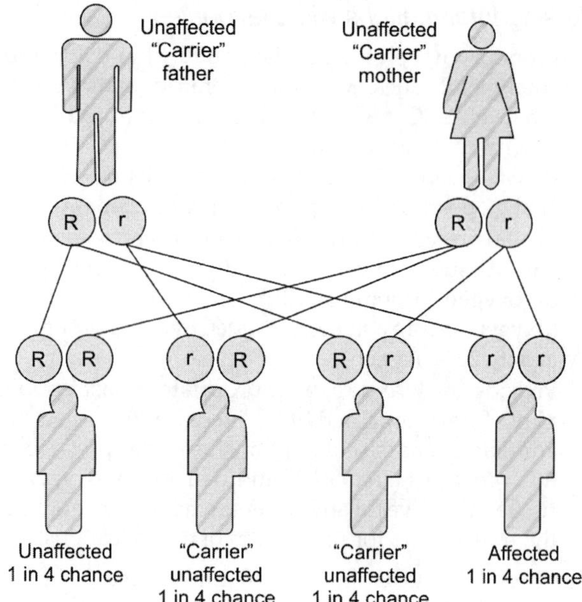

Fig. 15.4: Genetic trait of thalassemia

Thalassemias are not Contagious

While there are many different types of thalassemias, the main two are:

Alpha thalassemia: When the body has a problem producing alpha globin. The hemoglobin molecule is composed of two proteins which are alpha globin and beta globin. When the genes are missing or mutated, alpha thalassemia occurs and is related to the alpha globin protein.

Beta thalassemia (when the body has a problem producing beta globin): When the gene that controls the production of either of these proteins is missing or mutated, it results in that type of thalassemia.

Thalassemia minor: The individual with thalassemia minor has only one copy of the beta thalassemia gene (together with one perfectly normal beta-chain gene). The person is said to be heterozygous for beta thalassemia.

Thalassemia major: The child born with thalassemia major has two genes for beta thalassemia and no normal beta-chain gene. The child is homozygous for beta thalassemia. This causes a striking deficiency in beta-chain production and in the production of Hb A. Thalassemia major is a significant illness.

Pathophysiology

All cells have a nucleus at their center, and the nucleus contains DNA (deoxyribonucleic acid), a long, spiral-shaped molecule that stores the genes that determine different traits of individual. DNA, along with genes and the information they contain, is passed down from parents to their children during reproduction. Each cell has many DNA molecules, but because cells are very small and DNA molecules are long, the DNA is packaged very tightly in each cell. These packages of DNA are called chromosomes, and each cell has 46 of them. Each package is arranged into 23 pairs — with one of each pair coming from the mother and one from the father. When someone has beta thalassemia, there is a mutation in chromosome 11.

Beta thalassemia can be mild to severe and it occurs when the gene that controls the production of beta globin is defective. Beta globin is made on chromosome 11 (beta globin, along with alpha globin, is one of the proteins that makes up hemoglobin). So, if one of the genes that tells chromosome 11 to produce beta globin is altered, less beta globin is made. This abnormality of the beta-polypeptide chain in hemoglobin synthesis affects and decreases the ability of red blood cells to transport oxygen around the body. The body's natural response to a reduction in circulating hemoglobin is to attempt more and more production of erythrocytes. Progressive disease constantly stimulates the bone marrow but body perceives its inability to meet up the need for erythrocytes. As a result erythropoiesis from the extramedullary sites begins. So it is a chronic state of production and destruction RBCs, with a resulting state of inadequate amount of normal circulating hemoglobin. The bones become thin and fragile from excessive erythropoiesis.

Complications may also occur for those with thalassemia. The most prominent complication is iron overload (hemosiderosis) that is caused directly from this disease or through too many blood transfusions. Normally small amount of iron is absorbed from the intestines. Iron is necessary for production of RBCs, and it is a by-product of the hemolysis of RBCs. Hemosiderosis (deposition of excess amounts of iron in tissue) is developed in thalassemic children during their second decade of life. It is caused due to following reasons:

- Body absorbs more iron to meet up the need of more erythrocytes production.
- Increased absorption of iron combined with increased iron from the breakdown of RBCs.
- Blood transfusion for therapeutic reason also increases iron into the circulation.

In case of thalassemia, hepatosplenomegaly occurs as a result of erythropoiesis from the extramedullary sites. When there is an excess of iron in the body there is risk of damaging the heart, liver and endocrine system. Also, when patients have blood transfusions they develop an elevated risk for blood-borne infections such as hepatitis which can cause even more damage to the liver.

Manifestations

Some children with mild thalassemia have no symptoms at all. The signs and symptoms of beta thalassemia vary depending on the type that a child has and how severe it is. Those with beta thalassemia major and intermedia may not show any symptoms at birth, but usually develop them in the first 2 years of life.

Babies who begin to show symptoms of beta thalassemia after a few healthy months may fail to grow normally; have trouble feeding; and have episodes of fever, diarrhea, and other intestinal problems.

In children who do, symptoms of thalassemia can range from mild to severe. Some children with symptoms have only mild anemia. They may feel tired or irritable; be short of breath, dizzy or lightheaded; or have pale skin, lips or nail beds compared to their normal color. In more severe cases, they may also have these symptoms:

- Enlarged bones, mainly in the cheeks and forehead. Prominent zygoma leads to depression of nasal bridge and mongoloid slant of eyes giving a mongoloid appearance (Figs 15.5A and B).
- The skin shows dirty brown pigmentation due to iron deposition.
- A thalassemic child has extremely poor musculature and little fat due to hypercatabolic state.
- The abdomen becomes protuberant due to enlargement of spleen and liver.
- Coagulopathy may result from impaired hepatic synthesis of clotting factors.
- These children are prone to recurrent infections, gallstone formation, pathological fractures and chronic nonhealing leg ulcers.
- Inadequately treated patients may develop poor cardiac and hepatic function due to hemosiderosis.
- *Slowed growth:* Which may include later puberty—due to anemia. At the time of puberty, a thalassemic child may fail to grow further in height and show lack of development of secondary sexual characteristics.
- Dark urine
- Over time, thalassemia may play a part in other health problems that can cause symptoms, such as heart disease, infections and weak, osteoporosis.

Diagnostic Evaluation

In most cases, beta thalassemia is diagnosed before a child's second birthday. Characteristics of children with beta thalassemia major may be a swollen abdomen or symptoms of anemia or failure to thrive.

A series of lab tests can be conducted to determine the presence of thalassemia.

- *Complete blood count (CBC):* Complete blood count test shows the amount of different kinds of cells in child's blood. Having fewer red blood cells and less hemoglobin are signs of thalassemia. Blood tests can also give the details about the size of the cells.

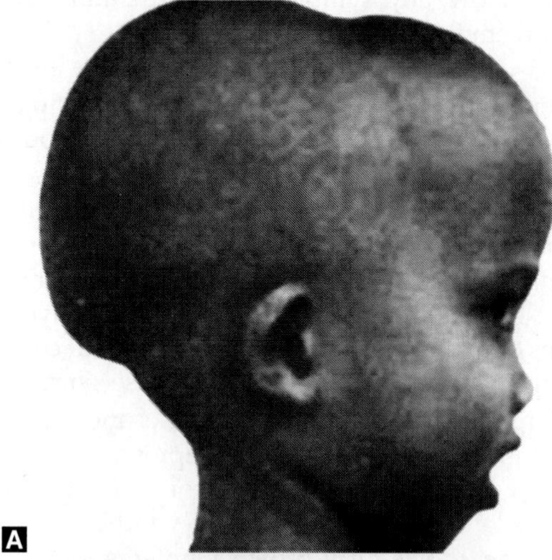

A

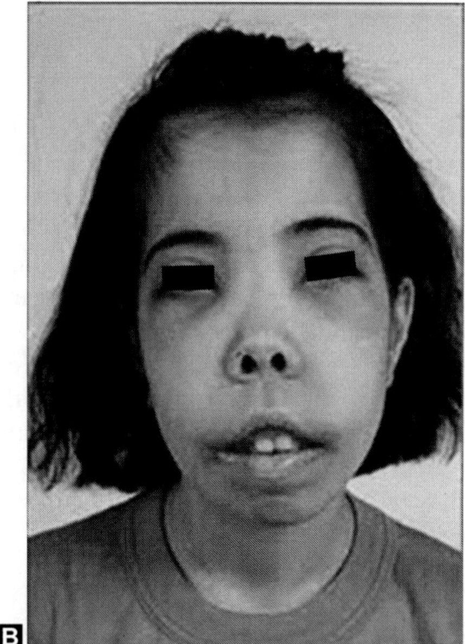

B

Figs 15.5A and B: Classical features of thalassemia seen in these children

People with thalassemia trait tend to have smaller red blood cells.

- *Red cell indices:* It includes the MCV (mean corpuscular volume) which is the measurement of the red blood cells. A low MCV is often one of the first indications for thalassemia (when iron-deficiency has been ruled out).
- *Blood smear:* When a thin layer of blood is examined through a series of stains microscopically. The white and red blood cells and platelets are evaluated for normal and mature structure. If thalassemia is present, the red blood cells are usually microcytic and can also be hypochromic, varying in size and shape, have nucleuses or look like a bull's eye under the microscope.
- *Hemoglobinopathy (Hb):* The red blood cells are evaluated in this test to measure the type and relative amounts of hemoglobin that is present.
- *DNA analysis:* DNA testing is done for abnormal hemoglobin genes. This test investigates the genes to see if there are mutations or deletions in the alpha and beta globin producing genes. It can also be conducted to evaluate carries in the family. Rarely, amniotic fluid testing is conducted.

  If both parents are carriers of the beta thalassemia disorder, tests may be done on a fetus before birth. This is done through either:
  - Chorionic villus sampling, which takes place about 11 weeks into pregnancy and involves removing a tiny piece of the placenta for testing.
  - Amniocentesis, which is usually done about 16 weeks into the pregnancy and involves removing a sample of the fluid that surrounds the fetus.

If one parent carries a beta thalassemia gene and the other carries a different gene that also affects beta globin, such as a sickle gene, their child could have a significant blood disorder. Therefore, people who carry beta thalassemia genes should seek genetic counseling if they are considering having children.

Treatment

The treatment depends on the severity and type of thalassemia. For patients with minor thalassemia, treatment is rarely needed and may be managed through avoiding excessive iron, eating a healthy diet and trying to avoid infections. With minor thalassemia one may need a blood transfusion after surgery to help manage and reduce any thalassemia complications.

The amount of treatment that beta thalassemia requires depends on how severe the symptoms are. For most children with beta thalassemia trait, whose only symptom may be mild anemia from time-to-time, no medical treatment will be necessary.

However, the blood counts in beta thalassemia trait look a lot like the blood counts in iron deficiency anemia, which is a very common disorder. It is important to know when children have beta thalassemia trait so that they do not treat them with iron if it is not needed.

Folic acid supplement is recommended for children with moderate cases of anemia to help boost production of new red blood cells.

The management of beta-thalassemia includes three techniques—(1) erythrocytes transfusion, (2) chelation therapy, and (3) splenectomy.

Some children with moderate anemia may require an occasional blood transfusion, particularly after surgery. Those with severe cases of beta thalassemia major, on the other hand, may require regular blood transfusions (preferably erythrocytes/neocytes transfusion) their entire lives to keep them healthy. In thalassemia patients, packed cell transfusions have improved survival. The purpose of a transfusion for a child with thalassemia is to give the child healthy red blood cells and hemoglobin. This helps their bodies get the oxygen they need. Theoretically, neocytes administration provides erythrocytes with a longer life and increases time between transfusions and decreases overall transfusion. Usually hemoglobin is maintained at approximately 11g/dL, to prevent the severe side effects and bony changes associated with the disease.

Transfused blood contains iron. Patients with severe thalassemia cannot use this iron to make their own blood cells, so after many transfusions the iron builds up in some of their organs. This is called iron overload or hemosiderosis. The iron build-up can harm the heart, liver and glands that make hormones. So the child's iron level is checked. If it starts to get too high, child will need a treatment called chelation therapy to remove the excess iron. This involves chelation therapy with deferoxamine (Deseferol) which is administered subcutaneously or IV. This drug binds to iron, so it can leave the body in urine. This therapy can be given by continuous subcutaneous infusion (by pump) over an 8 to 12 hours period at night. Therapy is continued until iron comes to an acceptable level.

Splenectomy

Thalassemia patients do suffer from splenomegaly because of extramedullary hematopoiesis, increased RBC (Fig. 15.6) destruction, repeated blood transfusions and iron overload. Splenectomy is indicated if there is increasing blood transfusion requirement increases to 1.5 times normal or more than 250 mL/kg/year of packed red cells or more than 400 mL/kg/year of whole blood, gross splenomegaly causing hypersplenism or if there are pressure symptoms on surrounding organs. There is also an increased appreciation of the adverse effects of splenectomy on blood coagulation. In general, splenectomy should be avoided unless absolutely indicated.

Splenectomy should be delayed till the age of 5 year as there is a greater risk of sepsis. All the thalassemic children needing splenectomy should receive pneumococcal vaccine, *H. influenzae* vaccine and meningococcal vaccine 4 weeks prior to treatment.

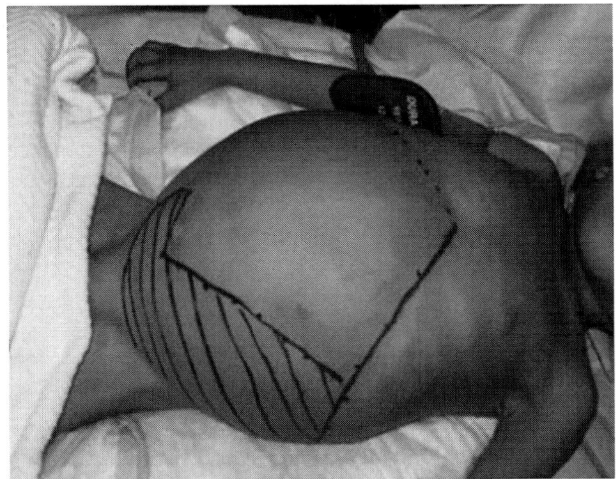

Fig. 15.6: Splenomegaly in thalassemia patient

Penicillin prophylaxis should be continued lifelong and any episode of infection should be treated as splenectomized patients are at an increased risk (200 times) of getting infection as compared to normal children.

Aspirin has been advocated to prevent pulmonary microemboli owing to platelet aggregation due to thrombocytosis after splenectomy.

After splenectomy, a dramatic increase in the Hb level occurred. All the patients had Hb >8g% with an average of 10g%. Most of the patients had a decrease in blood transfusion requirement with 96% of patients having blood transfusion requirements < 150 mL/kg/year. The frequency of blood transfusion requirement also decreases. Quality of life improved after splenectomy because of improved hemoglobin. Patients felt less fatigue and were able to carry out their daily activity in a better way. Decreasing blood transfusion requirement helped them to reduce the hospital visits.

Research into treating beta thalassemia with experimental gene therapies is ongoing, but for now it can only be cured by a procedure called a bone marrow transplant. Bone marrow, which is found inside bones, produces blood cells. In a bone marrow transplant, children are first given high doses of radiation or drugs to destroy the defective bone marrow. The bone marrow is then replaced with cells from a compatible donor, usually a healthy sibling or other relative. Bone marrow transplants carry many risks, so they usually are done only in the most severe cases of thalassemia.

Hemophilia

Hemophilia is an inherited bleeding diseases passed on to children from defective genes located on the X chromosome. Children with hemophilia have problems with bleeding because of low levels or complete absence of specific proteins, called 'factors,' in their blood that are necessary for prevention of excessive bleeding. The most common forms of hemophilia result from deficiencies of clotting factor proteins, factor VIII and factor IX. Both Factors VIII and IX are necessary to form a clot. Moreover, absence of additional two coagulation factors (factors IX and XI), has been associated with a constellation of symptoms similar to factor VIII deficiency.

- *Hemophilia A:* Hemophilia A is an X-linked, recessive disorder caused by deficiency of functional plasma clotting factor VIII (FVIII), which may be inherited or arise from spontaneous mutation. It is caused by a missing or reduced amount of the blood clotting protein Factor VIII.
- *Hemophilia B:* It is caused by a missing or reduced amount of the blood clotting protein factor IX.

Etiology and Incidence

Hemophilia A and B are present at birth and are usually inherited (Figs 15.7A and B). The defective genes located on the X chromosomes are passed from a parent to the child. A woman may carry and pass the gene that causes hemophilia, but not have hemophilia. Only males can have the disease, but females can carry the gene that causes it. Males (XY) have hemophilia when the gene for clotting factor VIII (hemophilia A) or clotting factor IX (hemophilia B) on the single X chromosome is affected. A female carrier of hemophilia has the hemophilia gene on one of her X chromosomes and the normal gene on her other X chromosome.

When a woman with hemophilia gene carrier becomes pregnant, there is a 50% chance that the child will get the X chromosome with the hemophilia gene. If the gene is passed onto the daughter, she will be a carrier.

If the father has hemophilia and the mother does not carry the hemophilia gene, then none of her sons will have hemophilia disease (because the mother has donated a normal X chromosome and the father has donated a normal Y chromosome). However in this scenario, all of the daughters will be carriers because the mother donates her normal X chromosome and the father has donated his abnormal X chromosome with the abnormal gene present. In about one-third of the children with hemophilia, there is no family history of the disorder. A new gene mutation, it is believed may be the cause of the disorder.

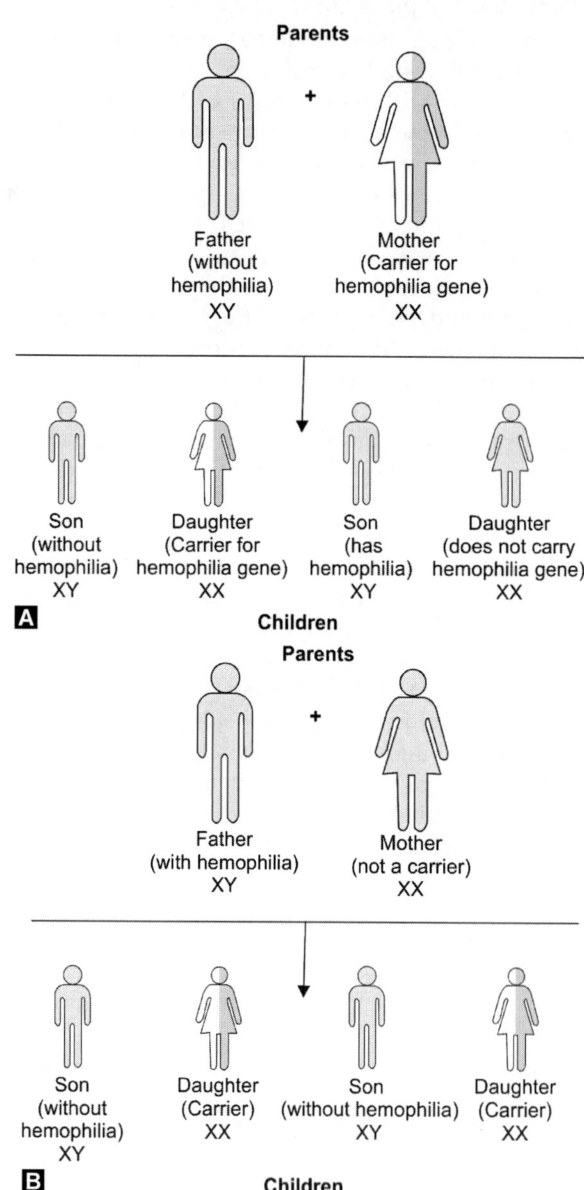

Figs 15.7A and B: Genetic inheritance of hemophilia shown in both ways (affected mother/father)

Manifestations

Following are the signs that can indicate the onset of this bleeding disorder:

- It is rare to diagnose hemophilia in children below six months of age as they are unlikely to suffer an injury that could lead to bleeding. But the child may develop bruises at the immunization site. When baby starts to crawl or walk, they get bruises on the stomach, chest, buttocks and back. The most common type of bleeding in hemophilia involves muscles and joints. So a child with hemophilia might refuse to use or move the affected joint due to swelling and pain. Recurrent joint bleeding can also lead to chronic damage too.

- Sometimes the disorder is diagnosed after circumcision, at which time prolonged bleeding may be observed.
- For a little older kids may show prolonged nosebleeds, excessive bleeding from biting down on the lips or tongue, excessive bleeding following a tooth extraction or loss of a tooth, excessive bleeding following surgery, etc.
- The most common symptom of hemophilia is excessive, uncontrollable bleeding. Patients with hemophilia do not bleed faster than normal children; they bleed for a longer time. The severity of symptoms in children with hemophilia depends on the severity of the disease. Hemophilia can be mild, moderate, or severe. This is based on the amount of clotting factor or the kind of bleeding episodes child has. A bleeding episode is bleeding that lasts longer than several minutes. Bleeding episodes can occur suddenly with or without injury.

Pathophysiology

Hemophilia is a bleeding disorder caused by a problem in blood's ability to form a clot. Hemophilia causes child to bleed more and longer than normal. Certain blood cells and substances normally form clots and stop child from bleeding too much. These include platelets, clotting factors, vitamin K, and fibrinogen. Platelets are a type of blood cell that helps form blood clots. Clotting factors are proteins that work with platelets to clot the blood. More than 10 factors in the blood work in sequence to produce blood clotting. Hemophilia A and hemophilia B are caused due to the two missing or defective constituents in the blood, i.e. factor VIII (antihemophilic factor) and factor IX (plasma thromboplastin). Hemophilia usually occurs only in boys, and two disorders are inherited in same ways and have same manifestations. Normal factor activity is described a percentage means level of factors remain in the blood. Normal levels of factors VIII and IX are 50% and 150% respectively. The severity of disorder is discussed below. Hemophilia can be mild, moderate, or severe. This is based on the amount of clotting factor or the kind of bleeding episodes child has. A bleeding episode is bleeding that lasts longer than several minutes. Bleeding episodes can occur suddenly with or without injury. Severe hemophilia is when factor VIII or IX clotting factor activity is less than 1%. Moderate hemophilia is when factor VIII or IX clotting factor activity is 1–5%. Mild hemophilia is when factor VIII or IX clotting factor activity is 6–40%.

Severe Hemophilia

- Spontaneous bleeding can occur unrelated to injury and is most dangerous when it occurs in the head.
- Joint bleeding is common. Hemarthrosis and joint destruction are characteristic of hemophilia.

Moderate Hemophilia

- Bleeding episodes are usually related to injury
- Joint bleeding can occur.

Mild Hemophilia

Episodes of bleeding are usually related to surgery or dental extractions.

- Joint bleeding is uncommon.

Other symptoms of hemophilia include:

- Bruising
- Soft tissue bleeding
- Bleeding from the nose, gums or mouth
- Pain, swelling and limited mobility in the joints and muscles
- Blood found in the urine or stool, or vomiting blood
- Excessive bleeding following circumcision.

Hemarthrosis and joint destruction in Hemophilia (Fig. 15.8)

Hemophilia is an inherited disorder of clotting factor deficiencies resulting in musculoskeletal bleeding, including hemarthroses, leading to musculoskeletal complications. Joint damage is the hallmark of the disease. The articular problems of hemophiliac patients begin in infancy. Patients with hemarthrosis commonly feel a tingling sensation—the 'aura'—before the episode of intra-articular bleeding. The joint becomes warm, swollen, very painful and with an antialgic position in flexion. The most commonly affected joints are the ankle, the knee, the elbow, and the hip. The correct management of hemophilic hemarthrosis should include prompt diagnosis, adequate hematological treatment, joint aspiration, physiotherapy and avoidance of rebleeding.

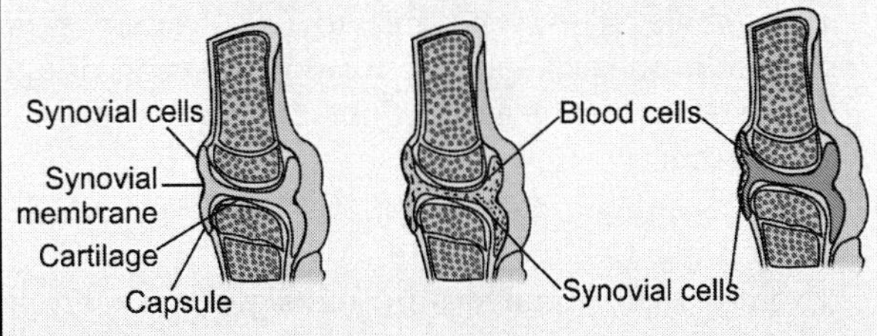

Fig. 15.8: Hemarthrosis and joint destruction in hemophilia

Diagnostic Evaluation

A complete medical and family history is taken and a physical examination is performed. To diagnose the condition a series of blood test like a complete blood count (CBC), prothrombin time (PT), activated partial thromboplastin time (PTT), and factors VIII and IX levels are done.

Expected laboratory values for suspected hemophilia are as follows:

- *Hemoglobin/hematocrit:* Normal or low
- Platelet count: Normal
- *Bleeding time and prothrombin time:* Normal
- *Activated partial thromboplastin time (aPTT):* Significantly prolonged in severe hemophilia, but may be normal in mild or even moderate hemophilia.

Normal values for FVIII assays are 50–150%. Values in hemophilia are described as mild: >5%, moderate: 1–5% and severe: < 1%.

Imaging studies for acute bleeds are chosen on the basis of clinical suspicion and anatomic location of involvement such as CT scan of head, MRI and USG of joints affected by acute or chronic effusions, etc.

Testing for inhibitors is indicated when bleeding is not controlled after adequate amounts of factor concentrate are infused during a bleeding episode. Inhibitor concentration is titrated using the Bethesda method, as follows:

- Positive result: Over 0.6 Bethesda units (BU)
- Low-titer inhibitor: Up to 5 BU
- High-titer inhibitor: Over 5 BU.

Treatment

While a cure for hemophilia is not currently available, the disorder may be managed effectively to prevent excessive bleeding and tissue damage by supplying the body with the missing or ineffective clotting factors.

- Treat bleeds early and appropriately. Bleeding is treated with RICE methodology means rest, ice, compression, and elevation. Children with mild hemophilia A may be able to use desmopressin acetate intranasal spray as it stops bleeding due to its vasoconstricting action. Sometimes aminocaproic acid (Amicar) or
- Get an annual comprehensive check up at the hemophilia treatment center.
- Exercise to maintain healthy joints
- Early treatment of bleeds is important and can be done by intravenous clotting factor replacement. This can even be done at home. Factor replacement prevents serious complications and allows children to live active lives.
- The goal of factor replacement is to stop or prevent bleeding by increasing the level of the missing or decreased factor VIII or IX. Both factors VIII and IX are available as natural or synthetic (recombinant) powders that can be diluted in sterile fluid and infused directly into a vein.
- Factor replacement therapy: In this treatment method, periodic infusion of the deficient clotting factor is sent into the child's bloodstream intravenously. Once the clotting factor is infused, it begins to work quickly and helps prevent joint damage. Although these treatments are effective, they are also expensive. Between 14% and 25% of children with severe hemophilia develop inhibitors (antibodies to the clotting factor). Their bodies view the clotting factor as a foreign substance and develop antibodies that block its clotting action. This can make the hemophilia difficult to treat. One method of overcoming the inhibitors is to increase the body's tolerance to the clotting factor by carefully infusing increasing amounts of the clotting factor over time. In severe cases, a child may need to get treatment for hemophilia on a regular schedule. In less severe cases, a child may need to get factors only when he has a bleeding problem.
- Medications: Medication like recombinant factor VII helps to deal with inhibitors. It activates another part of the coagulation process directly and bypasses the deficiencies.

Immune Thrombocytopenic Purpura

Immune thrombocytopenic purpura (ITP) is an acquired bleeding disorder characterized by immune-mediated destruction of platelets. Immune thrombocytopenic purpura is usually idiopathic and occasionally may be secondary to an autoimmune process such as lupus, rheumatoid arthritis, or lymphoproliferative disorders (lymphomas or chronic lymphocytic leukemia). Infection with HIV, *hepatitis B* and *C* and helicobacter pylori may also be associated with immune thrombocytopenic purpura. Bleeding is rare despite severely low platelet count due to the presence of functional platelets. It is usually a diagnosis of exclusion. Presence of adequate or increased number of megakaryocytes in the bone marrow with no other explanation confirms immune thrombocytopenic purpura. The initial treatment is typically steroids. Intravenous immunoglobulin, rituximab, and splenectomy are other treatment modalities.

Etiology and Incidence

The exact cause of ITP is not known and referred to as idiopathic. It is known, however, that in people with idiopathic thrombocytopenic purpura, the immune system malfunctions and begins attacking platelets as if they were foreign substances. In most children with ITP, the disorder follows a viral illness, such as the mumps or the flu. It may be that an infection sets off the immune system, triggering it to malfunction.

ITP usually results from development of an autoantibody directed against a structural platelet antigen. In childhood ITP, the autoantibody may be triggered by viral antigens. Immunoglobulin G (IgG) autoantibodies on the platelet surface. The immune system destroys platelets in the circulation and at the same time attacks bone marrow megakaryocytes, thereby reducing platelet production.

Other causes of isolated thrombocytopenia (e.g. drugs, lymphoproliferative disorders, other autoimmune diseases, viral infections) need to be excluded.

In children with acute ITP, distribution is equal between males (52%) and females (48%). Peak prevalence occurs in children aged 2 to 4 years. Approximately 40% of all patients are younger than 10 years. Spontaneous remission occurs in more than 80% of cases in children but is uncommon in adults.

Platelet count, cells/μL	*Signs and symptoms*
≥ 50,000	No major symptoms, although bleeding time may be increased
25,000–50,000	Petechiae and bruising with minor trauma
10,000–25,000	Spontaneous petechiae and bruising greater on the lower extremities and menorrhagia and epistaxis
< 10,000	Prominent bruising, mucosal bleeding (epistaxis, gum bleeding, gastrointestinal or genitourinary bleeding, and increased risk of central nervous system bleeding)

Pathophysiology

ITP is primarily a disease of increased peripheral platelet destruction, with most patients having antibodies to specific platelet membrane glycoproteins. The spleen and other organs of the reticuloendothelial system subsequently destroy these antibody coated platelets. Acute ITP often follows an acute infection and has a spontaneous resolution within 2 months. Chronic ITP persists longer than 6 months without a specific cause. Relative marrow failure may contribute to this condition, since studies show that most patients have either normal or diminished platelet production.

Manifestations

Children with ITP show the sudden onset bruising and petechiae and bleeding manifestations (Fig. 15.9). The type and the severity of bleeding is to be evaluated to exclude other causes of bleeding. Common signs,

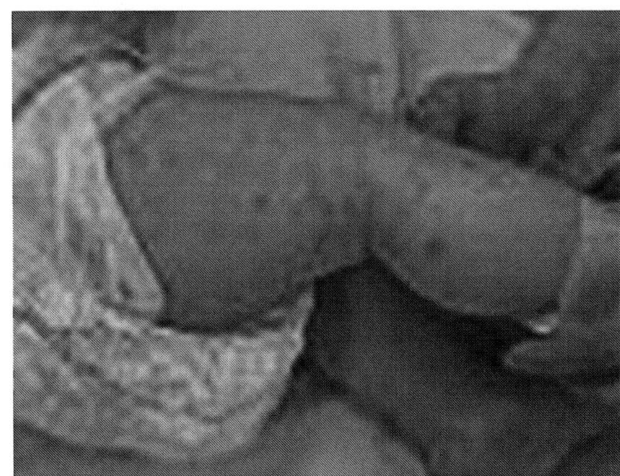

Fig. 15.9: A child with idiopathic thrombocytopenic purpura

symptoms, and precipitating factors of ITP include the following:

- Nonpalpable petechiae, which mostly occur in dependent regions:
- Hemorrhagic bullae on mucous membranes
- Purpura
- Gingival bleeding
- Signs of GI bleeding
- Retinal hemorrhages
- Evidence of intracranial hemorrhage, with possible neurologic symptoms
- *Nonpalpable spleen:* The prevalence of palpable spleen in patients with ITP is approximately the same as that in the non-ITP population (i.e. 3% in adults, 12% in children).

  Spontaneous bleeding when platelet count is less than 20,000/mm^3.

Diagnostic Evaluation

Blood test for CBC: A complete blood cell count (CBC) is the key laboratory finding. The white blood cell (WBC) count and hemoglobin level typically are normal in ITP, unless severe hemorrhage has occurred. On peripheral smear, truly giant platelets suggest congenital thrombocytopenia.

Therapeutic Management

- Prehospital care focuses on the ABCs, which include providing oxygen, controlling severe hemorrhage, and initiating intravenous (IV) fluids to maintain hemodynamic stability.
- Prehospital airway control may be necessary for a large intracranial hemorrhage.

- EMS providers should be aware of the potential for serious bleeding complications in patients with idiopathic thrombocytopenic purpura (ITP).

Disseminated Intravascular Coagulation (DIC)

DIC is an acquired disorder in which normal hemostatic balance is disturbed. There is excessive thrombin formation leading to fibrin deposition in microcirculation and consequent ischemic organ damage. It is characterized by hemorrhage and microvascular thrombosis.

Etiology and Incidences

Normally when you are injured, certain proteins in the blood become activated and travel to the injury site to help stop bleeding. However, in persons with DIC, these proteins become abnormally active. This often occurs due to inflammation, infection, or cancer.

Small blood clots form in the blood vessels. Some of these clots can clog up the vessels and cut off blood supply to various organs such as the liver, brain, or kidney. These organs will then be damaged and may stop functioning.

Over time, the clotting proteins are consumed or 'used up'. When this happens, then the person is at risk for serious bleeding, even from a minor injury or without injury. This process may also break up healthy red blood cells.

Risk factors for DIC include blood transfusion reaction, infection in the blood by bacteria or fungus, liver disease, recent surgery or anesthesia, sepsis, severe tissue injury (as in burns and head injury).

Pathophysiology

DIC is a complex pathophysiological disorder in which there is an unregulated thrombin explosion leading to release of free thrombin in the circulation resulting in widespread microvascular thrombosis. In order to counter this, there is release of free plasmin in the circulation. It involves activation of the procoagulant and fibrinolytic systems along with inhibitor consumption. Although hemorrhagic manifestations are more obvious, yet it is the diffuse thrombosis that leads to end organ damage and is responsible for most of its associated morbidity and mortality. DIC is thus defined as a systemic thrombo-hemorrhagic disorder seen in association with well-defined clinical conditions and laboratory evidence of (*i*) procoagulant activation, (*ii*) fibrinolytic activation, (*iii*) inhibitor consumption, and (*iv*) biochemical evidence of end organ damage or failure.

DIC occurs when the normal hemostatic balance is disturbed primarily by excessive thrombin formation. It is a dynamic process triggered by a variety of conditions causing activation of the clotting cascade and generation of excess thrombin within

Contd...

Contd...

the vascular system, which in turn leads to deposition of fibrin in the microcirculation. This definition implies that microclot formation and consequent ischemic organ failure and/or a hemorrhagic diathesis may occur.

The subsequent consumption of coagulation factors and platelets, enhanced fibrinolysis, and fibrin deposition result in the clinical picture of DIC of a bleeding diathesis accompanied by thrombosis that may lead to end organ damage. Bleeding is a more common manifestation of DIC but most of the morbidity and mortality of DIC is due to microvascular thrombosis. Routinely performed tests for DIC such as platelet count and prothrombin time may be normal in chronic DIC.

Manifestations

Hemorrhage is the commonest presentation characterized by spontaneous bruising, muscle oozing, bleeding from venipuncture sites, and secondary hemorrhage into surgical wounds. Usually bleeding is associated with varying degrees of shock, which is often out of proportion to the degree of blood. Bleeding occurs possibly from multiple sites in the body.

- Blood clots
- Bruising
- Drop in blood pressure.

Diagnostic Evaluation

The following tests may be done:

- Complete blood count with blood smear examination
- Fibrin degradation products
- Partial thromboplastin time (PTT)
- Platelet count
- Prothrombin time (PT)
- Serum fibrinogen.

Screening tests: Peripheral blood film examination–showing low platelets and schistocytes, platelet count–thrombocytopenia, prothrombin time (PT)–prolonged, activated partial thromboplastin time (APTT)–prolonged, thrombin time (TT)—prolonged, fibrinogen levels – low.

Therapeutic Management

Treatment should primarily focus on addressing the underlying disorder. DIC can result from numerous clinical conditions, including sepsis, trauma, obstetric emergencies, and malignancy. The goal is to determine and treat the cause of DIC. The disease causing DIC should be vigorously treated to reverse the process. For example, in case of sepsis, antibiotics should be started, and if a snake bite is the precipitating factor, antisnake venom should be initiated. Tissue perfusion and respiratory function must be maintained by replacing intravenous fluid and providing hemostatic support (replacement therapy).

In patients who have low levels of platelets, fibrinogen and other clotting factors as shown by prolonged PT, APTT, TT, replacement of these factors is useful. Although there have been some concerns that this replacement provides 'fuel to the fire', there are no clinical data to support these concerns. Replacement therapy is not indicated if there is no clinical bleeding and no invasive procedures are planned. If a patient is bleeding or a procedure is required, then an attempt to restore hemostatic capacity by replacing platelets and coagulation factors is indicated.

Blood clotting factors may be replaced with plasma transfusions. Platelet transfusions can raise the blood count. Heparin, a medication used to prevent clotting, is sometimes used to interrupt clotting events.

ABO Incompatibility and Hemolytic Disease of Newborn

The most common maternal-fetal blood group incompatibility is ABO incompatibility and the most common cause of hemolytic disease of the newborn (HDN). It is a common and generally mild type of hemolytic disease in babies. The term hemolytic disease means that red blood cells are broken down more quickly than usual which can cause jaundice, anemia and in very severe cases can cause death. Rh incompatibility, another hemolytic disease of the newborn, is associated with poorer fetal outcomes. During pregnancy, this breakdown of red blood cells in the baby may occur if the mother and baby's blood types are incompatible and if these different blood types come into direct contact with each other and antibodies are formed.

The important risk factors associated with ABO incompatibility are:

- Maternal blood type is O, while fetal blood type is A, B, or AB.
- Fetal-maternal hemorrhaging, allowing the blood of the fetus to commingle with that of the mother.
- Trauma to the abdomen that may lead to hemorrhaging.

So three conditions must exist for development of HDN. These are:

- Mother's and fetal erythrocytes are antigenically incompatible.
- If maternal-fetal antibodies commingle, it can launch a maternal immune response, thus creating antibodies that attack the foreign (or fetal) red blood cells.
- In ABO HDN maternal *IgG* antibodies with specificity for the *ABO blood group system* pass through the *placenta* to the *fetal* circulation where they can cause *hemolysis* of fetal *red blood cells* which can lead to fetal *anemia* and HDN. About half of the cases of ABO HDN occur in a firstborn baby. In contrast to Rh disease, ABO HDN does not become more severe after further pregnancies.

Significant problems with ABO incompatibility occur mostly with babies whose mothers have O blood type and where the baby is either A or B blood type. Premature babies are much more likely to experience severe problems from ABO incompatibility, while healthy full-term babies are generally only mildly affected. Unlike hemolytic disease that can result in subsequent babies when a mother has a negative blood group, ABO incompatibility can occur in first-born babies and does not become more severe in further pregnancies.

Etiology and Incidences

ABO incompatibility is a common and generally mild type of hemolytic disease in babies. Anti-A and anti-B antibodies are usually *IgM* and do not pass through the placenta, but some mothers 'naturally' have *IgG* anti-A or IgG anti-B antibodies, which can pass through the placenta.

A major cause of HDN is an incompatibility of the Rh blood group between the mother and fetus and most commonly, hemolytic disease is triggered by the D antigen. Pregnancies at risk of HND are those in which an Rh D-negative mother becomes pregnant with an RhD-positive child (the child having inherited the D antigen from the father). The mother's immune response to the fetal D antigen is to form antibodies against it (anti-D). These antibodies are usually of the IgG type, the type that is transported across the placenta and hence delivered to the fetal circulation.

Pathophysiology

During a pregnancy, mixing of maternal and fetal blood does not occur very often—the blood circulation of both mother and fetus are separated by the placental barrier, which does not often allow blood to commingle. Several reasons have been proposed to account for lack of intrauterine hemolysis due to ABO incompatibility. However, some circumstances can cause the two blood types to mix, such as miscarriage, trauma and birth, and sometimes they may mix for reasons unknown. Antibodies against the foreign blood types A and B may be formed. These antibodies could then pass across the placental membrane into the baby's circulation and may result in the destruction of some of the baby's red blood cells. The destruction of fetal red blood cells by these antibodies leads

Contd...

Contd...

to an increase of **bilirubin**—a waste product of red blood cells normally excreted by the liver— in fetal blood circulation.

The exposure of the Rh-negative mother to Rh-positive red cells occurs as a result of asymptomatic fetomaternal hemorrhage during pregnancy. After sensitization, maternal anti-D antibodies cross the placenta into fetal circulation and attach to Rh antigen on fetal RBCs, which form rosettes on macrophages in the reticuloendothelial system, specially in the spleen. These antibody-coated RBCs are lysed by lysosomal enzymes released by macrophages and natural killer lymphocytes and are independent of the activation of the complement system.

Manifestations

Jaundice: Most babies who have ABO incompatibility are born with higher than normal levels of bilirubin which can lead to newborn jaundice. This is unconjugated bilirubin, formerly excreted through maternal circulation.

Anemia: Many newborns who are affected by ABO incompatibility may develop issues with anemia after several weeks. This anemia is due to the increased amounts of breakdown of the red blood cells in response to maternal antibodies. These antibodies may persist in the newborn's body for several weeks following delivery.

Hepatosplenomegaly: It is resulting from anemia and the sequestration of erythrocytes.

Hydrops fetalis: This is an overwhelming condition of fetal edema and cardiovascular collapse caused by the above-mentioned processes.

The most important reason that ABO incompatibility does not cause hydrops fetalis is that naturally occurring anti-A and anti-B antibodies are IgM and thus do not cross the placenta.

Diagnostic Evaluation

As part of routine prenatal or antenatal care, the blood type of the mother (ABO and Rh) is determined by a blood test. A test for the presence of atypical antibodies in the mother's serum is also performed. At present, Rh D incompatibility is the only cause of HDN for which screening is routine.

After birth there are two options for testing for ABO incompatibility:

- *Coombs' test:* The cord blood of all babies whose mothers have an O blood group and the father either type A or B blood is tested. The direct Coombs' test evaluates for the presence of maternal antibody already attached to fetal erythrocytes. The theory behind this approach is that if the baby is type A or B and they test positive in direct antiglobulin tests (DAT), the baby can then be followed closely for jaundice.
- The alternate approach is to screen any baby who becomes significantly jaundiced (particularly within the first 24 hours).

Therapeutic Management

The antibodies in ABO HDN cause anemia due to destruction of fetal red blood cells and jaundice due to the rise in blood levels of bilirubin a by-product of hemoglobin breakdown. If the anemia is severe, it can be treated with a blood transfusion, however this is rarely needed. On the other hand, neonates have underdeveloped livers that are unable to process large amounts of bilirubin and a poorly developed *blood-brain barrier* that is unable to block bilirubin from entering the brain. This can result in kernicterus if left unchecked. If the bilirubin level is sufficiently high as to cause worry, it can be lowered via phototherapy in the first instance or an *exchange transfusion* if severely elevated.

While ABO incompatibility does not generally symptoms that require major medical treatment, treatment options can include the following:

Most neonates require phototherapy and adequate hydration to treat jaundice. Neonates with ABO incompatibility rarely does need an exchange transfusion. The best treatment for Rh incompatibility is prevention, which is done with immunoglobulin (RhoD).

Antihistamines to treat *allergic reactions* (if they occur).

Steroids to reduce swelling and inflammation.

IV Fluids

Exchange transfusions, replacing fetal blood with donated blood, are only performed in extreme cases and in specialized medical centers.

It is important to note that the anemia that may be caused by ABO incompatibility of the newborn is often negligible, and requires no treatment.

- Exchange transfusion should be considered in newborns born at more than 38 weeks' gestation with a bilirubin-to-albumin ratio of 7:2 and in newborns born at 35 to 37 weeks' gestation with a bilirubin-to-albumin ratio of 6:8. Exchange transfusion is not free of risk, with the estimated morbidity rate at 5% and the mortality rate as high as 0.5%. Apnea, bradycardia, cyanosis, vasospasm, and hypothermia with metabolic abnormalities (e.g.

hypoglycemia, hypocalcemia) are the most common adverse effects.

- IVIG has been shown to reduce the need for exchange transfusion in hemolytic disease of the newborn due to Rh or ABO incompatibility. The number needed to treat to prevent one exchange transfusion was noted to be 2:7 and was estimated to be 10, if all the infants with strongly positive direct Coombs' test were to receive the medication. In addition, it also reduced the duration of hospital stay and phototherapy. Although it was very effective as a single dose, multiple doses were more effective in stopping the ongoing hemolysis and reducing the incidence of late anemia.

Hyperbilirubinemia

A condition in which there is too much bilirubin in the blood is called hyperbilirubinemia. It is the condition of yellow discoloration of the skin, sclera, and mucous membranes due to elevated bilirubin as a result of abnormal bilirubin metabolism and/or excretion. Neonatal jaundice is caused by increased bilirubin production, decreased bilirubin clearance, or increased enterohepatic circulation.

When red blood cells breakdown, a substance called bilirubin is formed. Infants are not easily able to get rid of the bilirubin and it can build up in the blood and other tissues and fluids of the baby's body. This is called hyperbilirubinemia. Some jaundice is normal in neonates. Depending on the cause of the hyperbilirubinemia, jaundice may appear at birth or at any time afterward. Neonatal jaundice is caused by increased bilirubin production, decreased bilirubin clearance, or increased enterohepatic circulation.

Etiology and Incidences

During pregnancy, the placenta excretes bilirubin. When the baby is born, the baby's liver must take over this function. There are several causes of hyperbilirubinemia and jaundice, including the following:

Physiologic jaundice*:* Visible jaundice is developed in children due to elevation of unconjugated bilirubin concentration during their first week. This common condition is called physiological jaundice. Physiologic jaundice occurs as a 'normal' response to the baby's limited ability to excrete bilirubin in early days of life as low activity of the enzyme glucuronosyltransferase which normally converts unconjugated bilirubin to conjugated bilirubin. This enzyme is actively down-regulated before birth, since bilirubin needs to remain unconjugated in order to cross the placenta to avoid being accumulated in the fetus. After birth, it takes some time for this enzyme to gain function.

Infants are born with elevated levels of red blood cells. As their body begins to remove the old red blood cells immediately after birth, a yellow pigment called bilirubin is created. Typically, the yellow skin discoloration caused by bilirubin fades on its own as the maturing liver breaks the pigment down and it is removed in infant's urine and stool.

Furthermore, newborn babies have more red blood cells than adults, and thus more are breaking down at any one time; as well many of these cells are different from adult red cells and they do not live as long. All of this means more bilirubin will be made in the newborn baby's body. If the baby is premature, or stressed from a difficult birth, or the infant of a diabetic mother, or more than the usual number of red blood cells are breaking down (as can happen in blood incompatibility), the level of bilirubin in the blood may rise higher than usual levels.

Breastfed infants who fail to consume enough milk may suffer prolonged jaundice (breast milk jaundice), as the bilirubin stalls in the system due to inadequate nutrition. The reasons why healthy infants who adapt well to breastfeeding become jaundiced remain unknown. It is speculated that substances in breast milk may block the proteins in the liver responsible for breaking down bilirubin. About 2% of breastfed babies develop jaundice after the first week. It peaks about two weeks of age and can persist up to 3 to 12 weeks.

Not-enough-breastmilk jaundice: Higher than usual levels of bilirubin or longer than usual jaundice may occur because the baby is *not getting enough milk*. This may be due to the fact that the mother's milk takes longer than average to 'come in' (but if the baby feeds well in the first few days this should not be a problem), or because hospital routines limit breastfeeding or because, most likely, the baby is poorly latched on and thus not getting the milk which is available. When the baby is getting little milk, bowel movements tend to be scanty and infrequent so that the bilirubin that was in the baby's gut gets reabsorbed into the blood instead of leaving the body with the bowel movements.

Jaundice from hemolysis: Jaundice may occur with the breakdown of red blood cells due to hemolytic disease of the newborn (Rh disease), or from having too many red blood cells that breakdown naturally and release bilirubin.

Jaundice related to inadequate liver function: Jaundice may be related to inadequate liver function due to infection or other factors.

Pathophysiology

Neonatal physiologic jaundice results from simultaneous occurrence of the following 2 phenomena:

- Bilirubin production is elevated because of increased breakdown of fetal erythrocytes. This is the result of the shortened lifespan of fetal erythrocytes and the higher erythrocyte mass in neonates.
- Hepatic excretory capacity is low both because of low concentrations of the binding protein ligandin in the hepatocytes and because of low activity of glucuronyl transferase, the enzyme responsible for binding bilirubin to glucuronic acid, thus making bilirubin water soluble (conjugation).

Aged or damaged fetal RBCs are removed from the circulation by reticuloendothelial cells, which convert heme to bilirubin (1 g of Hb yields 35 mg of bilirubin. When red blood cells have completed their lifespan, or when they are damaged, their membranes become fragile and prone to rupture. RBCs travel intravascularly to cells of the reticuloendothelial system (spleen and liver primarily), its cell membrane ruptures and cellular contents, including hemoglobin, are subsequently released into the blood. The hemoglobin is phagocytosed by macrophages and split into its heme and globin. The globin portion, a protein, is degraded into amino acids and plays no role in jaundice.

Two reactions then take place with the heme molecule. The first oxidation reaction takes place by catabolic enzymes, heme oxygenase and results in biliverdin (green color pigment), iron and carbon monoxide. A second reaction catalyzed by biliverdin reductase converts biliverdin to unconjugated bilirubin. This bilirubin is insoluble in water and thus is bound to albumin and transferred to the liver. Once it arrives at the liver, it is conjugated with glucuronic acid to become more water soluble and able to be excreted from the body through the urinary and intestinal tracts. Conjugated bilirubin cannot be reabsorbed by the intestines.

Neonates lack proper intestinal bacteria for oxidizing bilirubin to urobilinogen in the gut. They, however, have sterile digestive tracts. They do have the enzyme β-glucuronidase, which deconjugates the conjugated bilirubin, which is then reabsorbed by the intestines and recycled into the circulation. Feedings invoke the gastrocolic reflex, and bilirubin is excreted in stool before most of it can be deconjugated and reabsorbed. However, in many neonates, the unconjugated bilirubin is reabsorbed and returned to the circulation from the intestinal lumen (enterohepatic circulation of bilirubin), contributing to physiologic hyperbilirubinemia and jaundice.

Manifestations

Neonatal jaundice first becomes visible in the face and forehead. If a finger lightly pressed on a baby's skin, blanching reveals the underlying yellow color. Jaundice then gradually becomes visible on the trunk and extremities (cephalocaudal progression). Jaundice disappears in the opposite direction. The explanation for this phenomenon is not well-understood but clinically useful because, visible jaundice in the lower extremities strongly suggests the need to check the bilirubin level either in the serum or noninvasively via transcutaneous bilirubinometry.

In most infants, yellow color is the only finding on physical examination. More intense jaundice may be associated with drowsiness. The baby develops a fever of over 100 °F yellow coloring deepens the baby is feeding poorly, appears listless or lethargic, and making high-pitched cries.

Severe jaundice also increases the risk of bilirubin passing into the brain, which can cause permanent brain damage. Overt neurologic findings, such as changes in muscle tone, seizures, or altered cry characteristics, in a significantly jaundiced infant are danger signs and require immediate attention to prevent kernicterus.

Hepatosplenomegaly, petechiae, and microcephaly may be associated with hemolytic anemia, sepsis, and congenital.

Diagnostic Evaluation

The serum bilirubin level required to cause jaundice varies with skin tone and body region, but jaundice usually becomes visible on the sclera at a level of 2 to 3 mg/dL (34 to 51μmol/L) and on the face at about 4 to 5 mg/dL (68 to 86 μmol/L). With increasing bilirubin levels, jaundice seems to advance in a head-to-foot direction, appearing at the umbilicus at about 15 mg/dL (258 μmol/L) and at the feet at about 20 mg/dL (340 μmol/L). Slightly more than half of all neonates become visibly jaundiced in the first week of life.

The total bilirubin level (conjugated plus unconjugated) 13 mg/dL or higher in premature neonates with clinical jaundice or in term neonates should be evaluated for cause of jaundice. Generally total bilirubin level remains higher in breastfed neonates than in bottle-fed neonates.

Direct Coombs', blood typing with Rh factor, reticulocyte counts can be done as other diagnostic test.

Therapeutic Management

It is critically important to identify the underlying cause of jaundice so that appropriate treatment can be initiated as soon as possible. In addition, treatment for hyperbilirubinemia itself may be necessary.

Physiologic jaundice usually is not clinically significant and resolves within 1 week. Breastfeeding mothers are to be encouraged to nurse at least 8 to 12 times a day. Frequent formula feedings can reduce the incidence and severity of hyperbilirubinemia by increasing GI motility and frequency of stools, thereby minimizing the enterohepatic circulation of bilirubin. Prevention of hyperbilirubinemia includes preventing the neonate from becoming dehydrated.

Breastfeeding jaundice may be prevented or reduced by increasing the frequency of feedings. If the bilirubin level continues to increase > 18 mg/dL in a term infant with early breastfeeding jaundice, a temporary change from breast milk to formula may be appropriate; phototherapy also may be indicated at higher levels. Stopping breastfeeding is necessary for only 1 or 2 days, and the mother should be encouraged to continue expressing breast milk regularly so she can resume nursing as soon as the infant's bilirubin level starts to decline. She also should be assured that the hyperbilirubinemia has not caused any harm and that she may safely resume breastfeeding. It is not advisable to supplement with water or dextrose because that may disrupt the mother's production of milk.

Definitive treatment involves:

- Phototherapy
- Exchange transfusion.

Phototherapy

This treatment remains the standard of care, most commonly using fluorescent white light, ideally 420–470 nm. (Blue light is most effective for intensive phototherapy.) Phototherapy is the use of light to photoisomerize unconjugated bilirubin into forms that are more water soluble and can be excreted rapidly by the liver and kidney without glucuronidation. It provides definitive treatment of neonatal hyperbilirubinemia and prevention of kernicterus. Phototherapy is an option when unconjugated bilirubin is > 12 mg/dL (> 205.2 μmol/L) and may be indicated when unconjugated bilirubin is > 15 mg/dL at 25 to 48 h, 18 mg/dL at 49 to 72 h, and 20 mg/dL at > 72 h. It is provided continuously with short breaks of child care like feeding, diadring, etc. Phototherapy is not indicated for conjugated hyperbilirubinemia. Because visible jaundice may disappear during phototherapy though serum bilirubin remains elevated, skin color cannot be used to evaluate jaundice severity. Blood taken for bilirubin determinations should be shielded from bright light, because bilirubin in the collection tubes may rapidly photo-oxidize.

Exchange Transfusion

Specific indications for exchange transfusion are serum bilirubin ≥ 20 mg/dL at 24 to 48 h or ≥ 25 mg/dL at > 48 h and failure of phototherapy to result in a 1 to 2 mg/dL decrease within 4 to 6 h of initiation or at the first clinical signs of kernicterus regardless of bilirubin levels. If the serum bilirubin level is > 25 mg/dL when the neonate is initially examined, preparation for an exchange transfusion should be made in case intensive phototherapy fails to lower the bilirubin level. An alternative approach uses the weight of the neonate in grams divided by 100 to determine the bilirubin level (in mg/dL) at which exchange transfusion is indicated. Thus, a 1000 g neonate would receive an exchange transfusion at a bilirubin level of ≥ 10 mg/dL, and a 1500 g neonate would receive an exchange transfusion at a bilirubin level of ≥ 15 mg/dL.

This treatment can rapidly remove bilirubin from circulation and is indicated for severe hyperbilirubinemia, which most often occurs with immune-mediated hemolysis. Small amounts of blood are withdrawn and replaced through an umbilical vein catheter to remove partially hemolyzed and antibody-coated RBCs as well as circulating Igs. The blood is replaced with uncoated donor RBCs. Only unconjugated hyperbilirubinemia can cause kernicterus, so if conjugated bilirubin is elevated, the level of unconjugated rather than total bilirubin is used to determine the need for exchange transfusion.

Most often, 160 mL/kg (twice the infant's total blood volume) of packed RBCs is exchanged over 2 to 4 h; an alternative is to give 2 successive exchanges of 80 mL/kg each over 1 to 2 h. To do an exchange, 20 mL of blood is withdrawn and then immediately replaced by 20 mL of transfused blood. This procedure is repeated until the total desired volume is exchanged. For critically ill or premature infants, aliquots of 5 to 10 mL are used to avoid sudden major changes in blood volume. The goal is to reduce bilirubin by nearly 50%, with the knowledge that hyperbilirubinemia may rebound to about 60% of pretransfusion level within 1 to 2 h. It is also customary to lower the target level by 1 to 2 mg/dL in conditions that increase the risk of kernicterus (e.g. fasting, sepsis, acidosis). Exchange transfusions may need to be repeated if bilirubin levels remain high. Finally, there are risks and complications with the procedure, and the success of phototherapy has reduced the frequency of exchange transfusion.

> **Kernicterus (Bilirubin Encephalopathy)**
>
> *Kernicterus is brain damage caused by unconjugated bilirubin deposition in basal ganglia and brainstem nuclei.* Normally, bilirubin bound to serum albumin stays in the intravascular space. However, bilirubin can cross the blood-brain barrier and cause kernicterus when serum bilirubin concentration is markedly elevated; serum albumin concentration is markedly low (e.g. in preterm infants); or bilirubin is displaced from albumin by competitive binders (e.g. sulfisoxazole, ceftriaxone, and aspirin).

Contd...

Contd...

In preterm infants, kernicterus may not cause recognizable clinical symptoms or signs. Early symptoms in term infants are lethargy, poor feeding, and vomiting. Opisthotonos, oculogyric crisis, seizures, and death may follow. Kernicterus may result in intellectual disability, choreoathetoid cerebral palsy, sensorineural hearing loss, and paralysis of upward gaze later in childhood. It is unknown whether minor degrees of kernicterus can cause less severe neurologic impairment (e.g. perceptual-motor problems, learning disorders).

There is no reliable test to determine the risk of kernicterus, and the diagnosis is made presumptively. A definite diagnosis can be made only by autopsy.

There is no treatment once kernicterus develops; it can be prevented by treating hyperbilirubinemia.

Nursing care of a Child with Hematologic Disorders

Nursing Diagnosis

- Activity intolerance, related to weakness and fatigue.
- Impaired gas exchange, related to decreased hemoglobin.
- *Nutrition:* Less than body requirements, related to poor nutritional intake and anorexia.
- Low platelet count/risk for injury related to decreased platelets.
- Ineffective tissue perfusion related to inadequate blood volume or hematocrit.
- Ineffective therapeutic regimen management, related to lack of knowledge about appropriate nutrition and medication regimen.

Expected Outcomes

- Within 1 month patient will be able to perform hygiene, dressing, and grooming activities without needing to rest between activities.
- Within 2 months patient will be able to carry out usual daily activities without shortness of breath or fatigue.
- Patient will eat three nutritious meals, containing sufficient iron, folic acid, vitamin C, and protein daily.
- Patient will not experience episodes of bleeding.
- Patient will verbalize understanding of dietary and medication regimen within 1 week.

Nursing Intervention

It is based on an understanding of the particular kind of anemia affecting the patient. Anemia from blood loss presents problems quite different from those related to chronic, and possibly incurable aplastic or hemolytic anemia.

For any patient with anemia severe enough to cause fatigue, assist with daily living activities, and provide planned rest periods. Encourage resting between care activities and encourage to perform ADLs in small segments. Assist patient/parents to follow a progressive plan of rest, activity, and exercise and prioritize activities. It prevents undue fatigue, and conserves energy.

For patients with anemias that interfere with clotting and that tend to cause bleeding episodes, nursing actions are directed toward preventing the episodes.

Monitor CBC and platelet counts which will detect further decrease in platelets. Instruct to report oozing of blood from the gums. Alert the patient/parents about potential causes for impending bleeding episode. Instruct to observe stool and urine for signs of bleeding. Administer stool softener to prevent constipation. Soft stool will not injure rectal mucosa, causing bleeding. Instruct to use soft toothbrush.

Patients with acute blood loss or severe hemolysis may have decreased tissue perfusion from decreased blood volume or reduced circulating RBCs. Transfusions or intravenous fluids (as prescribed), based on the symptoms and the laboratory findings is to be administered to replace lost volume. Supplemental oxygen may be necessary, but it is rarely needed on a long-term basis unless there is underlying severe cardiac or pulmonary disease as well. Monitor vital signs closely; other medications, such as antihypertensive agents, may need to be adjusted or withheld accordingly.

Nursing functions include administering blood, iron, vitamin B_{12}, and folic acid, and monitoring for desired effects. Patients are educated about needed dietary adjustments. Patients should be taught that iron is absorbed more readily if vitamin C is simultaneously present in the gastrointestinal (GI) system. Taking iron medication with orange juice provides the necessary vitamin C. Analgesia for headache or joint pain is given as ordered, and the patient is monitored for adverse side effects.

Develop meal plan that promotes optimal nutrition and maintain adequate amounts of iron, vitamins, and protein from diet or supplements. Adhere to nutritional supplement therapy when prescribed. Encourage the patient/parents to verbalize their understanding of rationale for using recommended nutritional supplements.

For patients with anemia, medications or nutritional supplements are often prescribed to alleviate or correct the condition. These patients/parents need to understand the purpose of the medication, how to take the medication and over what time period, and how to manage any side effects of therapy. To enhance compliance, the nurse can assist patient in developing ways to incorporate the therapeutic plan into their lives, rather than merely giving the patient a list of instructions. For example, many patients have difficulty taking iron supplements because of related gastrointestinal effects. Rather than seeking assistance from a health care provider in managing the problem, some of these patients simply stop taking the iron. Abruptly stopping some medications can have serious consequences, as in the case of high-dose corticosteroids to manage hemolytic anemia.

Nursing management: Preventive education is important, because iron deficiency anemia is common in women and children. Food sources high in iron include organ meats, other meats, beans, leafy green vegetables, raisins, and molasses. Taking iron-rich foods with a source of vitamin C enhances the absorption of iron. The nurse helps the patient to select a healthy diet. Nutritional counseling can be provided for those whose usual diet is inadequate. Patients with a history of eating fad diets or strict vegetarian diets are counseled that such diets often contain inadequate amounts of absorbable iron. The nurse encourages patients to continue iron therapy as long as it is prescribed, although they may no longer feel fatigued. Because iron is best absorbed on an empty stomach, patients should be advised to take the supplement an hour before meals. Most patients can use the less expensive, more standard forms of ferrous sulfate distributed in the hospitals. Tablets with enteric coating may be poorly absorbed and should be avoided.

CHAPTER 16

The Child with Neurologic Alterations

Chapter Outline

- Anatomy and Physiology of Neural System
- Brief Introduction of Nervous System
- Management and Nursing Interventions of Different Disorders
  - Infection of CNS
  - Acute Flaccid Paralysis
  - Neural Defects and CNS Circulation Problems
  - Disorders of Neural Tube Development
  - Seizure Disorders
  - Injury – Head and Spinal Cord

The vertebrate nervous system consists of the central nervous system (CNS) and the peripheral nervous system (PNS) (Flowchart 16.1). CNS comprises the brain (cerebrum, cerebellum, and brainstem) and the spinal cord. PNS is composed of nerves leading to and from the CNS, often through junctions known as ganglia. PNS includes sensory neurons, which link sensory receptors on the body surface, as well as in specialized receptor structures like the ear, with processing circuits in the CNS. The motor portion of the PNS consists of two components. Motor axons that connect the brain and spinal cord to skeletal muscles make up the somatic motor division of the PNS. The visceral or autonomic motor division consists of cells and axons that innervate smooth muscles, cardiac muscle, and glands.

Neural development is one of the earliest systems to begin and the last to be completed after birth. This development generates the most complex structure within the embryo and the long time period of development. The early CNS begins as a simple neural plate that folds to form a groove then tube, open initially at each end. By the 4th week of gestation, the neural

Flowchart 16.1: Detail of central and peripheral nervous system

Nervous system (NS)
- Peripheral NS
  - Autonomic NS
    - Sympathetic NS
    - Parasympathetic NS
  - Somatic NS
- Central NS
  - Brain
    - Forebrain
      - Telencephalon → Cerebral cortex, Basal ganglia, Hippocampus, Amygdala
      - Diencephalon → Thalamus, Hypothalamus
    - Midbrain
      - Mesencephalon → Tectum, Cerebellum
    - Hindbrain
      - Metencephalon → Pons, Cerebellum
      - Myelencephalon → Medulla
  - Spinal cord

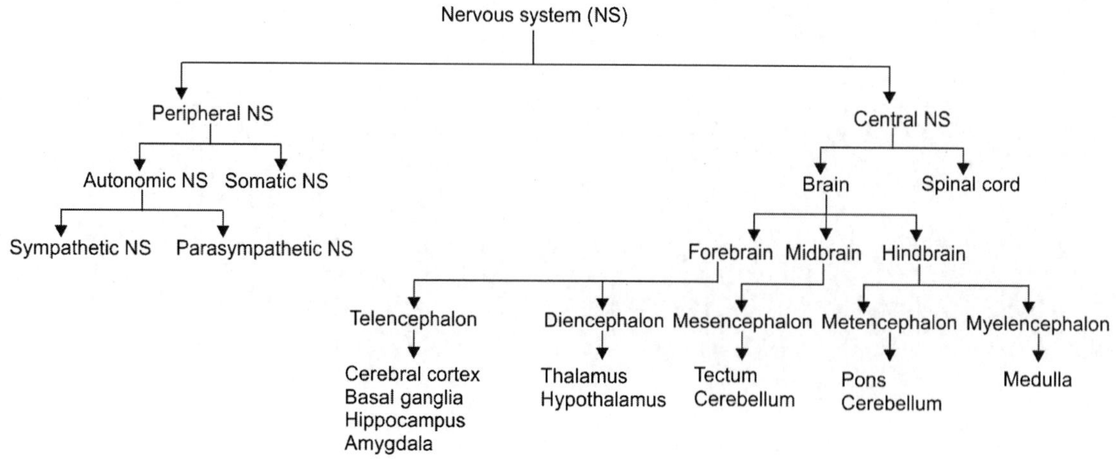

tube has closed to the anterior end to form the brain and at the posterior end to form the spinal cord. Failure of these opening to close contributes a major class of neural abnormalities (neural tube defects).

Within the neural tube stem cells generate the two major classes of cells that make the majority of the nervous system—neurons and glia. Both these classes of cells differentiate into many different types generated with highly specialized functions and shapes. The brain becomes the prominent body structure during second month of gestation. Rapid brain cell growth appears to occur twice during gestation. Number of neurons significantly increases between 15th to 20th weeks of gestation and again it rapidly grows at 30th weeks and continued through 1 year. Growth of brain occurs until approximately the 5th year of life.

THE AXIAL SKELETON

The axial skeleton protects the underlying structures of the CNS. The brain is encased in the skull, and protected by the cranium. The cranial vault is formed by the frontal, parietal, temporal, and occipital bones. The floor of the cranial vault has three components or fossa. The anterior fossa houses the frontal lobe of the brain, the middle fossa holds, the upper brainstem and pituitary gland, the posterior fossa contains the lower brainstem. Through the foramina blood vessels and cranial nerves enter and leave the skull.

The spinal cord is continuous with the brain and lies caudally to the brain, and is protected by the vertebra. The spinal cord reaches from the base of the skull, continues through or starting below the foramen magnum, and terminates roughly level with the first or second lumbar vertebra, occupying the upper sections of the vertebral canal. Microscopically, there are differences between the neurons and tissue of the CNS and the PNS. The CNS is divided in white and gray matter. This can also be seen macroscopically on brain tissue. The white matter constitutes of axons and oligodendrocytes, while the gray matter chiefly constitutes of neurons.

The Myelin Sheath

Myelin is the fatty material that forms a layer, the myelin sheath, usually around only the axon of a neuron (Fig. 16.1). It is essential for the proper functioning of the nervous system. It is an outgrowth of a type of glial cell. The production of the myelin sheath is called myelination. In humans, myelination begins in the 14th week of fetal development. The insulating envelope of myelin that surrounds the core of a nerve fiber or axon and that facilitates the transmission of nerve impulses,

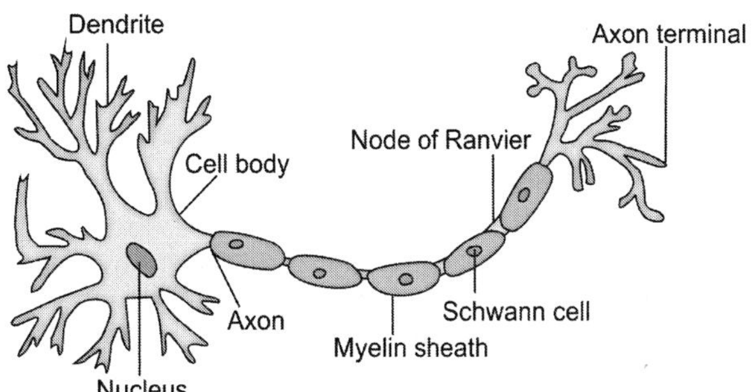

Fig. 16.1: The structure of neuron, building blocks of neural system

formed from the cell membrane of the Schwann cell in the PNS and from oligodendroglia cells. It is also called *medullary sheath.* Myelinated axons are white in appearance, hence the 'white matter' of the brain. The main purpose of a myelin layer is to increase the speed at which impulses propagate along the myelinated fiber. Coordination of fine and gross motor skills progresses with the deposition of myelin sheath. Disease, drugs and aging process can destroy myelin sheath.

The neural system develops multiple circuits that subserve similar functions in the perspective of broader behavioral purposes.

The most general functional definition divides neural systems into sensory systems like vision or hearing that acquire and process information from the environment, and motor systems that allow the organism to respond to such information by generating movements. There are, however, large numbers of cells and circuits that lie between these relatively well-defined input and output systems. These are collectively referred to as *associational systems*, and they carry out the most complex and least well-characterized brain functions. Coordination between various organs and systems of the body is crucial to homeostasis. The two systems that maintain homeostasis are the neural system and the endocrine system. The neural system is for quick coordination of nerve impulses. Each function is under the control of a specific area of the brain. The right hemisphere of the brain controls the left side of the body and is concerned with the social aspects of perception, intuition and experience. The left hemisphere of brain controls the right side of the body and is concerned with language acquisition and use of logical and verbal reasoning.

The Meninges

The meninges are the membranes that envelop the CNS. The meninges consist of three layers—the dura mater, arachnoid mater, and pia mater. These layers cover the brain and spinal cord with the primary function of protecting and nourishing the CNS. Dura mater, the thick outermost durable fibrous membrane is responsible for keeping the cerebrospinal fluid (CSF), and for surrounding and supporting the dural venous sinuses that carry blood from the brain to the heart. The dura mater has two layers having meningeal components. Between the periosteum of the bone and the dura mater lies the epidural space.

The arachnoid mater is the middle layer of the meninges, and is named from its spider web-like appearance. It is a delicate, avascular serous membrane loosely covering the brain. It provides a cushioning for the CNS. The pia mater is the innermost layer of the meninges. It envelopes and firmly attaches to the surface of the brain and spinal cord. The pia mater contains blood vessels and capillaries that are responsible for nourishing the brain.

The innermost layer is called the pia mater. But right in between the arachnoid layer and the pia mater, there is 'a space' named the '*subarachnoid space*.' This subarachnoid space houses the brain's *cisterns* ('pools' of CSF) as well as cerebral arteries and veins.

So main functions of the meninges include:

- Protecting the brain and spinal cord form mechanical injury.
- Providing blood supply to the skull and to the hemispheres.
- Providing a space for the flow of CSF.

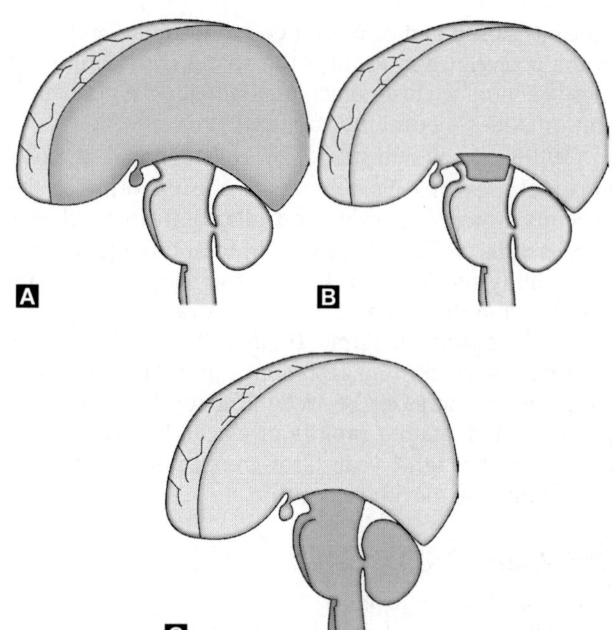

Figs 16.2A to C: Graphical representation of brain areas. **A.** Forebrain; **B.** Midbrain; **C.** Hindbrain

The Brain

The brain is located in the head, usually close to the primary sensory organs for such senses as vision, hearing, balance, taste, and smell. The brain is the most complex organ in a vertebrate's body. The three sections of brain are the cerebrum, cerebellum and brain-stem (Figs 16.2A to C). In a typical human, the cerebral cortex is estimated to contain 15 to 33 billion neurons, each connected by synapses to several thousand other neurons (Fig. 16.1). These neurons communicate with one another by means of long protoplasmic fibers called axons, which carry trains of signal pulses called action potentials to distant parts of the brain or body targeting specific recipient cells.

It is said that the brain is like a committee of experts. All the parts of the brain work together, but each part has its own special properties. The brain can be divided into three basic units—the forebrain, midbrain, and hindbrain.

The upper part of the spinal cord, the brainstem, and a wrinkled ball of tissue called the cerebellum form the hindbrain, which controls the body's reflexes and crucial basic life functions such as heart rate, breathing, and blood pressure. It also regulates when man feels sleepy or awake. The cerebellum coordinates movement. The uppermost part of the brainstem is the midbrain, which controls some reflex actions and is part of the circuit involved in the control of eye movements and other voluntary movements.

The forebrain is the largest part of the brain which has two hemispheres. It is most highly developed part of the human brain consists primarily of the cerebrum and the structures hidden beneath it. Although the two hemispheres seem to be mirror images of each other, they are different. For instance, the ability to form words seems to lie primarily in the left hemisphere, while the right hemisphere seems to control many abstract reasoning skills. The distinctive, deeply wrinkled outer surface is the *cerebral cortex*, which consists of gray matter. Beneath this lies the white matter.

The brain has centralized control over the other organs of the body. It is done by a complex of structures like *thalamus* and *hypothalamus*. The thalamus acts as a relay station for incoming nerve impulses from around the body that are then forwarded to the appropriate brain region for processing. The hypothalamus controls hormone secretions from the nearby *pituitary gland*. These hormones govern growth and instinctual behavior such as eating, drinking, sex, anger, and reproduction. The hypothalamus, for instance, controls when a new mother starts to lactate.

THE CRANIAL NERVES

Twelve pairs of nerves—the cranial nerves—lead directly from the brain to various parts of the head, neck, and trunk. Some of the cranial nerves are involved in the special senses (such as seeing, hearing, and taste), and others control muscles in the face or regulate glands. The nerves are named and numbered (according to their location, from the front of the brain to the back) (Table 16.1).

Table 16.1: The names, types and functions of the cranial nerves

Nerves	*Type*	*Function*
I Olfactory	sensory	Olfaction (smell)
II Optic	sensory	Vision (Contain 38% of all the axons connecting to the brain.)
III Oculomotor	motor	Eyelid and eyeball muscles
IV Trochlear	motor	Eyeball muscles
V Trigeminal	mixed	Sensory: Facial and mouth sensation Motor: chewing
VI Abducens	motor	Eyeball movement
VII Facial	mixed	Sensory: Taste Motor: Facial muscles and salivary glands
VIII Auditory	sensory	Hearing and balance
IXGlossopharyngeal	mixed	Sensory: Taste Motor: Swallowing
X Vagus	mixed	Main nerve of the parasympathetic nervous system (PNS)
XI Accessory	motor	Swallowing: moving head and shoulder
XII Hypoglossal	motor	Tongue muscles

The Spinal Cord

The spinal cord is a cylindrical-shaped bundle of nerve fibers that is connected to the brain at the brainstem. The spinal cord runs down the center of the protective spinal column extending from the neck to the lower back. It is about 45 cm in length, extends from the foramen magnum, where it is continuous with the medulla oblongata, to the level of the first or second lumbar vertebra.

Below that level, the vertebral canal is occupied by spinal nerve roots and meninges.

The spinal cord, like the brain, is surrounded by the three meninges. From and to the spinal cord are projections of the PNS in the form of spinal nerves. The nerves connect the spinal cord with skin, joints, muscles, etc. and allow for the transmission of efferent motor as well as afferent sensory signals and stimuli. The axons that link the spinal cord to the muscles and the rest of the body are bundled into 31 pairs of spinal nerves, each pair with a sensory root and a motor root that make connections within the gray matter. This allows for voluntary and involuntary motions of muscles, as well as the perception of senses.

- Cervical spinal nerves (C1 to C8) control signals to the back of the head, the neck and shoulders, the arms and hands, and the diaphragm.
- Thoracic spinal nerves (T1 to T12) control signals to the chest muscles, some muscles of the back, and parts of the abdomen.
- Lumbar spinal nerves (L1 to L5) control signals to the lower parts of the abdomen and the back, the buttocks, some parts of the external genital organs, and parts of the leg.
- Sacral spinal nerves (S1 to S5) control signals to the thighs and lower parts of the legs, the feet, most of the external genital organs, and the area around the anus.
- The single coccygeal nerve carries sensory information from the skin of the lower back.

Cerebrospinal Fluid (CSF)

CSF is a clear colorless bodily fluid found in the brain and spine. It is produced in the choroid plexus of the brain (within two lateral ventricles). It acts as a cushion or buffer for the brain's cortex, providing a basic mechanical and immunological protection to the brain inside the skull, and it serves a vital function in cerebral autoregulation of cerebral blood flow.

The CSF occupies the subarachnoid space (the space between the arachnoid mater and the pia mater) and the ventricular system around and inside the brain and spinal cord. It constitutes the content of the ventricles, cisterns, and sulci of the brain, as well as the central canal of the spinal cord. CSF returns to the vascular system by entering through the arachnoid villi into the venous sinuses.

Cerebral Blood Flow

The movement of blood through the network of blood vessels supplying the brain is called cerebral circulation. The arterial cerebral circulation is normally divided into anterior cerebral circulation and posterior cerebral circulation and supplied by internal carotid arteries and vertebral arteries. The arteries deliver oxygenated blood, glucose and other nutrients to the brain and the veins carry deoxygenated blood back to the heart, removing carbon dioxide, lactic acid, and other metabolic products. Approximately 17% of cardiac output and 20% of body oxygen are transported to the brain. The brain has high metabolic demand and requires approximately 10 times the oxygen used by the rest of the body. The brain also has sinuses or veins. These carry waste and carbon dioxide away from the cranium. The brain also has a structure called the blood-brain barrier across which nutrients and waste are exchanged. This barrier protects the brain.

APPROACH TO THE CHILD WITH NEUROLOGICAL PROBLEM

Clinical history: The mode of onset (trauma, infection) gives information about the etiology of the ailment.

Developmental history: It is necessary to identify whether the ailment has impact on neurodevelopment of the child or not.

Physical examination: The child's posture, gait, symmetry and strength of spontaneous movement, behavior, orientation, hyperkinesis are to be observed. The child may show involuntary movements such as tremors, convulsions, athetosis, chorea, etc. The reflexes of the child are to be checked.

A neurological examination includes:

- Mental status and changes in mood and behavior
- Motor skills
- Sensory skills like hearing, speech, vision
- Balance and coordination
- Reflexes
- Functioning of the nerves.

Items including a tuning fork, flashlight, reflex hammer, ophthalmoscope, and needles are used to help diagnose brain tumors, infections such as encephalitis and meningitis, and diseases such as Parkinson's disease, Huntington's disease, amyotrophic lateral sclerosis (ALS), and epilepsy. Some tests require the services of a specialist to perform and analyze results.

Common Neurological Diagnostic Tests

Diagnostic tests and procedures are vital tools to rule out the presence of a neurological disorder or other medical condition. Researchers and physicians use a variety of diagnostic imaging techniques and chemical and metabolic analyses to detect, manage, and treat neurological disease. Some procedures are performed in specialized settings, conducted to determine the presence of a particular disorder or abnormality.

Electromyography (EMG)

EMG is used to diagnose nerve and muscle dysfunction and spinal cord disease. It assesses the health of the muscles and the nerves controlling the muscles. It records the electrical activity from the brain and/or spinal cord to a peripheral nerve root (found in the arms and legs) that controls muscles during contraction and at rest.

During an EMG, very fine wire electrodes are inserted into a muscle to assess changes in electrical voltage that occur during movement and when the muscle is at rest. In an EMG, a needle electrode is inserted through the skin into the muscle. The electrical activity detected by the electrode is displayed on an oscilloscope. After placement of the electrodes, the child may be asked to contract the muscle (e.g. by bending the arm). The waveform produced on the oscilloscope provides information about the ability of the muscle to respond when the nerves are stimulated. The electrodes are attached through a series of wires to a recording instrument. EMG testing helps to differentiate primary muscle conditions from muscle weakness caused by neurological disorders.

Nerve Conduction Velocity Test

A nerve conduction velocity test is usually performed in conjunction with an EMG. This test evaluates the speed of conduction of impulses through a nerve. The nerve is stimulated, usually with electrodes that are placed on the skin. One electrode stimulates the nerve with a very mild electrical impulse. The resulting electrical activity is recorded by the other electrodes. The distance between electrodes and the time it takes for electrical impulses to travel between electrodes are used to calculate the nerve conduction velocity. This test is used to diagnose nerve damage or destruction. Abnormal results can indicate peripheral neuropathy, damage to the spinal cord and other conditions.

Electroencephalogram (EEG)

EEG is a painless, risk-free test which monitors brain activity through the skull. An EEG test is used to help diagnose the presence and type of seizure disorders, head injuries, tumors, infections, degenerative diseases, causes of confusion, and metabolic disturbances that affect the brain. EEGs are also used to evaluate sleep disorders, monitor brain activity when a patient has been fully anesthetized or loses consciousness, and confirm brain death.

In an EEG, electrodes are placed on the scalp over multiple areas of the brain to detect and record patterns of electrical activity and check for abnormalities. The leads are attached to wires and carry the electrical energy of the brain to a machine for reading. A very low electrical current is sent through the electrodes and the baseline brain energy is recorded. Patients are then exposed to a variety of external stimuli—including bright or flashing light, noise or certain drugs—or are asked to open and close the eyes, or to change breathing patterns. The electrodes transmit the resulting changes in brain wave patterns. Since movement and nervousness can change brain wave patterns, patients usually recline in a chair or on a bed during the test, which takes up to an hour. Testing for certain disorders requires performing an EEG during sleep, which takes at least 3 hours.

Lumbar Puncture (LP)

LP is done to collect CSF, which protects the brain and spinal cord. The fluid is tested to detect any bleeding or brain hemorrhage, diagnose infection to the brain and/ or spinal cord, identify some cases of multiple sclerosis and other neurological conditions, and measure intracranial pressure.

Lumbar puncture is a procedure used to measure the pressure inside the head (intracranial pressure). During a lumbar puncture, a small hollow needle is inserted in the space between the lumbar (low back) vertebrae below the level of the spinal cord, and fluid is removed or pressure measurements are taken. A lumbar puncture can be performed using any of the L3-L4, L4-L5, or L5-S1 interspaces (Figs 16.3A and B). Lumbar puncture testing helps to determine if headaches or vision concerns are related to increased pressure or to test for causes of developmental problems.

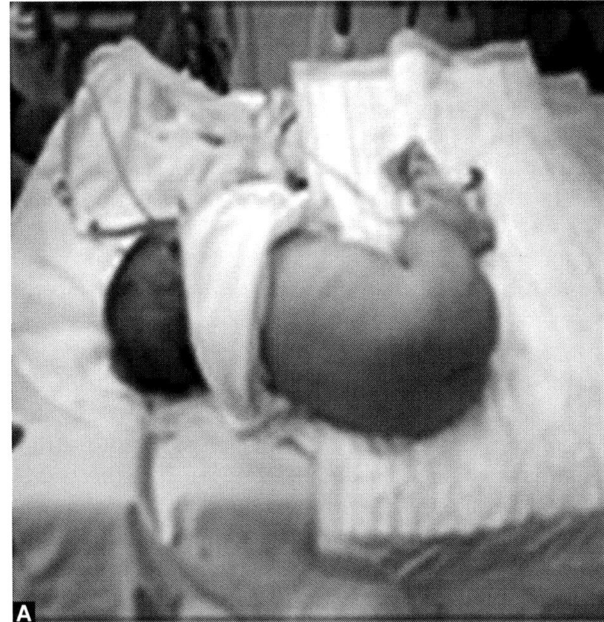

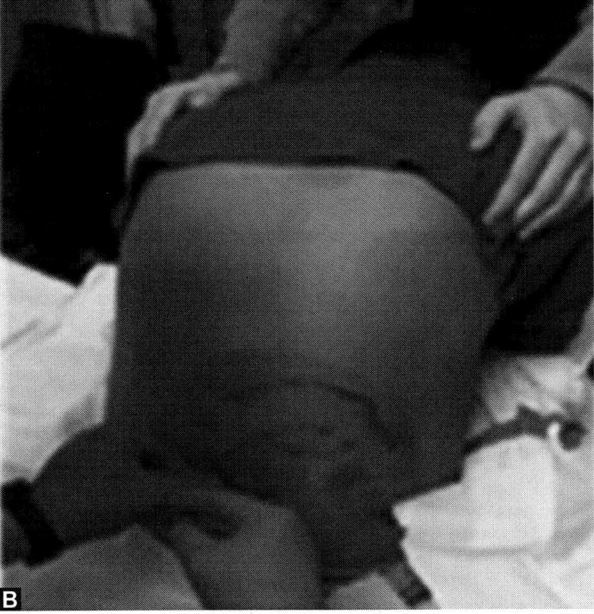

Figs 16.3A and B: Position of child is maintained to collect CSF

Sleep Tests

A sleep study (also called a polysomnogram) is a test that records your child's physical state during various stages of sleep and wakefulness. It provides data that are essential in evaluating sleep and sleep-related complaints, such as identifying sleep stages, body position, blood oxygen levels, respiratory events, muscle tone, heart rate and general sleep behavior. This information may be used to help diagnose causes of headaches, restless leg syndrome, muscle weakness, or fatigue.

Radiology Tests

Radiology tests (also known as imaging tests) are studies that produce pictures of what is going on inside the body. These tests use different forms of energy (X-rays, sound waves, radioactive particles, or magnetic fields) that are passed through the body and converted into images on a machine. These images can show normal body structure and function as well as abnormalities caused by diseases.

Genetic Tests

Genetic tests can often resolve uncertainty about genetic risks and confirm a diagnosis. For most patients, testing involves taking only a blood sample. A few tests involve taking hair, skin or other tissue samples. Genetic testing can identify many neurological disorders, including spina bifid. Genetic tests include the following:

- *Amniocentesis,* usually done at 14 to 16 weeks of pregnancy. Testing of a sample of the amniotic fluid in the womb for genetic defects (the fluid and the fetus have the same DNA) is done. Under local anesthesia, a thin needle is inserted through the woman's abdomen and into the womb. About 20 mL of fluid is withdrawn and sent to a lab for evaluation. Test results often take 1 to 2 weeks.
- *Chorionic villus sampling* or CVS, is performed by removing and testing a very small sample of the placenta during early pregnancy. The sample, which contains the same DNA as the fetus, is removed by catheter or fine needle inserted through the cervix or by a fine needle inserted through the abdomen. It is tested for genetic abnormalities and results are usually available within 2 weeks. CVS should not be performed after the 10th week of pregnancy.

Brain scans are imaging techniques used to diagnose tumors, blood vessel malformations, or hemorrhage in the brain. These scans are used to study organ function or injury or disease to tissue or muscle. Types of brain scans include computed tomography, magnetic resonance imaging, and positron emission tomography.

Computed tomography, also known as a CT scan, is a noninvasive, painless process used to produce rapid, clear two-dimensional images of organs, bones, and tissues. Neurological CT scans are used to view the brain and spine. They can detect bone and vascular irregularities, certain brain tumors and cysts, herniated disks, epilepsy, encephalitis, spinal stenosis (narrowing of the spinal canal), a blood clot or intracranial bleeding in patients with stroke, brain damage from head injury, and other disorders. Many neurological disorders share certain characteristics and a CT scan can aid in proper diagnosis by differentiating the area of the brain affected by the disorder.

Evoked potentials measure the electrical signals to the brain generated by hearing, touch, or sight. These tests are used to assess sensory nerve problems and confirm neurological conditions including multiple sclerosis, brain tumor, acoustic neuroma, and spinal cord injury. Evoked potentials are also used to test sight and hearing (specially in infants and young children), monitor brain activity among coma patients, and confirm brain death.

This test is painless and risk-free. Two sets of needle electrodes are used to test for nerve damage. One set of electrodes, which will be used to measure the electrophysiological response to stimuli, is attached to the patient's scalp using conducting paste. The second set of electrodes is attached to the part of the body to be tested. The physician then records the amount of time it takes for the impulse generated by stimuli to reach the brain. Under normal circumstances, the process of signal transmission is instantaneous.

DISORDERS OF CNS

Infection of CNS

Meningitis

Meningitis is an inflammation of the delicate membrane, meninges which cover the brain and spinal cord. The inflammation may be caused by infection with viruses, bacteria, or other microorganisms. Meningitis can be life-threatening because of the inflammation's proximity to the brain and spinal cord; therefore, the condition is classified as a medical emergency.

In bacterial meningitis, bacteria reach the meninges by one of two main routes—through the bloodstream or through direct contact between the meninges and either the nasal cavity or the skin. In most cases, meningitis follows invasion of the bloodstream by organisms that live upon mucous surfaces such as the nasal cavity. This is often in turn preceded by viral infections, which breakdown the normal barrier provided by the mucous surfaces.

The causative organism enters the bloodstream, crosses the blood-brain barrier, and triggers an inflammatory reaction in the meninges. Independent of the causative agent, inflammation of the subarachnoid and pia mater occurs. Increased intracranial pressure (ICP) results.

Meningeal infections generally originate in one of two ways—either through the bloodstream from other infections (cellulitis) or by direct extension (after a traumatic injury to the facial bones).

Pathophysiology

Once bacteria have entered the bloodstream, they enter the subarachnoid space in places where the blood-brain barrier is vulnerable—such as the choroid plexus. The current assumption is that high-grade bacteremia precedes meningitis and that bacteria invade from the bloodstream to the CNS. Alternatively, direct accesses to the CNS through dural defects or local infections are potential entrance routes.

By production and/or release of virulence factors into and stimulation of formation of inflammatory cytokines within the CNS, meningeal pathogens increase permeability of the blood-brain barrier, thus allowing protein and neutrophils to move into the subarachnoid space. There is then an intense subarachnoid space inflammatory response, which leads to many of the pathophysiologic consequences of bacterial meningitis, including cerebral edema and increased intracranial pressure.

Bacterial or meningococcal meningitis also occurs as an opportunistic infection in patients with acquired immunodeficiency syndrome (AIDS) and as a complication of Lyme disease. Bacterial meningitis is the most significant form. The common bacterial pathogens are *N. meningitidis* (meningococcal meningitis) and *S. pneumoniae*, accounting for 80% of cases of meningitis in adults. *H. influenzae* was once a common cause of meningitis in children, but, because of vaccination, infection with this organism is now rare in developed countries.

Types

Meningitis is either infectious (contagious) or noninfectious. Infectious meningitis is classified as viral, bacterial, fungal, depending on the type of organism causing the infection.

Viral meningitis, also called aseptic meningitis, is the most common type. It is rarely fatal and usually resolves with treatment. Meningitis develops in less than 1 in 1000 people who are infected with one of the viruses associated with the condition.

Bacterial meningitis is often severe and is considered a potential medical emergency. If left untreated, bacterial meningitis may be fatal or cause serious long-term complications. Because bacterial meningitis can progress rapidly, it is important to identify the bacteria and begin antibiotic treatment as soon as possible.

Bacterial infection in the ears, mouth, or sinuses can spread directly to the brain and spinal cord. Some types of bacteria are transmitted from person to person through secretions from the mouth and nose. Special features of different types of bacterial meningitis are—

- *Meningococcal meningitis:* Several different bacteria can cause meningitis. *N. meningitidis* is the one with the potential to cause large epidemics. In children and teens, meningococcus is the most common cause of bacterial meningitis. In adults, it is the second most common cause. Twelve serogroups of *N. meningitides* have been identified, six of which (A, B, C, W135, X and Y) can cause epidemics.

  Meningococcal bacteria may cause infection in a part of the body—the skin, gastrointestinal tract, or respiratory tract, for instance. For unknown reasons, the bacteria may then spread through the bloodstream to the nervous system. When it gets there, it causes meningococcal meningitis. Bacteria can also enter the nervous system directly after severe head trauma, surgery, or infection.

  The bacteria are transmitted from person-to-person through droplets of respiratory or throat secretions from carriers. The average incubation period is 4 days, but can range between 2 and 10 days.

  Meningococcemia, like many gram-negative blood infections, can cause disseminated intravascular coagulation (DIC), which is the inappropriate clotting of blood within the vessels. DIC can cause ischemic tissue damage when upstream thrombus obstructs blood flow and hemorrhage because clotting factors are exhausted. Small bleeds into the skin that cause the characteristic petechial rash. Rash appear with the 'star-like' shape. This is due to the release of toxins into the blood that breakdown the walls of blood vessels.

  The most important form of prevention is a vaccine against *N. meningitidis*. Different countries have different strains of the bacteria and therefore use different vaccines. Five serogroups, A, B, C, Y and W135 are responsible for virtually all cases of the disease in humans. Vaccines are currently available against all five strains, including the newest vaccine against serogroup B. The first vaccine to prevent meningococcal serogroup B (meningitis B) disease was approved by the European Commission on 22nd January, 2013.
- *Pneumococcal meningitis:* Pneumococcal meningitis is caused by bacteria called *S. pneumoniae*. These bacteria do not always cause meningitis. In some cases, they may cause other illnesses such as bacteremia, ear infections, pneumonia, sinus infections. Pneumococcal meningitis is transmitted from person-to-person. The bacteria are spread through the tiny droplets from an infected person's mouth, throat, or nose.
- *Staphylococcal meningitis:* It is caused by *Staphylococcus* bacteria (*S. aureus*). *S. epidermidis* bacteria, it usually develops as a surgery complication or an infection spread through the blood from another site. Risk factors include infections of heart valves, past infection of the brain, otitis media, pneumonia, septic lesions in scalp or skin, past meningitis due to spinal fluid shunts, recent brain surgery, spinal fluid shunt, trauma. Neonatal staphylococcal meningitis is often associated with umbilical sepsis, pyoderma or septicemia.

  Antibiotics should be started as soon as possible. Vancomycin is the first choice for suspected staphylococcal meningitis. Nafcillin is sometimes used. Often, treatment will include a search for, and removal of, possible sources of bacteria in the body. These include shunts or artificial heart valves.
- *H. influenzae* type b is a gram-negative bacterium that causes meningitis and acute respiratory

infections, mainly in children. In both developed and developing countries, it is an important cause of nonepidemic meningitis in young children, and is frequently associated with severe neurological sequelae, even if antibiotics are given promptly. There are six identifiable types of *H. influenza* bacteria, the most common one is *H. influenzae* type b, or Hib. Transmission occurs through direct contact with respiratory droplets from nasopharyngeal carrier. Neonates can acquire infection by aspiration of amniotic fluid or contact with genital tract secretions containing the bacteria. It is frequent in children between the ages of 3 and 12 months.

H. influenzae produces beta-lactamases, and it is also able to modify its penicillin-binding proteins, so it has gained resistance to the penicillin family of antibiotics. In severe cases, cefotaxime and ceftriaxone delivered directly into the bloodstream are the elected antibiotics, and, for the less severe cases, an association of ampicillin and sulbactam,cephalosporins of the second and third generation, or fluoroquinolones are preferred.

Macrolide antibiotics (e.g. clarithromycin) may be used in patients with a history of allergy to beta-lactam antibiotics. To protect infants and young children:

- HIB immunizations for infants and children are recommended by the American Academy of Pediatrics and the Advisory Committee on Immunization Practices.
- Several types of HIB vaccine are available for children ages 2 months and older.

• *Tuberculous meningitis (TBM):* TBM is caused by *Mycobacterium tuberculosis* (*M. tuberculosis*) and is the most common form of CNS tuberculosis (TB). TBM is associated with a high frequency of neurologic sequelae and mortality if not treated promptly.

The infection usually begins elsewhere in the body, usually in the lungs, and then travels through the bloodstream to the meninges where small abscesses (called microtubercles) are formed. When these abscesses burst, TB meningitis is the result. The clinical features of TBM are the result of basilar meningeal fibrosis and vascular inflammation. Classic features of bacterial meningitis, such as stiff neck and fever, may be absent. By the time treatment begins, there may be damage to brain tissue as well as nerves and blood vessels in the area around the brain. If treatment begins before the patient shows signs of brain damage, there is a good chance of making a full recovery. When allowed to progress without treatment, coma and death almost always ensue. In survivors of TBM, neurologic sequelae may occur that include mental retardation in children, sensorineural hearing loss, hydrocephalus, cranial nerve palsies, stroke-associated lateralizing neurological deficits, seizures, and coma.

In areas where TB prevalence is high, TB meningitis is most common in children aged 0 to 4 years. Diagnosis of TB meningitis is even more difficult than with other forms of bacterial meningitis. This is because it does not come on suddenly with classic meningitis symptoms.

TBM is treated with antitubercular drug (rifampicin, pyrazinamide, ethambutol and isoniazide). Treatment generally lasts for about a year, involving intensive treatment with three or four antibiotics at first and continually with two antibiotics for about 10 more months.

To prevent the development of TB meningitis, TB infections must be controlled. In communities where TB is common, the BCG (Bacillus Calmette-Guérin) vaccine can be used to control the spread of the disease. This vaccine is effective for controlling TB infections in young children.

Fungal meningitis develops in patients with conditions that compromise the effectiveness of their immune systems (e.g. HIV/AIDS, lupus, diabetes). Fungal meningitis occurs in 10% of patients with AIDS. *Cryptococcus neoformans* and *Candida albicans* are commonly involved in fungal meningitis.

Noninfectious meningitis may develop as a complication of another illness (e.g. mumps, tuberculosis, syphilis). A break in the skin and/or bones in the face or skull (caused by birth defect, brain surgery, head injury) can allow bacteria to enter the body.

Clinical Features

Early clinical features of bacterial meningitis are nonspecific and include fever, malaise and headache; and later on, meningismus (neck stiffness), photophobia, phonophobia and vomiting develop as signs of meningeal irritation. The infant may have projectile vomiting, shrill cry and a bulging frontanel. Seizures are a common symptom and may occur at the onset or during the course of the illness. There is generalized hypertonia and marked neck rigidity.

Small children often do not exhibit the aforementioned symptoms, and may only be irritable and look unwell (vacant stare). Persistent vomiting with fever, refusal to suck, poor cry, shock may be present in the neonates. The fontanel can bulge in infants aged up to 6 months. Other features that distinguish meningitis from less severe illnesses in young children are leg pain, cold extremities, and an abnormal skin color and maculopapular skin rashes.

The infection may trigger sepsis, a systemic inflammatory response syndrome of falling blood pressure, fast heart rate, high or abnormally low temperature, and rapid breathing. Seizures may be focal seizures, persistent seizures, late-onset seizures. Sometimes it is difficult to control with medication indicate a poorer long-term outcome.

Other signs of the disease include the presence of positive Kernig's sign or Brudziński sign.

Kernig's sign is assessed with the person lying supine, with the hip and knee flexed to 90°. In a person with a positive Kernig's sign, pain limits passive extension of the knee.

A positive Brudzinski's sign occurs when flexion of the neck causes involuntary flexion of the knee and hip.

'Jolt accentuation maneuver' helps determine whether meningitis is present in those reporting fever and headache. A person is asked to rapidly rotate the head horizontally; if this does not make the headache worse, meningitis is unlikely.

Laboratory Tests

The key to the diagnosis of bacterial meningitis is the proof of bacteria in the CSF by Gram staining or a positive bacterial culture. Detection rates in the CSF may be as high as 90%, while about 50% positive results are observed in blood cultures.

Management

Someone with bacterial meningitis will require urgent treatment in hospital. If they have severe meningitis, they may need to be treated in an *intensive care unit (ICU)*. A range of antibiotics can treat the infection, including penicillin, ampicillin, chloramphenicol and ceftriaxone, cefatoxime.

Initial therapy usually starts with third generation cephalosporins such as ceftriaxone (100 to 150 mg/kg/day/12 hourly) or cefatoxime (150 to 200 mg/kg/day 8 hourly) intravenously. If fever or signs of meningitis persist after 48 hours of therapy, CSF should be repeated and antibiotics reviewed. Antibiotic therapy is given 7 to 14 days depending upon the type of organisms. In case of Gram-negative bacteria the antibiotic treatment is continued up to 3 weeks. At the same time, patient may also be given oxygen, intravenous fluids. Monitoring of neurological status, management of raised intracranial pressure, fever and headache are important steps of treatment.

In meningococcal or pneumococcal meningitis, penicillin 4 to 5 lacs units/kg/day 6 hourly is also effective.

In staphylococcal meningitis, vancomycin may be the drug of choice, if penicillin resistance is suspected.

In *pseudomonas* infection, a combination of ceftazidime and an aminoglycosides (gentamycin, amikacin) is administered.

Management of seizure: Intravenous phenobarbitone 10 to 15 mg/kg is given to control seizure. Dilantin (7 mg/kg body weight) can also be used. Diazepam (2.5 μg – 0.3 mg may be given to reduce restlessness.

Adjuvant therapy: Adjuvant treatment with corticosteroids (usually dexamethasone) has shown some benefits, such as a reduction of hearing loss, and better short-term neurological outcomes. The likely mechanism is suppression of overactive inflammation.

Corticosteroids are recommended in the treatment of pediatric meningitis if the cause is *H. influenzae*, and only if given prior to the first dose of antibiotics (at least 15 minutes before). This helps to reduce sensorineural deafness and possibly internal hydrocephalus, and other behavioral disturbances. There is no role of dexamethasone in neonatal meningitis and other uses are controversial.

Encephalitis and Encephalopathy

Encephalitis is the medical term used for describing inflammation, irritation and swelling of the brain parenchyma due to an infection. It is a medical emergency that can be life-threatening without proper treatment. Encephalitis is manifested by neurologic dysfunction (e.g. altered mental status, seizures, behavior, motor or sensory deficits; speech or movement disorders; hemiparesis; or paresthesias).

Causes and Types

Encephalitis, in most cases, is caused by a viral infection. Exposure to viruses can occur through breathing in respiratory droplets from an infected person, contaminated food or drink, mosquito, tick, and other insect bites, skin contact.

Some common viruses known to cause the condition include polio, rabies virus, varicella zoster, mumps and rubella. Other groups of viruses include adenovirus, cytomegalovirus, West Nile virus and echovirus. Depending on the virus causing the disease and the mode of its transmission, encephalitis has been identified as different types:

- *Herpes simplex encephalitis:* It is caused by the herpes simplex virus (HSV1).

- *Japanese encephalitis:* It is caused by flavivirus, named after the yellow fever virus and was first identified in Japan. It is mainly transmitted through Culex mosquitoes.
- *West Nile encephalitis:* It is caused by a virus belonging to the Flaviviridae family and is spread through mosquitoes. Its main characteristic is high fever.
- *Tick-borne encephalitis:* Any virus that spreads through ticks to cause encephalitis is called tick-borne encephalitis.

Other causes of encephalitis include:

- Allergies to vaccination.
- Autoimmunity.
- Parasitic infection (roundworm, toxoplasma infection).
- The causes of encephalopathies may be hypoxia (brain tissue is deprived of oxygen and there is global loss of brain function).

The causes of encephalopathy are both numerous and varied such as infectious (bacteria, viruses, parasites), anoxic, metabolic (abnormalities of the water, electrolytes, vitamins, and other chemicals that adversely affect brain function), many types of toxic chemicals (mercury, lead, or ammonia), alterations in pressure within the brain (often from bleeding, tumors, or abscesses), renal failure and poor nutrition (inadequate vitamin B_1 intake), post- vaccinal reaction, hyperbilirubinemia in neonates, etc. Besides that hyperpyrexia, heat stroke, allergy, mercury or lead poisoning causes encephalopathies.

Risk Factors

Anybody can suffer from encephalitis, from children to elderly. But the risk is greater during the first few years of life. Additionally, people with a compromised immune system and those who have increased level of autoantibodies in them are at a greater risk.

Clinical Features

The virus reaches the brain tissue and causes inflammation. It causes swelling of the brain tissue and can even destroy the neurons. Sometimes, brain hemorrhage or bleeding is also seen.

The following symptoms may occur headache, confusion, disorientation, stiffness in the neck and the back. Papilledema, bulging fontanel, distended scalp veins, hyperventilation, Cheyne-Stokes respiration and bradycardia may develop due to sudden and severe rise of ICP. Other emergency symptoms may be:

- Loss of consciousness, poor responsiveness, stupor, coma.
- Muscle weakness or paralysis.
- Seizures.
- Severe headache.
- Sudden change in mental functions:
  - 'Flat' mood, lack of mood, or mood that is inappropriate for the situation.
  - Impaired judgment.
  - Inflexibility, extreme self-centeredness, inability to make a decision, or withdrawal from social interaction.
  - Less interest in daily activities.
  - Memory loss (amnesia), impaired short-term or long-term memory.

Pathophysiology

Normal neuronal activity requires a balanced environment of electrolytes, water, amino acids, excitatory and inhibitory neurotransmitters, and metabolic substrates. In addition, normal blood flow, normal temperature, normal osmolality, and physiologic pH are required for optimal brain function. Complex systems, such as those mediating arousal and awareness, and those involved in higher cognitive functions, are more likely to malfunction when the local milieu is deranged.

The inflammation causes the brain to swell, which leads to changes in the child's neurological condition, including mental confusion and seizures. The pathological changes occur in these cerebral conditions are nonspecific except HSV encephalitis and rabies, etc. Characteristic pathological changes found in Falciparum malaria. Diffuse cerebral edema, congestion and hemorrhages may be present in encephalitis. The neurons may show necrosis, and degeneration associated with neurophagocytosis. Meningial congestion, glial proliferation may be found with perivascular tissue necrosis and myelin breakdown. According to the type of infection demyelination, vascular and perivascular destruction, cerebrocortical involvement may occur.

Diagnosis

Most patients with encephalitis are diagnosed clinically. Usually it is manifested as neurologic dysfunction (e.g. depressed or altered level of consciousness, lethargy, seizure, ataxia, focal neurologic findings) and CNS inflammation. Emergency symptoms form the basis of suspecting encephalitis. But to diagnose its root cause, different tests might be needed. Diagnosis involves a combination of clinical examination with the help of brain scans mainly magnetic resonance imaging (MRI), blood examination for sugar, urea, electrolytes, metabolic products, electroencephalogram (EEG) along with the study of CSF. To exclude the exact cause and pathology of encephalitis toxicologic study, virology study, CT scan, urine examination can be done.

- Some viral encephalitis like herpes simplex encephalitis and Japanese encephalitis do have definitive diagnostic tests. Some of them can be detected by serological testing, where the presence of antibodies against the virus is detected. Tests that detect antibodies to a virus (serology tests).
- Test that detects tiny amounts of virus DNA (polymerase chain reaction (PCR)).

Treatment

The key to treatment of any encephalitis and encephalopathy is to understand the basic cause and thus design a treatment scheme to reduce or eliminate the cause(s). The goal of the treatment is to provide supportive care, which help the body to fight infection. Management includes:

- *Care of airway:* Airway clearance by maintaining position and suctioning is important. Moreover, patient needs administration of oxygen and cardiopulmonary insufficiency patient needs mechanical ventilation.
- *Maintenance of fluid-electrolyte balance:* Hydrotherapy is given to reduce hyperpyrexia. Dopamine may be used to combat shock. Sometimes mannitol or glycerol is used to decrease ICP.
- *Use of drugs:* Medications may include:
  - *Antiviral medications, such as acyclovir (Zovirax) and foscarnet (Foscavir)*: To treat herpes encephalitis or other severe viral infections (however, no specific antiviral drugs are available to fight encephalitis). Acyclovir 30 mg/kg/day in three divided doses is administered.
  - *Antibiotics*: If the infection is caused by certain bacteria.
  - *Antiseizure (such as phenytoin)*: To prevent seizures.
  - *Steroids (such as dexamethasone)*: To reduce brain swelling (in rare cases).
  - *Sedatives*: To treat irritability or restlessness.
  - *Acetaminophen*: For fever and headache.
  - *Antidote*: Specific antidote is administered in case of lead or other poisoning.
- *Physical care:* It includes eye, oral, skin, and bladder care.
- *Special care:* As the child recovers, physical, occupational, or speech therapy may be necessary to help the child regain muscle strength and/or speech skills.

  The extent of the problem is dependent on the severity of the encephalitis and the presence of other organ system problems that could affect the child. In severe cases, a breathing machine may be required to help the child breathe easier.

Prevention

Prevention is the best way to control outbreaks. Vaccination is available against tick-borne and Japanese encephalitis and should be considered by individuals who are at high-risk. Most of these viruses are spread by mosquito bites, so control of mosquitoes breeding is very important. In India the monsoon season is the encephalitis season.

Vaccinate animals to prevent encephalitis caused by the rabies virus.

Human vaccinations that are available include A vaccination to prevent a form of viral encephalitis, viz. herpes zoster, measles.

ACUTE FLACCID PARALYSIS (AFP)

Flaccid paralysis is a clinical manifestation characterized by weakness or paralysis and reduced muscle tone without other obvious cause (e.g. trauma). WHO defines AFP syndrome as 'characterized by rapid onset of weakness of an individual's extremities, often including weakness of the muscles of respiration and swallowing, progressing to maximum severity within 1 to 10 days. The term 'flaccid' indicates the absence of spasticity or other signs of disordered CNS motor tracts such as hyperflexia, clonus, or extensor plantar responses' (World Health Organization 1993 WHO/MNH/EPI/93.3. Geneva).

Common causes of AFP in India include poliomyelitis, Guillain–Barré syndrome, transverse myelitis and traumatic neuritis. The differential diagnosis of acute flaccid paralysis includes paralytic poliomyelitis, Guillain-Barré syndrome and transverse myelitis and less common traumatic neuritis. Distinguishing characteristics of paralytic polio and others are given in Table 16.2.

AFP Surveillance

Surveillance is the collection, analysis, interpretation and dissemination of information about a selected health event. Health officials use the information to plan, implement and evaluate health programs and activities. All cases of AFP cases should be reported, regardless of the final diagnosis. According to WHO the role of the laboratory in AFP surveillance.

- To confirm polio by virus isolation. Isolation and identification of poliovirus from feces is the best current method to confirm the diagnosis of poliomyelitis.

Table 16.2: Differential diagnosis of acute flaccid paralysis

Signs and symptoms	*Poliomyelitis*	*Guillain–Barré syndrome*	*Transverse myelitis*	*Traumatic neuritis*
Progression of paralysis	24 to 28 hours onset to full paralysis	From hours to 10 days	From hours to 4 to 5 days	From hours to days
Fever	Yes (at onset of AFP), gone the following days	Not common	Rarely present	Yes. Present before, during and after AFP
Flaccidity	Acute, asymmetrical. More proximal than distal	Acute, symmetrical and distal	Acute, lower limbs, symmetrical	Acute, asymmetric limb
Sensory sign and symptoms	No sensory change, severe myalgia and backache	Weakness, cramp, tingling, paresthesia of palms and soles	Anesthesia of lower limbs with sensory level	Pain in gluteal region
Muscle tone	Diminished	Diminished	Diminished in lower limbs	Diminished in limb
Deep tendon reflexes	Decreased or absent	Absent	Absent early, hyper-reflexia late	Decreased or absent
Cranial nerve	Only in case of bulbar and bulbospinal	Often present, affecting VII, IX, X, XI, XII cranial nerves	Absent	Absent
Respiratory difficulties	Only in case of bulbar and bulbospinal	In severe cases	Sometimes	Absent
CSF	High WBCs Normal or slightly increased protein	Less WBCs High protein	Normal WBCs Normal or slightly increased protein	Normal WBCs and protein
Bladder dysfunction	Rare	Transient	Present	Never
EMG: 3 weeks	Abnormal	Normal	Normal	Normal

- To trace the origin of a case. Molecular techniques are available to characterize fully the poliovirus. Maintaining reference bank of the molecular structure of known viruses allows the geographic origin on new isolates to be traced. The laboratory will also determine whether isolated viruses are wild or vaccine-like.
- To certify that polio has been eradicated. In addition to AFP surveillance, this may include stool surveys of healthy children in high-risk areas and environmental surveillance.
- To assess vaccine potency and efficacy the laboratory can perform potency tests on polio vaccine if circumstances indicate possible failure. A laboratory might participate in epidemiological serosurvey if knowledge of the antibody status of the population is important.

AFP surveillance focuses on children below 15 years because poliomyelitis rarely occur in older children. Steps of AFP surveillance include immediate, weekly and monthly reporting of AFP cases, including zero reports, case investigation, stool specimen collection and outbreak response immunization.

Special effort is made to obtain 2 stool samples (at least 24 hours apart) from AFP cases within 14 days of paralysis onset. Adequate specimen can be said as adequate volume (8–10 g) arriving WHO accredited laboratory in good conditions. Good condition means no desiccation, no leakage, adequate documentation, and evidence that the cold chain was maintained (presence of ice in collecting box). The specimens should be sent by the fastest, most reliable means of transport available. Specimens must arrive at the laboratory within 72 hours of collection, or they should be frozen at –20 °C.

Poliomyelitis

Discussed chapter 20.

Guillain–Barré Syndrome (GBS)

(Infective Polyneuritis)

Guillain–Barré syndrome is a disorder causing demyelization and axonal degeneration resulting in acute, ascending and progressiv neuropathy, characterized by weakness, paresthesia and hyporeflexia.

GBS is a disorder in which the body's immune system attacks part of the PNS. Guillain-Barré is called a syndrome rather than a disease because it is not clear that a specific disease-causing agent is involved. It is an acute polyneuropathy, a disorder affecting the PNS. GBS can be described as a collection of clinical syndromes that manifests as an acute inflammatory polyradiculoneuropathy with resultant weakness and diminished reflexes. The disease is usually triggered by an infection (2 to 4 weeks after viral infection). GBS can affect anybody, but common age group is 5 to 12 years. It can strike at any age and both sexes are equally prone to the disorder.

Causes

All forms of Guillain–Barré syndrome are autoimmune diseases, due to an immune response to foreign antigens that mistargets host nerve tissues through a mechanism known as molecular mimicry. Neurological manifestations usually begin postviral infection such as Epstein-Barr virus infection (infectious mononucleosis), mumps, measles, and those caused by echo, coxsackie and influenza viruses, rabies virus. Administration of neural vaccine for rabies can cause GBS. Severe form of acute motor axonal neuropathy has strong association with Campylobacter infection.

Pathophysiology

The disorder is most likely an autoimmune process. When Guillain-Barré is preceded by a viral or bacterial infection, it is possible that the virus has changed the nature of cells in the nervous system so that the immune system treats them as foreign cells. Damage results when the body's attempt to defend itself produces antibodies that strip away the myelin that covers and protects the nerves. Sensitized T-lymphocytes cooperate with B-lymphocytes to produce antibodies to fight the virus have taken on a new attack of not only the virus, but also of the myelin sheath. Due to molecular mimicry of the myelin and virus components, the body tends to react against itself as a cross reaction to the infecting organism. It may contribute to a nerve-conduction block leading to muscle paralysis, which may be accompanied by sensory or autonomic disturbances.

In diseases in which the peripheral nerves' myelin sheaths are injured or degraded, the nerves cannot transmit signals efficiently. That is why the muscles begin to lose their ability to respond to the brain's commands, commands that must be carried through the nerve network. The brain also receives fewer sensory signals from the rest of the body, resulting in an inability to feel textures, heat, pain, and other sensations. Alternately, the brain may receive inappropriate signals that result in tingling, 'crawling-skin,' or painful sensations. Because the signals to and from the arms and legs must travel the longest distances they are most vulnerable to interruption. Therefore, muscle weakness and tingling sensations usually first appear in the hands and feet and progress upwards. In mild cases, nerve axon function remains intact and recovery can be rapid if

Contd...

Contd...

remyelination occurs. In severe cases, axonal damage occurs, and recovery depends on the regeneration of this important tissue.

Physiologic effects of the disease include inflammation, demyelination of peripheral nerves, loss of granular bodies and degeneration of the basement membrane of the Schwann cell. The myelin is made up of Schwann cells and these cells will rejuvenate, but may take from several months to a year to completely recover.

Clinical Features

Ascending paralysis, weakness beginning in the feet and hands and migrating towards the trunk, diminished reflexes, and paresthesia, are the most typical symptoms, and some subtypes cause change in sensation or pain, as well as dysfunction of the autonomic nervous system. Most patients complain of paresthesias, numbness, or similar sensory changes. Paresthesias generally begin in the toes and fingertips, progressing upward but generally not extending beyond the wrists or ankles. Pain associated with GBS is most severe in the shoulder girdle, back, buttocks, and thighs and may occur with even the slightest movements. The pain is often described as aching or throbbing in nature.

These symptoms can increase in intensity until certain muscles cannot be used at all, and when severe, the person is almost totally paralyzed. In these cases the disorder is life-threatening—potentially interfering with breathing (the respiratory muscles are affected) and, at times, can include the following tachycardia, bradycardia, facial flushing, paroxysmal hypertension, orthostatic hypotension, anhidrosis and/or diaphoresis, urinary retention.

Respiratory insufficiency may occur if the intercostal muscles are paralyzed. Typical respiratory complaints in GBS include dyspnea on exertion, shortness of breath, difficulty swallowing, slurred speech.

Diagnosis

The diagnosis of GBS depends on findings such as rapid development of muscle paralysis, areflexia, absence of fever, and a likely inciting event. Cerebrospinal fluid analysis shows a characteristic albumin—cytological dissociation. The protein is elevated equal or more than 45 mg/dL. In almost 80% patients but cell number is normal. As opposed to infectious causes, this is an elevated protein level (100–1000 mg/dL), without an accompanying increased cell count (absence of pleocytosis). A sustained increased white blood cell count may indicate an alternative diagnosis such as infection.

Several disorders have symptoms similar to those found in Guillain-Barré, so it should be distinguished from others. Signs and symptoms of poliomyelitis (asymmetric paralysis), polymyositis, transverse myelitis, etc. need to be elicited. The quickness with which the symptoms appear (in other disorders, muscle weakness may progress over months rather than days or weeks). In Guillain-Barré, reflexes such as knee jerks are usually lost. Because the signals traveling along the nerve are slower, a nerve conduction velocity (NCV) test can give a clue to aid the diagnosis.

Blood examination for sugar, urea, electrolytes, liver function tests (LFTs), creatine phosphokinase (CPK) level, erythrocyte sedimentation rate (ESR) and metabolic products are useful guideline for confirmation of the diagnosis.

Management

All patients who have GBS should be admitted to a hospital for close observation for respiratory compromise, cranial nerve dysfunction, and autonomic instability. Autonomic nervous system dysfunction may manifest as fluctuations in blood pressure, cardiac dysrhythmias, gastrointestinal pseudo-obstruction, and urinary retention. Prophylaxis for deep venous thrombosis should be provided because patients frequently are immobilized for many weeks.

The care of a patient with GBS is challenging for the health care team. By incorporating both physical and psychological care in a patient with GBS, the critical care nurse can adapt to the changing plan of care that accompanies this diagnosis. Because the disease normally starts with a motor weakness and ends with the patient requiring months or even years of rehabilitation, the patient should be prepared for this extended period of treatment. It is only by collaboration of the entire health care team that such tasks as diagnosis, treatment, therapy, and pharmaceutical interventions are performed in such a way to help the patient regain a previous level of independence. Treatments for GBS include:

- Good nursing care
- Physiotherapy
- Plasmapheresis
- Immunoglobulins
- Counseling/support.

Supportive care is the cornerstone of successful management of the patients with acute condition.

Physiotherapy—Often, even before recovery begins, passive exercises are of the patient's limbs are needed to help keep the muscles flexible and strong and to prevent venous sludging (the build up of red blood cells in veins, which could lead to reduced blood flow) in the limbs which could result in deep vein thrombosis.

Subsequent treatment consists of attempting to reduce the body's attack on the nervous system, either by plasmapheresis, filtering antibodies out of the bloodstream. Plasmapheresis hastens recovery when used within two weeks of the onset of symptoms. In case of respiratory failure, assisted ventilation may be warranted.

Administering intravenous immunoglobulins (IVIg is done in GBS, to neutralize harmful antibodies and inflammation causing disease. IVIg has equivalent efficacy to plasmapheresis when started within two weeks of the onset of symptoms, and has fewer complications. IVIg is usually used first because of its ease of administration (300 to 400 mg/kg/day for 5 days) and safety profile. Its use is not without risk; occasionally it causes hepatitis, or in rare cases, renal failure if used for longer than 5 days. These two treatments are equally effective and a combination of the two is not significantly better than either alone.

Glucocorticoids have not been found to be effective in GBS.

Other treatment: All patients should be given subcutaneous fractionated or unfractionated heparin and support stockings until they are able to walk independently to prevent deep vein thrombosis. If a prolonged bedridden period is anticipated and a tracheostomy has already been performed, oral anticoagulant treatment with warfarin Coumadin can be started.

Pain and sensory symptoms are reported in majority of patients with GBS which may be treated effectively with opioid analogues though sedation and bowel hypomotility may become a problem. Other drugs, such as gabapentin, carbamazepine, acetaminophen, NSAIDs, and tricyclic antidepressants also can be tried.

Few patients develop respiratory failure due to paralysis of the diaphragm, the muscle most important for breathing. Any patients exhibiting clinical signs of respiratory compromise to any degree also should be admitted to an ICU. Admission to the ICU should be considered for all patients with labile dysautonomia, a forced vital capacity of less than 20 mL/kg, or severe bulbar palsy. Competent intensive care includes the following features:

- *Respiratory therapy:* Ineffective breathing pattern, ineffective airway clearance, related to respiratory muscle weakness or paralysis, decreased cough reflex, immobilization. Intensive care observation includes early initiation and insertion of an airway should the patient's ventilatory strength decline. An emergency tracheostomy kit should be placed at the bedside of a patient with potential respiratory complications due to paralysis ascending to the abdominal and thoracic muscles. Maintain airway patency and provide for ventilator and tracheostomy care. The level of sensory and motor function and/or deficit needs to be monitored on an ongoing basis to determine possible progression of the syndrome.

- *Cardiac monitoring:* Life-threatening paralysis of the respiratory muscles is often punctuated by the presence of cardiac involvement. This ranges from variations in blood pressure to involvement of the myocardium and potentially fatal arrhythmias. It is necessary to recognize the potentially fatal cardiovascular complications associated with the GBS and treat them accordingly.
- *Safe nutritional supplementation:* Nasogastric or gastric tube feeding should be instituted early and slowly. High energy (40 to 45 nonprotein kcal) and high protein diet (2 to 2.5 g/kg) have been recommended so has to reduce muscle wasting and assist respiratory weaning. Continuous enteral feeding seems to be better tolerated than bolus feeding in these patients.
- Monitoring for infectious complications (e.g. pneumonia, urinary tract infections, septicemia).

Counseling and support: Emotional problems also need to be addressed. This is why a specialized nursing facility is utilized rather than a typical nursing home. The beginning stages of this syndrome can be very frightening. Most patients with GBS were typically healthy. To find themselves paralyzed and helpless, being constantly monitored by machines and tubes, can be emotionally overwhelming. Counseling can help relieve the emotional difficulties an individual is feeling because of sudden paralysis and dependence on others. Counseling often is suggested to reassure individuals diagnosed with GBS or CIDP (chronic inflammatory demyelinating polyradicalneuropathy) and to help individuals with GBS feel positive about their treatment and recovery. Both victims and families often greatly benefit from support groups. It is helpful for both patient and family to know that most GBS patients get better. Most patients eventually walk and many can ultimately resume a normal life.

Following the acute phase, treatment often consists of rehabilitation with the help of a multidisciplinary team to focus on improving activities of daily living (ADLs). Recovery is complete in most cases, but may take 6 months to 2 years for restoration of full functions. Occupational therapists may offer equipment (such as wheelchair and special cutlery) to help the patient achieve ADL independence. Physiotherapy helps in helping patients with GBS to regain strength, endurance, and gait quality, as well as helping them prevent contractures, bedsores, and cardiopulmonary difficulties. Speech and language therapists help regain speaking and swallowing abilities, specially if the patient was intubated or received a tracheostomy.

What is Plasmapheresis?

Plasmapheresis is called plasma exchange. Plasmapheresis may speed the recovery GBS if done within 2 weeks of diagnosis. The process of plasmapheresis works like this: fresh plasma is given to the patient in an effort to dilute the insulting antibodies and give the nerve fibers a rest from 'attack,' allowing them to begin to regenerate. This technique seems to reduce the severity and duration of the Guillain-Barré episode. This may be because plasmapheresis can remove antibodies and other immune cell-derived factors that could contribute to nerve damage. The patient is typed and screened for the plasma and the nurse would follow basic guidelines for giving plasma and watching for a possible transfusion reaction as with any other blood products.

Nursing Interventions

The natural course of GBS is generally self-limited with gradual recovery in majority of the subjects. There is no specific treatment for GBS. Treatment must be based on the presented symptoms. The main nursing goals are to provide optimal supportive care and to anticipate and prevent complications. These patients are vulnerable to rapid deterioration and needs hospitalization for observation. The nursing interventions include:

- Turn and reposition the patient, and encourage coughing and deep breathing.
- Monitor for signs of respiratory distress; If respiratory failure becomes imminent, take necessary steps to establish an emergency airway with an endotracheal tube.
- Assess for extent of involve paralysis; perform passive range of motion exercises within the patient's pain limits. Passive range of motion 3 to 4 times per day is most advantageous for the immobilized patient. In acute phase it should include individual program of gentle exercises involving isometric, isotonic, isokinetic, and manual resistive and progressive resistive exercises. Rehabilitation should be focused on proper limb positioning, posture, orthotics.

- Give meticulous skin care to prevent skin-breakdown and contractures. It is needed to prevent pressure sores, related to muscle weakness, paralysis, impaired sensation, changes in nutrition, incontinence.
- Imbalanced nutrition, less than body requirements related to difficulty chewing, swallowing, fatigue, limb paralysis. Assess for swallowing difficulties. To prevent aspiration, test the gag reflex and elevate the head of the bed before giving the patient anything to eat.
- To prevent thrombophlebitis, apply antiembolism stockings and give prophylactic anticoagulants as ordered.
- If the patient has facial paralysis, give eye and mouth care every 4 hours.
- Monitor fluids and electrolytes as needed; bed pan is to be offered every 3 to 4 hours to monitor intake and output regularly. Prevention/ correction of constipation is important. Evaluate precautions to prevent complications; provide physical/ psychological support as needed.
- Mental support (with the purpose to reduce anxiety and depression) as well as education through all stages of the recovery depend on the needs of the patient and the patient's family. Excellent communication skills are required to relay empathy, accurately assess pain and recognize patients' capabilities.
- Provide diversions for the patient, such as televisions, family visits, or listening to the radio. Provide emotional support to the patient and his family.

Prognosis

Guillain-Barré syndrome can be a devastating disorder because of its sudden and unexpected onset. Most people reach the stage of greatest weakness within the first 2 weeks after symptoms appear, and by the third week of the illness 90% of all patients are at their weakest. The recovery period may be as little as a few weeks or as long as a few years. About 30% of those with Guillain-Barré still have a residual weakness after 3 years. About 3% may suffer a relapse of muscle weakness and tingling sensations many years after the initial attack. They may have some residual disability and handicaps.

NEURAL TUBE DEFECTS AND CSF CIRCULATION PROBLEM

Hydrocephalus

The term hydrocephalus is derived from the Greek words 'hydro' meaning water and 'cephalus' meaning head. As the name implies 'water on the brain', is a medical condition in which there is an abnormal accumulation of CSF in the ventricles, or cavities, of the brain. This may cause increased intracranial pressure inside the skull and progressive enlargement of the head. This widening creates potentially harmful pressure on the tissues of the brain. It is more common in infants, although it can occur in older adults.

CSF is formed by the choroid plexus of the four ventricles and by filtration from capillaries. Normally, CSF flows through the ventricles (through the foramen of Monro to 3rd ventricle, through the aqueduct of Sylvius to 4th ventricle). By way of the foramina of Luschka and foramen of Magendie CSF exits into cisterns of subarachnoid space (closed spaces that serve as reservoirs) at the base of the brain, bathes the surfaces of the brain and spinal cord, and then reabsorbs into the bloodstream. CSF has three important life-sustaining functions: (1) to keep the brain tissue buoyant, acting as a cushion or 'shock absorber'; (2) to act as the vehicle for delivering nutrients to the brain and removing waste; and (3) to flow between the cranium and spine and compensate for changes in intracranial blood volume.

Pathophysiology

CSF continuously circulates through the brain, its ventricles and the spinal cord and is continuously drained away into the circulatory system. About 20 mL of CSF is secreted in an hour and its turnover is 3 to 4 times in a day. The balance between production and absorption of CSF is critically important. Because CSF is made continuously, medical conditions that block its normal flow or absorption will result in an over-accumulation of CSF. Subarachnoid hemorrhage, meningitis, head injuries, and elevated levels of CSF protein all cause scarring and fibrosis in the subarachnoid space. Ventricles are dilated, at times unevenly. Periventricular oozing starts due to disruption in ependymal lining of ventricles, and subependymal edema occurs and white matter is compressed. Compression of the brain by the accumulating fluid eventually may cause neurological symptoms such as convulsions, intellectual disability and epileptic seizures. Cortex generally preserved till late but cortical atrophy may occur. The resulting pressure of the fluid against brain tissue is what causes hydrocephalus.

Generally infant's skull enlarges due to accumulation of fluid in the ventricles since the sutures are not closed, and the bones are soft and yielding under pressure. The pressure upon the brain tends to decrease due to cranial enlargement.

Causes

Hydrocephalus can be caused by impaired cerebrospinal fluid flow, reabsorption, or excessive CSF production. Hydrocephalus may result from inherited genetic abnormalities (such as the genetic defect that causes aqueductal stenosis) or developmental disorders (such as those associated with neural tube defects including spina bifida and encephalocele).

- The most common cause of hydrocephalus is CSF flow obstruction, hindering the free passage of cerebrospinal fluid through the ventricular system and subarachnoid space (e.g. stenosis of the cerebral aqueduct or obstruction of the interventricular foramina) secondary to tumors, hemorrhages, infections (meningitis, toxoplasmosis, cytomegalovirus) or congenital malformations.
- Hydrocephalus can also be caused by overproduction of cerebrospinal fluid (relative obstruction) (e.g. choroid plexus papilloma, villous hypertrophy).

Based on its underlying mechanisms, hydrocephalus can be classified into communicating and non-communicating (obstructive). Both forms can be either congenital or acquired.

Types

Communicating hydrocephalus, also known as non-obstructive hydrocephalus—communicating hydrocephalus occurs when the flow of CSF is blocked after it exits the ventricles. This form is called communicating because the CSF can still flow between the ventricles, which remain open. It has been theorized that impaired CSF reabsorption is due to functional impairment of the arachnoidal granulations (Pacchioni's granulations), which are located along the superior sagittal sinus and is the site of CSF reabsorption back into the venous system. Various neurologic conditions may result in communicating hydrocephalus, including subarachnoid/ intraventricular hemorrhage, meningitis and congenital absence of arachnoid villi. Scarring and fibrosis of the subarachnoid space following infectious, inflammatory, or hemorrhagic events can also prevent resorption of CSF, causing diffuse ventricular dilatation.

Noncommunicating hydrocephalus, also called 'obstructive' hydrocephalus—occurs when the flow of CSF is blocked along one or more of the narrow passages connecting the ventricles. One of the most common causes of hydrocephalus is 'aqueductal stenosis.' In this case, hydrocephalus results from a narrowing of the aqueduct of Sylvius, a small passage between the 3rd and 4th ventricles in the middle of the brain. This block may be partial or complete, and results accumulation of CSF within the ventricles. This condition is called internal hydrocephalus and it results in increased CSF pressure. The production of CSF continues, even when the passages that normally allow it to exit the brain are blocked. Consequently, fluid builds inside the brain, causing pressure that dilates the ventricles and compresses the nervous tissue. Compression of the nervous tissue usually results in irreversible brain damage. If the skull bones are not completely ossified when the hydrocephalus occurs, the pressure may also severely enlarge the head.

Noncommunicating hydrocephalus may occur due to congenital reasons or it may be acquired.

- Congenital causes include – stenosis of aqueduct of Sylvius.
  - The foramina of Magendie and Luschka may be occluded.
  - (Dandy-Walker syndrome).
  - Meningomyelocele.
  - Arnold-Chiari malformation.
- Acquired causes include complications of premature birth such as:
  - Intraventricular hemorrhage.
  - Diseases such as meningitis, tumors (medullo-blstoma, craniopharyngioma, astrocytoma).
  - Traumatic head injury, or subarachnoid hemorrhage, which block the exit of CSF from the ventricles to the cisterns or eliminate the passageway for CSF into the cisterns.

Clinical Features

Symptoms of hydrocephalus vary with age (fontanelle open/closed, cranial sutures fused/not), type of disease and its progression, and individual differences in tolerance to the condition.

In infancy, the most obvious indication of hydrocephalus is often a rapid increase in head circumference or an unusually large head size. Widen fontanelles and sutures become widely separated (Figs 16.4A and B). Children may also exhibit the Macewen sign, in which a 'cracked pot' sound is noted on percussion of the head. Other symptoms may include high pitch cry, vomiting, sleepiness, irritability and seizures. The infant becomes increasingly helpless and less able to raise his head. The neck muscles are underdeveloped due to lack of use. The eyes may have a wide bridge between them. The eyes become little protruded and shows downward deviation (also called 'sunsetting' eyes), The sclera are visible above the iris, since the upper lid is retracted by the taut skin over the bulging forehead. These infants have little resistance to infection. Affect and normal responses may be diminished.

Older children may experience different symptoms because their skulls cannot expand to accommodate the build up of CSF. Symptoms may include headache (on awakening in the morning), vomiting, nausea, papilledema

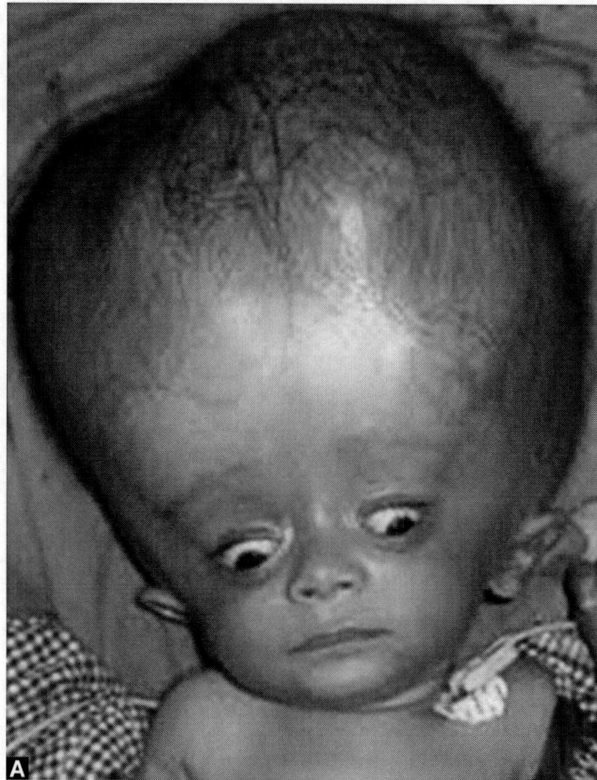

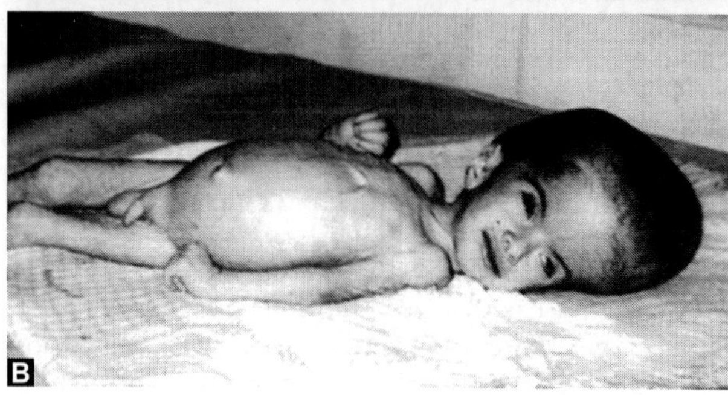

Figs 16.4A and B: Child with hydrocephalus

(swelling of the optic disk which is part of the optic nerve), blurred or double vision, sunsetting of the eyes, problems with balance, poor coordination, gait disturbance, urinary incontinence, slowing or loss of developmental progress, lethargy, drowsiness, irritability, or other changes in personality or cognition including memory loss. As the child's condition deteriorates, his body becomes emaciated, often weighing less than the head.

Diagnostic Evaluation

Head circumference measurements, repeated over time, may show that the head is getting bigger.

A head CT scan is one of the best tests for identifying hydrocephalus. CT scan and MRI confirms hydrocephalus and reveal ventricular enlargement or any structural defect, if present. Other tests that may be done include:

- Arteriography
- Brain scan using radioisotopes
- Cranial ultrasound (an ultrasound of the brain). Echoencephalopathy is exclusively done for neonates, because of open fontanelle
- Lumbar puncture and examination of the cerebrospinal fluid (rarely done)
- *Skull X-rays:* It shows a large skull with wide cranial sutures.

Treatment

- The goals of treatment are:
  - To reduce intracranial pressure
  - To reduce or prevent brain damage by improving the flow of CSF
  - To prevent and manage complications.

Medical treatment in hydrocephalus is used to delay surgical intervention. It may be tried in premature infants with posthemorrhagic hydrocephalus (in the absence of acute hydrocephalus). Normal CSF absorption may resume spontaneously during this interim period. Medical treatment is not effective in long-term treatment of chronic hydrocephalus. It may induce metabolic consequences and thus should be used only as a temporizing measure. Medications affect CSF dynamics by the following mechanisms:

- *Decreasing CSF secretion by the choroid plexus:* Acetazolamide and furosemide.
- *Increasing CSF reabsorption:* Isosorbide (effectiveness is questionable).

Since the causes of noncommunicating hydrocephalus are mechanical, treatment is surgery to remove a blockage. Modern surgery bypasses the point of obstruction by attempting to shunt the CSF to another area where it will be absorbed and finally excreted.

Nursing Care of a Child with Increased ICP (Table 16.3)

Shunt Insertion

In most cases, a shunt is surgically inserted. The shunt is a drainage system made of a long tube with a valve. The valve helps CSF flow at a normal rate and in the right direction. The most common treatment now in use is a shunt from one lateral ventricle into the circulating blood by way of the internal jugular vein to the right atrium of the heart or superior vena cava just proximal to it. Sometimes one

Table 16.3: Nursing care of a child with increased ICP		
Nursing diagnosis	*Nursing outcome*	*Nursing intervention with rationale*
Rise of ICP and prone to infection	The patient will not show further complication The patient will maintain and improve current level of consciousness (LOC) The patient will remain free from signs and symptoms of infection	Assess head circumference, fontanelles, cranial sutures, papillary reaction, reflexes, cranial nerve function and LOC. Vital signs to be checked in regular interval (15 min–2 h). Rise of temperature may increase the ICP, so early reporting and steps to reduce temperature are needed
Acute pain	The patient will exhibit no signs of pain or agitation.	Pain management by administration of analgesics. Environmental management: Alleviation of pain or a reduction in pain to a level of comfort that is acceptable to the patient. Manipulation of the patient's surroundings for promotion of optimal comfort
Imbalanced nutrition: Less than body requirements	The patient will show no signs of malnutrition	• Give small, frequent feedings to decrease the risk of vomiting. • Fix the feeding schedule. To avoid vomiting, necessary care should be given before feeding. Avoid movement, after the infant has been fed. Upright position and proper holding of the head during feeding is important. Assisting with or providing a balanced dietary intake of foods and fluids. Place the child on his side to prevent aspiration of vomitus
Risk for infection as the child is unable to move or lift head	Free from infection (chest, skin, etc.) The patient will remain free from signs and symptoms of infection	• Monitor vital signs and skin condition. Frequent change of position to avoid hypostatic pneumonia, and pressure lesion (head and ears). • Place the head on water pillow or pad (lamb's woolm or sponge rubber). • If pressure areas develop, great care to be given to prevent infection (infants debilitated condition might result in septicemia).
Impaired gas exchange	The patient will maintain adequate ventilation and oxygenation	Respiratory monitoring, oxygen therapy, airway management; collection and analysis of patient data to ensure airway patency and adequate gas exchange; administration of oxygen and monitoring of facilitation of patency of air passages
Risk of trauma due to huge head and poor neck muscles	The patient will remain free from accidental hazard	Carefully support the head during lifting to avoid trauma. Head and body to be rotated together, bringing no strain upon the neck
Anxiety	Family members will identify measures to reduce anxiety	• Minimizing apprehension, dread, foreboding, or uneasiness related to an unidentified source or anticipated danger by proper counseling. • Explain diagnostic procedures to the parents. • Encourage them to help in the infant's care.

end of the tube is inserted in the brain, and the other end is typically inserted into the abdomen. Excess fluid then drains from the brain and out the other end of the tube, where it is more easily absorbed. The shunt is typically needed permanently and has to be monitored regularly.

Shunt and Insertion of Shunt

A shunt is a mechanical device, made up of silicone elastomer (plastic) and are often impregnated with barium, designed to transport the excess CSF from or near the point of obstruction to a reabsorption site and it is implanted under the skin. The shunt performs two functions. It allows fluid to go only in one direction and the valve allows fluid to flow out only when the pressure in the head has exceeded some value (usually referred to as the 'opening pressure'). This system regulates the amount of the CSF in the body so that not too much is taken, nor too little.

The shunt has 3 components (Fig. 16.5). The first portion is called the shunt catheter or proximal portion of the shunt. This is a small narrow tube (catheter), which is implanted into the ventricle of the brain, above where the obstruction has occurred. It is then connected to the valve and reservoir. The valve controls how much fluid is withdrawn from the brain, it is then stored in the reservoir until it is released to drain down the distal (bottom) end. The distal end is a small, narrow piece of tubing (catheter) which leads to the point where

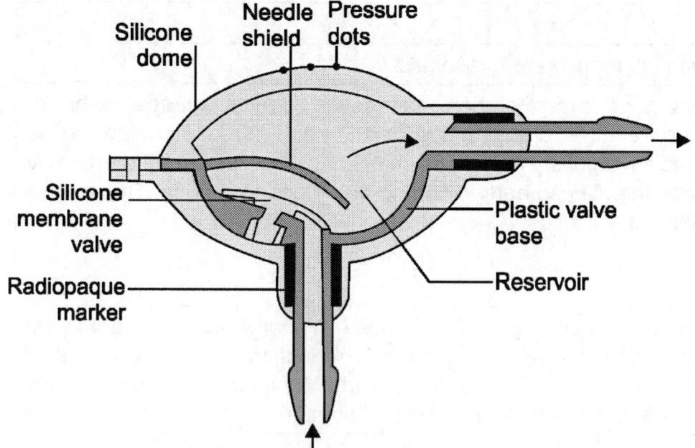

Fig. 16.5: Different parts of shunt

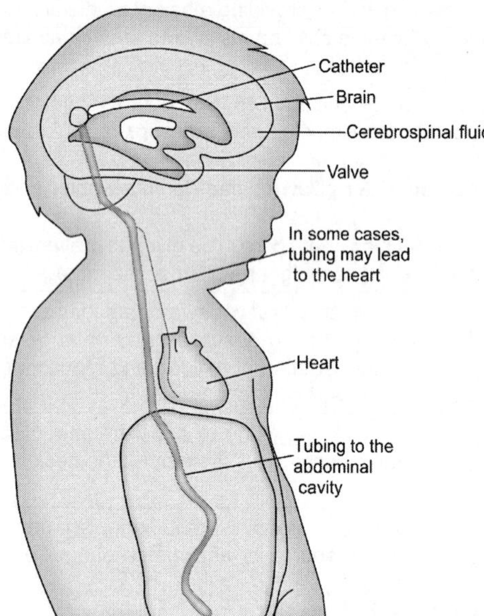

Fig. 16.6: Shunt and insertion of shunt

the excess CSF will drain and be absorbed by the body (Fig. 16.6).

The steps of insertion of shunt:

1. An area of hair on the head is shaved. This may be behind the ear or on the top or back of the head.
2. The surgeon makes a U-shape cut behind the ear. Another small surgical cut is made in the belly.
3. A small hole is drilled in the skull. A thin tube called a catheter is passed into a ventricle of the brain. This can be done with or without a computer as a guide. It can also be done with an endoscope that allows the surgeon to see inside the ventricle.
4. Another catheter is placed under the skin behind the ear. It is sent down the neck and chest, and usually into the belly area. Sometimes, it stops at the chest area. The doctor may make a small cut in the neck to help position it.
5. A valve is placed underneath the skin behind the ear. The valve is connected to both catheters. When extra pressure builds up around the brain, the valve opens, and excess fluid drains through the catheter into the belly or chest area. This helps lower intracranial pressure.
6. The patient is taken to a recovery area and then moved to a hospital ward.

Common complications of VP shunt include shunt malfunction or blockage, kinking, separation of shunt tube and infection. Malfunction may be related to growth and the shunt will need to be replaced with a longer catheter. Symptoms of shunt malfunction or infection include headache, fever, drowsiness, convulsions, increased head circumference and bulging fontanelle.

Antibiotics are given if there are signs of infection. Severe infections may require the shunt to be removed.

Nursing Care of a Child with Shunt (Table 16.4)

Other treatments may include:

Endoscopic Third Ventriculostomy (ETV)

A procedure called a ventriculostomy can be performed as an alternative to having a shunt inserted. *An endoscope being used to make a hole in the ventricle so the patient can avoid needing a shunt.*

For a small number of children, an endoscopic third ventriculostomy (ETV) surgery may be a treatment option. Most often it is done in children who have aqueductal stenosis. Depending on child's age and brain structures (typically be dilatation of the lateral ventricles, ballooning of the 3rd ventricle, and a relatively small 4th ventricle), ETV is done instead of putting in a shunt.

The technique consists of the creation of a single burrhole in the frontal region followed by ventricular cannulation and insertion of a 3 or 4 mm wide neuroendoscope into the lateral ventricle. The 3rd ventricle is then negotiated via the foramen of Monro and a hole is then made in the floor of the 3rd ventricle between the infundibulum of the pituitary gland and the mammillary bodies. This creates a CSF fistula between the 3rd ventricle and the subarachnoid space in front of the brainstem. The hole is made with a small electrode and enlarged with a balloon dilator, such that a very exciting close up view of the basilar artery is unveiled.

Table 16.4: Care of a child after insertion of shunt

Nursing diagnosis	*Nursing outcome*	*Nursing intervention with rationale*
Risk of infection due to shunt placement	The child will remain free from infection, as evidenced by being afebrile, clean and dry implant site, no ICP, can tolerate feeding	• Monitor vital signs every 15 mins until the child is reactive • Assess the neurological status and LOC frequently • Check the shunt valve 8 hourly, and to make certain that the fluid is fluctuating and draining • Monitor for swelling or redness along the shunt tract • Observe the dressing sites (head, abdomen or chest) • Administer the antibiotics as prescribed • Maintenance of strict aseptic technique when handling shunt drainage system
	Maintenance of desired flow of CSF through the shunt drainage system from the ventricles to the drainage site (abdomen or atrium)	Place the child in flat position to prevent rapid CSF drainage and on unoperated site to avoid pressure on the valve of shunt. Rapid CSF drainage (fontanel become depressed quickly) may cause subdural hematoma due to tearing of the vessels secondary to cerebral cortex pulling away from dura mater. Assess the head circumference regularly. Notify physician if the fontanelle depresses too rapidly. Lower the head end of the bed to prevent subdural hematoma
Acute pain related to surgery	Pain relieved as evidenced by no cry and restlessness, restful sleep	Assess the child's pain level, activity and irritability and administer drugs as prescribed. Distract the child by holding, cuddling and talking. Pain relief is necessary to stop crying, because crying increases ICP, metabolic demands
Peritoneostomy done (VP shunt implanted), vulnerable to GI complication	Free from GI complications as evidenced by no abdominal distension, vomiting, symptom of dehydration	• Observe and record the symptoms of abdominal distension and discomfort, if present or complained by the child • Maintain NPM in immediate postoperative period • Maintain intake–output as fluid is restricted for first 24 hours after surgery • Nasogastric suctioning is done to handle abdominal distension • 4 to 6 hourly mouth care is needed to treat the dry mouth • Give clear fluid as soon as child can tolerate it
Knowledge deficit of parent about caring the child with shunt or other surgical intervention	Parent will able to describe the care of the child as evidenced by an ability to demonstrate care the child, to identify rise of ICP and infection	• Determine the knowledge of parent about purpose and function of shunt • Teach parent to observe the child for rise of ICP • Teach parent to observe the child for patency of shunt or infection of the shunt • To demonstate them about basic care of the child like positioning, holding, feeding, skin care, etc. • Encourage the parents to provide as normal lifestyle as possible
Delayed growth and development	The patient will achieve age-appropriate growth, behaviors, and skills to the fullest extent possible	Developmental care: Structuring the environment and providing care in response to the behavioral cues and states of the preterm infant. Environmental management: Manipulation of the patient's surroundings for therapeutic benefit

Choroid Plexus Cauterization

Removing or cauterizing the parts of the brain that produce CSF.

Sometime, when child's body does not absorb CSF well, a choroid plexus cauterization (CPC) may be a treatment option. This is done during the same surgery as ETV. It is done to decrease the amount of CSF made in child's brain. This may help avoid the need for a shunt in the future.

In CPC, a flexible endoscope is used to reach the choroid plexus in the lateral ventricles each side of the brain and cauterization is done so it does not make as much CSF. CPC may lower the level of fluid enough that child's body can keep up with absorbing it.

The child will need regular check-ups to make sure there are no further problems. Tests are regularly done to check the child's developmental and for intellectual, neurological, or physical problems.

Visiting nurses, social services, support groups, and local agencies can provide emotional support and assist with the care of a child with hydrocephalus who has significant brain damage.

Nursing Intervention

The hydrocephalus is among the most important and frequent neurosurgical diseases, due to its clinical, surgical and social implications (Table 16.3). Nursing intervention is challenging both in the care during the clinical/surgical procedures and in the guidance and strengthening of the bond of the child with its family. The nurse plays an active role in counseling the family about the management required for the disorder.

- Treatment is surgical by direct removal of an obstruction and insertion of shunt to provide primary drainage of the CSF to an extracranial compartment, usually peritoneum (ventriculoperitoneal shunt).
  - The major complications of shunts are infections and malfunction (Table 16.4).
  - Other complications include subdural hematoma caused by a too rapid reduction of CSF, peritonitis, abdominal abscess, perforation of organs, fistulas, hernias and ileus.
- A third ventriculostomy/choroid plexus cauterization is a new nonshunting procedure used to treat children with hydrocephalus.

Disorder of Neural Tube Development

Spina Bifida

Spina bifida literally means 'split spine.' It is a developmental congenital disorder caused by the incomplete closing of the embryonic neural tube and covering mesoderm and ectoderm. Spina bifida is a malformation of the spine in which the posterior portion of the laminae of the vertebrae fails to close. It may occur anywhere in the spine, but the most common site is lumbosacral region. If the opening is large enough, this allows a portion of the spinal cord to protrude through the opening in the bones. Spina bifida happens when a baby is in the womb and the spinal column does not close all of the way.

Causes

No one knows for sure. Scientists believe that genetic and environmental factors act together to cause the condition.

The etiological factors associated with spina bifida are:

Genetic: Chromosomal abnormalities including Trisomy 13 and 15 have been reported.

Maternal factor: Maternal malnutrition, specially decreased folate levels is an important risk factor. Other factors include maternal age (more than 35 years, and below 20 years), alcohol, IDDM, valproate and carbamazepine.

Environmental: Radiation exposure increases the risk of defective neural tube development.

> **Pathophysiology**
>
> Spina bifida (SB) is a neural tube defect caused by the failure of the fetus's spine to close properly during the 1st month of pregnancy. Infants born with SB sometimes have an open lesion on their spine where significant damage to the nerves and spinal cord has occurred. The lesion results in varying degree of paralysis of the lower limbs, or other sensory defects. Club feet, scoliosis, and contracture and dislocation of the hips may also be associated with the defect. Even when there is no lesion present there may be improperly formed or missing vertebrae and accompanying nerve damage. In addition to physical and mobility difficulties, most individuals have some form of learning disability.

Type

Spina bifida malformations fall into three categories—spina bifida occulta, spina bifida cystica with meningocele, and spina bifida cystica with myelomeningocele (Fig. 16.7).

SB occulta, is the mildest form, in which one or more vertebrae are malformed and covered by a layer of skin. It is often called 'hidden spina bifida' because about 15% of healthy people have it and do not know it. In occulta, the outer part of some of the vertebrae is

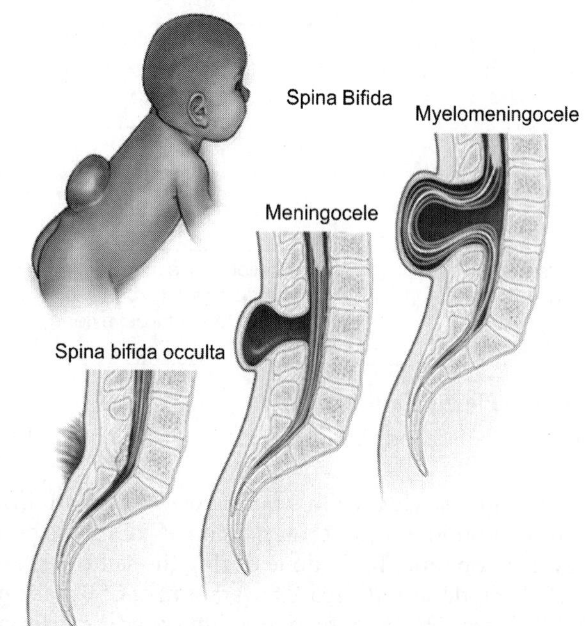

Fig. 16.7: Types of spina bifida: Spina bifida occulta, spina bifida cystica with meningocele and spina bifida cystica with mylomeningocele

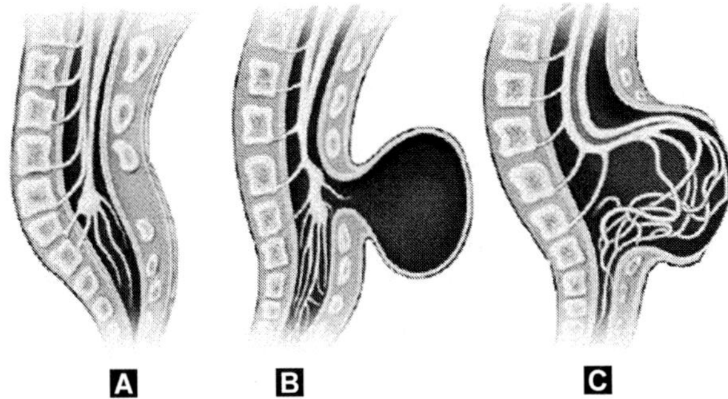

Figs 16.8A to C: A. Spina bifida occulta; **B.** Meningocele; **C.** Meningomyelocele

not completely closed. The splits in the vertebrae are so small that the spinal cord does not protrude. The skin at the site of the lesion may be normal, or it may have some hair growing from it; there may be a dimple in the skin, or a birthmark. Spina bifida occulta usually does not cause harm, and has no visible signs (Fig. 16.8).

In meningocele, the spinal cord develops normally but the meninges and spinal fluid) protrude from a spinal opening. A meningocele causes part of the spinal cord to come through the spine like a sac that is pushed out. A thin and translucent or membranous layer covers the sac which contains meninges and CSF (Figs 16.7 and 16.8). There is usually no nerve damage. Individuals with this condition may have minor disabilities.

Myelomeningocele is the most severe form of spina bifida. It is a sac-like protrusion of spinal cord, CSF and meninges through spinal cleft (Figs 16.7 and 16.8). It causes nerve damage and other disabilities. It is also known as open spinal dysraphism, or spina bifida aperta. Hydrocephalus develops in 70 to 90% of children with this condition. The most common location of the malformations is the lumbar and sacral areas, because the lumbar segment of spinal cord is the last part of neural tube to close during embryonic life.

Spina bifida meningocele and myelomeningocele are among the most common birth defects, with a worldwide incidence of about 1 in every 1000 births. The occulta form is much more common, but only rarely causes neurological symptoms. Myelomeningocele is the most significant and common form, and this leads to disability in most affected individuals. The terms spina bifida and myelomeningocele are usually used interchangeably.

Visible features of spina bifida occulta can sometimes be seen on the newborn's skin above the spinal defect, includes an abnormal tuft of hair, a collection of fat, a small dimple or birthmark. There is no hole or opening on the back. The spinal cord and nerves are usually normal but there are small spaces between a few of spine bones. Later in life, the person may have some small nerve problems (back ache). Many people who have spina bifida occulta do not even know it, unless the condition is discovered during an X-ray or other imaging test done for unrelated reasons.

Meningocele

In this form an external cystic defect can be seen at the back. The protective membranes around the spinal cord (meninges) push out through the opening in the vertebrae. Because the spinal cord develops normally, there is seldom evidence of weakness of legs or disturbances in bladder in bowel.

Myelomeningocele

Also known as open spina bifida, myelomeningocele is the most severe form—and the form people usually mean when they use the term 'spina bifida.'

In myelomeningocele, the baby's spinal canal remains open along several vertebrae in the lower or middle back. Because of this opening, both the membranes and the spinal cord protrude at birth, forming a sac on the baby's back (mainly at lumbosacral region). Loss of motor control and sensation occurs below the lesions. A sacral lesion leads to weakness to the lower lower limbs, a lower thoracic lesion may cause total flaccid paralysis.

In some cases, skin covers the sac. Usually, however, tissues and nerves are exposed, making the baby prone to life-threatening infections.

Neurological impairment is common, and higher the deformity the more neurological deficits will be present. The symptoms include:

- Muscle weakness of the legs, sometimes involving paralysis.
- Bowel and bladder problems like bladder and bowel control problems, including incontinence, urinary tract infections, and poor renal function.
- Seizures, specially if the child requires a shunt.
- Orthopedic problems—such as club foot, hip dislocation and a curved spine (scoliosis).
- Pressure sores and skin irritation.
- Abnormal eye movement.

Many children with spina bifida may have an associated abnormality of the cerebellum, called the Arnold-Chiari II malformation. In affected individuals, the back portion of the brain is displaced from the back of the skull down into the upper neck. In about 90% of the people with myelomeningocele, hydrocephalus also occurs because the displaced cerebellum interferes with the normal flow of CSF, causing an excess of the fluid to accumulate.

Diagnostic Evaluation

Prenatal diagnosis includes determining alpha-fetoprotein levels in blood at 16 to 18 weeks of gestation. Amniocentesis and fetal ultrasound testing are done if AFP level is high.

Diagnosis after birth includes transillumination test (shining light through the sac) confirms meningocele, MRI or a computed tomography (CT) scan to get a clearer view of the spinal cord and vertebrae. If hydrocephalus is suspected, a CT scan and/or X-ray of the skull to look for extra cerebrospinal fluid inside the brain. CT scan and MRI determine bony deformities and spinal cord herniation. These tests also diagnose the presence of hydrocephalus or Arnold-Chiari malformation.

Management

Treatment depends on the type and severity of the disorder. Generally, children with the mildest form need no treatment, although some may require surgery as they grow. The key early priorities for treating myelomeningocele are to prevent infection from developing in the exposed nerves and tissue through the spinal defect, and to protect the exposed nerves and structures from additional trauma. Early operation is advocated therefore to prevent further deterioration of neural tissue. Typically, a child born with spina bifida will have surgery to close the defect and minimize the risk of infection or further trauma. Surgery for SB cystica is laminectomy and closure of the defect or removal of the sac which is done within the first few days of life.

Prenatal microsurgical closure of meningomyelocele, performed at approximately 19 to 25 weeks of gestation to decrease the severity of Chiari II malformation and incidence of hydrocele. The surgery is considered experimental and there are risks to the fetus as well as to the mother. The major risks to the fetus are those that might occur if the surgery stimulates premature delivery, such as organ immaturity, brain hemorrhage, and death. Risks to the mother include infection, blood loss leading to the need for transfusion, gestational diabetes, and weight gain due to bed rest.

The nerve tissue that is damaged cannot be repaired, nor can function be restored to the damaged nerves, So children need lifelong management of neurological, orthopedic, bladder and bowel problem. Urodynamic studies are done early and a bladder emptying program is initiated, with close monitoring of the child's infection status.

Some individuals with spina bifida require assistive devices such as braces, crutches, or wheelchairs. The location of the malformation on the spine often indicates the type of assistive devices needed. Children with a defect high on the spine will have more extensive paralysis and will often require a wheelchair, while those with a defect lower on the spine may be able to use crutches, leg braces, or walkers. Beginning special exercises for the legs and feet at an early age may help prepare the child for walking with those braces or crutches when he or she is older.

Nursing Management

The objectives of nursing care are to prevent infection and injury of the sac, to help preserve whatever function is present orthopedically and urologically, to help the child for provision of adequate nutrition (Table 16.5).

Prognosis

Children with spina bifida can lead active lives. Prognosis, activity, and participation depend on the number and severity of abnormalities and associated personal and environmental factors. Most children with the disorder have normal intelligence and can walk, often with assistive devices. If learning problems develop, appropriate educational interventions are helpful.

SEIZURE DISORDER

Epilepsy

A seizure is associated with a paroxysmal burst of electrical activity within the CNS. Epilepsy is a brain disorder in which clusters of nerve cells, or neurons, in the brain sometimes signal abnormally causing strange sensations, emotions, and behavior, or sometimes convulsions, muscle spasms, and loss of consciousness. Epilepsy is a condition of recurring seizures that are unprovoked by an immediate identified cause. These seizures are episodes that can vary from brief and nearly undetectable to long periods of vigorous shaking. In epilepsy, seizures tend to recur, and have no immediate underlying cause. Epilepsy is not a specific disease entity in itself but rather a variety of recurrent seizure patterns are included in it.

Table 16.5: Care of a child with meningocele, mylomeningocele

Nursing diagnosis	*Nursing outcome*	*Nursing intervention with rationale*
Prone to infection due to open sac and operative procedure	The patient will remain free from signs and symptoms of infection as evidenced by normal temperature, no meningeal irritation, no leakage from the sac, normal WBC count	Assess head circumference, fontanelles, cranial sutures, reflexes, cranial nerve function.Monitor vital signs and WBC count. Note signs of infection along with irritability, cry, lethargy, or nuchal rigidity. Observe the sac or operated site for redness or oozing (clear/ purulent). Sterile normal saline dressing/petroleum gauze is to be applied over the sac or incision site
Risk for impaired skin integrity related to neuro-motor deficit	Intact skin of the child evidenced by no pressure areas or ulcerations	• The newborn is placed on abdomen until the operation is done. Frequent change of position and assessment of skin is important. Special bedding or bedframe can be used for alleviating pressure points, maintaining anatomic position of the hip and feet; and to prevent contamination of the sac with urine and stool, as it may pass between the sections of the frame • Stoma adhesive may be used on each side of the sac to anchor the dressing. It can minimize the skin irritation
Altered bladder and bowel function related to neurological deficit	Free from complication as evidenced by no sign of UTI or bowel problem	• Record the degree of continence, whether there is retention of urine or fecal impaction. If evidence of urinary infection occurs, culture should be done to determine the antibiotics. Intermittent catheterization may be needed in case of incontinence • Consult dietitian to be sure the diet provide adequate fluid and fiber. Medications like stool softener, suppositories may be used
Ineffective thermoregulation related to surgery	Effective thermoregulation as evidenced by no sign of hypothermia	• Keep the child warm, using warmer or incubator • Monitor vital signs • Avoid unnecessary exposure of the child
Altered nutrition less than body requirement related to disease process	Proper nutrition as evidenced by absence of dehydration, restlessness and cry	• Administer intravenous fluid as prescribed • Begin oral feeding in side lying position as it is tolerated by the child • Watch for abdominal distention as it can interfere feeding
Risk of complications related to disease process	Absence of complications	• Keep the child in prone position with legs abducted. A pillow or pad is placed between the knees to counteract the hip subluxation • Postoperatively the child may be placed in low Trendelenburg position to prevent CSF pressure or leakage from the incision site • Elevate head end if hydrocephalus is suspected • Provide passive range of exercises to prevent chest complication and to develop contractures
Impaired physical mobility due to neuromuscular deficit and use of cast after operation		Record activity of the legs
Knowledge and skill deficit in parents related to giving care to their child	Parents	

Etiology

Approximately 50% of childhood seizures are idiopathic. Epilepsy can have both genetic and acquired causes, with interaction of these factors in many cases.Many possible causes may disturb the normal pattern of neuron activity, from illness to brain damage to abnormal brain development—can lead to seizures. It can be categorized as primary or secondary.

Primary seizure is associated with genetic predisposition which includes febrile seizure and benign seizures of newborn; but structural abnormality in the brain is not found in this case. Secondary epilepsy or symptomatic seizures are usually provoked by brain damage from other disorders including brain tumors, strokes, and heart attacks. Epilepsy is also associated with a variety of developmental and metabolic disorders, anoxia, trauma, infections, toxic disturbances, etc. Other causes include head injury, prenatal injury, and poisoning. The causes of convulsion according to age of child are:

Early neonatal period: Birth asphyxia, trauma, intraventricular hemorrhage, metabolic disorder, hypoglycemia, hyponatremia, hypocalcemia in newborns and infants: birth trauma, congenital conditions genetic factors, fever/infection, metabolic or chemical imbalances in the body, progressive brain disease.

Other possible causes of seizures may include the following:

- Brain tumor
- Neurological problems
- Drug withdrawal
- Medications.

Our society has created insignificant myths about epilepsy which is one of the reasons for not availing treatment.

Myth: Epilepsy is because of possession by evil spirit and hence sorcery is the treatment.

Fact: Epilepsy is a neurological disorder and there are drugs to treat.

Myth: People with epilepsy are possessed by spirits and hence should be worshipped/shunned.

Fact: Epilepsy is due to transient electrical disturbances in the brain and the individuals should be treated like any other person.

Myth: Epilepsy is contagious, so one should not come in contact with a person with epilepsy.

Fact: It is not contagious.

Myth: People with epilepsy are below normal in their intelligence.

Fact: Epilepsy does not affect intelligence or memory. If the attacks are frequent or the person is taking large doses of antiepileptic drugs, this may affect the memory temporarily.

Myth: Marriage cures epilepsy.

Fact: OFF COURSE NOT! MEDICINES DO.

Pathophysiology

A seizure occurs when part(s) of the brain receives a burst of abnormal electrical signals that temporarily interrupts normal electrical brain function. The brain consists of millions of nerve cells, and electrical impulses are sent through many of these cells by neurotransmitters. Epilepsy may develop because of an abnormality in brain wiring, an imbalance of nerve signaling chemicals called neurotransmitters, or some combination of these

Contd...

Contd...

factors. People with epilepsy have an abnormally high level of excitatory neurotransmitters (glutamate, aspartate) that increase neuronal activity, while others have an abnormally low level of inhibitory neurotransmitters that decrease neuronal activity in the brain. Either situation can result in too much neuronal activity and cause epilepsy. One of the most-studied neurotransmitters that plays a role in epilepsy is GABA, or gamma-aminobutyric acid, which is an inhibitory neurotransmitter (Fig. 16.9). Several types of epilepsy have now been linked to defective genes for ion channels, the 'gates' that control the flow of ions in and out of cells and regulate neuron signaling.

Normally brain's electrical activity is nonsynchronous. In epileptic seizures, due to structural or functional problems within the brain, a group of neurons begin firing in an abnormal, excessive, and synchronized manner. This results in a wave of depolarization known as a paroxysmal depolarizing shift. The result of these discharges is activation of associated motor and sensory organs. This leads to seizure.

Classifications

Many types of seizures exist. The International Classification of seizures is used to divide seizures into two major groups—focal or partial and generalized (Flowchart 16.2).

Focal or Partial Seizures

Focal seizures may also be called partial seizures, usually last just a few seconds. Focal seizures take place

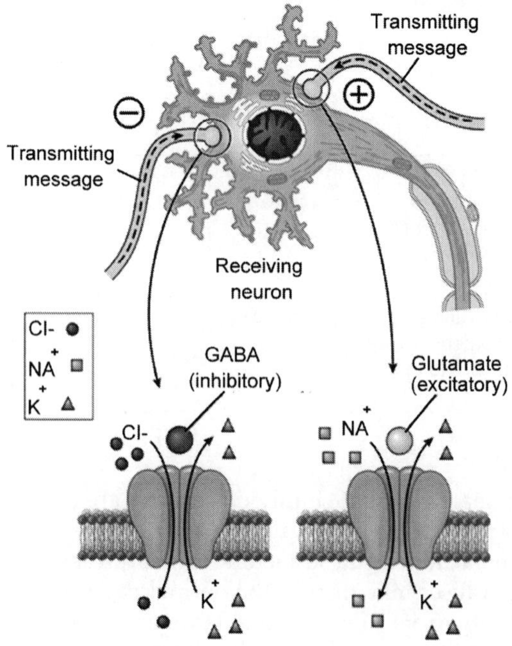

Fig. 16.9: Neurotransmitters involved in epilepsy

Flowchart 16.2: Seizure classification

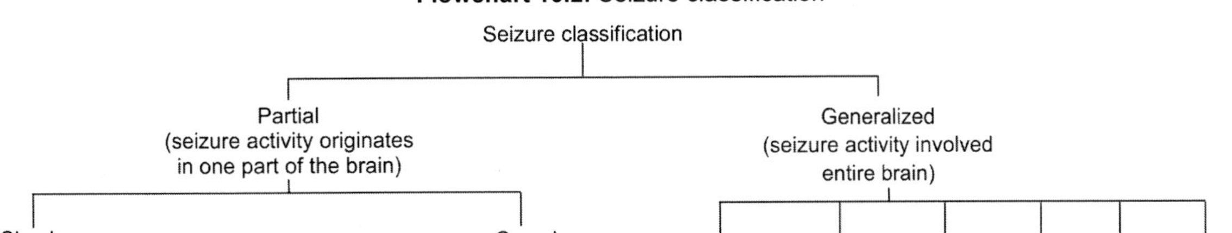

when abnormal electrical brain function occurs in one or more areas of one hemisphere of the brain. As a result symptoms are seen on only one side of the body. Partial seizures begin focally but it may become generalized when the electrical impulses are passed across the corpus callosum to the other hemisphere. People having a complex focal seizure may display strange, repetitious behaviors such as blinks, twitches, mouth movements, or even walking in a circle. These repetitious movements are called automatisms.

Focal seizures, particularly with complex focal seizures are often preceded by certain experiences, known as an aura. An aura is a strange feeling which include sensory (visual, hearing or smell), psychic, autonomic, or motor phenomena. Jerking activity may start in a specific muscle group and spread to surrounding muscle groups in which case it is known as a Jacksonian march. Two types of focal seizures include the following:

Simple Focal Seizures

Simple focal seizures consists of motor, autonomic, or sensory symptoms.The person may show different symptoms depending upon which area of the brain is involved. If the abnormal electrical brain function is in the occipital lobe, sight may be altered, but muscles are more commonly affected. The person's muscles are typically more commonly affected. The seizure activity is limited to an isolated muscle group, such as the fingers, or to larger muscles in the arms and legs. Consciousness is not lost in this type of seizure. This type of seizure may last 20 seconds to several minutes. Symptoms may include odd smell, odd taste in the mouth, abdominal discomfort, unexplained fear or dread. The person may also experience sweating, nausea, or become pale.

Complex Focal Seizures

This type of seizure commonly occurs in the temporal lobe of the brain, the area of the brain that controls emotion and memory function.This seizure usually lasts between 1 and 2 minutes. Consciousness is usually lost during these seizures and a variety of behaviors can occur. These behaviors may range from gagging, lip smacking, scratching or pulling of shirt buttons, running, screaming, crying, and/or laughing. Some people with focal seizures, specially complex focal seizures, may experience auras—unusual sensations that warn of an impending seizure. These auras are actually simple focal seizures in which the person maintains consciousness. The symptoms an individual person has, and the progression of those symptoms, tend to be stereotyped, or similar every time. When the person regains consciousness, the person may complain of being tired or sleepy after the seizure. This is called the postictal period.

Generalized Seizures

Generalized seizures are a result of abnormal neuronal activity on both sides of the brain. It starts at any age. There are 6 main types of generalized seizures—tonic-clonic, tonic, clonic, myoclonic, absence, and atonic seizures. They all involve loss of consciousness and typically happen without warning. These seizures may cause loss of consciousness, falls, or massive muscle spasms.

Tonic, Clonic, and Tonic- Clonic seizures: Tonic seizures cause stiffening of muscles of the body, generally those in the back, legs, arms including diaphragm; and it lasts a few seconds. The clonic seizure is symmetric, and rhythmic cause repeated jerking movements of muscles on both sides of the body (alternate contraction and relaxation of major muscle group). Tonic-clonic seizures present with a contraction of the limbs followed by their extension along with arching of the back which lasts 10 to 30 seconds (the tonic phase). A cry may be heard due to contraction of the chest muscles. Tonic-clonic seizures cause a mixture of symptoms, including stiffening of the body and repeated jerks of the arms and/or legs as well as loss of consciousness.

This phase usually ends spontaneously in less than 5 minutes. Respirations are irregular and the child may have stridor. Tonic-clonic seizures are sometimes referred to by an older term: grand mal seizures. Loss of bowel or bladder control may occur during a seizure.

The tongue may be bitten at either the tip or on the sides during a seizure. After the shaking has stopped it may take 10 to 30 minutes for the person to return to normal; this period is called the 'postictal phase'. During the postictal period, the person may be sleepy, have problems with vision or speech and may have a bad headache, fatigue.

Grand mal seizure (generalized tonic-clonic (GTC) seizures) is characterized by 5 distinct phases that occur. The body, arms, and legs will flex (contract), extend (straighten out), and tremor (shake), followed by a clonic period (contraction and relaxation of the muscles) and the postictal period.

Atonic Seizure

With atonic seizures, there is a sudden loss of postural tone (muscle tone) and the person may fall from a standing position or suddenly drop his or her head. The patient may show impairment in consciousness, confusion and lethargy. During the seizure, the person is limp and unresponsive. The atonic seizure is also called drop attacks.

Myoclonic Seizure

Myoclonic seizures cause jerks or twitches of the upper body, arms, or legs. This type of seizure refers to quick movements or sudden jerking of a group of muscles. These seizures may occur singly or in clusters, meaning that they may occur several times a day, or for several days in a row and can occur on both sides of the body. Myoclonic seizures are brief, random contractions of a muscle group, followed by loss of muscle tone and forward falling. Impairment of consciousness may occur during this seizure. Myoclonic seizure disorder occurs in infants before 6 months of age is called *infantile spasm,* those that occur during adolescence is called *juvenile myoclonic epilepsy.*

Absence Seizures

Absence seizures cause momentary lapses of consciousness , formerly called petit mal seizure. No muscle activity occurs except for eyelid fluttering, twitching, or head bobbing. These seizures almost always begin in childhood or adolescence, and they tend to run in families, suggesting that they may be at least partially due to a defective gene or genes. Some people with absence seizures have purposeless movements during their seizures, such as a jerking arm or rapidly blinking eyes. Others have no noticeable symptoms except for brief times when they are 'out of it', or shows a blanck facial expression. It lasts for 5 to 10 seconds. Immediately after a seizure, the person can resume whatever he or she was doing. However, these seizures may occur so frequently that the person cannot concentrate in school or other situations. Childhood absence epilepsy usually stops when the child reaches puberty. Absence seizures usually have no lasting effect on intelligence or other brain functions.

Diagnostic Evaluation

The diagnosis of epilepsy is typically made based on the description of the seizure and the underlying cause. An electroencephalogram and neuroimaging are also usually part of the workup.

Medical History

Taking a detailed medical history, including symptoms and duration of the seizures, is still one of the best methods available to determine if a child has epilepsy and what kind of seizures he or she has. The diagnosis of epilepsy is based on history of two or more seizures. The questions are asked about the seizures and any past illnesses or other symptoms the child may have had, and in that case caregivers' accounts of the seizure (before, during and after the episode) are vital to this evaluation.

EEG

An EEG records brain waves detected by electrodes placed on the scalp. This is the most common diagnostic test for epilepsy and can detect abnormalities in the brain's electrical activity. People with epilepsy frequently have changes in their normal pattern of brain waves, even when they are not experiencing a seizure. While this type of test can be very useful in diagnosing epilepsy, it is not foolproof. Some people continue to show normal brain wave patterns even after they have experienced a seizure. In other cases, the unusual brain waves are generated deep in the brain where the EEG is unable to detect them. Many people who do not have epilepsy also show some unusual brain activity on an EEG. Whenever possible, an EEG should be performed within 24 hours of a patient's first seizure. Ideally, EEGs should be performed while the patient is sleeping as well as when he or she is awake, because brain activity during sleep is often quite different than at other times.

Video monitoring is often used in conjunction with EEG to determine the nature of a person's seizures. It also can be used in some cases to rule out other disorders such as cardiac arrhythmia or narcolepsy that may look like epilepsy.

Brain Scans

One of the most important ways of diagnosing epilepsy is through the use of brain scans. The most commonly used brain scans include CT, positron emission tomography (PET) and MRI. CT and MRI scans reveal the structure of the brain, which can be useful for identifying brain tumors, cysts, and other structural abnormalities. PET and an adapted kind of MRI called functional MRI can be used to monitor the brain's activity and detect abnormalities in how it works. SPECT (single photon emission computed tomography) is a relatively new kind of brain scan that is sometimes used to locate seizure foci in the brain.

The newer imagings is magnetoencephalogram (MEG does not require electrodes) can detect signals from deeper in the brain (detects the magnetic signals generated by neurons) than an EEG. Magnetic resonance spectroscopy (MRS) can reveal abnormalities in the brain's biochemical processes and near-infrared spectroscopy, a technique that can detect oxygen levels in brain tissue.

Blood Tests

The blood samples are often screened for metabolic or genetic disorders that may be associated with the seizures of the child. They also may be used to check for underlying problems such as infections, lead poisoning, anemia, and diabetes that may be causing or triggering the seizures.

Other Tests

Kidney and liver function test, lumbar puncture.

Developmental, Neurological, and Behavioral Tests

Some tests are devised to measure motor abilities, behavior, and intellectual capacity as a way to determine how the epilepsy is affecting that child. These tests also can provide clues about what kind of epilepsy the child has.

Therapeutic Management

Most epilepsy seizures can be controlled with just one drug at the optimal dosage. It is given to reduce the level of neuronal excitability below seizure threshold or to prevent its spread. Combining medications usually amplifies side effects such as fatigue and decreased appetite, so in most of the cases monotherapy is used. Combinations of drugs are sometimes prescribed if monotherapy fails to effectively control a patient's seizures.

The goal of seizure management is to control, stop, or decrease the frequency of the seizures without interfering with the normal activities of daily living (ADLs). The major goals of seizure management include the following:

- Proper identification of the type of seizure
- Using medication specific to the type of seizure
- Using the least amount of medication to achieve adequate control
- Maintaining appropriate medication levels.

The number of times a person needs to take medication each day is usually determined by the drug's half-life, or the time it takes for half the drug dose to be metabolized or broken down into other substances in the body. Some drugs, such as phenytoin and phenobarbital, only need to be taken once a day, while others such as valproate must be taken two or three times a day.

There are a number of medications available. Phenytoin, carbamazepine and valproate appear to be equally effective in both focal and generalized seizures. The least expensive anticonvulsant is phenobarbital. The World Health Organization gives it a first-line recommendation in the developing world and it is commonly used there. Access however may be difficult as some countries label it as a controlled drug.

Surgery

Another treatment option for seizures is surgery. Surgery may be considered in a person who:

- has seizures that are unable to be controlled with medications.
- has seizures that always start in one area of the brain.
- has a seizure in a part of the brain that can be removed without disrupting important behaviors such as speech, memory, or vision.

Surgery for epilepsy and seizures is a very complicated surgery, and common procedures include cutting out the hippocampus via an anterior temporal lobe resection, removal of tumors, and removing parts of the neocortex. The operation may remove the part of the brain where the seizures are occurring, or, sometimes, the surgery helps to stop the spread of the bad electrical currents through the brain.

A person may be awake during the surgery. The brain itself does not feel pain. With the person awake and able to follow commands, the surgeons are better able to make sure that important areas of the brain are not damaged.

Other Treatment

A low-carbohydrate, adequate-protein (ketogenic) diet appears to decrease the number of seizures by half in about 30 to 40% of children. It is a reasonable option in those who have epilepsy that is not improved with medications and for whom surgery is not an option. About 10% stay on the diet for a few years due to issues of effectiveness and tolerability. Side effects include stomach and intestinal problems in 30%, and there are long-term concerns of heart disease. Less radical diets are easier to tolerate and may be effective. It is unclear why this diet works.

Vagus Nerve Stimulation (VNS)

Some people, whose seizures are not being well-controlled with seizure medications, may benefit from a procedure called vagus nerve stimulation (VNS). VNS is currently only used for persons over the age of 12 who have partial seizures that are not controlled by other methods.

VNS attempts to control seizures by sending small pulses of energy to the brain from the vagus nerve, which is a large nerve in the neck. This is done by surgically placing a small battery into the chest wall. Small wires are then attached to the battery and placed under the skin and around the vagus nerve. The battery is then programmed to send energy impulses every few minutes to the brain. When the person feels a seizure coming on, he or she may activate the impulses by holding a small magnet over the battery. In many cases, this will help to stop the seizure.

There are some side effects that may occur with the use of VNS. These may include, but are not limited to, hoarseness, pain or discomfort in the throat, change in voice.

Avoidance Therapy

Avoidance therapy consists of minimizing or eliminating triggers. For example, in those who are sensitive to light, using a small television, avoiding video-games or wearing dark glasses may be useful.

Nursing Intervention

The primary goal of care is to minimize the impact of seizure disorders on the lives of individuals with developmental disabilities.

Emergency Care During Seizure

- Roll the child on his or her side to prevent choking on any fluids or vomit. Be sure that the child is not face down to prevent suffocation.
- Do not try to stop the child's movements or hold them down.
- Cushion the child's head by placing a pillow, blanket, jacket, or other soft, preferably flat object.
- Loosen any tight clothing around the neck.
- Keep the child's airway open. If necessary, grip the child's jaw gently and tilt his or her head back.
- Do not restrict the child from moving unless he or she is in danger.
- Do not put anything into the child's mouth, not even medicine or liquid. These can cause choking or damage to the child's jaw, tongue, or teeth.
- Remove any sharp or solid objects that the child might hit during the seizure.
- Note how long the seizure lasts and what symptoms occurred so nurse can tell a doctor or emergency personnel if necessary.
- Stay with the child until the seizure ends.
- Do not shake the child or shout. Do not restrain the child during seizures.
- Stay with the child until he or she is completely alert.

If a seizure lasts longer than 5 minutes or if there are more than two seizures in an hour without a return to normal between them it is considered a medical emergency known as status epilepticus. This may require medical help to keep the airway open and protected.

After the seizure, do not offer food or fluid until the patient is fully awake, able to sit upright, and can swallow easily. The child may need to reorient to the day, time and surroundings. Temporary amnesia may occur with seizures, so handing over the child to his or her family is important.

INJURY

- Head injury
- Spinal cord injury.

Head Injury

The scalp is rich with blood vessels, so even a minor cut there can bleed profusely. The 'goose egg' or swelling that may appear after a head blow is the result of the scalp's veins leaking fluid or blood into (and under) the scalp. It may take days or even a week to disappear.

Fortunately, most childhood falls or blows to the head result in injury to the scalp only, which is usually more frightening than threatening. An internal head injury could have more serious implications because it may result in bleeding or bruising of the brain.

Head injuries fall into following categories:

- **External** (usually scalp) injuries in which no break occurs in the integrity of the barrier between the intracranial cavity and the outside environment. The scalp is rich with blood vessels, so even a minor cut there can bleed profusely. The 'goose egg' or swelling that may appear after a head blow is the result of the scalp's veins leaking fluid or blood into (and under) the scalp. It may take days or even a week to disappear.

- **Internal** head injuries, which may involve the skull, the blood vessels within the skull, meninges or the brain. This is penetrating injury which breaks the integrity of the barrier between intracranial cavity and outside environment; infection is a major concern.

  The brain is cushioned by cerebrospinal fluid, but a severe blow to the head may knock the brain into the side of the skull or tear blood vessels, and damage to the brain itself—can be serious and possibly life-threatening.
- *Coup and contrecoup injury:* In head injury, a coup injury occurs directly below the site of impact with an object, and a contrecoup injury occurs on the side opposite the area that was impacted, caused by the rapid movements of the semisolid brain within the cranial cavity. Coup and contrecoup injuries are associated with cerebral contusions (Fig. 16.10). When a moving object impacts the stationary head, coup injuries are typical, while contrecoup injuries are produced when the moving head strikes a stationary object.

  CSF plays a major role in coup and contrecoup injuries to the brain. A blow to a stationary but moveable head causes acceleration, and the brain floating in CSF lags behind, sustaining an injury directly underneath the point of impact (coup injury). When a moving head hits the floor, sudden deceleration results in an injury to the brain on the opposite side (contrecoup injury).
- *Missile injury:* Penetrating head injury of the skull involves 'a wound in which an object breaches the cranium but does not exit it.' In contrast, a perforating head injury is a wound in which the object passes through the head and leaves an exit wound.

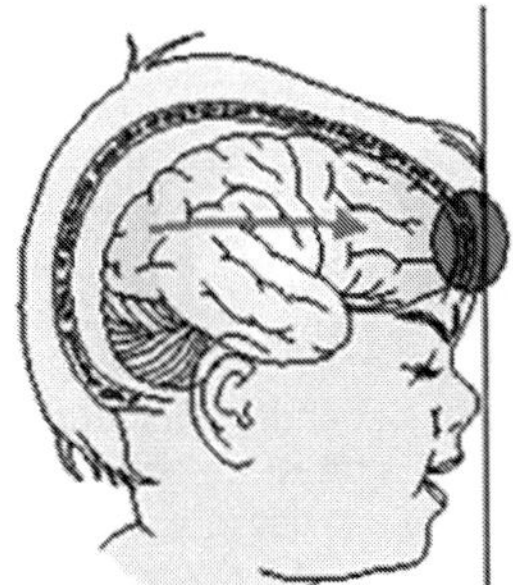
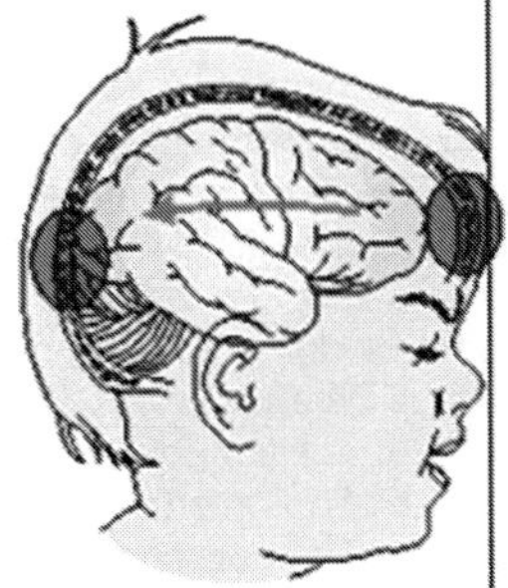

Fig. 16.10: Coup and contrecoup head injury

Skull Fractures

A skull fracture is a break in one or more of the eight bones that form the cranial portion of the skull, usually occurring as a result of blunt force trauma. The causative forces and fracture pattern, type, extent, and position are important in assessing the sustained injury. A closed fracture, also called a simple fracture, is one in which the skin is not broken or cut. C**ompound fracture**, an open fracture is one in which the skin is broken and the bone emerges from it.

Linear fracture: Linear skull fractures are breaks in the bone that transverse the full thickness of the skull from the outer to inner table. They are usually fairly straight with no bone displacement. The common cause of injury is blunt force trauma where the impact energy transferred over a wide area of the skull.

Depressed Fracture

This refers to a fracture that causes the skull to be depressed or to extend into the brain cavity. These fractures have the highest risk of tearing the dura, damaging the underlying brain, or both.

Basal Fracture

A basal fracture occurs in the floor of the skull. This is any area around the eyes, ears, nose, or back, near the spine. This fracture includes symptoms like battle sign, raccoon eyes, rhinorrhea, otorrhea and hemotympanum.

Concussion

A concussion is a type of traumatic brain injury (TBI) that happens when the brain is shaken hard enough to bounce against the skull. It is a transient and reversible neurotonal dysfunction, with instantaneous loss of awareness and responsiveness.

Contusion

Other types of TBIs are a contusion, which is a bruise on the brain that can cause swelling, and a hematoma, which is bleeding in the brain that collects and forms a clot. Contusions can occur with open or closed injuries and can impair a wide range of brain functions, depending on contusion size and location. Larger contusions may cause brain edema and increased intracranial pressure (ICP). Contusions may enlarge in the hours and days following the initial injury and cause neurologic deterioration.

In addition to the above types, fractures can further be classified as *greenstick* (incomplete), or *comminuted* (broken into three or more sections).

Intracranial Hemorrhage

Intracranial bleeding occurs when a blood vessel within the skull is ruptured or leaks. If intracranial hemorrhage occurs, a hematoma within the skull can put pressure on the brain. A localized collection of blood outside the blood vessels, usually in liquid form within the tissue is called hematoma.

Epidural hematomas (EDH) are collections of blood between the skull and dura mater and are less common than subdural hematomas. EDH usually result from a skull fracture that tears an artery coursing through the skull (Fig. 16.11). Epidural hematomas that are large or rapidly expanding are usually caused by arterial bleeding, classically due to damage to the middle meningeal artery by a temporal bone fracture. Patients may experience a brief black out when the injury first occurs and then regain full consciousness. Without intervention, patients with arterial epidural hematomas may rapidly deteriorate, and die. As the hemorrhage develops rapidly, patient begins to experience a progressive headache, slip into a coma and even die. Small, venous epidural hematomas are rarely lethal. However, if they receive prompt surgical care, patients with even the largest EDH can make a good recovery.

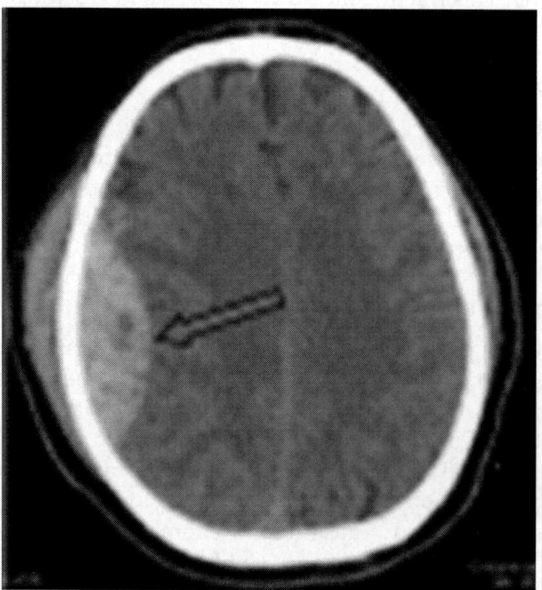

Fig. 16.11: Epidural hematomas after head trauma

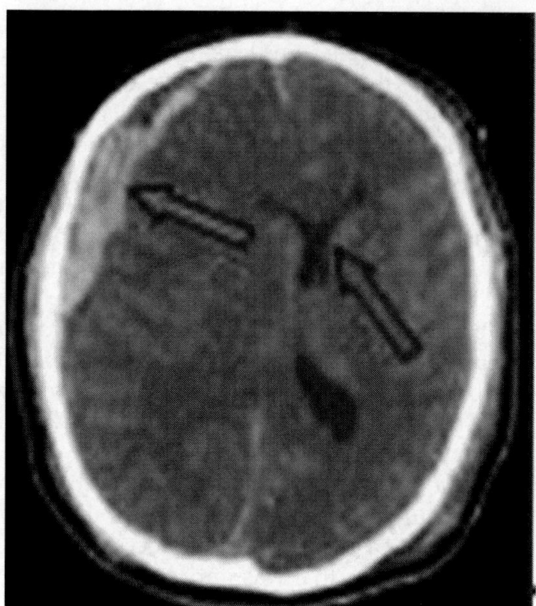

Fig. 16.12: Subdural hematomas after head trauma

Subdural hematomas are collections of blood between the dura mater and the cerebrum (Fig. 16.12). Acute subdural hematomas arise from laceration of cortical veins or avulsion of bridging veins between the cortex and dural sinuses. They often occur with head trauma from falls and motor vehicle crashes. Compression of the brain by the hematoma and swelling of the brain due to edema or hyperemia can increase ICP. Complications include focal neurologic deficits depending on the site of hematoma and brain injury, increased intracranial pressure leading to herniation of brain and ischemia due to reduced blood supply and seizures. When these processes occur, mortality and morbidity can be high.

Pathophysiology

Brain function may be immediately impaired by direct damage of brain tissue. Further damage may occur shortly thereafter from the cascade of events triggered by the initial injury. TBI of any sort can cause cerebral edema and decrease brain blood flow. The cranial vault is fixed in size (constrained by the skull) and filled by noncompressible CSF and minimally compressible brain tissue; consequently, any swelling from edema or an intracranial hematoma has nowhere to expand and thus increases ICP. Cerebral function depends on adequate supply of nutrition, oxygen and other substrates; an abnormal increase of ICP interferes with the balance and delivery of those nutrients. The secondary damage is influenced by changes in cerebral blood flow (hypo- and hyperperfusion), impairment of

Contd...

Contd...

cerebrovascular autoregulation, cerebral metabolic dysfunction and inadequate cerebral oxygenation. Cerebral blood flow is proportional to the cerebral perfusion pressure (CPP), which is the difference between mean arterial pressure (MAP) and mean ICP. When ICP increases or MAP decreases, CPP decreases. When CPP falls below 50 mm Hg, the brain may become ischemic. Ischemia and edema may trigger various secondary mechanisms of injury (e.g. release of excitatory neurotransmitters, intracellular Ca, free radicals, and cytokines), causing further cell damage, further edema, and further increases in ICP. Systemic complications from trauma (e.g. hypotension, hypoxia) can also contribute to cerebral ischemia and are often called secondary brain insults. Excessive ICP initially causes global cerebral dysfunction. If excessive ICP is unrelieved, it can push brain tissue across the tentorium or through the foramen magnum, causing herniation and increased morbidity and mortality.

Classification

Severity of head injury is assessed in following ways:

- Glasgow coma scale (GCS) (Table 16.6): A 3 to 15 point scale used to assess a patient's level of consciousness and neurologic functioning ; scoring is based on best motor response, best verbal response, and eye opening (e.g. eyes open to pain, open to command).
- Duration of loss of consciousness: Classified as mild (mental status change or loss of consciousness [LOC] < 30 min), moderate (mental status change or LOC 30 min to 6 hr), or severe (mental status change or LOC >6 hr).
- Post-traumatic amnesia (PTA): The time elapsed from injury to the moment when patients can demonstrate continuous memory of what is happening around them.

Diagnostic Evaluation

Physical examination begins with assessing the ABCs (airway, breathing, circulation) to make certain that the patient is stable and does not need emergent life-saving interventions. This is specially important in those patients who are unconscious and may not be able to maintain their own airway or breathe on their own.

For the unconscious patient the level of coma is assessed by the Glasgow coma scale. The Glasgow coma scale number is useful in tracking whether the patient is improving or declining in function over time.

The skull may be examined for signs of trauma, including contusion and hematoma. Palpating or feeling the skull may find evidence of a fracture. If a laceration

Table 16.6: Glasgow coma scale

The Glasgow Coma Scale (GCS) defines the severity of a TBI within 48 hours of injury	*Classification of severity of head injury based on Glasgow coma scale (within 48 hours) is as follows*	*Ranchos Los Amigos scale of cognitive functioning*
Eye opening Spontaneous = 4 To speech = 3 To painful stimulation = 2 No response = 1 **Motor response** Follows commands = 6 Makes localizing movements to pain = 5 Makes withdrawal movements to pain = 4 Flexor (decorticate) posturing to pain = 3 Extensor (decerebrate) posturing to pain = 2 No response = 1 **Verbal response** Oriented to person, place, and date = 5 Converses but is disoriented = 4 Says inappropriate words = 3 Says incomprehensible sounds = 2 No response = 1 **Total score = 15**	Critical head injury = GCS of 3 to 4 Severe head injury = GCS of 5 to 8 Moderate head injury = GCS of 9 to 13 or loss of consciousness of 5 minutes and more Mild head injury = GCS of 14 or 15 plus amnesia or brief LOC (less than 5 min) Minimal head injury = GCS of 15 with no loss of consciousness and amnesia	The severity of deficit in cognitive functioning can be defined by the Ranchos Los Amigos scale level I = No response level II = Generalized response level III = Localized response level IV = Confused-agitated level V = Confused-inappropriate level VI = Confused-appropriate level VII = Automatic-appropriate level VIII = Purposeful-appropriate

is present, it is important to know if there is a broken bone beneath it. The face may be examined as well, since the face provides protection to the front of the head.

The health care professional may also examine the patient for evidence of a basilar skull fracture, in which an injury has occurred to the bones that support the brain. Signs of this type of fracture include bruising of the tissues around the eyes (called raccoon eyes), bruising behind the ear (Battle's sign), bleeding from the ear canal, or cerebrospinal fluid leaking from the ear or nose.

The neurologic exam may include evaluation of the cranial nerves, the short nerves that leave the brain and control the face muscles, eye movements, swallowing, hearing, and sight, among other functions.

The exam may include evaluation of muscle tone and strength of the arms and legs; sensation in the extremities (including light touch, pain, and vibration); and if the neck is determined not to be injured, the patient's ability to walk may be assessed.

The diagnosis of brain injury involves CT scans looking for signs for brain injury, bleeding in the brain either through CAT scan, MRIs and X-rays to measures various areas of person's speech, movement, and thought. CT scan is the investigation of choice. It reveals bony injury, hematoma (appears hyperdense when compared to brain parenchyma), evidence of cerebral edema (hypodense compared to normal brain parenchyma and isodense compared to CSF) or mass effect (midline shift). Some time a small lesion in vital areas of brain may not be seen on CT but seen on MRI. MRI is usually reserved for later detailed evaluation after acute problem has been addressed.

It is important to remember that injuries to other parts of the body may also be present, and the evaluation of the head injury may occur at the same time as the evaluation of other injuries.

Therapeutic Management

In any child with brain injury should be treated in a pediatric trauma center or, failing that, a tertiary care hospital with pediatric trauma care capability. Hypoxia must be treated appropriately; the child needs prompt attention to airway, breathing and circulation. Pediatric patient with head injury may be brought unconscious, posturing (decerebrate or decorticate), or actively convulsing. All patients should be presumed to be full stomach and oxygen therapy should be initiated. Comatose patients need to be intubated with rapid sequence intubation technique, with due attention to cervical spine stabilization. A cervical spine collar should be placed until cervical spine X-rays are obtained to rule out a fracture or dislocation.

The basic aim of treatment is to minimize the primary injury and prevent secondary insult to the brain. Treatment remains supportive. As discussed in pathogenesis the key to management of a head injured patient with cerebral edema or diffuse axonal injury is to maintain cerebral perfusion pressure by control of ICP and hemodynamic status.

The treatment of a head injury depends upon the type of injury. For patients with minor head injuries (concussions), nothing more may be needed other than observation and symptom control. Headache may require pain medication. Nausea and vomiting may require medications to control these symptoms.

Neurosurgical Management

Neurosurgical management includes operative removal of extradural (epidural) hematoma or subdural hematomas, as soon as possible after the diagnosis is made. ICP monitor needs to be placed in most cases for ICP and CPP monitoring and further management in the pediatric intensive care unit (PICU).

Cerebral perfusion pressure (CPP) is defined as the difference between the mean arterial pressure (MAP) and the intracranial pressure (ICP). This represents the pressure gradient driving cerebral blood flow (CBF) and hence oxygen and metabolite delivery. The normal brain autoregulates its blood flow to provide a constant flow regardless of blood pressure by altering the resistance of cerebral blood vessels. In brain injury, cerebral perfusion pressure may be maintained by raising the mean arterial pressure or by lowering the intracranial pressure. In practice ICP is usually controlled to within normal limits (< 20 mmHg) and MAP is raised therapeutically.

Bleeding

Intracerebral bleeding or bleeding in the spaces surrounding the brain are neurosurgical emergencies, although not all bleeding requires an operation. The decision to operate will be individualized based upon the injury and the patient's medical status. One option may include craniotomy, drilling a hole into the skull or removing part of one of the skull bones to remove or drain a blood clot, and thereby relieve pressure on brain tissue.

Other times, the treatment is supportive, and there may be a need to monitor the pressure within the brain. The neurosurgeon may place a pressure monitor through a drilled hole through the skull to monitor the pressure.

Supportive care is often required for those patients with significant amounts of bleeding in their brain and who are in coma. Many times, the patient requires intubation to help control breathing and to protect them from vomiting and aspirating vomit into the lungs. Medications may be used to sedate the patient for comfort and to prevent injury if the bleeding causes combativeness. Medications may also be used to try to control swelling in the brain if necessary.

Seizure Control

Midazolam may be used to control seizures in patients with status epilepticus. Propofol or thiopentone may also be used, however hypotension associated with the use of these agents should be treated with fluid therapy.

Phenytoin should be initiated in patients with post-traumatic seizures, although use of prophylactic phenytoin in all head injured children is not supported by clinical evidence. In patients who are sedated and muscle relaxed, EEG should be monitored and nonconvulsive seizures should be controlled to reduce the cerebral oxygen consumption.

Sedation and Muscle Relaxation

Sedation and muscle relaxation is recommended for adequate control of ICP. Fentanyl, midazolam and vecuronium infusion is a good combination as long as hypotension is avoided. Subject to availability, phenobarbitone, propofol may be used. Intermittent thiopentone and intravenous lidocaine is recommended to blunt raised ICP response while suctioning the endotracheal tube. Alternatively instillation of lidocaine in the endotracheal tube may be as effective.

Fluid Therapy

Initial resuscitation should be done with normal saline or Ringer's lactate solution to support hemodynamic status in a hypotensive patient. A central line should be placed to guide fluid therapy by central venous pressure monitoring. Glucose should be maintained at normal level. Hypoglycemia should be avoided in infants and neonates. More commonly, due to stress of the head injury, serum glucose is high, glucose containing fluids should be avoided initially. Ringer's lactate or half normal saline may be used. Hypertonic saline has been used by some centers in presence of hyponatremia due to cerebral salt wasting syndrome.

Mannitol can reduce ICP by two machanisms. Reduction of viscosity which is transient, and dependent upon autoregulation being intact. More potent action, however is by its osmotic effect.

Mannitol in dosages of 0.5 to 1 gm/kg may be used intravenously at 6 hourly interval with monitoring of serum osmolality (to be kept under 320). Mannitol should not be used if serum osmolality is >330, patient is hypotensive, patients with renal failure. Rapid pushes of mannitol can transiently increase ICP by causing transient systemic hypertension, therefore should be avoided. Mannitol has a theoretical risk of enlarging a hematoma by rapid shrinkage of brain and tearing of bridging veins. Therefore a CT may be necessary to rule out a hematoma before mannitol therapy is initiated.

Induced Hypothermia

Prevention of iatrogenic hyperthermia and prompt treatment for fever is very important to keep cerebral metabolic oxygen requirements down.

Nutritional Need

Early institution of enteral feeds is recommended if there is no associated intraabdominal injury to major organs such as liver, spleen, or duodenal hematoma.

Spinal Cord Injury

A spinal cord injury (SCI) is an injury to the spinal cord resulting in its vascular or venous drainage. This injury causes either temporary or permanent changes in the cord's normal motor, sensory, or autonomic function.

Causes

Common causes of damage are trauma (car accident, gunshot, falls, sports injuries, etc.) or disease (transverse myelitis, polio, spina bifida, Friedreich's ataxia, etc.)

Pathophysiology

The spinal cord is a bundle of nerves that runs down the middle of the back. It carries signals back and forth between the body and the brain. A spinal cord injury disrupts the signals. Spinal cord injury occurs when the bony protection surrounding the cord is damaged by way of fractures, dislocation, burst; compression, hyperextension or hyperflexion. Most injuries do not cut through the spinal cord. Instead, they cause damage when pieces of vertebrae tear into cord tissue or press down on the nerve parts that carry signals. The cord may be crushed, stretched beyond tolerance, or completely divided. Spinal cord injuries can be complete or incomplete. With a complete spinal cord injury, the cord cannot send signals below the level of the injury. As a result, paralysis is developed below the injury. With an incomplete injury, some movement and sensation below the injury may be present.

Contd...

Contd...

An incomplete injury means that the ability of the spinal cord to convey messages to or from the brain is not completely lost; some sensation and movement is possible below the level of injury. A complete injury is indicated by a total lack of sensory and motor function below the level of injury.

Manifestations

Injury to the spine can cause problems with voluntary motor control. The muscles may contract uncontrollability, become weak, or be completely paralyzed. Manifestations of SCI include loss of some or all sensation and movement below the level of injury. The location of the spinal cord injury dictates the parts of the body that are affected, and respiratory depression or apnea, hypotension and bradycardia, hypothermia, neck pain, loss of bladder and bowel control may occur. The exam may include evaluation of muscle tone and strength of the arms and legs; sensation in the extremities (including light touch, pain, and vibration); and if the neck is determined not to be injured, the patient's ability to walk may be assessed.

Diagnostic Evaluation

A radiographic evaluation using an X-ray, MRI or CT scan can determine if there is any damage to the spinal cord and where it is located. A neurologic evaluation incorporating sensory testing and reflex testing can help determine the motor function of a person with a SCI.

Treatment

A spinal cord injury is a medical emergency. Immediate treatment can reduce long-term effects. The first stage in the management of a suspected spinal cord injury follows the basic life support principles of resuscitation. It needs to look after the airway plus add cervical spine control. As a basic principle, the head should be maintained in the neutral position, where spine is neither flexed, extended, latterly flexed to either side or rotated. The head should be supported with manual inline support to maintain this position.

Treatments may include medicines, braces or traction to stabilize the spine, and surgery. Inflammation can cause further damage to the spinal cord, and patients are sometimes treated with drugs to reduce swelling. Corticosteroid drugs (30 mg/kg followed by 5 mg/kg of body weight) are used by continuous infusion within 8 hours of the injury. Surgery may also be necessary to remove any bone fragments from the spinal canal and to stabilize the spine. Until permanent surgical stabilization can be performed, other measures can be adopted. The patient may be placed in halo traction and Gardner-Wells tongs as temporary stabilization method.

Later treatment usually includes medicines and rehabilitation therapy. Mobility aids and assistive devices may help the child to get around and do some daily tasks.

CHAPTER 17

The Child with Malignancy

Chapter Outline

- Review of Cancer
- Diagnostic Tests and Procedures, Therapies of Cancer
- Management and Nursing Interventions of Different Conditions
  - Leukemia
  - Tumors
  - Different Lymphomas
  - Bone Cancers

'Childhood cancer is more than chemo and no hair. It is about resilience, strength, hope, courage, love, cuddies, and bravery....'

Cancer in children and adolescents is rare and biologically very different from cancer in adults. Childhood cancer often is difficult to detect in its early stages because the associated signs and symptoms are nonspecific, insidious in onset, and mimic more common disorders. Despite the ongoing global effort to prevent, cure, and control cancer, the specific needs of children and young people are often overlooked. Although 80% of childhood cancers are potentially curable with current treatments, every day around 250 children worldwide lose their lives to cancer.

In India cancer is the 9th common cause for the deaths among children between 5 to 14 years of age. The proportion of childhood cancers relative to all cancers reported by Indian cancer registries varied from 0.8 to 5.8% in boys, and from 0.5 to 3.4% in girls.

The most common types of cancer diagnosed in children and adolescents are leukemia (34%), brain and central nervous system tumors (23%), lymphoma (12%), rhabdomyosarcoma (3%), neuroblastoma (7%), Wilms tumor (5%), bone cancer (3%). The time from onset of symptoms to diagnosis of pediatric cancer is variable and ranges from a median time of 21 days for neuroblastoma to 72 days for Ewing's sarcoma.

REVIEW OF CANCER

In modern medicine, the term *tumor* means a neoplasm that has formed a lump. Neoplasm refers to an abnormal mass of tissue arising from an abnormal proliferation of cells (neoplasia) (Fig. 17.1). These cells do not behave like normal cells, as they usually divide at a faster rate and do not die when they are supposed to. Normally, cells undergo many processes which control their rate of growth and cell division, thus maintaining their natural size. Cells also die naturally in the process known as apoptosis. In a neoplasm, however, these processes are absent, leading to the larger than normal growth of the tissue (lump/tumor). A tumor can be cancerous or benign.

Benign neoplasms are noncancerous forms of tissue proliferation such as skin moles, lipomas or uterine fibroids. These neoplasms do not become cancerous and mainly cause problems due to their space-occupying nature.

Potentially malignant neoplasms include carcinoma in situ. The earliest form of precancer is dysplasia. The cells proliferate only in their site of origin and do not spread invade and destroy. However, dysplasia may become high-grade and transform into carcinoma in situ.

Malignant neoplasms are commonly called cancer. DNA damage is considered to be the primary underlying

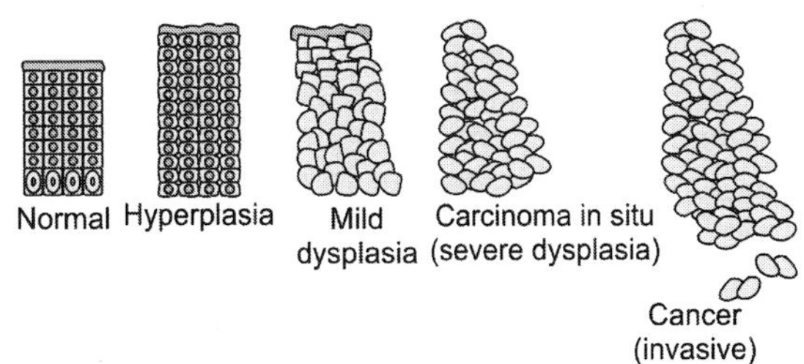

Fig. 17.1: Changes in abnormal cell growth

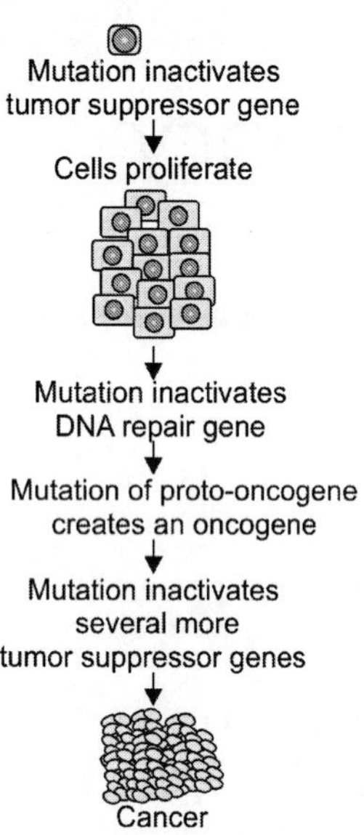

Fig. 17.2: Transformation of normal cells into cancer cells

cause of malignant neoplasms known as cancers. The fast growing cancer cells loss the ability to perform their intended functions because changes in the cell's deoxyriboneuclic acid (DNA) cause wrong information to be transmitted (Fig 17.2). They invade and destroy the surrounding tissue, compress vascular structures and vital organs, which results in symptoms. The neoplasms are described as cancerous when they have following distinct features:

Abnormal Cell Growth

- Capacity to invade other tissues
- Capacity to spread to distant organs via blood vessels or lymphatic channels (metastasis).

In leukemia, a cancer of the blood that starts in the bone marrow, these abnormal cells very rarely form a solid tumor. Instead these cells crowd out other types of cells in the bone marrow. This prevents the production of normal red blood cells, other white blood cells, and platelets.

The process used to find out if cancer has spread within the lymph system or to other parts of the body is called staging. Cancer can spread through tissue, the lymph system, and the blood. Tumor staging describes a cancer, such as where it is located, if or where it has spread, and whether it is affecting other parts of the body. Diagnostic tests and in some cases surgical interventions are needed to find out the cancer's stage, so staging may not be complete until all of the tests are finished. There are different stage descriptions for different types of cancer. Knowing the stage helps to decide what kind of treatment is best and can help predict a patient's prognosis.

Pathophysiology of Cancer

Cancer is not a singular, specific disease but a group of variable tissue responses that result in uncontrolled cell growth and spread of cell. Healthy tissues are composed of cells which have a specific size, structure, function and growth rate that best serves the needs of the tissues they compose. Cancer is fundamentally a disease of tissue growth regulation failure. In order for a normal cell to transform into a cancer cell is regulated by proteins produced by the genetic material in cells. Genetic material can be altered or mutated by environmental factors, errors in genetic replication or repair processes, or by tumor viruses. The affected genes are divided into two broad categories.

- Oncogenes—oncogenes are genes which promote cell growth and reproduction. Altered or mutated genes are called oncogenes, and it is these oncogenes that allow uncontrolled growth in cells the genes which regulate cell growth and differentiation must be altered.
- Tumor suppressor genes—tumor suppressor genes are genes which inhibit cell division and survival. Cancer cells growth is caused by the under-expression or disabling of tumor suppressor genes.

Cellular growth rates are regulated by proteins produced by the genetic material in cells. Genetic material can be altered or mutated by environmental factors, errors in genetic replication or repair processes, or by tumor viruses. Altered or mutated genes are called oncogenes, and it is these oncogenes that allow uncontrolled growth in cells *Replication of the enormous amount of data contained within the DNA of living cells will probably result in some errors (mutations). Complex error correction and prevention is built into the process, and safeguards the cell against cancer. If significant error occurs, the damaged cell can 'self-destruct' through programmed cell death, termed apoptosis. If the error control processes fail, then the mutations will survive and be passed along to daughter cells. Moreover, some environments make errors more likely to arise and propagate. Such environments can include the presence of disruptive substances called carcinogens, repeated physical injury, heat, ionizing radiation, or hypoxia. Cancers are caused by a series of mutations (errors). Each mutation alters the behavior of the cell somewhat in following manner:*

- *A mutation in the error-correcting machinery of a cell might cause that cell and its children to accumulate errors more rapidly.* The epigenetic deficiencies in expression of DNA repair genes, in particular, likely cause an increased frequency of mutations, some of which then occur in oncogenes and tumor suppressor genes.
- *A further mutation in an oncogene might cause the cell to reproduce more rapidly and more frequently than its normal counterparts.*
- *A further mutation may cause loss of a tumor suppressor gene, disrupting the apoptosis signalling pathway and resulting in the cell becoming immortal.*
- A further mutation in signaling machinery of the cell might send error-causing signals to nearby cells.

The transformation of normal cell into cancer is akin to a chain reaction caused by initial errors, which compound into more severe errors, each progressively allowing the cell to escape the controls that limit normal tissue growth. This rebellion-like scenario becomes an undesirable survival of the fittest, where the driving forces of evolution work against the body's design and enforcement of order. Once cancer has begun to develop, this ongoing process, termed clonal evolution drives progression towards more invasive stages.

Contd...

Contd...

Cardinal signs of cancer in children
Cancer can be hard to detect in children. Children with cancer may experience the following symptoms or signs. Sometimes, children with cancer do not show any of these symptoms. Or, these symptoms may be caused by a medical condition that is not cancer. Many of the symptoms can be described using an acronym provided by The Pediatric Oncology Resource Center.
C Continued, unexplained weight loss, headaches, often with early morning vomiting
I Increased swelling or persistent pain in the bones, joints, back, or legs
L Lump or mass, specially in the abdomen, neck, chest, pelvis, or armpits
D Development of excessive bruising, bleeding, or rash
C Constant, frequent, or persistent infections
A A whitish color behind the pupil
N Nausea that persists or vomiting without nausea
C Constant tiredness or noticeable paleness
E Eye or vision changes that occur suddenly and persist
R Recurring or persistent fevers of unknown origin

Incidence of childhood cancer (globally):

Childhood: 14.9 per 100,000 < 15 years of age
16.4 per 100,000 < 20 years of age

Adult: 470.1 per 100,000

Causes of Childhood Cancers

In a small percentage of childhood cancers, familial or genetic factors are thought to predispose the child to cancer. Familial and genetic factors are identified in 5 to 15% of childhood cancer cases. In < 5 to 10% of cases, there are known environmental exposures and exogenous factors, such as prenatal exposure to tobacco, X-rays, or certain medications. For the remaining 75 to 90% of cases, however, the individual causes remain unknown. In most cases, as in carcinogenesis in general, the cancers are assumed to involve multiple risk factors and variables.

Aspects that make the risk factors of childhood cancer different from those seen in adult cancers include:

- Different, and sometimes unique, exposures to environmental hazards. Children must often rely on adults to protect them from toxic environmental agents.
- Immature physiological systems to clear or metabolize environmental substances.
- The growth and development of children in phases known as 'developmental windows' result in certain 'critical windows of vulnerability'.

According to another controversial opinion cancer develops as immune system cannot distinguish between normal and abnormal cells. Factors that affect tumor growth and development include the status of an individual's immune system, the rate the tumor cells are growing, the number of tumor cells actively spreading, and the rate that the normal tissues are being destroyed by the tumor. Several factors affect normal immune function, including stress, malnutrition, advancing age, and chronic diseases. Cancer itself appears to suppress the immune system both early and late in the disease process.

Diagnostic Tests and Procedures for Children

Test	*Description*	*Rationale*	*Nursing considerations*
Bone marrow aspiration	The usual site of bone marrow aspiration is the anterior or posterior iliac crests, (the tibia is sometimes used in infants)	It shows the presence, absence and ratio of cells that are specific to and diagnostic of certain diseases like leukemia, aplastic anemia, specific vitamin deficiencies, neoplastic disorders	• Counseling of the child and parents regarding the test is to be done Take consent • Sedative, anesthetic agents or combination of sedative and analgesic is administered to the child according to the protocol of the institute • Keep the child in prone position with a small pillow under the hips to facilitate access to the posterior iliac crest. Diversion and if necessary, restraining is to be done during aspiration • Apply pressure dressing (if platelet count is below 50,000/ mm^3)/ dressing on the aspiration site Monitor vital signs until stable, and monitor the puncture site for bleeding and signs of infection later

The procedures related to childhood cancer are:

Biopsy: A biopsy is a test in which a small piece of the tissue will be removed and studied under a microscope to see if there are any cancer cells. The initial process for obtaining the specimen is called a biopsy. A biopsy is usually considered a 'small' operation; most of the time it does not require an overnight stay in the hospital. There are different ways that a specimen of the tumor can be obtained:

- *A percutaneous needle biopsy:* In this procedure, a needle is placed through the skin into the tumor and a small piece of the tumor is removed inside the needle. Sometimes this procedure is done using an ultrasound or CT scan to guide the person doing the biopsy. This procedure is usually not done with anesthesia, although intravenous sedation may be required depending on the site of the tumor and age of the child. Depending on the location of the tumor, this procedure may or may not be safer than one of the procedures discussed below. A needle biopsy is able to provide an adequate specimen to make a correct diagnosis about 90% of the time.
- *An open incisional biopsy:* In this procedure, which is almost always done under anesthesia, a small cut is made in the skin through which a small piece of the tumor is removed. This procedure provides an adequate specimen to make a correct diagnosis about 100% of the time.
- *An open excisional biopsy:* In this procedure, which is almost always done under anesthesia, a cut is made in the skin and an attempt is made to remove the entire tumor. This is a bigger operation than either of the two other procedures. This operation is appropriate for children whose tumors have been fully imaged if the surgeon believes that the entire tumor can be removed and doing so will not result in either a functional deficit (i.e. if a calf tumor could be taken out without doing an amputation or otherwise compromising the ability to ambulate), or a cosmetic defect (i.e. if a tumor of the sinuses could be taken out without producing a big facial scar or facial deformity).

Central line: This is commonly referred to as 'PORT'. A small container, about the size of a coin, and about a centimeter thick, attached to a long catheter, is implanted onto the chest, below the collar bone, and that tube is tunneled below the skin and inserted into a large central vein, wither in the lower neck (internal jugular vein), or below the collar bone (subclavian vein). So the container is bang below the skin, and the tube is in the vein. Special right angled, winged needles are available, which are inserted into the container and drugs are delivered. This is the system of choice, is very convenient for the patient, who already has undergone so many pricks for tests and so on, and wherever possible and feasible, must be used.

Kidney test: Some chemotherapy drugs are nephrotoxic. The kidneys breakdown and remove these chemotherapy drugs from the body. When chemotherapy drugs break-down, they make products that can damage cells in the kidneys, ureters and bladder. The potential for kidney damage varies with the type of chemotherapy drug used (cisplatin, mitomycin, nitrosureas, high dose methotrexate).

The kidney functioning is monitored by few tests like creatinine clearance test, BUN, GFR, etc.

Renal and liver function test: The levels of serum creatinine reflect the function of the kidneys. Standard values differ slightly from lab-to-lab, but on an average, the upper limit of serum creatinine is 1.3 mg%. Similarly, the liver function is reflected by the levels of serum bilirubin (must be less than 1.0 mg%), the enzymes SGOT and SGPT, and prothrombin time. This renal and liver function assessment is important, as majority of chemotherapy agents are metabolized and excreted by the liver or kidney, and if the function is deranged, an adjustment in the dosage of the chemotherapy agent will be needed.

CG and 2D Echocardiogram with Doppler studies: These tests give an idea of the function of the heart, both structural as well as functional. Common drugs like doxorubicin and epirubicin have a definite effect on the heart as well, and before giving these drugs, we have to ensure a normal heart function. If the heart function is deranged, we might have to consider giving other chemotherapy agents.

Lumbar puncture: A lumbar puncture is a procedure for taking a sample of fluid from around the spine. A long, thin spinal needle is inserted through the skin, and then through the space between the vertebrae until it enters the space that contains the CSF. The needle is usually inserted between the 3rd and 4th or 4th and 5th lumbar vertebrae (Fig. 17.3). The needle does not enter the spinal cord because the test is done in the lower back, below the level to which the spinal cord extends.

In case of cancer, lumbar puncture is done to find out if there are cancer cells in the fluid surrounding the brain and spinal cord. Chemotherapy medicines may be injected into the CSF at the time a child is having their lumbar puncture.

Pulmonary function test: Pulmonary function testing (PFT) is performed on survivors of childhood cancer. Bleomycin (chemo drug), pulmonary radiotherapy and pulmonary surgery are all associated with pulmonary function impairment. Pulmonary radiotherapy, specially in combination with bleomycin or surgery, is the most important risk factor. This emphasizes the need for adequate counseling and follow-up for this patient population.

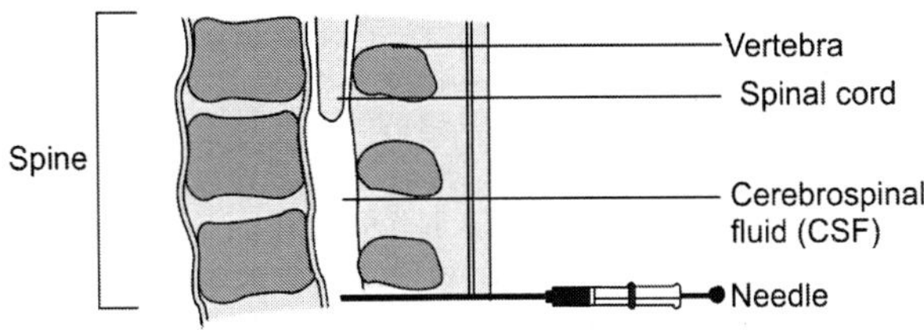

Fig. 17.3: Aspiration of cerebrospinal fluid

Blood Test

Blood studies: A complete blood count is a must before every chemotherapy cycle. One must see the hemoglobin (must be more than 10 gm%, ideally more than 12 is desirable), the WBC count (must be more than 4000/cu.mm), the absolute neutrophil count (ANC) (must be more than 1800), and the platelet count (must be more than 100000). WBC or the white blood cell count reflects the resistance power of the body. 'Neutrophils' are most important first-line defense mechanism of the body. CT should only be given if the WBC and ANC counts are above the desired number. Platelets are important for the first part of clotting of blood, and if the platelets decrease, there is a bleeding tendency. Hence this count must also be normal.

Checking red blood cells (RBC), white blood cell (WBC) and platelet count is necessary before treatment. If RBC is too low child may need a blood transfusion. If either, WBC or platelet count is too low, having more treatment could push them down to a dangerous level.

Bone marrow aspiration and biopsy	A procedure in which a needle is placed into the cavity of a bone, usually the hip or breast bone, to remove a small amount of bone marrow for examination under a microscope.

Imaging Test

CT scan: CT scans are considered one of the greatest medical innovations in the last 50 years. The powerful tests can diagnose internal injuries from major accidents and illnesses in the internal abdomen area that physicians cannot see during a check-up. In childhood cancer it is used to diagnose the stage of cancer, monitor response to treatment for cancer.

SPECT scan: Single photon emission computed tomography (SPECT) scans are similar to PET scans. They use a special camera to make 3-dimensional images of inside the body. SPECT scans are effective for getting information about blood flow to tissues and chemical reactions in the body. SPECT scans are often used for diagnosing and monitoring treatment for brain tumors and cancers affecting bones.

SPECT scans are done by injecting a small amount of radioactive isotope, or tracer, into a vein. The tracer travels to places in the body where there is tumor activity. After the tracer is injected the child will have to lie very still on the SPECT scanner table while pictures are taken.

Nuclear Medicine Scans

Bone scans: A bone scan is a test that can find damage to the bones, find cancer that has spread to the bones, and watch problems such as infection and trauma to the bones. A bone scan can often find a problem days to months earlier than a regular X-ray test.

Find bone cancer or determine whether cancer from another area, such as the breast, lung, kidney, thyroid gland, or prostate gland, has spread metastasized to the bone.

PET scan: Positron emission tomography scan is a procedure to find malignant tumor cells in the body. A small amount of radioactive glucose (sugar) is injected into a vein. The PET scanner rotates around the body and makes a picture of where glucose is being used in the body. Malignant tumor cells show up brighter in the picture because they are more active and take up more glucose than normal cells do. Sometimes a PET scan and a CT scan are done at the same time. If there is any cancer, this increases the chance that it will be found.

Gallium scan: A gallium scan is a nuclear medicine imaging test that uses gallium citrate Ga 67, a radioactive isotope to look for areas of inflammation or infection in the body. The first part of the test involves an injection of a chemical called gallium citrate into the bloodstream. Gallium citrate behaves rather like iron and some of it attaches to proteins in human blood, particularly to the protein called transferrin. It then circulates around the body with blood, and begins to collect in different parts of the body.

A special camera takes images of the body's tissues. Areas of inflammation or rapidly dividing cells show up specially well because they 'take up' more gallium than normal tissue. Gallium emits gamma rays, a type of radioactive wave, which are detected by the gamma camera, are converted into an electrical signal, and sent to a computer. The computer builds a picture by converting the differing intensities of radioactivity emitted into different colors (red spots/hot spots, blue spots/cold spots, etc.) or shades of gray. It can take several days for the gallium to build up, which is why the second part of the scan is done a few days later.

This imaging is done to diagnose and stage certain cancers like lymphoma, lung, osteosarcoma, Ewing's sarcoma, soft tissue sarcoma, rhabdomyosarcoma, and to evaluate how well cancer treatment is working.

MIBG scan: Metaiodobenzylguanidine (MIBG) scans help locate and diagnose certain types of tumors in the body. MIBG is a substance that gathers in some tumors, particularly neuroblastoma tumors. When MIBG is combined with radioactive iodine (tracer) and it is administered through an IV, it provides a way to identify primary and metastatic disease. Pictures are then taken under a scanner that is similar to a CT scan and look for bright spots on the scan, which indicate cancer cell. The scans may occur 24, 48, or 72 hours after the tracer is given. MIBG scans are helpful for locating both bone and soft tissue tumors.

An MIBG scan does not hurt, but it may be difficult or uncomfortable for a child to lie still for the test. Young children may be given a sedative to help them lie still for the entire test. A special medicine is given to protect the thyroid gland from the radioactive substance in the tracer.

Approach to the Child with Cancer

The treatment of childhood cancer depends on several factors, including the type and stage of cancer, possible side effects, the family's preferences, and the child's overall health. Treatment options might include surgery, radiation therapy, chemotherapy, and/or other types of treatment. In many cases, more than one of these treatments is used. The most common types of cancer treatment are as follows:

- Chemotherapy
- Radiation therapy
- Surgery
- Bone marrow transplant (or stem cell transplant)
- Immunotherapy
- Targeted therapy
- Others.

There are exceptions, but childhood cancers usually respond well to chemotherapy because they tend to be cancers that grow fast. (Most forms of chemotherapy affect cells that are growing quickly.) Children's bodies are also generally better able to recover from higher doses of chemotherapy than are adults' bodies. Using more intensive treatments gives a better chance of treating the cancer effectively, but it can also lead to more short- and long-term side effects. It needs a balance between intensive treatments and to limit side effects as much as possible. The child's care plan includes treatment for symptoms and side effects, an important part of cancer care. Treating childhood cancer requires a very specialized approach, and so does the care and follow-up after treatment. The earlier any problems can be recognized, the more likely it is they can be treated effectively.

Chemotherapy

Chemotherapy is a general term for medications (antineoplastic agents) used to destroy or stop the growth of cancer cells. Each drug has its own mode of action and side effect profile. Treatment plan of child with cancer uses the best medicine or combination of medicines available to most effectively combat the child's specific type and stage of cancer. This treatment may be given orally, intravenously, intramuscularly, subcutaneously or intrathecally. Chemotherapy non-selectively kills rapid growing cells (such as cells of the hematopoietic system, GI tract and integumery system) and the side effects of the drugs represent challenges to the caregivers. The early side effects include:

Bone marrow depression: Adverse effects of chemotherapeutic agents on hemopoietic system results in neutropenia, anemia, thrombocytopenia. The child faces threat of opportunistic infections due to neutropenia. Existing bacteria on the skin and gut enter into the blood- stream and leads to life-threatening infection. The usual responses of inflammation (erythema, edema, swelling) is absent as there is markedly decreased WBCs. The health care providers and family must remain acutely aware of elevated body temperature and breaks of skin during acute phase of neutropenia.

GI upset: The noxious stimulus of chemotherapy triggers nausea and vomiting, which is treated with nonsedating antiemetic drugs called 5-HT3 serotonin antagonists (ondensetron, kytril, zofran).

Some chemotherapeutic drugs cause sloughing of the mucosal tissue and leads to the development of mucositis and esophagitis. This extremely painful situation precipitates poor nutrition and bacterial infection may occur if bacteria, yeast of the gut enter into the blood through the damaged mucous membrane. Poor intake, decreased activity and pain medication may contribute constipation. Passage of hard stool through the rectum may cause abrasion and again bacterial infection due to entry of microorganisms via break integument.

Alopecia: Chemotherapy drugs are powerful medications that attack rapidly growing cancer cells. Unfortunately, these drugs also attack other rapidly growing cells in body including those in hair roots. Fortunately, most of the time hair loss from chemotherapy is temporary. Regrow of hair occurs 3 to 10 months after the treatment ends, though new hair may temporarily be a different shade or texture. Hair loss has a tremendous psychological effect, specially on the school age and adolescent population.

Common Late Effects of Chemotherapy

Late side effects experienced by childhood cancer survivors include:

Learning disabilities: Cognitive and memory impairments appear to be more common in children who were younger than years at the time of treatment and in those who received chemotherapy directly in the spine or radiation to the head and neck area. The chemotherapeutic drugs, like methotrexate and cytarabine (Ara-C), also can interfere with learning.

Learning difficulties range from mild to severe, and may show up soon after treatment or several years later. Common learning difficulties include problems with memory, processing speed, and multitasking. Children who are at risk of learning disabilities should be evaluated after their cancer treatment ends.

Abnormal bone growth: Radiation therapy may cause *abnormal bone growth*. Children who undergo radiation treatment may be at risk for stunted bone growth later on, specially in the area where the radiation was targeted. Chemotherapy has a similar effect, and even though there may be a period of catch-up growth after treatment, some children would not grow past a certain height.

Growth disorders also can be caused by treatment's effect on the glands and hormones of the endocrine system, the system in the body that regulates growth and development. Children younger than 5 years or those who were in puberty at the time of treatment seem to be most susceptible. They also may be at risk for developing osteoporosis or scoliosis.

Thyroid problems: The thyroid gland controls metabolism of body. It may be damaged by radiation to the head or neck. The result is typically hypothyroidism, which results in fatigue, weight gain, thinning hair, and dry skin.

Hearing loss: Chemotherapy, radiation to the brain, and even certain antibiotics can lead to high-frequency hearing loss, tinnitus (ringing in the ears), or dizziness.

Vision problems: Blurred or double vision, glaucoma, or cataracts are more likely in children who were treated for tumors near the eye or received radiation to the brain.

Dental problems: Very young children who have had radiation to the brain may have short dental roots, delayed teeth, or missing teeth. All children who have received chemotherapy are at risk for tooth decay and gum disease.

Lung, liver, or kidney problems: Childhood cancer treatments have been linked to several types of organ damage later in life, although the severity varies widely depending on the type of cancer and treatment.

Heart problems: Children who had chemotherapy with antibiotic drug anthracycline or underwent chest and spinal radiation are at increased risk for heart problems up to 20 years or longer after treatment. The severity of the problem depends on how much chemotherapy or radiation was given during treatment, what part of the body the radiation was delivered to, and the child's age at the time of treatment. Family genetics, weight, and cholesterol level also have an impact regarding heart problems.

Delayed sexual development and fertility issues: Both chemotherapy and radiation can cause fertility problems. These late effects may be from damage to the endocrine system or to the sexual organs themselves.

Because of the risk, special measures are taken prior to or during treatment to preserve the reproductive organs. For example, during radiation the ovaries and testicles are shielded from treatment. The good news is that despite these potential risks, many childhood cancer survivors can go on to have healthy children of their own.

Increased risk of future cancers: Childhood cancer survivors have a slightly increased risk of developing a second cancer at some point in their life, even if the original cancer does not recur. The factors which affect this risk are type of the first cancer, the treatments given, and any genetic predisposition.

Radiation Therapy

Radiation therapy uses high-energy radiation from X-rays, gamma rays, or fast-moving subatomic particles (called particle or proton beam therapy) to kill cancer cells and shrink tumors by damaging their DNA, the genetic material in a cell. When DNA is damaged, cells either stop dividing or die. It is the single most effective cancer-treating agent. Radiation may be used for curative purpose, to eradicate cancer cells or palliatively (in low doses) to prevent further growth of the tumor. Types of childhood cancer treated with radiation therapy include brain tumors, Wilms tumor, and head and neck cancers. Total body irradiation is given before some stem cell transplant attempts, which helps to iradicate microscopic disease and promote bone marrow suppression.

Radiation therapy is delivered one of three ways:

- External-beam radiation therapy uses a machine (linear accelerator) that directs specific amount of high-energy beams of radiation at cancerous tumors or diseased areas of the body.
- Internal radiation therapy, also called brachytherapy, delivers radiation either inside a body cavity or within body tissue.
- Systemic radiation, which involves swallowing or receiving an injection of a substance, such as radioactive iodine or radioactive material bound to a monoclonal antibody,that travels through the blood to locate and kill tumor cells.

Most children receive only external radiation therapy, and which also sometimes given in hyperfractionated doses (daily dose is split into smaller doses). The split doses are administered frequently to minimize side effects and increase tumor kill by decreasing time repair between doses.

Receiving radiation therapy for cancer treatment is not a one-time deal; children visit the hospital 4 to 5 days a week for several weeks. Receiving small daily doses of radiation helps to protect the normal cells from damage, while weekend breaks help them recover from the trauma of radiation. The preparation of the child and family is done through counseling and simulation which includes education about the process and side effects of the treatment. Simulation is the process of measuring child's body and marking the skin to help direct the beams of radiation safely and exactly to the intended locations. The child will lie on an X-ray table while a radiation therapist uses an X-ray machine (called a simulator) to define the treatment area. The radiation oncologist controls the depth and peripheral margins of the radiation site, and marked as 'tattoo', which should not be wiped off because it helps to position the radiation for each treatment. Sometimes it is difficult to keep the younger children still during treatment, in that cases, the children may wear a custom body cast or be sedated to help immobilize them. To prevent unnecessary radiation exposure, parents are not allowed in the treatment room, but can still be there for their child during therapy.

Although the main purpose of radiation is to destroy cancer cells, it also can damage healthy cells. The physical side effects of radiation therapy depend on the dose of radiation, the location where it was received, and whether the radiation was internal or external. The early side effects of radiation are:

Erythema: The most common side effect is the erythema within the radiated area. This area may be red, sensitive, or easily irritated in the days, weeks, and months during and after treatment. The skin may swell or droop or the texture may change, which should go away 2 to 3 weeks after treatment ends.

Fatigue: Both during treatment and after, fatigue (tiredness) often begins within a few weeks of the start of treatment and lasts for 4 to 6 weeks after it is completed. Encourage your child to rest and sleep as often as possible, even if it does not immediately result in more energy. In the long run, rest helps the body recover from radiation treatment.

GI upset: Children may have gastrointestinal problems (such as loss of appetite, diarrhea, nausea, and vomiting) if they received radiation treatment to the pelvis or abdomen. Some who receive radiation therapy to the head and neck also may have nausea and vomiting.

Bone marrow suppression: Radiation therapy may cause low levels of platelets, red blood cells, and white blood cells. Bone marrow suppression depends on the dose and site of therapy.

Radiation therapy as a treatment modality is not without risk. In general, radiotherapy is used more sparingly in children than in adults because developing tissues and organs are more vulnerable to its late adverse effects. Radiation therapy in children below 3 years is devastating as it effects in brain tissue development and may alter cognitive potential. Bone growth of child is altered if it is delivered to areas of growth potential like growth plates of long bones, spine, and facial bone.

Surgery

Surgery has an integral role in treating most childhood cancers. Surgery is used to treat cancer in a variety of ways, including diagnosis, tumor removal, or to support a child undergoing cancer treatment or performing reconstructive surgery. The role that surgery plays in the treatment depends upon the type, location, and extent of the cancer. In case of cancer, the diagnosis is made by biopsy. The purpose of a biopsy is to obtain a small piece of the tumor for microscopic test. The test result confirms the tumor type and influences therapy decisions. The goal of surgery is to remove the entire tumor and the margin (tissue around the tumor), leaving a negative margin (no cancer in the healthy tissue). For most childhood tumors, there is microscopic tumor left after surgery, and then doctors will recommend chemotherapy, radiation therapy, or other treatments.

There are two main types of surgery:

Open (conventional) surgery: A specific part of the body is accessed by making an incision in the body. Cancerous tumors are often removed through open surgery.

Minimally invasive surgery: Surgeons will perform the same operation they would in an open surgery, but do so using small incisions and instruments specially designed to fit through the small incisions. If the child is having a minimally invasive surgical procedure, the surgeon will make a series of small incisions (about half an inch each), rather than one large incision. Because it uses much smaller incisions than traditional surgery, minimally invasive methods usually mean less pain, easier recovery, less scarring or disfiguring, and more normal growth after surgery. Minimally invasive surgery is less common for cancer patients than for other types of diseases.

In cancer treatment, surgeries are further classified according to the purpose that they serve in treatment.

Primary surgery: Primary surgery removes all or most of the tumor at one time. In some cases, the tumor is too big, or is in an area of the body where it cannot be safely removed. In these cases, chemotherapy or radiation may be given before surgery to help shrink the tumor and make it easier to remove.

Second look (exploratory) surgery: Second look or exploratory surgery is performed to see how well treatments (chemotherapy, radiation therapy) have worked in killing cancer cells. Sometimes, surgeons are able to remove remaining tumor(s) during this surgery.

Supportive care surgery and procedures: Supportive care surgery or procedures are done to cope with cancer treatments. Examples of supportive care surgery include:

- Putting a central venous line into a vein in the chest. A central venous catheter is a central line placed to provide easy access to the venous system. The line will allow treatments to be given and blood samples taken without being 'stuck' with a needle.
- Putting a gastrostomy tube (G-tube) into the child's stomach. If the child is not able to take food by mouth for an extended period of time, the G-tube can be used to feed the child until he or she is able to eat food by mouth again.

Side effects of surgery depend on the location and type of the tumor and whether it has metastasized.

Bone Marrow Transplant (Stem Cell Transplant)

Bone marrow contains the youngest type of blood cells known as hematopoietic stem cells. As a hematopoietic stem cell ages, it becomes a white cell, red cell, or platelet. A bone marrow transplant (BMT) replaces diseased or damaged cells with noncancerous stem cells that can grow healthy, new cells. BMT is usually used when cancer treatments have destroyed normal stem cells in the bone marrow. The stem cells can be replaced through BMT. A BMT is also performed when the chances for cure with chemotherapy alone are low. There are two major types of BMT.

Allogenic type of transplant: This type of transplant is used for patients with leukemias, some lymphomas. Here bone marrow or blood cells are received from donor other than the patient. The donor is selected through tissue typing called human lymphocyte antigens (HLA). These antigens are found on the surface of white blood cells. If a related donor is not available, then a search for a compatible, unrelated donor is performed. Unrelated donor cells can come from a living donor or frozen cord blood.

The autologous type of transplant: This is performed for patients who has solid tumors such as neuroblastoma, Hodgkin's disease, and brain tumors. Here the patient's own bone marrow or blood cells are used for transplant. In autologous transplant peripheral stem cells are usually collected, but stem cells from the bone marrow also can be used. These are collected either before the patient has chemotherapy or following a course of chemotherapy. To collect peripheral stem cells, the patient receives medications such as granulocytes cells stimulating factor (G-CSF and/or GM-CSF) to increase the number of peripheral blood stem cells available.

By the process of apheresis stem cells are collected. An *apheresis machine* has a circuit that will collect blood, separate, and remove white blood cells containing stem cells, and then return red blood cells to the patient. This process takes about 4 hours and may need to be repeated for 2 or 3 days in a row. For certain diseases, the peripheral blood stem cells may be treated with anticancer medications to prevent tumor cells from being placed into back into the patient's body.

Preparation and the Transplant

Before transplant the child will undergo testing to make sure he/she is healthy enough to withstand the rigors of transplant. Testing will include evaluation of the heart function with ECG and lung function, kidney and liver function, and infection status. Depending upon the disease, a bone marrow aspirate and spinal tap may be performed.

The child will be given preparative treatment, called 'conditioning' before the transplant. Conditioning includes high doses of chemotherapy and sometimes, radiation of the whole body. The objectives of 'conditioning' are:

- Elimination of the cancer
- Making space in the bone marrow for new cells to grow.
- Suppression of the immune system so that new cells may be accepted.

Commonly used drugs include cyclophosphamide, melphalan, busulfan, etoposide, thiotepa, carboplatin.

Once conditioning is complete, stem cells are given through a catheter (preferably through central line).

It can take between 14 and 30 days for enough blood cells, particularly white blood cells, to be created so the body can fight infection. The identification of new blood cells and an increase in white blood cells following BMT is called engraftment. Until then, the child will be at a high risk for infection, anemia, and bleeding.

Infection is very common before, during, and after transplant as the child's immune system has already been eliminated during conditioning. Protection of the child from infection and proper use of antibiotic is must. Anemia and thrombocytopenia are corrected with transfusion of red blood cells and platelets. IV fluids or nutrition and pain medicines are used to help with symptoms like nausea, loss of appetite and mucositis. These problems usually improve as the new cells grow in the patient.

Graft vs. host disease (GVHD): This occurs only in an allogeneic blood or marrow transplant. Certain types of donor cells, called T-lymphocytes react to the patient's body and recognize it as 'antigen'. Medicines are given post-transplant to prevent this complication, but it may occur despite this.

- *Acute graft vs. host disease:* Most commonly occurs within 3 months of transplant and skin, liver, and intestines of patient may be affected. Skin involvement occurs as a red rash that may be itchy or develop blisters. Liver involvement may cause jaundice or elevation of other liver tests. Intestinal involvement may cause very severe diarrhea. Medicines such as steroids are used to treat GVHD and are often successful in controlling it.
- *Chronic graft vs. host disease:* It may occur months or even years after the transplant. Most commonly it is a continuation of acute GVHD. Many different parts of the body may be affected. Skin is the most common organ affected—patients may have red, scaly skin or skin that is thickened and tough. There may also be changes in the mucous membrane lining of mouth, dry eyes, dry mouth, joint stiffness, lung restriction, and difficulty absorbing nutrients from foods. In addition, patients are at risk for infection because of the medications needed to control the GVHD as well as the effect of GVHD upon the immune system.

Organ toxicity: Conditioning and prior cancer treatment may damage the lungs, liver, kidneys, and heart. These effects are unpredictable and not all children recover from organ toxicity.

Late effects: There is a very good chance that there will be long-term effects following BMT that may not be identified until years after treatment. These include:

- **Growth** and other endocrine gland problems may develop depending upon the type of conditioning used.
- **Sterility** is common for most patients in later life.
- **Organ damage** like liver, kidneys, lungs, or heart may occur.
- **Cataracts** may develop and affect vision.

Immunotherapy

Immunotherapy is sometimes referred to as either biotherapy or biological therapy. The biologic response modifiers are the recent additions in cancer therapy. Immunotherapy uses the body's own immune system to fight cancer cells. It is also used to help control side effects from other cancer treatments.

In immunotherapy, the substances that naturally occur in the body are used to boost the functioning of the immune system. As a result, the body is able to destroy cancer cells more effectively. As immunotherapy uses naturally occurring substances, so it can lessen the side effects of cancer treatments and help the body replace normal cells that have been damaged or destroyed. The spread of cancer cells in the body is also prevented by immunotherapy.

The immune system which is a network of organs and cells that work to protect the body against disease; looks for cells that are not normal, such as bacteria, viruses, and cancer cells, and tries to destroy them.

During this therapy, patients are given substances called biological response modifiers (BRMs). Normally body creates these BRMs to fight cancer and other diseases. BRMs enhance the body's natural immune system and destroy cancer cells. BRMs can also change the way the body reacts to a tumor.

There are two primary ways that BRMs work in immunotherapy:

- *Active immunotherapies:* Stimulating the body's natural immune system responses to work harder and more efficiently.
- *Passive immunotherapies:* Giving substances, such as man-made proteins, to supplement a patient's immune system to help it work more effectively.

Four common BRMs used to treat cancer are:

- Cytokines
- Interleukins
- Colony-stimulating factors
- Monoclonal antibodies.

Most often immunotherapy is given in addition to other cancer treatments such as chemotherapy. Treatments are generally injected into a vein through an IV, but there are also tablets and injection that can be given at home.

The side effects depend upon the type of treatment performed. It is common for patients treated with immunotherapy to get flu-like symptoms. Side effects generally go away at the end of treatment.

Common side effects are changes in blood pressure, chills, diarrhea, easy bruising or bleeding, fever, loss of appetite, muscle aches, nausea, skin rash, vomiting, weakness.

Targeted Therapy

Targeted therapies are a newer approach to cancer treatment and a major focus for research. These therapies use medications or other substances to stop the growth and spread of cancer.

Targeted therapies work by focusing on the ways cancer cells act differently from healthy cells and interrupting these processes. They 'target' processes that play an important role in cancer growth so that cancer cells are unable to increase. An example of this would be stopping blood vessels that 'feed' cancer cells, or interfering with signals that the cancer cells need for growth. While each type of targeted therapy works differently, they all aim to disrupt the way cancer cells duplicate and interact with other cells.

Targeted therapies can be used alone or in combination with other treatments, such as chemotherapy and radiation. When used in combination, targeted therapies can improve the effectiveness of other treatments.

Side effects of targeted therapies vary widely among the different types of medications. When side effects do occur, they are generally milder than side effects from other cancer therapies and go away at the end of treatment. In rare cases, patients have had allergic reactions to some therapies.

Other Management

Management of Tumor Lysis Syndrome (TLS)

Chemotherapy may cause the cancer cells to breakdown very quickly. This can cause chemical imbalances in the blood that affect the kidneys and the heart. This is called tumor lysis syndrome (TLS).

Where WBCs count is very high, the Tumor lysis syndrome may occur after chemotherapy. When chemo kills these cells, they break open and release their contents into the bloodstream. This can overwhelm the kidneys, which are not able to get rid of all of these substances at once. Excess amounts of certain minerals may also affect the heart and nervous system. This problem can be prevented by making sure the child gets lots of fluids during treatment and by giving certain drugs, such as bicarbonate, allopurinol, and rasburicase, which help the body get rid of these substances.

LEUKEMIA

Leukemia is a hematological malignancy. It is developed in the bone marrow, the spongy center of the bones that makes blood cells. It accounts for approximately 30 to 35% of all childhood cancers; approximately 1 in 1000 children will be diagnosed with leukemia by the age of 19, although it is more common in children under the age of 10. The most common types in children are acute lymphocytic leukemia (ALL) and acute myelogenous leukemia (AML).

In leukemia, abnormal white blood cells divide out of control and crowd out the normal cells in the bloodstream (Fig. 17.4). These immature WBCs (blasts) compete with normal cells for space and nutrition. The abnormal white blood cells are not mature, and therefore cannot carry out their infection-fighting function in the blood. These cells crowd out healthy white blood cells, as well as the red blood cells which carry oxygen to the body and the platelets which cause the blood to clot. As the bone marrow production of normal cells is suppressed the child may show leukopenia, anemia, and thrombocytopenia at diagnosis.

Previously leukemia was fatal, but today child with ALL (most common form of leukemia) can almost always achieve remission and survival rate is about 85%.

Etiology and Incidence

The causes of childhood leukemia are not well understood. It accounts for 30% of all cancers diagnosed in children under 15 years of age in industrialized countries. Most cancers in children, like those in adults,

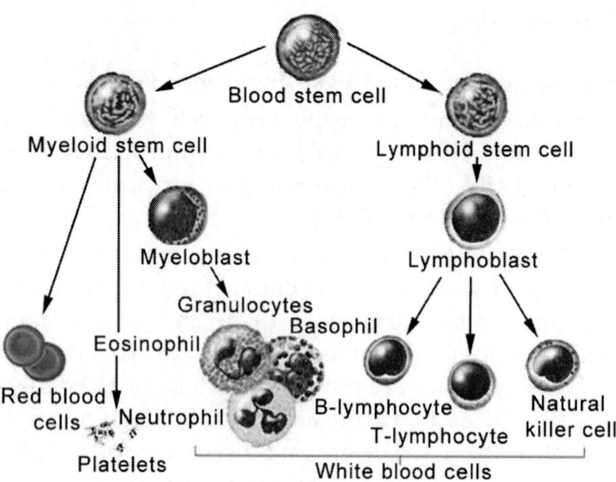

Fig. 17.4: Normal hemopoietic system

are thought to develop as a result of mutations in genes that lead to uncontrolled cell growth and eventually cancer. Genetic risk factors, associated with the part of DNA, are most often inherited from parents. While some genetic factors increase the risk of childhood leukemia, most cases of leukemia are not linked to any known genetic causes.

In the majority of cases of childhood leukemia, the cause is unknown. While a number of causes and highly suspected risk factors have been identified, reviews stress that these are responsible for only a very small number of cases. The known and highly suspected causes include genetic factors (2 to 3% of cases are associated with Down syndrome) and exposure to ionizing radiation in utero and after birth. Infectious diseases are likely to have a role in the etiology of childhood leukemia, specially ALL. Delayed exposure to infection during early infancy could result in an abnormal response, leading to development of leukemia. Leukemia could also be a rare response to a specific although unidentified infectious agent. (*WHO 2009*).

Exposure to high levels of radiation is a risk factor for childhood leukemia. Japanese atomic bomb survivors had a greatly increased risk of developing AML, usually within 6 to 8 years after exposure. If a fetus is exposed to radiation within the first months of development, there may also be an increased risk of childhood leukemia, but the extent of the risk is not clear.

Many studies have shown that exposure to ionizing radiation can damage DNA, which can lead to the development of childhood leukemia and possibly other cancers. For example, children and adolescents who were exposed to radiation from the World War II atomic bomb blasts had an elevated risk of leukemia.

Children who are getting intensive treatment to suppress their immune function (mainly organ transplant patients) have an increased risk of certain cancers, such as lymphoma and ALL.

Leukemia represents about 40% of all childhood cancers, peak incidence of ALL occurs between ages 2 and 6 years and it is common in boys than girls. Overall incidence of ALL is about 80% and AML accounts for 15% of all cases of leukemia.

Pathophysiology

Leukemia is a group of malignant diseases in which genetic abnormalities in a hemopoietic cell give rise to an unregulated clonal proliferation of cells. These cells have advantage of increased rate of replication and decreased rate of apoptosis. It leads to formation of immature cells, or blast cells in the bone marrow, which crowd out other normal cells production. This results in disruption of normal marrow function and, ultimately, bone marrow failure. In leukemia, normal bone marrow is replaced by malignant blast cells. The child becomes anemic and thrombocytopenic as RBC and platelet production is affected as the blast cells take over the bone marrow. The symptoms of the disease reflect bone marrow failure and organ infiltration.

Clinical Manifestations

A child with leukemia may seem to be struggling to keep up their typical activity level or they may not have the energy to do even their favorite activities. Children with leukemia may have more viral or bacterial infections than usual as their WBCs are defective. They also may become anemic because leukemia affects the bone marrow's production of RBCs. This makes them appear pale, and they may become abnormally tired and short of breath while playing. Bone marrow suppression causes thrombocytopenia and children with leukemia might bruise and bleed very easily, experience frequent nosebleeds, or bleed for an unusually long time after even a minor cut. Other clinical manifestations of leukemia include:

- Pain in the bones or joints, sometimes causing a limp
- Easy bruising, unusual bleeding, frequent nosebleeds, bleeding gums, petechiae
- Swollen lymph nodes (sometimes called swollen glands) in the neck, groin, or elsewhere
- An abnormally tired feeling
- Poor appetite
- Fevers with no other symptoms and lasts for several days

- Abdominal pain (caused by abnormal blood cells building up in organs like the kidneys, liver, or spleen)
- Night sweats, irritability.

Occasionally, the spread of leukemia to the brain can cause headaches, seizures, balance problems, or abnormal vision. If ALL spreads to the lymph nodes inside the chest, the enlarged mass can crowd the trachea and important blood vessels, leading to breathing problems, and interfere with blood flow to and from the heart.

Diagnostic Evaluation

The diagnosis is often established from a history of the clinical manifestations and an initial CBC. Then, depending on the results of the medical history, physical exam and preliminary blood tests, the child might need a bone marrow aspiration and biopsy. For the confirmatory test of leukemia, the marrow sample is examined under microscope to look for abnormal cells. A lumbar puncture is done, and examined for evidence of blast cells in spinal fluid. This shows whether the leukemia has spread to the central nervous system or not. Imaging studies, such as X-rays, ultrasounds, CT scans, or MRIs are also performed.

Therapeutic Management

Leukemia is treated by combination chemotherapy and sometimes radiation. According to protocol, the particular drugs are used and their dose, route and scheduling are determined on the basis of specific type of leukemia. Some of the drugs commonly used to treat childhood leukemia include:

Vincristine (oncovin), daunorubicin, also known as daunomycin (cerubidine), doxorubicin (adriamycin), cytarabine, also known as cytosine arabinoside or ara-C (cytosar), L-asparaginase (elspar), PEG-L-asparaginase, etoposide, teniposide (vumon), 6-mercaptopurine (purinethol), 6-thioguanine, methotrexate, mitoxantrone, cyclophosphamide (cytoxan), prednisone, dexamethasone (decadron, others).

Children with leukemia probably get several of these drugs at different times during the course of treatment, but they do not get all of them in one point of time. The 5-year survival rate for children diagnosed with leukemia and subsequently treated is approximately 70%.

Treatment extends over a 2-year period. Before induction of chemotherapy the child is treated for presenting signs which may include sepsis, anemia, hemorrhage, and metabolic abnormalities. To ensure metabolic stability, the serum electrolytes levels are determined. Where WBCs count is very high, the tumor lysis syndrome may occur after chemotherapy. (discussed above).

The diagnosis of acute lymphocytic leukemia (ALL) is made on the basis of a bone marrow biopsy and its treatment is divided into phases like induction, consolidation and maintenance.

Phase I is called induction. The goal of induction is to bring about a *remission*. This means to reduce blast cells in the bone marrow less than 5%, the normal marrow cells return, and the blood counts become normal. To induce remission, patients are given 4 or 5 drugs over a period of several weeks, usually while hospitalized. Approximately 98% of children achieve remission within 1 month of treatment.

Phase II is consolidation, when the children undergo 6 to 9 months of intensive chemotherapy, usually as outpatients. The goal of this phase (also called *intensification*) is to get rid of leukemia cells in hidden places. Several drugs are used, depending on the child's risk category. *Some children may benefit from a stem cell transplant at this time.*

Phase III is maintenance. Then they move on to 18 months of outpatient maintenance therapy.

Periodic spinal taps to administer chemotherapy into the spinal fluid and surveillance bone marrow biopsies are performed throughout the 2-year period.

As with ALL, the diagnosis of acute myelogenous leukemia (AML) is made through bone marrow biopsy. In AML, remission is brought about with a combination of 3 chemotherapy drugs given to hospitalized patients. Follow-up chemotherapy is administered for 4 to 6 months. Patients require frequent hospitalizations throughout this period. By examining the chromosomes of leukemia cells at the time of diagnosis, it is determined which patients are likely to stay in remission and which are not.

If the leukemia comes back during or after treatment, the child will again be treated with chemo. This may include the same or different drugs, depending on how long the remission lasted. A stem cell transplant may be considered for children whose leukemia comes back soon after starting treatment, specially if there is a brother or sister who is a good match. Some children have a relapse in which leukemia cells are found in one part of the body (such as the cerebrospinal fluid or the testicles) but are not found in the bone marrow. These children may have intense chemo, sometimes along with radiation or surgery to the affected area.

A *stem cell transplant may* be required for children whose leukemia has returned or has not responded to standard treatments. Patients with acute leukemia at high risk for relapse or patients with chronic leukemia are advised to undergo a bone marrow or stem cell transplant from a matched sibling or unrelated donor in their first remission. Stem cell transplant may also be used for other children who relapse after a second course of chemo. Patients in other groups usually do not undergo transplantation unless they relapse. Stem cells, which are immature blood cells, are taken from the bone marrow of the patient before cancer treatment (autologous), or from a donor whose marrow most closely matches the patient (allogeneic).

Stem cells may also be collected from a newborn's umbilical cord and placenta and used for a cord blood transplant. These cells are used to replace diseased stem cells destroyed by cancer treatment, creating a new 'blood factory' that will hopefully produce healthy, mature white blood cells.

Radiation therapy may be used when leukemia has affected the brain and central nervous system or is likely to spread to these areas. Beams of radiation are precisely aimed at the treatment area from outside the body.

Nursing Management (Table 17.1)

Nursing Diagnosis

Risk for infection during acute phases of disease/treatment, due to immune-suppressed state of the child.

Table 17.1: Care of a child with leukemia

Nursing interventions	*Rationale*
• Place the child in private room. Screen/limit visitors as indicated • Require good hand-washing protocol for all personnel and visitors • Use sterile techniques to change any dressings and IV lines • Monitor vital signs 4 hourly and as necessary. Observe for fever associated with tachycardia, hypotension, subtle mental changes • Prevent chilling. Force fluids, administer tepid sponge bath. Administer acetaminophen for fever • Encourage frequent turning and deep breathing. • Auscultate breath sounds, noting crackles, rhonchi; inspect secretions for changes in characteristics; e.g. increased sputum production or change in sputum color. Observe urine for signs of infection; e.g. cloudy, foul-smelling, or presence of urgency or burning with voids • Inspect skin for tender, erythematous areas; open wounds. Cleanse skin with antibacterial solutions • Inspect oral mucous membranes. Provide good oral hygiene. Use a soft toothbrush, or swabs for frequent mouth care • Handle client gently. Keep linens dry/wrinkle- free • Promote good perianal hygiene. Examine perianal area at least daily during acute illness. Avoid rectal temperatures, use of suppositories • Coordinate procedures and tests to allow for uninterrupted rest periods • Encourage increased intake of foods high in protein and fluids with adequate fiber • Fresh fruits and vegetables are to be washed or peeled before giving to the patient • Avoid/limit invasive procedures (e.g. venipuncture and injections) as possible • In general, the child should not be given live virus or live bacterial vaccines • Monitor intake of fluid of the child and his output. Note decreased urine output in presence of adequate intake. Measure urine specific gravity and pH. Weigh daily, monitor BP and HR, evaluate skin turgor, capillary refill, and general condition of mucous membranes • Note presence of nausea, fever • Encourage fluids as per need of the child • Administer IV fluids as indicated • Administer medications as indicated, like antibiotics, Antiemetics: 5-HT_3 receptor antagonist drugs such as ondansetron (Zofran) or granisetron (Kytril)	• Protect client from potential sources of infection. These children are prone to infection as they have profound bone marrow suppression, neutropenia, and receive chemotherapy • Prevents cross-contamination/reduces risk of infection • Although fever may accompany some forms of chemotherapy, and fever occurs in most leukemia clients. Septicemia may occur without fever • Hydrotherapy reduces fever, which contributes to fluid imbalance, discomfort, and CNS complications • Changing positions prevent stasis of respiratory secretions, reducing risk of atelectasis or pneumonia. • Early intervention is essential to prevent sepsis or septicemia in immunosuppressed person • The oral cavity is an excellent medium for growth of organisms and is susceptible to ulceration and bleeding • Wrinkle-free bed prevents sheet burn/skin excoriation • May indicate local infection • Note: Open wounds may not produce pus because of insufficient number of granulocytes • Promotes cleanliness, reducing risk of perianal abscess; enhances circulation and healing. Perianal abscess may be fatal in immunosupressed clients • Conserves energy for healing, cellular regeneration • Good nutrition promotes healing and prevents dehydration. Constipation prevention is necessary as it potentiates retention of toxins and risk of rectal irritation/tissue injury • Avoid/limit invasive procedures as possible • The live vaccines could produce infection in the severely immunocompromised child • Tumor lysis syndrome occurs when destroyed cancer cells release toxic levels of potassium, phosphorus, and uric acid. Elevated phosphorus and uric acid levels can cause crystal formation in the renal tubules, impairing filtration and leading to renal failure • So maintenance of adequate hydration is necessary to promote urine flow, to prevent uric acid precipitation, and thus to enhance clearance of antineoplastic drugs. • A decreased platelet count increases the risk of hemorrhage, so prevention of tissue injury and early detection of the symptoms can avoid the hazard

Contd...

Contd...

Nursing interventions	*Rationale*
• Allopurinol (Zyloprim); potassium acetate or citrate, sodium bicarbonate; stool softener • Inspect skin/mucous membranes for petechiae, ecchymotic areas; note: bleeding gums, frank or occult blood in stools and urine, oozing from invasive line sites • Implement measures to prevent tissue injury/bleeding • Gentle brushing of teeth or gums with soft toothbrush, or sponge-tipped applicator; avoiding forceful nose blowing • Needle sticks when possible; using sustained pressure on oozing puncture/IV sites • Limit oral care to mouth rinse if indicated (e.g. a mixture of 1/4th tsp baking soda and 1/8th tsp salt in 8 oz water; may use hydrogen peroxide in water or saline for bleeding or infected oral tissue) • Provide soft diet • Monitor laboratory studies; platelets, Hb/Hct, clotting • Administer RBCs, platelets, clotting factors as directed • Maintain external central vascular access device (subclavian or tunneled catheter or implanted port) • Assess the pain site of the child by using pain scale (use FLACC Pain Scale 0 to 10) • Monitor vital signs, note nonverbal cues; e.g. cry, movement muscle tension, restlessness • Provide quiet environment and reduce stressful stimuli; e.g. lighting, noise, constant interruptions • Maintain comfortable position and support joints, extremities with pillows/padding • Frequent change of position and encourage/assist with gentle ROM exercises • Provide nonpharmacologic measures (comfort measures [e.g. massage, cool packs)] and psychologic support (e.g. encouragement, talking, presence, if possible to allow parent) • Evaluate and support child's coping mechanisms • Encourage use of stress management technique like (Fig. 17.5), relaxation/deep-breathing exercises, guided imagery, visualization, therapeutic touch • Assist with/provide diversional activities, suitable play therapy • Monitor uric acid level as appropriate • Administer medications as prescribed • Analgesics/opioids/antianxiety agents • Physical health status is to be noted. Reports of fatigue, inability to participate in activities or ADLs are to be evaluated • Encourage the child to keep a diary of daily routines and energy levels, noting activities that increase fatigue • Provide quiet environment and uninterrupted rest periods. Encourage rest periods before meals • Implement energy-saving techniques; e.g. sitting, rather than standing, use of stool at bath time. Assist with ambulation/ other activities as indicated • Recommend small, nutritious, high-protein meals and snacks throughout the day. Schedule meals around chemotherapy. Give oral hygiene before meals • Provide supplemental oxygen • Review pathology of specific form of leukemia and various treatment options	• The nose is the one of the most common sites of bleeding. Blood loss can be reduced through avoidance of nose bleeds • The mucous membranes are fragile, potential sites of infection and easily affected by chemotherapy and irradiation. • Additional pressure may be needed to stop bleeding if the platelet count is low • Helpful in assessing need for intervention; may indicate developing complications • Verbal reactions is useful to assess effectiveness of interventions • Promotes rest and enhances coping abilities • Bone or joint discomfort may be decreased • Improves circulation in the tissues and facilitates joint mobility • Need for medication may be minimized • Successful management of pain needs involvement of the child. Use of effective techniques provides positive reinforcement, promotes sense of control, and prepares child for interventions to be used after discharge • Using own learned perceptions/behaviors to manage pain can help client cope more effectively • Facilitates relaxation, augments pharmacologic therapy, and enhances coping abilities • Helps with pain management by redirecting attention • Rapid turnover and destruction of leukemic cells during chemotherapy can elevate uric acid, causing swollen painful joints in some clients. Massive infiltration of WBCs into joints can also result in intense pain • Given for mild pain not relieved by comfort measures. Aspirin-containing products is to avoided because they may potentiate hemorrhage • Use pain relieving drug around-the-clock, rather than PRN, when pain is severe • Effects of leukemia, anemia, and chemotherapy may be cumulative (specially during acute and active treatment phase), necessitating assistance • Record of patient's energy level helps to prioritize activities and arrange them around fatigue pattern • Restores energy needed for activity and cellular regeneration/tissue healing • Maximizes available energy for self-care tasks like taking bath • Smaller meals require less energy for digestion than larger meals. Increased intake provides fuel for energy • Maximizes oxygen available for cellular uptake, improving tolerance of activity • Treatments can include various antineoplastic drugs, transfusions, peripheral progenitor (stem) cell transplant or bone marrow transplant

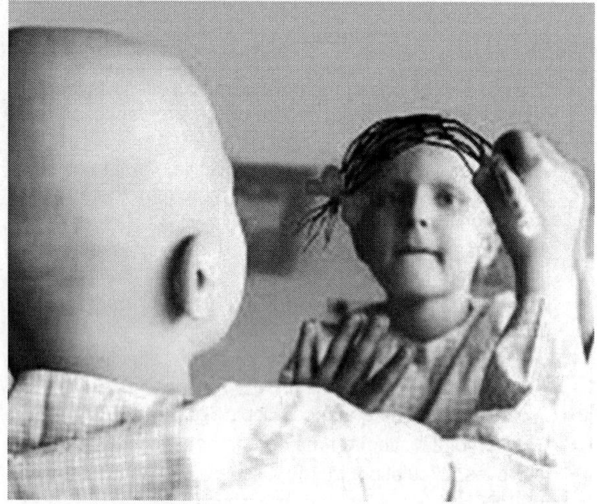

Fig. 17.5: Being bald is part of her new body image, she is conscious and tries to alter it

Expected Outcome

The child will out of signs of infection as evidenced by an afebrile state, no signs and symptoms of infection around the site central venous catheter and negative culture report.

Nursing Diagnosis

Risk for deficient fluid volume and imbalanced nutrition; less than body requirement due to vomiting, hemorrhage, diarrhea, mucositis, taste change, etc.

Expected Outcome

Demonstrate adequate fluid volume, as evidenced by stable vital signs; normal urine output. Improved nutritional status of the child as evidenced that child can eat food with appropriate nutrients for growth.

Nursing Diagnosis

Acute pain related to enlarged organs/lymph nodes, bone marrow packed with leukemic cells, and/or due to antileukemic treatments and/or anxiety, fear.

Expected Outcome

Pain level (NOC) as evidenced that the child is relaxed and able to sleep/rest appropriately.

Nursing Diagnosis

Activity intolerance may be related to generalized weakness; reduced energy stores, increased metabolic rate from massive production of leukocytes, and/or imbalance between oxygen supply and demand (anemia or hypoxia), and/or effect of drug therapy.

Expected Outcome

Increase in activity tolerance as evidenced by participation in ADL; demonstrate a decrease in physiological signs of intolerance; e.g., pulse, respiration, and BP remain within child's normal range.

Nursing Diagnosis

Deficient knowledge and understanding regarding disease, treatment, self-care, prognosis and discharge need.

Expected Outcome

Improved knowledge and understanding of the child and parents as evidenced by their ability to verbalize disease process, potential complications and therapeutic needs.

Brain Tumors

Brain and central nervous system tumors are the second most common cancers in children (next to leukemia), making up about 21% of childhood cancers. Brain tumors are a diverse group of tumors described by their tissue origin, location inside the brain, and rate of growth. It can directly destroy brain cells (Fig. 17.6). They can also indirectly damage cells by pushing on other parts of the brain. Malignant brain tumors are likely to grow quickly and spread into other brain tissue but are confined to the brain and spine and rarely metastasize to bone marrow and other organs. But it may recur after treatment. Sometimes, brain tumors that are not cancer are called malignant because of their size and location and the damage they can do to vital functions of the brain.

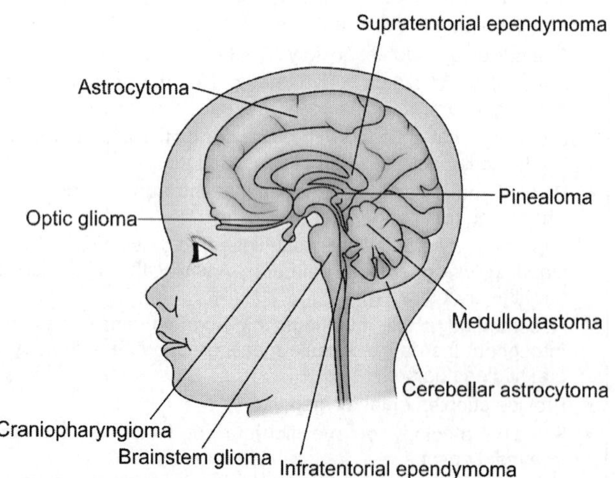

Fig. 17.6: Types of tumor in the brain

Etiology and Incidence

The causes of most childhood brain tumors are not known. Brain tumors can occur at any age. Brain tumors that occur in infants and children are very different from adult brain tumors, both in terms of the type of cells and the responsiveness to treatment. Tumors can occur at any age. Many tumors are more common at a certain age. In general, brain tumors in children are very rare. There are many types of brain tumors, and the treatment and for each is different.

The majority of brain tumors have abnormalities of genes involved in cell cycle control, causing uncontrolled cell growth. These abnormalities are caused by alterations directly in the genes, or by chromosome rearrangements which change the function of a gene.

Patients with certain genetic conditions (i.e. neurofibromatosis, retinoblastoma) also have an increased risk to develop tumors of the central nervous system. There have also been some reports of children in the same family developing brain tumors who do not have any of these genetic syndromes.

Research has been investigating parents of children with brain tumors and their past exposure to certain chemicals. Some chemicals may change the structure of a gene that protects the body from diseases and cancer. Children who have received radiation therapy to the head as part of prior treatment for other malignancies are also at an increased risk for new brain tumors.

CNS tumors represent 35% of solid tumor malignancies diagnosed in children. Most brain tumors in children start in the lower parts of the brain, such as the cerebellum or brainstem. Adults are more likely to develop tumors in upper parts of the brain. Spinal cord tumors are less common than brain tumors in both children and adults.

Pathophysiology

Brain tumors are classified based on the exact site of the tumor, the type of tissue involved, whether it is cancerous.

Gliomas

The most common type of brain tumor is a glioma. Gliomas begin from glial cells, which are the supportive tissue of the brain. There are several types of gliomas, categorized by where they are found and the type of cells that originated the tumor. The following are the different types of gliomas:

Astrocytomas are the most common type of childhood brain tumor, approximately about 40%. Astrocytomas are glial cell tumors that are derived from connective tissue cells called astrocytes. These cells can be found anywhere in the brain or spinal cord. Astrocytomas are usually noncancerous, slow-growing tumors. They commonly develop in children ages 5

Contd...

Contd...

through 8 and called low-grade gliomas. Astrocytomas are generally subdivided into high-grade or low-grade tumors. High-grade astrocytomas are the most malignant of all brain tumors.

Brainstem Gliomas

Brainstem gliomas are tumors found in any portion of the brainstem. About 11 to 15% of brain tumors in children are brainstem gliomas. Most brainstem tumors cannot be surgically removed because of the remote location and delicate and complex function this area controls. Brainstem gliomas occur almost exclusively in children; the group most often affected is the school-age child. The child usually does not have increased intracranial pressure, but may have problems with double vision, movement of the face or one side of the body or difficulty with walking and coordination.

Ependymomas

Ependymomas are also glial cell tumors, which constitute 10% of brain tumors in children. They are slow growing supratentorial tumors, usually develop in the lining of the ventricles or in the spinal cord. It arises from the cells that support, nourish, make myelin and line the ventricles that cerebrospinal fluid flows through. Most common place they are found in children is near the cerebellum. The tumor often blocks the flow of the CSF causing increased intracranial pressure. This type of tumor mostly occurs in children younger than 10 years of age.

Optic Nerve Gliomas

Optic nerve gliomas are found in or around the nerves that send messages from the eyes to the brain. They are frequently found in persons who have neurofibromatosis, a condition a child is born with that makes the child more likely to develop tumors in the brain. Persons usually experience loss of vision, as well as hormone problems, since these tumors are usually located at the base of the brain where hormonal control is located. These are typically difficult to treat due to the surrounding sensitive brain structures.

Medulloblastomas

Medulloblastomas are one type of primitive neuroeclIodermal tumors occur in the midline of the cerebellum. About 25% of pediatric brain tumors are medulloblastoma. This tumor is rapidly growing and often blocks drainage of the CSF, causing symptoms associated with increased ICP. Medulloblastoma cells can metastasize to other areas of the central nervous system, specially around the spinal cord. A combination of surgery, radiation and chemotherapy is usually needed to control these tumors.

Craniopharyngioma

Craniopharyngioma are benign tumors occur adjacent to structure containing pituitary gland and optic nerve. Most persons with this type of brain tumor develop symptoms before the age of 20 years. Symptoms include headaches, as well as problems with vision. Hormonal imbalances are common, including poor growth and short stature. Symptoms of increased intracranial pressure may also be seen. Although these tumors are benign, they are hard to remove due to the sensitive brain structures that surround them.

Manifestations

As with most childhood cancers, the symptoms of brain tumors are diffuse and confusing, and are often initially attributed to viruses, neurological problems, or even emotional problems. Most parents of children diagnosed with brain tumors report variations of the symptoms listed below, symptoms that had no apparent cause and may have lasted for several months.

When a tumor grows into or presses on an area of the brain, it may stop that part of the brain from working the way it should. This leads to swelling and increased pressure inside the skull. Since the brain controls learning, memory, senses (hearing, visual, smell, taste, touch), emotions, muscles, organs, and blood vessels, the presentation of symptoms varies accordingly. Symptoms vary depending upon which part of the brain the tumor is found.

More than 50% of pediatric CNS tumors develop in the posterior fossa, the lower part of brain that contains both the cerebellum and the brainstem. They can cause headaches, nausea, vomiting, blurred or double vision, strabismus, nystagmus, dizziness, ataxia and trouble in handling objects.

Sometimes ICP may be increased due to tumor mass itself or, more commonly, by the tumor obstructing the normal flow of CSF. They may be irritable, be lethargic, feed poorly and have increased head circumference and bulging fontanel.

Loss of developmental milestones, poor academic performance of school-aged children, change of personality, fatigue and symptoms of vague intermittent headache are important symptoms which need to explore during physical examination and history taking of the child.

The brainstem involvement leads to cranial nerve deficits and hemiparesis. The characteristics of supratentorial tumors are headaches, seizures or focal neurological deficits.

Symptoms of brain tumors in the cerebrum (front of brain) may include seizures, visual changes, slurred speech, paralysis or weakness on half of the body or face, increased intracranial pressure, drowsiness or confusion, personality changes.

Diagnostic Evaluation

The following tests and procedures may be used:

- *Physical exam and history:* An exam of the body to check general signs of health, including checking for signs of disease, such as lumps or anything else that seems unusual. A history of the patient's health habits and past illnesses and treatments will also be taken.
- *Neurological exam:* A series of questions and tests to check the brain, spinal cord, and nerve function. The exam checks a person's mental status, coordination, and ability to walk normally, and how well the muscles, senses, and reflexes work. This may also be called a neuro exam or a neurologic exam.
- *MRI with gadolinium:* A procedure that uses a magnet, radio waves, and a computer to make a series of detailed pictures of the brain and spinal cord. A substance called gadolinium is injected into a vein. The gadolinium collects around the cancer cells so they show up brighter in the picture. This procedure is also called nuclear magnetic resonance imaging (NMRI).
- *Serum tumor marker test:* A procedure in which a sample of blood is examined to measure the amounts of certain substances released into the blood by organs, tissues, or tumor cells in the body. Certain substances are linked to specific types of cancer when found in increased levels in the blood. These are called tumor markers.

Therapeutic Management

Treatment depends on the size and type of tumor and the child's general health. The goals of treatment may be to cure the tumor, relieve symptoms, by minimally disturbing the surrounding brain tissue and improve brain function or the child's comfort.

Surgery is needed for most primary brain tumors. Some tumors may be completely removed. In cases where the tumor cannot be removed, surgery may help reduce pressure and relieve symptoms. Chemotherapy or radiation therapy may be used for certain tumors. Usually radiation therapy is avoided in children younger than 3 years because of the toxic effects on the developing brain. Therapy depends on the type of tumor, its location, the amount of residual tumor after surgery and age of the child.

- *Astrocytoma:* Surgery to remove the tumor is the main treatment. Chemotherapy and/or radiation therapy may also be necessary.
- *Brainstem gliomas:* Surgery is usually not possible because of the tumor's location in the brain. Radiation is used to shrink the tumor and prolong life.
- *Ependymomas:* Treatment includes surgery. Radiation and chemotherapy may be necessary.
- *Medulloblastomas:* Surgery alone does not cure this type of tumor. Chemotherapy with or without radiation is often used in combination with surgery.

Medicines used to treat primary brain tumors in children include:

- *Corticosteroids:* Corticosteroids decrease brain edema. In central nervous system tumors, corticosteroids have been found not only to reduce peritumoral and vasogenic brain edema, but also reduce increased intracranial pressure and, decrease CSF production. The primary corticosteroid used to control cerebral edema is dexamethasone to reduce edema in brain swelling.
- *Diuretics:* Diuretics to reduce brain edema and pressure. Usually diuretics such as urea or mannitol is administered to reduce brain swelling and pressure.
- *Anticonvulsants:* Children with supratentorial tumors are at risks of seizures from the tumor itself or from scar tissue formation after surgery. These children need anticonvulsants with monitoring of therapeutic level.
- Pain medicines.

Some of the chemo drugs used to treat children with brain tumors include carboplatin, carmustine (BCNU), cisplatin, cyclophosphamide, etoposide, lomustine (CCNU), methotrexate, temozolomide, thiotepa, vincristine.

These drugs may be used alone or in various combinations in cycles, depending on the type of brain tumor. Each cycle generally lasts about 3 to 4 weeks and is followed by a rest period to give the body time to recover.

The child with brain tumor needs comfort measures, safety measures, physical therapy, occupational therapy, and other such steps may be required to improve quality of life. Counseling, support groups, and similar measures can help the family cope.

Nursing Management

Nurses can help to recognize brain tumor early in the disease and initiate the diagnostic process. As part of a multidisciplinary team, nurses can provide postoperative care, initiate and manage chemotherapy, manage disease-and treatment-related symptoms, promote health, provide psychosocial care, and improve the quality of life for patients with brain tumor.

Nursing Diagnosis and Planning

The following nursing diagnosis and expected outcomes may be appropriate for the child with brain tumor and the child's family.

- Headaches are usually the result of increased intracranial pressure, a consequence of cerebral edema, tumor growth, or intracranial hemorrhage.

Expected outcome: The child will say a decrease in the severity of pain.

- Cancer-related fatigue is persistent tiredness or exhaustion, out of proportion to recent activities, that is caused by cancer or cancer treatment.

Expected outcome: The child will gain energy, participate in daily care and show interest in environment.

- Susceptible to infection chemotherapy, radiation therapy, and corticosteroids are all forms of immunotherapy that suppress the immune system.

Expected outcome: The child will remain free from infection as evidenced by normal body temperature, laboratory pictures.

- Anxiety and depression of child and parents related to the disease, surgery and prognosis.

Expected outcome: The child and parents will show less anxiety about the courses of the disease, as evidenced by expressing less anxiety and an ability to solve problem.

- Disturbed body image related to shaved head and neurological symptoms.

Expected outcome: The child will able to overcome it and will participate in social interaction.

Nursing Intervention

Nursing intervention focuses on controlling acute symptoms (pain, nausea and vomiting, fatigue, visual problem, lack of coordination; i.e. [symptoms according to site of tumors], preparation for surgery and post-operative care. Brain tumor and its treatment create a variety of problems for patients, their families, and loved ones. Present sufferings, treatment and proposed surgery, and prognosis are substantial burdens and increase the risk for anxiety, depression, and other mental health problems. If information and support are not given, psychological and behavioral problems can affect a patient's memory, decision making, and participation in the plan of care. The child should be oriented about anesthesia and the intensive care unit.

Implement measures to prepare the child for surgery. Shaving the head (may be traumatic for the child) before surgery and a large dressing covering the head are to be done. These children are prone to infection, protect the child from potential sources of infection. Monitoring vital signs, maintaining hydration, administering preoperative drugs, to note the patient's complaints(if anything new), any adverse drug reaction seen, etc.

Postoperatively, concerns about pain, hemorrhage, infection and monitoring for signs and symptoms of increased ICP are important nursing activities. Position the head on the unaffected side or otherwise directed. Level of consciousness, airway, vital signs, edema of head and neck are to be checked in regular interval. Increased ICP is a risk in the postsurgery period related to cerebral edema, hydrocephalus, hemorrhage, obstruction of VP shunt. Check and record vital signs, neurological status, mental status of the child frequently after coming from OT. The child should not be placed in Trendelenburg's position as it increases ICP and the risk of bleeding. Prompt reporting regarding increased ICP is necessary, which may need further evaluation through MRI or CT scan.

In brain tumor operation VP shunt is attached temporarily for drainage of CSF and thus to decrease the ICP. Nursing actions related to VP shunt includes maintaining its level, to measure the amount, color of the fluid. Normal CSF is colorless, bloody or discolored drainage is to be reported immediately, as it can be sign of contamination or bleeding.

Assessment for functional deficits is to be done, which may results from surgery or damage to normal brain tissue. If the deficits are significant, rehabilitative therapy may be necessary to help the child to regain function (see the long-term disabilities of child above).

Parents should be aware about potential as well as actual side effects of chemotherapy and radiation therapy. They should also know the early symptoms of increased ICP and other probable complications.

MALIGNANT LYMPHOMAS

Malignant lymphomas are neoplasm of lymphoid tissues that make at least 30% of childhood cancers. These cancers start in certain cells of the immune system called *lymphocytes*. They most often grow in lymph nodes and other lymph tissues (Fig. 17.7), like the tonsils or thymus.

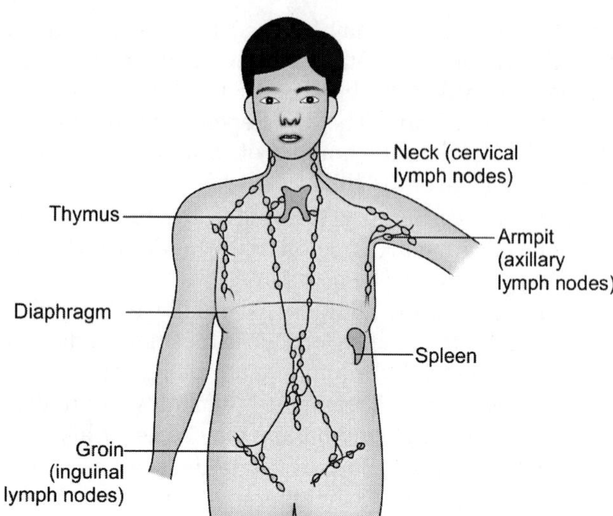

Fig. 17.7: The lymphatic system is made up of organs such as the bone marrow, thymus, spleen and lymph nodes

They can also affect the bone marrow and other organs, and can cause different symptoms depending on where the cancer is. Based on biologic behavior and current management, it is convenient to classify lymphomas in children in two broad categories—Hodgkin's and non-Hodgkin's lymphoma.

Both types occur in children and adults. The two are distinguished by cell type. They share similar symptoms such as painless swelling of the lymph nodes, fever and fatigue. Non-Hodgkin's lymphomas are more common with at least 15 different types.

Hodgkin's lymphoma accounts for about 4% of childhood cancers. It is more common, though, in bimodal incidence curve: early adulthood (age 15 to 40 years, usually people in their 20s) and late adulthood (after age 55 years). Hodgkin's lymphoma is rare in children younger than 5 years of age. This type of cancer is very similar in children and adults, including which types of treatment work best.

Non-Hodgkin's lymphoma makes up about 6% of childhood cancers. It is more likely to occur in younger children than Hodgkin's lymphoma, but it is still rare in children younger than 3 years. The most common types of non-Hodgkin's lymphoma in children are different from those in adults. These cancers often grow quickly and require intensive treatment, but they also tend to respond better to treatment than most non-Hodgkin's lymphomas in adults.

The diagnosis of Hodgkin's or non-Hodgkin's lymphoma typically is made on the basis of a lymph node biopsy. Treatment involves chemotherapy, radiation therapy or both. The nature of the therapy depends on the type of lymphoma and the extent of its spread in the body. When a patient is diagnosed with lymphoma, a treatment plan is formulated. Patients whose lymphoma has relapsed are candidates for bone marrow transplantation.

Non-Hodgkin's Lymphomas

Non-Hodgkin's lymphoma is a cancer that starts in the cells called lymphocytes, which are part of the body's immune system. NHL is one of the most rapidly growing cancers in children. Because lymph tissue is found throughout the body, childhood non-Hodgkin's lymphoma can begin in almost any part of the body. Cancer can spread to the liver and many other organs and tissues. Once a malignancy begins in one part of the lymph system, it often spreads throughout the rest of the system before it is detected.

The difference between HL and NHL is based on clinical behavior, pathology, mode of metastasis and responsiveness to therapy. The disease differs greatly from adult NHL. The rapid clinical course and early spread of bone marrow and CNS resembles ALL which sometimes makes it difficult to distinguish between lymphoma and leukemia in children. In general, people with lymphoma have no or only minimal bone marrow involvement, whereas those with leukemia have extensive bone marrow involvement.

Etiology and Incidence

Different factors like viral, genetic, immunologic and environmental may cause NHL. Exposure to Epstein-Barr virus has been associated with B-cell lymphoma. Although the exact cause is unknown, a link to the immune system is thought to exist. The children with immunodeficiency syndrome or acquired immunodeficiency syndrome or those children on long immunosuppressive drugs (after organ transplant) are at higher risk of NHL or other lymphoproliferative disorders.

Manifestations

In most cases of non-Hodgkin's lymphoma, a painless, firm swelling in the neck, the armpit, or the groin lymph nodes is present. Since extranodal sites are often involved, other less specific signs like swelling of the face, weakness, tiredness, sweating, specially at night, unexplained fever, unexplained weight loss may occur. Gastrointestinal tract involvement leads to abdominal pain, jaundice, diarrhea, gastrointestinal bleeding, and constipation. If the spleen or liver are involved, they are enlarged. If the bone marrow is involved, neutropenia, fatigue, bleeding or bruising occurs. In mediastinal disease breathing difficulties, occasional cough, sometimes difficulties in swallowing and possibly significant tracheal deviation are seen.

Diagnostic Evaluation

Physical examination looks for enlarged lymph nodes and hepatosplenomegaly along with extensive laboratory works to confirm NHL. Complete blood count (CBC) and chest X-ray are necessary to rule out a lot of other things, specially lung diseases and leukemia.

If initial tests confirm that the child may have a lymphoma, the doctor may refer the child to a pediatric hematologist/oncologist, who may do a biopsy of any lumps or tumor to confirm what type of lymphoma it is. Also, a bone marrow aspiration may be ordered and CT scans, and possibly other tests as needed in the child's individual situation.

Lymphomas are usually treated by a combination of chemotherapy, radiation, and/or bone marrow transplants. The cure rate varies greatly depending on the type of lymphoma and the progression of the disease.

More than 90% of non-Hodgkin's lymphoma (NHL) in childhood can be grouped into one of three histologic subtypes—lymphoblastic, undifferentiated, and diffuse large cell type. Lymphoblastic lymphomas most commonly present with mediastinal involvement. The majority of nonlymphoblastic lymphomas arise within the abdomen. Because of the tendency of NHL for extralymphatic dissemination, systemic therapy is always required.

Therapeutic Management

Treatment of childhood lymphoma is largely determined by histology and *staging*. Staging is a way to categorize or classify patients according to how extensive the disease is at the time of diagnosis.

Children who have non-Hodgkin's lymphoma are considered to be at one of these stages:

Stage I non-Hodgkin's lymphoma applies to children who have non-Hodgkin's lymphoma in only one area or lymph node, and that area or node is not in the abdomen or chest.

Stage II non-Hodgkin's lymphoma applies to children who have any one of these:

Disease in only one area, including the lymph nodes in the area.

Disease in 2 or more areas or lymph nodes, with all the cancer either above or below the diaphragm, disease that started in the stomach or intestines and that was completely removed through surgery.

For children with stage I or stage II non-Hodgkin's lymphoma, chemotherapy may take between 2 and 6 months. This depends on the subtype of the disease. About 90 to 100% of children with non-Hodgkin's lymphoma are cured with this treatment.

Stage III non-Hodgkin's lymphoma applies to children who have any one of these:

Disease on both sides of the diaphragm, disease that started in the chest, disease in 2 or more areas in the abdomen, disease around the spine.

Stage IV non-Hodgkin's lymphoma applies to children who have non-Hodgkin's lymphoma in their bone marrow, brain, spine or cerebrospinal fluid.

Children with stage III or stage IV non-Hodgkin's lymphoma will need more intense chemotherapy treatment. This may last from 6 months to 2 years.

Chemotherapy is the primary form of treatment for all types of lymphoma. In certain cases, radiation may also be used. In non-Hodgkin's lymphoma, radiation is rarely used. They may use it as an emergency treatment to reduce the size of a tumor in the chest if the tumor is in the way of breathing or blood flow from the heart. They may also use radiation along with chemotherapy to treat non-Hodgkin's lymphoma that has spread to the central nervous system or the testicles.

Children whose lymphoma comes back after treatment may have high doses of chemotherapy medicines combined with a hematopoietic cell, or stem cell, transplant. The chemotherapy medicines are designed to kill cancer cells that remain in the child's body. Before stem cell infusion high dose chemotherapy is administered and to damage the bone marrow, so the marrow cannot make new stem cells that would become blood cells. This hematopoietic cell transplant may be autologous or allogeneic stem cell transplant.

Significant improvements in survival rates have resulted from the development of effective combination chemotherapy programs. Cure rates in excess of 90% can be expected in children with localized disease.

Hodgkin's Lymphomas

Hodgkin's lymphoma is a type of lymphoma, which is a malignant process originating from lymphoreticular system. This cancer of the immune system is marked by the presence of a type of cell called the Reed-Sternberg cell. Hodgkin's lymphoma is named for Dr Thomas Hodgkin's, who described several cases of the cancer within the lymph system in 1832.

Etiology and Incidence

The cause of Hodgkin's disease is unknown. However, several serologic studies suggest that infectious agents such as Epstein- Barr virus, herpes virus, cytomegalovirus may be involved in occurrence of this disease. The Reed-Sternberg cells are readily infected by EBV and this infection can precede the initiation of malignant clone. But this phenomenon cannot be demonstrated in all cases.

In USA, approximately 1,700 kids and teens younger than 20 years are diagnosed with lymphomas each year. In younger children, non-Hodgkin's lymphoma is more common than Hodgkin's lymphoma, but in teens, Hodgkin's lymphoma is more common.

Pathophysiology

Hodgkin's lymphomas are malignant cell infiltrations of the lymphatic system which originate in a single lymph node or a group of lymph nodes in the same anatomic region. This disease is characterized by a large cell with multiple or multilobuled nuclei called Reed-Sternberg cells (Fig. 17.8). This cell type is considered the hallmark of Hodgkin's lymphomas. The Reed-Sternberg cell is clonal in origin and arises from the germinal center of body. These cells are thought to represent activated B-and T-lymphocytes. Hodgkin's lymphomas appears to arise in lymphoid tissue and spreads to adjacent lymph glands in a relatively orderly fashion. Hematogenous spread is occur from lymph nodes to nonnodal sites such as spleen, liver, bone, bone marrow, lungs, mediastinum, and/or brain and is usually associated with systemic symptoms.

Clinical Manifestations

The most common symptom of Hodgkin's is the painless enlargement of one or more lymph nodes, or lymphadenopathy (in the neck, chest, underarm, or groin). The nodes may also feel rubbery and swollen when examined. The nodes of the neck and shoulders (cervical and supraclavicular) are most frequently

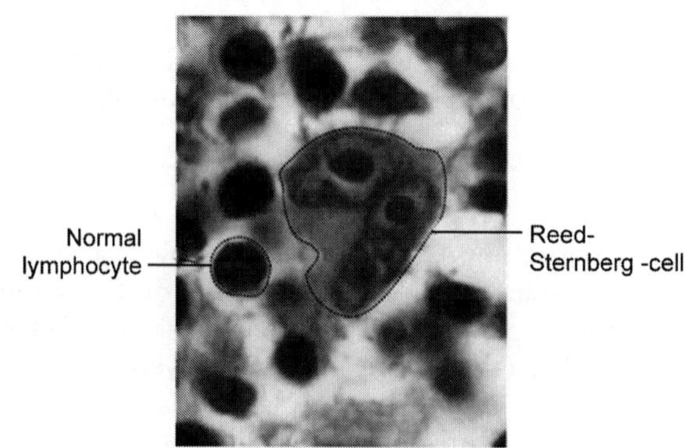

Fig. 17.8: Presence of specific blood cells in blood picture of Hodgkin's lymphoma

involved (80 to 90% of the time, on average). The lymph nodes of the chest are often affected, and these may be noticed on a chest radiograph. Other symptoms are:

- Persistent fatigue
- Fever and chills
- Night sweats
- Unexplained weight loss — as much as 10 % or more of your body weight
- Loss of appetite
- Itching
- Splenomegaly occurs in about 30% of people with Hodgkin's lymphoma. The enlargement, however, is seldom massive and the size of the spleen may fluctuate during the course of treatment.
- Hepatomegaly due to liver involvement, is present in about 5% of cases.

Diagnostic Evaluation

- Physical exam and history taking.
- CT scan
- PET scan
- Chest X-ray
- Complete blood count (CBC) and ESR
- Blood chemistry studies
- *Lymph node biopsy:* The removal of all or part of a lymph node. The lymph node may be removed during a thoracoscopy, mediastinoscopy, or laparoscopy. One of the following types of biopsies may be done:
  - *Excisional biopsy:* The removal of an entire lymph node.
  - *Incisional biopsy*: The removal of part of a lymph node.
  - *Core biopsy:* The removal of tissue from a lymph node using a wide needle.
  - *Fine-needle aspiration (FNA) biopsy:* The removal of tissue from a lymph node using a thin needle.

Therapeutic Management

Approximately 90 to 95% of children with Hodgkin's lymphoma can be cured, prompting increased attention to devising therapy that produces less long-term morbidity for these patients. Combined modality therapy regimens have resulted in excellent treatment outcomes and reduced the incidence of treatment sequelae by utilizing lower doses and smaller volumes of radiation therapy and fewer cycles of less toxic chemotherapy in clinically-staged children. Prognostic factors used in determining chemotherapy intensity include stage, presence or absence of B symptoms (fever, weight loss, and night sweats), and/or bulky disease. The staging is the same for both Hodgkin's as well as non-Hodgkin's lymphomas.

Nursing Management of Patient with Lymphoma

Nursing Diagnosis

Risk for ineffective airway clearance/breathing pattern due to tracheobronchial obstruction: enlarged mediastinal nodes and/or airway edema (Hodgkin's and non-Hodgkin's); superior vena cava syndrome (non-Hodgkin's).

Anxiety of (parents and child) regarding disease, treatment and prognosis; as they have deficient knowledge about it (Table 17.2).

Neuroblastoma

A *blastoma* is a type of cancer, more common in children, that is caused by malignancies in precursor cells, often called blasts. Examples are nephroblastoma, medulloblastoma and retinoblastoma. The suffix '-blastoma' is used to imply a tumor of primitive, incompletely differentiated (precursor) cells, e.g. chondroblastoma is composed of cells resembling the precursor of chondrocytes. Blastomas usually occur in children.

Neuroblastoma is a cancer that develops from immature nerve cells found in several areas of the body. It is a solid, malignant tumor which manifests as a lump or mass in the abdomen or around the spinal cord. Neuroblastoma most commonly arises in and around the adrenal glands, which have similar origins to nerve cells and sit atop the kidneys. However, neuroblastoma can also develop in other areas of the abdomen and in the chest, neck and near the spine, where groups of nerve cells exist. It can also cause bone pain and fever.

Etiology and Incidence

The cause of neuroblastoma is unknown. Its prevalence is similar in various parts of the world, which suggests that environmental factors do not cause the disease. This type of cancer occurs in infants and young children. It is rarely found in children older than 10 years. It accounts for 5 to 7% of all childhood malignancies; about 1 in 6000 children will be diagnosed with neuroblastoma by the age of 5 years. It is more common in boys than girls.

Table 17.2: Nursing care of a patient with lymphoma

Nursing interventions	*Rationale*
Assess and monitor respiratory rate, depth, rhythm. Dyspnea and use of accessory muscles, nasal flaring, altered chest excursion are to be noted and reported	Tachypnea, dyspnea, use of accessory muscles may indicate progression of respiratory involvement and compromise requiring prompt intervention
Place patient in position of comfort (upright position), usually weight supported on arms, feet dangling	Maximizes lung expansion, decreases work of breathing, and reduces risk of aspiration
Reposition and assist with turning periodically	Promotes aeration of all lung segments and mobilizes secretions
Instruct and assist with deep-breathing techniques, pursed-lip or abdominal diaphragmatic breathing if indicated	Helps promote gas diffusion and expansion of small airways. Provides patient with some control over respiration, helping to reduce anxiety
Observe for neck vein distension, headache, dyspnea, and stridor, dizziness, periorbital and facial edema	Non-Hodgkin's's patients are at risk for superior vena cava syndrome, which may result in tracheal deviation and airway obstruction, representing an oncologic emergency
Determine specific pathophysiology, illness, surgery or trauma involved and impact on the child. Provide factual information	Patient's perception about this illness is crucial to planning interventions that will be appropriate to patient and family. This also decreases anxiety of the parents and promotes trust in caregivers
Discuss potential complications relative to specific therapeutic regimen	Possible side effects and long-term physical complications of radiation (direct or indirect) and some chemotherapy agents include pneumonitis, hypothyroidism, pericarditis, cardiomyopathy
Strict maintenance of fluid and electrolytes	It is necessary to minimize tumor lysis syndrome. TLS causes restlessness, irritability, and changes in the sensorium of the child
Emphasize need for ongoing medical follow-up	Following treatment, there is increased risk of secondary malignancies (thyroid, myeloid leukemia, non-Hodgkin's's lymphoma) in addition to other complications listed above

Pathophysiology

Neuroblastoma starts in early forms of nerve cells found in a developing embryo or fetus. Neuroblastoma normally is a cancer of the sympathetic nervous system and adrenal medulla. Cells proliferate and begin to form a solid mass. These cells are immature and nonfunctional. The tumor infringes and infiltrates into adjacent normal tissue and organs. Metastesis may occur in the bone marrow, bone, liver, skin and rarely in the lung and brain.

Clinical Manifestations

Most malignant solid tumors, such as neuroblastoma, produce swelling or pain. The symptoms of neuroblastoma vary because the location of the tumor determines the symptoms that are noticed by the parents. Most neuroblastomas are found in the abdomen. Parents may feel a lump or mass while dressing or bathing their child. A tumor in the abdomen may cause the child to feel 'full', experience stomach pain, loss of appetite, constipation and difficulty urinating. Other primary sites can include the head or neck/chest. The lump or mass may found in the chest, neck, or pelvis.

Tumors located in the head and neck may present as a mass. The child may have 'black eyes', much like bruises, a droopy eyelid, a pupil that does not constrict properly, vision problems. Chest tumors may cause pain, difficulty breathing, or a persistent cough. Tumors that grow in spinal areas may cause the child to have pain, numbness of the lower extremities, constipation and difficulty urinating.

Symptoms sometimes appear with less specific characteristics such as loss of appetite, nausea, weight loss, stomach pain, constipation, difficulty urinating, fever, or other vague feelings of ill health, and therefore any unusual signs or symptoms for which there are no apparent causes should be investigated.

Diagnostic Evaluation

Tests and procedures used to diagnose neuroblastoma include physical examination and history taking. Urine tests may be used to check for high levels of certain markers that result from the neuroblastoma cells producing excess catecholamines. These chemicals are normally found in urine, but are found in higher levels in 95% of the children diagnosed with this disease. A simple 24-hour urine collection is done to detect these abnormal levels. Urine catecholamines levels (homovanillic acid [HVA] andvanillymandelic acid [VMA] are elevated in 95% of patients with neuroblastoma. These two markers HMA and VMA are serially monitored during treatment and for follow up when treatment is complete.

Imaging tests may reveal a mass that can indicate a tumor. Imaging tests may include X-ray, ultrasound, computerized tomography (CT) scan, metaiodobenzylguanidine (MIBG) scan and magnetic resonance imaging (MRI), among others. Imaging tests used to stage cancer include X-rays, bone scans, and CT, MRI and MIBG scans, among others. Definite diagnosis is made by biopsy. Tumor samples are sent to special reference laboratories to look at the genetic makeup of the tumor. The genetic information is helpful in determining treatment plan and the disease prognosis.

Therapeutic Management

Treatment will be determined by many factors, including the stage of the disease at diagnosis and the child's age. Neuroblastoma is often present at birth, but is most often diagnosed much later when the child begins to show symptoms of the disease. The average age at diagnosis is 2 years. About 25% of newly diagnosed neuroblastomas are found in children under the age of 1 year. This age group has the best prognosis, with cure rates as high as 90%. It is not yet known why children under the age of 1 year do so much better. The International Staging System for Neuroblastoma is used to compare patients and their treatments.

- Stage I: Neuroblastoma at this stage is localized, meaning it is confined to one area, and may be completely removed with surgery. Lymph nodes connected to the tumor may have signs of cancer, but other lymph nodes do not have cancer.
- Stage IIA: Neuroblastoma at this stage is localized, but may not be as easily removed through surgery.
- Stage IIB: Neuroblastoma at this stage is localized and may or may not be easily removed through surgery. Both the lymph nodes connected to the tumor and the lymph nodes nearby contain cancer cells.
- Stage III: Neuroblastoma at this stage is considered advanced, and it is not possible to remove the tumor through surgery. The tumor may be a larger size at this stage. Lymph nodes may or may not contain cancer cells.
- Stage IV: Neuroblastoma at this stage is considered advanced and has spread (metastasized) to other parts of the body.

Children with advanced disease may need radiation therapy on the tumor sites and systemic chemotherapy for several months. Peripheral blood stem cell transplant after myeloablative chemotherapy is part of the risk based treatment for advanced stage diseases. After transplantation oral 13-cis-retinoic acid may be administered to the high-risk group of children.

Nursing Management

Assessment

Decreased activity and appetite are often reported by the parents about the child with neuroblastoma. Assess the location of the tumor (in abdomen, chest, spinal cord, eye) and effect of its compression. Compression-related symptoms are to be assessed, i.e. pain, bleeding, condition of chest, edema in face and periorbital area (when compression is on superior vena cava), movement and functioning of bladder and bowel (when compression is on spinal cord) of the child. To explore, whether the child suffers impaired range of mobility with pain and limping, or not.

Nursing Diagnosis

Acute pain related to tumor pressure.

Anxiety and depression of parents related to diagnosis, surgery and prognosis.

Deficient knowledge about the disease and its management.

Nursing Interventions

Education, information and support to the family will help them to cope with the crisis. Attending nurse should explain more about what to expect from the parents.

Pain management is necessary in both pre-and post-operative period with prescribed medicine and other nonpharmacologic measures.

Special care for the wound is needed. Assess the wound carefully for bleeding and signs of infection.

Usually bowel habit changes because of pain, immobility, medications, surgery and alterations of nutrition; so appropriate steps are to be taken to eliminate toxins from the body.

Management of the airway is of concern if the child has any mediastinal disease. Characteristics of the respiration (effort, rate, color of the skin, use of extra muscle) are to be explored along with monitoring of the pulse. Maintaining position of the child and oxygenation can improve the situation.

Evaluation

Does the child rest quietly for an uninterrupted period?

Has the child's cry and irritability decreased?

Are the parents asking questions related to the treatment and care of the child?

Bone Cancers

Primary bone cancers occur most often in older children and teens, but they can develop at any age. They account for about 4% of childhood cancers.

Primary bone cancer is different from *metastatic* bone cancer, which is cancer that started somewhere else in the body and has spread to the bone. Metastatic bone cancer is more common than primary bone cancer because many types of cancer can spread to the bone.

Two main types of primary bone cancers occur in children are osteosarcoma and Ewing's sarcoma.

Osteosarcoma

Osteosarcoma, the most common type of primary malignant bone tumor, is defined by the presence of malignant mesenchymal cells producing osteoid or immature bone. Osteosarcoma is most common in teens, and usually develops in areas where the bone is growing quickly, such as near the ends of the long bones in the legs or arms. It often causes bone pain that gets worse at night or with activity. It can also cause swelling in the area around the bone.

Osteosarcoma is one of the most common types of bone cancer in children and accounts for nearly 3% of all childhood cancers. The disease usually occurs in the long bones, such as the distal end of femur, the proximal end of tibia and the proximal of humerus, and pelvis. Osteosarcoma affects children most often between 10 and 25 years of age. Osteogenic sarcoma cancer cells can also metastasize to other areas of the body. Most commonly, these cells spread to the lungs. However, bones, kidneys, the adrenal gland, the brain, and the heart can also be sites of metastasis.

Etiology and Incidence

The cause of osteosarcoma is unknown, although associations have been made between the exposure to ionizing irradiation associated with radiation therapy for other types of cancer (i.e. Hodgkin's and non-Hodgkin's disease) and osteosarcoma. Genetics may play an important role in developing osteosarcoma as familial tendencies are involved in it.

Osteogenic sarcoma is one of the most common types of bone cancer in children and accounts for nearly 3% of all childhood cancers. This cancer is also more prevalent in males than in females, possibly because of the rapid growth rate at this age. Prior to adolescence, the percentage of affected males and females is equal.

Pathophysiology

Osteosarcoma is the most common type of cancer that develops in bone. Like the osteoblasts in normal bone, the cells that form this cancer make bone matrix. But the bone matrix of an osteosarcoma is not as strong as that of normal bones.

An association has been made that repeated trauma to an area may be a risk factor for developing this type of cancer. It is uncertain whether trauma is a cause or effect of the disease. Cancer lesions in the bone can make that area of the bone weaker, thus, making injury more likely. However, repeated injuries to a certain area of the bone may lead to an increased production of osteoid tissue to repair the damaged area. The rapid production of osteoid tissue may lead to the malignancy. Osteosarcoma occurs from bone producing cells that invade the medullary canal of the bone and form a solid tumor. Commonly it involves the rapidly growing bones mentioned above. A possible association of rapid and repeated bone growth to malignant transformation may be suggested.

Manifestations

Osteosarcoma includes the following symptoms:

- Pain in a bone
- Swelling or tenderness around a bone or joint
- Interference with normal movements
- Weak bones, leading to fractures
- Fatigue, fever, weight loss, anemia.

Bone pain is the most common symptom. Sometimes a lump can be felt on the bone, or the tumor will interfere with normal movements. What often happens is that a child injures themselves while playing, and the pain persists long after the injury should have healed. So, assuming that a bone is broken, the parents take the child to the doctor for evaluation, at which time X-rays reveal a bone tumor.

Diagnostic Evaluation

In addition to a complete medical history and physical examination of the child, diagnostic procedures for osteogenic sarcoma may include:

- *X-rays:* Initially the X-rays of the primary site and chest are taken
- *Bone scans:* This nuclear imaging method is used to detect bone diseases and tumors, determine the cause of bone pain or inflammation and rule out any infection or fractures.
- *Magnetic resonance imaging (MRI):* It is a diagnostic procedure that uses a combination of large magnets, radiofrequencies, and a computer to produce detailed images of organs and structures within the body. This test is done in case of osteosarcoma to identify abnormalities of the bones.

- *Computer-assisted tomography scan (CT or CAT scan)*: It is a diagnostic imaging procedure that uses a combination of X-rays and computer technology to produce cross-sectional images (often called slices), both horizontally and vertically, of the body. A CT scan shows detailed images of any part of the body, including the bones, muscles, fat, and organs. CT scans are more detailed than general X-rays.
- *Complete blood count (CBC):* It is a measurement of size, number and maturity of different blood cells in a specific volume of blood.
- *Blood tests, including blood chemistries*: The blood is tested for alkaline phosphatase and lactate dehydrogenase (LDH). A large amount of alkaline phosphatase can be found in the blood when the cells that form bone tissue are very active, as in growing children and adolescents, or when a broken bone is mending, or when bone cancer is present.
- *Biopsy of the tumor:* Which uses invisible electromagnetic energy beams to produce images of internal tissues, bones, and organs onto film.
- *Bone marrow aspiration and/or biopsy*: This procedure involves taking a small amount of bone marrow fluid (aspiration) and/or solid bone marrow tissue (called a core biopsy), usually from the hip bones, to be examined for the number, size, and maturity of blood cells and/or abnormal cells.

Therapeutic Management

Specific treatment for a bone tumor is determined on child's age, overall health, and medical history, type, location, and size of the tumor, extent of the disease. Different treatment options of osteosarcoma is given below:

- *Surgery:* Surgery is an integral part of treatment for patients with localized osteosarcoma as well as select patients with metastatic or recurrent osteosarcoma. The main goal of surgery is to remove all of the cancer. This limb-sparing surgery consists of local removal of the cancer, including wide margins of healthy tissue in order to ensure that most of the cancer was removed. If even a small number of cancer cells are left behind, they might grow and multiply to make a new tumor. To lower the risk of this happening, surgeons remove the tumor plus some of the normal tissue that surrounds it. This is known as *wide excision*.

  The removed tissue is examined under a microscope to see whether the margins (outer edges) contain cancer cells or not. If cancer cells are seen at the edges of the tissue, the margins are called *positive*. Positive margins can mean that some cancer was left behind. When no cancer cells are seen at the edges of the tissue, the margins are said to be *negative, clean,* or *clear*. A wide excision with clean margins helps limit the risk that the cancer will grow back where it started.

  The type of surgery done depends on the location of the tumor. Although all operations to remove osteosarcomas are complex, tumors in the limbs are generally not as hard to remove as those at the base of the skull, in the spine, or in the pelvis.

  Sometimes the surgeons will graft (add on) bone or tissue (from either the patient or a donor) to replace diseased bone and tissue that have been removed. An artificial bone, called an implant, may also be used.
- *CyberKnife therapy:* The CyberKnife system is the world's first and only robotic radiosurgery system designed to treat tumors throughout the body noninvasively. It provides a pain-free, non-surgical option for patients who have inoperable or surgically complex tumors, or who may be looking for an alternative to surgery. The treatment – which delivers high doses of radiation to tumors with extreme accuracy – offers new hope to patients who have inoperable or surgically complex tumors, or who may be looking for a nonsurgical option.
- *Chemotherapy:* Multimodality treatment consisting of surgery and chemotherapy are conducted in osteosarcoma cases. Chemo is an important part of the treatment for patients with osteosarcoma (although some patients with low-grade osteosarcoma might not need it). Chemotherapy can either be administered before, i.e. preoperative, induction or neoadjuvant chemotherapy or after surgery, i.e. postoperative or adjuvant chemotherapy. Most current protocols employ chemotherapy both before and after surgery.

  Most osteosarcomas are treated with chemo before surgery as *neoadjuvant chemotherapy* for about 10 weeks and then again after surgery as *adjuvant chemotherapy* for up to a year. Patients with high-grade osteosarcomas that responded well to chemo before surgery usually get the same chemo drugs after surgery. Patients whose tumors responded poorly usually get different chemo after surgery.

  Usually, 2 or more drugs are given together. Some common combinations of drugs include:
  - High-dose methotrexate, doxorubicin, and cisplatin (sometimes with ifosfamide)
  - Doxorubicin and cisplatin

- Ifosfamide and etoposide
- Ifosfamide, cisplatin or carboplatin, and epirubicin.

Different research studies on this disease found that 90% of patients developed recurrent disease after surgery alone. Therefore chemotherapy is continued to eradicate the microscopic presence of the disease in anywhere in the body.

- *Radiation therapy:* Radiation therapy can be useful in some cases where the tumor cannot be removed completely by surgery. For example, osteosarcoma can start in hip bones or in the bones of the face, particularly the jaw. Radiation therapy is used only for palliative pain control in advanced stage of disease as osteosarcoma in generally unresponsive to irradiation.
- *Amputation:* Before the mid-1970s, patients with high-grade osteosarcoma were treated with surgery only, which was usually an amputation as there were limitations in imaging modalities and the incipient advances in molecular medicine and pharmacology made to assess the real size of the tumors and the grade of extension beyond the cortices. It is still necessary in some cases. Favorable tumor location allows specially trained orthopedic surgeons to perform complex limb-salvage procedure.
- Resections for metastases, such as pulmonary resections of cancer cells in the lung—surgical resection of lung metastases is widely accepted in osteosarcoma patients. The unique characteristics of osteosarcoma, including metastatic affinity for the lung, make pulmonary metastasectomy a central component of therapy for this disease. Pulmonary metastasectomy in osteosarcoma is also thought to lead to long-term survival.

Rehabilitation including physical and occupational therapy, and psychosocial adaptation.

Prosthesis fitting and training

Antibiotics to prevent and treat infections.

Continual follow-up care to determine response to treatment, detect recurrent disease, and manage late effects of treatment.

Nursing Management

Initially, the nurse should explain all the diagnostic tests and procedures. Adolescents and their parents need to provide information and support to decrease their anxiety and apprehensiveness about the disease osteosarcoma and plan of treatment.

Focus of the nursing care is to keep the child comfortably and management of pain related to disease process and procedure.

Preparation of the child for surgery as it is primary treatment in case of osteosarcoma. Nurse should be available to answer questions and clarify what the physician has explained about surgery, amputation, prosthesis, and postoperative management.

Careful evaluation of the patient is necessary, as in some instances metastatic pulmonary lesions are not visualized, and there may be micrometastatic lesions.

Physical therapy starts as soon as the patient recovers from surgery. In addition to the usual postoperative care, management of pain, infection, potential hemorrhage and pneumonia (child with pulmonary metastasis), stump care with phantom limb pain; are nursing concerns.

If chemotherapy drugs are continued for the patient, the nurse should ensure that the patient receives 1 and 1½ to 2 maintenance hydration to overcome tumor lyses syndrome (see nursing care of leukemia).

Preparation of patient for discharge includes helping the child to verbalize and to adjust with the change of body image. The child may need wheelchair or crutches until the healing process is complete, some adaptation may need to made in the home.

Allow the child to express their anger, or they may show depression which is the part of the grieving process, i.e. grief over the lost limb. The nurse should encourage a visit/meeting if another adolescent with a similar problem is available as a resource person.

Follow up care need to include a careful assessment of psychosocial adjustment. Social interactions, school attendance, behavioral changes (if any) of the child are to be explored and necessary support to be given.

Outcome—does the child complain of discomfort? Has his pain decreased? Is he afebrile? Are the family and child discussing fears and anxiety related to the disease and treatment?

Prognosis

The prognosis depends on the location of the tumor and whether or not it has spread; generally a 5-year survival rate of 70% is given for childhood bone cancers.

Ewing's Sarcoma

Ewing's sarcoma is a primary bone cancer that affects mainly children and adolescents. Ewing's sarcoma is a less common type of bone cancer, which can also

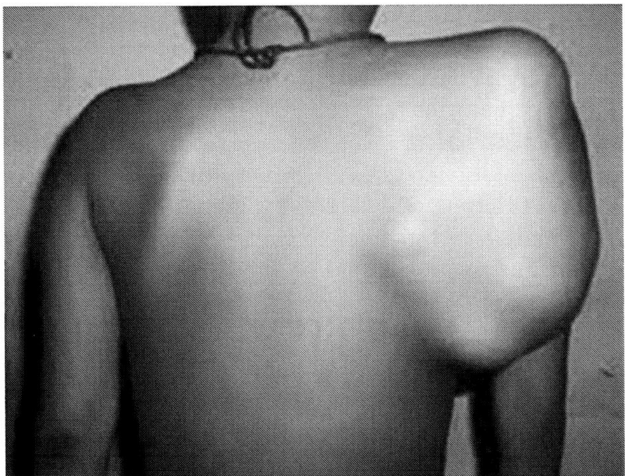

Fig. 17.9: The child with Ewing's sarcoma

cause bone pain. Ewing's tumors that grow in bone are typically found in the long bones of the legs and arms (Fig. 17.9), or bones in the chest, trunk, pelvis, back, or head. In addition to the classic Ewing's tumor, which is named for the doctor who first described it, James Ewing's, there are 2 other types of bone tumor that belong to the Ewing's family of tumors. One is called primitive neuroectodermal tumor or PNET. This tumor often times arises in the brain. The other is known as an Askin's tumor, which usually arises in the chest wall.

Etiology and Incidence

The cause of Ewing's sarcoma is not known. It is not inherited as pre-existing congenital chromosomal abnormalities are not associated; rather it occurs after the child is born. This change can be tested for in the biopsy specimen used to confirm the diagnosis.

It is the second most common bone cancer in children, but it is also relatively uncommon. It accounts for only 1% of all childhood cancers. Although it can occur at any age, it very rarely occurs in adults over the age of 30 years.

Manifestations

In Ewing's sarcoma, the following symptoms may be present:

- Swelling and soreness around the tumor area (commonly mistaken for a sports injury or the 'bumps and bruises' every child gets).
- A low fever that at first may seem to be caused by an infection.
- Bone pain, specially pain that worsens during exercise or at night.
- Limping, which is caused by a tumor on a leg bone.
- Weight loss, anorexia, malaise, and fatigue.

Diagnostic Evaluation

The diagnostic workup is the same as for osteosarcoma. Biopsy is also required to differentiate Ewing's sarcoma from other neoplastic processes.

Therapeutic Management

Even when a Ewing's sarcoma is very small, it may have spread. For this reason, Ewing's always requires treatment across the child's entire body.

- Treatment almost always starts with chemotherapy to destroy the tumor cells and prevent the cancer from spreading.
- Surgery, radiation or a combination of both are used along with chemotherapy. (see osteosarcoma).
- Most children respond very well to chemotherapy.
- The 5-year cure rate for localized Ewing's sarcoma (cancer that has not spread from the primary site) is 70 to 80%.

Nursing Intervention

Nursing care is similar to that for children with osteosarcoma, with the addition of care for the child receiving radiation therapy.

Rhabdomyosarcoma

A *rhabdomyosarcoma,* is a type of cancer, specifically a sarcoma, in which the cancer cells are thought to arise from skeletal muscle progenitors. It starts in cells that normally develop into skeletal muscles. Rhabdomyosarcoma is a fast-growing, highly malignant soft tissue sarcoma which arises in undifferentiated striated muscle cells. This type of cancer can occur in a variety of places in the body—the head, neck, and around the eyes; the extremities; in the pelvic region and genitourinary tract; and in the chest and lungs.

Etiology and Incidence

This is the most common type of soft tissue sarcoma in children. It makes up about 3% of childhood cancers. Although these tumors can arise almost anywhere, the most common locations for these tumors to develop are in the structures of the head and neck (nearly 40% of all cases), the male or female genitourinary tract (about 25% of all cases), and the extremities (about 20% of all cases). Rhabdomyosarcoma accounts for 5 to 8% of childhood cancers and usually affects children the ages of 2 to 6 years and 15 to 19 years.

Pathophysiology

Rhabdomyosarcoma tumors arise from a cell called a 'rhabdomyoblast', which is a primitive muscle cell. Instead of differentiating into striated muscle cells, the rhabdomyoblasts grow out of control. Since this type of muscle is located throughout the body, the tumors can appear at numerous locations. The 4 major sites in which rhabdomyosarcoma is found are:

Depending on the 'histology' of the cells, the tumors are classified in 4 groups:

- *Embryonal rhabdomyosarcoma*: Most common type, usually found in children under 15 years and in the head and neck region and genitourinary tract. It accounts 50 to 60% of the tumors and has the best prognosis.
- *Botryoid type*: A variant of the embryonal type; the tumor arises as a grape-like lesion in mucosal-lined hollow organs such as the vagina and urinary bladder.
- *Alveolar type*: A more aggressive tumor which usually involves the muscles of the extremities or trunk (about 20%), and has a less favorable prognosis. This disease is most often found in the adolescent age group.
- *Pleomorphic type*: Usually seen in adults and arises in muscles of the extremities.

Manifestations

Symptoms depend on the location of the tumor, and pain may be present. Typical presentations of nonmetastatic disease, by location, are as follows:

- Lump or swelling, firm and painless to touch, in the extremities, the groin area, or the vaginal area
- Drooping eyelids, swelling of the eye, protruding eyeball, rapid vision changes
- Hoarseness, difficulty in swallowing
- Abdominal pain that persists for more than a week.

Keep a close eye on child for small lumps which do not disappear in a week or so, but instead keep growing larger. Specially watch the pelvic region and the arms and legs. Also watch for any changes in the eyes. Rhabdomyosarcoma is a rapidly growing tumor and the sooner treatment begins, the more favorable is the prognosis.

Diagnostic Evaluation

- *Complete blood count (CBC):* Anemia may be present because of inflammation, or pancytopenia may be present from bone marrow involvement.
- *Liver function tests (LFT):* Including lactic acid dehydrogenase (LDH), aspartate aminotransferase (AST), alanine aminotransferase (ALT), alkaline phosphatase, and bilirubin levels; metastatic disease of the liver may affect values of these proteins.
- *Renal function tests (RFT):* Including blood urea nitrogen (BUN) and creatinine levels.
- *Urinalysis:* Hematuria may indicate involvement of the genitourinary tract.
- *Blood electrolyte and chemistry:* Including sodium, potassium, chlorine, carbon dioxide, calcium, phosphorous, and albumin values.

Liver and renal function, as well as blood electrolytes and chemistry, must be assessed before chemotherapy.

Genetic studies: Fluorescent in situ hybridization (FISH), reverse transcriptase–polymerase chain reaction (RT-PCR) assay: When FISH is unavailable or uninformative.

Imaging studies: Plain radiography, computed tomography (CT) scanning, magnetic resonance imaging, bone scanning, ultrasonography, echocardiography.

Biopsy: Open or core needle biopsy: To obtain tissue sampling for diagnosis and molecular studies.

Bone marrow aspiration and biopsy: To assess for metastatic spread to bone marrow.

Treatment

Treatment for children with RMS focuses on achieving 'local control' and 'systemic control.' Local control refers to the permanent eradication of the 'primary tumor.' This is usually accomplished by surgical removal or irradiation of the tumor (or both) and any involved nearby areas, in addition to chemotherapy treatment. Systemic control refers to the permanent control of invisible 'micrometastases' or visible 'metastases', generally by chemotherapy (sometimes with additional surgery or radiation therapy).

All children with RMS are treated with chemotherapy. Depending upon the size and location of the primary tumor, and how much of it can be surgically removed, most children will also receive some combination of radiation therapy and surgery.

Prognosis

Survival rates depend upon the site and stage of the cancer; current statistics state a 5-year survival rate of 60% overall for this type of cancer.

Wilms' Tumor

Wilms' tumor is a type of kidney cancer that was named after Dr Max Wilms, who first described it. Wilms' tumor or nephroblastoma starts in one, or rarely, both kidneys. It is most often found in children about 3 to 4 years old, and is uncommon in children older than age 6 years. It can show up as a asymptomatic swelling or lump in the abdomen.

Wilms' tumor is a cancerous tumor on the kidney, although it is totally unrelated to adult kidney cancer. It occurs in about 8 in 1 million children under age 14 years; it is more common in children under age 7 years. Wilms' tumor is best treated when it is found early, before it has spread to other areas of the body. Prognosis is related to stage of disease at diagnosis, histopathologic features of the tumor, and age of patient.

Etiology and Incidence

In most children, the causes of Wilms' tumor are unknown. In 1 to 2% of children in whom Wilms' tumor develops, have a family history of this disease. Very rarely, people who develop Wilms' tumor have other congenital malformations. These include aniridia (the lack of an iris in the eye), cryptorchidism, hypospadius and a condition where one side of the body is slightly larger than the other (hemihypertrophy).

Wilms' tumor represents 5 to 6% of childhood cancers and the mean age of diagnosis is 2 to 5 years.

Pathophysiology

It is thought to come from very specialized cells in the embryo known as *metanephric blastema*. These cells are involved in the development of the child's kidneys while they are in the womb. The cells usually disappear at birth, but in many children with Wilms' tumor, cells called *nephrogenic rests* can still be found. Initially this disease is local, but metastasis to other organs occasionally occurs. The lungs are the most common site of metastasis.

Clinical Features

Common symptoms of Wilms' tumor are abdominal swelling and/or pain, nausea, vomiting, constipation, loss of appetite, fever of unknown origin, night sweats, abnormal urine color or blood in the urine, malaise, hypertension.

The child may show some or all of the above symptoms. The symptoms are the result of the tumor on the kidney. The lump of the tumor itself can sometimes be felt, but it may not always be detectable. The kidneys are located toward the back of the abdomen and the lump may be growing on the back of the kidneys or toward the inside and it may not be as easily detected. Sometimes these symptoms are attributed to a common kind of stomach flu, and are therefore left untreated by. The child may complain pain in leg, at the top of thigh. As a general rule, parent should contact physician if any time symptoms of nausea, fever, stomach pain, vomiting last longer than several days, it is a cause for concern.

Diagnostic Evaluation

A variety of tests and investigations may be needed to diagnose a Wilms' tumor.

USG: An abdominal ultrasound scan is usually the first thing that is done to identify tumor.

MRI and/or CT scan—MRI and/or CT scan of the abdomen and chest. These scans help to identify exactly where the tumor is, and whether it has spread beyond the kidney. This is known as staging. Other tests—the blood test, urine test, and X-ray are effective at properly diagnosing a Wilms' tumor. Urine and blood samples will also be taken to check your child's kidney function and general health.

Biopsy: Most children will go on to have a biopsy, where a sample of tissue is taken from the tumor to confirm the diagnosis.

Therapeutic Management

Treatment for Wilms' tumor is based mainly on the stage of the cancer and whether its histology is favorable or unfavorable. In the United States, doctors prefer to use surgery as the first treatment in most cases, and then give chemotherapy (and possibly radiation therapy) afterward. In Europe, doctors prefer to start the chemotherapy before surgery. The results seem to be about the same.

Most often, the stage and histology of the cancer are actually determined when surgery is done to remove the cancer, because the true extent of the tumor often cannot be determined by imaging tests alone. The findings from surgery are then used to guide further treatment. But sometimes it is clear that the cancer has already spread beyond the kidney even before surgery is done, based on imaging tests. This can affect the order in which treatments are given, as well as the extent of surgery.

Stage I

The tumor is only affecting the kidney and has not begun to spread. It can be completely removed with surgery. The tumor along with the entire kidney, nearby structures, and some nearby lymph nodes are removed.

Children younger than 2 years with small tumors (weighing less than 550 g) may not need further treatment, such as chemo. If the cancer does come back, the chemo drugs actinomycin D (dactinomycin) and vincristine (and possibly more surgery) are very likely to be effective at this point.

For children older than 2 years who have larger tumors, for children of any age who have tumors with unfavorable histology surgery is usually followed by chemo with actinomycin D and vincristine. If the tumor cells have certain chromosome changes, the drug doxorubicin (adriamycin) may be given as well. The chemo is given for several months.

Stage II

The tumor has begun to spread beyond the kidney to nearby structures, but it is still possible to remove all possible signs of cancer by surgery. After surgery, standard treatment is chemo with actinomycin D and vincristine is administered in case of favorable histology. If the tumor cells have certain chromosome changes, the drug doxorubicin (adriamycin) may be given as well. The chemo is given for several months.

Unfavorable histology with focal anaplasia: When the child recovers from surgery, radiation therapy is given over several weeks. Chemotherapy with above combination is given for about 6 months.

Unfavorable histology with diffuse (widespread) anaplasia: After surgery, these children get radiation over several weeks. This is followed by a more intense type of chemo using the drugs vincristine, doxorubicin, etoposide, cyclophosphamide, and carboplatin, along with mesna (a drug that protects the bladder from the effects of cyclophosphamide), which is given for about 6 months.

Stage III

These tumors were not removed completely with surgery because of their size or location or for other reasons. In some cases, surgery to remove the tumor may be postponed until other treatments are able to shrink the tumor first (see below). The tumor has spread beyond the kidney; either because the tumor has burst before or during the operation, has spread to lymph glands (nodes), or has not been completely removed by surgery.

Favorable histology: Treatment is usually surgery if it can be done, followed by radiation therapy over several days. Then chemo with 3 drugs (actinomycin D, vincristine, and doxorubicin). If the tumor cells have certain chromosome changes, the drugs cyclophosphamide and etoposide may be given as well. Chemo is given for about 6 months.

Unfavorable histology with focal (only a little) anaplasia: Treatment starts with surgery if it can be done, followed by radiation therapy over several weeks. This is followed by chemo, usually with 3 drugs (actinomycin D, vincristine, and doxorubicin) for about 6 months.

Stage IV

These tumors have already spread to distant parts of the body at the time of diagnosis. As with stage III tumors, surgery to remove the tumor might be the first treatment, but it might need to be delayed until other treatments can shrink the tumor. Either in favorable or unfavorable histology, surgery to remove the tumor is the first treatment if it can be done, followed by radiation therapy. This is followed by chemo with the drugs vincristine, doxorubicin, etoposide, cyclophosphamide, and carboplatin, along with mesna given for about 6 months.

For stage IV cancers that have spread to the liver, surgery may be an option to remove any liver tumors that still remain after chemo and radiation therapy.

Stage V

Treatment for children with tumors in both kidneys is unique for each child, although it typically includes surgery, chemo, and radiation therapy at some point.

If not enough functioning kidney tissue is left after surgery, a child may need to get dialysis. If there is no evidence of any cancer after a year or two, a donor kidney transplant may be done.

Nursing Intervention

The goals of nursing management of WT include:

- Assessing for presence of WT
- Provide emotional care for the parents and child
- Preparing the child and the parents for diagnostic procedures and treatment
- Assisting in therapeutic management
- Planning for discharge.

Assessing for Presence of WT

Abdominal mass/enlarged abdomen is often reported by parents, who detect the condition during giving care to the child. Nurse should be familiar with the clinical features of WT as well as other possible causes of an enlarged abdomen. If the possibility of WT exists, prompt referral to a physician is indicated.

Bed warning against palpation of abdomen of child must be put up, as there is risk of rupturing the protective capsule of the tumor. Excessive manipulation can cause seeding of the tumor and spread of cancerous cells.

Provide Emotional Care for the Parents and Child

Frequently they feel guilty for not noting earlier the presence of the tumor and its symptoms. The parents are to be reassured that nothing they have or have not done will alter the outcome for the child.

Support and reassurance throughout the treatment and follow up is important for the parents and child to minimize their anxiety related to loss of one kidney.

Preparing the Child and the Parents for Diagnostic Procedures and Treatment

Explanation regarding diagnostic procedure should be clear and concise. Some written material with graphics may be helpful to understand the procedure and treatment.

Assisting in Therapeutic Management

Monitor the renal status by observing weight changes, intake and output and circulatory overload. Other postoperative monitoring includes GI activity, bowel sounds, abdominal distension (child is prone to intestinal obstruction), signs and symptoms of infection, hemorrhage and BP of the patient.

Assessing the output from the remaining kidney and nasogastric tube drainage, fluid requirement of the child is calculated and administered to the child. Another IV solution may be hung so that the amount lost by NG output in last 4 hours is replaced over the next 4 hours. The replacement fluid usuall contains potassium as gastric contents are potassium rich. Moreover, serum electrolytes levels are checked every 8 to 12 hours during this process.

Planning for Discharge

Parents must understand the importance of treatment (continued care of chemotherapy and radiotherapy) and follow up care, they can verbalize the early signs of complications. Information and support to the parents can help to allay their anxiety as well as to support them regain some control over their child's life.

Retinoblastoma (RB)

RB is a cancer of the eye. RB develops from the immature cells of a retina, the light-detecting tissue of the eye and is the most common malignant tumor of the eye in children. RB is usually found because an observant parent notices a child's eye looks unusual. Normally when a light is shined in a child's eye, the pupil looks red because of the blood in vessels in the back of the eye. In an eye with RB the pupil often looks white or pink. This white glare (leukocoria) of the eye may be noticed after a flash picture is taken.

Etiology and Incidence

RB is a rare malignant tumor of the embryonic neural retina. It is thought to result from a sequence of genetic mutation, which starts sporadically, occurring within a single retinal cell that then multiplies to form the tumor. So identifying the RB gene mutation that led to a child's retinoblastoma can be important in the clinical care of the affected individual and in the care of (future) siblings and offspring. It accounts for about 3% of childhood cancers. It usually occurs before the age of 5, around the age of 2; and can occur in one or in both eyes and is hereditary in some cases.

A higher incidence is noted in developing countries, this has been implicated to lower socioeconomic status and the presence of human papilloma virus sequences in the retinoblastoma tissue. In the developed world, RB has one of the best cure rates of all childhood cancers (95 to 98%), with more than 9 out of every 10 sufferers surviving into adulthood.

Manifestations

The most common and obvious sign of RB is an abnormal appearance of the retina as viewed through the pupil, called leukocoria, also known as amaurotic cat's eye reflex. Other signs of RB are deterioration of vision, a red and irritated eye with glaucoma, faltering growth or delayed development. Some children with retinoblastoma can develop a squint, commonly referred to as 'cross-eyed' or 'wall-eyed' (strabismus).

RB presents with advanced disease in developing countries and eye enlargement is a common finding.

Diagnostic Evaluation

Depending on the position of the tumors, they may be visible during a simple eye exam using an ophthalmoscope to look through the pupil. Leukocoria or strabismus is often detected by parent. A positive diagnosis is usually made only with a fundoscopic examination under anesthetic (EUA). A white eye reflection is not always a positive indication of retinoblastoma and can be caused by light being reflected badly or by other conditions such as Coats' disease.

The presence of the photographic fault red eye in only one eye and not in the other may be a sign of retinoblastoma. A more clear sign is 'white eye' or 'cat's eye' leukocoria. Screening for retinoblastoma should be part of a 'well baby' screening for newborns during the first 3 months of life, to include:

Screening for RB should be part of a 'well baby' screening for newborns during the first 3 months of life.

The red reflex: Checking for a normal reddish-orange reflection from the eye's retina with an ophthalmoscope or retinoscope from approximately 30 cm or 1 foot, usually done in a dimly lit or dark room.

The corneal light reflex/Hirschberg test: Checking for symmetrical reflection of beam of light in the same spot on each eye when a light is shined into each cornea, to help determine whether the eyes are crossed. If the eye examination is abnormal, further testing may include imaging studies, such as computerized tomography (CT), magnetic resonance imaging (MRI), and ultrasound CT and MRI can help define the structure abnormalities and reveal any calcium depositions. Ultrasound can help define the height and thickness of the tumor. Bone marrow examination or lumbar puncture may also be done to determine any metastases to bones or the brain.

Therapeutic Management

The goal of current treatment of RB is to save the life of child's life preserve the eye and its vision at optimal level. The various treatment modalities for RB are given below:

- *Enucleation of the eye:* The patients with unilateral disease present with advanced intraocular disease, have no chance for useful vision even if the tumor is destroyed; usually undergo enucleation, which results in a cure rate of 95%. In bilateral RB, enucleation is usually reserved for eyes that have failed all known effective therapies or without useful vision.
- *External beam radiotherapy (EBR):* This is another treatment modality that can be administered for multifocal disease.The most common indication for EBR is for the eye in a young child with bilateral RB who has active or recurrent disease after completion of chemotherapy and local therapies. However, patients with hereditary disease who received EBR therapy are reported to have a 35% risk of second cancers.
- *Brachytherapy:* Brachytherapy involves the placement of a radioactive implant (plaque), usually on the sclera adjacent to the base of a tumor. It used as the primary treatment or, more frequently,in patients with small tumors or in those who had failed initial therapy including previous EBR therapy.
- *Thermotherapy:* Thermotherapy involves the application of heat directly to the tumor, usually in the form of infrared radiation. It is also used for small tumors.
- *Laser photocoagulation and cryotherapy:* Laser photocoagulation or cryotherapy is recommended only for small posterior tumors. This therapy is used to coagulate all the blood supply to the tumor.
- *Systemic chemotherapy:* Systemic chemotherapy has become forefront of treatment in the past decade, in the search of globe preserving measures and to avoid the adverse effects of EBR therapy. The common indications for chemotherapy for intraocular RB include tumors that are large and that cannot be treated with local therapies alone in children with bilateral tumors. It is also used in patients with unilateral disease when the tumors are small but cannot be controlled with local therapies alone.

Nursing Management

Assessment

Nurses work in the hospital and community should be able to recognize the early signs of RB and their importance. If parents make comment about an unusual gleam in their child's eye or a change in facial expression, should be promptly referred to an ophthalmologist. Nurse can assess for strabismus, esotropia, exotropia, or decreased vision.

Nursing diagnosis

- Anxiety of the child and family related to the diagnosis and enucleation or fear of blindness.
- Disturbed visual perception related to visual changes caused by the tumor or enucleation.
- Deficient knowledge about the disease and treatment.

Interventions

Preparing the family members and the child for diagnostic and treatment modalities. They should know that treatment is based on staging and the Reese staging system is used to classify RB. Explaining about available treatment modalities, and reason to choose the specific treatment for the child, its prognosis; can minimize the anxiety of the family members.

Postoperatively the child will wear a patch over the socket for 1 week approximately. The enucleated orbit needs special care like special observation for infection, hemorrhage and edema. The shape of the orbit is maintained by a conformer and then prosthesis is placed at about 5 to 6 weeks. Nursing interventions include teaching the parents how to remove, clean and reinsert first the conformer then the prosthesis. The child should learn to use protective eyewear during play and other hazardous activities.

Family must know the importance of follow up care and do the retinal examination under anesthesia and by CT is indicated. Genetic counseling is the primary mode of prevention of RB. The siblings of the genetically inherited patient should be periodically examined.

Patients with genetic RB have a chance of developing second malignancy (osteosarcoma) later in life. Although no specific investigation is recommended, signs and symptoms should be carefully evaluated with a high index of suspicion.

Prognosis

Good prognosis depends upon early presentation of the child in health facility. Late presentation of the child in hospital is associated with poor prognosis.

CHAPTER 18

The Child with an Endocrine or Metabolic Disorder

Chapter Outline

- Review of the Endocrine System
- Inborn Errors of Metabolism
- The Clinical Picture and Management of Hypothyroidism versus Hyperthyroidism
- Nursing Consideration of a Child with Endocrine Disorder
- Endemic Cretinism (Environmental Disease)
- Comparison of Signs and Symptoms and Management among Hypoglycemia, Hyperglycemia and Ketoacidosis

REVIEW OF THE ENDOCRINE SYSTEM

The endocrine system is an intricate collection of hormone-producing glands scattered throughout the body (Table 18.1). Once a hormone is secreted, it travels through the blood stream from the endocrine gland that produced it to the cells designed to receive its message. These cells are called target cells. Along the way to the target cells, special proteins bind to some of the hormones. These proteins act as carriers that control the amount of hormone that is available for the cells to use. The target cells have receptors that latch onto only specific hormones, and each hormone has its own receptor, so that each hormone will communicate only with specific target cells that have receptors for that hormone. When the hormone reaches its target cell, it locks onto the cell's specific receptors and these hormone-receptor combinations transmit chemical

Table 18.1: Location and functions of endocrine glands in body (Fig. 18.1)

Name of the gland	*Location of the gland and hormone produced*	*Functions*
Hypothalamus	Lower central part of the brain releasing hormones for the pituitary gland	• Stimulates or suppresses the release of hormones in the pituitary gland to control water balance, sleep, temperature, appetite and blood pressure. Serves as the primary link between the endocrine and nervous systems.
Pituitary	Base of the brain under the hypothalamus. ACTH, ADH, corticotropin, luteinizing hormone (LH), FSH, human growth hormone (hGH), oxytocin, prolactin, thyrotropin	• Controls the activity of other endocrine glands (thyroid, ovaries, adrenal). • Helps with functions such as the growth of long bones, muscles, and viscera; body water balance; utilization of nutrients and minerals; sensitivity to pain. • In females, it helps stimulate egg production, prepares the uterus for pregnancy, triggers uterine contraction during labor, activates lactation. • In men, it helps to stimulates sperm production.
Thyroid	Front portion of the lower neck Thyroxine, triiodothyronine, calcitonin	• Helps to regulate metabolism (including weight control and energy levels), the body's calcium • Balance, muscle strength, emotions, the ability to tolerate heat or cold, and the development of the brain and nervous system in children. Thyroid hormone is essential in development as well as many aspects of homeostasis and metabolism

Contd...

Contd...

Adrenal	Above of each kidney Catecholamines (adrenaline or epinephrine); mineralocorticoids (like aldosterone); glucocorticoids (like cortisol); steroid hormones (like androgen)	• Help control metabolism, kidney function, blood pressure, cardiovascular function, • The body's response to stress, the immune system, and sexual development and function. • Help balance the effects of insulin in breaking down sugar for energy. • Glucocorticoids, such as cortisol, are important both in growth and nutrient supply and are also modulators of immune function
Pancreas	Behind the stomach Insulin, gastrin, glucagon, somatostatin	• Regulates the level of sugar in the bloodstream and keeps the muscles supplied with glucose
Para-thyroid	Above and below the thyroid Parathyroid hormone	• Regulate calcium and phosphorous concentrations in the bloodstream
Pineal	Middle of the brain Melatonin	• Helps regulate the wake-sleep cycle
Thymus	In the chest just under the breastbone Thymosin	• Development of the body's immune system
Gonads	Female ovaries—on each side of the uterus Male testes—in the scrotum Ovaries—estrogen and progesterone Testes—androgens (testosterone)	• Regulate puberty and fertility • Ovaries—induce female sexual characteristics such as breast growth, the accumulation of body fat around the hips and thighs, and the growth spurt that occurs during puberty. Both estrogen and progesterone are also involved in regulating the menstrual cycle and pregnancy. • Testes—induce male sexual characteristics such as maturation of the penis, deepening of the voice, development of muscles, increase in facial and body hair and the growth spurt that occurs during puberty. They also regulate sex drive and are involved in production of sperm cells.

instructions to the inner workings of the cell. Endocrine glands influence almost every cell, organ, and function of our bodies, helping to control mood, metabolism, growth, tissue function, and sexual development.

Endocrine Disorders in Children

The endocrine glands are a group of small organs and body tissues that produce, store and secrete hormones, chemical substances that regulate various body functions (Figs 18.1 and 18.2). Hormones play a vital role in metabolism, growth and development, digestion, sexual function, reproduction and other body functions. They also affect mood. While men and women have the same hormones, the levels of certain hormones are different.

Endocrine diseases can be complex and involve many body systems and structures because hormones are powerful. A tiny amount can cause big changes in cells or even the whole body, and too much or too little of a certain hormone can cause serious health problems.

The symptoms of the endocrine disorders are different in children than in adults, although the children have the same endocrine system problems. Endocrine system disorder means that the levels of the hormones of the specific gland are disturbed. The common endocrine disorders of children are given below:

- *Disorder of pancreas:* Diabetes is one of the endocrine system disorders that can occur in children. Even though the type 1 diabetes mostly occurs in

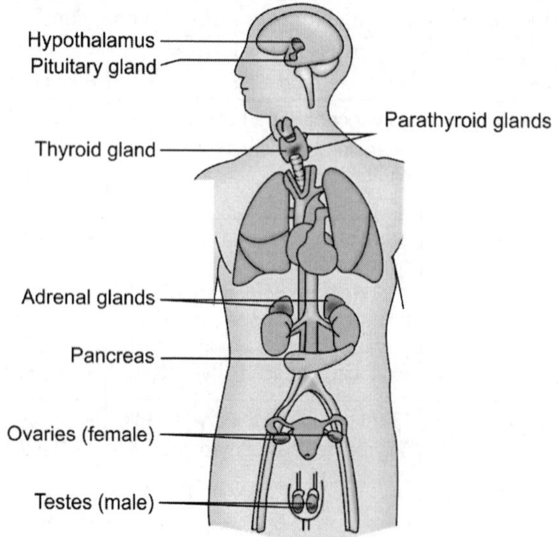

Fig. 18.1: Distribution of endocrine glands in human body

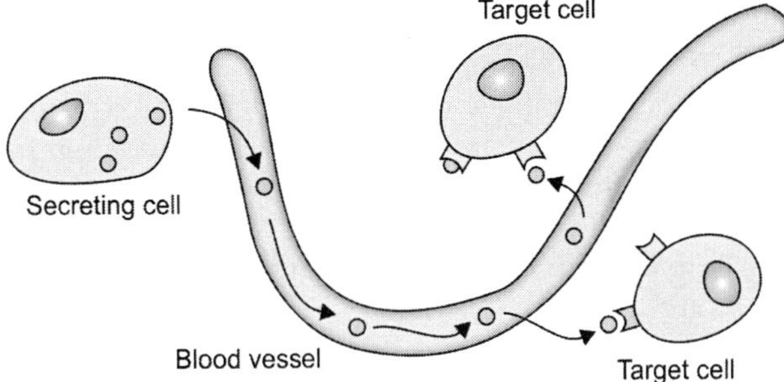

Fig. 18.2: Secretion of hormone and latched by target cells

children, which is, by the way, also called juvenile diabetes, they may also develop type 2 diabetes. When the level of hormone insulin is imbalanced, diabetes occurs. While in type 1 diabetes mellitus there is an immune-mediated disorder, and there is clinical overlap with a range of other autoimmune disorders, in type 2 diabetes the body's cells do not recognize insulin.

- *Disorder of the pituitary gland:* The pituitary gland creates the human growth hormone and abundance of this hormone leads to gigantism, a condition marked by an extremely big body size for the child's age. On the other side, when the levels of the human growth hormone are decreased, the child will stay dwarf, extremely small in size.
- *Disorder of thyroid gland:* Hyperthyroidism and hypothyroidism occur in children. The child who suffers from hyperthyroidism has extremely high levels of the hormones of the thyroid gland, while on the other hand, the child who has the problem with hypothyroidism has very low levels of the thyroid hormones.
- *Disorder of gonads:* Generally, the girls enter puberty at about 10 years of age, while in boys it happens at about 12 years of age. Precocious puberty, the consequence of hypothalamus malfunction may occur when children enter puberty earlier than 7 years (girls) and 9 years (boys) of age respectively.
- *Disorder of the adrenal gland:* The main disorder of the adrenal glands is called Cushing's syndrome, which is developed when these glands create extremely high levels of the hormone called cortisol.

Each of these endocrine system disorders has its own characteristic warning signs and when the parents notice them in their children, it is important to take immediate medical attention in order to treat the disorder promptly.

Diagnostic Tests and Procedures (Table 18.2)

Diagnostic tests and procedures are done for several reasons, including:

- To measure the levels of various hormones in a patient's body
- To learn if the endocrine glands are working correctly
- To determine the cause of an endocrinological problem
- To confirm an earlier diagnosis.

Disorders in Endocrine System

Neonatal hypoglycemia—*See* High-risk Newborn (Chapter 28)

Hypocalcemia—*See* High-risk Newborn (Chapter 28)

Phenylketonuria

Phenylketonuria (PKU) is a condition that prevents body from breaking down phenylalanine. PKU is characterized by a deficiency of phenylalanine hydroxylase, the enzyme needed to convert phenylalanine to tyrosine. Phenylalanine is found in many foods, such as meat, poultry, fish, eggs, milk, cheese, beans, nuts, and seeds. When phenylalanine is not broken down properly, it builds up in the body. PKU is a genetic metabolic disorder that results in central nervous system (CNS) damage from toxic levels of phenylalanine in the blood. It can cause brain damage and lead to serious growth and learning problems, such as mental retardation.

Table 18.2: Diagnostic tests and procedures are done to measure the level of various hormones

Test	*Description*	*Normal value*	*Indications*	*Preparation and nursing considerations*
GH	An agent (such as insulin, arginine, clonidine) is given to stimulate release of GH	Peak value >7 – 10 ng/mL	Evaluate GH production, and GH deficiency	NPO after mid night. The specimen must be drawn in specific time. Notify doctor if hypotension, hypoglycemia develops.
Cortrosyn	Tests adrenal gland function. At first baseline data is taken and 1hr. Later cortrosyn (ACTH) given	Cortisol should rise atleast double the baseline data. Cortisol <18 ug/dL suggests adrenal insufficiency	To identify congenital adrenal hyperplasia (CAH) in infants.	Time specific; samples must be drawn before and 1 hour after Cortrosyn.

Etiology and Incidences

PKU is caused by a defect in the gene that makes the enzyme needed to break down phenylalanine. The enzyme that breaks down phenylalanine may be present only in small amounts, or it may be absent. Both parents must pass on the defective gene in order for a baby to have the condition. This is called an autosomal recessive trait (means the child has inherited two identical genes for a specific trait) (Fig. 18.3).

The mean incidence of PKU varies widely in different human populations. United States Caucasians are affected at a rate of 1 in 10,000. In India, incidence rate is 1:18,300.

Pathophysiology

PKU is caused by a mutated gene for the enzyme phenylalanine hydroxylase (PAH), which converts the amino acid phenylalanine (Phe) to other essential compounds in the body, in particular tyrosine. Tyrosine is a 'nonessential' amino acid, which is essential for PKU patients because without PAH it cannot be produced in the body through the breakdown of phenylalanine. Tyrosine is necessary for the production of neurotransmitters like epinephrine, norepinephrine, and dopamine. Excessive levels of phenylalanine tend to decrease the levels of other amino acids in the brain. However, as these amino acids are necessary for protein and neurotransmitter synthesis, Phe build-up hinders the development of the brain, causing intellectual disability. Most of this process takes place during first decade of life.

Phenylalanine plays a role in the body's production of melanin, the pigment responsible for skin and hair color. Therefore, infants with the condition often have lighter skin, hair, and eyes than brothers or sisters without the disease.

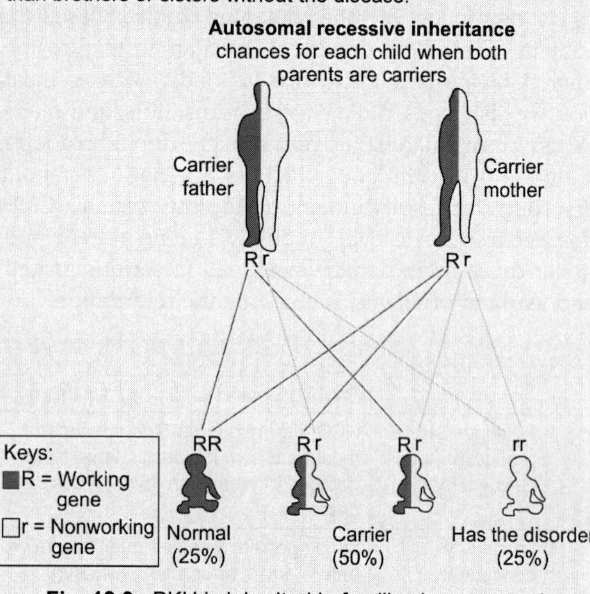

Fig. 18.3: PKU is inherited in families in autosomal recessive pattern

Manifestations

A child with PKU may look normal and completely healthy for the first few months of life. If left untreated, signs and symptoms may appear between 3 and 6 months of age. The first sign may be digestive problems with vomiting. Child may be less active and develop more slowly than other children. He may lose interest in the things around him.

Other symptoms may include:

- Delayed mental and social skills, learning, speech, or behavior problems
- Short length and head size significantly below normal
- Hypertonia, and hyperactive behavior
- Jerking movements of the arms or legs
- More irritable, fussy, or restless than normal
- Vomiting, muscle stiffness, or seizures
- Skin rashes, infantile eczema
- Tremors
- Unusual positioning of hands.

If the condition is untreated or foods containing phenylalanine are not avoided, a 'mousy' or 'musty' odor may be detected on the breath and skin and in urine. The unusual odor is due to a buildup of phenylalanine substances in the body.

Diagnostic Evaluation

Blood tests are usually done during your child's first days of life. Because the test shows the accumulation of phenylalanine, screening done before the third day of life has a higher risk of a false negative outcome. Screening for PKU is done with bacterial inhibition assay (Guthrie test), immunoassays (fluorometric, chromatographic). Measurements done using MS/MS determine the concentration of Phe and the ratio of Phe to tyrosine, both of which will be elevated in PKU. PKU is characterized by serum phenylalanine levels greater than 20 mg/dL.

Genetic tests may be needed to check your child's genes. This test may also help your child's healthcare providers decide on a treatment plan.

Therapeutic Management

PKU is not a curable disease but a treatable disease, and best results may be obtained with early treatment. However, if PKU is diagnosed early enough, an affected newborn can grow up with normal brain development and live a normal life in terms of educational achievement, career success, etc. by managing and controlling Phe levels through diet, or a combination of diet and medication. Treatment involves a diet that is extremely low in phenylalanine, particularly when the child is growing. A dietitian can carefully calculate a sparing amount of breast milk or regular formula to be mixed with the phenylalanine-free formula. The diet must be strictly followed. This requires close supervision by a registered dietitian, nurse and doctor, and cooperation of the parent and child. Those who continue the diet into adulthood have better physical and mental health.

Phenylalanine occurs in significant amounts in milk, eggs, and other common foods. The artificial sweetener (aspartame) also contains phenylalanine. Any products containing aspartame should be avoided. Supplementary 'protein substitute' formulas are typically prescribed for classic PKU patients (starting in infancy) to provide the amino acids and other necessary nutrients that would otherwise be lacking in a low-phenylalanine diet. In addition, tyrosine, which is normally derived from phenylalanine and which is necessary for normal brain function, is usually supplemented. A special infant formula called Lofenalac is made for infants with PKU. It can be used throughout life as a protein source that is extremely low in phenylalanine and balanced for the remaining essential amino acids. The goal of therapy is to keep the serum phenylalanine level at 2–6 mg/dL in infants and 2–15 mg/dL in children older than 12 years.

Taking supplements such as fish oil to replace the long chain fatty acids missing from a standard phenylalanine-free diet may help improve neurologic development, including fine motor coordination. Other specific supplements, such as iron or carnitine, may be needed.

A safe amount of phenylalanine differs for each person with PKU and can vary over time. In general, the idea is to consume only the amount of phenylalanine that's necessary for normal growth and body processes, but no more. A safe amount can be determined through:

- Regular review of diet records, growth charts and blood levels of phenylalanine
- Frequent blood tests that monitor PKU levels as they change over time, especially during childhood growth spurts and pregnancy
- Other tests that may be done to assess growth, development and health.

INBORN ERRORS OF METABOLISM

Congenital Adrenal Hyperplasia

This condition occurs when the adrenal glands do not produce enough corticosteroids. The symptoms of adrenal insufficiency may include weakness, fatigue, abdominal pain, nausea, dehydration, and skin changes. Adrenal insufficiency is treated with medications to replace corticosteroid hormones.

Disorders of Pituitary Gland

The pituitary gland, located at the base of the brain, is known as the 'master gland' because it secretes hormones that influence nearly all the systems of the body.

While roughly the size of a pea, the pituitary gland produces hormones that regulate many body functions, including energy and metabolism, sexual development and functioning, bone mass, blood pressure, body growth, and the production of breast milk in women.

Disorders in Children

Diabetes Insipidus (Table 18.3)

Diabetes is a Greek word meaning 'siphon'; and .' *Insipidus* is a Latin word meaning 'without taste.' In contrast to diabetes mellitus, which involves the excretion of sweet urine, diabetes insipidus (DI) involves the passing of urine that is tasteless because of its relatively low sodium content.

DI is a rare disorder of vasopressin or ADH, a hormone that helps the kidneys regulate the amount of water in the body. Normally, the pituitary gland releases vasopressin to decrease the amount of urine the kidneys send to the bladder, thus keeping person from getting dehydrated. In child with DI, there is either not enough vasopressin or his kidneys cannot respond to it normally, which means the body gets rid of more water in the urine than it should. This can be dangerous.

Etiology

DI is due either to (1) deficient secretion of arginine vasopressin (AVP)—also known as antidiuretic hormone (ADH)—by the pituitary gland (central or neurogenic DI) or (2) renal tubular unresponsiveness to ADH (nephrogenic DI). Between two basic kinds of DI central diabetes insipidus occurs when the body does not produce or release enough vasopressin. It is usually a result of a problem in the brain or central nervous system. It is by far the most common form of DI, affecting almost all of the children with the condition. With medication it is easily treatable. Nephrogenic diabetes insipidus occurs when there is a genetic or other problem that does not allow the kidneys to respond normally to vasopressin. This type of DI is much less common, and is more difficult to treat.

Table 18.3: Hormones secreted by anterior pituitary gland, its action and related disorders

Hormone	*Action*	*Condition related to hormonal deficit/ increased secretion*	*Disorder*
Growth hormone (GH)	GH stimulates normal growth of bones and tissues throughout the body	GH deficiency leads to a decrease in muscle mass, central obesity and impaired attention and memory. Children experience growth retardation and short stature	Dwarfism (low GH level) Acromegaly (high GH level)
Adrenocorticotropic hormone (ACTH)	ACTH stimulates the two adrenal glands, each placed close to a kidney. ACTH triggers these adrenal glands to release hormones, including adrenaline (epinephrine) and cortisol, which regulate many aspects of metabolism, immune function, and blood pressure.	ACTH deficiency leads to a lack of production of glucocorticoids such as cortisol by the adrenal gland. If the problem is chronic, symptoms consist of fatigue, weight loss, failure to thrive (in children), delayed puberty (in adolescents), hypoglycemia, anemia and hyponatremia	Adrenal insufficiency Cushing's syndrome (high level)
Thyroid-stimulating hormone (TSH)	TSH is a hormone that stimulates production and secretion of thyroid hormones from the thyroid gland. Thyroid hormone regulates the body's metabolism and is essential for growth and brain development	TSH deficiency leads to typical symptoms of tiredness, intolerance to cold, constipation, weight gain, hair loss and slowed thinking, as well as a slowed heart rate and low blood pressure. In children, hypothyroidism leads to delayed growth and in extreme inborn forms to a syndrome called cretinism.	Hypothyroidism (low T4 and T3) Cretinism is a condition of severely stunted physical and mental growth due to untreated congenital deficiency of thyroid hormone (congenital hypothyroidism) usually due to maternal hypothyroidism.
Luteinizing hormone (LH) and follicle-stimulating hormone (FSH)	LH and FSH together referred to as the gonadotropins. are hormones that control sexual development and function in males and females	Lack of LH/FSH in children is associated with delayed puberty	
Prolactin (PRL)	PRL is a hormone that stimulates milk production and female breast growth for lactation	PRL plays a role in breastfeeding, and inability to breastfeed may point at abnormally low prolactin levels	

Pathophysiology

The basis of water loss in DI is distinct from that of water loss caused by diabetes mellitus. The renal tubular collecting ducts are unable to concentrate urine secondary to ADH deficiency or resistance.

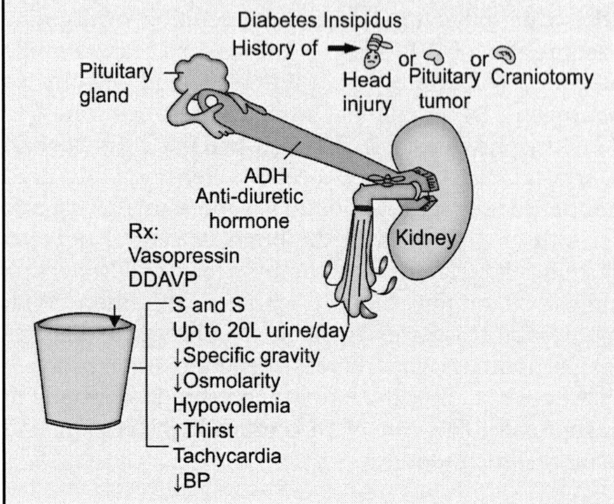

The collecting duct concentrates urine by reabsorbing water, a function controlled by the posterior pituitary gland via secretion of AVP (i.e. ADH). Reabsorption of sugars, amino acids, and virtually all electrolytes is completed by the time the urine has reached this segment of the nephron. Thus, the inability to conserve water by reabsorption in the collecting duct depletes body water but leaves sodium unaffected. The net result is an extremely diluted, increased urine output resulting in hypernatremia. Polydipsia follows, as the thirst mechanism urges replenishment of body water.

Secretion of ADH occurs in the posterior pituitary gland and is regulated at the paraventricular and supraoptic nuclei, which sense changes in osmolality. Destruction of the paraventricular or supraoptic nuclei or of the posterior pituitary by tumor, pressure, or surgical ablation results in decreased ADH secretion and central DI. Alternatively, DI may be idiopathic or inherited as either an autosomal dominant or an autosomal recessive trait.

Nongenetic causes of DI include injuries. Typical injuries include head trauma, tumor, and neurosurgical procedures. At all ages, destructive lesions of the pituitary, the hypothalamus, or both are the most common cause of DI.

Diagnostic Evaluation

Diagnosis of DI may be difficult in infants and children because of nonspecific presenting features such as poor feeding, failure to thrive, irritability. Accordingly, a high index of suspicion is necessary.

At its earliest sign the child with DI shows a vigorous suck with vomiting, fever without apparent cause, constipation, and excessively wet diapers from urination. In older infants and young children, irritability is generally due to a borderline state of dehydration coupled with hypernatremia and, sometimes, fever. Nocturia is common and expected because of increased urine production. Central DI tends to develop suddenly.

The typical examination reveals an irritable infant with a dripping wet diaper, along with detectable signs of dehydration (e.g. dry mucous membranes, diminished skin turgor, decreased tearing, tachycardia). Often, skin turgor is not diminished in individuals with hypernatremic dehydration despite significant dehydration. In severely dehydrated patients, the pulse may be thready and rapid. Hypotension may be present because of hypovolemic shock. Mobile fecaliths may be palpable in the abdomen.

Treatment

For central (neurogenic) DI, the treatment of choice is the synthetic ADH analogue desmopressin. Other useful medications include chlorpropamide and thiazide diuretics. Nephrogenic DI cannot be effectively treated with desmopressin, because the receptor sites are defective and the kidney is prevented from responding. Thiazide diuretics, amiloride, and indomethacin or aspirin are useful when coupled with a low-solute diet.

Parents must be educated regarding water replacement in infants and young children who cannot express thirst or access fluids without assistance. Gastrointestinal illnesses that cause decreased intake, increased stool losses, or both must receive early and serious attention to prevent life-threatening electrolyte and fluid balance abnormalities

Syndrome of Inappropriate Antidiuretic Hormone

The syndrome of inappropriate antidiuretic hormone secretion (SIADH) is defined by the hyponatremia and hypo-osmolality resulting from inappropriate, continued secretion or action of the hormone, which results in impaired water excretion.

Etiology

It is usually caused by diseases affecting the central nervous system such as meningitis, head injury, brain tumors. Surgery of brain tumors may precipitate the child to have transient SIADH.

Pathophysiology

In general, the plasma Na^+ concentration is the primary osmotic determinant of AVP release. Excessive ADH results in the kidney reabsorbing too much free water. In persons with SIADH, the nonphysiological secretion of AVP results in enhanced water reabsorption, leading to dilutional hyponatremia, high urine specific gravity. While a large fraction of this water is intracellular, the extracellular fraction causes volume expansion and then some degree of accompanying potassium excretion (kaliuresis). Eventually, a steady state is reached and the amount of Na^+ excreted in the urine matches Na intake. Ingestion of water is an essential prerequisite to the development of the syndrome; regardless of cause, hyponatremia does not occur if water intake is severely restricted.

In addition to the inappropriate AVP secretion, persons with this syndrome may also have an inappropriate thirst sensation, which leads to an intake of water that is in excess of free water excreted. This increase in water ingested may contribute to the maintenance of hyponatremia. Once the sodium level falls below 125 mEq/L, the child shows manifestations of hyponatremia.

Manifestations

Manifestations that occur with SIDAH include decreased urine output, increased urine specific gravity ((>1.030), fluid retention, weight gain, hyponatremia, and increased urine osmolality. Manifestations of hyponatremia may present as:

- Confusion, disorientation, delirium
- Generalized muscle weakness, myoclonus, tremor, asterixis, hyporeflexia, ataxia, dysarthria, Cheyne-Stokes respiration, pathologic reflexes
- Generalized seizures, coma.

Diagnosis

SIADH is best defined by the classic Bartter-Schwartz criteria which include hyponatremia with corresponding hypo-osmolality, continued renal excretion of sodium, urine less than maximally dilute, absence of clinical evidence of volume depletion, absence of other causes of hyponatremia, correction of hyponatremia by fluid restriction. The laboratory tests include serum sodium, potassium, chloride, and bicarbonate, plasma osmolality, serum creatinine, blood urea nitrogen, blood glucose, urine osmolality, serum uric acid, serum cortisol, TSH.

Imaging studies that usually be considered include chest radiography (for detection of an underlying pulmonary cause of SIADH), computed tomography (CT) or magnetic resonance imaging (MRI) of the head (for detection of cerebral edema occurring as a complication of SIADH, for identification of a CNS disorder responsible for SIADH, or for helping to rule out other potential causes of a change in neurologic status.

Treatment

Initial treatment is correction of underlying cause. The goal is to correct hyponatremia at a rate that does not cause neurologic complications, and aim at maximum serum sodium level of 125–130 mEq/L. A child with severe hyponatremia may need intravenous (IV) infusion of sodium chloride. In case of transient SIDAH drug therapy is usually not indicated. In case of management of chronic SIDAH medications such as lithium and demeclocycline is used to block the action of ADH at the renal collecting tubules. Management of hyponatremia include the following:

- Three percent hypertonic saline (513 mEq/L)
- Loop diuretics with saline
- Vasopressin-2 receptor antagonists (aquaretics, such as conivaptan)
- Water restriction.

Precocious Puberty

Puberty is the process of physical maturation manifested by an increase in growth rate and the appearance of secondary sexual characteristics. Puberty starts on average in girls between ages 8–13 and in boys between ages 9–14. Precocious puberty has most commonly been defined as the onset of puberty (appearance of any sign of secondary sexual maturation) before the age of 8 years in girls and before the age of 9 years in boys. Traditionally it involves early physical changes of puberty and also linear growth acceleration and acceleration of bone maturation, which leads to early epiphyseal fusion and short adult height compared with genetic height potential.

Body changes associated with puberty may occur at an abnormally young age in some children if the pituitary hormones that stimulate the gonads to produce sex hormones rise prematurely. By definition, males who have precocious puberty must develop secondary sexual characteristics when younger than 9 years. The classic definition of sexual precocity for girls is the onset of secondary sexual characteristics prior to age 8 years. The current guidelines recommend the evaluation of any girl younger than 8 years who has an advanced bone age or a rapid progression through puberty.

Etiology

If the pituitary glands release hormones that stimulate the gonads to produce sex hormones too early, some kids may begin to go through puberty at a very young age. This condition is called precocious puberty. The exact mechanism of sexual pseudoprecocity is not fully understood; however, TRH-induced TSH excess is thought to be the common stimulator of the follicle-stimulating hormone (FSH) receptor.

Flowchart 18.1: Algorithm of etiologies of precocious puberty.

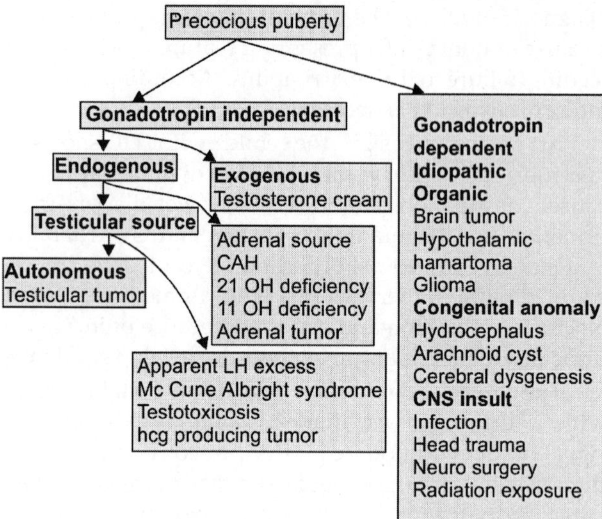

Precocious puberty can be idiopathic or caused by CNS tumors, head trauma, or radiation in the cranium (Flowchart 18.1).

This condition may occur without any specific cause; some cases are thought to be caused by the genetic problems, changes in the brain, tumors that may release hormones. This condition may be caused due to:

- Hypothalamic hamartoma
- McCune-Albright syndrome
- Congenital adrenal hyperplasia
- Tumors releasing LCG hormone
- Disorders of adrenal glands
- Disorders of ovaries
- Disorders of testicles.

This syndrome is thought to be a malfunctioning or damage in the brain that may cause hypothalamus send a message to the body to start the puberty.

Pathophysiology

The onset of puberty is caused by the secretion of gonadotropin-releasing hormone (GnRH) by the hypothalamus. This stimulates the pituitary gland to release LH and FSH and subsequently maturation to the gonads and gonadal activity. In girls, FSH stimulates formation of ovarian follicle and to produce estrogen; which is necessary to develop secondary sex characteristics. LH is involved in the process of ovulation and production of progesterone.

- The exact mechanism of sexual pseudoprecocity is not fully understood; however, TRH-induced TSH excess is thought to be the common stimulator of the follicle-stimulating hormone (FSH) receptor.

Contd...

Contd...

- Serum FSH and luteinizing hormone (LH) levels are elevated into the pubertal range. Mounting evidence suggests that increased serum levels of prolactin produce resistance to LH stimulation of the gonads, perhaps leading to hypothalamic gonadotropin-releasing hormone (GnRH) production and stimulation of pituitary LH and FSH release.

High-amplitude pulses of GnRH cause pulsatile increases in the pituitary gonadotropin-luteinizing hormone (LH) and follicle-stimulating hormone (FSH). Increased LH levels stimulate production of sex steroids by testicular Leydig cells or ovarian granulosa cells. Pubertal levels of androgens or estrogens cause the physical changes of puberty, including penile enlargement and sexual hair in boys and breast development and maturation of the vagina and labia in girls. These levels also mediate the pubertal growth spurt. Increased FSH levels cause enlargement of the gonads in both sexes and eventually promote follicular maturation in girls and spermatogenesis in boys.

CNS abnormalities associated with precocious puberty include tumors (e.g. astrocytomas, gliomas, germ cell tumors secreting human chorionic gonadotropin [hCG]), hypothalamic hamartomas, acquired CNS injury caused by inflammation, surgery, trauma, radiation therapy, or abscess, congenital anomalies (e.g. hydrocephalus, arachnoid cysts, suprasellar cysts).

Manifestations

Most children with precocious puberty grow faster than their peers at first, but finish growing before reaching their anticipated height.

Children with this disorder may have psychosocial difficulties as they may not be emotionally prepared for the physical changes of puberty and may feel self-conscious about these changes. It is an abnormal syndrome that may lead to different physical and social discomforts. This syndrome may occur in girls if they experience any of the symptoms before age of 8 years:

- Faster growth
- Beginning of menstruation
- Development of breasts
- Maturation of outer genitals
- Growth of pubic and armpit hair.

Signs of precocious puberty in boys: Boys, who suffer from this condition, may begin to experience these following symptoms before age of 9 years:

- Growth of penis and testes
- Development of pubic hair
- Development of armpit hair
- Growth of facial hair
- Growth of upper lip hair
- Growth of muscles
- Change in quality of voice
- Deepening of voice.

Diagnosis

Diagnosis of precocious puberty starts with thorough history taking including onset of sexual characteristics and the physical examination. Blood tests are done to check the level of hormones and other underlying reasons of this syndrome. Some medical tests for the diagnosis of this condition may include:

Blood hormone testing: It is done to evaluate the raised level of estrogen, testosterone, LH, FSH. GnRH stimulation test is a definitive test to delineate between central gonadotropin dependent and peripheral gonadotropin dependent precocious puberty. Synthetic GnRH is administered IV or subcutaneously and serial blood samples (obtained over a period of two hours) are drawn to assay FSH and LH. The FSH peak is higher before puberty than the LH peak. With the onset of puberty, the LH peak is higher than the FSH peak. Early morning testosterone in boys is higher in early puberty.

Pubertal levels of sex steroid are found in gonadotropin-independent precocious puberty.

Hand and wrist X-rays for bone age: If bone age is within one year of chronological age, either puberty has not started or has only just started. If the bone age is two years advanced then puberty has probably been present for at least a year or is progressing rapidly. Bone scan is not routinely required but is useful with suspected McCune-Albright syndrome (MAS).

- *CT scan and MRI of brain:* These are more accurate to visualise tumors.

Abdominal and pelvic ultrasound: They are beneficial in diagnosing adrenal tumors and ovarian tumors or cysts. Pelvic ultrasound is essential in precocious pseudopuberty (gonadotropin-independent precocious puberty) to detect ovarian tumors or cysts. Although not required in CPP, it will demonstrate changes in ovaries and uterus.

Other ultrasound: Testicular and adrenal ultrasound can help to establish diagnosis of tumors, but much better imaging is ultimately achieved with MRI for adrenal tumors.

- *MRI of abdomen:* It also provides evidence of pubertal changes in the uterus and ovaries.

Treatment

- The goal of treatment for precocious puberty is to stop, and possibly reverse, the onset of puberty and to maximize adult height. Treatment of this disorder may include use of medicines to stop this process before time as well as curing of underlying conditions. Currently GnRH agonist is administered in case of central precocious puberty. GnRH blockers inhibit the binding of GnRH to the pituitary gland, causing decreased production of pubertal hormones. At children's, usually synthetic luteinizing-hormone-releasing hormone (LHRH) is used. It slows or reverses sexual development. GnRH can be administered either intranasally or by monthly intramuscular injection. After initiation of the therapy GnRH secretion suppresses within 2–4 weeks and symptoms of secondary sexual characteristics, accelerated growth rate and bone maturation will regress within one year of treatment. Treatment compliance is highly needed otherwise it can promote pubertal changes rather than suppress puberty. No evidence suggests that GnRH agonist therapy interferes with the child's reproduction in future. The pubertal progression starts when therapy cessased.

So, Medical treatments include:

- Gonadotropin-releasing hormone (GnRH) agonists are used in CPP, as well as for other etiologies, including McCune-Albright syndrome (MAS) and testotoxicosis.
- Glucocorticoids are used for congenital adrenal hyperplasia (CAH).
- Testolactone is an inhibitor of steroid biosynthesis. It is used most commonly for MAS but also in testotoxicosis.
- Tamoxifen may be used in McCune-Albright syndrome (MAS).
- Ketoconazole may be used to inhibit steroid biosynthesis in testotoxicosis.
- Cyproterone acetate may be used for anti-androgen action. Flutamide is also used to counter androgen excess.
- Medroxyprogesterone (a progesterone analogue) may also be used.

For children with peripheral precocious puberty, it is really important to treat the cause. Sometimes surgery is also required to remove the tumors from human body.

Complications

Children with early sexual development are more likely to suffer from psychological and social disorders. Most of the kids suffering from precocious puberty are embarrassed to face the people as they receive negative remark/behavior. Young people are not able to hold the inferiority complex at a time when their body is going through hormonal changes, such people have low esteem and sometimes they start taking Alcohol, drugs and other illegal things due to depression of their abnormal appearance.

Congenital Adrenal Hyperplasia (CAH)

Congenital adrenal hyperplasia (CAH) affects adrenal glands, a pair of walnut-sized organs located above the kidneys. CAH is a collection of genetic conditions that limit adrenal glands' ability to make certain vital hormones. In most cases of congenital adrenal hyperplasia, the adrenal glands do not produce enough cortisol. CAH is caused by a defect in the enzymes pathway of adrenal steroidal production. Diminished glucocorticoids production prompts increased production of ACTH, further increasing adrenal androgen excess.

The production of two other kinds of hormones also may be affected, including mineralocorticoids (aldosterone) and androgens (testosterone). Mineralocorticoid production may be normal or low. Infants waste salt through kidneys when there is diminished production of mineralocorticoid. As a result it causes 'salt wasting' and leads to hypovolemia, low serum sodium levels and hyperkalemia.

The cause of congenital adrenal hyperplasia is an inherited genetic defect that limits production of one of the many enzymes the adrenal glands use to make cortisol. The enzyme most commonly lacking in congenital adrenal hyperplasia is 21-hydroxylase. Congenital adrenal hyperplasia may sometimes be called 21-hydroxylase deficiency. Signs and symptoms of congenital adrenal hyperplasia are worst when the enzyme deficiency is severe.

Most of the problems caused by classic congenital adrenal hyperplasia are related to a lack of cortisol, which plays an important role in regulating blood pressure, maintaining blood sugar and energy levels, and protecting body against stress.

Congenital adrenal hyperplasia can cause problems with normal growth and development in children including normal development of the genitals. It affects both males and females.

Manifestations

A child with classic congenital adrenal hyperplasia may be identified with

- **A lack in the adrenal glands' production of aldosterone.** This can lead to low blood pressure, lower sodium level and higher potassium level. Sodium and potassium normally work together to help maintain the right balance of fluids in body, transmit nerve impulses, and contract and relax muscles.

- **Excess production of the male sex hormones (androgens such as testosterone).** It is marked by ambiguous genitalia of the female child; and postnatal virilisation in both sexes. This can result in short height, early puberty in boys, abnormal genital development in girls and severe acne. Signs and symptoms may vary, depending on which specific gene is defective.

The condition is passed along in an inheritance pattern called autosomal recessive. Children who have the disorder have two parents who either have the condition themselves or who are both carriers of the genetic mutation that causes the condition.

Diagnostic Evaluation

- *Physical exam.* Appropriate evaluation of electrolytes, carbon dioxide levels and physical examination of newborn infants may avert salt wasting crisis of CAH. The finding in ambiguous genitalia raise the suspicion of congenital adrenal hyperplasia, the next step is to confirm the diagnosis with blood and urine tests.
- *Blood and urine tests.* Tests used to diagnose congenital adrenal hyperplasia measure levels of hormones manufactured by the adrenal glands cortisol, aldosterone and androgens. A diagnosis can be made by elevated values of 17-hydroxyprogesterone, a glucocorticoid precursor. Elevated level of rennin indicates mineralocorticoid deficiency.

Karyotyping: This is genetic blood tests which can analyze chromosomes, called karyotyping, to determine the sex of the child. A karyotype test is required to determine genetic sex depending on the degree of genital ambiguity.

USG: A pelvic ultrasound can be used to produce images of female reproductive structures, the cervix, uterus and fallopian tubes, to confirm whether the child is a girl.

Therapeutic Management

- *Medications:* In most cases, replacement hormone medication is prescribed to boost the levels of deficient hormones in child and restore them to normal levels. Treatment for the child with CAH involves lifelong treatment. Usually child may be given an oral drug—such as hydrocortisone or dexamethasone to replace cortisol and fludrocortisone to replace aldosterone on a daily basis. The dosage is prescribed on the basis of body size and is given two or three times per day in either suspension or tablet form. Mineralocorticoid replacement therapy is needed in case of child with salt wasting CAH. At times, children with congenital adrenal hyperplasia need multiple drugs, with even higher doses prescribed during periods of illness or severe stress, including surgery.

Steroid-type replacement medications may cause side effects, particularly if the doses are high and are used long-term. Side effects of medication, such as the loss of bone mass and impaired growth are monitored by regular interval, and medications are adjusted accordingly. Therapy is monitored with serum electrolytes, 17-hydroxyprogesterone levels, and rennin levels. Regular check up of child's progress, including monitoring changes in height, weight and blood pressure is important.

Treatment for girls with classic congenital adrenal hyperplasia involves a careful balance of the right amount of cortisone medications. Adequate cortisone replacement is needed to suppress androgens, allowing for normal height and minimizing masculine characteristics. However, too much cortisone may cause Cushing's syndrome.

Surgery: In some infant girls who have ambiguous external genitalia, reconstructive surgery is recommended to correct the appearance and function of the genitals. This procedure may involve reduction of the clitoris size and reconstruction of the vaginal opening. The surgery is typically performed between 2 and 6 months of age.

Growth Hormone Deficiency

Growth hormone is an anterior pituitary hormone whose main effect is to promote growth of body tissues. Pituitary growth hormone secretion is stimulated by growth hormone–releasing hormone (GHRH) from the hypothalamus. Growth hormone deficiency may result from disruption of the growth hormone axis in the higher brain, hypothalamus, or pituitary causing poor growth and short stature.

Etiology and Incidence

Although most instances of isolated growth hormone deficiency are idiopathic, specific etiologies cause most growth hormone deficiency associated with other pituitary deficiencies. Growth hormone deficiency dysfunction can be congenital or acquired. Hypopituitarism may be congenital, resulting from abnormal formation of the pituitary or hypothalamus before the child is born, or acquired, stemming from damage to the pituitary or hypothalamus during or after birth. Congenital hypopituitarism is present at birth, although it may not be apparent for many months. Congenital growth hormone deficiency may be associated with an abnormal pituitary gland or may be part of other pituitary deficiencies (hypopituitarism), optic nerve hypoplasia, and absence of the septum pellucidum; it occurs with an incidence of about 1 in 50,000 births.

Acquired hypopituitarism may become evident any time during infancy or childhood, and may occur after severe head injury or a serious illness such as meningitis or encephalitis. Many cases of acquired hypopituitarism result from a tumor called craniopharyngioma. This tumor may press on the hypothalamus or pituitary, causing one or more hormone deficiencies. Deficiency consists of surgical removal of the tumor, which usually results in permanent hypopituitarism.

Manifestations

The history in patients with suspected growth hormone deficiency (GHD) should focus on the following issues:

Birth weight and length: Intrauterine growth retardation is an issue in the differential diagnosis and should be apparent from the birth history.

Symptoms of GH deficiency in children include the following:

- Short stature
- Low growth velocity for age and pubertal stage
- Increased amount of fat around the waist
- The child may look younger than other children his or her age
- Delayed tooth development.

Many teens with GHD experience low self-esteem due to their developmental delays. Short stature and/or a slow rate of maturing as in young women who have not developed breasts or young men whose voices have not changed may be especially troubling.

Diagnosis

The child with growth hormone deficiency is often small, with an immature face and chubby body build. The rate of growth of all body parts is slow, so that the child's proportions remain normal. Intelligence is normal. A thorough physical examination, and an X-ray of the hand and wrist may be obtained to see how bone development compares to height and chronologic age.

Height and Weight Measurement

The best way to evaluate height or weight measurements is to plot the points on a growth chart. A growth chart depicts the child's growth over time, allows comparison of the height or weight to other children, and graphically depicts changes in growth or growth velocity.

Pubertal status—calculate stage of puberty using the Tanner staging system.

'Provocative tests' is done by using an agent (such as insulin) to provoke a pituitary to release a burst of growth hormone. The peak growth hormone level is measured 20–30 minutes later. The amount of insulin-like growth hormone-I (IGF-I) in the blood may be measured. IGF-I is the 'middle-man' in the growth process. Growth hormone stimulates the liver and other body tissues to produce IGF-I, which then acts as the link between growth hormone in the blood and the machinery inside cells that causes growth. The amount of IGF-I in the blood provides an indirect measure of the amount of growth hormone present.

Both IGF-1 and IGFBP-3 are growth hormone–dependent. Low values of IGF-1 and IGFBP-3 suggest growth hormone deficiency. If the peak growth hormone level is less than 10 mcg/mL in children or less than 3 mcg/mL in adults, growth hormone deficiency is diagnosed.

Persons with growth hormone deficiency may have increased total cholesterol, low-density lipoprotein (LDL) cholesterol, and triglyceride levels.

Karyotype—girls with otherwise unexplained short stature should have a karyotype study to rule out Turner syndrome. Boys in which there is clinical suspicion of a possible genetic etiology of the growth disorder have about the same likelihood of having an abnormal karyotype as is seen in girls being evaluated for Turner syndrome.

Other tests that may be performed include a CT scan and/or MRI of the brain and/or bones. Images from these tests may reveal tumors. Reduced bone density can be evaluated by a DEXA or bone density scan.

Test for thyroxine and thyroid-stimulating hormone: Hypothyroidism should be excluded as a cause of growth failure and short stature.

Therapeutic Management

The goals of treatment are to increase growth in children and restore energy, metabolism, and body composition. They may be given growth hormone, which is called somatropin (humatrope, genotropin) (Table 18.4). The drug is given as shots six or seven times a week subcutaneously.

GH deficiency is treated by replacing GH with daily injections under the skin or into muscle. Until 1985, growth hormone for treatment was obtained

Table 18.4: Growth hormone disorders

	Dwarfism	*Acromegaly*
Diagnostic test	• Growth hormone stimulation test • MRI • Radiographic studies	• Serum growth hormone levels are measured
Treatment	• Children—administration of growth hormone • Surgery	• Bromocriptine (parlodel) • Octreotide (sandostatin) • Hypophysectomy or radiation • Lifelong replacement of thyroid hormone, corticosteroids, and sex hormones
Nursing management	Assessment of mental status, ability to cope with the effects of the disorder, and understanding the treatment plan.	Assess safely in relation to impaired eyesight, chewing, swallowing, and sleep apnea monitor serum glucose levels

by extraction from human pituitary glands collected at autopsy. Since 1985, recombinant human growth hormone (rHGH) is a recombinant form of human GH produced by genetically engineered bacteria, manufactured by recombinant DNA technology.

Although growth hormone is normally secreted in multiple peaks during the day and mostly at night, a single daily injection of recombinant growth hormone can provide physiologic replacement. In order for growth hormone replacement to be effective, other pituitary deficiencies should be treated. Response to growth hormone therapy is measured (every 3–6 months) by sequential height determinations and by occasional bone age determinations.

Treatment is continued as long as potential for growth exists and the child is responding to therapy. With early diagnosis and a good response to treatment, children with growth hormone deficiency can expect to reach normal adult height. Treatment is continued until the child's growth plates closed (14 years of age for girls and 17 years for boys) or the child reaches an acceptable height.

Because growth hormone deficiency can cause a lack of energy and strength, patients should eat a balanced diet, get regular exercise, and get plenty of sleep.

PSYCHOLOGICAL SUPPORT OF SHORT STATURE CHILD

Children who are short for their age sometimes have problems and face negative reactions from the society. Some of these problems may be helped by frank and open discussion with teachers and classmates. It is very important to provide emotional support for the child with GH deficiency and to emphasize the child's many good and valuable characteristics, so that the child's stature does not limit his horizons. More about psychosocial adaptation to short stature can be learned from parents of short children and from health care professionals.

Pituitary Tumors may Require Surgery

Other Therapy

Radiation therapy to the pituitary gland may be required, if surgery for tumor removal cannot be safely accomplished.

Disorder of Thyroid Gland

A little butterfly or bow tie shaped thyroid gland remains under the skin sitting in the center of the front of the neck over the windpipe and just above the collar bone (Fig. 18.4). The major hormones that the thyroid makes and releases into the bloodstream are called T4 or **thyroxine** and T3 or **triiodothyronine**. Pituitary thyrotropin regulates thyroid hormone production. TSH synthesis and secretion are stimulated by thyrotropin-releasing hormone (TRH) of hypothalamus. Serum T4 concentration modulates secretion of both TRH and TSH by means of a classic negative feedback loop. Thyroid hormone synthesis absolutely requires iodine. The recommended dietary allowance of iodine is 40-50 mcg daily in infants, 70–120 mcg daily for children, and 150 mcg daily for adolescents and adults.

The thyroid is a different type of structure from the small round lymph nodes which are easily felt on the sides of every child's neck. The lymph nodes are there to protect against infection. The thyroid gland is there to make thyroid hormone, a body chemical needed by all cells so that they will work properly and at the right speed. The hypothalamus produces a hormone called TRH which travels down to command certain cells in the pituitary to make another hormone called TSH. TSH in turn directs the thyroid to make thyroid hormone (thyroxine) also called T4. If the thyroid makes too much T4, then the hypothalamus and pituitary, will cut

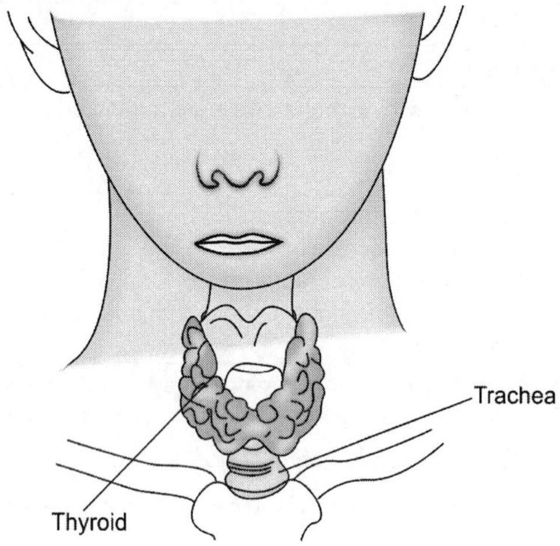

Fig. 18.4: Location of thyroid gland in human body

down the production of TRH and TSH. If the thyroid makes too little T4, then the level of TSH rises to drive the thyroid to get bigger and to make more thyroid hormone (T4).

So disorder of thyroid gland functioning can be classified as hypothyroidism and hyperthyroidism. Hypothyroidism is a condition in which levels of thyroid hormones in the blood are abnormally low. Thyroid hormone deficiency slows the body's metabolic needs. Thyroid hormone deficiency slows body processes and kids and teens with this condition may also grow more slowly and reach puberty at a later age. Hyperthyroidism is a condition in which the levels of thyroid hormones in the blood are excessively high. In children, the condition is usually caused by Graves' disease, an autoimmune disorder in which specific antibodies produced by the immune system stimulate the thyroid gland to become overactive.

Congenital Hypothyroidism

Hypothyroidism is a condition in which the levels of thyroid hormones in the blood are very low. A baby can have hypothyroidism from birth if he or she is born without a thyroid gland or if the thyroid did not develop completely before birth. And sometimes a baby's thyroid is fully developed at birth but just can't make enough thyroid hormone.

Incidence

Hypothyroidism can be congenital. Thyroid dysgenesis affects 1 per 4000 newborns worldwide.

> **Pathophysiology**
> Hypothyroidism is among the most common endocrine diseases. Congenital hypothyroidism most commonly results from agenesis, dysplasia, or ectopy of the thyroid; however, it is also caused by autosomal recessive defects in the thyroid hormone synthesis and defects in other enzymatic steps in T4 synthesis and release.

Manifestations

Most infants with congenital hypothyroidism are asymptomatic during the neonatal period or display subtle and nonspecific symptoms of thyroid hormone deficiency.

The lack of symptoms initially may result, in part, from an ectopic thyroid gland with clinically significant reserve function, partial defects in thyroid hormone synthesis, or to the moderate amount of maternal T4 that crosses the placenta and is able to boost fetal levels within 25–50% of normal levels observed at birth.

Detection of congenital hypothyroidism based on signs and symptoms alone may be delayed until age 6–12 weeks or older because of the protean clinical presentation and requires a high index of suspicion by the health care provider. The following are among the earliest signs of hypothyroidism:

- Prolonged gestation
- Elevated birth weight
- Delayed stooling after birth, constipation
- Prolonged indirect jaundice
- Large fontanelles
- Myxedema of the eyelids, hands, and/or scrotum
- Large protruding tongue (secondary to accumulation of myxedema in the tongue)
- Hypothermia
- Poor feeding, poor management of secretions
- Bradycardia
- Delayed relaxation of deep tendon reflexes (the achilles tendon reflex appears to be most sensitive to effects of hypothyroidism
- Decreased activity level
- Noisy respirations
- Hoarse cry.

Diagnosis

Congenital hypothyroidism is usually revealed by new born screening. Ideally, TSH test should be done at 2–6 days of age. If this test is performed before that a false interpretation may come out, because of the rise in TSH immediately after birth is a part of normal transition of newborn. Thyroid scan is also done to identify the functioning tissue of thyroid gland.

Therapeutic Management

Congenital hypothyroidism is treated with thyroid hormone replacement, usually in the form of levothyroxine. Usually a single oral daily dose is given which varies with weight and age. The therapy targets to maintain normal TSH and thyroxine (T4) level through titration of dosage.

Acquired Hypothyroidism

CLT (i.e. autoimmune thyroiditis, Hashimoto thyroiditis) is the most common cause of acquired hypothyroidism and goiter in children living in iodine-sufficient areas. An increased frequency of CLT occurs in children with trisomy 21 syndrome, Ulrich-Turner syndrome, Klinefelter syndrome, or other autoimmune diseases, including type 1 diabetes mellitus. CLT appears to require both an environmental trigger and a genetically determined defect in immune surveillance.

Etiology and Incidence

Hashimoto's thyroiditis is an immune system problem that often causes problems with the thyroid and blocks the production of thyroid hormone. Hashimoto's thyroiditis, which results from an autoimmune process that damages the thyroid and blocks thyroid hormone production, is the most common cause of hypothyroidism in children. Infants can also be born with an absent or underdeveloped thyroid gland, resulting in hypothyroidism. Less frequently decreased secretion by the pituitary glands (TSH) or decreased thyrotropin releasing hormone (TRH) secretion by the hypothalamus causes hypothyroidism.

Pathophysiology

Hashimoto's thyroiditis, which results from an autoimmune process that damages the thyroid and blocks thyroid hormone production, is the most common cause of hypothyroidism in kids. Evidence suggests that the disease develops secondary to a defect in cell-mediated immunity whereby suppressor T lymphocytes fail to destroy forbidden clones of thyroid-directed T lymphocytes, which form as part of random immunologic differentiation. The attack on the thyroid involves natural killer cells and the complement cascade. Various thyroid autoantibodies (antithyroglobulin antibody, antithyroid peroxidase antibody) are demonstrable in the serum but are not believed to play a role in the pathogenesis of chronic lymphocytic thyroiditis (CLT).

Manifestations

Thyroid hormone deficiency slows body processes and may lead to fatigue, a slow heart rate, dry, thick skin, weight gain, and constipation. It also includes goiter (one lobe frequently larger than other), cold intolerance, weight gain, decreased linear growth, edema of face, eyes, and hands and menstrual problems (delayed or irregular menses) and delayed osseous maturation.

Diagnostic Evaluation

A simple blood test for TSH and T4 measurement is done to see the thyroid gland functioning. This also checks to ensure the medication dosage is the correct amount.

In children with hypothyroidism, an X-ray of the hand and wrist (knee in infants) may be taken to determine the degree of delayed bone growth.

It is usually unnecessary to perform ultrasounds of the thyroid unless the enlargement is uneven, a lump or a nodule is suspected. If there is a nodule, an ultrasound will help to tell if it is fluid-filled or solid.

A thyroid scan uses a very safe weak radioactive material to see if the thyroid behaves in a normal way by taking up the radioactivity evenly. A spot with no uptake of radioactivity may be described as 'cold' and could be a tumor. In some cases a thyroid biopsy, using a small needle may be done.

The needle is placed in the thyroid to remove some cells for examination under a microscope. Older children tolerate this procedure well without sedation. If they are scared, a hand held by a parent and some anesthetic cream helps.

Therapeutic Management

It can be treated with oral thyroid hormone replacement.

ENDEMIC CRETINISM (ENVIRONMENTAL DISEASES)

Children with endemic cretinism suffer from hypothyroidism that begins at conception because the dietary iodine deficiency prevents synthesis of normal levels of thyroid hormones symptoms include—mental retardation that can be profound spastic dysplasia problems with gross and fine motor control resulting from damage to both the pyramidal and the extrapyramidal systems. Children with endemic cretinism suffer from hypothyroidism that begins at conception because the dietary iodine deficiency prevents synthesis of normal levels of thyroid hormones. It is more severe than that seen in congenital hypothyroidism because the deficiency occurs much earlier in development and results in decreased brain thyroid hormone exposure both before and after the time the fetal thyroid begins functioning. Damage occurs both to structures such as the corticospinal system that develop relatively early

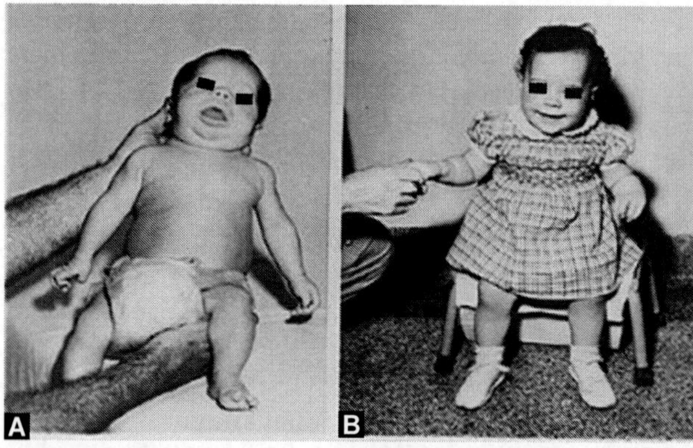

Figs 18.5A and B: Cretinism before treatment and after treatment

in the fetus and structures such as the cerebellum that develop predominantly in the late fetal and early neonatal period. If postnatal hypothyroidism is present, there is growth retardation and delayed or absent sexual maturation (Fig. 18.5).

Hyperthyroidism (Graves Disease)

Hyperthyroidism is a condition in which the levels of thyroid hormones in the blood are very high. In kids and teens, the condition is usually caused by Graves' disease, an immune system problem that causes the thyroid gland to become very active. Hyperthyroidism is treated with medications, surgery, or radiation treatments.

Hyperthyroidism is a condition in which the levels of thyroid hormones in the blood are excessively high. Symptoms may include—weight loss, nervousness, tremors, excessive sweating, increased heart rate and blood pressure, protruding eyes, and a swelling in the neck from an enlarged thyroid gland (goiter). In children, the condition is usually caused by Graves' disease (Fig. 18.6), an autoimmune disorder in which specific antibodies produced by the immune system stimulate the thyroid gland to become overactive. The disease may be controlled with medications or by removal or destruction of the thyroid gland through surgery or radiation treatments.

Pathophysiology

In some children thyroid stimulating immunoglobulins (TSIs) are produced in their thyroid gland. But the cause of antibody production is not known. The thyroid gland is stimulated by circulating autoantibodies (TSI) to make T3 and T4. Excessive thyroid hormone is secreted as these TSI bind to the TSH receptor sites on the thyroid gland. In newborns, through placenta the maternal TSI are transferred to the fetus. Neonatal hyperthyroidism is caused as TSI bind to the receptor of TSH.

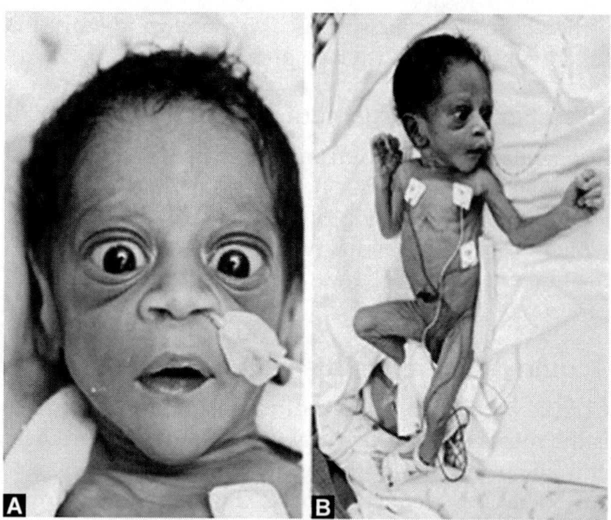

Figs 18.6A and B: A child with grave disease

Manifestations

Diarrhea, weight loss, nervousness, muscle weakness, tremors, excessive sweating, increased heart rate and blood pressure, heat intolerance, exophthalmos (protruding eyes), and a swelling in the neck from an enlarged thyroid gland (goiter). Poor attention span, and behavior or school problems are common in Graves disease. Hyperthyroidism in neonates is characterized by tachycardia, hypertension, irritability, voracious appetite with poor weigh gain, prominent eyes, and thyroid enlargement. Though, these are self limiting signs, but cardiac failure and death can occur if the signs are not recognised or poorly treated.

Diagnostic Evaluation

Physical Examination

The above mentioned signs and symptoms of hyperthyroidism, suggest Graves disease.

Blood Test

One common test for Graves' disease is a blood test to measure the amount of thyroid-stimulating hormone (TSH) in the body. Elevated serum T4 levels, little TSH may indicate hyperthyroidism.

Another blood test for Graves disease measures molecules (antibodies/TSIs) that bind specifically to pieces of the thyroid peroxidase and thyroglobulin proteins from the thyroid gland. High levels of these antibodies indicate Graves disease or another autoimmune thyroid disease.

Thyroid Scan

Thyroid uptake of radioactive iodine is increased.

Therapeutic Management

Graves disease is the most common form of hyperthyroidism in childhood. Current treatment options include antithyroid medications, surgery, and radioactive iodine.

Antithyroid drugs of the thiourea class have been available since the late 1940s, and their uses and limitations have been well defined. The two agents available for use are methimazole (tapazole) and propylthiouracil (PTU). These drugs inhibit the production of TSI. This immunosuppressive effect may explain the reduction in thyroid gland size often observed during therapy with the thioamide drugs. Methimazole has a longer half-life in serum than PTU and, therefore, can be administered as a once- or twice-daily dose. PTU is usually administered three times daily.

Both agents have a rather significant array of adverse effects. The most common adverse effect is a pruritic skin rash. Both agents can induce autoimmune or allergic responses ranging from skin rashes and fever to arthralgia, arthritis, and frank lupus like findings with positive ANAs and vasculitis. Leukopenia may be induced by both drugs and may be dose related. There is a small risk of serious adverse reactions that include hepatic failure and bone marrow suppression.

RAI (radioactive iodine) treatment of thyrotoxicosis has proved efficacious for 50 years. Sometimes, the child has a serious reaction to anti-thyroid drugs, or if the drug doesn't help eliminate symptoms, radioactive iodine may be another treatment option. This oral medication destroys part or all of the thyroid gland, blocking the production of thyroid hormone.

When radioactive iodine is used at appropriate doses, there is a very high cure rate without increased risks of thyroid cancer or genetic damage. Radioactive iodine (^{131}I) is given as an oral solution, and used in children older than 10 years.

Subtotal thyroidectomy was the treatment of choice for Graves disease before experience with RAI developed. Medical management of the candidate for subtotal thyroidectomy preoperatively and postoperatively is very important. Therefore, pretreatment with antithyroid thioureylene drugs until a euthyroid state is reached and 10 days to 2 weeks of treatment with daily potassium iodide drops (Lugol's solution), decreases gland's vascularity. Total thyroidectomy is associated with very high cure rates and a small risk of hypoparathyroidism and recurrent laryngeal nerve damage. Calcium level is monitored after surgery. It is common after thyroidectomy for the child to require thyroid hormone replacement to avoid hypothyroidism.

Nursing Consideration—A child with Endocrine Disorder (Table 18.5)

Endocrine disorder, if not identified at birth the disorder is usually detected when a child comes for routine checkup for example child's height and weight are measured and found to be above or below, a typical measurement for that age. For example, acute loss in weight, often first symptoms of type 1 diabetes mellitus (T1D); over weight is related to thyroid deficiency. Pituitary difficulties are usually related to short/tall stature; extreme thirst has relation to diabetes insipidus, extreme appetite may have relation with T1D. UTI can cause frequent micturations but excessive urination may be resulted due to pituitary difficulties or diabetic mellitus. Other symptoms like poor muscle tone, scaling or dry or darkening skin, exophthalmoses, early or late pubertal changes; are all indications of endocrine disorders.

History of one day activity of child can give clues of decreased endocrine functions. A quiet child lies down after school and plays with videogame or reads story book, whereas ill child lies down and sleep. The healthy child may go constantly but can sit through for favourite cartoons in television or meal. The child with increased thyroid hormone production may be unable to sit quietly at all.

Nursing Implications

Advise parents to seek medical examination and to do laboratory tests, as prescribed. Retina test, fundoscopic examination, neurological testing, nutritional assessment are all associated tests and examinations. Nurse should aware the child and the family members about the procedures and to meet up the queries related to that.

Nursing assessment of a child with endocrine diseases includes history taking, physical examination, obtaining laboratory and diagnostic tests. Clinical manifestations of endocrine disorders are diverse and occur as a result of the altered control of the body processes, normally regulated by different hormones.

History Taking

Family history of endocrine disorder (familial trait), and growth and development problem.

Maternal Factor

Take prenatal history, discuss maternal factors like taking drug or alcohol during pregnancy, history of illness like diabetes, hypothyroidism.

Birth History

Type of delivery, birth asphyxia, trauma, birth size.

Childhood History

Feeding difficulty, disease, treatment received (any external steroids).

Physical Examination

Observation and inspection: Note a fatigue appearance, poor muscle tone, sweatiness, faintness, nervousness

Table 18.5: Nursing process related to endocrine disorders of child

Nursing diagnosis	*Outcome*	*Interventions*
Delayed growth and development	Nutritional status will improve, the child will show improvement in nutritional status, gain weight	• Monitor growth parameters using standard growth chart • Encourage favorite foods (within prescribed diet restrictions if present) to maximize oral intake • Supplement diet, if indicated • Compliance of hormone supplementation to enhance ability to achieve appropriate growth • Provide care related to fluid and electrolyte imbalance or diarrhea due to complication of disorder • Offer age appropriate toys/play to develop gross motor activities and further development • Provide support to the families with developmental delay: growth and development may be slowly achieved, need ongoing motivation
Disturbed body image related to changes in physical appearance and abnormal growth and development due to hormonal dysfunction as evidenced by verbalization of dissatisfaction with the child's look	Appropriate self-esteem is demonstrated by the child in relation to his/her body image	• Explore the feeling, allow to ventilate feeling is associated with less body image disturbance • Relate to child on age level, not appearance level • Involve the child in decision making process, a sense of control will improve body image • Allow to spend time with peers with same endocrine disorders. Peers opinion is more accepted • Refer to counseling or support groups for further support to the child
Deficient knowledge of the child and family regarding the disorder as evidenced by questions about disease, treatment	The child and family gain sufficient knowledge and skills for self management	• Assess the child's development level and family's ability to absorb instruction; the nurse will understand how she can start session for the family • Organize awareness program based on teaching plan, written material on disease, treatment, care and follow-up • Conduct return demonstration to develop skill on self-care
Disruption of family processes of the child due to hospitalization and as evidenced by missed work, demonstration of inadequate coping	Family's functional system will be maintained and the child and family will demonstrate adequate coping, adaptation to new situations, asking questions, seeks supports	• Encourage to verbalize their queries and concerns • Explain procedures, treatment, child's behavior, plan of care • Identify support systems • Provide family with information, about support groups, financial resources, special clinics • Involve parents in child care as they will feel needed and valued and give them a sense of control over their child's health
Nutritional imbalance (less than or more than boy requirement) related to the endocrine disorder as evidenced by growth parameters excessively less or more than expected age	Nutritional status is balanced, adhere to nutritional guidelines, demonstrate adequate growth and development	• Determine weight and height norm for age or the child's pre-treatmental measurements; it is necessary to determine the gal to workout • Enquire food preferences and provide favored food within diet restrictions • Dietician may be consulted for more detailed information and assistance • Vitamins and minerals may be prescribed to attain/maintain vitamins and minerals in the body

Contd...

Contd...

Nursing diagnosis	*Outcome*	*Interventions*
Deficit or excess fluid volume related to the endocrine disorder as evidenced by sign and symptom of dehydration or edema and excessive urine output	Adequate fluid volume maintenance as evidenced by normal skin and mucous membrane, urine output, absence of edema	• Assess hydration status (skin turgor, pink and moist oral mucus membrane, presence of tears and edema present or not; urine output mL/kg/hour; vital signs in normal range for age or not) every 4–8 hours. Assess serum electrolyte and serum hormone levels. These assessments are necessary to evaluate and maintain adequate fluid volume. • Assess adequacy of urine output to evaluate end organ perfusion. • Maintenance of strict I/O to evaluate effectiveness of rehydration. • Monitor daily weight, as it is one of the best indicators of fluid volume status in children • For maintenance of fluid balance, administer special hormone, fluid, electrolyte as ordered • In case of fluid volume deficit, maintain IV line and administer IV fluid as ordered to maintain fluid volume • In case of fluid volume excess, maintain fluid restriction as ordered to restore homeostasis
Noncompliances of therapy	Compliance of therapy will improve, the child and the family will follow therapy schedule, ask questions regarding therapy and its prognosis.	• Listen nonjudgementally the causes of non-compliance • Easy planning of treatment and care which suits with the family schedule • Giving written material regarding treatment is helpful, the child and family can comply the therapy • Establish follow-up visits to fit family's situation to promote compliance • Team approach can enhance compliance • Help the child in their behavioral changes, which may precipitate due to chronic nature of illness.

or confusion. Note hair texture, protuberant tongue, drooping eyelids, exophthalmoses. Cardiopulmonary assessment, any labored respiration like kussmaul respiration in diabetic ketoacidosis.

Laboratory Diagnosis

- Tests and procedures serum and urine
- Hormone and other levels
- Evaluation bone maturation
- Genetic studies
- Radio imaging tests like MRI, CT, etc.

Diabetes Mellitus

The word 'diabetes' means 'to run through' or 'to siphon' in Greek. In the 17th century, doctors found that people with diabetes had sweet urine. They added the Latin word 'mellitus,' meaning honey. This is how we got the name diabetes mellitus. Diabetes is a disease caused when the body does not produce or properly use insulin. It is a metabolic disorder during which the body has none at all (or reduced ability) to produce the hormone insulin or the insulin is inactivated (insulin resistance).

Diabetes is a disease caused when the body does not produce or properly use insulin, an anabolic hormone. Insulin is produced by the beta cells of the islets of Langerhans located in the pancreas, and the absence, destruction, or other loss of these cells results in type 1 diabetes. Most pediatric patients with diabetes have type 1 diabetes mellitus (T1DM) and a lifetime dependence on exogenous insulin. The number of people living with diabetes is estimated at 382 million and is expected to rise to 592 million by 2035 (*International Diabetes Federation*).

Type 1 diabetes is usually diagnosed in children and young adults, and only 5% of people with diabetes have this form of the disease. Type 1 diabetes mellitus, formerly known as insulin-dependent diabetes or juvenile diabetes is a form of diabetes mellitus that results from the autoimmune destruction of the insulin-producing beta cells in the pancreas. So, pancreas is unable to produce and secret insulin. Normally, the body's immune system fights off foreign invaders like viruses or bacteria. But for unknown reasons, in people with type 1 diabetes, the immune system attacks various cells in the body, destroy the cells of the pancreas that produce insulin. This results in a complete deficiency of the insulin hormone.

Type 2 diabetes—unlike type 1 diabetes, in which the body cannot produce normal amounts of insulin, in type 2 diabetes the body cannot respond to insulin normally. Children with the condition tend to be overweight. Children can control their blood sugar level with dietary changes, exercise, and oral medications, but many will need to take insulin injections like people with type 1 diabetes.

Some people develop a type of diabetes called secondary diabetes, which is similar to type 1 diabetes, but the beta cells are not destroyed by the immune system; rather, they are destroyed by some other factor, such as cystic fibrosis or pancreatic surgery.

Etiology and Incidence

The exact cause of type 1 diabetes is unknown. Most likely it is an autoimmune disorder. Type 1 diabetes mellitus (T1DM) is an autoimmune disorder that occurs when the immune system mistakenly attacks and destroys healthy tissue of pancreas which produce insulin. While its causes are not yet entirely understood, scientists believe that both genetic predisposition and an environmental factor or viral trigger initiate the autoimmune destructive process. Its onset has nothing to do with diet or lifestyle. Present research targets on identifying specific genes that may affect person's susceptibility to T1DM. There is nothing to do to at present to prevent T1DM, nothing man can do to get rid of it. However, several different means of islet cell transplantation are being experimented and are quite promising. Children with T1DM are prone to develop other auto immune disorders like Hashimoto disease, Grave disease, celiac disease. The tendency to develop autoimmune diseases, including type 1 diabetes, can be passed down through families.

Pathophysiology

Normally, the hormone insulin is secreted by the pancreas in low amounts. When man takes meal, sugar (glucose) from food stimulates the pancreas to release insulin. The amount that is released is proportional to the amount that is required by the size

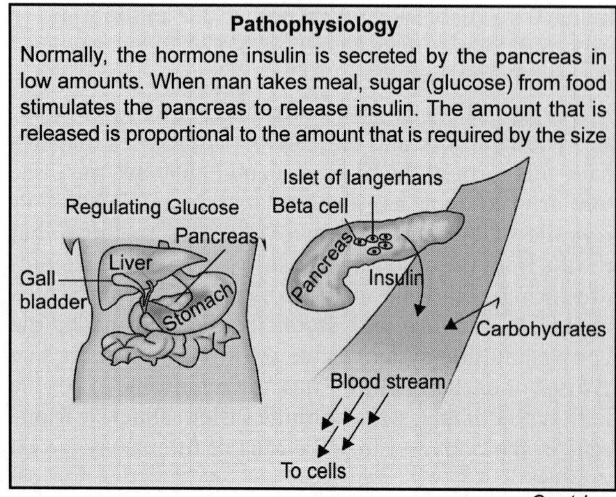

Contd...

of that particular meal. Glucose is the primary source of energy for body cells. Insulin's main role is to help move certain nutrients, especially sugar—into the cells of the body's tissues. Cells use sugars and other nutrients from meals as a source of energy to function. The amount of sugar in the blood decreases once it enters the cells. Normally, that signals the beta cells in the pancreas to lower the amount of insulin secreted so that persons don't develop hypoglycemia.

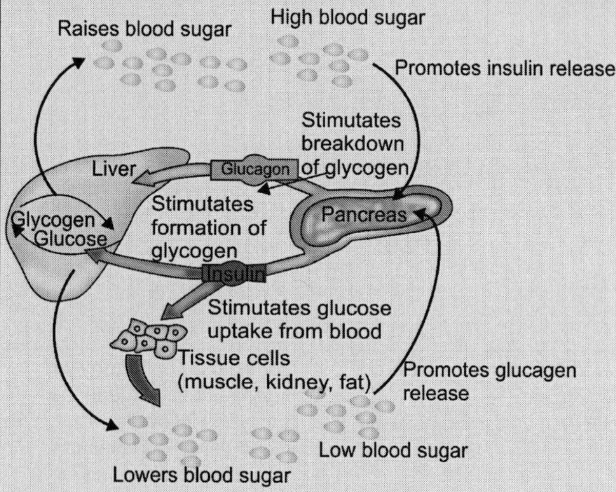

Diabetes is a disorder in which the body cannot make energy from food as it should. This is because the body does not produce enough insulin, or else the insulin produced is not working properly. Insulin is needed for body's cells to take up sugar from food. Sometimes cells do not respond to insulin. Causes are mystery still, but it seems both genetics and environmental factors like lack of exercise and obesity play a role in it.

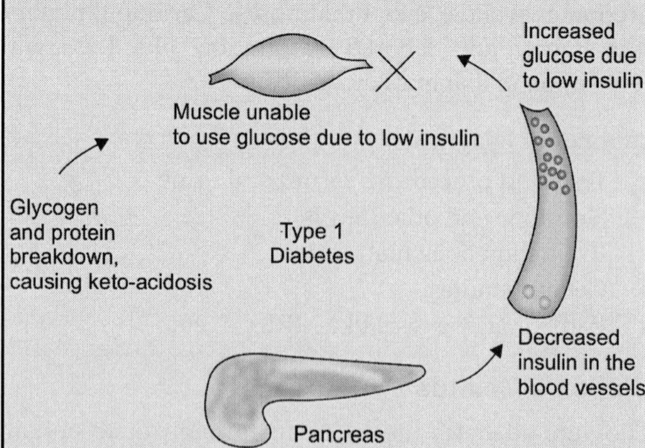

Type 1 diabetes is characterized by the body's inability to produce insulin due to the autoimmune destruction of the beta cells in the pancreas. The destruction of the beta cells that occurs with type 1 diabetes throws the entire process into disarray.

In people with type 1 diabetes, sugar is not moved into the cells, because insulin is not available. The subsequent lack of insulin leads to increased blood and urine glucose. When sugar builds up in the blood instead of going into cells, the body's cells starve for nutrients and other systems in the body must provide energy

Contd...

Contd...

for many important bodily functions. As a result, high blood sugar develops and can cause:

- *Dehydration:* The build-up of sugar in the blood can cause an increase in urination (to try to clear the sugar from the body). When the kidneys lose the glucose through the urine, a large amount of water is also lost, causing dehydration.
- *Weight loss:* The loss of sugar in the urine means a loss of calories; therefore, many people with high sugars lose weight. (Dehydration also contributes to weight loss.)
- *Diabetic ketoacidosis (DKA):* Without insulin and because the cells are starved of energy, the body breaks down fat cells. Products of this fat breakdown include acidic chemicals called ketones that can be used for energy. Levels of these ketones begin to build-up in the blood, causing an increased acidity. The liver continues to release the sugar it stores to help out. Because the body cannot use these sugars without insulin, more sugar piles into the bloodstream. In the absence of insulin, however, severe hyperglycemia, dehydration, and ketone production contribute to the development of DKA. The most serious complication of DKA is the development of cerebral edema, which increases the risk of death and long-term morbidity. Very young children at the time of first diagnosis are most likely to develop cerebral edema.
- *Damage to the body:* Uncontrolled diabetes can damage child's nerves, veins, and arteries. Long-term high blood sugar levels may damage other body tissue and organs over time, such as child's eyes and kidneys.

Diabetes is life-threatening if it is not controlled. Even with treatment, child may be at an increased risk of thyroid or Celiac disease. Certain medicines used to treat diabetes may increase the risk of pancreas or thyroid problems.

Manifestations

The classical symptoms of type 1 diabetes include: polyuria, polydipsia, xerostomia (dry mouth), polyphagia, fatigue, weight loss and blurred vision.

- *Frequent urination:* Because the body tries to get rid of the extra blood sugar by passing it out of the body in the urine.
- *Extreme thirst:* The build-up of sugar in the blood can cause an increase in urination. When the kidneys lose the glucose through the urine, a large amount of water is also lost, causing dehydration.
- *Increased appetite:* Eat a lot because the body is hungry for the energy it cannot get from sugar.
- *Sudden weight loss:* Loss of body weight despite increased food intake. It begins as it starts to use fat and muscle for fuel because body cannot use sugar normally. The loss of sugar in the urine means a loss of calories; the person loses weight. Dehydration also contributes to weight loss.
- Feel tired a lot because the body cannot use sugar for energy.
- *Sudden vision changes:* Over time, the high sugar levels in the blood may damage the nerves and small blood vessels of the eyes.

Many type 1 diabetics are diagnosed when they present with diabetic ketoacidosis. The signs and symptoms of diabetic ketoacidosis include xeroderma (dry skin), rapid deep breathing with fruity odor on the breath, drowsiness, abdominal pain, and vomiting, drowsiness and lethargy then stupor or unconsciousness. Without insulin and because the cells are starved of energy, in an attempt to nourish the starving cells, the liver makes sugar from the body stores of protein and fat. Products of this fat breakdown include acidic chemicals called ketones that can be used for energy. Levels of these ketones begin to build-up in the blood, causing an increased acidity. The liver continues to release the sugar it stores to help out. Because the body cannot use these sugars without insulin, more sugar piles into the bloodstream. The combination of high excess sugars, dehydration, and acid buildup is known as 'ketoacidosis' and can be life-threatening if not treated immediately.

Hypoglycemia (Table 18.6) can develop quickly in people with diabetes who are taking insulin. Symptoms usually appear when a person's blood sugar level falls below 70 milligrams per deciliter (mg/dL). The symptoms of hypoglycemia include:

- Headache
- Hunger
- Nervousness
- Palpitations
- Shaking
- Sweating
- Weakness.

Diagnostic Evaluation

Diabetes is diagnosed with the following blood tests:

- *Random blood sugar:* A blood sample will be taken at a random time. Blood sugar values are expressed in milligrams per deciliter (mg/dL) or millimoles per liter (mmol/L). Regardless of when person last ate, a random blood sugar level of 200 mg/dL (11.1 mmol/L) or higher suggests diabetes, especially when coupled with any of the signs and symptoms of diabetes, such as increased thirst, urination, and fatigue (this must be confirmed with a fasting test).
- *Fasting blood glucose level:* A fasting blood sugar level from 100 to 125 mg/dL (5.6 to 6.9 mmol/L) is considered prediabetes. Diabetes is diagnosed if it is higher than 126 mg/dL two different times.

Table 18.6: Comparison of hypoglycemia, hyperglycemia and ketoacidosis

Descriptor	*Hypoglycemia*	*Hyperglycemia*	*Ketoacidosis*
Onset	Rapid	Slow	Slow
Signs and symptoms	Palpitation, trembling, pallor, sweating, cold skin	Increased urination and thirst, weight loss, fatigue, blurred vision	Signs of hyperglycemia, abdominal pain, vomiting, dehydration, Kussmaul breathing and acetone breath odor, dry skin and mucus membrane, decreased urination
Sensorium	Neuroglycopenic symptoms, personality change, slurred speech, irritability,decreased level of consciousness unconsciousness, seizure activity	Headache, hunger and emotional lability	Increasing lethargy, decreasing level of consciousness, coma
Causes	Too much insulin, missed or delayed meal, too much activity without taking eating extra sugar	Increased food intake, little or no exercise, less insulin, increased physical or mental stress	Excessive stress, inadequate insulin
Laboratory findings	Blood glucose less than 70 mg/dL	Blood glucose more than 160 mg/dL	Blood glucose more than 300 mg/dL, Urine ketones and serum ketones–positive. Serum pH less than 7.25
Treatment	Carbohydrate replacement therapy (oral/ intravenous), measure for seizure activity, IM/IV glucagon injection	Insulin, exercise and increased oral fluid	IV fluids, insulin, replacement of electrolytes, other supportive care

- *Oral glucose tolerance test:* Diabetes is diagnosed if the glucose level is higher than 200 mg/dL 2 hours after you drink a special sugar drink.
- *Glycosylated hemoglobin (A1C) test:* This blood test indicates the child's average blood sugar level for the past two to three months. It works by measuring the percentage of blood sugar attached to hemoglobin, the oxygen-carrying protein in red blood cells. Diabetes is diagnosed if the result of the test is 6.5% or higher.
- *Autoantibody testing:* If a child receives a diagnosis of diabetes, blood tests are done to check for autoantibodies that are common in type 1 diabetes. These tests help to distinguish:
- Between type 1 and type 2 diabetes.
- Ketone testing is also used sometimes. The ketone test is done using a urine sample or blood sample. Ketone testing may be done when the blood sugar is higher than 240 mg/dL, and nausea and vomiting occur. The presence of ketones—by products from the breakdown of fat in urine also suggests type 1 diabetes, rather than type 2.

Therapeutic and Nursing Management

Living with T1DM is a constant challenge. People with this disease must measure their blood glucose level and carefully balance insulin doses with eating and other activities throughout the day and night. It means the child is to achieve near normal glycosylated hemoglobin (that is A1C levels be below 7%, which translates to an estimated average glucose of 154 mg/dL (8.5 mmol/L). Despite this constant attention, people with T1DM still run the risk of dangerous high or low blood glucose levels, both of which can be life threatening. The diabetes management also facilitates the appropriate growth of child and to maintain an age appropriate lifestyle.

Children who have type 1 diabetes they need to:

- Check their blood sugar levels often by pricking their fingers a couple of times a day
- Give themselves insulin shots, have someone help give them shots, or use an insulin pump
- Follow a healthy eating plan so they can keep blood sugar levels under control and grow normally
- Correct deficient fluid volume related to hypergly-cemia evidenced by polyuria and polydipsia
- Prevent injury related to hypoglicemia or hypergly-cemia
- Exercise regularly
- Have regular checkups in health care set up so they can stay healthy and get treatment for any diabetes problems.

Insulin and Other Medications

Insulin lowers blood sugar by allowing it to leave the bloodstream and enter cells. Anyone who has type 1 diabetes needs lifelong insulin therapy. Insulin must be injected under the skin using a syringe, insulin pen, or insulin pump. It cannot be taken by mouth because the acid in the stomach destroys insulin.

For controlling blood sugar levels and reduce the risk of developing diabetes problems, children need regular injections of insulin. After starting the insulin therapy there may be a 'honeymoon' period, during which blood sugar is controlled with little or no insulin. This phase is characterized by hypoglycemia and a decreased need of insulin. However, this phase may exist from a few weeks to one year or more. Misconception that diabetes is 'going away' is to be addressed properly and the child and family must learn to recognise and treat hypoglycemia.

Types of insulin are many and include:

Types	*Onset*	*Peak*	*Effect*
Rapid-acting insulin	5–10 min	30–90 min	5 hours
Short-acting insulin	20–60 min	2–3 hours	5–8 hours
Intermediate options (NPH/ Lente)	2–4 hours	4–10 hours	10–18 hours
Long acting	3–5 hours	10–16 hours	18–24 hours
Mixed type (70/30) it has 70% intermediate acting and 30% rapid acting insulin.			

The choice of insulin types and schedule of injections is determined on the basis of the child's need, i.e. based on age, body weight, and pubertal status. The injection schedule is individually prescribed according to the child's glycemic targets. The peak actions of the chosen insulin are timed to correspond to the child's usual mealtimes and snack times to minimise the possibility of hypoglycemia. A combination of rapid acting analogue with a long acting peak less insulin is a recent option for the basal/bolus insulin.

As insulin is a protein it cannot be given orally, administered by subcutaneous injection into the adipose tissue over large muscle masses. Subcutaneous insulin injection sites are abdomen, arms, hips and thighs (most rapid to low absorption sites); although almost any area on the body may be used for insulin injection. A 45 degree angle is maintained with ½ inch needle or 90 degree angle with 5/16 inch needle to avoid injecting into the muscles and vascular space. Rotation of injection sites helps prevent adipose hypertrophy, which absorb insulin poorly.

Even at a very young age, children with diabetes can play a part in the daily management of their diabetes. Blood glucose meters are simple to use. Insulin pens are also available, making giving insulin easy and convenient. Pump therapy is an alternative for managing child's diabetes. Some parents and children with their health care team may choose an insulin pump over injections to deliver insulin. An insulin pump is a beeper-size device that can be worn on or under clothing or on a waistband/belt. It provides a steady supply of insulin through a tiny tube placed under the skin. When child eats, additional insulin to cover the meal is provided by pushing buttons. Pumps have many advantages over injections, including providing more flexibility and eliminating the need to carry insulin pens or vials.

Child's insulin regimen should provide flexibility, convenience, and good blood glucose control. Children and with diabetes and their parents need to know how to adjust the amount of insulin they are taking when they exercise, when they are sick, when they will be eating more or less food and calories, when they are travelling.

Using a method called carbohydrate counting is the easiest way to achieve this. A carbohydrate-to insulin ratio provided by health care team to enable parent and child to use this method, providing a variety of food choices while achieving good blood sugars.

Diet

Since children with diabetes have the same nutritional needs for growth and development as other children, they do not need to be on a special diet. Moreover they need to achieve the goals, 'diabetes control' so as to prevent or delay different complications of diabetes. Child's meal plan is one of the most important parts of managing diabetes. It can also be one of the most challenging for children and their families. Dieticians assist in making meal planning healthful and to accommodate the child's and family's individual food preferences and meal schedule. The daily meal plan is tailored to an individual's needs. It is likely to include three meals and two or three snacks eaten at set times each day using the diabetic exchange list. It should include 55% carbohydrate, 30% fat and 15% protein.

What is Food Exchange list ?

The exchange lists group foods together because they are alike. Foods on each list have about the same amount of carbohydrate, protein, fat and calories. In the amounts given, all choices on each list are equal. Any food on the list can be exchanged or traded for any other food on the list. The lists are grouped into groups: carbohydrate group; milk exchange, vegetable exchange, fruit exchange, bread exchange, meat and meat substitute group; and fat group. Grouping foods this way allows for more convenient exchange among these lists and more flexibility in choosing foods.

A good diet for children with diabetes at all ages is the same as that recommended for everyone. This includes: plenty of complex carbohydrates, such as whole-grain breads, pastas, potatoes, beans, and peas; unprocessed foods, such as bran cereals, oatmeal, and fresh fruits and vegetables. Snacks are important since most children require frequent feedings to supply necessary calories for growth. Snacks may also be necessary in active children to avoid hypoglycemia. Good snack choices include fresh fruit, dried fruit, cheese crackers, peanut butter crackers, yogurt, grain crackers, if strenuous exercise is planned. These snacks also are used for treating mild symptoms of hypoglycemia after initial treatment with orange juice or glucose tablets to raise blood sugar quickly. Desserts that are good for all members of the family include fresh fruit, low-fat yogurt, pudding, and Jell-O.

Fluid

Correction of deficient fluid volume related to hyperglycemias evidenced by polyuria and polydipsia. Monitor blood glucose levels, electrolyte levels. Observe vital signs which alter due to dehydration and for signs and symptoms of dehydration. Administer insulin as ordered, maintain intake and output chart record.

Injury Prevention

Prevent injury of a child with DM related to hypoglycemia or hyperglycemias. Prepare the child and family to prevent injury related to hypoglycemia or hyperglycemias. The child should wear medical identification band, carry some sweets such as candy at hand always. He/she should be alert for signs for hypoglycemia especially before meal, during exercises. The child or family needs to monitor blood glucose levels to prevent hazards. Glucagon injection (as prescribed) may need to administer if child is unconscious.

The steps to prevent hyperglycemias include monitoring of blood glucose and urine ketones level daily especially on sick days; no discontinuation of insulin intake irrespective of food intake; if the RBS is above 250 mg/dL or the child is having fever or undergone surgery, is to be informed to the physician immediately.

These children have the risk for impaired skin integrity related to vascular changes associated with DM. Care of the cut and wounds are essential, daily foot care and sole are to be given. The peripheral pulses and sensations are to be checked and recorded, because the child is prone to develop peripheral neuropathy after 5 years of diagnosis. More insulin may be required when there is an infection. The site of injections is to be rotated to avoid lipodystrophy.

Self-care

Having children participate as much as possible in their care gives them some measure of control. Children under age three can choose which finger to stick for blood sugar tests or which place to use for the insulin injection.

Parents should handle treatment with a matter-of-fact yet affectionate attitude, and the American Academy of Pediatrics suggests that all adults in the family share responsibility for insulin injections and blood tests. Children four to seven years old can help with monitoring blood sugar and with injections.

Play and Activity

Exercise enhances the action of insulin in lowering blood glucose levels and promotes a greater sense of well being. There is no difference in the need for play and exercise between normal children and diabetic children. The child with diabetes should be encouraged to participate in age appropriate sports/game. Parent must teach them about prevention and management of hypoglycemia:

- Before exercise child must take food
- If exercise/gym is planned before meal, he/she should take snack in between
- In case of strenuous exercise, child should eat carbohydrate and protein rich food like milk or sandwich
- Avoid exercising during insulin peak
- Add extra 15 to 30 g carbohydrate snacks for each 45–60 minutes of exercise.

Child Care and School

Child care and school personnel need to know about diabetic students, their insulin schedule, and their snack needs. School personnel also need to be able to recognize and treat hypoglycemia. They need to know how to test blood sugar and have guidelines for giving insulin and testing for urine ketones.

Support

The more parents understand about diabetes and deal with it matter-of-fact, the better the chance that the child will do well. The tools and resources currently available make it possible for parents and their child, along with health care team, to manage the disease. With better blood glucose control, parents will reduce their child's risk for eye, kidney, nerve, and cardiovascular complications, and allow their child to grow up and lead productive, fulfilling lives (Fig. 18.7).

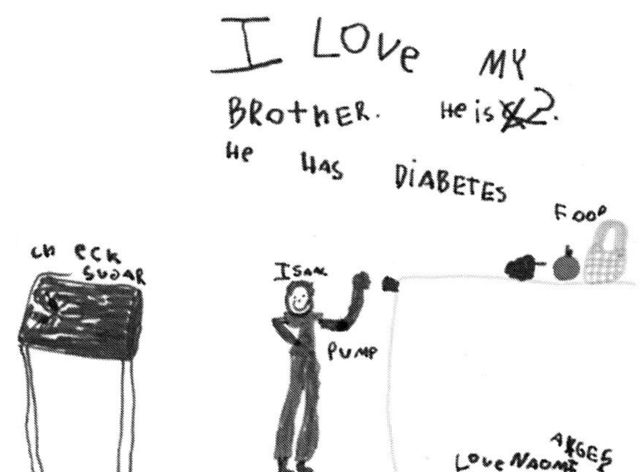

Fig. 18.7: Family support is important to a diabetic child

Mental Health

Emotional support for the entire family is very important. Depression and depressive symptoms are generally more common in people living with type 1 diabetes. Different studies show that the prevalence rate of depression is more than three times higher in diabetics than non-diabetics; recent evidence has suggested that reduced pre-frontal cortical thickness is associated with depression in people with type 1 diabetes. These neurological changes may be caused by long-term reduced glycemic control and may increase risk of depression.

CHAPTER 19

Cardiovascular System

Chapter Outline

- Review of the Heart and Circulation
- Cyanotic Heart Diseases
- Acyanotic Heart Diseases
- Obstructive Heart Diseases
- Nursing Care of the Family and Child with Congenital Cardiac Diseases
- Acquired Heart Diseases
- Arrhythmias
- Hypertension
- Kawasaki Disease
- Shock

REVIEW OF THE HEART AND CIRCULATION

Heart and arteries are parts of the cardiovascular system (Fig. 19.1). The heart is completely developed in the first eight weeks of intrauterine life. The cardiovascular system distributes blood throughout human body. The heart is an amazing muscle that moves blood to and from the heart and lungs, and throughout the body, with the help of four valves (the tricuspid, pulmonary, mitral, and aortic) that open and close with each beat of the heart, controlling the direction of blood flow.

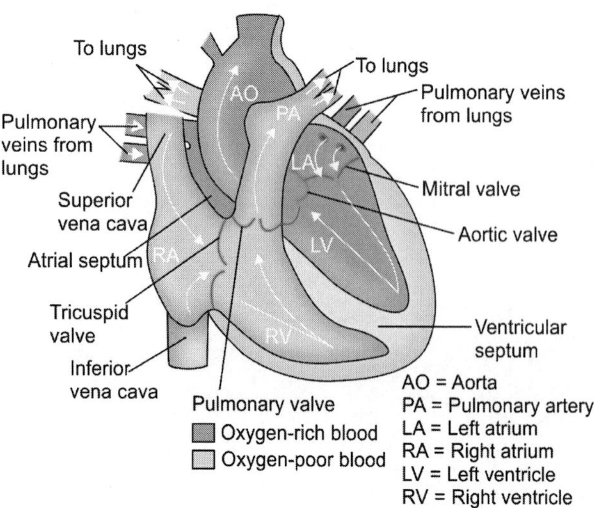

Fig. 19.1: Normal heart

It is a closed system and blood never leaves the network of arteries, veins and capillaries. Blood and lymph move through the circulatory system. The lymph is essentially recycled blood plasma after it has been filtered from the blood cells and returned to the lymphatic system. The blood and the lymphatic system collectively make up the circulatory system.

Fetal Circulation

Fetal circulation is propelled by the fetal heart through the fetus, umbilical cord, and placental villi. The fetal circulation is markedly different from the adult circulation. In the fetus, gas exchange does not occur in the lungs but in the placenta and thus relies on the maternal circulation to carry out gas, nutrient and waste exchange. The fetal and maternal blood never mix, instead they interface at the placenta. Consequently, the liver and the lungs are non-functional, and a series of shunts exist in the fetal circulation so that these organs are almost completely by-passed (Fig. 19.2). The fetal cardiovascular system is designed in such a way that the most highly oxygenated blood is delivered to the myocardium and brain. These circulatory adaptations are achieved in the fetus by both the preferential streaming of oxygenated blood and the presence of intracardiac and extracardiac shunts. Thus, the fetal circulation can be defined as a 'shunt-dependent' circulation (*See* Chapter 5: Newborn).

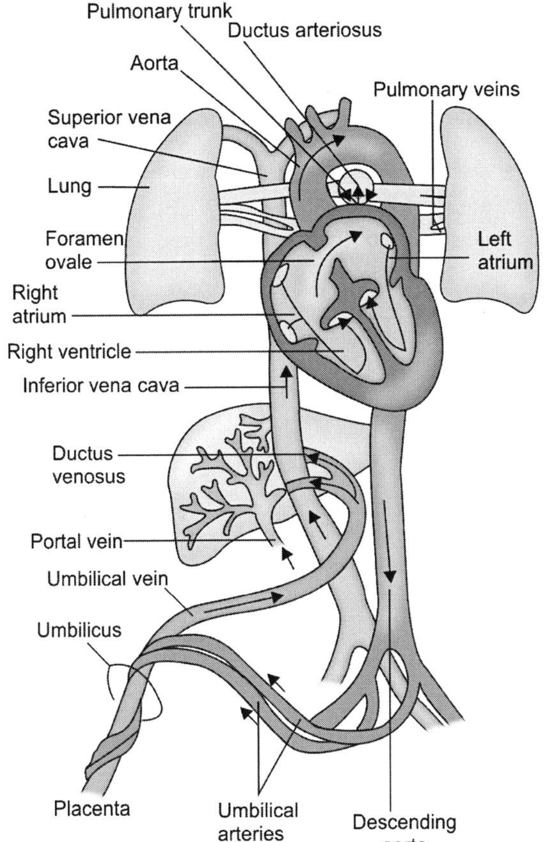

Fig. 19.2: Schematic diagram of fetal circulation

Salient Features of Fetal Circulation

- In the fetus, gas exchange occurs in the placenta
- The fetal circulation is 'shunt-dependent'
- Cardiac output in the fetus is defined in terms of combined ventricular output
- Despite low oxygen partial pressure, the presence of fetal hemoglobin and a high CVO help maintain oxygen delivery in the fetus.

Common Diagnostic Tests

- An electrocardiogram (ECG or EKG) is a test that measures the electrical activity of the heartbeat. An ECG gives two major kinds of information. First, by measuring *time intervals on the ECG*, means, how long the electrical wave takes to pass through the heart. Finding out how long a wave takes to travel from one part of the heart to the next shows if the electrical activity is normal or slow, fast or irregular. Second, by measuring the *amount of electrical activity passing through the heart muscle*, a cardiologist may be able to find out if parts of the heart are too large or are overworked.
- The chest X-ray gives the cardiologist information about *lungs and the heart's size and shape.* The amount of radiation from a chest X-ray is extremely small and does not cause any long-term side effects.
- An echocardiogram is an ultrasound movie of the inside of the heart. It can detect nearly every congenital heart defect or any problem of the *heart muscle function*. The test is often performed by a specialized technician called a sonographer, or by a physician. The test requires placing a few stickers, like those used for the ECG, on chest. The sonographer will place a special ultrasound device called a probe on the front of chest, upper abdomen and the root of the neck to record pictures of the heart. Many adjustments in the ultrasound machine is made during the study to get the clearest pictures possible. An echocardiogram usually takes 40–60 minutes to perform.
- A cardiac catheterization is a procedure that allows to get direct information about the *blood pressures and patterns of blood flow within the heart*. An angiogram is an X-ray movie that is taken while contrast, a special fluid that's visible by X-ray, is injected into a cardiac chamber or major blood vessel. Since a catheterization and angiogram require special X-ray equipment the test is usually scheduled in advance.

Sometimes a heart defect is treated during the cardiac catheterization. This is called an interventional or therapeutic catheterization. These treatments include opening up a hole in the wall between the upper chambers, opening up a blocked valve or vessel, plugging off the unnecessary vessel or closing unnecessary holes in the heart.

- Magnetic resonance imaging (MRI) is another way to take clear pictures of the heart and measure heart function. The MRI uses painless magnet waves to evaluate the heart and the blood vessels connected to the heart and lungs. MRI is a non-invasive test that uses a magnetic field and radiofrequency waves to create detailed pictures of organs and structures inside the body. It can be used to examine the heart and blood vessels, and to identify areas of the brain affected by stroke. MRI is also sometimes called nuclear magnetic resonance (NMR) imaging.
- In pediatric cases MRI scans are done to diagnose many differential conditions such as heart valve disorders, regurgitation, congenital heart problems, etc. and to evaluate the success of surgical repair.

- The CT scan uses multiple X-ray images to take an X-ray movie of the heart and lungs without placing catheters into the circulation. Like the MRI, this test sometimes takes clearer pictures than an angiogram. The test only requires a simple IV in the hand, and it can be done more quickly than an MRI. Unlike MRI imaging, the CT scan uses about the same amount of X-ray as is needed for an angiogram.
- *Holter monitoring:* Holter monitoring is also called ambulatory electrocardiography which continuously records heart rate and rhythm for 24 hours. Electrodes and leads are attached to the child, who wears a compact recorder. Parents need to maintain a diary along with the monitor. Recording the times of activities, symptoms, or other events in a diary is necessary, and that to be returned with the monitor.
- *Pulse oximetry:* Pulse oximeters are medical devices that monitor the level of oxygen saturation in a child/ patient's blood and alert the health care worker if oxygen levels drop below safe levels, allowing rapid intervention. The extremity needs to be relatively motion free for accurate reading. All nail polish must be removed.

Disorders of Cardiovascular System

The disorders of cardiovascular system, seen in children are:

- Congenital disorders
- Other disorders.

Congenital Heart Diseases

Congenital heart diseases are related to heart defects that develop during pregnancy and are present at birth (congenital). Congenital heart defects are the most common type of birth defect, affecting one of every 150 babies is born with some form of congenital heart disease. While congenital heart defects are common, not all cases are serious enough to require treatment. In cases where treatment is necessary, advances in medical technology and practice are making it possible for more patients than ever to not only survive into adulthood but to do so with a high quality of life. Congenital heart disease refers to problems of the heart and major arteries that are present at birth. Those problems can relate to:

- Heart structure, such as abnormal openings in heart walls
- Irregular heart rhythm
- Heart muscle deterioration.

Structural problems with the heart's wall and valves can often be corrected through surgery or, in some case, newer minimally invasive procedures. Narrowed arteries can be opened through a procedure called angioplasty and through the insertion of stents, tubes to hold the artery open.

Classification of congenital cardiac anomalies:

Cyanotic Heart Diseases

- Tetralogy of Fallot
- Transposition of the great arteries
- Tricuspid atresia
- Pulmonary atresia
- Persistent truncus arteriosus.

Acyanotic Heart Diseases

(left to right shunt)

- Ventricular septal defect
- Atrial septal defect
- Patent ductus arteriosus
- Atrioventricular septal defect.

Obstructive

- Pulmonic stenosis
- Aortic stenosis
- Aortic coarctation
- Hypoplastic left heart syndrome.

Child with Cyanosis

Cyanosis refers to a blue or purple hue to the skin due to an increased concentration of deoxygenated hemoglobin in the capillary bed, results from a variety of conditions, many of which are life-threatening. It is most easily observed on the lips, tongue and fingernails, ear lobes, mucous membranes, and locations where the skin is thin. Cyanosis indicates there may be decreased oxygen in the blood stream. It may suggest with the problem with the lungs but most often is a result of mixing red and blue blood due to the defects of the heart or great vessels. Cyanosis is a finding based on observation, not a laboratory test.

Two mechanisms result in cyanosis: Systemic arterial oxygen desaturation and increased oxygen extraction by the tissues. Based upon these mechanisms, two types of cyanosis are described as central cyanosis and acrocyanosis.

Central Cyanosis

Central cyanosis is evident when systemic arterial concentration of deoxygenated hemoglobin (Hb) in the blood exceeds 5 gm/dL (oxygen saturation ≤ 85%). *Of note, cyanosis cannot be detected by observation in patients with severe anemia (Hb* <5 gm/dL [3.1 mmol/L]).

Central cyanosis refers to the presence of cyanosis on the 'central' parts of the body, including lips, mouth, head and torso. Central cyanosis is never normal and is always associated with a decrease level of oxygen in the blood. It is due to problem of the heart, lung or blood.

Acrocyanosis

Acrocyanosis refers to the presence of cyanosis in the extremities particularly the palms of the hands and soles of the feet, it can also be seen on the skin around the lips. Acrocyanosis is often normal in babies, provided it is not accompanied with central cyanosis.

Mechanism of cyanosis: Alveolar hypoventilation, diffusion impairment, ventilation-perfusion mismatch, right-to-left shunting at the intracardiac great vessels or intrapulmonary level, hemoglobinopathy (including methemoglobinemia) that limits oxygen transport.

Patients with peripheral cyanosis have a normal systemic arterial oxygen saturation. However, increased oxygen extraction results in a wide systemic arterio-venous oxygen difference and increased deoxygenated blood on the venous side of the capillary beds. The increased extraction of oxygen results from sluggish movement of blood through the capillary circulation. Causes include vasomotor instability, vasoconstriction caused by exposure to cold, venous obstruction, elevated venous pressure, polycythemia, and low cardiac output.

This is relatively common in young infants, and is generally a physiologic finding due to the large arteriovenous oxygen difference that results during slow flow through peripheral capillary beds.

CYANOTIC HEART DISEASES

Tetralogy of Fallot (TOF)

It is a most complex congenital heart defect which is classically understood to involve four anatomical abnormalities of the heart.

- The first component is a narrowing of the pulmonary valve. The pulmonary valve is the entrance to the pulmonary artery found in the right ventricle. Because of this narrowing, less blood is pumped from the right ventricle into the lungs.
- The second component is a large VSD, which is a hole between the ventricles. This allows large amounts of unoxygenated blood from the right ventricle to pass into the left ventricle without going to the lungs. The body is supplied with blood that is depleted of oxygen.
- Another component is the increased musculature of the right ventricle in comparison to the left because of the increased effort required to get blood through the narrowed pulmonary valve.
- The last component is the displacement of the aorta, over ridding of aorta. The aorta lies directly over the VSD.

Pathophysiology and Altered Hemodynamics

In TOF blood returns normally from systemic circulation into the right atrium and then reaches the right ventricle. The pulmonary stenosis and right ventricular outflow tract obstruction seen with TOF usually limits blood flow to the lungs. When blood flow to the lungs is restricted, the combination of the ventricular septal defect and overriding of aorta allows oxygen poor blood returning to the right atrium and right ventricle to be pumped out the aorta to the body. The' shunting 'of oxygen-poor blood from the right ventricle to the body results in a reduction in the arterial oxygen saturation, so that babies appear cyanotic. The extent of cyanosis is dependent on the amount of narrowing of the pulmonary valve and right ventricular out flow tract.

The body attempts to compensate for unoxygenated blood by developing polycythemia. The resulting increased viscosity of blood causes decreased circulation and possibly thrombophlebitis, emboli and cerebrovascular disease.

Clinical Features

Tetralogy of Fallot symptoms vary, depending on the extent of obstruction of blood flow out of the right ventricle and into the lungs. Signs and symptoms may include:

- Cyanosis is an important sign of tetralogy of Fallot. Cyanosis is a bluish tint to the skin, lips, and fingernails. Low oxygen levels in the blood cause cyanosis. Shortness of breath and rapid breathing, especially during feeding.

Babies who have unrepaired TOF may have 'tet spells' during first 24 months of life and may lasts from few minutes to hours. These spells happen in response to an activity like crying or having a bowel movement. Sudden drop of oxygen in blood level precipitates tet spell. This causes the baby to become very blue. The baby also may:

- Have a hard time breathing, gasp for breath
- Become very tired and limp
- Not respond to a parent's voice or touch
- Become very fussy
- Pass out.

Short episode of tet spell may be followed by sleep but prolonged episodes lead to unconsciousness, convulsions or even death. Tet spell results in hypoxia and metabolic acidosis.

Loss of consciousness: Exercises cause dyspnea in TOF children. Toddlers or older children may instinctively squat when they are short of breath. Squatting increases blood flow to the lungs. If TOF was not treated in infancy children would get very tired during exercise and could faint.

A heart murmur: Another common sign of TOF is a heart murmur. A heart murmur is an extra or unusual sound that health personal might hear while listening to the heart. The sound occurs because the heart defect causes abnormal blood flow through the heart.

Clubbing of fingers and toes: An abnormal, rounded shape of the nail bed.

Poor weight gain: Babies who have TOF may tire easily while feeding. Thus, they may not gain weight or grow as quickly as children who have healthy hearts. Also, normal growth depends on a normal workload for the heart and normal flow of oxygen-rich blood to all parts of the body.

Diagnosis

These may include blood tests, a chest X-ray of the heart, echocardiography, electrocardiogram.

Chest X-ray: It shows a small boot-shaped heart due to RVH and poorly vascularized lung bed. The pulmonary artery is small and aorta is larger than normal size. There may be right aortic arch, clear hilar areas of lung.

Electrocardiogram: ECG records the electrical activity of the heart to show the rate and rhythm. In case of TOF ECG shows right axis deviation and RVH.

Electrocardiography: The VSD, overriding aorta and pulmonary stenosis can be visualized by color flow 2D echo and continuous wave doppler.

Cardiac catheterization: It shows systolic hypertension in right ventricle with rapid fall in pressure as the catheter goes into the pulmonary artery.

Therapeutic Management

- Once TOF is diagnosed, the immediate management focuses on determining whether the child's oxygen levels are in a safe range. If oxygen levels are critically low soon after birth, a prostaglandin infusion is usually initiated to keep the ductus arteriosus open which will provide additional pulmonary blood flow and increase the child's oxygen level.
- The medical management of TOF includes constant monitoring of child's condition, oxygen therapy, correction of dehydration and anemia, antibiotic therapy, and other supportive care.
- If the child has tet spells, place the child in a knees-to-chest position. This position adjusts the pressure and blood flow in the heart. The enhanced systemic venous return helps to dilate the right ventricle thereby decreasing right ventricular pressure leading to right to left shunting.
- To reduce the pulmonary and valve spasm, propranolol is usually administered in a dose of 1 mg/kg body weight up to four times in a day.

Surgical management: Most children with this kind of heart defect have it repaired during a single surgery when they are very young (usually not recommended during neonatal period). Sometimes more than one surgery is needed. Complete repair consists of closing the ventricular septal defect with a patch and enlarging the right ventricular outflow tract. The latter usually requires incision across the pulmonary valve annulus and placement of a patch of synthetic material to widen the outflow tract at all levels of obstruction. Palliative procedures is done to increase pulmonary blood flow or a definitive intra-cardiac repair.

Transposition of the Great Arteries

Transposition of the great arteries (TGA) is a ventriculoarterial discordant lesion in which the aorta arises from the right ventricle and the pulmonary artery from the left ventricle. The most common form of TGA is the dextro type (referred to as D-TGA).Transposition of the great arteries (TGA) is an embryologic defect accounts for approximately 5% of all CHD and occurs predominantly in male babies.

Pathophysiology and Altered Hemodynamics

Normally, the right side of the heart collects the unoxygenated blood and pumps it to the lungs via the pulmonary artery. The left side of the heart receives the blood from the lungs and pumps it out to the body via the aorta. With transposition, the aorta connects to the right ventricle (rather than the left), so instead of the right ventricle pumping blood to the lungs, it pumps it back to the body. On the left side of the heart, the pulmonary artery connects to the left ventricle, which pumps the blood that returns from the lungs back to the lungs. There are two separate circuits at work. One handles and recirculates the unoxygenated blood from and to the body; the other handles and recirculates the oxygenated blood from and to the lungs. In this way life can only be maintained if some communication is provided with VSD, ASD, PDA or co-lateral circulation resulting mixing of oxygenated and deoxygenated blood causing cyanosis. .Babies with transposition of the great vessels need the patent foramen ovale (PFO) and PDA to remain open so there is mixing of oxygenated blood with unoxygenated blood.

Transposition of the great arteries symptoms include:

- Blue or purple tint to lips, skin and nails (cyanosis). Cyanosis may be mild if mixing of blood occurs through a large VSD or PDA. It may be severe if ventricular septum is intact or PDA is closing.
- Dyspnea, metabolic acidosis and severe hypoxia. Afterwards CCF is found
- Lack of appetite

- Poor weight gain
- Clubbing may develop in few months
- The condition may complicated with multiorgan ischemia, cardiomegaly and growth failure.

Diagnosis

- *Examination:* Cyanosis is the major indication that there is a problem with newborn. Heart murmur is usually associated during a physical examination. In this case, a heart murmur is a noise caused by the turbulence of blood flowing through the openings that allow the blood to mix, such as the ventricular septal defect or patent ductus arteriosus.
- *Echocardiogram (also called 'echo' or ultrasound):* Sound waves create an image of the heart. This procedure evaluates the structure and function of the heart by using sound waves recorded on an electronic sensor that produce a moving picture of the heart and heart valves.
- *Electrocardiogram (ECG):* A record of the electrical activity of the heart
- *Chest X-ray:* This test uses invisible X-ray beams to produce images of internal tissues, bones, and organs onto film.
- *Pulse oximetry:* A non-invasive way to monitor the oxygen content of the blood
- *Cardiac catheterization:* A cardiac catheterization is an invasive procedure that gives very detailed information about the structures inside the heart. Under sedation, a small, thin, flexible tube (catheter) is inserted into a blood vessel in the groin, and guided to the inside of the heart. Blood pressure and oxygen measurements are taken in the four chambers of the heart, as well as the pulmonary artery and aorta. Contrast dye is also injected to more clearly visualize the structures inside the heart.
- *Cardiac MRI:* A three-dimensional image shows the heart's abnormalities.

Management

The baby will immediately receive a medicine called prostaglandin through an IV (intravenous line). This medicine helps keep a blood vessel called the ductus arteriosus open, allowing some mixing of the two blood circulations. Besides that the situation is managed with digoxin, diuretics, and iron therapy.

Transposition of the great arteries is unpredictable. Approximately one-third of newborns with TGA have extremely low oxygen levels that can harm their bodies and will require an urgent intervention, called a balloon atrial septostomy (BAS), within hours after birth. A procedure using a long, thin flexible tube (balloon atrial septostomy) may be needed to create a large hole in the atrial septum to allow blood to mix. This is a life-saving procedure, which creates or enlarges a hole between the upper chambers of the heart to allow red and blue blood to mix.

These above steps may allow doctors to delay surgery until the baby grows larger and is more stable, which can improve the outcome of surgery.

A surgery called an arterial switch procedure is used to permanently correct the problem within the baby's first week of life. This surgery switches the great arteries back to the normal position and keeps the coronary arteries attached to the aorta.

Surgery

Corrective surgery requires heart-lung bypass and is done in the newborn period after the baby has been given a couple days to adjust to life outside the uterus. The surgical repair is aimed at returning the arteries back to their normal position. Postoperative hospital stay averages 1 to 2 weeks.

Tricuspid Atresia

Tricuspid atresia is a heart defect present at birth in which one of the valves (tricuspid valve) between two of the heart's chambers is not formed. Instead, there is solid tissue between the chambers.

Pathophysiology and Altered Hemodynamics

Atresia means blockage. In tricuspid atresia, the right side of the heart cannot properly pump blood to the lungs because the tricuspid valve, located between the upper right chamber (atrium) and the lower right chamber (ventricle), is missing. Instead, a solid sheet of tissue blocks the flow of blood from the right atrium to the right ventricle. As a result, the right ventricle is usually very small and underdeveloped (hypoplastic) and an atrial septal defect or patent foramen ovale is present.

This defect may be seen with a single ventricle, which means instead of a left and right ventricle, there is just one large ventricle. The survival of an infant with tricuspid atresia depends upon communication between the right and left atriums via an atrial septal defect, as well as a ventricular septal defect, if there are two ventricles. Because of the lack of an A-V connection, an atrial septal defect (ASD) must be present to maintain blood flow. Also, since there is a lack of a right ventricle there *must* be a way to pump blood into the pulmonary arteries, and this is accomplished by a ventricular septal defect (VSD). The left ventricle receives the mixed blood and pump into the systemic circulation. While the infant is in utero, or before he or she is born, there is a natural connection between the atriums called the PFO or patent foramen ovale. This is a normal structure in fetal circulation. This structure will need to remain open even after delivery.

Symptoms

Tricuspid atresia symptoms become evident soon after birth, and can include:

- Blue tinge to the skin and lips (cyanosis). In 90% cases of tricuspid atresia, pulmonary blood flow is decreased and presented as early onset cyanosis.
- Difficulty breathing (dyspnea)
- Tiring easily, especially during feedings
- Slow growth.

Some babies with tricuspid atresia may also develop symptoms of heart failure, including:

- Fatigue and weakness
- Shortness of breath
- Swelling (edema) in the legs, ankles and feet
- Swelling of the abdomen (ascites)
- Sudden weight gain from fluid retention
- Irregular or rapid heartbeat.

Diagnosis

Cardiac examination: Murmurs, associated with VSD and PDA.

Chest X-ray: The heart size may be normal or increased. The pulmonary vascularity is usually decreased.

Electrocardiogram: ECG reveals left and right atrial enlargement, decreased or absent ventricular pressures and left ventricular hypertrophy.

Echocardiogram: 2D electrocardiograph identifies the cardiac anomalies like absence of tricuspid valve, size of right ventricle, VSD, etc. Because this test tracks blood flow, it can measure the amount of blood moving through holes in the walls between the right and left sides of the heart. In addition, an echocardiogram can identify associated heart defects, such as an atrial septal defect or a ventricular septal defect.

Management

The baby may require oxygen, and a medication called prostaglandin to maintain adequate oxygen level in the blood. Prostaglandin is an intravenous medication that keeps open the connection between the pulmonary artery and the aorta. This connection, called PDA or patent ductus arteriosus, is open in the fetus, and closes soon after birth. When the PDA closes, some babies with tricuspid atresia turn quite blue/cyanosed. An infusion of prostaglandin can re-open the PDA and is a life-saving intervention. *Not all babies with tricuspid atresia require prostaglandin.*

If the baby has labored breathing or poor effort, he or she may need help with a breathing machine or ventilator. It is not uncommon for babies to have poor respiratory effort or apnea while on prostaglandin infusion.

Surgery

Palliative surgery—Blalock-Taussig shunt

Babies who require prostaglandin to maintain adequate oxygen level will require surgery soon after birth. The surgery involves creation of a 'shunt,' which is a tube that connects one of the branches of the aorta and the pulmonary artery, and thus replaces the PDA. This operation is called the Blalock-Taussig shunt or BT shunt. Many babies with tricuspid atresia are well enough to be discharged home soon after birth. However, some of these babies may require the 'shunt' operation at a few weeks of life if the level of oxygen in their blood is decreasing.

Some babies with tricuspid atresia are too 'pink' or have too much blood-flow to the lungs, and will require an operation called 'pulmonary artery banding' to narrow the pulmonary artery and regulate blood flow to the lungs. Babies with tricuspid atresia and transposition of great arteries may require the 'Norwood operation' if the aorta is too small.

Pulmonary Atresia

Atresia means blockage. Pulmonary atresia is a congenital malformation of the pulmonary valve in which the valve orifice fails to develop. The valve is completely closed thereby obstructing the outflow of blood from the heart to the lungs. The pulmonary valve is the entrance in the right ventricle to the pulmonary artery. The pulmonary artery carries blood from the right ventricle to the right and left lungs. With the disease pulmonary atresia, the flap-like openings are completely covered by a layer of tissue, thus preventing the ability of blood flow to the lungs to become oxygenated. The body requires oxygenated blood for survival.

Pulmonary atresia is not threatening to a developing fetus however, because the mother's placenta provides the needed oxygen since the baby's lungs are not yet functional.

Once the baby is born its lungs must now provide the oxygen needed for survival, but with pulmonary atresia there is no opening on the pulmonary valve for blood to get to the lungs and become oxygenated and the only source of pulmonary blood flow is a patent ductus arteriosus. Due to this, the newborn baby is blue in color and pulmonary atresia can usually be diagnosed within hours or minutes after birth. Pulmonary atresia accounts for less than 1% of all CHD.

> **Pathophysiology and Altered Hemodynamics**
>
> When pulmonary stenosis (PS) is present, resistance to blood flow causes right ventricular hypertrophy. If right ventricular failure develops, right atrial pressure will increase, and this may result in a persistent opening of the foramen ovale, shunting of unoxygenated blood from the right atrium into the left atrium, and systemic cyanosis. If Pulmonary Stenosis is not severe, congestive heart failure occurs, and systemic venous engorgement will be noted. An associated defect such as a patent ductus arteriosus partially compensates for the obstruction by shunting blood from the left ventricle to the aorta then back to the pulmonary artery (as a result of the higher pressure in the left ventricle) and back into the lungs.

Pulmonary valve stenosis signs and symptoms may include:

- *Heart murmur:* An abnormal whooshing sound heard using a stethoscope, caused by turbulent blood flow
- Shortness of breath, especially during exertion
- Chest pain
- Loss of consciousness (fainting)
- Fatigue
- Palpitations.

Treatment

Surgical intervention is called valvotomy, to separate fused leaflets in the pulmonary valve. Another option includes the surgical placement of a valve called a pulmonary homograft, which is a donated pulmonary valve and artery. This valve may grow with the child and blood-thinners are not required.

Persistent Truncus Arteriosus

Truncus arteriosus accounts for less that 1% of all CHD. This malformation combines the aorta and pulmonary artery into one large arterial vessel rather than two. This large, single vessel usually sits above a large VSD. There are usually valve abnormalities associated with this combined vessel.

The result of the common aorta and pulmonary artery is unrestricted left-to-right blood flow, which causes congestive heart failure. The heart works harder than it normally would to oxygenate the body. CHF is a condition in which the heart is unable to keep up with the energy requirements of the body.

Treatment

Treatment is with neonatal surgical repair. The ventricular septal defect is closed with a patch. The pulmonary arteries are then detached from the common artery (truncus arteriosus) and connected to the right ventricle using a tube (a conduit or tunnel). There have been cases where the condition has been diagnosed at birth and surgical intervention is an option. A number of these cases have survived well into adulthood.

ACYANOTIC HEART DISEASES (Left to Right Shunting Lesions Cause Increased Pulmonary Blood Flow)

Ventricular Septal Defect (VSD)

With a VSD, there is a hole in the septum (wall between the right and left ventricles) (Fig. 19.3). In the normal heart, the right side handles unoxygenated blood, and the left side handles blood rich in oxygen. The ventricular septum consists of an inferior muscular and superior membranous portion and is extensively innervated with conducting cardiomyocytes.

Membranous ventricular septal defects are more common than muscular ventricular septal defects, and are the most common congenital cardiac anomaly. It accounts for 20 to 25% of all congenital heart disease and disorders.

These defects can vary greatly in size, but they all allow oxygen rich blood in the left ventricle to mix with blood depleted of oxygen in the right ventricle.

Four different septal defects exist, with perimembranous most common, outlet, atrioventricular, and muscular less commonly.

- Membranous VSDs are located near the heart valves. These VSDs can close at any time.

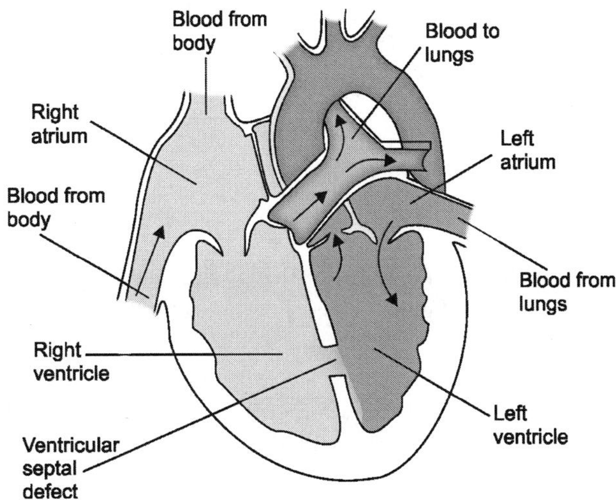

Fig. 19.3: Ventricular septal defect (VSD)

- Muscular VSDs are found in the lower part of the septum. They are surrounded by muscle, and most close on their own during early childhood.
- Inlet VSDs are located close to where blood enters the ventricles. They are less common than membranous and muscular VSDs.
- Outlet VSDs are found in the part of the ventricle where blood leaves the heart. These are the rarest type of VSD.

Pathophysiology and Altered Hemodynamics

During ventricular contraction, or systole, some of the blood from the left ventricle crosses the VSD and leaks into the right ventricle. From there it returns to pulmonary circulation and reenters the left ventricle via the pulmonary veins and left atrium. The shunt is left to right. This has two net effects. First, the circuitous refluxing of blood causes volume overload on the left ventricle. Second, the leakage of blood into the right ventricle therefore elevates right ventricular pressure and volume, as the left ventricle normally has a much higher systolic pressure (~120 mmHg) than the right ventricle (~20 mmHg), causing pulmonary hypertension with its associated symptoms.

In some advanced situations, the pulmonary arterial pressure can reach levels that equal the systemic pressure. This reverses the left to right shunt, so that blood then flows from the right ventricle into the left ventricle, resulting in cyanosis, as blood is bypassing the lungs for oxygenation.

In larger defects it is observable, who may present with breathlessness, poor feeding and failure to thrive in infancy. Patients with smaller defects may be asymptomatic.

Sign and Symptoms

The symptoms and physical findings associated with ventricular septal defects (VSDs) depend on the size of the defect and the magnitude of the left-to-right shunt, which, in turn, depends on the relative resistances of the systemic and pulmonary circulations. Common symptoms include:

- Fatigue
- Sweating
- Rapid breathing
- Heavy breathing
- Congested breathing
- Disinterest in feeding, or tiring while feeding
- Poor weight gain.

Treatment

Many times observation is the only treatment, needed with regular checkups with the cardiologist. Usually 75–80% of small VSD and 5–10% of larger VSDs will spontaneously close during the first 2 years of life. Small VSD does not require surgery, antibiotics may be administered to prevent endocarditis.

Babies who develop signs of CCF, treated with diuretics to get rid of extra fluid in the lungs. To increase the strength of the heart, digoxin is used. Sometimes antihypertensive is added to decrease the workload of the heart.

In babies who are failing to thrive because it is too difficult for them to eat, a high calorie formula , a fortified breast milk will be added to help the baby to grow.

Surgery

Surgical repair of a ventricular septal defect usually involves open-heart surgery. Surgical repair of a ventricular septal defect usually involves open-heart surgery, which is done under general anesthesia. The surgery requires a heart-lung machine and an incision in the chest. The doctor uses patches or stitches to close the hole.

- *Catheter procedure:* This method may be used to close some ventricular septal defects. Patching during catheterization does not require opening the chest. Rather than opening the chest, the doctor inserts a thin tube (catheter) into a blood vessel in the groin and guides it to the heart. A small mesh patch or plug is used to close the hole.
- *Hybrid procedure:* A hybrid procedure uses surgical and catheter-based techniques. Access to the heart is usually through a small incision and the procedure may be performed without stopping the heart and using the heart-lung machine. A plug is delivered to close the VSD via a catheter placed through the small hole that the surgeon created. Recovery from this procedure is quicker than with standard surgery.

After repair, regular medical follow-up is necessary to ensure that the ventricular septal defect remains closed. Frequency of medical checkup depends on the size of the ventricular septal defect and the presence or absence of any other problems.

Surgery to close a ventricular septal defect generally has excellent long-term results.

Atrial Septal Defect (ASD)

A 'hole' exists in the wall that separates the top two chambers of the heart (Fig. 19.4). This defect allows oxygen-rich blood to leak into the oxygen-poor blood chambers in the heart. ASD is a defect in the septum between the heart's two upper chambers (atria). The septum is a wall that separates the heart's left and right sides.

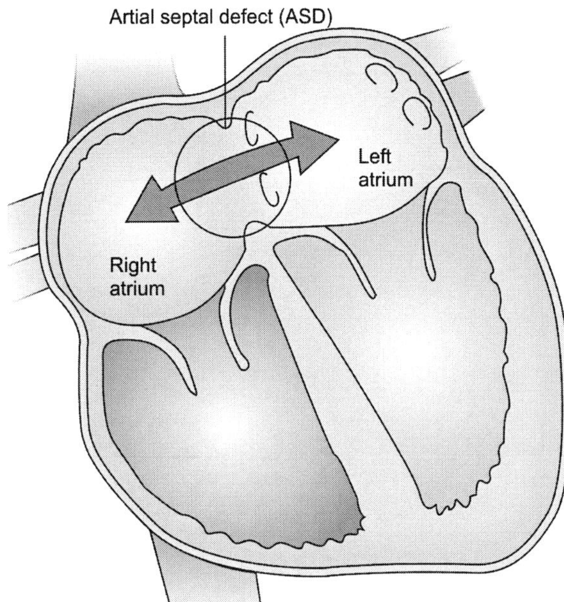

Fig. 19.4: Atrial septal defect (ASD)

Incidence and Types

Atrial septal defect accounts for approximately 5 to 10% of all congenital heart disease. Because it is difficult to differentiate a PFO from an ASD, the exact incidence is difficult to establish.

The three major types of ASDs are:

1. *Ostium secundum:* This defect is in the middle of the atrial septum. It is the most common form of ASD. About 8 out of every 10 babies born with ASDs have secundum defects. At least half of all secundum ASDs close on their own. However, this is less likely if the defect is large.
2. *Ostium primum:* This defect is in the lower part of the atrial septum. It often occurs along with problems in the heart valves that connect the upper and lower heart chambers. Primum defects are not very common, and they do not close on their own.
3. *Sinus venosus:* This defect is in the upper part of the atrial septum, adjacent to superior venacava, and is commonly associated anomalous connection of the right pulmonary vein to the right atrium or right superior venacava. Sinus venosus defects are rare, and they do not close on their own.

Pathophysiology and Altered Hemodynamics

ASDs vary in size. As oxygenated blood in left atrium is under high pressure it is forced through the defect into right atrium. They all allow oxygen-rich blood from the left side of the heart to mix with blood headed to the lungs to become oxygenated. This shunting of blood does not produce cyanosis. This makes for very inefficient function and too much blood going to the right side and then being pumped into the lungs. The right side can become dilated or enlarged. The larger the size of the ASD, the greater the effects on heart and lung function. Extra blood flowing into the right atrium through an ASD can cause the atrium to stretch and enlarge. Over time, this can lead to arrhythmias (irregular heartbeats). Arrhythmia symptoms may include palpitations or a rapid heartbeat.

Diagnosis

Heart sounds, like soft systolic flow murmurs are heard best at the left upper sterna border in ostium secundum ASD. It is preceded by a loud first sound and may radiated to the apex and back. Pulmonary second sound P_2 is widely slit and fixed. In ostium primum ASD, systolic murmur heard best at the lower left sterna border because of mitral regurgitation.

Right atrial and ventricular dilation and increased pulmonary markings are seen in chest X-rays. ECH shows right ventricular hypertrophy and right axis deviation. Associated problems and complications can be detected through Doppler echocardiogram and color flow mapping and cardiac catheterization.

Clinical Features

Many babies who are born with atrial septal defects (ASDs) have no signs or symptoms. When signs and symptoms do occur, heart murmur is the most common. Ostium secundum and sinus venosus ASDs are usually asymptomatic. In case of ostium primum ASD, child may have recurrent chest infections, breathlessness on exertion, bulging of chest, easy fatigability, poor weight gain, cardiac enlargement.

Over time, if a large ASD is not repaired, the extra blood flow to the right side of the heart can damage the heart and lungs and cause heart failure. This does not occur until adulthood. Signs and symptoms of heart failure include:

- Fatigue (tiredness)
- Tiring easily during physical activity
- Shortness of breath
- A buildup of blood and fluid in the lungs
- A buildup of fluid in the feet, ankles, and legs.

Treatment

Child with ASD may not require treatment if he or she has few or no symptoms, or if the defect is small. However, medical management usually is done with digoxin and diuretics. If bacterial endocarditis is there, it is managed with antibiotics and other methods of preventing infection.

- Cardiac catheterization may be recommended in severe cases.
- An umbrella-shaped patch is closed and inserted into the damaged area through a small tube, called a catheter. The umbrella patch is then opened to cover the hole.
- It requires a small incision, avoiding the need for open-heart surgery.

Surgery

- It may be option if child cannot have a cardiac catheterization.
- Surgeons stitch or patch the hole in the wall.
- Child will be connected to a heart-lung machine, which will do the work of the heart during surgery.

Patent Ductus Arteriosus

Patent ductus arteriosus (PDA) is a congenital disorder in the heart wherein a neonate's ductus arteriosus fails to close after birth. The ductus arteriosus (DA) is a normal fetal blood vessel that closes soon after birth. In a PDA, the vessel does not close and connection remains 'patent' (open) resulting in irregular transmission of blood between two of the most important arteries close to the heart, the aorta and the pulmonary artery.

Within minutes or up to a few days (5–7 days) after birth, the DA is supposed to close. This change is normal in newborns. If the closure of the DA does not occur even after two to three weeks of age it is called as PDA (Fig.19.5).

Incidence: PDA is common in neonates with persistent respiratory problems such as hypoxia, and has a high occurrence in premature children. In hypoxic newborns, too little oxygen reaches the lungs to produce sufficient levels of bradykinin and subsequent closing of the DA. Premature children are more likely to be hypoxic and thus have PDA because of their underdeveloped heart and lungs.

Pathophysiology and Altered Hemodynamics

A PDA allows a portion of the oxygenated blood from the left heart to flow back to the lungs by flowing from the aorta (which has higher pressure) to the pulmonary artery. If this shunt is

Contd...

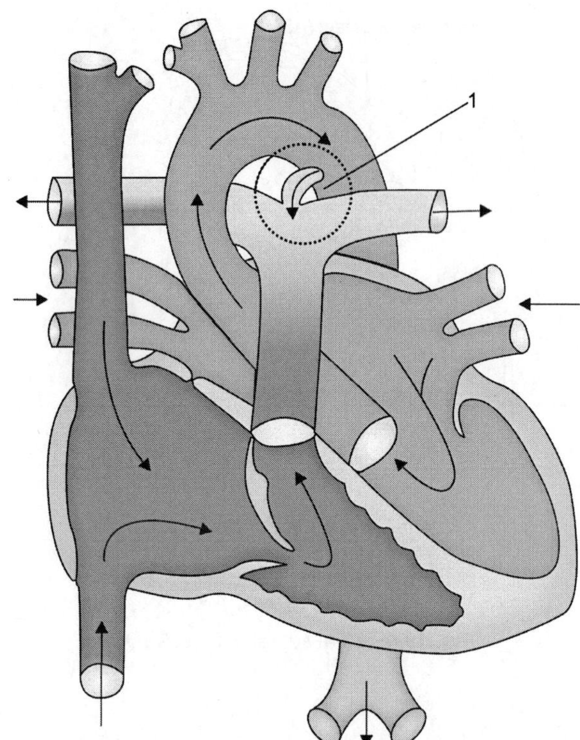

Fig. 19.5: Patent ductus arteriosus (PDA)

Contd...

substantial, the neonate becomes short of breath. The additional blood is re-circulated through the lungs and returned to the left atrium and left ventricle. This causes increased workload on the left side of the heart and increased pulmonary vascular congestion and possibly resistance, and potentially increased right ventricular pressure and hypertrophy. The additional fluid returning to the lungs increases lung pressure to the point that the neonate has greater difficulty inflating the lungs. This uses more calories than normal and often interferes with feeding in infancy. This condition, as a constellation of findings, is called congestive heart failure.

In some cases, such as in transposition of the great vessels (the pulmonary artery and the aorta), a PDA may need to remain open. In this cardiovascular condition, the PDA is the only way that oxygenated blood can mix with deoxygenated blood. In these cases, prostaglandins are used to keep the DA open.

Clinical Features

The symptoms of PDA depend on the size of the DA and how much blood flow it carries. Babies with a large PDA might experience symptoms such as a bounding (strong and forceful) pulses result from runoff of blood from the aorta to the pulmonary artery, fast breathing, poor feeding habits, shortness of breath, sweating while feeding, tiring very easily, poor growth.

Patients may be asymptomatic or show signs of CHF. They are at risk for bacterial endocarditis and pulmonary vascular obstructive disease in later life due to chronic excessive pulmonary blood flow.

Therapeutic Management

The three treatment options for PDA are medication, catheter-based procedures, and surgery. Administration of indomethacin (prostaglandin inhibitor) has proved successful in closing PDA in premature infants and in some newborns. It is usually given orally or intravenously in dose of 0.2 mg/kg of body weight and before the age of ten days. The dose may be repeated up to three times, at an interval of 12 to 24 hours.

Catheter based procedure: A catheter (a thin, flexible tube) is fed through their veins using special X-rays until it reaches the heart. A special plug is then inserted across the PDA to block blood flow to the heart. The plug will remain in position within the ductus. This is called 'transcatheter device closure.' Sometimes it is done on small PDAs to prevent the risk of infective endocarditis, an infection of the lining of the heart, valves, or arteries. The procedure lasts approximately two hours and child will be able to go home the same day.

Surgery

Surgery of PDA is done if the size of the opening is large enough that the lungs could become overloaded with blood, a condition that can lead to an enlarged heart. A PDA also might be closed to reduce the risk of developing a heart infection known as endocarditis, which affects the tissue lining the heart and blood vessels.

Atrioventricular Septal Defect

An atrioventricular septal defect (AVSD) is a birth defect of the heart in which important parts at the center of the heart are not fully formed. There are holes between chambers of the heart, and the valves that control the flow of blood between these chambers may not be formed correctly. This means that blood flows where it normally should not be able to, and extra blood flows to the lungs. This defect is also known as atrioventricular canal (AV canal) defect or endocardial cushion defect.

In AV septal defect, there is a hole in the wall between the right and left atria. There is also a hole in the septum between the right and left ventricles.

In addition, the two atrioventricular valves are not formed correctly. A baby with AV septal defect may have just one larger valve opening in the middle, instead of one on each side of the heart.

Together these problems may create a hole in the center of the baby's heart. As a result, blood does not flow the way it should between the chambers. So the heart has to work harder to pump blood to the lungs and the rest of the body.

This condition is also known as atrioventricular canal defect or endocardial cushion defect.

Clinical Features

Usually these patients have moderate to severe CHF. There is a characteristic murmur. Mild cyanosis is observed, which increases in crying. These children are at high risk for developing pulmonary vascular obstructive disease.

Treatments

All AVSDs, both partial and complete types, usually require surgery. Surgery depends on how sick the child is and the specific structure of the AVSD. If possible, surgery should be done before there is permanent damage to the lungs. As short-term method medication may be used to treat congestive heart failure, but it is only a short-term measure until the infant is strong enough for surgery.

During surgery, any hole in the septa is closed using patches. Sometimes the mitral valve does not close completely, allows blood to flow backwards and make the heart work harder to get enough blood to the rest of the body. This leaky mitral valves need to be repaired or replaced. For a complete AVSD, the common valve is separated into two distinct valves—one on the right side and one on the left. With proper treatment, most babies with AVSD grow up to lead healthy, productive lives.

OBSTRUCTIVE HEART DISEASES

In an obstructive disorder, the blood flow is restricted or completely blocked. This blockage or narrowing can occur in any of the four heart valves or above or below the valve. The blockage (atresia) or narrowing (stenosis) can occur in vessels returning blood to the heart (veins) or in vessels pumping blood out of the heart (arteries).

Unfortunately, even the most impressive structures, such as the heart, can have problems. Valves do not always work the way they should. If a valve is not formed properly from birth **(congenital valve disease)** or if it is damaged at some point after birth from age or disease **(acquired valve disease),** then vital organs, such as the brain and kidneys, may not get the oxygen-rich blood they need to function.

Heart valve disease (sometimes called **valvular heart disease)** can strain the heart, too. But when the valves are defective or do not work the way they should, it can put the heart and other organs at risk. Valve disease can affect one or more of the four valves in the heart (mitral, aortic, tricuspid, and pulmonary). Most often it causes one or both of the following problems:

Regurgitation: The valves tissue flaps, or leaflets, that control the flow and direction of the blood, do not fully close, which causes blood to leak back into the heart.

Stenosis: The leaflets cannot open fully to allow enough blood to flow through.

The heart has to work harder to compensate for the faulty valve, which can weaken the heart and increase the risk of **heart failure** (a condition where the heart does not fill up with enough blood or pump enough blood to supply the body with the oxygen and nutrients that it needs) or sudden cardiac arrest (when the heart stops beating). A heart valve problem can also increase the risk of blood clots, which can cause stroke.

Valve defects

Defective valves may be caused by:

- **Stenosis (narrowing):** The valve is not able to open completely. As a result, the heart has to work harder to pump blood through it.
- **Regurgitation:** The valve does not close correctly and allows blood to leak backward.
- **Atresia:** The valve is missing a hole for the blood to pass through. This is considered a more complex defect.

Pulmonary Stenosis

Pulmonary stenosis accounts for approximately 5 to 8% of all CHD. Pulmonary stenosis is a narrowing at the entrance to the pulmonary artery (pulmonary valve), and the pulmonary blood flow is decreased. The pulmonary valve is within the heart's right ventricle. Because of the narrowing of the valve, the right ventricle needs to work harder to get blood past the blockage and get hypertrophied.

Pulmonary atresia is the extreme form of PS in which the pulmonary valve orifice fails to develop. The valve is completely closed thereby obstructing the outflow of blood from the heart to the lungs. The right ventricle may be hypoplastic.

Pathophysiology and Altered Hemodynamics

The main pathophysiological consequence of PS is RV strain and an increase in RV pressure. The cellular effect on the RV depends on the timing of obstruction and on the size of obstruction. If the obstruction is present in a fetus or neonate, the myocardial response is hyperplasia and an increase in vascularity. There is an increase in myocyte size (hypertrophy) without an increase in capillary network when the obstruction develops within mature myocardium.

Generally children with mild to moderate obstruction are hemodynamically well tolerated and are not associated with cyanosis or cardiac symptoms. In the severe to critical form of PS, right ventricular pressure increases and causes thickening of right ventricular wall. Right atrial pressure increases if the RV hypertrophy is severe, resulting to right to left shunting through foramen of ovale. Cyanosis becomes apparent when there is a right-to-left shunt at the atrial level via an atrial septal defect and exaggerated by limited blood flow to the pulmonary vascular bed. If there is no atrial or ventricular level shunt, sudden death may ensue due to compromised cardiac output.

Clinical Manifestations

The most obvious symptom is blue, or cyanotic skin in a newborn which can be noted shortly after birth or several weeks later as the ductus arteriosus closes. Clinical symptoms such as dyspnea, heart murmur, exercise intolerance, cyanosis, and syncope may occur. In severe PS, the RV will eventually fail as the myocardium becomes unable to support the enhanced work load imposed by the stenosis, and patients develop jugular venous distension, peripheral edema, pleural effusion, ascites, and hepatomegaly. Severe and critical PS may be differentiated clinically by the presence of cyanosis (more pronounced with critical PS) and symptoms of profound heart failure (present with critical PS).

Diagnosis

Cardiac examination: A systolic ejection murmur is heard best at upper sterna border.

Electrocardiogram: The ECG may be normal or show right ventricular hypertrophy with mild to moderate PS. In severe PS, the ECG shows right ventricular hypertrophy and enlargement of right atrium.

Chest radiograph: Chest X-ray shows right ventricular hypertrophy and post-stenotic pulmonary artery dialatation.

Echocardiogram: The structure of the pulmonary valve, the location and severity of the narrowing (stenosis), and the size of the RV and its out flow tract can be visualized.

Other imaging tests: Magnetic resonance imaging and CT scans are sometimes used to confirm the diagnosis of pulmonary valve stenosis.

Cardiac catheterization: During the procedure blood pressure and oxygen measurements are taken in the four chambers of the heart, as well as the pulmonary artery and aorta. Contrast dye is also injected to more clearly visualize the structures inside the heart. This test is generally only done when child will need balloon valvuloplasty to treat pulmonary valve stenosis because that procedure can be done at the same time as cardiac catheterization.

Management

Some cases of pulmonary stenosis are mild and do not require treatment except for routine checkups. However, if case is more serious child will most likely be admitted to the intensive care unit (ICU) or special care nursery once symptoms are noted. Initially, child may be placed on oxygen, and possibly even on a ventilator, to assist his or her breathing. IV medications may be given to help the heart and lungs function more efficiently. An IV medication called prostaglandin E1 is used for treatment of pulmonary atresia, as it stops the ductus arteriosus from closing, allowing mixing of the pulmonary and systemic circulations. But prostaglandin E1 can be dangerous as it can cause apnea. Another example of preliminary treatment is heart catheterization to evaluate the defect or defects of the heart; this procedure is much more invasive.

Surgery

Surgical repair may be needed for child. The procedure aims at relieving the obstruction of blood flow through the pulmonary valve. This procedure requires heart-lung bypass. Postoperative hospital stay averages 5 to 7 days.

Child may need either balloon valvuloplasty or open-heart surgery. The decision to perform a balloon valvuloplasty or open-heart surgery depends on the extent to which the pulmonary valve is obstructed. Pulmonary stenosis is classified as mild, moderate or severe, depending on a measurement of the blood pressure difference between the right ventricle and pulmonary artery.

Ultimately, however, the patient will need to have a series of surgeries to improve the blood flow permanently. The first surgery will likely be performed shortly after birth. A shunt can be created between the aorta and the pulmonary artery to help increase blood flow to the lungs. As the child grows, so does the heart and the shunt may need revised in order to meet the body's requirements.

The type of surgery recommended depends on the size of the right ventricle and the pulmonary artery.

If they are normal in size and the right ventricle is able to pump blood, open heart surgery can be performed to make blood flow through the heart in a normal pattern.

If the right ventricle is small and unable to act as a pump, doctors may perform another type of operation called the Fontan procedure. In this three-stage procedure, the right atrium is disconnected from the pulmonary circulation. The systemic venous return goes directly to the lungs, by-passing the heart.

Another treatment option involves the electrosurgical puncture of the atretic valve using a wire introduced into the patient percutaneously. The puncture is then dilated using a balloon catheter to allow blood flow from the right ventricle into the pulmonary artery.

The outcome varies for every child. If the condition is left uncorrected it may be fatal, but the prognosis has greatly improved over the years for babies with pulmonary atresia. Some factors that affect, how well the child does include how well the heart is beating, the condition of the blood vessels that supply the heart, and how leaky the other heart valves are. Most cases of pulmonary atresia can be helped with surgery. If the patient's right ventricle is exceptionally small, many surgeries will be needed in order to help stimulate normal circulation of blood to the heart.

Aortic Stenosis

Aortic stenosis accounts for approximately 5% of all CHD. It is more common in males than females. The aorta is the large artery that supplies oxygen-rich blood to the body. The aortic valve is within the heart's left ventricle and acts as the entrance to the aorta. Narrowing of the aortic valve, which controls blood flow between left ventricle and aorta, is known as aortic stenosis. Depending on the severity of the stenosis, the symptoms at birth can vary from none to decreased blood flow and decreased oxygenation to the body. As the PDA closes, the symptoms usually become more acute.

Aortic stenosis is three types:

1. The commonest valvular type is the stricture of aortic valve
2. In subvalvular type, the narrowing remains below the aortic valve
3. In supravalvular, the stenosis remains above the aortic valve.

Pathophysiology and Altered Hemodynamics

The human aortic valve normally consists of three leaflets (trileaflets) and has an orifice of 3.0–4.0 square centimeters. In aortic stenosis, the opening of the aortic valve becomes narrowed or constricted (stenotic).

As a consequence of this stenosis, the left ventricle must generate a higher pressure with each contraction to effectively move blood forward into the aorta. Increased pressure in the LV has direct correlation with the degree of obstruction in aortic valve. Initially, the LV generates this increased pressure by thickening its muscular walls (myocardial hypertrophy).

The type of hypertrophy usually seen in aortic stenosis is known as concentric hypertrophy, in which the walls of the LV are (approximately) equally thickened. In the later stages, the left ventricle dilates, the wall thins, and the systolic function deteriorates (resulting in impaired ability to pump blood forward). Heart failure can develop due to this heavy workload. In severe cases, pulmonary edema may occur as a result of increased left ventricular pressure that may cause a backflow of blood into the lungs.

Sometimes, a percutaneous balloon valvuloplasty (opening of a valve) can effectively relieve the valve obstruction. This procedure involves a special catheter (tube) containing a balloon being passed through the aortic valve. The surgeon inflates the balloon to stretch the valve open. The surgical repair aims to relieve the obstruction of blood flow through the aortic valve. This procedure requires heart-lung bypass. Postoperative hospital stay averages 7 to 10 days.

Clinical Manifestation

Less severe forms of the disease may be 'silent'—causing no visible symptoms—until later in life. As the child grows older, increased physical growth requires additional cardiac output. Children may present the following symptoms in severe obstruction.

- Fatigue and exercise intolerance
- Having pain, pressure or tightness in their chest
- Exertional dyspnea
- Fainting or feeling weak or dizzy when active
- Having palpitations

Babies born with severe aortic stenosis may have to work hard to breathe, have poor appetite or trouble feeding, and failure to thrive.

They may also show signs of shock because their heart cannot pump enough blood to the rest of their body. Signs of cardiogenic shock include less frequent urination, cool limbs, increased heart rate, fussiness, poor feeding, rapid breathing, lethargy, mottled skin. They have decreased perfusion and pulmonary congestion.

Diagnosis

Cardiac examination: A harsh systolic murmur, click, or other abnormal sound is almost always heard at the upper right sternal border, radiating to the upper left sternal border and neck. A vibration or movement can be felt when placing a hand over the heart. There may be a faint pulse or changes in the quality of the pulse in the neck.

Electrocardiogram: The ECG may be normal or demonstrate left ventricular hypertrophy.

Chest radiograph: Usually normal heart size is seen. In severe case of stenosis, dilatation of ascending aorta may be seen.

Echocardiogram: Type of stenosis as well as presence of other cardiac defects can be seen. The function of left ventricle and thickness of its wall is also assessed.

Management

Regular checkups by a health provider may be all that is needed if there is no symptoms or only mild symptoms. The health care provider should ask about child's health history, do a physical exam, and perform an echocardiogram.

People with severe aortic stenosis may be told not to play competitive sports, even if they have no symptoms. If symptoms do occur, strenuous activity must often be limited.

Medicines are used to treat symptoms of heart failure or abnormal heart rhythms (most commonly atrial fibrillation). These include diuretics, nitrates, and beta-blockers. High blood pressure should also be treated. If aortic stenosis is severe, this treatment must be done carefully so blood pressure does not drop to dangerously low levels.

Treatment may be done in the *cardiac catheterization lab* using a balloon procedure. A balloon is inserted across the valve. When the balloon is inflated, the valve is stretched open. Then the balloon is removed. This is called balloon valvuloplasty.

Some children need surgery to replace their aortic valve with an artificial valve. In some cases the child's own pulmonary valve can be used to replace the damaged aortic valve.

Aortic Coarctation

Coarctation of the aorta is a narrowing of some portion of the aorta (Fig. 19.6A). This narrowing is usually found just past the arch of the aorta, opposite the area of the PDA. Coarctation of the aorta accounts for approximately 8% of all CHD, it is more commonly found in male and may accompany other congenital defects like VSD, PDA, tubular hypoplasia of the aortic isthmus and bicuspid aortic valve.

There is a common association between CoA and Turner syndrome.

Altered Hemodynamics

The aorta is the large artery that supplies blood to the whole body. The left ventricle pumps blood through the aortic valve into the aorta and eventually to the body. The narrow aortic lumen may exist as preductal or postductal obstruction depending upon the position of the obstruction in relation to the ductus arteriosus. The narrowing of the aortic lumen can vary in severity from a mild constriction to total occlusion. This impedes circulation to the lower parts of the body, creating increased pressure proximal to the obstruction. As a result pressure in the upper part of the body is increased and pressure in the lower part is decreased. Collateral vessels grow and by pass the coarctation to perfuse the lower body parts. The condition produces an obstruction to the blood flow through the aorta causing increased pressure and workload of the left ventricle.

Clinical Manifestation

The clinical features depend upon the type of obstruction and usually become evident after the closure of PDA. The presenting features of neonates are severe CCF, poor perfusion, tachypnea, acidosis and absence of femoral pulse. The older children's growth and development may be normal without symptoms, but overgrowth of upper extremities and hypertension, absence of femoral pulse may be suggestive of CoA. The symptoms may include:

- Increased BP in the upper part of the body, resulting in headache, dizziness, fainting, epistaxis and later CVA, encephalopathy.
- Child may occasionally complaints of weakness and pain in legs after exercise. The femoral and pedal pulse may be absent or diminished, and legs may be cooler than arms.
- Other manifestations are fatigue, cramps, exertional dyspnea, feeding problem, poor weight gain, irritability and tachycardia.

Diagnosis

Diagnosis is confirmed by cardiac examination, chest X-ray, barium swallow, electrocardiogram, M mode echocardiography, cardiac catheterization and angiocardiography. Specific ' E' sign in barium swallow is very suggestive of CoA. The first arch of the 'E' is formed due to dilatation of aorta before the coarctation, the second arch due to poststenotic dilatation, and middle notch due to the coarctation.

Management

Medical management of CoA is done with PGE1 infusion, antibiotics and prevention and treatment of complications.

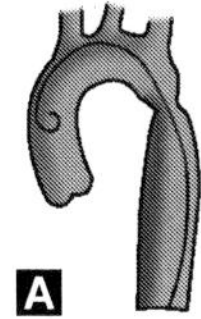

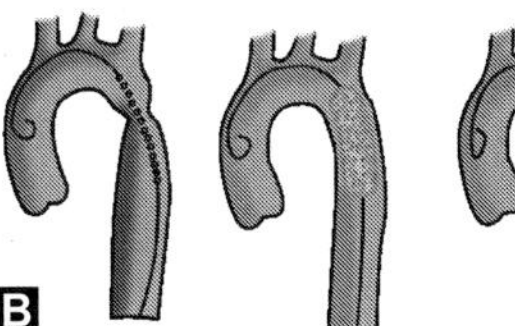

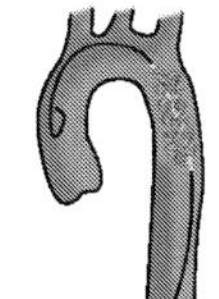

Figs 19.6A and B: A. Coarctation of the aorta; **B.** Correction of coarctation of the aorta

Surgical correction of CoA (Fig. 19.6B)

- Individualized to anatomy of CoA
- Plan to include treatment of any additional cardiac defects.

Child, Adolescent: Repair is done at 2 to 3 years of age upon diagnosis.

Surgery: Four common types of repair—regardless of technique, usually performed via a left thoracotomy incision. End-to-end anastomosis was done in 1954 by Crawford and Nylin.

Excision of CoA area, circumferential anastomosis is completed with interrupted sutures anteriorly.

NURSING CARE OF THE FAMILY AND CHILD WITH CONGENITAL CARDIAC DISEASES

The diagnosis of a chronic condition in any family member causes much distress. When an infant is born with a heart defect, the parents may grieve over the loss of the healthy newborn they had anticipated and experience shock, denial, guilt, anger, despair or confusion on learning that their infant has a cardiac defect. Some parents may be unable at first to respond to their newborn. Even greater stress may occur if the condition is one that requires surgical intervention. The nurse should become familiar with parents reaction and nursing intervention require to:

Help family to adjust to the disorder: A birth of a baby with severe cardiac anomaly is a shock to the family, parents always suffer with high anxiety and fear that their child will not survive. Here role of nurse is to support the family in their stress, assessing their level of understanding and to provide information as needed (thorough but simple in language). She also helps the other members of the health team to understand the parents' reaction.

The nurse needs to support the family in their great pain and emotional investment. She can foster parent-infant attachment and encourage parents to hold, touch and look at their child.

Teach the parent to care the child which can minimize their anxiety and fear.

Introduce parents to other families with similarly affected children. It can help them to adjust to their daily stress.

Counseling of family about the disorder and its care: Before describing the defect a review of the basic structure and function of heart is important. Picture, diagram, models are to be used for better understanding of CHD.

Increasingly, families are collecting information from different sources. It is important to inform the families about authentic internet sites and medical literature. Parents must know that information from general sources or other families might not be applicable to their own situation.

Prepare Child and Family for Surgery

Some heart defects need repair soon after birth. For others, it is better to wait months or years. Certain heart defects may not need to be repaired. The surgery is needed for the child's well-being.

In general, symptoms that indicate that surgery is needed are blue or gray skin, lips, and nail beds (cyanosis). These symptoms mean there is not enough oxygen in the blood (hypoxia). Difficulty breathing because the lungs are 'wet,' congested, or filled with fluid (heart failure). Child suffers with problems of heart rate or heart rhythm (arrhythmias). Child shows feeding or sleeping problem and lack of growth and development.

The three most common clinical presentations are:

1. A Murmur
2. Cyanosis
3. Respiratory difficulty.

Nursing Assessment

Cardiovascular assessment is an important nursing skill in the assessment and management of acutely ill children and children with chronic conditions. Assessment for cardiac problems is described in Table 19.1.

Look for signs of cardiovascular problems:

- Inspection
- Palpation
- Percussion
- Auscultation.

The general objectives of nursing care for the child with CHD include prevention of physical and emotional fatigue, provision of adequate fluid and nutrition, prevention of infection and care and support to the parents and child to cope with the problems that precipitates before and after surgery.

Nursing diagnosis: Impaired gas exchange related to disturbed pulmonary blood flow or pulmonary hypertension.

Expected outcome: Patient maintains optimal gas exchange as evidenced by normal ABGs and alert responsive mental condition or no further reduction in mental status.

Nursing Intervention

Patient is to be placed in *semi-upright position which facilitates breathing*. Position with proper body alignment for optimal respiratory functioning (if tolerated, head of bed at 45 degrees). *This promotes lung expansion and improves air exchange.*

Routinely check the patient's position so he or she does not slide down in bed. This would cause the

Table 19.1: Assessment of ill children with cardiac problems

Taking history	*Physical examination*	*Review of vital signs*
• Chief complaint • Prenatal, perinatal and family history • Feeding patterns • Fatigue • Edema • Dyspnea/tachypnea • Cyanosis • Growth and development • Medications • Psychosocial history, sleep pattern	• General appearance • Size for age, level of consciousness and activity level, anthropometric measurements • Physical characteristics suggesting chromosomal defects • Skin and mucous membrane - • Note pallor, cyanosis, mottling or edema • Temperature of extremities and diaphoresis • Clubbing • Chest wall size and shape	• Assessing vital signs, skin color, oxygen saturation • Upper extremities are the preferred site of BP taking • Document location and be consistent • Four extremity blood pressure should be obtained during initial assessment • Assessing heart rate • Listen with stethoscope to apical pulse for 1 minute • Listen for fast rates, slow rates or an irregular rhythm • Palpate pulse for 1 minute • Brachial pulse for infants • Radial pulse for children, capillary refill

abdomen to compress the diaphragm, which would cause respiratory embarrassment.

- Patient may need help if he/she is unable to effectively clear the airway. Periodic oral and nasal secretions is to be suctioned if needed
- Monitor oxygen saturation and administer oxygen if required
- Prevention of aspiration, with continuous monitoring of respiratory pattern
- Administer drugs like diuretic and bronchodialators
- Analysis of blood gas analysis.

Nursing diagnosis: Low cardiac output related to reduced myocardial functions.

Expected outcome: Cardiac output and activity tolerance of child is improved.

Nursing Intervention

- Bed rest, minimum exercise (care in the bed, indoor play, and other activities of daily living)
- Administer prescribed drugs like digoxin, diuretics, antihypertensives which improve cardiac output
- Organize medication and nursing schedule to provide periods of uninterrupted sleep
- Monitor child's condition (heart sound, vital signs).

Nursing diagnosis: Activity intolerance related to hypoxia.

Expected outcome: The child is able to do age appropriate activity.

Nursing Intervention

- Oxygen therapy and continuous monitoring of oxygen saturation by pulse oximetry. Pulse oximetry is a useful tool to detect changes in oxygenation. O_2 saturation should be maintained at 90% or greater. A higher liter flow of oxygen is generally required for activity versus rest (e.g. 2 L at rest, and 4 L with activity).
- Uninterrupted period of rest and sleep
- Advice parents to do activities of daily living for the child so that child's energy can be conserved
- Providing timely feeding, changing diaper and tactile stimulation prevents cry of the child and saves energy expenditure. Prevent excessive crying, provide diversional activities, prevent constipation.

Nursing diagnosis: Altered nutrition, less than body requirements related to excessive energy demands needed by increased cardiac workload.

Expected Outcome: Normal nutritional status of child.

Nursing Intervention

- Feed in semi-erect position
- Nasogastric feeding may be started if the child is unable to take oral feeds or get cyanosed while feeding
- Provide small frequent feedings
- Provide foods with high nutritional value (24 kcal/oz formula)
- Determine child's likes and dislikes
- Monitor input and output
- *Daily weight monitoring:* Maintaining a healthy weight is important for cardiac health. Restricting intake of salt can also help lessen fluid retention and improve symptoms related to heart valve disease.
- Assess the child for developmental milestones.
- *Nursing diagnosis:* Increased potential for infection related to poor nutritional status.
- *Expected outcome:* No infection.

Nursing Intervention

- Prevent exposure to communicable diseases. Early detection and treatment of upper respiratory and GI infection.
- Immunizations should be up-to-date
- Handwashing should be observed. Maintaining general cleanliness and hygienic measure are important.
- Be certain that the child receives prophylactic medication for infective endocarditis.

Congestive Cardiac Failure (CCF)

Every cardiac patient has a potential for developing CCF. Congestive cardiac failure (CCF) by itself is not a diagnosis. It is a clinical syndrome caused by different anatomical and or pathological conditions, which is the primary diagnosis.

CCF is a term defined as 'inability of the heart to pump enough blood out to the rest of the body, at rest or during stress, necessary for the metabolic needs of the body (systolic failure) and inability to receive blood into the ventricular cavities at low pressure during diastole (diastolic pressure)'.

Etiology

The etiology of pediatric heart failure may be cardiac or noncardiac and can occur at any age. The predominant etiology during infancy is congenital heart disease. VSD is the commonest defect presenting with heart failure. Myocardial disease especially myocarditis is commonest cause HF in children under 5 years. Rheumatic fever and rheumatic heart disease continue to be an important cause of suffering and HF among children above 5 years. Among noncardiac disease, severe anemia can be a condition to cardiac decompensation at any age.

In children, cardiac failure is most often caused by congenital heart disease (left to right shunts) and cardiomyopathy.

Altered Hemodynamics

Heart failure is the clinical condition in which the heart fails to meet the metabolic and circulatory demands of the body and can result from worsening systolic and/or diastolic dysfunction. In systolic dysfunction, the stroke volume decreases, thereby reducing cardiac output. Subsequently, the heart responds with 3 compensatory mechanisms: (i) increasing left ventricular volume and elasticity (ii) increasing contractile state of activation of circulating catecholamines, or (iii) increasing filling or preload. Each compensatory mechanisms is limited, so in an untreated patient, the heart fails, leading to HF.

In diastolic dysfunction, stroke volume is decreased from decreased ventricular filling. To compensate, left ventricular end-diastolic pressure is increased. Diastolic dysfunction may be caused by conditions such as hypertension (causing ventricular hypertrophy).

Particularly in children, one of many congenital abnormalities may lead to dysfunction of the heart, causing increased compensatory mechanisms and the HF. The mechanism for HF include volume overloading (from right to left sided shunting, for example), valvular incompetence, increased overload (such as valvular stenosis or coarctation), and others.

Heart failure is often separated into two categories; right sided and left sided failure. **In right sided failure**, the right ventricle is unable to pump blood effectively into the pulmonary artery resulting in increased pressure in the right atrium and systemic venous circulation. Systemic venous hypertension causes Hepatosplenomegaly and occasionally edema.

In left sided failure, the left ventricle is unable to pump blood into the systemic circulation resulting in increased pressure in the left atrium and pulmonary veins. The lungs become congested with blood, causing elevated pulmonary pressure and pulmonary edema.

Clinical Features

The child with CCF may become suddenly dyspneic, cyanotic. A young child may develop abdominal pain, fever, anorexia, dyspnea, cough suddenly. Dyspnea, orthopnea or paroxysmal nocturnal dyspnea can be reported by parent. Sometimes a mother may complaint of palpitation, tachycardia and profuse sweating, pallor or peripheral cyanosis and cold extremities of child.

Symptoms are different for children of different age, in babies regardless of the cause of CCF the end result of significant heart failure is poor growth. Slow weight gain is related to two factors. Because of easy fatigability baby takes small feed and there is an excessive loss of calories from increased work of breathing associated with CCF. In addition, as the lungs fill with fluid, it becomes more difficult for babies to breathe and they will use more of the muscles of their chest and belly to compensate. The baby breathes too fast during feeding and become very sweaty as of the extra work needed to eat.

Uncommonly, there may be an unusual weight gain due to collection of water, manifesting as facial puffiness or as rarely as edema on the feet. The baby may be brought with the complaints of persistent hoarse crying, breathes too fast with wheezing and excessive perspiration, restlessness.

Diagnosis

Physical examination: A child with CCF may present tachycardia, tachypnea, Gallop rhythm, dyspnea, decreased peripheral pulse and mottling of the extremities, delayed capillary refill, failure to thrive, decreased activity tolerance, sweating, etc. (Table 19.2).

Chest X-ray: Very commonly X-ray shows cardiomegaly. The heart dialates or hypertrophy occurs both in presence of volume and pressure overload, cardiomyopathy or dysrhythmias. It may gives clues to certain structural heart diseases, and also to right versus left sided heart involvement. Pulmonary markings are often increased, showing pulmonary congestion.

ECG: Usually abnormal, and although not useful in assessing HF, may give diagnostic clues for the underlying pathology of heart failure.

Urine test: In chronic HF, proteinuria and high specific gravity of urine are common.

Blood test: As renal function decreased due to decreased perfusion in CCF, an increase in blood urea nitrogen and creatinine levels may be present. CBC, differential may give clues to anemia and infection causing or complicating HF. Atrial blood gas analysis is important.

Echocardiogram: This test is valuable for evaluating cardiac function and ruling out structural heart disease.

Other tests: Thyroid, renal and hepatic function tests are also valuable.

Table 19.2: Signs of CCF in children

Left sided failure	*Right sided failure*
Tachypnea	Hepatomegaly
Tachycardia	Facial edema
Cough	Jugular vein engorgement
Wheezing	Edema on feet
Rales	

Abbreviation: CCF = Congestive cardiac failure

Therapeutic and Nursing Management of CCF

The October 2007 cardiovascular medicines section of the WHO Essential Medicines List for children (EMLc) contains digoxin, frusemide, spironolactone and, on the complementary list, dopamine. The goals of management are to:

- Reducing cardiac work
- Augmenting myocardial contractility
- Remove accumulated fluid and sodium
- Improve tissue oxygenation and decreased oxygen consumption.

Reducing cardiac work: The workload on the heart is reduced when metabolic needs are kept to a minimum. This is accomplished by limiting physical activities (bed rest) preserving body temperature, treating any infection, reducing the effort of breathing (semi Fowler's position) and using medication to sedate an irritable child.

Supplemental cool humidified oxygen is usually provided to increase the amount of oxygen during inspiration.

Baby with CCF is kept in bed rest with minimal handling. The propped up position with an incline of about 30 degree is maintained. It may help the work of breathing by pooling the edema fluid in the dependent areas and to reduce the collection of fluid in lungs. Administration of humidified oxygen (40–50% concentration) improves impaired oxygenation secondary to pulmonary congestion, thus reducing the work of heart by reducing requirements of cardiac output.

Administration of Morphine sulfate (0.05 mg/kg SC) or other sedative (Diazepam) may be needed if the child is restless or dyspneic. These drugs reduce anxiety and lower the catecholamine secretion, thus reducing physical activity, the respiratory rate and the heart rate. The workload of heart comes down as the oxygen demand of the body tissues goes down. The sedative also helps in keeping the child in bed.

Management of fever, anemia and infection is necessary to reduce the workload of heart. At a temperature of 36 to 37 °C, the overall circulatory and metabolic needs are minimal, thus reducing work of heart. Anemia causes tachycardia and hyperkinetic circulatory state to meet up oxygen demand of the body. Correction of anemia results in decreased cardiac work. If transfusion is indicated, 3 to 5 mL packed red cells/kg body weight can be given every 12 hours. Worsening of CCF by transfusion can be prevented, the patient can be given frusemide.

CCF can be managed by use of vasodialators. It reduces the arteriolar and venous vasoconstriction, reduce the work of heart. The use of ACE inhibitors is now well-established in infants and children (captopril dose is 1 mg/kg 8 hourly and can be given increased up to 6 mg/kg/day). ACE inhibitors suppress rennin angiotensin/aldosterone system, thus reducing vasoconstriction as well as sodium and water retention. They prevent potassium loss and hence reduce arrhythmias. These drugs suppress catecholamines and thus its ill effect on myocardium as well as arrhythmias.

Augmenting myocardial contractility: Iontropic drugs improve cardiac output. In infants and children digitalis glycosides [digoxin (lanoxin)] is used which decreases heart rate and increases myocardial contractility. It has rapid onset of action and also eliminated quickly.

Besides digitalis, catecholamine ionotropic agents like dopamine has been found to be useful. In a patient with CCF if the blood pressure is low, dopamine may be used. At a dose of less than 5 µg/kg/min of Dopamine causes peripheral vasodilation, increases myocardial contractility and renal blood flow resulting in natriuresis (Table 19.3).

Remove accumulated fluid and sodium: Treatment consists of diuretics, possible fluid restriction and possible sodium restriction. Diuretic is used to eliminate excess water and salt to prevent re-accumulation. It reduces total body sodium, thus reducing the blood pressure and peripheral vascular resistance. The potent oral diuretics frusemide is administered which starts its action within 20 minutes. Frusemide interferes with the sodium reabsorption mechanism in descending limb of loop of Henle. Patient on frusemide should be given potassium supplement.

Studies suggest that it is preferable to combine frusemide with potassium sparing diuretic. The combination is more useful in preventing potassium and magnesium loss, thus reducing arrhythmias as against the combination of frusemide and potassium supplement.

ACE inhibitor I drug can be combined with frusemide, if indicated. The patient on ACE I should neither be given potassium supplements or potassium

Table 19.3: Rational for use of digoxin in heart failure
• Inotropic effects
• Slowed heart rate, improving balance of oxygen supply and demand
• Inhibition of sympathetic nervous system
• Inhibition of renin release

sparing diuretics like triamterene, amiloride or aldactone even in combination with frusemide.

Nursing Diagnoses

- Impaired gas exchange related to altered pulmonary blood flow or oxygen deprivation
- Activity intolerance related to decreased cardiac output due to structural defect and myocardial dysfunction
- *Altered nutrition:* Less than body requirements related to the excessive energy demands required by increased cardiac workload
- Fluid volume excess related to fluid accumulation (edema)
- Increased potential for respiratory infection secondary to pulmonary vasculature overloading, and other infection related to poor nutritional status
- Anxiety related to diagnostic procedures and hospitalization
- Developmental delay related to decreased energy, inadequate nutrition, physical limitations and social isolation
- Alteration in parenting related to parental perception of the child as vulnerable.

Nursing Intervention and Outcome

Impaired gas exchange related to altered pulmonary blood flow or oxygen deprivation.

Goal of nursing action: The patient will exhibit improved respiratory function.

Nursing intervention includes placing the child in inclined posture of 30 to 45 degree. Tilt mattress support of incubator, place older infant in sent (Fowler's position). Avoid any constricting clothing or restraints around abdomen and chest. Administer humidified O_2 as prescribed.

Expected Outcome:

Respirations remain with normal limits; color is good and child rest quietly.

Activity intolerance related to decreased cardiac output due to structural defect and myocardial dysfunction (Table 19.4).

Goal of nursing action: The patient will exhibit improved cardiac output.

Nursing intervention includes administration of digoxin (lanoxin) at regular interval (usually every 12 hours). Nursing established precaution to prevent toxicity. Often an ECG rhythm strip is taken to assess cardiac status before administration. Ensure adequate intake of K. Monitor serum potassium levels (decrease enhances digoxin toxicity). Administer medications to decrease over load as ordered. Check blood pressure. Observe for signs of hypotension. Monitor electrolyte levels.

Table 19.4: Symptoms of CCF

Criteria for impaired myocardial function	*Criteria for pulmonary congestion*	*Criteria for systemic venous congestion*
• Tachycardia • Decreased urine output • Weakness • Anorexia • Cool extremities • Decreased blood pressure • Sweating • Fatigue • Restlessness • Pale • Weak peripheral pulses • Cardiomegaly	• Tachycardia • Retraction (infants) • Exercise intolerance • Cough • Wheezing • Dyspnea • Flaring nares • Orthopnea • Cyanosis • Grunting	• Weight gain • Peripheral edema • Neck vein dysfunction • Hepatomegaly • Ascitis

Expected outcome:

Heartbeat is strong, regular and within normal limits for age. Peripheral perfusion is adequate.

Goal (2): The patient will experience reduction of anxiety.

Nursing intervention:

Employ flexible feeding schedule. Handle child gently. Hold and comfort the infant. Employ comfort measures found effective in individual cases. Encourage family to provide comfort.

Expected outcome:

Infant rests quietly and breath easily.

Altered nutrition: Less than body requirements related to the excessive energy demands required by increased cardiac workload.

Goal of nursing action: The patient will able to conserve energy and increase total intake.

Nursing Intervention:

- A child with CCF needs small frequent feeds, as he/she has problem in sucking and swallowing and breathing simultaneously.

- Anticipate the child's hunger and give feed before energy is spent in crying.
- Feed small volumes or frequent intervals using the nipple soft and free flowing, to ensureless energy expenditure in sucking. Implement gavage feeding if infant becomes fatigues before taking an adequate amount.
- The food preference of the older child is to be considered and provide food according to his likes and dislikes.

Expected outcome: Increased appetite and maintain nutritional status.

Fluid volume excess related to fluid accumulation (edema).

Goal: The patient will exhibit no evidence of fluid excess.

Nursing Intervention

Administer diuretics as prescribed, maintain fluid restriction if ordered, provide skin care for children with edema, change position frequently, use resilient mattress or mattress cover.

Expected outcome: Infant exhibits evidence of fluid loss, frequent urination, and weight loss.

Increased potential for respiratory infection secondary to pulmonary vasculature overloading, and other infection related to poor nutritional status.

Goal of Nursing Intervention

To protect the child from infection.

Nursing intervention

- It is safe to keep the child away from any source of infection. Follow aseptic technique in caring this child.
- Maintain neutral thermal environment. Place newborn in an incubator or under warmer. Keep infant warm and treat fever promptly.
- Provide skin care for children with edema. Change position frequently. Use resilient mattress or mattress cover.
- Prophylactic antibiotic may be administered, if prescribed.

Expected outcome: Free from infection.

Anxiety related to diagnostic procedures and hospitalization.

Goal of nursing action: To allay anxiety.

Nursing Intervention

- To meet up queries of parents and family
- To orient about the hospital set up, functioning protocol
- To introduce with other parents whose child has gone under same procedure.

Expected outcome: Less anxiety and better participation in the procedure.

Developmental delay related to decreased energy, inadequate nutrition, physical limitations and social isolation.

Goal of nursing action: To promote normal growth and development.

Nursing intervention

- Monitoring growth and development
- Maintenance of nutrition and hydration of patient
- Taking care of the co-morbid conditions.

Expected outcome: The child is progressing to his/her normal level of growth and development.

The goals of treatment are to:

- *Improve cardiac function:* Through administration of digitalis glycosides [digoxin (lanoxin)].
- *Remove accumulated fluid and sodium:* Treatment consists of diuretics, possible fluid restriction and possible sodium restriction. Diuretics to eliminate excess water and salt; and thus to prevent re-accumulation of fluid.
- *Decrease cardiac demands:* The workload on the heart is reduced when metabolic needs are kept to a minimum. This is accomplished by limiting physical activities (bed rest) preserving body temperature, treating any infection, reducing the effort of breathing (semi Fowler's position) and using medication to sedate an irritable child.
- *Improve tissue oxygenation and decreased oxygen consumption:* Supplemental cool humidified oxygen is usually provided to increase the amount of oxygen during inspiration.

ACQUIRED HEART DISEASES

Rheumatic Fever (RF)

Rheumatic fever causes chronic progressive damage to the heart and its valves and is the most common cause of pediatric heart disease in the world. Until 1960, it was a leading cause of death in children and a common cause of structural heart disease. The disease has been known for many centuries. Dramatic declines in the incidence of rheumatic fever are thought to be largely due to antibiotic treatment of streptococcal infection in the late 1940.

Rheumatic fever (RF) is an illness which arises as a complication of untreated or inadequately treated strep throat infection. Rheumatic fever can seriously damage the valves of the heart.

Throat infection with a member of the Group A streptococcus (strep) bacteria is a common problem among school-aged children. It is easily treated with a ten-day course of antibiotics by mouth. However, when such a throat infection occurs without symptoms, or when a course of medication is not taken for the full ten days, there is a 3% chance of that person developing rheumatic fever. Other types of strep infections (such as of the skin) do not put the patient at risk for RF.

Children between the ages of five and fifteen are most susceptible to strep throat, and therefore most susceptible to rheumatic fever. Other risk factors include poverty, overcrowding, and lack of access to good medical care. Just as strep throat occurs most frequently in fall, winter, and early spring, so does rheumatic fever.

Etiology and Incidences

Two different theories exist as to how a bacterial throat infection can develop into the disease called rheumatic fever. One theory, less supported by research evidence, suggests that the bacteria produce some kind of toxin. This toxin is sent into circulation throughout the bloodstream, thus affecting other systems of the body.

Research seems to point to a different theory, however. This theory suggests that the disease is caused by the body's immune system acting inappropriately. It is interesting to note that members of certain families seem to have a greater tendency to develop rheumatic fever than do others. This could be related to the above theory, in that these families may have cell antigens which more closely resemble streptococcal antigens than do members of other families.

RF is most often seen in susceptible children between the ages of 5 and 15 years; and however is still the most common cause of heart disease in children in many developing countries.

Pathophysiology

The body produces antibodies, which are specifically designed to recognize and destroy invading agents; in this case, streptococcal bacteria. The antibodies are able to recognize the bacteria because the bacteria contain special markers called antigens. Group A beta hemolytic streptococci located in pharyngeal area triggers an abnormal humoral and cell mediated immunologic response in children who have RF. Due to a resemblance between Group A streptococcus bacteria's antigens and antigens present on the body's own cells, the antibodies mistakenly attack the body itself. The strep bacterium contains a protein similar to one found in certain tissues of the body. Therefore, immune system cells that would normally target the bacterium may treat the body's own tissues as if they were

Contd...

Contd...

infectious agents, particularly tissues of the heart, joints, skin and central nervous system. This immune system reaction results in inflammation. Inflammation caused by rheumatic fever may last for a few weeks (self-limiting) to several months. In some cases, the inflammation may cause long-term complications like permanent damage to cardiac valve tissue.

Clinical Manifestations

In addition to fever, in about 75% of all cases of RF one of the first symptoms is arthritis. The joints (especially those of the ankles, knees, elbows, and wrists) become red, hot, swollen, shiny, and extraordinarily painful. Unlike many other forms of arthritis, the arthritis may not occur symmetrically. The arthritis of RF rarely strikes the fingers, toes, or spine. The joints become so tender that even the touch of bedsheet or clothing is terribly painful.

A peculiar type of involuntary movement, coupled with emotional instability, occurs in about 10% of all RF patients. The patient begins experiencing a change in coordination, often first noted by changes in handwriting. The arms or legs may flail or jerk uncontrollably. The patient seems to develop a low threshold for anger and sadness. This feature of RF is called Sydenham's chorea or St. Vitus' Dance.

A number of skin changes are common to RF. A rash called erythema marginatum develops (especially in those patients who will develop heart problems from their illness), composed of pink splotches, which may eventually spread into each other. It does not itch. Bumps the size of peas may occur under the skin. These are called subcutaneous nodules; they are hard to the touch, but not painful. These nodules most commonly occur over the knee and elbow joint, as well as over the spine.

Diagnosis

Jones Criteria for Diagnosis of Rheumatic Fever

In 1944, the 'Jones criteria' provided guidelines for the diagnosis of rheumatic fever. The guidelines, which have been revised and modified, are still used today (Table 19.5). In addition to previous infection with streptococcus (positive throat culture, and rising ASO titer), the diagnosis of rheumatic fever requires the presence of 2 major Jones criteria or 1 major plus 2 minor Jones criteria.

Tests are also performed to provide evidence of recent infection with group A streptococcal bacteria. A swab of the throat can be taken, and smeared on a substance in a petridish, to see if bacteria will multiply

Table 19.5: Jones criteria for diagnosis of rheumatic fever	
Major Jones criteria	*Minor Jones criteria*
• Carditis • Polyarthritis (arthritis in two or more joints) • Chorea • Erythema marginatum • Subcutaneous nodules	• Arthralgia—joint pain without swelling • Fever of 101–102 °F • Previous rheumatic fever or rheumatic heart disease • Laboratory findings including elevated erythrocyte sedimentation rate, elevated C-reactive protein, elevated white blood cell count • Prolonged PR interval on an ECG

and grow over 24–72 hours. These bacteria can then be specially processed, and examined under a microscope, to identify streptococcal bacteria. Other tests can be performed to see if the patient is producing specific antibodies; that are only made in response to a recent strep infection.

- Listening to the heart for abnormal rhythms, murmurs or muffled sounds that may indicate inflammation of the heart.
- Conducting a series of simple movement tests to detect-indirect evidence of inflammation of the central nervous system.

Tests for Strep Infection

If your child was already diagnosed with a strep infection, your doctor may not order any additional tests for the bacterium. If your doctor orders a test, it will most likely be a blood test that can detect antibodies to strep bacteria circulating in the blood. The actual bacteria may no longer be detected in your child's throat tissues or blood.

Electrocardiogram (ECG or EKG)

An electrocardiogram—also called an ECG or EKG—records electrical signals as they travel through your child's heart. Your doctor can look for patterns among these signals that indicate inflammation of the heart or poor heart function.

Echocardiography

An echocardiogram uses sound waves to produce live-action images of the heart. In most cases, the diagnosis of mitral stenosis is most easily made by echocardiography, which shows left atrial enlargement, thick and calcified mitral valve with narrow and 'fish-mouth'-shaped orifice and signs of right ventricular failure in advanced disease.

Damage to heart valves is not likely to occur early in the disease, but an echocardiogram can show such problems. This test may need to be repeated in the future in a patient who has had rheumatic fever to reassess the heart valves based on symptoms or changes in the physical exam.

The goals of treatment for rheumatic fever are to destroy any remaining group A streptococcal bacteria, relieve symptoms, control inflammation and prevent recurring episodes of rheumatic fever.

Treatments used for rheumatic fever include:

- *Antibiotics:* Your child's doctor will prescribe penicillin or another antibiotic to eliminate any remaining strep bacteria that may exist in your child's body.
  After your child has completed the full antibiotic treatment, your doctor will begin another course of antibiotics to prevent recurrence of rheumatic fever. This preventive treatment usually continues until your child is at least 21 years old. If an older teenager has had rheumatic fever, he or she may continue taking the antibiotics past age 20 to complete a minimum five-year course of preventive treatment. People who experienced inflammation of the heart when they had rheumatic fever may be advised to take the preventive antibiotic treatment much longer or even for life.
- *Anti-inflammatory treatment:* Your doctor will prescribe a pain reliever, such as aspirin or naproxen (Anaprox, Naprosyn, others), to reduce inflammation, fever and pain. If symptoms are severe or your child is not responding to the anti-inflammatory drugs, your doctor may prescribe a corticosteroid, such as prednisone.
- *Anticonvulsant medications:* If the involuntary movements of Sydenham chorea are severe, your doctor may prescribe an anticonvulsant, such as valproic acid (Depakene) or carbamazepine (Carbatrol, Equetro, others).
  Bed rest is recommended for the child and his or her activities are restricted until inflammation, pain and other symptoms have improved. If inflammation is present in heart tissues, doctor may recommend strict bed rest for a few weeks to a few months, depending on the degree of inflammation.

Treatment

A 10-day course of penicillin by mouth, or a single injection of penicillin G is the first line of treatment for RF. Patients will need to remain on some regular dose of penicillin to prevent recurrence of RF. This can mean a small daily dose of penicillin by mouth, or an injection every three weeks. Some practitioners keep patients on this regimen for five years, or until they reach 18 years of age (whichever comes first).

Arthritis quickly improves when the patient is given a preparation containing aspirin, or some other anti-inflammatory agent (ibuprofen). Mild carditis will also improve with such anti-inflammatory agents, although more severe cases of carditis will require steroid medications. A number of medications are available to treat the involuntary movements of chorea, including diazepam for mild cases, and haloperidol for more severe cases.

Prognosis

The long-term prognosis of an RF patient depends primarily on whether he or she develops carditis. This is the only manifestation of RF which can have permanent effects. Those patients with no or mild carditis have an excellent prognosis. Those with more severe carditis have a risk of heart failure as well as a risk of future heart problems, which may lead to the need for valve replacement surgery.

Prevention

Prevention of the development of RF involves proper diagnosis of initial strep throat infections, and adequate treatment within 10 days with an appropriate antibiotic. Prevention of RF recurrence requires continued antibiotic treatment, perhaps for life. Prevention of complications of already-existing RF heart disease requires that the patient always take a special course of antibiotics when he or she undergoes any kind of procedure (even dental cleanings) that might allow bacteria to gain access to the bloodstream.

Rheumatic Heart Disease

Rheumatic heart disease is permanent damage to the heart caused by the inflammation of rheumatic fever. Problems are most common with the valve between the two left chambers of the heart (mitral valve), but the other valves may be affected. The damage may result in one of the following conditions:

- *Valve stenosis:* This condition is a narrowing of the valve, which results in decreased blood flow. Almost all cases of mitral stenosis are due to disease in the heart secondary to rheumatic fever and the consequent rheumatic heart disease. When the mitral valve area goes below 2 cm^2, the valve causes an impediment to the flow of blood into the left ventricle, creating a pressure gradient across the mitral valve. This gradient may be increased by increases in the heart rate or cardiac output. The constant pressure overload of the left atrium will causes the left atrium to increase in size. As the left atrium increases in size, it becomes more prone to develop atrial fibrillation.

Symptoms of mitral stenosis include heart failure symptoms, such as dyspnea on exertion, orthopnea and paroxysmal nocturn dyspnea, palpitations, chest pain, hemoptysis, thromboembolism.

Treatment

The treatment options for mitral stenosis include medical management, mitral valve replacement by surgery, and percutaneous mitral valvuloplasty by balloon catheter. Medical management includes administration of digitalis and diuretics. Digitalis helps in reducing the heart rate and left ventricular filling.

Valve Regurgitation

This condition is a leak in the valve, which allows blood to flow in the wrong direction. Aortic regurgitation is leakage of the aortic valve each time the left ventricle relaxes.

A leaking (or regurgitant) aortic valve allows blood to flow in two directions. Oxygen-rich blood either flows out through the aorta to the body—as it should—or it flows backwards from the aorta into the left ventricle when the ventricle relaxes.

Aortic insufficiency often has no symptoms for many years. Symptoms may occur slowly or suddenly. Bounding pulse, chest pain (pain increases with exercise and goes away with rest), fainting, fatigue, palpitations, shortness of breath with activity or when lying down, swelling of the feet, legs, or abdomen, uneven, rapid, racing, pounding, or fluttering pulse, weakness, more often with activity.

Diagnosis

It may require some tests like pulse oximetry, chest X-ray, echocardiogram, (also called 'echo' or cardiac ultrasound)—ultrasound waves create an image of the heart and can show the size, shape and movement of the heart's valves and chambers as well as the flow of blood through the heart, electrocardiogram (ECG)—a record of the electrical activity of the heart.

Exercise stress test, Cardiac MRI: A three-dimensional image shows the heart's abnormalities, cardiac catheterization—a thin tube is inserted into the heart through a vein and/or artery in either the leg or through the umbilicus ('belly button') if the regurgitation is moderate or severe.

Valvoplasty

Surgery to repair or to replace the aortic valve is often necessary in severe cases. Depending on the age, gender and particular needs of your child, as well as the valve anatomy, surgeons may attempt to repair the valve, or at least improve its function, with a surgery called a valvuloplasty.

Artificial Valves

Another option to treat aortic regurgitation includes the use of mechanical (artificial) valves as replacement valves. If this is the case, your child may need to stay on blood-thinning medicines for the rest of his or her life to lower the risk of developing blood clots.

- *Damage to heart muscle:* The inflammation associated with rheumatic fever can weaken the heart muscle, resulting in poor pumping function.

  Damage to the mitral valve, other heart valves or other heart tissues can cause problems with the heart later in life. Resulting conditions may include:
  - **Atrial fibrillation,** an irregular and chaotic beating of the upper chambers of the heart (atria)
  - **Heart failure,** an inability of the heart to pump enough blood to the body.

Infective Endocarditis

Infective endocarditis (IE) is a microbial infection of the endothelial surface of the heart. It is a life-threatening infection in which the inner lining of the heart, particularly the heart valves, becomes inflamed. The commonest site of infection is generally a diseased valve from where the infection can spread to the mural endocardium or the vascular endothelium. Infective organisms may be other than bacteria, like fungi or rickettsia, etc.

Predisposing Factors

IE predominantly occurs in a diseased heart. In children the common underlying disease could be congenital heart disease like: Ventricular septal defect (VSD), VSD with aortic regurgitation, Fallot's tetralogy. IE occurs over the mitral valve or the aortic valve in rheumatic heart disease. Patients with prosthetic valves or those who have had a recent cardiac surgery. Other infections like boils, tooth abcess, UTI, ear/dental infection.

Pathophysiology

A normal heart has a smooth lining, making it difficult for bacteria to stick to it. However, persons with congenital heart disease may have a roughened area on the heart lining caused by pressure from an abnormal opening or a leaky valve. Damaged or denuded endothelium is a potent inducer or thrombogenesis and provides a nidus to which bacteria can adhere and eventually form an infected vegetation. The infection generally starts at a jet leision, that is, where the high pressure jet in a VSD or aortic stenosis hits endocardium or the endothelium. In children with heart disease, the sheer force associated with an abdominal high-velocity jet stream of blood can damage the endothelium. Thrombogenesis at such a site results in the deposition of sterile clump of platelets, fibrin, and occasionally red blood cells, and the formation of nonbacterial thrombotic endocarditis (NBTE). NBTE also can produce in children with indwelling intravenous catheters positioned in the right side of the heart.

Bacterimia occurs when bacteria enter the bloodstream and lodge inside the heart, where they multiply and cause infection, initiates endocarditis. The commonest organisms are streptococcus viridance, enterococci, Pseudomonas aeroginosa and some gram negative bacteria.

Clinical Features

The symptoms of infective endocarditis can either develop slowly or come on suddenly. These can include feeling generally unwell, tired and inactive; having a fever; and/or: shivering and sweating at night, loss of appetite, weight loss, arthalgia, and diffuse myalgia, rigors.

The clinical findings of IE in children relate to 4 underlying phenomena: bacteremia (or fungemia), valvulitis, immunologic responses, and emboli. Valvulitis may result in changing cardiac auscultatory findings or the development of congestive heart failure. Extracardiac manifestations of IE e.g. petechiae, hemorrhages.

On occasion, the presentation may be fulminant, with rapidly changing symptoms and high, spiking fevers. These children are acutely ill, and some require urgent intervention.

Diagnosis

In addition to a complete medical history and physical examination of your child, diagnostic procedures may include:

Complete blood count (CBC): A measurement of size, number, and maturity of different blood cells in a specific volume of blood.

Blood culture: Blood cultures are indicated for all patients with fever of unexplained origin and a pathological heart murmur, a history of heart disease, or previous endocarditis. Usually, 3 blood cultures are obtained by separate venipunctures (sets of blood cultures have been obtained from separate venipunctures, and ideally spaced over 30 to 60 minutes) on the first day, and if there is no growth by the second day of incubation, 2 more may be obtained. It has been seen that these set of blood culture would detect 95% of cases. The commonest cause for negative blood cultures is previous antibiotic therapy.

Echocardiography: This test is of immense help in identification of culture negative endocarditis. Echocardiography can determine the site of infection and extent of valvular damage, and cardiac function also can be serially monitored. Color Doppler is a sensitive modality for detection of valvular insufficiency. The severity of valvular flow disturbances can be roughly estimated and may influence surgical and medical treatment decisions.

Treatment

Principles of treatment are: (i) identification of the organism; (ii) finding out the antibiotic sensitivity; (iii) using heavy doses of bactericidal antimicrobial agents. Usually, in patients who are not acutely ill and whose blood cultures are still negative, antibiotics may be withheld for ≥48 hours while additional blood cultures are obtained. A prolonged course of therapy (at least 2 weeks and often 4 to 8 weeks) is necessary for several reasons. Organisms are embedded within the fibrin-platelet matrix and exist in very high concentrations with relatively low rates of bacterial metabolism and cell division, which results in decreased susceptibility to β-lactam and other cell wall-active antibiotics.

Prolonged parenteral therapy is the only way to achieve bactericidal serum levels for the time needed to kill all the bacteria present in a vegetation of endocarditis. Treatment generally ranges from 4–8 weeks

S aureus bacteremia may persist for 3 to 5 days with β-lactam antistaphylococcal therapy and for 5 to 10 days with vancomycin therapy. Blood cultures should be repeated to assess the adequacy of treatment and to document the cessation of bacteremia. Additional blood cultures should be performed once or twice in the 8 weeks after completion of antibiotic treatment to ensure cure. Recommendations for antibiotic treatment.

ARRHYTHMIAS

An arrhythmia (also called dysrhythmia) is an abnormal rhythm of the heart. An irregular heartbeat is an arrhythmia. The most common irregularity occurs during breathing. When a child breathes in, the heart rate normally speeds up for a few beats. When the child breathes out, it slows down again. This variation with breathing is called sinus arrhythmia. It is completely normal.

There are many kinds of arrhythmia that affect different chambers of the heart in different ways. Some are harmless, and some are serious.

Arrhythmia is an abnormal heartbeat. Typically this means a child's heart is beating too fast or too slow for the activity they are doing. In some children an abnormal heartbeat causes symptoms. But in many cases, it causes no problem.

The normal heart rate is controlled by sinus node of the heart, known as the 'pacemaker'. It makes the heart beat slower during times of rest or sleep and beat faster with exercise or when you are scared or excited. In an arrhythmia, abnormal electrical signals through the heart muscle may cause the heart to beat too fast, too slow, or in an irregular manner. In any of these situations, the heart may not be able to pump an adequate amount of blood to the body with each beat. Regardless of why the heart is not pumping well, the effects on the body are often the same, and include poor oxygen and blood delivery to all the tissues of the body. Electrical abnormalities of the heart are the underlying cause of an arrhythmia. These abnormalities can lead to a heartbeat that is too fast (tachycardia) or too slow (bradycardia).

There are many causes of arrhythmia in children, affect different chambers of the heart in different ways. Some may be present at birth, and others are acquired, such as after an infection of the heart or heart surgery.

Supraventricular tachycardia (SVT) and long Q-T syndrome (LQTS) are examples of arrhythmias that a child may be born with. SVT is the most common cause of a fast heartbeat and is usually not life threatening. LQTS, however, can be linked with life-threatening arrhythmias triggered by exercise, startle or fright.

After heart surgery, the normal electrical system of the heart may become scarred and not function normally. It may cause very rapid heartbeats or, more commonly, a heartbeat that is too slow for the child's level of activity.

Symptoms

The following are the most common symptoms of arrhythmias (Table 19.6). However, each child may experience symptoms differently. Symptoms may include weakness, fatigue, heart palpitations, low blood pressure, dizziness, fainting, difficulty feeding.

Table 19.6: Brief description of few cardiac conditions	
Atrial arrhythmias	*Ventricular arrhythmias*
Sinus arrhythmia: It is a benign condition in which the heart rate varies with breathing. Sinus arrhythmia is commonly found in children.	**Premature ventricular contractions (PVCs):** A condition in which an electrical signal originates in the ventricles and causes the ventricles to contract before receiving the electrical signal from the atria. PVCs are not uncommon and typically do not cause symptoms or problems. However, if the frequency of the PVCs increases significantly, symptoms such as weakness, fatigue, dizziness, fainting, or palpitations may be experienced.
Sinus tachycardia: A condition in which the heart rate is faster than normal for the child's age because the sinus node is sending out electrical impulses at a rate faster than usual. Most commonly, sinus tachycardia occurs as a normal response of the heart to exercise when the heart rate increases to cope with increased energy requirements. Sinus tachycardia can be completely appropriate and normal, such as when a child is exercising vigorously. However, it may cause symptoms, such as weakness, fatigue, dizziness, or palpitations if the heart rate becomes too fast to pump an adequate supply of blood to the body. Sinus tachycardia is often temporary, occurring when the body is under stress from exercise, strong emotions, fever, or dehydration, to name a few causes. Once the stress is removed, the heart rate will return to its usual rate.	**Ventricular tachycardia (VT):** A life-threatening condition in which an electrical signal is sent from the ventricles at a very fast but often regular rate. If the heart rate is sustained at a high rate for more than 30 seconds, symptoms such as weakness, fatigue, dizziness, fainting, or palpitations may be experienced. A person in VT may require an electric shock or medications to convert the rhythm to back normal sinus rhythm.
	Ventricular fibrillation (VF): A condition in which many electrical signals are sent from the ventricles at a very fast and erratic rate. As a result, the ventricles are unable to fill with blood and pump. This rhythm is life-threatening because there is no pulse and complete loss of consciousness. A person in VF requires prompt defibrillation to restore the normal rhythm and function of the heart. It will result in sudden cardiac death if not treated within seconds.
Premature supraventricular contractions or premature atrial contractions (PAC): A condition in which an atrial pacemaker site above the ventricles sends out an electrical signal early. The ventricles are usually able to respond to this signal, but the result is an irregular heart rhythm. PACs are common and may occur as the result of stimulants such as coffee, tea, alcohol, cigarettes, or medications.	**Wolff-Parkinson-White Syndrome (WPW):** A condition in which an electrical signal may arrive at the ventricle too fast due to an extra conduction pathway or a shortcut from the atria to the ventricles. Tachycardia is a common symptom.
Supraventricular tachycardia (SVT), paroxysmal atrial tachycardia (PAT): A condition in which the heart rate speeds up due to a series of early beats from an atrial or junctional pacemaker site above the ventricles. PAT usually begins and ends rapidly, occurring in repeated periods. This condition can cause symptoms such as weakness, fatigue, dizziness, fainting, or palpitations if the heart rate becomes too fast. This condition is the most common type of abnormal tachycardia in children, and is sometimes referred to as paroxysmal supraventricular tachycardia (PSVT).	
Atrial flutter: A condition in which the electrical signals come from the atria at a fast but regular rate, often causing the ventricles to contract faster and increase the heart rate. When the signals from the atria are coming at a faster rate than the ventricles can respond to, the ECG pattern develops a signature 'sawtooth' pattern, showing two or more flutter waves between each QRS complex. The number of waves between each QRS complex is expressed as a ratio, i.e. a two-to-one atrial flutter means that two waves are occurring between each QRS.	
Atrial fibrillation: A condition in which the electrical signals come from the atria at a very fast and erratic rate. The ventricles contract in an irregular manner because of the erratic signals coming from the atria.	

An atrial arrhythmia is an arrhythmia caused by abnormal function of the sinus node or the atrioventricular node, or by the development of another atrial pacemaker within the atrium that takes over the function of the sinus node. A ventricular arrhythmia is an arrhythmia caused by an abnormal electrical focus within the ventricles, resulting in abnormal conduction of electrical signals within the ventricles. The sinus node and atrioventricular node may function normally.

Arrhythmias can also be classified as slow (bradyarrhythmia) or fast (tachyarrhythmia). 'Brady-' means slow, while 'tachy-' means fast.

Some of the more common arrhythmias are listed in Table 19.6.

Diagnosis

A complete medical history and physical examination:

- *Electrocardiogram (ECG):* An ECG can indicate the presence of arrhythmias or other types of heart conditions. There are several variations of the ECG test, including the following:
  - *Resting ECG:* The child is lying down during this ECG.
  - *Exercise ECG, or stress test:* However, rather than lying down, the child exercises by walking on a treadmill or pedaling a stationary bicycle while the ECG is recorded. This test is done to assess changes in the ECG during stress such as exercise.
  - *Holter monitor.* An ECG recording done over a period of 24 or more hours. Holter monitoring may be done when an arrhythmia is suspected but not seen on a resting ECG. Arrhythmias may be short-lived in nature and not seen during the shorter recording times of the resting ECG.
  - *Continuous recording:* The ECG is recorded continuously during the entire testing period.
  - *Event monitor, or loop recording:* The ECG is recorded only when the person starts the recording when symptoms are felt or when an abnormal rhythm is detected.
- *Electrophysiologic study (EPS):* An invasive test in which a small catheter is inserted in a large blood vessel in the leg or arm and advanced to the heart. This gives the doctor the capability of finding the site of the arrhythmia's origin within the heart tissue, thus determining how to best treat it. Another procedure called an **esophageal electrophysiologic study** may be ordered where a soft, thin flexible plastic tube is inserted in the nostril and placed in the esophagus (which is close to the atria) to provide a more precise ECG recording.
- *Tilt table test:* A test that may be recommended for children who have frequent fainting (syncope) episodes. The test displays how the heart rate and blood pressure respond to a change in position-lying down to standing up. During this test, medication may be given intravenously to help prevent a fainting episode once the cause has been identified by the doctor.

Treatment

- *Lifestyle modifications:* Factors such as stress, caffeine, or alcohol can provoke arrhythmias
  - *Medication:* Many rhythm disorders, especially tachycardias, respond to medications. It will be determined by the type of arrhythmia, other conditions which may be present, and other medications already being used by child. These drugs cannot cure the arrhythmia, but they can improve symptoms. They do this by preventing the episodes from starting, decreasing the heart rate during the episode or shortening how long the episode lasts. Some children must take medication every day; others need medications only when they have a tachycardia episode. Some children need hospital admission to begin the medication as those have serious side effects.

Other Treatments

- *Defibrillators:* Like a pacemaker, a defibrillator can deliver electrical impulses to the heart. A small battery-operated implantable cardioverter defibrillator (ICD) can be implanted near the left collarbone through a surgical procedure. Wires run from the defibrillator to the heart. It senses if the heart has developed a dangerously fast or irregular rhythm and delivers an electrical shock to restore a normal heartbeat.
- *Catheter ablation:* Some tachycardias are life-threatening or significantly interfere with a child's normal activities. These problems may warrant more permanent treatment. 'Ablation' literally means removal or elimination. In the case of catheter ablation, a catheter (a long, thin wire) is guided through a vein in the leg to the heart. Arrhythmias are often caused by microscopic defects in the heart muscle. Once the problem area of the heart is pinpointed, the catheter heats or freezes the muscle cells and destroys them. The small area of the heart is altered, so electrical current would not pass through the tissue.

- *Surgery:* Surgery is usually recommended only if all other options have failed. In this case, the child is put under anesthesia, the chest is opened, and the heart is exposed. Then, the tissue causing the arrhythmia is removed.
- *Artificial pacemaker:* A variety of rhythm disorders can be controlled with an artificial pacemaker. Slow heart rates, such as heart block, are the most common reason to use a pacemaker. An artificial pacemaker is a small device (1 to 2 ounces, 1.5 by 1.5 inches). It is put inside the body and connected to the heart with a thin wire. It works by sending small, painless amounts of electricity to the heart to make it beat.

  Inserting a pacemaker is a simple operation. The wires are attached to the heart, and the pacemaker is placed in the abdomen (belly) or under the skin of the chest wall. Sometimes only one wire is attached to the heart. In other cases two wires are used. Many different models and brands of pacemakers exist. Some can sense when child is active and increase the heart's beating to keep up with exercise.

HYPERTENSION

High blood pressure is a common condition in which the force of the blood against artery walls is high enough that it may eventually cause health problems, such as heart disease. Hypertension is defined as an average systolic and diastolic blood pressure that exceeds or is equal to the 95th percentile for age, sex and height on the basis of measurements obtained on at least three occasions. Prehypertension, which is diagnosed when a child's average BP is above the 90th percentile but below the 95th; prehypertension in adolescent is defined whose BP is greater or equal than 120/80 mmHg. Normal BP is defined as systolic or diastolic pressure that is less than the 90th percentile for age and sex (National High Blood Pressure Education Program Working Group on high Blood Pressure in children and Adolescents [NHBPEP], 2004).

Stage I hypertension is diagnosed if a child's BP is greater than the 95th percentile but less than or equal to the 99th percentile plus 5 mmHg. Stage II hypertension is diagnosed if a child's BP is greater than the 99th percentile plus 5 mmHg.

Hypertension is classified as either primary (essential) hypertension or secondary hypertension. About 90–95% of cases are categorized as primary hypertension, defined as high blood pressure with no obvious underlying cause. The remaining 5–10% of cases are categorized as secondary hypertension, defined as hypertension due to an identifiable cause, such as chronic kidney disease, narrowing of the aorta or kidney arteries, or an endocrine disorder such as excess aldosterone, cortisol, or catecholamines.

Etiology and Incidence

Risk factors for high blood pressure in children include obesity and a family history of high blood pressure. Other risk factors may include medical problems such as sleep apnea or other sleep disorders.

Pathophysiology

So BP is determined by the balance between cardiac output and vascular resistance. A rise in either of these variables, in the absence of a compensatory decrease in the other, increases mean BP, which is the driving pressure. Under normal conditions, the amount of sodium excreted in the urine matches the amount ingested, resulting in near constancy of extracellular volume. Retention of sodium results in increased extracellular volume, which is associated with an elevation of BP. In a child who is obese, hyperinsulinemia may elevate BP by increasing sodium reabsorption and sympathetic tone.

In a hypertension, however, the blood pushes too hard against the blood vessels, which can cause damage to blood vessels, the heart, and other organs. Increased arterial BP (hypertension) over time may precipitate cardiac enlargement, cerebrovascular disease, renal disease, subsequent renal failure.

Clinical Manifestations

- Signs and symptoms that should alert the care giver to the possibility of hypertension in neonates include the following:
- Failure to thrive
- Seizure
- Irritability or lethargy
- Respiratory distress
- Congestive heart failure.

Signs and symptoms that should alert the care giver to the possibility of primary hypertension in older children include all of the above, as well as the following:

- Headache
- Fatigue
- Blurred vision
- Epistaxis
- Bell's palsy.

Diagnosis

A comprehensive medical history, physical examination and laboratory tests can differentiate from primary to secondary hypertension. Taking BP on all four extremities and repeated twice if elevated, is needed. Complete blood cell count, BUN, creatinine, uric acid, and electrolyte levels, echocardiography, USG kidneys, arteriography, and urine analysis can rule out the causes of secondary hypertension.

Management

Primary Hypertension

In children with mild or moderate hypertension, non-pharmacologic therapy may suffice to lower BP to within normal limits. It emphasises risk factor modification through lifestyle counseling. In general, treating high blood pressure in children is not that different from treating it in adults. This non-pharmacologic therapy avoids the need for drugs that have adverse effects and that require a degree of compliance difficult to achieve in children. General management plan for a child with hypertension is given below:

- *DASH eating plan:* The dietary approaches to stop hypertension (DASH) diet plan includes eating less fat and saturated fat as well as eating more fresh fruits and vegetables and whole-grain foods. Limiting salt intake can also help lower a child's blood pressure.

  Potassium supplementation can decrease BP and reduce ventricular hypertrophy in adults. How potassium supplementation affects children with hypertension remains to be determined. However, avoiding potassium depletion (e.g. from diuretic therapy) and prescribing a potassium-rich diet in patients without renal insufficiency appear reasonable.

  A low-fat diet is recommended for all patients with a high BP; a low-salt diet is also recommended for all such patients, though it may yield only a 4% reduction of the elevated pressure.
- *Weight reduction:* Being overweight increases the risk of developing high blood pressure. Weight reduction should be a goal in all overweight children with hypertension, regardless of etiology. Following the DASH eating plan and getting regular exercise can help child lose weight. Obesity and hypertension are closely correlated, particularly in adolescents.

  Aerobic and isotonic exercises have a direct beneficial effect on BP. They help in reducing excess weight or maintaining appropriate body weight. Encourage participation and organization in sports. Limit the amount of time child spends playing video games and watching TV. Only patients with severe uncontrolled hypertension or cardiac abnormalities that require exercise restriction are exempt from aerobic and isotonic exercises.

  Stress-reducing activities (e.g. meditation, yoga, biofeedback) can reduce BP when performed on a regular basis. However, this effect is lost when the activity is discontinued.
- *Prevention from tobacco smoke:* Tobacco smoke can make blood pressure rise; it can also directly damage child's heart and blood vessels. Protection of the child from tobacco smoke is important, even from passive smoking.

Pharmacologic Measure

Indications for pharmacologic treatment include symptomatic hypertension, secondary hypertension, hypertensive target-organ damage, diabetes, and hypertension that persists despite nonpharmacologic measures. It may take a while to find a combination of drugs that works best to control high blood pressure with the least side effects. Drugs used to treat high blood pressure include:

- Diuretics to reduce the amount of fluid in the blood by helping the body rid itself of extra sodium.
  - ACE inhibitors, alpha-blockers, and calcium channel blockers help keep the blood vessels from tightening up. Angiotensin-converting enzyme (ACE) inhibitors, angiotensin II receptor blockers (ARBs), and calcium-channel blockers have the strongest data to support their use in pediatric patients. The task force on blood pressure control in children, recommends the use of ACE inhibitors or ARBs only for children with diabetes and microalbuminuria or proteinuric renal disease and recommends beta-blockers or calcium-channel blockers for children with hypertension and migraine headaches. A low dose of 1 drug should be started first. If this dose is unsuccessful, it should be titrated upward.
- Beta-blockers prevent the body from making the hormone adrenaline. Adrenaline is a stress hormone. It makes the heart beat harder and faster. It also makes blood vessels tighten. All of this makes blood pressure higher.
  - When sleep-disordered breathing is discovered, weight loss, tonsillectomy and adenoidectomy, or use of continuous positive airway pressure may improve the patient's sleep and secondarily improve BP.

Secondary Hypertension

Effective treatment of the underlying cause will often result in control of secondary hypertension.

KAWASAKI DISEASE

Kawasaki disease is an autoimmune disease in which the medium-sized blood vessels throughout the body become inflamed. The disorder was first described in 1967 by Tomisaku Kawasaki in Japan. It is also known as Kawasaki syndrome, lymph node syndrome and mucocutaneous lymph node syndrome.

Kawasaki disease is largely seen in children under five years of age. It is an illness that involves the skin, mouth, and lymph nodes. The cause is unknown, but if the symptoms are recognized early, kids with Kawasaki disease can fully recover within a few days. Untreated, it can lead to serious complications that can affect the heart, where it can cause fatal coronary artery aneurysms in untreated children. Without treatment, mortality may approach 1%, usually within six weeks of onset.

Clinical Manifestations

The first phase, which can last for up to 2 weeks, usually involves a persistent fever higher than 104 °F (39 °C) and lasts for at least 5 days. The conjunctivae and oral mucosa, along with the skin, become red and inflamed, red, dry, cracked lips, swollen tongue with a white coating and big red bumps, sore, irritated throat (Fig. 19.7). Edema is often seen in the hands and feet. One or more cervical lymph nodes are often enlarged. In untreated children, the febrile period lasts on average approximately 10 days, but may range from five to 25 days. Other symptoms that typically develop include a rash on the stomach, chest, and genitals.

During the second phase, which usually begins within 2 weeks of when the fever started, the skin on the hands and feet may begin to peel in large pieces. The child also may experience joint pain, diarrhea, vomiting, or abdominal pain.

Diagnosis

No single test can detect Kawasaki disease, it can only be diagnosed clinically (i.e. by medical signs and symptoms). There exists no specific laboratory test for this condition. Most kids diagnosed with Kawasaki disease will have a fever lasting 5 or more days and at least four of these symptoms:

- Redness in both eyes
- Changes around the lips, tongue, or mouth
- Changes in the fingers and toes, such as swelling, discoloration, or peeling
- A rash in the trunk or genital area
- A large swollen lymph node in the neck
- Red, swollen palms of hands and soles of feet.

Many other serious illnesses can cause similar symptoms, and must be considered in the differential diagnosis, including scarlet fever, toxic shock syndrome, juvenile idiopathic arthritis, and childhood mercury poisoning (infantile acrodynia), allergic drug reaction. If Kawasaki disease is suspected, the tests to monitor heart function (such as an echocardiogram) is usually done.

Treatment

It should begin as soon as possible, ideally within 10 days of when the fever begins. Usually, a child is treated with:

- **Intravenous immunoglobulin** (IVIG) is a product derived from human blood that is made of antibodies that fight infection and inflammation. Treatment is given in the hospital **intravenously** (through a vein).
- High doses of **aspirin** may be given, followed by a course of low-dose aspirin after the fever resolves. The length of treatment depends on whether coronary aneurysms are found.
- In severe cases not responsive to IVIG, **corticosteroids** (medications used to reduce inflammation) or other anti-inflammatory medications may be used.

  Follow-up care: Children need close follow-up once they are discharged from the hospital.
- Cardiologists will order echocardiograms at regular intervals to look for coronary aneurysms and decide the length of treatment with aspirin.
- IVIG can interfere with vaccines, especially the **MMR** (measles-mumps-rubella) and **Varicella** (chickenpox) vaccines. It may be recommended to withhold vaccines for 11 months following IVIG.
- Because aspirin can have serious effects in children who get chickenpox or influenza, parents must notify

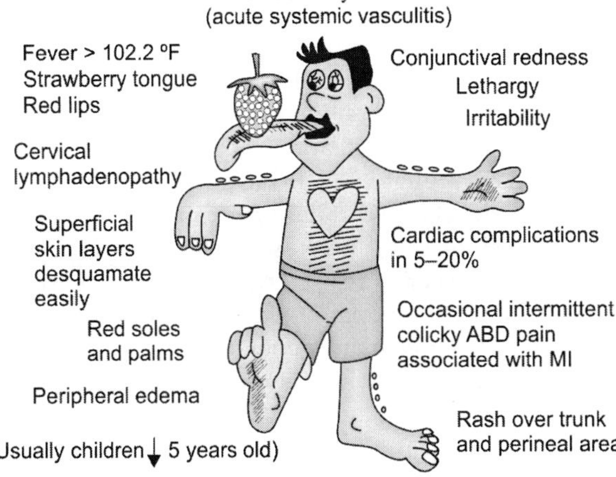

Fig. 19.7: Kawasaki syndrome

their physician immediately if they are exposed to influenza or varicella or have any symptoms.

Cardiomyopathy in Children

Cardiomyopathies are disease of heart muscles. The muscle becomes abnormally thick, stiff or enlarged, affecting the heart's ability to fill or pump blood and maintain its rhythm. It is a serious condition in which the heart muscle is weak and incapable of pumping as much blood as it should. Common symptoms are dyspnea and peripheral edema. Cardiomyopathies are relatively rare in children.

Etiology

When children develop cardiomyopathies, there is often not an identifiable factor such as another illness. Sometimes the cardiomyopathy is inherited, may be a heart infection called myocarditis. It occurs as a consequence of a viral infection such as *coxsackie*. This can cause an inflammation of the heart known as acute (sudden) myocarditis. When the inflammation settles, heart function may slowly return to normal but, in some cases, it persists and is then indistinguishable from dilated cardiomyopathy. These viral infections can even occur in the womb and, if the damage does not resolve itself, the infant may be born with dilated cardiomyopathy. In many cases, a cause is never found.

It is a protein abnormality in the heart muscle, toxicity of chemotherapy drugs, metabolic disorders or muscle disorders are among the factors that can cause cardiomyopathy in a child or teenager. Other secondary causes of cardiomyopathy are hemochromatosis, Kawasaki disease, thyroid dysfunction, collagen diseases, Duchenne muscular dystrophy.

There are different types of cardiomyopathies, including:

- *Dilated cardiomyopathy:* The most common type in both adults and children. It results when the pumping chambers (ventricles) of the heart are abnormally enlarged and weakened. Some children who have a dilated heart have no symptoms while others develop heart failure (difficulty breathing, difficulty eating, excessive sweating and poor growth). There are many different causes of dilated cardiomyopathy. Some families have many members, across many generations, with this type of cardiomyopathy, which is known as familial dilated cardiomyopathy.
- *Hypertrophic cardiomyopathy:* Occurs when one or more pumping chambers (ventricles) in your child's heart become unusually thickened or 'muscle-bound.' This may affect the left ventricle, which pumps blood to the body, or both the left and right ventricles (the right ventricle pumps blood to the lungs). This type of cardiomyopathy is often associated with abnormal heart rhythms, which can lead to sudden death. Hypertrophic cardiomyopathy may run in families; members of affected families are encouraged to undergo screening.
- *Restrictive cardiomyopathy:* The rarest type of cardiomyopathy in children. The chambers of the heart become stiff, resulting in improper heart muscle relaxation, so that your child's heart cannot fill with blood adequately. Abnormal heart rhythms may also occur with this disease. There are no medicines that are known to improve patients with restrictive cardiomyopathy, and a heart transplant is often recommended for children with this condition.
- *Noncompaction cardiomyopathy:* Characterized by a spongy appearance of the heart muscle on echocardiography. Noncompaction cardiomyopathy is thought to be caused by incomplete heart cell maturation. It can exist alone or along with structural heart disease; it can be part of an underlying syndrome or occur idiopathically (with no identifiable cause).

The blood waiting to get into the heart develops a high pressure and this can cause fluid to leak out of the blood vessels into the lung (pulmonary edema). The amount of blood that the heart can pump is severely reduced and this is even more of a problem on exercising. In some cases the heart of a child who has a cardiomyopathy will become progressively weaker and the child will end up in a stage of heart failure (difficulty breathing, difficulty eating, excessive sweating and poor growth) advanced enough to require transplantation. However, in some cases, cardiomyopathies can be treated with medications and the child's health may improve.

Diagnosis

Several tests are organized after taking child's history and examining the child. These will usually comprise an electrocardiogram (ECG) to measure the electrical activity of the heart and a chest X-ray to visualize the heart and lungs. The diagnosis is made by echocardiography. Detailed images of the heart are assessed by cardiac magnetic resonance imaging (MRI).

Some blood and urine tests may also be necessary to attempt to find a cause.

In the long term, repeated echocardiograms will be performed to assess the cardiac function and assess recovery.

Symptoms of Cardiomyopathy

Sometimes infants have symptoms of cardiomyopathy shortly after birth. They can include:

- Breathlessness
- Difficulty in feeding and sweating while nursing or taking a bottle
- Poor weight gain
- Irritability, lethargy or unresponsiveness.

Sometimes symptoms do not appear until the child is older. They can include:

- Heart murmur or other abnormal heart sounds
- Difficulty exercising, difficulty breathing and/or chest pains with exercise
- Dizziness or fainting
- General malaise
- Heart palpitations
- Vomiting and stomach pains
- Sudden collapse.

Treatment

The treatment aims to decrease the size of a dilated heart, relax the heart, increase the pumping strength, regulate the rhythm of the heart, to manage CHF. Often several medications are used in combination.

In mild cases:

- Diuretics to encourage the child to pass urine and reduce the water retention
- ACE inhibitors such as captopril, enalapril or lisinopril to make the work of the heart easier
- Beta blockers such as carvedilol may be used to slow the filling of the heart
- Digoxin may be used in addition to the above.

In severe cases:

In case of worst heart failure and signs of poor perfusion the IV dobutamine are useful.

Ventilation on an intensive care unit, oxygen therapy, IV afterload reduction agents (nitroprusside) are helpful.

Drugs to stimulate the heart (known as inotropes), such as adrenaline.

Pacemakers and implantable defibrillators help to control the heart rhythm so the heart does not beat too slowly or in an irregular pattern. The devices are implanted under the skin and connected to the heart with tiny wires called leads.

Heart transplantation: When an advanced stage of heart failure (symptoms that interfere with daily activities or growth in infants, and physical changes) results from a cardiomyopathy, heart transplant may be considered.

When the heart function is very poor and does not recover, a heart transplant may be considered.

If the condition is suspected to be acute myocarditis, immunoglobulins may be used.

Prognosis

Of those who are taken to the treatment with severe heart failure, approximately one third make a complete recovery, one third recover but remain on medicine to assist heart function and one third either die or require a heart transplant. Outpatient visits may be lifelong, with repeated echocardiograms to assess cardiac function.

SHOCK

Shock is a life-threatening medical condition as a result of insufficient blood flow throughout the body. Shock often accompanies severe injury or illness. Medical shock is a medical emergency. This circulatory failure is a complex clinical syndrome characterized by inadequate tissue perfusion to meet the metabolic demands of the body, resulting in cellular dysfunction (hypoxia) and can lead to other conditions such as heart attack (cardiac arrest) and eventual organ failure.

More than 10 million children die each year in the world. The highest mortality rates are observed in children under five years in developing countries. Shock is the result of various etiologies and the leading causes of shock in children younger than 5 years of age are: pneumonia, diarrhea, malaria, neonatal pneumonia or sepsis, preterm delivery, and asphyxia at birth. The early recognition of signs of shock and aggressive therapy to restore the intravascular volume and reverse the biochemical cascade is believed to improve outcome. It can damage any and all tissues and organ systems in the body. Delay in recognizing and quickly treating a state of shock results in a progression from compensated reversible shock to widespread multiple system organ failure to death.

Types of Shock

- **Anaphylactic shock** is a type of severe hypersensitivity or allergic reaction. Causes include allergy to insect stings, medicines, or foods (nuts, berries, sea food), etc.
- **Cardiogenic shock** happens when the heart is damaged and unable to supply sufficient blood to the body. This can be the end result of a heart attack or congestive heart failure.

- **Hypovolemic shock** is caused by severe blood and fluid loss, such as from traumatic bodily injury, which makes the heart unable to pump enough blood to the body, or severe anemia where there is not enough blood to carry oxygen through the body.
- **Neurogenic shock** is caused by spinal cord injury, usually as a result of a traumatic accident or injury.

Pathophysiology

In healthy child, the primary function of the cardiovascular system is to provide oxygen and other substrates to the cells for metabolic functioning. In early **compensated shock** several compensatory mechanism are activated. In the face of impending hypoperfusion, sympathetic nervous system stimulation increases heart rate and systemic vascular resistance (SVR) through the release of catecholamines from adrenal glands. Renin-angiotensin-aldosterone system is also activated, contributing to vasoconstriction, maintenance of SVR, and fluid retention through concentration of urine.

In children, vascular tone is maintained in low flow states of septic and cardiogenic shock. Therefore, children can often maintain their blood pressure until they are in profound shock. Compensatory vasoconstriction is often so pronounced that systemic blood pressure can be maintained within the normal range despite significant circulatory compromise. Hypotension is typically a late finding among children in shock. With vasoconstriction, causes poor glomerular filtration and blood flow is shunted away from skin and splanchnic bed (non-vital organs), to brain, heart, and lungs. As a result, extremities are cold and mottled, capillary refill is prolonged (Table 19.7), catecholamine-induced tachycardia occurs. In lack of tissue perfusion, oxygen is depleted in the tissue cells, causing them to revert to anaerobic metabolism, producing lactic acidosis. The acidosis places an extra burden on the lungs as they attempt to compensate for the metabolic acidosis by increased respiratory rate to remove excess carbon dioxide. If shock is left untreated, the compensatory mechanisms will fail and **uncompensated shock** develops.

Organ hypoperfusion manifests itself as early organ dysfunction with altered mental status, tachypnea, tachycardia, lethargy, decreased or absent urine output, and mottled extremities. *Failure of normalization of peripheral pulses, skin temperature, and capillary refill with treatment predicts death from shock.* Once the blood pressure falls, the patient will progress into **irreversible shock**. Irreversible shock, as the name implies, is the point of no return when the mortality rate is high irrespective of interventions.

Classification of Shock

- Compensated
  - Blood flow is normal or increased and may be maldistributed; vital organ function is maintained
- Uncompensated
  - Microvascular perfusion is compromised; significant reductions in effective circulating volume
- Irreversible
  - Inadequate perfusion of vital organs; irreparable damage; death cannot be prevented.

Diagnosis

At all stages the principal differentiating signs are observed in the (i) degree of tachycardia and perfusion to extremities (ii) level of consciousness, and (iii) Blood pressure. Additional signs may be present, depending on the type and etiology of the shock (Table 19.8).

Assessment of ABC: First assess airway patency, ventilation, then circulatory system, respiratory rate and pattern, work of breathing, oxygenation (color), level of alertness, heart rate, BP, perfusion, and pulses, liver size, CVP monitoring may be helpful.

Laboratory Investigations

These are needed to ascertain the cause of shock and to appraise the performance of other body organs/ systems. A baseline investigation should include complete blood count, platelet count, blood glucose level, serum electrolytes, arterial blood gases, blood culture, blood grouping, renal function tests, chest X-ray, ECG, etc.

Treatment

Early recognition and timely intervention are critical in treating shock and preventing progression of the shock cascade. Furthermore, early goal directed therapy has been shown to decrease mortality in adults and children. The goal of resuscitation is to reverse circulatory insufficiency and correct the hypoperfusion. The first step in clinical management is always ABCs. Airway is the first priority and may need to be protected or a definitive airway established particularly in children with altered mental status. Since functional residual capacity is smaller in pediatric patients compared to adults, early assisted ventilation might be required. In addition, endotracheal intubation may be indicated for hemodynamic instability alone since taking over the work of breathing will decrease oxygen consumption substantially. Care must be taken in selecting the appropriate induction agent for controlled pharmacological intubation to avoid hypotension and myocardial depression.

Follow-up of Response to Treatment

The most sensitive indicator of adequate cardiac output in children is the heart rate. Treatment should be

Table 19.7: Types of pediatric shock, mechanism, clinical features, and intervention

Types of shock	*Mechanism*	*Clinical features*	*Intervention*
Hypovolemic (absolute or relative depletion of blood volume)	• *CO:* Decreased, • *SVR:* Increased	Tachycardia, weak pulse, sunken eyes/fontanels, oliguria, capillary refill prolonged.	• *Oxygen:* Immediate venous access. • Arrest hemorrhage or fluid loss in burns by cling-film. Crystalloid bolus 20 mL/kg over 20 min; reassess and repeat 2 × if indicated. • Blood products for hemorrhagic shock. • Assess CVP to avoid over-transfusion and pulmonary oedema.
Cardiogenic shock	• *CO:* Decreased • *SVR:* Increased	Arrhythmia, often tachycardia, weak or absent pulse, hepatomegaly	Dopamine, dobutamine, epinephrine, milrinone. May give small fluid boluses 5–10 mL/kg under close monitoring. Urgent ECHO assessment
• Distributive • Anaphylactic • Neurogenic	• *CO:* Increased, then decreased SVR greatly decreased • *CO:* Normal • *SVR:* Decreased	Angioedema, respiratory distress due to narrowing of airways, stridor, wheezing, early hypotension, weak rapid pulse.	Adrenergic and fluid support, supra-therapeutic doses of inotropes if required. Support SVR with vasopressors, phenylephrine.
• Septic • Warm shock • Cold shock	• *CO:* Normal • *SVR:* Decreased • *CO:* Decreased • *SVR:* Increased	• Warm extremities, tachycardia, bounding pulse, wide pulse pressure, hypotension, hyperpnea, altered senses • Cold extremities, tachycardia, poor peripheral perfusion, diminished pulses, hyperpnea, altered senses.	Crystalloid bolus 20 mL/kg, repeat till stable. Consider albumin bolus. Drugs: dopamine or norepinephrine/adrenaline. Stabilize with crystalloid as above. Consider early dopamine/epinephrine under ECHO guidance.
Obstructive	• Preload decreased • *CO:* Decreased • *SVR:* Normal/raised	Tachycardia, hypotension, distended JVP, tracheal deviation if pneumothorax present, pulsus paradoxus in case of tamponade	• Rapidly fatal if underlying process not recognized. • Give fluid boluses while preparing for emergent drainage

Abbreviations: CO = cardiac output, SVR = systemic venous resistance, JVP = jugular venous pressure; ECHO = echocardiography

Table 19.8: Signs of shock

Early signs of shock	*Late sign of shock*	*Cardiovascular assessment*	
Sinus tachycardia Delayed capillary refill Fussy, irritable	• Bradycardia • Altered mental status (lethargy, coma) • Hypotonia, decreased DTR's Cheyne-Stokes breathing • Hypotension is a very late sign Lower limit of SBP = 70 + (2 × age in years)	• Heart Rate • Too high: 180 bpm • For infants • 160 bpm for children >1 year old • Blood Pressure • Lower limit of • SBP = 70 + (2 × age in years) • Peripheral pulses • Present/Absent • Strength (diminished, normal, bounding)	– Skin perfusion–capillary refill time – Temperature – Color – Mottling – CNS perfusion—recognition of parent – Papillary reaction – Muscle tone – Reaction to pain • Renal Perfusion • UOP more than 1 cc/kg/hour

modified as necessary based on monitored vital signs, exam findings and laboratory values. The earliest sign of reversal of shock is usually a decline in heart rate followed by improved blood pressure and increased urine output. The goals should be normalization of capillary refill (< 2 seconds), normal peripheral pulses, warm extremities, adequate urine output of greater than 1 mL/kg/hr, normal mental status.

CHAPTER 20

Common Communicable Diseases in Children

Chapter Outline

- Common Viral Infections
- Whooping Cough
- Measles
- Poliomyelitis
- Treatment of Residual Paralysis
- Chickenpox (Varicella–Zoster, Shingles)
- Dengue
- Rabies
- HIV Infection
- Common Bacterial Infection
- Tuberculosis
- Leprosy
- Common Parasitic Infections
- Kala-Azar
- Filariasis
- Helminthiasis
- Echinococcosis (Hydatid Disease)

INTRODUCTION

Communicable diseases spread from one person to another or from an animal to a person. The spread often happens via airborne viruses or bacteria, but also through blood or other bodily fluid. The terms infectious and contagious are also used to describe communicable disease.

Infectious disease results from the interplay between those few pathogens and the defenses of the hosts they infect. The appearance and severity of disease resulting from any pathogen, depends upon the ability of that pathogen to damage the host as well as the ability of the host to resist the pathogen. Infectious disorders are prevalent and remain a leading cause of death. Infectious diseases cause 63% of all childhood deaths and 48% of premature deaths. Most instances of the common communicable diseases, such as measles, chicken pox, and mumps, are encountered in childhood.

In light of this, it is clear that effective public health surveillance is critical for the early detection and prevention of epidemics due to communicable diseases (Fig. 20.1). There is a clear and urgent need for surveillance of (i) known existing communicable diseases, especially those with high epidemic potential, (ii) early recognition of new infection, and (iii) monitoring the growing resistance to antimicrobial drugs.

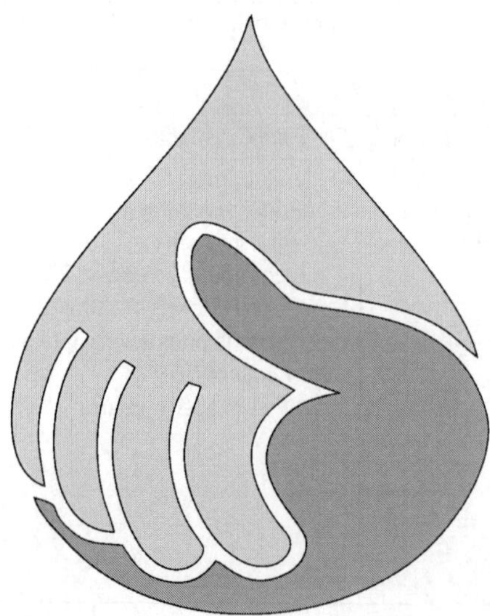

Fig. 20.1: Unite in the fight against communicable diseases

COMMON VIRAL INFECTIONS

Diphtheria

Diphtheria is an upper respiratory tract illness caused by *Corynebacterium diphtheria* which is Gram positive, non motile organism.

Incubation period: Usually from 2 to 6 days, occasionally longer.

Infectious period: Unless treated, the period of infectivity may vary from 14–28 days from the onset of the disease.

Transmission: By direct contact with carrier or disease or breathing the aerosolized secretions of infected individuals.

Immunity: Passive immunity from mother, natural disease. Active immunization increases resistance to infection. Vaccines consist of microorganisms or cellular components that act as antigens. Administration of the vaccine stimulates the production of antibodies with specific protective properties.

Season: Late autumn, winter.

Causes of the Disease

Diphtheria spreads through respiratory droplets of an infected person or someone who carries the bacteria but has no symptoms. The bacteria most commonly infects nose and throat. The throat infection causes a gray to black, tough, fiber-like covering, which can block the child's airways. In some cases, diphtheria infects skin first and causes skin lesions.

Once infected, the bacteria make dangerous substances called toxins. The toxins spread through bloodstream to other organs, such as the heart and brain, and cause damage.

Because of widespread immunization (vaccination) of children, diphtheria is now rare in many parts of the world.

Risk factors for diphtheria include crowded environments, poor hygiene, and lack of immunization.

Manifestations

Symptoms like fever of 38 °C (100.4 °F) or above, chills, fatigue, bluish skin coloration (cyanosis, sore throat, hoarseness, cough, headache, difficulty swallowing, painful swallowing, difficulty breathing, rapid breathing, foul-smelling blood stained nasal discharge and lymphadenopathy are seen in diphtheria. Thin, gray membranes appear on tonsils and pharynx (Fig. 20.2), causing 'bull neck', neck edema. The swollen throat is often accompanied by a serious respiratory condition, characterized by a brassy or 'barking' cough, stridor, hoarseness, and difficulty breathing, and referred as '*diphtheritic croup*' (extremely rare in countries where diphtheria vaccination is customary). Symptoms can also include cardiac arrhythmias, myocarditis, and cranial and peripheral nerve palsies.

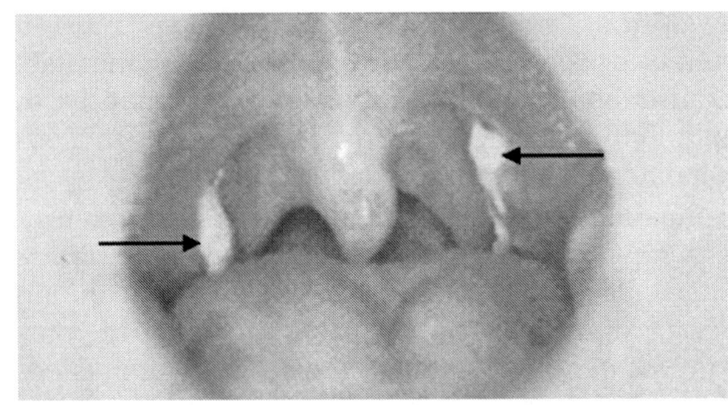

Fig. 20.2: Diphteria: Notice the pseudomembrane in the posterior pharynx. It can become very large and may obstruct in airway

Diagnosis

Diagnosis of diphtheria is usually made based on signs and symptoms. A swab specimen is taken from the throat to test for the bacteria. Tests used may include:

- Gram stain or throat culture to identify the diphtheria bacteria
- Toxin assay (to detect the presence of the toxin made by the bacteria)
- Electrocardiogram

Diphtheria treatment today involves:

- Using diphtheria antitoxin to neutralize the toxin produced by the bacteria
- Using antibiotics to kill and eliminate diphtheria bacteria

Diphtheria patients are usually kept in isolation, until they are no longer able to infect others—usually about 48 hours after antibiotic treatment begins. The disease is usually not able to be spread after the patient has been on antibiotics for 48 hours. At least 2 subsequent cultures taken 24 hours apart after cessation of therapy demonstrate negative results.

Repeat cultures are performed at a minimum of 2 weeks after completion of therapy in patients and carriers; if results are positive, an additional 10 days course of oral erythromycin should be administered and follow-up cultures performed.

Critical care needs and complications must be addressed. Mechanical ventilation may be inevitable because the combination of airway obstruction by the diphtheritic membrane and peripharyngeal edema pose a fatality risk in patients with diphtheria.

Antitoxin therapy: Specific antitoxin is the mainstay of therapy and should be administered on the basis of clinical diagnosis because it neutralizes free toxin only. Efficacy diminishes with elapsing time after the onset of mucocutaneous symptoms. Antitoxin is administered once at an empiric dose based on the degree of toxicity, site and size of the membrane, and duration of illness. Usually it is administered by intravenous (IV) route, with infusion over 30–60 minutes.

Antibiotic therapy: Penicillin and erythromycin are only recommended for treatment. Erythromycin is marginally superior to penicillin for eradication of nasopharyngeal infection. Erythromycin (orally or by injection) for 14 days (40 mg/kg per day with a maximum of 2 g/d).

Procaine penicillin G given intramuscularly for 14 days (300,000 U/d for patients weighing <10 kg and 600,000 U/d for those weighing >10 kg). Patients with allergies to penicillin G or erythromycin can use rifampin or clindamycin.

Nursing Considerations

The aims of therapy and nursing care are to inactivate toxin, to kill the organism, and to prevent respiratory obstruction. Nursing care of hospitalized child with diphtheria involves droplet precautions, monitoring of the child's respiratory status. So, nursing activities include:

- To keep the child in strict bed rest, strict isolation.
- To clean throat, gargle may be ordered.
- To give liquid or soft diet, gavage or parenteral fluid.
- To observe for respiratory obstruction (tracheotomy).
- To use suctioning as needed.
- To administer oxygen, if needed.
- To administer antitoxin against toxin, and broad spectrum antibiotic against diphtheria bacilli.
- To give toxoid to immunized contact.

The primary focus of nursing should be preventive, because diphtheria is a vaccine preventable disease. The incidence of diphtheria has drastically reduced through national immunization programs.

WHOOPING COUGH

Pertussis (whooping cough), is a highly contagious bacterial disease of respiratory tract, caused by *Bordetella pertussis*. Symptoms are initially mild, and then it is characterized by severe coughing spells, which produce the namesake high-pitched 'whoop' sound in infected babies and children when they inhale air after coughing (Fig. 20.3). Pertussis remains a significant cause of morbidity and mortality in infants younger than 2 years.

Worldwide, whooping cough is common and seen as endemic or epidemic form. It affects about 48.5 million people yearly. As of 2010 it caused about 81,000 deaths, down from 167,000 in 1990. This is despite generally high coverage with the DTP vaccine. Pertussis is one of the leading causes of vaccine-preventable deaths world-wide. Ninety percent of all cases occur in developing countries.

Causative agent: Bacterium *Bordetella pertussis,* which is rod shaped Gram negative bacillus.

Incubation period: From 6 – 20 days.

Infectious period: A person can spread the disease from the very beginning of the sickness (when he has cold-like symptoms) and for at least 3 weeks after the onset of paroxysmal stage. The catarrhal phase is the most infectious period.

Transmission: Direct contact or droplet infection, coughing and sneezing. Almost everyone who is not immune to whooping cough will get sick if exposed to it.

Immunity: Natural disease or vaccine.

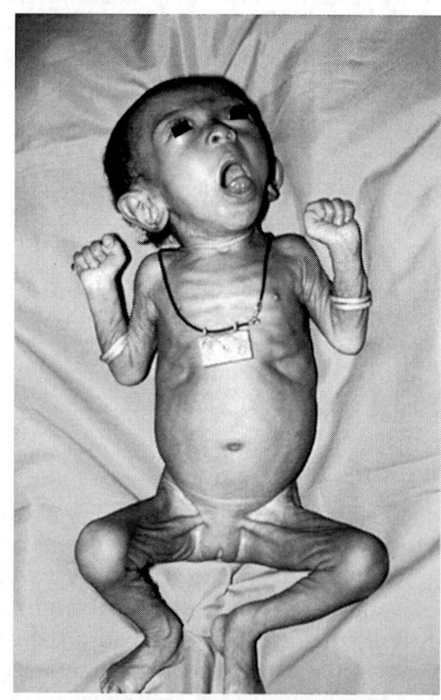

Fig. 20.3: Extreme sternal retractions in whooping cough

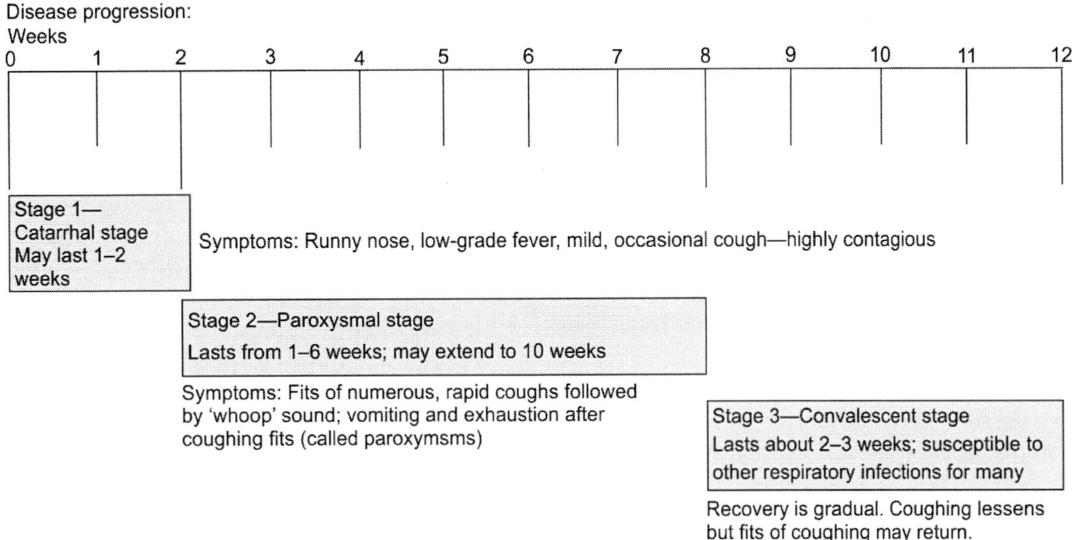

Fig. 20.4: Pertussis progresses through different stages

Season: Any time in the year, but more common in winter and springs.

Manifestations

Pertussis is divided into catarrhal, paroxysmal, and convalescent stages (Fig. 20.4). The detail of which is given below.

Catarrhal phase: Usually mild respiratory symptoms, mild coughing, sneezing, or runny nose, fever are seen in the catarrhal stage. Initially cough disturbs in night then it occurs both in day and night.

Paroxysmal phase: After one to two weeks, the coughing classically develops into uncontrollable fits, each with five to ten forceful coughs, followed by a high-pitched 'whoop' sound in younger children, or a gasping sound in older children, as the patient struggles to breathe in through half open glottis afterwards (paroxysmal stage). The whoop may be present with or without cyanosis and apnea and patient looks suffocated with red congested face, sweating, engorged neck and scalp veins. The child become confused and restless and fainting and/or vomiting after coughing may occur.

The cough from pertussis has been documented to cause subconjunctival hemorrhages, rib fractures, urinary incontinence, hernias, postcough fainting, and vertebral artery dissection. Violent coughing can cause the pleura to rupture, leading to a pneumothorax. If there is vomiting after a coughing spell or an inspiratory whooping sound on coughing, the likelihood almost doubles that the illness is pertussis. The coughing spells can occur on their own or can be triggered by yawning, stretching, laughing, eating or yelling; they usually occur in groups, with multiple episodes on an hourly basis throughout the day. This stage usually lasts two to eight weeks, or sometimes longer.

Convalescent phase: A gradual transition then occurs to the convalescent stage, which usually lasts one to two weeks. This stage is marked by a decrease in paroxysms of coughing, both in frequency and severity, and a cessation of vomiting. A tendency to produce the 'whooping' sound after coughing may remain for a considerable period after the disease itself has cleared up. Patient's general condition and appetite improve.

Diagnosis

The diagnosis of pertussis is made by throat swab culture and a polymerase chain reaction (PCR) test.

- The culture specimen should be obtained during the first 2 weeks of cough by using deep nasopharyngeal aspiration.
- For PCR testing, nasopharyngeal specimens should be taken at 0-3 weeks following cough onset.
- A combination of culture and PCR assay is recommended if a patient has a cough lasting longer than 3 weeks.
- Monitoring of white blood cell counts is also needed.

Therapeutic Management

Goals of therapy are:

- Primary prevention through immunization.
- Limit the number of paroxysms—it is done through antibiotic therapy. Antimicrobial agents can hasten the eradication of *B pertussis* and help

prevent spread. Erythromycin, clarithromycin, and azithromycin are the preferred agents for patients aged 1 month or older.

- Observe the severity of cough and provide assistance when necessary.
- Maximize nutrition, rest, and recovery.

Nursing Considerations

Nursing diagnosis: Ineffective breathing pattern due to airway edema, and a thick mucus.

Expected results: Children will able to maintain free airway breathing by reduced.

Intervention: Assess the respiratory status of children as often as possible or continuously review the signs and symptoms of increased difficulty breathing and respiratory obstruction (stridor, retraction, respirator rate, barking cough, cyanosis). If a child can tolerate, place him on high-Fowler's position.

The child can be kept in a tent and give the cool air, it helps in loosening the thick mucus. Give oxygen, if necessary. His respiratory status needs monitoring with a cardiopulmonary monitor and pulse oximeter.

Nursing diagnosis: The risk reduction associated with lowering volume of fluid through oral intake.

Expected outcome: The child will maintain fluid balance is characterized by good skin turgor and urine output of 1 to 2 mL/kg/hour.

Intervention: Assess the child's ability to tolerate liquid (swallow, choke, or cough).

Provide and monitor IV fluids, as instructed, monitor I/O carefully.

Assess for signs of dehydration. Small and frequent feedings may benefit the infant, feeding should not be exhaustive to the child.

Nursing diagnosis: Anxiety (children) are associated with respiratory distress and effect of hospitalization.

Expected results: Children will be reduced his anxiety is evidenced by periods of rest and enough sleep, respiratory status is stable.

Intervention: Let the child in a comfortable position during treatment of oxygen therapy. All examinations and procedures need not be made until the child's respiratory status improves. Encourage parents to stay with the children. Create tranquillity and calm atmosphere otherwise coughing paroxysms may triggered by noises or frightening experiences.

Nursing diagnosis: Anxiety (parents) are associated with lack of knowledge about the condition.

Expected outcome: Parents will express that anxiety is reduced and the increased understanding of the condition of children and reduced the fear of the procedure.

Intervention

Assess understanding of parents about the condition of their child; and the assessment allows nurse to develop her lesson plan which will help parents to understand the child's condition and treatment, and thus to reduce fear.

Explain all procedures, medication, and equipment.

Provide emotional support to parents during the child-patient stay in hospital.

MEASLES

Measles, also known as rubeola, is a viral infection of the respiratory system. The virus lives in the mucus of the nose and throat of people with this infection. Measles is a very contagious disease that can spread through contact with infected mucus and saliva. The coughing or sneezing of an infected person can release the virus into the air. The virus can live on surfaces for several hours. As the infected particles enter the air and settle on surfaces, e.g. on surfaces and door handles, anyone within close proximity can become infected with the measles virus. According to WHO measles is one of the leading causes of death among young children even though a safe and cost-effective vaccine is available (Fig. 20.5). In 2013, there were 1,45,700 measles deaths globally—about 400 deaths every day or 16 deaths every hour. Measles vaccination resulted in a 75% drop in measles deaths between 2000 and 2013 worldwide.

Causative agent: A specific measles virus, RNA virus of the genus Morbillivirus of paramyxoviridae family.

Incubation period: From 8 – 12 days.

Infectious period: Ranges from 3 to 5 days before the appearance of the rash to 4–5 days after appearance of the rash.

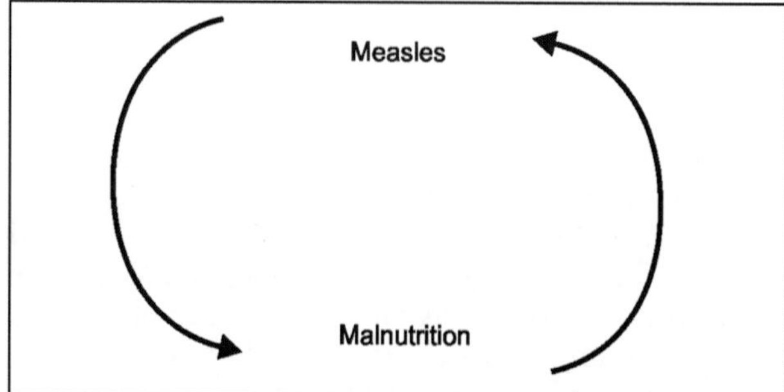

Fig. 20.5: The vicious cycle of measles and malnutrition

Transmission: Droplet infection in direct contact or less frequently by airborne spread.

Immunity: Natural disease or live vaccine. Children are protected by maternal antibody up to six months.

Season: Usually in late winter and spring, but may found in all seasons.

Manifestations

Signs and symptoms of measles are manifested in three stages means prodromal or pre-eruptive phase, eruptive phase, convalescent phase.

Prodormal or pre-eruptive phase: Measles virus enter the body and slowly spreads. This stage is usually starts after ten days of infection and lasts for 3–5 days. Prodorme phase is characterized by fever and 'the three C', corya (profuse running nose), cough (harsh dry or brassy) and conjunctivitis. Going off food, tiredness, and aches and pains are usual. Diarrhea and/or vomiting is common. Some children may have photophobia and lymphadenopathy. Koplik spots appear approximately 2days before the appearance of rash. Koplik spots are tiny grayish or bluish spots with a red base, cluster near the molar of buccal mucosa. These spots approximately last for three days, after that it sloughs off.

Eruptive phase: A red blotchy rash normally develops about 3–4 days after the first symptoms. It usually starts on the head and neck, and spreads down the body and extremities and to the feet (Fig. 20.6). It takes 2–3 days to cover most of the body. The rash often turns a brownish color and gradually fades over a few days. The duration of rash is 6–7 days. Fever usually rise again and regress gradually within 3 days. A fine superficial skin shedding occurs in face and body leaving browning discoloration of skin.

Convalescent phase: It means the disappearance of rash, fever and other constitutional symptoms. The child remains sick for number of days and lost weight. Due to poor resistance the child may develop other sicknesses caused by bacteria or viral infections.

Most children are better within 7–10 days. An irritating cough may persist for several days after other symptoms have gone. The immune system makes antibodies during the infection. These fight off the virus and then provide lifelong immunity.

Therapeutic Management

There is no prescription medication to treat measles. The virus and symptoms typically disappear within two to three weeks. However, symptomatic management includes:

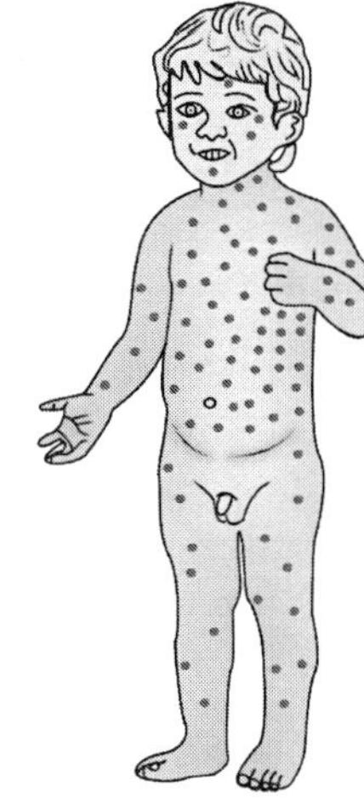

Fig. 20.6: Measles rash

- Acetaminophen to relieve fever and muscle aches
- Rest to help boost your immune system
- Plenty of fluids
- Humidifier to ease a cough and sore throat
- **Vitamin A supplements:** Vitamin A supplements have been shown to help prevent serious complications arising from a measles infection.
- Antibiotics do not kill the measles virus and so are not normally given. They may be prescribed if a complication develops, such as a secondary bacterial ear infection or secondary bacterial pneumonia.
- Cough remedies have little benefit on any coughs.

Complications

Measles can be a serious in all age groups. However, children younger than 5 years of age and adults older than 20 years of age are more likely to suffer from measles complications.

Common Complications

Common measles complications include ear infections and diarrhea. Ear infections occur in about one out of every 10 children with measles and can result in permanent hearing loss. Diarrhea is reported in less than one out of 10 people with measles. Some people may suffer from severe complications, such as pneumonia (infection of the lungs) and encephalitis (swelling of the brain). These children may need to be hospitalized and could die.

- As there is respiratory involvement, secondary bacterial infections such as bronchopneumonia, otitis media, croup can occur. As many as one out

of every 20 children with measles gets pneumonia, the most common cause of death from measles in young children.
- About one child out of every 1,000 who get measles will develop encephalitis that can lead to convulsions and can leave the child deaf or mentally retarded.

Prevention

Routine measles vaccination for children, combined with mass immunization campaigns in countries with high case and death rates, are key public health strategies to reduce global measles deaths. 0.5 mL live attenuated measles vaccine (subcutaneous injection) has been in use at 9–12 months of age. Two doses of the vaccine are recommended (second dose at 16–24 months) to ensure immunity and prevent outbreaks, as about 15% of vaccinated children fail to develop immunity from the first dose.

The measles vaccine is often incorporated with rubella and/or mumps vaccines in countries where these illnesses are problems. It is equally effective in the single or combined form. In 2013, about 84% of the world's children received 1 dose of measles vaccine by their first birthday through routine health services – up from 73% in 2000.

The fourth millennium development goal (MDG 4) aims to reduce global measles deaths by the end of 2015, by at least 95% compared with 2000 levels. By the end of 2020, to achieve measles and rubella elimination in at least five WHO regions.

The strategy focuses on the implementation of 5 core components:
- Achieve and maintain high vaccination coverage with 2 doses of measles- and rubella-containing vaccines.
- Monitor the disease using effective surveillance, and evaluate programmatic efforts to ensure progress and the positive impact of vaccination activities.
- Develop and maintain outbreak preparedness, rapid response to outbreaks and the effective treatment of cases.
- Communicate and engage to build public confidence and demand for immunization.
- Perform the research and development needed to support cost-effective action and improve vaccination and diagnostic tools.

Nursing Considerations

Measles is a killer disease in at-risk settings of overcrowding, population movement, displacement, conflict zones and areas with high HIV rates. It is a vaccine preventable disease with serious and potentially fatal consequences. Nurses save lives by conducting immunization programs in community as well as in community. They can also limit adverse outcomes by recognizing and appropriately responding to measles.
- Keep the child in bed rest, isolation is important until 5th day of rash.
- Keep a child in bed until fever and cough subside.
- Dim light, clean eyelid, irrigate eye with saline.
- Encourage fluid during fever.
- Increase humidity in child's room to relieve cough.
- Relieve itching of skin by tepid bath and soothing lotion.
- Immune serum or gamma-globulin may be given to modify illness and reduce complication.
- Antibacterial therapy given for treatment of complication, e.g. respiratory infection or gastroenteritis.

Supportive care for treating measles: Supportive care can include:
- IV fluids.
- Take axillary temperatures. These patients typically have sore mouths so oral thermometers may cause pain.
- Medications to control fever or pain. Generally paracetamol is given instead of aspirin (causes Reye's syndrome in children).
- Antibiotics to treat secondary infections from bacteria.
- Good nursing care includes eye care, oral care, skin care, fluid and nutrition to prevent malnutrition.

Vitamin A as part of measles treatment: In developing countries, malnutrition, vitamin A deficiency, and severe measles are common. For these situations, the treatment of measles should include vitamin A medication for two days, starting as soon as a measles diagnosis is made. This treatment has been shown to decrease the risk of blindness and death.

At the time of measles vaccination campaigns, all children 6 months to 5 years should be screened for malnutrition. Malnutrition is an important cause of postmeasles mortality.

POLIOMYELITIS

Poliomyelitis is a highly contagious disease caused by a virus that attacks the nervous system. Children younger than 5-year-old are more likely to contract the virus than any other group. The virus is transmitted through the fecal-oral route or, less frequently, by a common vehicle (e.g. contaminated water or food) and multiplies in the intestine, from where it can invade the nervous system and can cause paralysis. There is no cure for polio, it can only be prevented by immunization.

Agent: RNA enterovirus, called as poliovirus. Three serotypes of the virus are Burnhide (type 1), Lansing (type 2), Leon (type 3). They got their names from the cases in which they were first isolated. Type 1 is the type most often isolated from paralytic cases. Type 3 less so and type 2 least commonly.

Host: Man is the only reservoir and natural host of the virus. The most vulnerable age is between 6 months to 3 years. The virus can live in water for 4 months, and in a cold environment it can remain in stool for 6 months.

Incubation period: Usually from 7 to 14 days but may extend to 35 days.

Infectious period: The period between 7–10 days before and after onset of symptoms is most infectious period.

Transmission: Oro-fecal transmission. It may be transmitted through droplets in acute phase of disease, when the viruses remain in the throat and oropharyngeal secretions.

Immunity: Inactivated polio virus (IPV), and oral polio vaccine (OPV).

Season: Rainy season.

Case Classification

- *Confirmed:* Acute onset of a flaccid paralysis of one or more limbs with decreased or absent tendon reflexes in the affected limbs, without other apparent cause, and without sensory or cognitive loss; and in which the patient has a neurologic deficit 60 days after onset of initial symptoms; or has died; or has unknown follow-up status.
- *Probable:* Acute onset of a flaccid paralysis of one or more limbs with decreased or absent tendon reflexes in the affected limbs, without other apparent cause, and without sensory or cognitive loss.

Pathophysiology

The virus enters the mouth and multiplies in lymphoid tissues in the pharynx and intestine. The virus hijacks the host cell's own machinery, and begins to replicate. Poliovirus divides within gastrointestinal cells for about a week, from where it spreads to the tonsils, the intestinal lymphoid tissue (Peyer's patches), and the deep cervical and mesenteric lymph nodes, where it multiplies abundantly. Poliovirus can survive and multiply within the blood and lymphatics for long periods of time, sometimes as long as 17 weeks. In a small percentage of cases, it can spread and replicate in other sites, such as brown fat, the reticuloendothelial tissues, and muscle.

Contd...

Contd...

This sustained replication of virus causes a major viremia, and leads to the development of minor influenza-like symptoms. Rarely, this may progress and the virus may invade the central nervous system (CNS), and a local inflammatory response may also occur. In most cases, this causes a self-limiting inflammation of the meninges, which is known as non-paralytic aseptic meningitis. Penetration of the CNS provides no known benefit to the virus. Poliovirus spreads along certain nerve fiber (possibly through olfactory) pathways, preferentially replicating in and destroying motor neurons within the spinal cord, brain stem, or motor cortex The mechanisms by which poliovirus spreads to the CNS are poorly understood, but it appears to be primarily a chance event—largely independent of the age, gender, or socioeconomic position of the individual.

In brief, the virus, which enters the body through either ingestion or inhalation, has a preference for the CNS, affecting only certain cells, such as the anterior horn cells of the spinal cord.

Types of Poliomyelitis and Clinical Manifestations

Poliomyelitis may be classified according to its clinical manifestations:

Subclinical/asymptomatic poliomyelitis: Approximately 95% of polio cases are subclinical, and patients may not experience any symptoms. This form of polio does not affect the CNS.

Abortive Poliomyelitis

Polio can be a minor illness, as it is in 80–90% of clinical infections, chiefly in young children, and not involve the CNS. Due to viremia it may manifest as fever, headaches, gastrointestinal upset and sore throat. Polio virus can be isolated from throat washings and stool. It can be interpreted that polio viruses are growing in gut and throat lymphatic tissue and have not migrated to the spinal cord or brain. Postpolio syndrome (PPS) would be unlikely in these cases because of the lack of neurological involvement to any appreciable extent. Recovery occurs in 24–72 hours. This is termed the abortive type of polio.

Nonparalytic

This form, which does affect the CNS, produces only mild symptoms and does not result in paralysis. Symptoms are fever, severe headache, stiff neck and back, deep muscle pain, and sometimes areas of hyperesthesia (increased sensation) and paresthesia (altered sensation). There may be no further progression from this picture of viral meningitis or there be loss of tendon reflexes and weakness or paralysis of muscle groups. The patient may be febrile due to viremia and may complain of nausea and vomiting. Muscle strength

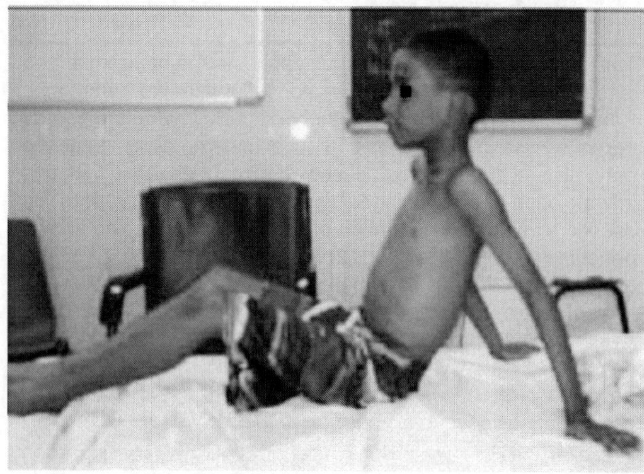

Fig. 20.7: The elicitation of the tripod sign: The child when asked to sit up tries to sit up by supporting himself with his hands placed behind him like a tripod

testing at this time and after fever breaks does not show weakness, however, there is probably undetectable permanent nerve damage to some extent. Theoretically PPS should be possible.

The signs need to be elicited are kiss the knee test, tripod sign, head drop sign and neck rigidity:

Kiss the Knee Test

The test is positive when the child fails to kiss his own knees without bending the knees. This occurs due to neck rigidity.

Tripod Sign

A nuchal-spinal sign in which the sitting position requires a rigid spine and both arms extended towardsthe back for support, typically seen in children with nonparalytic poliomyelitis (Fig. 20.7).

Head Drop Signs

By raising an infant's trunk at the shoulders; a head that dropsbackward suggests nuchal limpness typical of paralytic and non-paralytic poliomyelitis.

Paralytic Polio Myelitis

This is the rarest and most serious form of polio (in and around 1%) which produces full or partial paralysis in the patient. Types of paralytic polio vary only with the amount of neural damage and inflammation that occurs, and the region of the CNS affected. Spinal polio, bulbar polio (affects the brainstem), bulbo-spinal and encephalitic polio. Some areas which are not usually affected by the viruses are the white mater of the spinal cord, cerebellar hemispheres and nonmotor part of the cerebral cortex. According to the World Health Organization (WHO), one in 200 polio infections will result in permanent paralysis.

- *Spinal type:* The peak of paralysis is reached within the first week. In spinal poliomyelitis, viral replication occurs in the anterior horn cells of the spine, causing inflammation, swelling, and, if severe, destruction of the neurons. The large proximal muscles of the limbs are most often affected muscle pain, hyperaesthesia, tremors, diminished deep tendon reflexes precede asymmetrical flaccid paralysis. Flaccid paralysis is commonly developed in the lower limbs and it also affects the large muscles than small muscles. Involvement of diaphragm and intercostal muscles may cause respiratory difficulty. There is no sensory loss in affected part.
- Bulbar poliomyelitis results from viral multiplication in the brainstem. It is a severe form affecting the medulla oblongata, which may result in dysfunction of the swallowing mechanism, respiratory embarrassment, and circulatory distress. Atelectasis and pneumonia may develop due to regurgitation of fluid and aspiration of secretions. Shallow and irregular breathing, with diminished oxygen saturation, rapid, thread pulse, rise in blood pressure, dusky red and mottled skin are the outcome of the paralysis in the medullary centres. The child becomes restless, confused and unconscious.
- *Bulbospinal poliomyelitis:* Both the features of bulbar and spinal form of paralysis are present in this patient. About 25% cases of paralytic polio belong to this category of poliomyelitis.
- *Encephalitic poliomyelitis:* irritability, tremors, drowsiness, convulsions and unconsciousness are often seen in this polio. Paralysis may upper motor neuron type.

Postpolio syndrome is a complication that can occur after a person has caught and recovered from poliovirus. Symptoms of the syndrome can appear up to 35 years after the polio infection.

Diagnostic Evaluation

Polio is diagnosed through medical history, physical examination. Case classification is done in following ways:

Confirmed

Acute onset of a flaccid paralysis of one or more limbs with decreased or absent tendon reflexes in the affected limbs, without other apparent cause, and without sensory or cognitive loss; and in which the patient has a neurologic deficit 60 days after onset of initial symptoms; or has died; or has unknown follow-up status.

Probable

Acute onset of a flaccid paralysis of one or more limbs with decreased or absent tendon reflexes in the affected limbs, without other apparent cause, and without sensory or cognitive loss.

- The likelihood of poliovirus isolation is highest from stool specimens, intermediate from pharyngeal swabs, and low from blood or spinal fluid. The isolation of poliovirus from stool specimens contributes to the diagnostic evaluation. To increase the probability of poliovirus isolation, at least two stool specimens should be obtained 24 hours apart from patients with suspected poliomyelitis as early in the course of disease as possible (ideally within 14 days after onset).
- Isolation of virus from the cerebrospinal fluid (CSF) is diagnostic but is rarely accomplished (LP is best to avoid, as it may cause development of paralysis). Bacterial meningitis is excluded through CSF study which shows increase in cells and inconsistent elevation of protein.
- Isolation of wild poliovirus constitutes a public health emergency and appropriate control efforts must be initiated.

Therapeutic Management

Because there is no cure for polio, supportive therapy is the main treatment. Improving a child's chance of recovery is the main goal of treatment. This type of treatment helps minimize discomfort and prevent complications while the child recovers. Supportive treatment may include medications for polio symptoms, ventilators to help the person breathe, exercise, and a balanced diet.

Polio is not a treatable disease, yet it is almost completely preventable. Vaccination with the polio vaccine provides the most effective form of prevention. Childhood immunization programs protect from infection by the poliovirus.

Acute Stage

In the acute stage, the treatment is mainly medical means general supportive treatment for the pyrexia and irritation, for the prevention of secondary respiratory infection, and for the treatment of any respiratory paralysis are the main aspects of the treatment. The paralyzed legs are supported by plaster splints or pillows and sandbags to keep the hip joints in 5° of flexion and in neutral rotation. The knee joint is held at 5° of flexion, and the foot is supported in a 90° position. Splinting relieves pain and spasm and prevents the development of deformities.

Recovery Stage

Treatment in the recovery stage is mainly by the orthopedic department, involving physiotherapy and splinting. The aims of treatment are to assist in the recovery of paralyzed muscles by remedial exercises and to prevent deformities by the use of orthotic devices. At first the muscle power of the limbs, extent of contractures and deformities, method of ambulation, shortening of the limb are assessed by grading chart.

Efficient physiotherapy in the management of paralytic polio includes exercise therapy, hydrotherapy, and electrical stimulation of muscles, etc. Physical therapy includes exercises that strengthen the leg muscles, maintain the range of motion in knee and ankle, improve gait problems associated with foot drops.

Orthotic Treatment

Appropriate orthotic appliances are prescribed to prevent deformities due to muscle imbalance and to stabilize the joints. There are currently many various types of orthoses, and the range of devices available to the prescriber continues to increase with the advent of new materials such as carbon fiber, as well as advances in manufacturing techniques. Orthoses are available for all parts of the body and aid in conservative and definitive treatment for many deformities.

Many patients require revision of orthotic devices such as braces, canes, and crutches or may use new, lighter orthotic devices to treat new symptoms. Common issues include genu recurvatum, knee pain, back pain, degenerative arthritis, or arthralgia. Surgery for scoliosis or fractures may also be necessary to treat new conditions. Appropriate orthotic appliances are prescribed to prevent deformities due to muscle imbalance. Orthotic devices like ankle-foot orthosis'/ below-knee orthosis or caliper is used when the power of muscles controlling the hip and knee are normal and the weakness is only in the dorsiflexors or plantar flexors of the ankle or invertors or evertors of the foot. When the quadriceps power is low, the knee has to be stabilized and hence a knee-ankle-foot orthosis (full or above-knee caliper) is prescribed.

TREATMENT OF RESIDUAL PARALYSIS

The final aim should be for patients to return home and be accepted and integrated into their communities. Since overuse weakness is frequently present in these patients, the role of slowly progressive, nonfatiguing exercise in their rehabilitation is emphasized. New muscle weakness of a mild-to-moderate degree responds well to a nonfatiguing exercise program and pacing of activity, with rest periods to avoid muscle overuse. Generalized fatigue may be treated with energy conservation, weight-loss programs, and lower-extremity orthoses.

An orthosis is a device that externally supports an existing body part, with the objective of supporting, correcting, or compensating for skeletal deformity or weakness. There are currently many various types of orthoses (Fig. 20.8), and the range of devices available to the prescriber continues to increase with the advent of new materials such as carbon fiber, as well as advances in manufacturing techniques. Orthoses are available for all parts of the body and aid in conservative and definitive treatment for many deformities. The thermoplastic leaf spring AFO, or drop foot splint, is one good example of an orthosis commonly used. It assists dorsiflexion and uses 3-point pressure to stabilize the ankle joint.

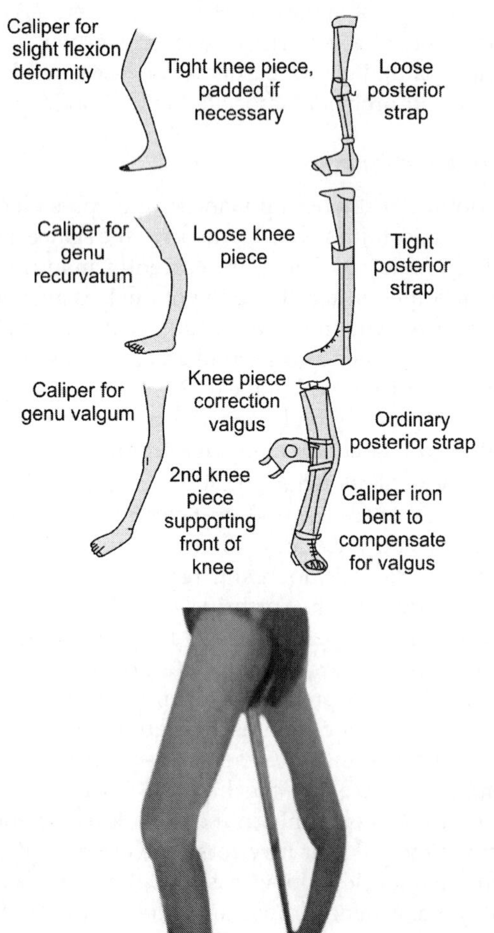

Fig. 20.8: Special supports for deformed knees in poliomyelitis

Prevention

The first safe, effective vaccine against polio used killed polioviruses to stimulate production and release of antibodies. It was developed under the direction of Dr Jonas E Salk, and was nicknamed the **Salk vaccine.** It was replaced by an oral preparation of attenuated viruses called **poliovirus vaccine live oral**, nicknamed the **Sabin vaccine** after its discoverer, Dr Albert Sabin. It does not induce intestinal immunity and so is not effective for poliovirus eradication in areas where wild-type polioviruses still exist in large numbers. However, it does not cause vaccine-associated paralytic poliomyelitis and so is preferred for routine immunization in areas where the risk of infection by a wild-type poliovirus is very low.

Current eradication strategies recommended by WHO have proved successful; these four strategies are:

1. High, routine infant immunization coverage with at least three doses of oral polio vaccine (OPV) (Fig. 20.9), plus a dose at birth in polio-endemic countries;
2. National immunization days (NIDs) targeting all children.
3. Acute flaccid paralysis (AFP) surveillance and laboratory investigations; and
4. Mop-up immunization campaigns to interrupt final chains of transmission.

Wild poliovirus has not been found in India since 13 January 2011 meaning that, from that date, India is no longer a country where polio is endemic. Three years of being polio free is a notable milestone for the country as a whole, but the success of the immunization and awareness campaign has had a wider impact. With this achievement, it is hoped that soon the entire WHO South-East Asia Region can be certified polio free. According to the forty-first World Health Assembly1988 resolution, no single country can be certified as polio

Fig. 20.9: Campaigning for polio vaccine

free; WHO Regions as a whole are certified as polio free. For certification, all countries in the WHO Region need to not register a case of wild polio for 3 years in the presence of high quality surveillance.

Nursing Considerations

Complete bed rest, and place the child on firm mattress with support for feet, change position frequently. Encourage a return to mild activity as soon as possible.

Maintain a patent airway, and keep a tracheotomy tray at the patient's bed side. In bulbar polio, therapy is directed at suctioning of pharynx, postural drainage, IV fluid, tracheostomy, oxygen, respirator.

Help the child in physiotherapy. Apply moist heat to decrease muscular pain. Provide good skin care, reposition.

Encourage oral intake of food and fluid. Provide tube feedings when needed.

Prevent fecal impaction by giving enough fluids to ensure an adequate daily urine output of low specific gravity. Catheterization of distended bladder may be necessary. Antibacterial prophylaxis may be ordered. Good disposal of stool because it is infectious.

Prolong rehabilitation may be necessary including braces, splint or surgery. Postpolio syndrome (PPS) is treated with rest and such supportive measures as powered wheelchairs, pain relievers, and medications to help the patient sleep. Children are also encouraged to simple work and play and take frequent rest.

There is hope that polio will follow smallpox as a disease that humankind has completely wiped out. Public health professionals hope that the vaccination campaigns that are underway by the nurses will clear the disease in the next few years.

Mumps

Causative agent: Paramyxovirus

Incubation period: Usually from 16 to 18 days but may extend to 25 days.

Infectious period: The virus may be found in the saliva for one to six days before the glands swell and for the duration of glandular enlargement (5–9 days).

Transmission: The disease is transmitted mainly by droplet infections, and after direct contact with an infected person.

Immunity: Natural, through disease, live attenuated virus. The presence of maternal antibodies typically protects infants younger than 1 year from the disease.

Season: Late winter, spring.

Manifestations

Subclinical infection is common. The prodromal period tends to be rather nonspecific and may include a low grade fever, anorexia, malaise, and headache. Parotitis (unilateral or bilateral) is the most common manifestation occurring in 30–40% of cases. Parotid swelling may occur with fever. Pain on chewing or swallowing, is one of the earliest symptoms. Sublingual or submandibular glands may also be affected.

Complications

Mumps is generally a disorder of parotid gland, but can affect other organs too. Complications include CNS involvement, orchitis, oophoritis, and deafness. Orchitis occurs in 20–30% of postpubertal males, usually unilaterally. Oophoritis in females occurs less often (5%) and may mimic appendicitis. Sterility is an extremely rare sequela.

The CNS is involved in about 15% of cases, either early or late in the disease, most often as aseptic meningitis (resolving in one to three days) and most often without sequelae. Hearing loss caused by mumps was relatively common in the pre-vaccine era and still occurs occasionally. Encephalitis is rare, occurring in 1–10% of patients manifested by a headache and stiff neck. Less common complications of mumps include arthralgia, pancreatitis (4% of cases), prostatitis, nephritis, myocarditis, mastitis, polyarthritis and lacrimal gland involvement.

Mumps during the first trimester of pregnancy may increase the rate of spontaneous abortion. There is no firm evidence that mumps during pregnancy causes congenital malformations.

Diagnostic Evaluation

During an epidemic, the clinical diagnosis of mumps is easy, however when cases are sporadic the clinical diagnosis is less reliable. The IgM antibodies are usually present at the onset of illness (when glands are swollen) and reach a maximum level one week later. They may be present for several weeks or months following the illness, and decline with time (usually four to eight weeks). Recent vaccination with mumps vaccine or MMR can elicit a mumps IgM antibody response. The IgG antibodies are also detectable at the onset of illness reaching a peak in convalescence, then slowly declining over many years or decades. Mumps IgM and IgG EIA serologic tests are most commonly available for laboratory diagnosis and confirmation of a suspect case. Recent data shows that mumps IgM antibody can be negative or indeterminate or the IgM response delayed in symptomatic individuals previously vaccinated with one or two doses of mumps-containing vaccine at the appropriate intervals. Mumps may also be confirmed by isolation of the virus in cell culture inoculated with throat washings (nasopharyngeal swab), saliva, urine or CSF, or by the detection of viral RNA by PCR in these samples.

Therapeutic Management

Generally, supportive therapy is indicated for uncomplicated mumps. There is no specific treatment for mumps. The disease is generally self-limiting, running its course before receding, with no specific treatment apart from controlling the symptoms with pain medication and substances to reduce fevers such as acetaminophen. Use of aspirin is to be avoided because of the potential risk of developing Reye syndrome. Warm saltwater gargles, soft foods, and extra fluids may also help relieve symptoms. However, hospitalization may be required if meningitis or pancreatitis develops.

Prevention

The most common preventative measure against mumps is a vaccination with a mumps vaccine, invented by American microbiologist Maurice Hilleman at Merck. The vaccine may be given separately or as part of the MMR immunization vaccine that also protects against measles and rubella. This principal strategy to prevent mumps needs to achieve and maintain high immunization levels, primarily in infants and young children. Universal immunization as part of good health care should be routinely carried out. Programs aimed at vaccinating children with MMR should be established and maintained in all communities. In addition, all other persons thought to be susceptible should be vaccinated, unless otherwise contraindicated. This is especially important for adolescents and young adults in light of the past observed increased risk of disease in these populations. Aware parents and educators to exclude infected children from large-population facilities, until 9 days after parotid swelling begins or until this swelling subsides.

Advise all children and adults to follow good hand washing practices.

CHICKENPOX (VARICELLA-ZOSTER, SHINGLES)

Varicella is an acute infectious disease. It is caused by varicella-zoster virus (VZV), which is a DNA virus that is a member of the herpes virus group. The disease is generally regarded as a mild, self-limiting viral illness with occasional complications. After the primary infection, VZV stays in the body (in the sensory nerve ganglia) as a latent infection. Primary infection with VZV causes varicella. Reactivation of latent infection causes herpes zoster (shingles). However, varicella is not totally benign even today. A significant number of varicella cases are associated with complications, among the most serious of which are varicella pneumonia and encephalitis.

Causative agent: Varicella-Zoster virus

Incubation period: 10–21 days.

Infectious period: One to two days before the onset of rash, and 4–5 days thereafter.

Transmission: Varicella is highly contagious. The virus spreads in the air when an infected person coughs or sneezes.

Immunity: Recovery from primary varicella infection usually provides immunity for life. In otherwise healthy people, a second occurrence of varicella is uncommon and usually occurs in people who are immunocompromised.

Season: Most cases occur during the winter and spring.

Manifestations

A mild prodrome of fever and malaise may occur 1–2 days before rash onset, particularly in adults. In children, the rash is often the first sign of disease. The rash is generalized and pruritic (itchy). It progresses rapidly from macules to papules to vesicular lesions before crusting. The rash usually appears first on the head, chest, and back then spreads to the rest of the body (pleomorphic rash) (Fig. 20.10). The lesions are usually most concentrated on the chest and back. The most common other presenting symptoms of varicella are complaints of abdominal pain by some children, headache, malaise, anorexia, cough and coryza, sore throat.

Diagnosis

In general, laboratory studies are unnecessary for diagnosis, because varicella is clinically obvious. However, some tests and procedures may be helpful in confirming the diagnosis or identifying complications. Imaging studies are typically not required for varicella unless secondary complications are a concern (e.g. chest radiography for varicella pneumonia).

Therapeutic Management

Treatment approaches include supportive measures, antiviral therapy, administration of varicella zoster

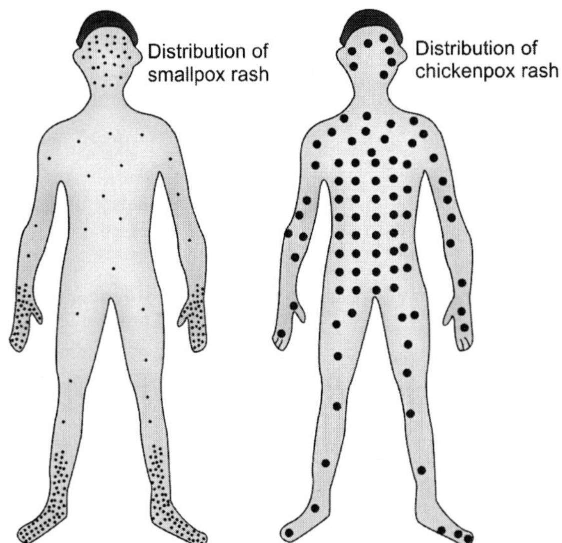

Fig. 20.10: Distribution of rash both in chickenpox and smallpox

immune globulin (VZIG), and management of secondary bacterial infection. Medications used in the treatment of varicella include antivirals, antipyretics, antihistamines, and immune globulin. Early recognition of secondary bacterial infection and appropriate follow-up are major issues. Failure to recognize occult infection may result in serious illness and even death.

Isolate patients with varicella because the disease is highly contagious and airborne spread can occur. Isolation is especially important if the hospital also admits patients who are immunocompromised because their exposure to the disease can be serious and even fatal.

Manage pruritus in patients with varicella with cool compresses and regular bathing. Discourage scratching to avoid scarring. Trimming the child's fingernails and having the child wear mittens while sleeping may reduce scratching.

Warm soaks and oatmeal or cornstarch baths may reduce itching and provide comfort. Topical calamine lotion may produce caking of lesions and excessive drying of the skin, causing the child to scratch. Oral antihistamines, such as diphenhydramine and hydroxyzine, are used for severe pruritus. Caution must be used with topical diphenhydramine; toxicity may occur from systemic absorption if it is applied to the entire body.

Because of the association of varicella and aspirin therapy leading to Reye syndrome, acetaminophen is recommended for use for the reduction of fever.

The routine use of acyclovir or valacyclovir in healthy children is recommended by the AAP if it can be given within 24 hours after the rash first appears in children older than 12 years, those with chronic cutaneous or pulmonary disorders, those on long-tern salicylate therapy, and children receiving corticosteroids. Intravenous acyclovir is recommended only for the treatment of varicella in immunocompromised children or in healthy children with varicella pneumonia or encephalitis. In some instances, acyclovir may be considered for teenagers and adults with otherwise uncomplicated varicella. Additionally, antiviral therapy should be considered for patients with recent steroid use or those with extensive eczema.

Varicella zoster immune globulin is indicated for high-risk individuals within 10 days (ideally within 4 days) of chickenpox exposure. This agent reduces complications and the mortality rate of varicella, not its incidence. It is used as postexposure prophylaxis in high-risk individuals; for immunologically normal patients, post-exposure prophylaxis using varicella vaccine is preferred. High risk groups include:

- Immunocompromised children and adults
- Newborns of mothers with varicella shortly before or after delivery
- Premature infants
- Infants less than one year of age

When maternal varicella has developed within 5 days before or 2 days after delivery, neonatal varicella is likely to be severe and disseminated. Prophylaxis or treatment is required with VZIG and acyclovir. Without these drugs, mortality rates may be as high as 30%. The primary causes of death are severe pneumonia and fulminant hepatitis.

If the onset of maternal varicella is more than 5 days ante partum, a full-term neonate will usually have only mild varicella. Treatment with VZIG is not recommended in such cases, but acyclovir may be used, depending on individual circumstance.

A high level of suspicion is necessary for early recognition and timely appropriate treatment of secondary infections. Suspect secondary infection if systemic manifestations do not improve in 3–4 days, the fever returns or worsens, or the child's condition deteriorates after initial improvement. Suspicion of secondary bacterial infection should prompt early institution of empirical antibiotic therapy until the results of culture studies become available.

Dietary measure: Advise parents to provide a full and unrestricted diet to the child. Some children with varicella have reduced appetite and should be encouraged to take sufficient fluids to maintain hydration. Adequate hydration is especially important if the child is receiving acyclovir because the drug can crystallize in the renal tubules if administered to dehydrated individuals.

The duration of the visible blistering caused by varicella zoster virus varies in children usually from 4 to 7 days, and the appearance of new blisters begins to subside after the 5th day. Chickenpox infection is milder in young children, and symptomatic treatment, with sodium bicarbonate baths or antihistamine medication may ease itching.

DENGUE

Dengue fever is caused by dengue virus infection, which is transmitted by *Aedes aegypti* or *Aedes albopictus* mosquitoes that carry one of the four serologically distinct DENV. There are an estimated 390 million new infections per year in tropical and subtropical regions. Usually incubation period is 3–10 days but may extend to 25 days. Infectious period is 7 days before swelling to 9–10 days after onset.

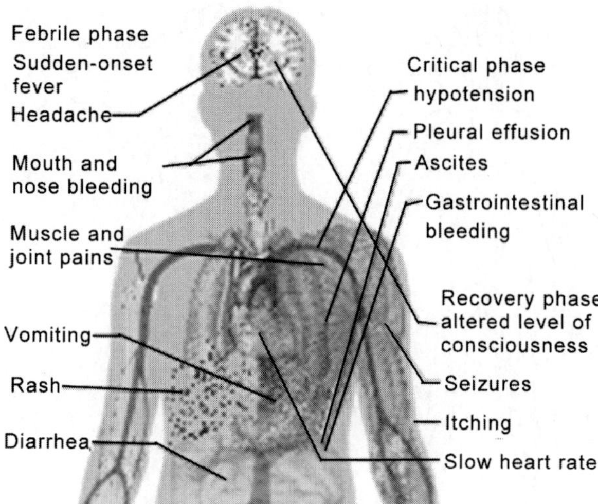

Fig. 20.11: Symptoms of dengue fever

Manifestations

Symptoms are usually begin 4–6 days after infection and last for up to 10 days. Clinically, high fever, rash, lethargy and severe joint and muscle pain are the most common presentations of DENV infection. Along with this, retro-orbital pain on eye movement or pressure and photophobia, nausea, vomiting, sore throat, chest pain, abdominal discomfort (Fig. 20.11). Skin rash usually appears 3–4 days after the onset of fever. The child generally recovers.

Sometimes symptoms are mild and can be mistaken for those of the flu or another viral infection. Younger children and people who have never had the infection before tend to have milder cases than older children and adults.

Dengue hemorrhagic fever: Early symptoms of dengue hemorrhagic fever are similar to those of dengue fever. But after several days the patient becomes irritable, restless, and sweaty. However, serious problems can develop. The dengue hemorrhagic fever, a rare complication characterized by high fever, damage to lymph and blood vessels, bleeding from the nose and gums, enlargement of the liver, and failure of the circulatory system. Bleeding appears as tiny spots of blood on the skin (petechiae) and larger patches of blood under the skin (ecchymoses). Minor injuries can cause bleeding. Epistaxis, hematemesis and malena may present. The Hess test (tourniquet) is usually positive. These symptoms are followed by a shock-like state or child may recover spontaneously. People with weakened immune systems as well as those with a second or subsequent dengue infection are believed to be at greater risk for developing dengue hemorrhagic fever.

Dengue shock syndrome (DSS): Shock syndrome is a dangerous complication of dengue infection and is associated with high mortality. Severe dengue occurs as a result of secondary infection with a different virus serotype. DSS is characterized by abdominal pain, hemorrhage and circulatory collapse. Shock occurs after 2–6 days with sudden collapse, cool clammy extremities, weak thready pulse, and blueness around the mouth (circumoral cyanosis). Increased vascular permeability, together with myocardial dysfunction and dehydration, contribute to the development of shock, with resultant multi organ failure. The symptoms may progress to massive bleeding, shock, and death. The only known effective treatment in DSS is timely and aggressive fluid resuscitation.

Diagnostic Evaluation

Diagnosis of dengue infection is easily and best accomplished by demonstration of specific IgM antibodies in blood.

Other tests may include arterial blood gases, blood tests (find signs of the virus in the blood), coagulation studies, electrolytes, hematocrit, liver enzymes, platelet count, Serum studies from samples taken during acute illness and convalescence (increase in titer to Dengue antigen), Tourniquet test (causes petechiae to form below the tourniquet), X-ray of the chest (may demonstrate pleural effusion).

Therapeutic Management

Current treatment strategies are mostly geared towards the alleviation of symptoms and the prevention of shock by fluid resuscitation with colloid or crystalloid solutions.

Because dengue hemorrhagic fever is caused by a virus for which there is no known cure or vaccine, the only treatment is to treat the symptoms.

- A transfusion of fresh blood or platelets can correct bleeding problems
- Intravenous fluids and electrolytes are also used to correct electrolyte imbalances
- Oxygen therapy may be needed to treat abnormally low blood oxygen
- Rehydration with IV fluids is often necessary to treat dehydration
- Supportive care in an intensive care unit/ environment.

Prevention

Mosquitoes carrying dengue viruses mainly breed in water containers in the house and on the environment. Control of this dengue vector can be accomplished by source reduction, which includes covering, emptying and cleaning the water storage containers regularly and eliminating containers or solid waste that may accumulate water for mosquito breeding. Alternatively, another effective strategy to control the spread of DENV is to kill the mosquito vector. Traditional methods of spraying with the insecticide dichlorodiphenyltrichloroethane (DDT) have been very effective for killing the mosquito vectors of DENV and malaria. However, due to the potential impact of DDT on human health and the environment, this chemical was banned by the Stockholm Convention on Persistent Organic Pollutants in 2004.

RABIES

Rabies is a viral disease, the deadly virus spread to people from the saliva of infected animals. Rabies causes acute inflammation of the brain in humans and other warm-blooded animals. Rabies causes about 26,000 to 55,000 deaths worldwide per year. More than 95% of these deaths occur in Asia and Africa.

Causative agent: Rhabdovirus

Incubation period: Incubation period is 2–12 weeks in humans. Incubation periods as short as four days and longer than six years have been documented, depending on the location and severity of the contaminated wound and the amount of virus introduced.

Infectious period: Ten days (if the animal is still healthy, rabies is unlikely)

Transmission: Rabies is transmitted to humans from infected animals bites (contaminated saliva) and scratches from claws of infected animals. Airborne transmission in laboratory setting, through transplantation of corneas from undiagnosed donors also may occur.

Most rabies cases in humans are the result of dog bites (more than 99% of cases), in the Americans, bat bites are the most common source of rabies infections in humans.

Immunity: Human diploid cell vaccine (HDCV).

Season: Can occur any time in the year.

Pathogenesis

After a typical human infection by bite, the virus enters the peripheral nervous system. It then travels along the afferent nerves toward the CNS. During this phase, the virus cannot be easily detected within the host, and vaccination may still confer cell-mediated immunity to prevent symptomatic rabies. When the virus reaches the brain, it rapidly causes encephalitis, the prodromal phase, and is the beginning of the symptoms. Once the patient becomes symptomatic, treatment is almost never effective and mortality is over 99%. Rabies may also inflame the spinal cord, producing transverse myelitis.

Manifestations

Rabies is a slowly developing infection. Initially, patient presents flu like symptoms. If the patient is left untreated, he/she may complain not feeling well, headache, sore throat, discomfort at the site of bite. Signs and symptoms may soon expand to hyper activity, muscle spasm or convulsions, slight or partial paralysis, anxiety, insomnia, confusion, agitation, abnormal behavior, paranoia, terror, and hallucinations, progressing to delirium. The person may have hydrophobia.

Hydrophobia: Hydrophobia ('fear of water') is the historic name for rabies. It refers to a set of symptoms in the later stages of an infection in which the patient has difficulty swallowing, shows panic when presented with liquids to drink, and cannot quench his or her thirst. Saliva production is greatly increased, and attempts to drink, or even the intention or suggestion of drinking, may cause excruciatingly painful spasms of the muscles in the throat and larynx. The decreased ability to swallow of patient results in drooling or aspiration. Death almost always occurs 2–10 days after first symptoms.

Diagnostic Evaluation

History of Bite or Scratch of Animals

Rabies is diagnosed by testing saliva, blood samples, spinal fluid, and skin samples. Multiple tests may be necessary. The tests rely on detection of proteins on the surface of the rabies virus, detection of the genetic material of the virus, or demonstration of an antibody (immune) response to the virus.

Therapeutic Management

Almost all human cases of rabies were fatal until a vaccine was developed in 1885 by Louis Pasteur and Émile Roux. Till today the focus of rabies management is preventive, i.e. to avoid touching and petting strange animals, proper vaccination of pets and keep them away from wild and outdoor animals. Vaccination against rabies is used in two distinct situations, where vaccination are the same, but the immunization schedule differs.

- To protect those who are at risk of exposure to rabies, i.e. pre-exposure vaccination;
- To prevent the development of clinical rabies after exposure has occurred, usually following the bite of an animal suspected of having rabies, i.e. post-exposure prophylaxis (Table 20.1).

Pre-exposure vaccination should be offered to people at high risk of exposure to rabies, such as laboratory staff working with rabies virus, veterinarians, etc. This vaccination consists of three full intramuscular (IM) doses of cell-culture- or embryonated-egg-based vaccine given on days 0, 7 and 21 or 28 (a few days' variation in the timing is not important). For adults, the vaccine should always be administered in the deltoid area of the arm; for young children (under 1 year of age), the anterolateral area of the thigh is recommended. Rabies vaccine should never be administered in the gluteal area: administration in this manner will result in lower neutralizing antibody titres.

Treatment is recommended if a health-care professional thinks that someone was exposed to a potentially rabid animal. Treatment after exposure can prevent the disease if administered promptly, generally within 10 days of infection. Strict adherence to the WHO-recommended guidelines for optimal postexposure rabies prophylaxis virtually guarantees protection from the disease. The administration of vaccine, and immunoglobulin if required, must be conducted by, or under the direct supervision of, a physician. Post-exposure prophylaxis depends on the type of contact with the confirmed or suspect rabid animal, as follows:

Wound Treatment

Thorough washing of the wound with soap/detergent and water, followed by the application of ethanol or an aqueous solution of iodine or povidone.

Passive Immunization

Human rabies immunoglobulin (HRIG) or equine rabies immunoglobulin (ERIG) should be used for category III exposures (Table 20.1). Passive immunization should be administered just before or shortly after administration of the first dose of vaccine given in the postexposure prophylaxis regimen. If it is not immediately available, passive immunization can be administered up until the seventh day after initiation of the primary series of postexposure prophylaxis (with cell-culture or embryonated-egg rabies vaccine).

Dosage and Administration

The dose for HRIG is 20 IU/kg body weight and for ERIG 40 IU/kg body weight. The full dose of rabies immunoglobulin, or as much as is anatomically feasible, should be administered into and around the wound site. Any remainder should be injected IM at a site distant from the site of active vaccine administration. Multiple needle injections into the wound should be avoided. If the correct dose of rabies immunoglobulin is too small to infiltrate all wounds, as might be true of a severely bitten individual, it can be diluted in physiological buffered saline to ensure greater wound coverage.

Active Immunization

Cell-culture- or embryonated-egg-based rabies vaccines should always be used for postexposure prophylaxis. They can be administered either IM or ID.

Intramuscular Regimens

Both a five-dose and a four-dose IM regimen are recommended for postexposure vaccination; the fivedose regimen is the more commonly used:

- The five-dose regimen is administered on days 0, 3, 7, 14 and 28 into the deltoid muscle.
- The four-dose regimen is administered as two doses on day 0 (one dose in the right and one in the left

Table 20.1: Type of contact, exposure and recommended postexposure prophylaxis of rabies

Category	*Type of contact with a suspected or confirmed rabid domestic or wild[a] animal or animal unavailable for testing*	*Type of exposure*	*Recommended postexposure prophylaxis*
I	Touching or feeding of animals Licks on intact skin	None	None, if reliable case history is available
II	Nibbling of uncovered skin Minor scratches or abrasions without bleeding	Minor	Administer vaccine immediately. Stop treatment if animal remains healthy throughout an observation period of 10 days[b] or is proved to be negative for rabies by a reliable laboratory using appropriate diagnostic techniques
III	Single or multiple transdermal bites or scratches, licks on broken skin Contamination of mucous membrane with saliva (i.e. licks) Exposure to bats	Severe	Administer rabies immunoglobulin and vaccine immediately. Stop treatment if animal remains healthy throughout an observation period of 10 days or is proved to be negative for rabies by a reliable laboratory using appropriate diagnostic techniques

[a]Exposure to rodents, rabbits and hares seldom, if ever, requires specific anti-rabies post-exposure prophylaxis.

[b]This observation period applies only to dogs and cats. Except in the case of threatened or endangered species, other domestic and wild animals suspected to be rabid should be humanely killed and their tissues examined for the presence of rabies antigen using appropriate laboratory techniques.

arm (deltoid muscles), and then one dose on each of days 7 and 21 into the deltoid muscle.

An alternative postexposure regimen for healthy, fully immunocompetent exposed people who receive wound care plus high-quality rabies immunoglobulin plus WHO-prequalified rabies vaccines consists of four doses administered IM on days 0, 3, 7 and 14.

Intradermal regimens: Intradermal administration of cell-culture- and embryonated-egg-based rabies vaccines has been successfully used in many developing countries that cannot afford the five- or four-dose IM schedules.

- *The two-site ID method:* One ID injection at two sites on days 0, 3, 7 and 28.

The volume per intradermal injection should be 0.1 mL with both purified Vero cell rabies vaccine, and purified chick embryo rabies vaccine.

> Induced Coma (Milwaukee protocol): In 2004, American teenager Jeanna Giese survived an infection of rabies unvaccinated. She was placed into an induced coma upon onset of symptoms and given ketamine, midazolam, ribavirin, and amantadine. Her doctors administered treatment based on the hypothesis that detrimental effects of rabies were caused by temporary dysfunctions in the brain and could be avoided by inducing a temporary partial halt in brain function that would protect the brain from damage while giving the immune system time to defeat the virus. After 31 days of isolation and 76 days of hospitalization, Giese was released from the hospital. She survived with all higher level brain functions, but an inability to walk and balance.

HIV INFECTION

HIV (human immunodeficiency virus) is the virus that causes an acquired cell mediated immunodeficiency disorder. The virus damages or destroys the cells of the immune system, leaving them unable to fight infections and certain cancers. AIDS (acquired immune deficiency syndrome) is the most advanced manifestation of illness. As defined by the US Centers for Disease Control and Prevention (US), a person has AIDS when HIV has drastically reduced his or her CD4 cell count, or when a person living with HIV is diagnosed with at least one opportunistic infection.

According to the WHO, an estimated 3.2 million children age 15 and under were living with AIDS at the end of 2013, and about 91% of infected children are residing at sub-Saharan Africa. An estimated 260,000 children were newly infected with HIV in 2012; further, nearly 700 children are newly infected with HIV every day.

(UNAIDS, *Global Report*, 2014).

Etiology

Most HIV infections in children are passed from mother to child during pregnancy, labor and delivery, or breastfeeding. The incidence of mother-to-child HIV transmission is decreasing. Since the mid-1990s, HIV testing and preventive drug regimens have started since the mid-1990s.

HIV is spread when blood, semen, or vaginal fluids from an infected person enter another person's body or adolescent's body, usually through sexual contact, from sharing needles when injecting drugs, or from mother to baby during birth. Other causes of child HIV include:

Blood transfusions: Using infected blood through blood transfusion or injections with unsterilized needles can lead to HIV infection in children. In the wealthier countries this problem has been virtually eliminated, but in developing countries this still occurs.

Illicit drug use: Injected drug use continues to spread HIV among young people living on the streets. High-risk behaviors, including sharing needles, have been among children as young as age 10 years.

Sexual transmission: Although, sexual transmission is not a main cause of HIV/AIDS among children, children may be infected with HIV if they become sexually active at an early age. Children may also become infected through sexual abuse or rape.

Pathophysiology

The immune system protects the body by recognizing antigens on invading bacteria and viruses and reacting to them. But HIV is more complicated, it starts to destroy CD4+ cells, with the help of RNA and an enzyme reverse transcriptase, this enzyme plays a key role in viral replication. HIV lifecycle includes six phases: binding and entry, reverse transcription, integration, replication, budding, and maturation.

Entry of HIV into CD4+ cell occurs by direct fusion of the envelope proteins and CD4+ cell receptors and coreceptors on the outside of CD4+ cells. The HIV membrane and the envelope proteins remain outside of the CD4+ cell, whereas the core of the virus enters the CD4+ cell. CD4+ cell enzymes interact with the viral core and stimulate the release of viral RNA and the viral enzymes reverse transcriptase, integrase, and protease.

Before incorporation into the DNA of the CD4+ cells the viral RNA must be converted to DNA. Reverse transcription i.e. conversion of viral RNA to DNA is mediated by the enzyme reverse transcriptage. As a result, a single strand of DNA is produced from viral RNA, which undergoes replication into double stranded HIV DNA.

This integrates with the CD4+ cells DNA with the help of the viral enzyme integrase. This new DNA causes the production of messenger DNA that initiates the synthesis of HIV proteins. The virus then uses the CD4+ cell to make more copies of HIV (replication).

The HIV proteins and viral RNA, all the components needed to make a new virus, assemble at the host cell's surface to form new viruses. These new viruses push through the different parts of the cell wall by budding and push through the wall of one CD4+ cell. These new viruses leave the CD4+ cell and contain all the components necessary to infect other CD4+ cells, but cannot do so until it has matured. During this process, the HIV protease enzyme cuts the long HIV proteins of the virus into smaller functional units that then reassemble to form a mature virus. The virus is now ready to infect other cells.

Contd...

Contd...

Struggle between HIV replication and the immune responses of the patient affect cell-mediated and immune-mediated reactions, as it causes cell incapacitation and death. The infected children will exhibit symptoms of viral or fungal infection. The result of this destruction is failure of T-cell production and eventual immune suppression. Immunoglobulins become nonfunctional, as a result the child become extremely vulnerable to bacterial infections.

Manifestations

Following may be the signs and symptoms of associated with immunodeficiency:

- Unusually frequent and severe occurrences of upper respiratory infection.
- Common childhood bacterial infections, such as otitis media, sinusitis, and pneumonia.
- Recurrent fungal infections, such as candidiasis (thrush), that do not respond to standard antifungal agents.
- Recurrent or unusually severe viral infections, such as recurrent or disseminated herpes simplex or zoster infection or cytomegalovirus (CMV).

Frequently present and somewhat suggestive signs.

- Growth failure, wasting
- Failure to thrive
- Chronic diarrhea
- *Failure to attain typical milestones:* Suggests a developmental delay; such delays, particularly impairment in the development of expressive language, may indicate HIV encephalopathy.
- Behavioral abnormalities (in older children), such as loss of concentration and memory, may also indicate HIV encephalopathy.
- *Physical examination:* Signs and symptoms of pediatric HIV infection found during physical examination include candidiasis, thrush in the oral cavity and posterior pharynx, linear gingival erythema and median rhomboid glossitis, parotid enlargement and recurrent aphthous ulcers, oral hairy leukoplakia.
- *Pneumocystis jiroveci* (formerly *P. carinii*) *pneumonia (PCP):* Most commonly manifests as cough, dyspnea, tachypnea, and fever.
- *Lipodystrophy:* Presentations include peripheral lipo-atrophy, truncal lipohypertrophy, and combined versions of these presentations; a more severe presentation occurs at puberty.
- *Digital clubbing:* As a result of chronic lung disease.
- Pitting or nonpitting edema in the extremities.
- Generalized cervical, axillary, or inguinal lymphadenopathy.

Diagnostic Evaluation

Detection of antibody to HIV is the usual first step in diagnosing HIV infection. Viral diagnostic tests like DNA, PCR, RNA assay precisely diagnose most HIV infected infants as early as one month of age to six months of age. Traditional antibody measurement tests like enzyme linked immunosorbent assay (ELISA) and Western blot assay is not accurate in infants younger than 18 months, because of the persistence of the maternal HIV antibody. Two positive virologic samples obtained on two separate occasions established positive diagnosis.

- Preferred virologic assays include HIV DNA polymerase chain reaction (PCR) and HIV RNA assays. The HIV PCR DNA qualitative test is usually less expensive.
- Further virologic testing in infants with known perinatal HIV exposure is recommended at 2 weeks, 4 weeks, and 4 months.

In older children and adults, an ELISA to detect HIV antibody, followed by a confirmatory Western blot (which has increased specificity), should be used to diagnose HIV infection.

Rapid HIV tests, which provide results in minutes, simplify and expand the availability of HIV testing. Their sensitivity is as high as 100%, but they must be followed with confirmatory Western blotting or immunofluorescence antibody testing, as with conventional HIV antibody tests.

Therapeutic Management

There is no cure for HIV infection. Early infant diagnosis is critical. When ART is administered as early as possible in the course of infection, it can help children living with HIV lead longer, healthier lives. Taken every day, these medicines can drastically reduce the concentration of HIV in the bloodstream and increase levels of CD4 cells, thereby slowing the progression of the disease. Classes of antiretroviral agents include the following:

- Nucleoside or nucleotide reverse transcriptase inhibitors (NRTIs)
- Protease inhibitors (PIs)
- Nonnucleoside reverse transcriptase inhibitors (NNRTIs)
- Fusion inhibitors.

Combination ART with at least 3 drugs from at least 2 classes of drugs is recommended for initial treatment of infected infants, children, and adolescents because it provides the best opportunity to preserve immune function and delay disease progression. Drug combinations for initial therapy in ART-naive children include a backbone of 2 NRTIs plus 1 NNRTI or 1 PI.

Initiation of treatment: All babies, below one year of age, who are infected with HIV should start HIV treatment immediately. This is also the case for babies who become infected with HIV through breastfeeding.

It is also recommended that HIV treatment should start to all children aged over twelve months when they are diagnosed as HIV.

Starting treatment at the right time can help reduce the risks of child becoming ill not only because of HIV but also with some other opportunistic infections.

Therefore children aged over twelve months are recommended to start HIV treatment when their CD4 cell count falls to a certain level. The level depends on the age of the child:

Aged 1–3 years: CD4 cell percentage below 25%, or a CD4 cell count below 1000.

Aged 3–5 years: CD4 cell percentage below 20%, or a CD4 cell count below 500.

Aged 5 years and above: CD4 cell count below 350.

In making a recommendation about starting HIV treatment, child's viral load is estimated. HIV treatment may be started earlier if child has a high viral load (above 100,000 copies/mL).

Patients aged one year or older with acquired immunodeficiency syndrome (AIDS) or significant symptoms should be aggressively treated regardless of $CD4^+$ percentage and count or plasma HIV RNA level.

In addition to antiretroviral drugs (ARDs), other types of medication are required as appropriate for specific infections or malignancies. For example, *P. jiroveci* pneumonia prophylaxis is recommended in patients who are HIV positive and younger than 1 year and in older children based on $CD4^+$ counts.

COMMON BACTERIAL INFECTION

Tetanus

Tetanus is an acute, often-fatal disease of the nervous system that is caused by nerve toxins produced by the bacterium *Clostridium tetani.* This bacterium is found throughout the world in the soil and in animal and human intestines. The tetanus bacteria often enter the body through a puncture wound, which can be caused by nails, splinters, insect bites, burns, any skin break, and injection-drug sites. The disease is characterized by muscular stiffness and painful paroxysmal spasms of the voluntary muscles caused by the powerful antitoxin of the causative bacteria.

Tetanus toxin can affect neonates within the first two weeks after birth to cause muscle spasms, inability to nurse, and seizures. It is one of the leading cause of neonatal death. This typically occurs in the premises of poor hand washing practice, unhygienic delivery practice, and can be associated with poor sanitation methods in caring for the umbilical cord stump of the neonate. The number of neonatal tetanus and childhood tetanus is declining because of tetanus vaccination programs. Worldwide, however, neonatal tetanus is still, unfortunately, common among the incompletely immunized women.

Causative agent: Tetanus is caused by a type of bacteria (*Clostridium tetani*), a gram positive, anerobic, spore bearing organism.

Incubation period: The incubation period between exposure to the bacteria in a contaminated wound and development of the initial symptoms of tetanus ranges from two days to two months, but it is commonly within 14 days of injury. The shorter the incubation period, the higher is the risk of death.

Infectious period: Not directly transmitted from person-person.

Transmission: Contamination of wound with tetanus spores

Immunity: An attack of tetanus does not give immunity to the patient against tetanus. Tetanus vaccine is necessary for prevention of tetanus. Active immunity of child develops by DTP, DT vaccines; passive immunity by tetanus toxoid injection.

Season: Any time in the year.

Pathophysiology

Tetanus begins when spores of '*Clostridium tetani*' enter into damaged tissue. The spores transform into rod-shaped bacteria and produce the neurotoxin tetanospasmin. The tetanus toxin affects the site of interaction between the nerve and the muscle that it stimulates. This region is called the neuromuscular junction. Tetanus toxin is taken up into terminals of lower motor neurons and transported axonally to the spinal cord and/or brainstem. The tetanus toxin blocks postsynaptic inhibition of spinal motor reflexes resulting in prolonged spasmodic contractions of the skeletal muscles. It means, the toxin amplifies the chemical signal from the nerve to the muscle, which causes the muscles to tighten up in a continuous ('tetanic' or 'tonic') contraction or spasm. This results in either localized or generalized muscle spasms. Tetanus affects skeletal muscle, the first muscles to be affected are the neck and masseter muscles, causing rigidity of the neck and spasms of the jaw (lock jaw/trismus). This is followed by generalized spasms of the muscles involved in swallowing, respiration muscles, or back muscles (opisthotonos: characteristic body shape). The other type of striated muscle, cardiac muscle, cannot be tetanized because of its intrinsic electrical properties. Renal failure can also occur due to muscle rigidity. Death results from exhaustion, respiratory failure, or cardiac arrest.

Manifestations

During a one- to seven-day period, progressive muscle spasms caused by the tetanus toxin in the immediate wound area may progress to involve the entire body in a set of continuous muscle contractions. Restlessness, headache, and irritability are common. The tetanus neurotoxin causes the muscles to tighten up into a continuous ('tetanic' or 'tonic') contraction or spasm. The jaw is 'locked' (Fig. 20.12) by muscle spasms, giving the name 'lockjaw' (also called 'trismus'). Muscles throughout the body are affected, including the vital muscles necessary for normal breathing. When the breathing muscles lose their power, breathing becomes difficult or impossible and death can occur without life-support measures (mechanical ventilation). Even with breathing support, infections of the airways within the lungs can lead to death.

In children and adults muscular stiffness in the jaw is a common first sign of tetanus. This symptom is followed by stiffness in the neck, difficulty swallowing, stiffness in the stomach muscles, muscle spasms, sweating, and fever. Newborn babies with tetanus are normal at birth, but stop sucking between three and 28 days after birth. They stop feeding and their bodies become stiff while severe muscle contractions and spasms occur. Death follows in most cases.

Therapeutic Management

The goals of treatment in patients with tetanus include supportive therapy, care of the wound to eradicate

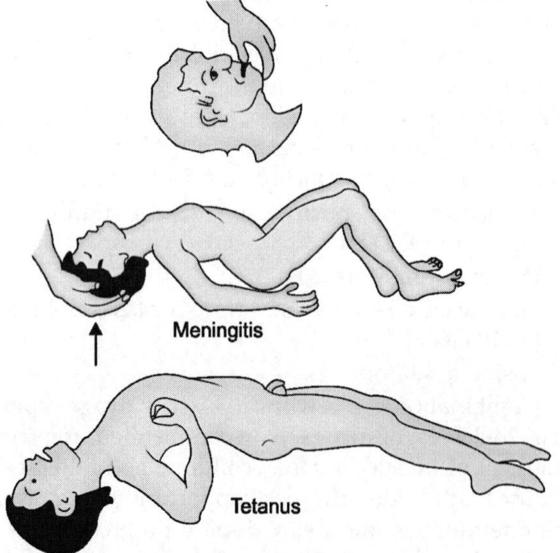

Fig. 20.12: Specific body spasms are seen in the disorders mentioned above

spores and alter conditions for germination, stopping the toxin production within the wound, neutralizing unbound toxin, control other symptoms, management of complications.

Supportive therapy: Patients should be kept in dark and quiet environment preferably in the ICU, to avoid the risk of reflex spasms. Unnecessary procedures and manipulations should be avoided.

Attempting endotracheal intubation may induce severe reflex laryngospasm; preparations must be made for emergency surgical airway control. Rapid sequence intubation techniques means with succinylcholine are recommended to avoid this complication.

Tracheostomy should be performed in patients requiring intubation for more than 10 days. Tracheostomy has also been recommended after onset of the first generalized seizure.

Recently acquired wounds should be explored, carefully cleansed, and properly debrided.

Elimination of toxin production: Antimicrobials are used to decrease the number of toxin producing of *C tetani* (vegetative forms) in the wound. Penicillin G was used widely for this purpose, but it is not the current drug of choice. Metronidazole (e.g. 0.5 g every 6 hours) has comparable or better antimicrobial activity, and penicillin is a known antagonist of gamma-aminobutyric acid (GABA), as is tetanus toxin. Metronidazole is also associated with lower mortality. Other antimicrobials that have been used are clindamycin, erythromycin, tetracycline, and vancomycin. Their role is not well established.

Neutralizing unbound toxin: Tetanus immune globulin (TIG) is recommended for treatment of tetanus to remove unbound tetanus toxin; but it cannot affect toxin bound to nerve endings. A single intramuscular (IM) dose of 3000–5000 units is generally recommended for children and adults, with part of the dose infiltrated around the wound if it can be identified.

The WHO recommends TIG 500 units by IM injection or intravenously (IV)—depending on the available preparation—as soon as possible; in addition, 0.5 mL of an age-appropriate tetanus toxoid-containing vaccine. Tetanus disease does not induce immunity; patients without a history of primary tetanus toxoid vaccination should receive a second dose 1–2 months after the first dose and a third dose 6–12 months later.

Control other symptoms: Benzodiazepines (diazepam) is the most frequently used drug in tetanus; it reduces anxiety, produces sedation, and relaxes muscles. Lorazepam is an effective alternative. High dosages of either may be required (up to 600 mg/day). If the spasms are not controlled with benzodiazepines, long-term neuromuscular blockade is required. Phenobarbital is also used every 2–4 hours to treat severe muscle spasms and provide sedation when neuromuscular blocking agents are used.

Management of complications: Fractures of the spine or other bones may occur as a result of muscle spasms and convulsions. Specific therapy for autonomic system complications and control of spasms should be initiated. Magnesium sulfate can be used alone or in combination with benzodiazepines for this purpose. It should be given IV in a loading dose of 5 g (or 75 mg/kg), followed by continuous infusion at a rate of 2–3 g/hour until spasm control is achieved.

Prevention

Immunizing infants and children with DTP or DT and adults with TT prevents tetanus. More recently, some countries have been using a combination vaccine that includes vaccines for diphtheria, tetanus, pertussis, vitamin A (HepB), and sometimes *Hemophilus inflenzae* type b (Hib).

Neonatal tetanus can be prevented by immunizing pregnant women with tetanus toxoid. This protects the mother and enables tetanus antibodies to be transferred to her baby.

Clean practices are especially important when a mother is delivering a child, even if she has been immunized. People who recover from tetanus do not have natural immunity and can be infected again and therefore need to be immunized.

WHO, UNICEF and UNFPA agreed to set the year 2005 as the target date for worldwide elimination of neonatal tetanus. This implies the reduction of neonatal tetanus incidence to below one case per 1000 live births per year in every district. This goal was reaffirmed by the United Nations General Assembly Special Session (UNGASS) in 2002. Because tetanus survives in the environment, eradication of the disease is not feasible and high levels of immunization have to continue even after the goal has been achieved.

To achieve the elimination goal, countries implement a series of strategies:

- Improve the percentage of pregnant women immunized with vaccines containing tetanus toxoid.
- Administer vaccines containing tetanus toxoid to all women of childbearing age in high-risk areas. This is usually implemented through a three round campaign approach.
- Promote clean delivery and childcare practices.
- Improve surveillance and reporting of neonatal tetanus cases.

Nursing Considerations for Tetanus

Nursing Diagnosis

- Ineffective airway clearance and difficulty in breathing related to the respiratory muscle fatigue.
- Increased body temperature related to the effects of toxins.
- Changes in nutrition, less than body requirements related to the mastication muscle stiffness.
- Apprehension of the child related to speech difficulties.
- Impaired daily need related to the condition of weak and frequent seizures.
- The risk of fluid and electrolyte imbalances related to low intake of fluid and oliguria.
- Risk of trauma and injury related to frequent seizures.
- Lack of knowledge of the family members about tetanus disease and its management.
- Deficient rest and sleep due to frequent seizures.
- Presence of complications due to severe infection of tetanus such as constipation, retention of urine, fever, high blood pressure, irregular heartbeats and difficulty in breathing.

Nursing Intervention

- Assess the frequency and pattern of breath, and symptoms related to respiratory muscle spasms. Give the tactile stimulation immediately after apnea.
- Perform cardiac and respiratory monitoring continuously. Suction airway and administer oxygen as needed.
- Assess the child's ventilator and neurologic status and provide respirator support as needed.
- Assess the status of the reflex with respect to feeding, sucking, swallowing and coughing.
- Monitor laboratory tests as indicated.
- Fluid, medications, electrolyte supplements as indicated.
- Review the signs of hypoglycemia, give parenteral nutrition.
- Make provision of drinking according to tolerance.
- Seizure precautions, quiet environment.
- Involve parents in child care to minimize fear and apprehension of the child.
- Information and support to the family members.
- Educate the child and family about immunizations.

TUBERCULOSIS

Tuberculosis is a single major infectious disease causing significant morbidity and mortality amongst all humans, including children. India has one of the highest tuberculosis burdens globally. Young children with TB, a vulnerable population, where lack of early diagnosis results in poor outcomes. TB is caused by a bacterium called *Mycobacterium tuberculosis*. TB bacteria are spread from person to person through the air. The TB bacteria are put into the air when a person with TB disease of the lungs or throat coughs, sneezes, speaks, or sings. However, children are less likely to spread TB bacteria to others. This is because the forms of TB disease most commonly seen in children are usually less infectious than the forms seen in adults. Among children, the greatest numbers of TB cases are seen in children less than 5 years of age, and in adolescents older than 10 years of age.

Causative agent: *Mycobacterium tuberculosis. It is an acid fast bacilli, grows in Ziehl-Neelsen media.*

It is rapidly inactivated by sunlight and ultraviolet light.

Incubation period: Average incubation period is 3–8 weeks.

Infectious period: Patients are infective as long as they remain untreated. Effective antimicrobial treatment reduces infectivity by 90% within 48 hours.

Transmission: Mainly droplet infection transmit the disease. The minuscule droplets can remain airborne for minutes to hours after expectoration. The number of bacilli in the droplets, the virulence of the bacilli, exposure of the bacilli to UV light, degree of ventilation, and occasions for aerosolization all influence transmission. Introduction of *M tuberculosis* into the lungs leads to infection of the respiratory system; however, the organisms can spread to other organs, such as the lymphatics, pleura, bones/joints, or meninges, and cause extrapulmonary tuberculosis. It may cause due to ingestion also. Trans-placental transmission may occur,causing congenital tuberculosis.

Immunity: Man has no inherited immunity against TB. It is acquired as a result of natural infection or BCG vaccination.

Season: Infection may occur in any time in the year.

Not everyone infected with TB bacteria becomes sick and two TB-related conditions exist: latent TB infection and TB disease. Once infected with TB bacteria, children are more likely to get sick with TB disease and to get sick more quickly than adults. In comparison to children, TB disease in adults is usually due to past TB infection, years later that becomes active, when a person's immune system becomes weak for some reason (e.g. HIV infection, diabetes).

Persons with latent TB infection:

- Usually have a skin test or blood test indicating TB infection;

- Have TB bacteria in their bodies, but the bacteria are not active;
- Are not sick and do not have symptoms;
- Cannot spread bacteria to others; and
- Are often given medicine to prevent them from developing TB disease.

If TB bacteria become active in the body and multiply, the person will get sick with TB disease. Persons with TB disease:

- Usually have a skin test or blood test indicating TB infection;
- Are sick from TB bacteria that are active (meaning that they are multiplying and destroying tissue in their body);
- Usually have symptoms of TB disease; and
- Must be given medicine to treat TB disease.

Pathophysiology

The tubercle bacilli establish infection in the lungs after they are carried in droplets small enough (5–10 microns) to reach the alveolar spaces (Figs 20.13A). Following deposition in the alveoli, *M tuberculosis* is engulfed by alveolar macrophages, but survives and multiplies within the macrophages. The infected macrophages produce cytokines and chemokines that attract other phagocytic cells, including monocytes, other alveolar macrophages and neutrophils, which eventually form a nodular granulomatous structure called the tubercle. Successful containment of TB is dependent on the cellular immune system, mediated primarily through T-helper cells (TH1 response). T cells and macrophages form a granuloma (Ghon focus) with a centre that contains necrotic material (caseous center), *M tuberculosis*, and peripheral granulation tissue consisting primarily of macrophages and lymphocytes. The granuloma, the Ghon focus usually shows slow healing with calcification and fibrosis and serves to prevent further growth and spread of *M tuberculosis*. These individuals are noninfectious and have latent TB infection; the majority of these patients will have a normal CXR and be tuberculin skin test positive. If the bacterial replication is not controlled, the tubercle enlarges and the bacilli enter local draining lymph nodes. This leads to lymphadenopathy, a characteristic clinical manifestation of primary tuberculosis (TB) (Figs 20.13A to C). The bacilli continue to proliferate until an effective cell-mediated immune (CMI) response develops, usually two to six weeks after infection. Failure by the host to mount an effective CMI response and tissue repair leads to progressive destruction of the lung.

Unchecked bacterial growth may lead to hematogenous spread of bacilli to other parts of the body like meninges, peritoneum, bones, joints, kidney, lymph nodes, to produce disseminated TB. Disseminated disease with lesions resembling millet seeds is termed miliary TB. Bacilli can also spread by erosion of the caseating lesions into the lung airways–and the host becomes infectious to others.

Manifestations

Signs and symptoms of TB disease in children include:

- Cough
- Feelings of sickness or weakness, lethargy, and/or reduced playfulness
- Weight loss or failure to thrive
- Fever
- Night sweats.

The most common form of TB disease occurs in the lungs, but TB disease can affect other parts of the body as well. Symptoms of TB disease in other parts of the body depend on the area affected. Infants, young children, and immune-compromised children (e.g.

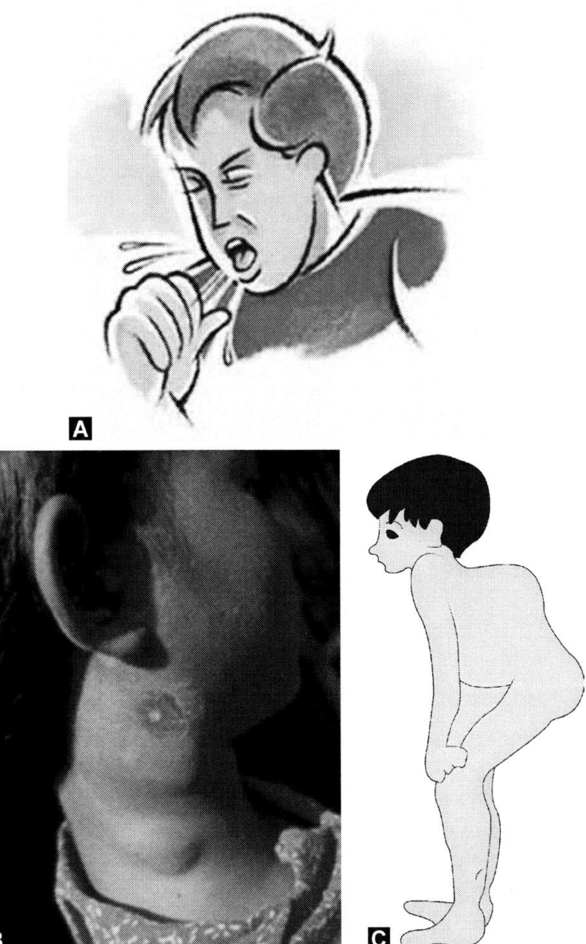

Figs 20.13A to C: A. Mode of TB transmission; **B.** Enlarged cervical gland commonly seen in child with TB infection; **C.** Caries spine

children with HIV) are at the highest risk of developing the most severe forms of TB such as TB meningitis or disseminated TB disease.

Diagnostic Evaluation

Confirming the diagnosis of TB disease in children is based on combination of the factors like (i) clinical signs and symptoms typically associated with TB disease, (ii) positive tuberculin skin test (TST) or positive TB blood test (IGRA), (iii) chest X-ray that has patterns typically associated with TB disease, and (iv) history of contact with a person with infectious TB disease. In case of children a laboratory test can be challenging because (i) it is difficult to collect sputum specimens from infants and young children; and (ii) the laboratory tests used to find TB in sputum are less likely to have a positive result in children; this is due to the fact that children are more likely to have TB disease caused by a smaller number of bacteria (paucibacillary disease). For these reasons, the diagnosis of TB disease in children is often made without laboratory confirmation.

Skin Test

TB skin testing is considered safe in children, and is preferred over TB blood tests for children less than 5 years of age.

Blood Test

A newer generation of tests which measure the production of interferon gamma by the peripheral mononuclear cells have been developed to identify the patients with TB disease or latent infection.

Chest X-rays

A chest X-ray is a necessary as additional criteria for the diagnosis of pulmonary tuberculosis.

Therapeutic Management

The therapeutic management of tuberculosis requires correct assessment of the patient with respect to the site of disease, bacteriological status, treatment type of patient and the severity of disease. After appropriately defining the disease, the patient is then categorized to receive appropriate anti-TB therapy and the drug dosages are already recommended.

A pediatric TB expert should be involved in the treatment of TB in children and in the management of infants, young children, and immunocompromised children who have been exposed to someone with infectious TB disease. It is very important that children or anyone being treated for latent TB infection or TB disease finish the medicine and take the drugs exactly as instructed.

Latent TB Infection

Treatment is recommended for children with latent TB infection to prevent them from developing TB disease. Infants, young children, and immunocompromised children with latent TB infection or children in close contact with someone with infectious TB disease, require special consideration because they are at increased risk for getting TB disease. Consultation with a pediatric TB expert is recommended before treatment begins. Isoniazid is the anti-TB medicine that is most commonly used for treatment of latent TB infection. In children, the recommended length of treatment with isoniazid is 9 months.

TB Disease

TB disease is treated by taking several anti-TB medicines for 6 to 9 months. It is important to note that if a child stops taking the drugs before completion, the child can become sick again. If drugs are not taken correctly, the bacteria that are still alive may become resistant to those drugs. TB that is resistant to drugs is harder and more expensive to treat, and treatment lasts much longer up to 18–24 months.

Vaccines

BCG, or bacille Calmette-Guerin, is a vaccine to prevent TB disease. BCG is used in many countries to prevent childhood TB disease. However, the BCG vaccine is not generally used in the United States, because of the low risk of infection with TB bacteria and the variable effectiveness of the vaccine. The BCG vaccine should only be considered for very select persons who meet specific criteria and in consultation with a TB doctor.

Nursing Consideration

Health care workers, especially community health nurses, must be knowledgeable about the transmission, pathogenesis, diagnosis, and treatment of this disease. Armed with this knowledge, an effective teaching program for nurses must be initiated to interrupt the spread of tuberculosis. Promptly identifying cases and treating appropriately are the focus of disease prevention.

Nursing Diagnosis

- Infection, risk for (spread/reactivation)
- Airway clearance, ineffective

- Compliance of therapy and thus to prevent drug resistance TB.

Desired Outcomes

- Identify interventions to prevent/reduce risk of spread of infection.
- Demonstrate techniques/initiate lifestyle changes to promote safe environment.
- Maintain patent airway. Expectorate secretions without assistance.

Nursing Actions

Instruct patient to cough or sneeze and expectorate into napkin and to refrain from spitting. Show proper disposal of tissue and good hand washing techniques. Behaviors necessary to prevent spread of infection (droplet).

Stress importance of uninterrupted drug therapy. Compliance with multidrug regimens for prolonged periods is difficult, so directly observed therapy (DOT) should be started.

Encouraged parents for selection and serving well-balanced meals for the children with TB. They should provide frequent small 'snacks' in place of large meals as appropriate.

Assess respiratory function noting breath sounds, and efforts. Note ability to expectorate mucus and cough effectively; document character, amount of sputum, presence of hemoptysis.

Place patient in semi or high-Fowler's position. Assist patient with coughing and deep-breathing exercises. Clear secretions from mouth and trachea; suction as necessary. Maintain fluid intake of at least 2500 mL/day unless contraindicated. Administer drugs as prescribed (mucolytic agent, or bronchodialator).

Aware parents about (a) individual risk factors for reactivation of tuberculosis and lowered resistance associated with malnutrition, noncompliance of AT drug schedule, use of immunosuppressive drugs (b) identification symptoms that should be reported to healthcare provider, i.e. hemoptysis, chest pain, fever, difficulty breathing, hearing loss (c) potential side effects of treatment (dryness of mouth, constipation, visual disturbances, headache, orthostatic hypertension) and its solution.

LEPROSY

Leprosy is a chronic disease caused by a slow multiplying bacillus, *Mycobacterium leprae*. The disease mainly affects the skin, the peripheral nerves, mucosa of the upper respiratory tract and also the eyes. It is a curable disease. Early diagnosis and treatment with multidrug therapy (MDT) remain key in eliminating the disease as a public health concern. Untreated, leprosy can cause progressive and permanent damage to the skin, nerves, limbs and eyes.

Leprosy, a disease as old a mankind, has been a public health problem in many developing countries including India. India with its 4 million cases of leprosy, accounts for one-third of the world's population of leprosy patients. One-fourth of them are below 15 years of age.

Agent

Leprosy is caused by the acid-fast, rod-shaped bacteria *Mycobacterium leprae*, which was discovered in 1873 by GA Hansen.

Incubation Period

M. leprae multiplies slowly and the incubation period of the disease is about 3–5 years or more in lepromatous casea. Symptoms can take as long as 20 years to appear.

Transmission

Although not highly infectious, it is transmitted via droplets, from the nose and mouth, during close and frequent contacts with untreated cases. Contact transmission may occur between infected person and others.

Immunity

Subclinical infections contribute active immunity.

Classification of Leprosy

WHO categorizes the disease based on the type and number of skin areas affected. They are:

- *Paucibacillary*: Five or fewer lesions with no bacteria detected in the skin smear (sample taken from the area).
- *Multibacillary*: More than five lesions or bacteria is detected in the skin smear, or both.

The **Ridley-Jopling system** is used internationally in clinical studies. It has six classifications based on severity of symptoms. These types are:

- *Intermediate leprosy*: A few flat lesions that sometimes heal by themselves and can progress to a more severe type
- *Tuberculoid leprosy*: A few flat lesions, some large and numb; some nerve involvement; can heal on its own, persist, or may progress to a more severe form
- *Borderline tuberculoid leprosy*: Lesions like tuberculoid but small and more numerous; less nerve

enlargement; may persist, revert to tuberculoid, or advance to another form

- *Mid-borderline leprosy*: Reddish plaques, moderate numbness, swollen lymph glands; may regress, persist, or progress to other forms
- *Borderline lepromatous leprosy*: Many lesions with flat lesions, raised bumps, plaques, and nodules, sometimes numb; may persist, regress, or progress
- *Lepromatous leprosy*: Many lesions with bacteria; hair loss; nerve involvement; limb weakness; disfigurement; does not regress.

Manifestations

Leprosy primarily affects the skin and the peripheral nerves. It may also strike the eyes and the thin tissue lining the inside of the nose. The main symptoms of leprosy include:

- Skin lesions that have decreased sensation to touch, temperature, or pain, do not heal after several weeks or month, are often less pigmented than the surrounding skin, though they may reddish or copper colored (Fig. 20.14A).
- Single or multiple skin lesions that are often found on cooler parts of the body such as the face, buttocks, and extremities.
- Thickening of the skin and peripheral nerves.
- Ulcerations of the skin due to loss of sensations (Fig. 20.14B).
- Peripheral nerve involvement leading to loss of sensation in the hands, arms, feet, and legs.
- Peripheral nerve involvement leading to muscle weakness—There is loss of muscles strength in the hands and feet. With severe nerve damage of the hands and feet, there is paralysis of the small muscles, leading to 'clawing' of the fingers and toes. Food drop, wrist drop, planter ulcers, etc.
- Hoarseness.
- Other symptoms in advanced cases are testicular involvement leading to sexual dysfunction or sterility.
- Eye involvement including eye pain, eye redness, inability to close the eyelids (lagophthalmos), corneal ulcers, and blindness. It can also cause dry eyes by decreasing tear production. Tears protect the eye by keeping it moist and healthy. Bacteria can invade the cooler part of the eye. Reactions may also involve the eye and may cause a painful 'red eye.'
- *Lagophthalmos*: Weakness of the eyelids, preventing proper closure of the lid which protects the eye. The ability to feel something in the eye may be lost, making it easier for damage to occur.

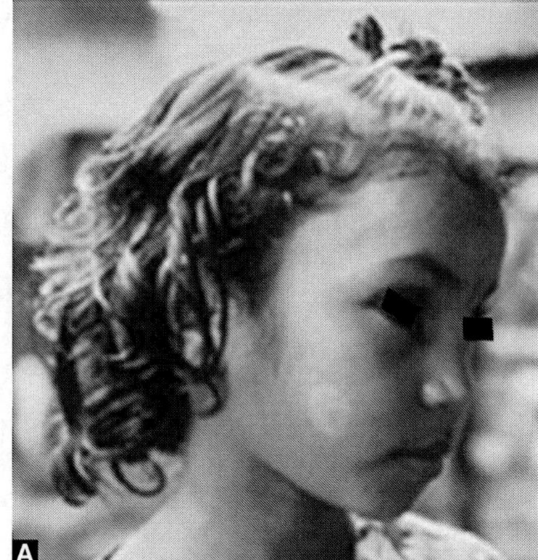

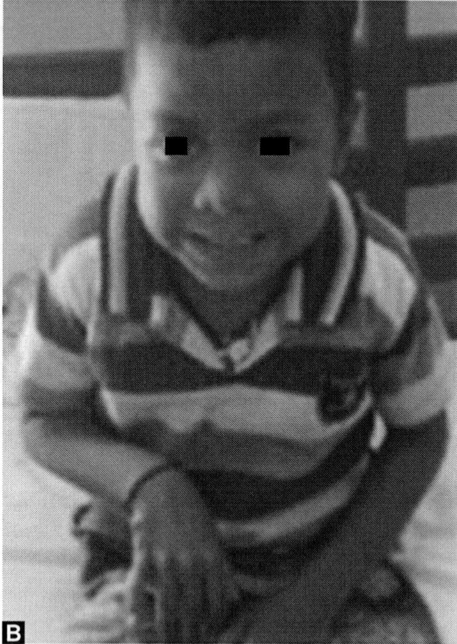

Figs 20.14A and B: A. Child with leprosy; **B.** Ulcers that come from injuries to the numb hand of the child due to leprosy

- Loss of eyebrows and eyelashes (madarosis)
- Destruction of the nasal cartilage (saddle nose): This results when the there is damage to the nasal cartilage by bacteria. This can lead to difficulty in breathing.

Leprosy damages the nerves in the cooler parts of the body, especially those near the skin that relate to the hands, feet and face. If treated during the early stages there will be no loss of sensation or paralysis but if the nerves are damaged, then feeling and movement will not return.

Diagnostic Evaluation

To recognize leprosy:

- Talk to the person
- Examine their skin
- Test the feeling in the skin patches
- Examine the hands and feet
- Feel the nerves
- Skin smear test.

Talk to the Person

Question	*Inference*
How long has the skin patch been there? How did it start? Has it changed?	Leprosy patches usually appear slowly.
Do the patches itch? Is there pain?	Leprosy patches do not itch and are not usually painful.
Does the person have unusual sensations in their hands or feet, such as numbness, tingling or a burning feeling?	Unusual sensations in the hands or feet can be a sign of leprosy.
Does the person think that their hands or feet have become weaker? Do they have problems with holding or lifting things and with moving their hands and feet?	Losing strength in hands or feet can be a sign of leprosy.

Examine their Skin

Examining of the skin is to be done from head to toe, and on the front of the body as well as the back. Leprosy patches are usually lighter than the surrounding skin; they may be reddish in color and can have a raised edge. Sometimes leprosy is seen as thickening of the skin and there are no skin patches. The skin can be shiny and dry to the touch. It may be redder than the surrounding skin. Some nodules, or lumps can be seen on the skin. They are usually a sign of a serious infection. A skin smear taken from a nodule will show a large number of leprosy bacilli.

Test the Feeling in the Skin Patches

Closing the eyes of the patient, it is done with a piece of cotton or tip of the pen. He/she is asked to point to the place where the examiner has touched the skin.

Examination of Hands and Feet

Four points on the both palm and sole are checked specially. If the person has lost feeling in their hand or foot, this may mean that they have leprosy.

Feel the Nerves

Enlarged nerves can be a sign of leprosy. Two nerves that are commonly enlarged can be felt quite easily. These are the ulnar and the peroneal nerves.

Skin Smear Test

This test is useful to confirm very infectious cases when it is difficult to be sure of diagnosis on clinical grounds alone. For example, if there is skin thickening or lumps and there are no obvious anesthetic patches. A negative skin smear means that although they have leprosy bacilli in their body, there are too few to be seen in the smear. Presence of leprosy bacilli in skin smear test means that the patient is heavily infected. This will affect the type of treatment to be given to the patient.

Therapeutic Management

World Health Organization (WHO) now focus on regimens with shorter duration both for tuberculoid (TT) or paucibacillary (PB) leprosy and for lepromatous (LL) or multibacillary (MB) leprosy.

The drugs that are more frequently used in the treatment of leprosy include rifampin, dapsone, clofazimine, ofloxacin, minocycline, and clarithromycin. Multidrug therapy is required in all cases to prevent antimicrobial resistance. The standard regimen according to WHO for MB leprosy is combination of rifampin, dapsone, and clofazimine. For PB leprosy, rifampin is usually prescribed in combination with dapsone. For single-lesion PB leprosy, a single dose of rifampin combined with single doses of ofloxacin and minocycline is recommended. Dosages and duration of treatment for different presentations of leprosy are given below:

Leprosy Treatment for Children (Table 20.2)

The dosage for children varies according to their age, but they must take the same drugs for the same length of time as an adult. That means 6 months for PB and 12 months for MB. As the Table 20.2 shows, clofazimine is only given for MB leprosy. The treatment for those aged 10–14 years is also available in blister packs.

Table 20.2: Leprosy treatment for children

MDT for children		*Below 10 years*	*10 –14 years*
Monthly dose	Rifampicin Dapsone	300 mg 25 mg	450 mg 50 mg
MB only	Clofazimine	100 mg	150 mg
Daily dose	Dapsone	25 mg	50 mg
MB only	Clofazimine	50 mg twice a week	50 mg every other day

The WHO has recommended that patients undergoing treatment for leprosy should be evaluated monthly. In addition, patients should be informed about the potential signs and symptoms of recurrences and be advised to seek medical care if any of them are observed after treatment or after the initial episode has been completed.

Other Therapeutic Measure

Because of the lack of sensation associated with leprosy, patients are usually at risk for significant injury associated with trauma or burns in hypoesthetic areas. Patients should be advised to protect areas at risk of injury.

Reconstructive surgery may be indicated in patients with soft tissue defects, particularly for plantar ulcerations in patients with leprosy.

COMMON PARASITIC INFECTIONS

Malaria

Malaria is a mosquito-borne infectious disease of humans and other animals caused by parasitic protozoans belonging to the genus *Plasmodium*. Children under five years of age are one of most vulnerable groups affected by malaria. There were an estimated 660,000 malaria deaths around the world in 2010, of which approximately 86% were in children under five years of age (WHO 2013).

In high transmission areas, partial immunity to the disease is acquired during childhood. In such settings, the majority of malarial disease, and particularly severe disease with rapid progression to death, occurs in young children without acquired immunity. Severe anemia, hypoglycemia and cerebral malaria are features of severe malaria more commonly seen in children than in adults.

Host

Man is the intermediate host (asexual lifecycle of malaria parasite takes place).

And mosquito is the definitive host (asexual life cycle of malaria parasite takes place).

Agent

The four *Plasmodium* species that infect humans *are Plasmodium falciparum, P. vivax, P.ovale,* and *malariae). P.vivax* causes 70% of all infections in India, and about 25-30% infection caused by *P. Falciparum*.

Incubation Period

The incubation period for malaria is the time between the mosquito bite and the release of parasites from the liver. This varies, depending on which malaria parasite is causing the disease. The period is usually not less than 10 days.

Period of Communicability

Malaria is communicable as long as mature, viable gametocytes exist in the circulating blood in sufficient density to infect vector mosquitoes.

Transmission

Infection is usually transmitted by anopheline mosquitoes.

Immunity

Immunity to malaria in humans is acquired only after repeated exposure over several years.

Season

Mostly seen in July to November. Prevalence of malaria increases in warm humid environment.

Pathophysiology

Malaria infection develops via two phases: one is exoerythrocytic phase (involves the liver), and other one is erythrocytic phase (involves RBCs). During a blood meal, an infected female *Anopheles* mosquito injects 8–15 malarial sporozoites, which rapidly migrate to the liver where they infect hepatocytes, multiplying asexually and asymptomatically for a period of 8–30 days. After a period of time, 30–40 thousand merozoites are released into the blood stream to penetrate erythrocytes after attaching via receptors cells to begin the erythrocytic stage of the life cycle. Some hepatic forms of schizonts persist and remain dormant in the hepatocytes and may cause relapse. The time period before merozoites enter the blood is designated the pre-patent period; this is between 7 and 30 days for *Plasmodium falciparum*.

Within the red blood cells, the parasites multiply further, again asexually (trophozoites and schizonts), periodically breaking out of their host cells to invade fresh red blood cells. Several such amplification cycles occur. Thus, classical descriptions of waves of fever (sometimes in periodicity) arise from simultaneous waves of merozoites escaping and infecting red blood cells. The rupture of erythrocytes releases toxins that induce the release of cytokines from macrophages, resulting in the symptoms of malaria. Some merozoites mature into larger forms called gametocytes, which reproduce sexually if they are ingested by a mosquito.

Sporozoites of some *P. vivax* do not immediately develop into exoerythrocytic-phase merozoites, but instead produce hypnozoites that remain dormant for periods ranging from several months (7–10 months is typical) to several years. After a period of dormancy, they reactivate and produce merozoites. Hypnozoites are responsible for long incubation and late relapses in *P. vivax* infections, although their existence in *P. ovale* is uncertain.

The parasite is relatively protected from attack by the body's immune system because for most of its human life cycle it resides within the liver and blood cells and is relatively invisible to immune surveillance. However, circulating infected blood

Contd...

Contd...

cells are destroyed in the spleen. To avoid this fate, the *P. falciparum* parasite displays adhesive proteins on the surface of the infected blood cells, causing the blood cells to stick to the walls of small blood vessels, thereby sequestering (the binding of mature trophozoites to the endothelium of small blood vessels) the parasite from passage through the general circulation and the spleen. The blockage of the microvasculature causes symptoms such as in placental malaria. Sequestered red blood cells can breach the blood–brain barrier and cause cerebral malaria.

Manifestations

Patients with *P. vivax* infection commonly present with paroxysmal fevers, chills, headaches, and myalgias. Three stages of malaria fever are described as cold stage, hot stage, and sweating stage and followed by an afebrile period. The symptoms of cold stage include irritability and drowsiness, with poor appetite and trouble sleeping. These symptoms are usually followed by chills and rigors within one hour. Then a fever with rapid pulse and breathing occurs and the patient complains other symptoms like severe headache, vomiting. In this hot stage the fever may either gradually increase over 1–2 days or may rise very suddenly to 105 °F (40.6 °C) or above with intense headache, excessive thirst and lasts for 2–6 hours. Then, as fever ends and body temperature quickly returns to normal, there's an intense episode of sweating. The skin become cool and moist, pulse rate comes down and patient sleeps for 2–4 hours. The same pattern of symptoms—chills, fever, sweating—may repeat at intervals of 2 or 3 days, depending on which particular species of malaria parasite is causing the infection. Chills and rigor may not be present in infancy and early childhood.

Patients with *P. falciparum* malaria present with high fever that may be accompanied by chills, rigors, sweats, and headache. Other common findings include generalized weakness, backache, myalgias, vomiting, and pallor. In chronically infected children, anemia and hypersplenism are common. Splenic rupture is a serious complication in children with hypersplenism.

Cerebral or malignant malaria: Initial presentation is usually fever followed by inability to eat or drink. The progression to coma or convulsion is usually very rapid within one or two days. Convulsions may be very subtle with nystagmus, salivation or twitching of an isolated part of the body. Effort should be given to exclude other treatable causes of coma (e.g. bacterial meningitis, hypoglycemia).

Severe Malaria

Children with hyperparasitemia due to acute destruction of red cells may develop severe anemia. Features of severe malaria are (i) cerebral malaria (unrousable coma), (ii) severe normocytic anemia (Hb <5 g/dL), (iii) renal failure (serum creatinine >3 mg/100 mL), (iv) pulmonary edema, (v) hypoglycemia (<40 mg/100 mL), (vi) circulatory collapse/shock (systolic blood pressure less than 50 mm Hg in children below 5 years), (vii) spontaneous bleeding/disseminated intravascular coagulopathy, (viii) repeated generalized convulsions, (ix) acidemia/acidosis.

Other manifestations are: (i) Impaired consciousness but rousable, (ii) Prostration, extreme weakness (inability to stand or sit), (iii) hyperparasitemia, (iv) jaundice (total serum bilirubin >3 mg/dL), (v) hyperpyrexia (axillary temperature > 39.5 °C).

Diagnostic Evaluation

Microscopic Examination

Light microscopy of well stained thick and thin films by a skilled microscopist has remained the 'gold standard' for malaria diagnosis. Thick films are nearly 10 times more sensitive for diagnosis of malaria as larger amount of blood are there in a given area as compared to thin films. Species identification is better with thin films as morphology of the parasite and RBC are well preserved. Timing of sample collection should be as soon as malaria is suspected. It can be collected any time irrespective of fever and not necessarily only at the height of fever. Collection should be before administration of antimalarials which causes detection of parasites difficult due to its morphologic alteration.

Routine Blood Examination

Hb% usually remains low, WBC counts shows leukopenia, both bilirubin and gammo globin remain remains raised.

Rapid Diagnostic Tests (RDTs)

These are immunochromatographic test (ICT) to detect plasmodium specific antigens in blood sample. Test employ monoclonal antibodies directed against targeted parasite antigens.

Other nonspecific laboratory abnormalities are common in patients with this disease, such as elevated C-reactive protein levels, elevated procalcitonin levels, thrombocytopenia, neutropenia, and elevated liver enzyme levels. Hyponatremia and hypoglycemia deserve special mention, because they are associated with more-severe morbidity and occur more commonly in children than in adults.

Therapeutic Management

Treatment for malaria must be selected on the basis of the infecting *Plasmodium* species, the severity of disease, the drug susceptibility of the infecting parasites, and the availability of medications and resources. *P. vivax* and *P. ovale* are usually susceptible to chloroquine (Table 20.3).

Primaquine is effective against the exoerythrocytic liver phase and is administered to prevent relapse, but occasional relapses may still occur, despite administration of appropriate therapy. As primaquine can cause hemolytic anemia in children with G6PD deficiency they should be preferably screened for the same prior to starting treatment. As infants are relatively G6PD deficient it is not recommended in this age group. Children who acquired malaria transplacentally or via a transfusion do not have hypnozoite forms of malaria and need not be treated with primaquine. This drug can be administered to patients on chemoprophylaxis after they have left the endemic area. It is not to be used until erythrocytic forms have been destroyed by another drug.

A toxic-appearing child with a history of malaria exposure should be admitted to an intensive care unit, and aggressive diagnosis and treatment should be pursued. Appropriate laboratory work must be performed, including blood smears for malaria parasites, and empirical parenteral antimalarial therapy must be initiated. If no parasites are seen on initial smears, follow-up smears should be obtained every 8 hours if there is continued concern about malaria.

Table 20.3: Recommended treatment in chloroquine sensitive malaria

Drug sensitivity	*Recommended treatment*
P. vivax and chloroquine sensitive	Chloroquine 10 mg base/kg stat followed by 5 mg/kg at 6, 24 and 48 hours OR
P. falciparum	Chloroquine 10 mg base/kg stat followed by 10 mg/kg at 24 hours and 5 mg/kg at 48 hours. (Total dose 25 mg base/kg) In case of vivax malaria to prevent relapse primaquine should be given in a dose of 0.25 mg/kg/day for 14 days. In case of falciparum malaria a single dose of primaquine (0.75 mg/kg) is given for gametocytocidal action.

(i) Chloroquine should not be given in empty stomach and in high fever. Bring down the temperature first. If vomiting occurs within 45 minutes of a dose of chloroquine that particular dose is to be repeated after taking care of vomiting by using domperidone/ Ondansetron.

Nursing Management

Temperature

Monitor the temperature trend. Rheumatic fever is caused by the effects of endotoxin in the hypothalamus and releases endorphins that pyrogen. In the state of hyperpyrexia, nurse should start hydrotherapy as it can rapidly bring the temperature down. Oral paracetamol (acetaminophen) is safe and effective for fever and should be used in doses of 10 mg/kg. This dose can be repeated 3–6 times a day, as required.

Anemia

Anemia develops in many children with malaria. Adequate food and fluid, standard hematinic therapy, prevention of infection, to provide rest and support are effective in this situation. Because the onset of anemia is gradual, children withstand a low level of hemoglobin quite well and blood transfusions are rarely needed. Packed red cell transfusion should be given cautiously when PCV is 12% or less, or hemoglobin is below 4 g%. Transfusion should also be considered in patients with less severe anemia in the presence of respiratory distress (acidosis), impaired consciousness or hyperparasitemia (>20% of RBCs infected).

Vomiting

Vomiting is common in malaria. An antiemetic such as domperidone can be used, and antimalarials should be continued. Vomiting stops when the malaria is cured. If dehydration develops due to repeated vomiting, the dehydration is to be corrected by appropriate parenteral fluids. The hypoglycemia sometimes accompanies severe malaria which is corrected with glucose–containing fluids.

Risk for infection related to decreased immune system – Standard protocol of infection prevention is to be followed.

Hospitalization in malaria: The child with malaria may need hospitalization if he/she has intractable vomiting and causing dehydration, altered consciousness and repeated convulsions, respiratory difficulty, oliguria or anuria.

In a child with malaria, impaired consciousness, respiratory distress, hypoglycemia, and jaundice are risk factors for death, so the child should be treated as an emergency. On the other hand, children with malaria who are fully conscious, who have fever (low to moderate), and who can tolerate oral hydration and nutrition nutrition can be treated on an outpatient basis. Increased fluid intake is necessary for the child with malaria. Co-existing infection is to be treated immediately to avoid a sudden deterioration.

KALA-AZAR

Leishmaniasis refers to the spectrum of infectious disease produced by species of the *Leishmania* parasite. It is a chronic and potentially fatal parasitic disease of the viscera, particularly the liver, spleen, bone marrow and lymph nodes, due to infection by the parasite called *Leishmania donovani. Leishmania donovani* is transmitted by the female phlebotomine sandfly bites. Kala-azar can cause no or few symptoms but typically it is associated with long duration fever, anorexia, fatigue, enlargement of the liver, spleen and nodes and suppression of the bone marrow (Fig. 20.15A).

The disease is also known as Indian leishmaniasis, visceral leishmaniasis, leishmania infection. The disease can present in three main ways as: cutaneous (CL), mucocutaneous (MCL), or visceral leishmaniasis (VL). The CL is the most common form, which causes an open sore at the bite sites, which heals in a few months to a year and half, leaving an unpleasant-looking scar. The MCL form presents with ulcers of the skin, mouth, and nose. The VL form starts with skin ulcers and then later presents with fever, low red blood cells, and enlarged spleen and liver. Leishmaniasis is considered one of the classic causes of a markedly enlarged (and therefore palpable) spleen; the organ, which is not normally felt during examination of the abdomen, may even become larger than the liver in severe cases.

The name '*Leishmania donovani*' honors two men: the British pathologist William Boog Leishman who in 1903 wrote about the protozoa that causes kala-azar and the researcher C. Donovan, who made the same discovery independently the same year.

Epidemiology

It affects as many as 12 million people worldwide, with 1.5–2.0 million new cases each year.

Causative agent: *Leishmania donovani,* an intracellular parasite. Infections in humans are caused by more than 20 species of *Leishmania.* The sand flies feed on animals and humans for blood, which they need for developing their eggs. Life cycle of the parasite completes in two different hosts, i.e. man and sandfly. The amastigote form or 'Leishmania bodies' are formed in human body and flagellated or promastigotes are developed in the insect body.

Incubation period: Usually from 10 days to 2 years, with an average of 1–6 months.

Transmission: Person to person by the bite of female phlebotomine sandfly.

Season: It is mostly seen during and after rains.

In India, endemic eastern states are Bihar, Jharkhand, Uttar Pradesh and West Bengal. Estimated 165.4 million population at risk in above mentioned 4 states. Mostly poor socioeconomic groups of population primarily living in rural areas are affected.

Manifestations

Initially, leishmania parasites cause skin sores or ulcers at the site of the bite. If the disease progresses, it attacks the immune system. The disease is characterized by gradual onset of:

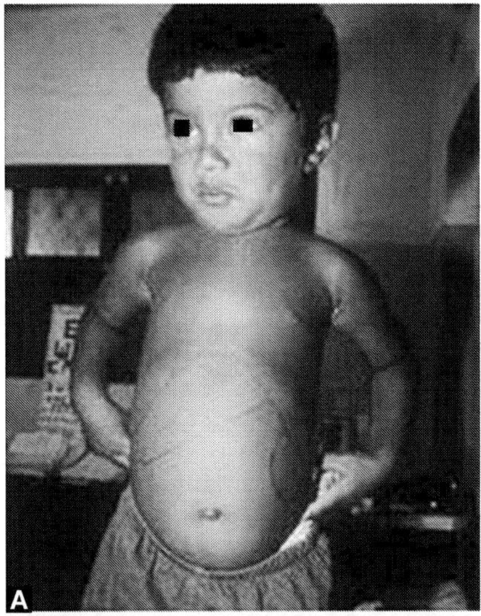

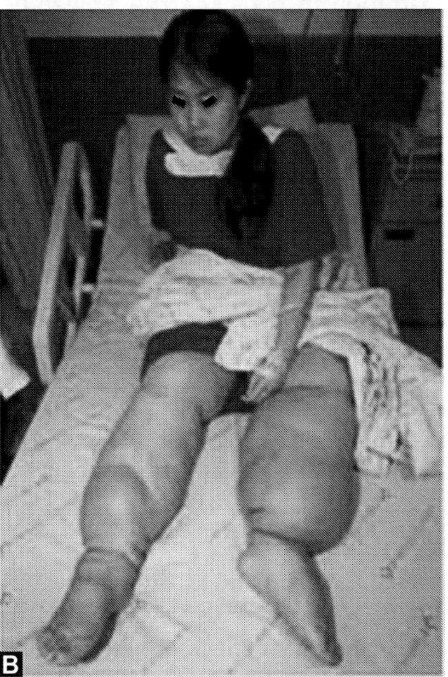

Figs 20.15A and B: A. A child with leishmaniasis infection; **B.** A girl with lymphatic filariasis

- Recurrent fever intermittent or remittent with often double rise.
- Headache, vomiting, malaise and toxic features.
- Loss of appetite, pallor and weight loss with progressive emaciation.
- Weakness.
- *Splenomegaly:* Spleen enlarges rapidly to massive enlargement (within 2 weeks), usually soft and nontender.
- *Liver:* Enlargement not to the extent of spleen, soft, smooth surface, sharp edge.
- *Lymphadenopathy:* It is not very common in India
- *Skin:* Dry, thin and scaly and hair may be lost. The term 'kala-azar' comes from India where it is the Hindi for black fever, and it is termed so, as patients show gray pigmentation of skin of hands, feet, abdomen and face.
- *Anemia:* It develops rapidly.

Anemia with emaciation and gross splenomegaly produces a typical appearance of the patients.

Diagnostic Evaluation

- *Clinical:* A case of fever of more than 2 weeks duration not responding to antimalarials and antibiotics. Clinical laboratory findings may include anemia, progressive leucopenia thrombocytopenia and hypergammaglobulinemia.
- *Laboratory:* Leishmanias is diagnosed in the hematology laboratory by direct visualization of the amastigotes (Leishman-Donovan bodies). Parasite demonstration in bone marrow/spleen/lymphnode aspiration or in culture medium is the confirmatory diagnosis. Amastigotes are seen with monocytes or, less commonly in neutrophils, of peripheral blood and in macrophages in aspirates.
- *Serology tests:* Variety of tests are available for diagnosis of kala-azar. The most commonly used tests include direct agglutination test (DAT), dipstick and ELISA, complement fixation test, PCR test, counter-immune electrophoresis. However all these tests detect IgG antibodies that are relatively long lasting. Aldehyde test of napire is commonly used but it is a nonspecific test. Anemia, leucopenia, reverse albumin and globulin ratio, increased ESR and IgG are seen in blood test.

Therapeutic Management

The treatment is determined by where the disease is acquired, the species of *Leishmania*, and the type of infection. There are different treatment options available for kala azar, with varying effectiveness and side effects. Pentavalent antimonials (sodium stibogluconate) are usually the first line of drugs. It is given as a 30 days course of intramuscular injection (20 mg/kg/day). The commonly used drugs are urea stibamine or neostigmine. While antimonials are quite toxic and present a risk to patients receiving treatment, those who are cured for kala-azar almost always develop immunity for life. When SSG fails to work amphotericin B 1 mg/kg body weight. IV infusion daily or alternate day for 15–20 infusions. Dose can be increased in patients with incomplete response with 30 injections.

Prevention

Leishmaniasis can be partly prevented by sleeping under nets treated with insecticide. Other measures include spraying insecticides to kill sandflies and treating people with the disease early to prevent further spread. Sanitary measures for elimination of breeding places of the parasites. An organized centrally sponsored control programme has been launched in endemic areas in India in 1990–91. Government of India provides kala-azar medicines, insecticides and technical support. The state governments implement the programme through primary health care system and district/zonal and State malaria control organizations and provide other costs involved in strategy implementation.

FILARIASIS

Lymphatic filariasis, commonly known as elephantiasis, is a neglected tropical disease caused by microscopic, thread like worms. Infection occurs when filarial parasites are transmitted to humans through mosquitoes. Infection is usually acquired in childhood causing hidden damage to the lymphatic system.

The painful and profoundly disfiguring visible manifestations of the disease, lymphoedema, elephantiasis and scrotal swelling occur later in life and lead to permanent disability. The patients with filaria are not only physically disabled, but suffer mental, social and financial losses contributing to stigma and poverty.

Lymphatic filariasis affects over 120 million people in 73 countries throughout the world. Worst affected countries are Bangladesh, Democratic Republic of Congo, Ethiopia, India, Indonesia, Myanmar, Nigeria, Nepal, Philippines and the United Republic of Tanzania.

Etiology and Transmission

Lymphatic filariasis is caused by infection with parasites classified as nematodes (roundworms) of the family Filarioidea. There are three types of these thread-like filarial worms: *Wuchereria bancrofti* (seen in 90% cases), *Brugia malayi*, and *B. timori*, which also cause the diseases.

Adult worms lodge in the lymphatic system and disrupt the immune system. The worms can live for an average of 6–8 years and, during their life time, produce millions of microfilariae (immature larvae) that circulate in the blood.

Microfilariae is transmitted to mosquito when they bite an infected host and ingest blood. Microfilariae mature into infective larvae within the mosquito. The mature parasite larvae are deposited on the skin, when infected mosquitoes bite people, from where they can enter the body. The larvae then migrate to the lymphatic vessels where they develop into adult worms, thus continuing a cycle of transmission. The disease is transmitted by different types of mosquitoes for example by the *Culex* mosquito, widespread across urban and semi-urban areas; Anopheles mainly in rural areas, and Aedes, mainly in endemic islands in the Pacific.

Clinical Manifestations

Lymphatic filariasis infection involves asymptomatic, acute, and chronic conditions, showing no external signs of infection. These asymptomatic infections still cause damage to the lymphatic system and the kidneys as well as alter the body's immune system. The most visible symptom of lymphatic filariasis is elephantiasis, i.e. edema with thickening of the skin and underlying tissues (Fig. 20.15B). Elephantiasis results when the parasites lodge in the lymphatic system. It was the first disease discovered to be transmitted by mosquito bites. This disease belongs to the group of diseases called helminthiasis.

Acute episodes of local inflammation involving skin, lymph nodes and lymphatic vessels often accompany the chronic lymphoedema or elephantiasis. Some of these episodes are caused by the body's immune response to the parasite. However most are the result of bacterial skin infection where normal defences have been partially lost due to underlying lymphatic damage.

When lymphatic filariasis develops into chronic conditions, it leads to lymphoedema or elephantiasis (skin/tissue thickening) of limbs and hydrocele. Involvement of breasts and genital organs is common.

Diagnostic Evaluation

A diagnosis of lymphatic filariasis should be considered in any patient with an appropriate exposure history who presents with characteristic signs and symptoms or unexplained eosinophilia. Definitive diagnosis can be made by detection of circulating filarial antigen (for *W. bancrofti* infection only), demonstration of microfilariae or filarial DNA in the blood, or of adult worms in the lymphatics.

The blood collection is usually done at night to coincide with the appearance of the microfilariae as they are nocturnally periodic, which means that they only circulate in the blood at night. Filariasis is usually diagnosed by identifying microfilariae on Giemsa stained, thin and thick blood film smears, using the 'gold standard' known as the finger prick test.

Serologic test techniques provide an alternative to microscopic detection of microfilariae for the diagnosis of lymphatic filariasis. Because lymphedema may develop many years after infection, lab tests are often negative with these patients.

Therapeutic Management

WHO's strategy of therapy is based on two key components:

- Stopping transmission through large-scale annual treatment of all eligible people in an area or region where infection is present
- Alleviating the suffering caused by lymphatic filariasis through increased morbidity management and disability prevention activities.

Mass Drug Administration

Prevention of lymphatic filariasis is possible by stopping the spread of the infection. Large-scale treatment involves a single dose of 2 medicines given annually to an entire at-risk population in the following way: albendazole (400 mg) together with ivermectin (150–200 mcg/kg) or with diethylcarbamazine citrate (DEC) (6 mg/kg). Ivermectin is the drug which acts directly on the microfilaria and in single doses of 200 to 400 µgm/kg keeps the blood microfilaria counts at very low levels even at the end of one year, like DEC.

These preventive chemotherapy medicines have a limited effect on adult parasites but effectively clear microfilariae from the bloodstream and prevent the spread of parasites to mosquitoes. Large-scale treatment conducted annually for 4–6 years, treating all persons living in areas where the infection is present can interrupt the transmission cycle.

The strategy that appears most suitable for elimination of filariasis in India is the administration of single annual dose of albendazole 400 mg along with

DEC 6 mg/kg body weight. This not only will prevent transmission of filariasis in the community by reducing the microfilaria levels, but also has the added benefit of clearing the intestinal helminths.

Morbidity Management

Morbidity management and disability prevention are vital for improving public health. Surgery can alleviate most cases of hydrocele. Clinical severity of lymphoedema and acute inflammatory episodes can be improved using simple measures of hygiene, skin care, exercise, and elevation of affected limbs.

HELMINTHIASIS

According to WHO, helminthiasis is infestation with one or more intestinal parasitic worms (roundworms (*Ascaris lumbricoides*), whipworms (*Trichuris trichiura*), or hookworms (*Necator americanus* and *Ancylostoma duodenale*) (Table 20.4).

Globally, more than 1 billion people are infected with one or more soil-transmitted helminth (STHs), mainly in areas with warm and moist climates where sanitation and hygiene are poor. STH infections are among the most common infections worldwide and affect the poorest and most deprived communities. Infected people excrete helminth eggs in their feces, which then contaminate the soil in areas with inadequate sanitation. Other people can then be infected by ingesting eggs or larvae in contaminated food, or through penetration of the skin by infective larvae in the soil (hookworms).

The main species that infect people are the roundworm (*Ascaris lumbricoides*), the whipworm (*Trichuris trichiura*) and the hookworms (*Necator americanus* and *Ancylostoma duodenale*.

Helminthiasis is associated with nutritional problems such as vitamin deficiencies, stunting, anemia, and protein-energy malnutrition, which in turn affect cognitive ability and intellectual development. Infestation can cause morbidity, and sometimes death, by compromising

Table 20.4: Helminthiasis is infestation with one or more following intestinal parasitic worms seen in human body

Agent	*Transmission*	*Manifestation*	*Diagnosis*	*Treatment*
Ascaris-lumbricoides (roundworm)	Oral-fecal route, iIngestion of eggs from contaminated food or fluid or soil. The eggs are transferred from fingers, toys and other vectors.	Pain abdomen, abdominal distension, nausea, cough, loss of weight, anemia, growth failure, vit.deficiencies, bruxism, voracious appetite. Pneumonitis, obstructive jaundice, intestinal obstruction may occur.	Fecal smear	Single dose albendazole (15 mg/kg), or mebendazole 100 mg BD × 3days, or single dose pyrante pamoate 10 mg/kg
Oxyuriasis (pin/ threadworm	Ingestation or inhalation of eggs, transfer from hands to mouth	Intense pruritus and (nocturnal), irritability, sleep disturbances	Microscopic examination, perineal swab test (tape test)	Single dose albendazole (15 mg/kg), or mebendazole 100 mg BD × 3days, or single dose pyrantale pamoate 10 mg/kg
Ancylostomiasis (hookworm)	Skin penetration from direct contact of contaminated soil, direct ingestion of larvae through foods	Progressive anemia, loss of appetite, epigastric pain, black stool, an irritant papulovesicular rash, pneumonitis	Examination of stool for hook worm ova and occult blood, eosinophilia	Single dose albendazole (10 mg/kg), or mebendazole 100 mg BD × 3days, or single dose pyrantel pamoate 10 mg/kg
Teniasis (tape-worm)	Consumption of infective cysticerci in improperly cooked meat (beef/pork)	Asymptomatic, abdominal pain and distension, nausea, anorexia, recurrent diarrhea, wt. loss, insomnia, segments of worms seen in stool. Cysticercosis in brain is manifested by convulsions, or inflammation, alteration of level of consciousness.	Fecal smear, microscopic examination	Praziquantel (PZQ) single dose (10 mg/kg)[safety in children under 4 years of age is not established]. In neurocysticurcosis-albendazole (15 mg/kg/day in three divided doses for 28 days OR PZQ 50 mg/kg/day in three divided doses for 2–3 weeks

nutritional status, affecting cognitive processes, inducing tissue reactions, such as granuloma, and provoking intestinal obstruction or rectal prolapse. Malnutrition due to helminths may directly affect cognition. This includeds low educational performances, decreased ability to focus, difficulty with abstract cognitive tasks. Anemia has also been associated with reduced stamina for physical labor, a decline in the ability to learn new information, and 'apathy, irritability, and fatigue'.

Prevention and control measures include: (1) use of clean water for personal and domestic uses; (2) sanitation and health education such as by promoting use of latrines; (3) awareness on personal hygiene such as hand washing and washing of food; (4) avoiding the use of uncomposted human faeces as fertilizer. In epidemic areas, mass deworming programs of school children is an important preventive method. Simple measures can be effective including constant wearing of shoes, soaking vegetables with bleach, adequate cooking of foods, handwashing at critical times (before contact with food and after use of the toilet), reducing open defecation, deworming of pet and proper disposal of their feces.

Control of helminthiasis is based on drug treatment, improved sanitation and health education.

Lifecycle of Helminths

Ascariasis: Ascaris lumbricoides is a nematode, commonly known as round worm, remains in intestine. It's size varies between 12–40 cm. Man is the only reservoir of infection. Each female ascaris produces eggs, which are excreted through feces and remain in external environment. On ingestion of mature eggs by human host, it hatches out in the duodenum to release larvae penetrates the wall of the duodenum and enters the blood stream. From there, it is carried via the portal, then systemic circulation to the lungs. The larva matures further in the lungs (10–14 days), penetrate the alveolar walls. In three weeks, the larva passes from the respiratory system to be coughed up, swallowed, and thus returned to the small intestine. Upon reaching the small intestine it matures to an adult male or female worm. Fertilization can now occur and the female produces as many as 2–2.5 lakh eggs per day for a year. These fertilized eggs become infectious after two weeks in soil; they can persist in soil for 10 years or more.

The eggs have a lipid layer which makes them resistant to the effects of acids and alkalis, as well as other chemicals. This resilience helps to explain why this nematode is such a ubiquitous parasite.

Oxyuriasis vermicularis (pinworm)—infection occurs by ingesting infective eggs.

Man is only natural or definitive host of pinworms. The larvae hatch from the egg in the small intestine.

Adults mature in the large intestine in about a month. The worm does not multiply inside the human body.

Gravid females move outside the anus during the night and deposit eggs in the perianal area. The larvae in the egg become infective in approximately 4 to 6 hours. Each egg matures after six hours in a larva, which can survive for about twenty days. The movement of the female worm and the eggs causes itching which makes it more likely for self-infection to occur.

ECHINOCOCCOSIS (HYDATID DISEASE)

Hydatid disease in man is caused mainly by infection by the larval stage of the dog tapeworm *Echinococcus granulosus*. It follows accidental ingestion of tapeworm eggs excreted in the feces of infected dogs. Hydatid disease is one of the most geographically widespread zoonoses. The natural hosts are canine predators, particularly domestic dogs and foxes and cattle, sheep and goats are intermediate host, man is an accidental intermediate host. Worldwide, four species of tapeworm are clinically important to man: *E. granulosus, Echinococcus multilocularis, Echinococcus vogeli* and *Echinococcus oligarthrus*, of which the first two are the most common and therefore the most important. The condition is complicated and expensive to treat, and may require extensive surgery and prolonged drug therapy. The WHO aims for an effective disease control strategy by 2018.

Echinococcus granulosus require two mammalian hosts for completion of their lifecycle. The tapeworm (a small one, about 5 mm long) lives in their gut of canid carnivores such as dogs and eggs are excreted with the stool to infect intermediate hosts (herbivores such as sheep, goats).

The egg hatches in the intermediate host and the larva invades the intestinal wall and is carried to the liver, lungs, brain and other organs, where it forms a hydatid cyst. Herbivores are then eaten by canid carnivores, where new adult tapeworms develop over about six weeks, and the cycle repeats.

Humans, especially children become infected by handling infected dogs. Hand to mouth transfer of eggs or by inhalation of dust contaminated with infected eggs causes the infection. In humans the cysts persist and grow for many years and can become very large. Infection is considered primary when spread by ingestion, and secondary when larval tissue proliferates after spread from the primary site—usually after trauma to the cyst.

Clinical Manifestation

- Most cysts causing symptoms are larger than 5 cm in diameter. Symptoms can include vague pains, cough, low-grade pyrexia and abdominal fullness. Later, as the mass presses on surrounding organs, symptoms become more specific.
- In the abdomen, where there is less restriction on growth through pressure from other organs, cysts may grow to several liters.
- The liver is the most commonly affected organ.
- In the liver, symptoms of obstructive jaundice and abdominal pain can develop. Pressure of the cyst on the biliary tract can cause biliary colic, jaundice, and urticaria. Vomiting of hydatid membranes (hydatid emesia) and passage of membranes in the stools (hydatid enterica) occur rarely.
- Involvement of the lungs may result in chronic cough, dyspnoea, pleuritic chest pain or hemoptysis. Expectoration of cyst membranes and fluid may be observed with intrabronchial rupture.

Diagnosis

History of residence and close association to dogs is to be explored.

- Ultrasound for abdominal cysts with fine-needle aspiration.
- CXR or CT scan for those in the lung.

Management

In general, human disease is treated by surgical removal of the cyst with supplementary chemotherapy (mebendazole or albendazole). Surgical removal may not prevent other cysts growing and causing further problems.

CHAPTER 21

The Child and Skin Conditions

Chapter Outline

- Review of Structure and Function of the Skin
- Nursing Care of Child with Skin Infection
- Herpes Simplex Virus Infection
- Burns
- Insect Bites and Stings

'The skin, or integument, is much more than a simple wrapping around our bodies. It is an active and versatile organ which is waterproof so that we do not dry up in the heat or melt in the rain, and it protects us from the damaging radiation of sunlight.'
—Ghaz

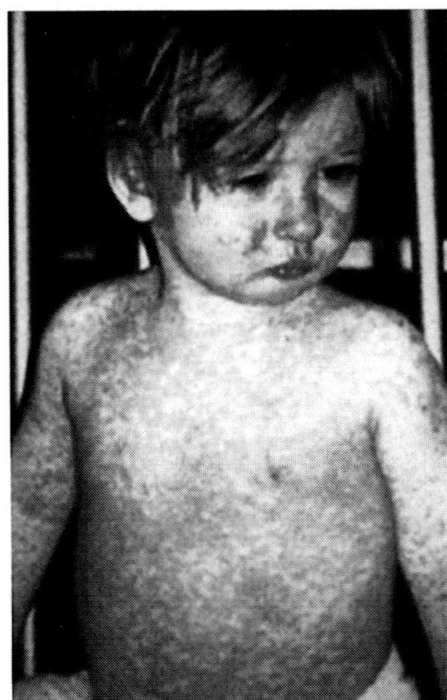

REVIEW OF STRUCTURE AND FUNCTION OF THE SKIN

The skin is an organ of the integumentary system made up of multiple layers of ectodermal tissue, and guards the underlying muscles, bones, ligaments and internal organs. The knowledge of structure and functions of skin is necessary to understand the changes that occur with different disorders. *The skin is made up of two principal layers of tissue—the epidermis and dermis. Both layers contain nerve endings which transmit sensations of pain, pressure, heat and cold. Under these layers is the subcutaneous layer, which is composed of largely adipose tissue (Fig. 21.1).*

The epidermis is nonvascular stratified epithelium. The outermost part—the epidermis consists of several layers of cells the lowest of which are called the mother cells. Constant cell division occurs here which move up to the surface, where they flatten, die and are transformed into a material called keratin. Keratin is a fibrous protein and, is also the principal component of nails and hair. It is finally shed as tiny, barely visible scales. It takes 3 to 4 weeks for a cell in the lowest layer to reach the skin surface. The lower most layer of epidermis is stratum basale, it anchors the epidermis to the dermis. *The*

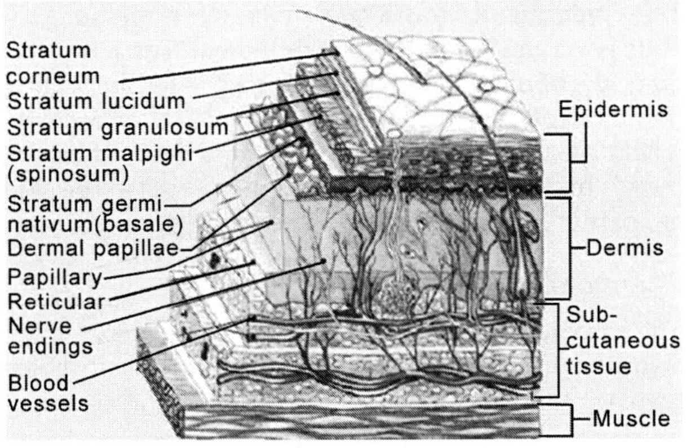

Fig. 21.1: Cross-section of skin

pigment-producing cells, melanocytes remain in this layer which gives skin its color.

Lying beneath the epidermis is another layer of the skin, known as the dermis. The *dermis* consists of connective tissue and cushions the body from stress and strain (that gives the skin its flexibility and strength). It contains nerves and lymphatics, hair follicles, sweat glands and sebaceous glands. The dermis is made up of important proteins—elastin and collagen. Moreover, tiny blood capillaries are also found in this layer, which provide a constant supply of oxygen and nutrients to the skin cells.

The sweat glands are vital in regulating the body's temperature, while the sebaceous glands lubricate the skin and hair. Each sweat gland is formed of a coiled tube of epidermal cells which leads into the sweat duct to open out on the skin surface. The sweat glands are controlled by the nervous system and are stimulated to secrete either by emotion or by the body's need to lose heat. *The apocrine glands develop at puberty and are a sexual characteristic.*

The skin's innermost layer is known as subcutaneous layer. This is where fat is deposited to act as an energy store as well as an insulator. The dermis insulate the body from heat and cold, provides protective padding, and serves as an energy storage area. The fat is contained in living cells, called fat cells, held together by fibrous tissue. The fat layer varies in thickness, from a fraction of an inch on the eyelids to several inches on the abdomen and buttocks in some people.

Functions of Skin

Skin is not just the largest, but also one of the most important organs of human body since it performs an array of various significant functions.

Protection

The epidermis acts as a barrier between our internal body parts and the external environment. Therefore, it is this layer of the skin which is responsible for preventing the entry of harmful foreign agents, such as bacteria, inside the body. Therefore, our skin is deemed as our body's first line of defense. Langerhans cells in the skin are part of the adaptive immune system.

Thermoregulation

The blood vessels of the dermis provide nutrients to the skin and help regulate body temperature. Skin helps body to maintain a constant internal temperature. When the temperature of the environment rises, the blood vessels present in the skin dilate. In this way, more heat is lost from the body. On the other hand, in response to a cold environment, these blood vessels constrict, thereby cutting down the body's heat loss.

Sweat glands present in the skin also play an important role in the regulation of temperature. More sweat is produced when the temperature of the surroundings rises. The evaporation of this sweat from the skin creates a cooling effect.

Hair not only contributes to a person's appearance but has a number of important physical roles, including regulating body temperature, providing protection from injury, and enhancing sensation. Moreover, hair follicles help maintain the body's temperature when it is exposed to a cold environment. When the hair stand on end, a phenomenon more commonly known as goose bumps, air is trapped between them acting as an insulator to prevent the loss of heat.

Moisture Retention

The epidermis acts as a barrier between our internal body parts and the external environment. Therefore, it is this layer of the skin which is responsible for preventing the entry of harmful foreign agents, such as bacteria, inside the body. Moreover, it contains a layer of cells known as melanocytes.

Removal of Toxins

Through the production of sweat, the skin helps our body get rid of toxins, such as urea. To maintain optimal health, it is necessary that a human being should have a healthy skin. If functions of skin are not performed properly because of illness or any other reason, the buildup of toxic material can cause loss of skin elasticity, increase in wrinkles or blemishes and cause skin cancer in some cases.

Vitamin D Production

Our skin contains a substance called ergosterol, which is responsible for the synthesis of vitamin D. On exposure to sunlight, ergosterol is converted into vitamin D_2 which is 1 form of 5 types of vitamin D. Vitamin D is a steroid vitamin and it promotes the absorption of calcium and phosphorous together with their metabolism.

Protection from ultraviolet rays–Moreover, it contains a layer of cells known as melanocytes.

Sensation

Skin contains a variety of nerve endings that jump to heat and cold, touch, pressure, vibration, and tissue injury. The nerve endings sense pain, touch, pressure, and temperature. Some areas of the skin contain more nerve endings than others. For example, the fingertips and toes contain many nerves and are extremely sensitive to touch.

Pediatric Difference

Thin skin: Pediatric skin is thinner than adult skin. It causes more water loss through skin.

Large surface volume ratio: The ratio of skin surface area to body volume is greater in children than in adults, results in greater absorption through skin (topical medications). Large skin surface area precipitates rapid fluid loss and heat loss, leads to hypothermia.

Immature eccrine glands: Children are less able to maintain thermoregulation through skin, because eccrine glands do not reach mature function before 2 to 3 years of age.

Lack of melanocytes: Increased photosensitivity occurs in infants as they have fewer melanocytes than adults.

Less IgA secretion: IgA secreted by the epithelial cells of mucous membrane, does not reach at adult level before 2 to 5 years. This makes the infant prone to infection.

Hormonal change: During adolescence sebum production is increased due to hormonal changes, which attributes to acne vulgaris.

Infections of the Skin

Diaper dermatitis, or diaper rash as it is more commonly known, is not a diagnosis but rather a category of skin conditions affecting the diaper area. There are four types of diaper dermatitis, including:

- Irritant contact dermatitis
- Overgrowth of yeast (*Candida albicans*)
- Allergic contact dermatitis
- Inflammatory skin conditions such as seborrheic dermatitis.

The most common type of diaper dermatitis is irritant contact dermatitis, associated with skin exposure to either urine or feces or both for a long period of time. Irritant contact dermatitis usually appears as bright red, sometimes slightly swollen, or even blister-like patches in the diaper area. Prolonged irritant contact dermatitis can increase the risk of infection in the affected area.

The primary treatment and prevention of irritant contact dermatitis includes barrier creams and ointments, most commonly containing zinc oxide. A mild topical steroid ointment or cream can also be very helpful in more quickly reducing the inflammation.

The next most common type of diaper dermatitis is the overgrowth of yeast, most commonly *Candida albicans*. The warm, moist, and often irritated environment of the diaper makes the skin more prone to an overgrowth of yeast. This condition generally develops on top of irritant contact dermatitis.

Usually, it appears as bright red bumps, patches, and sometimes pus-bumps that are found on the skin and in its folds. The condition can be treated with an over-the-counter topical antifungal cream such as clotrimazole (Mycelex), mycostatin (Nystatin), or with a prescription medication. A barrier cream, often containing zinc oxide, is also recommended to treat and prevent this skin condition. If irritant contact dermatitis is also present, sometimes an additional mild topical steroid is prescribed. If this condition is only treated with topical steroids, the yeast will spread.

Rarely, allergic contact dermatitis will occur. This condition is usually associated with a component of the diaper itself. Symptoms include redness and swelling with itchiness that continues to recur in the same area such as the near the diaper's adhesive tape, or around the leg where there is elastic in the diaper.

Treatment of allergic contact dermatitis is very similar to the treatment of irritant contact dermatitis: barrier creams and ointments, most commonly containing zinc oxide, or mild topical steroid ointment if necessary.

To prevent allergic contact dermatitis, parents need to identify the material that is causing the problem and avoid it.

Topical steroids require very careful use, specially in the diaper area to prevent potential side effects such as thinning of the skin and stretch marks. These effects can be prevented by using low potency topical steroids, such as hydrocortisone 1 to 2%, and applying topical steroids sparingly to the affected areas only twice daily as needed for no longer than 2 weeks at a time.

Impetigo

Impetigo is a highly-contagious bacterial infection of the surface layers of the skin, usually exhibited as painful and itchy blisters and sores around the mouth and nose (in very young children it can also occur in the nappy area). It is not serious, but it is sore and itchy in nature (Fig. 21.2). There are two types of impetigo. These are:

1. *Bullous impetigo* It causes large, painless, fluid-filled blisters that stay longer.
2. *Nonbullous impetigo*: It is more contagious and causes sores that quickly burst to leave a yellow-brown crust.

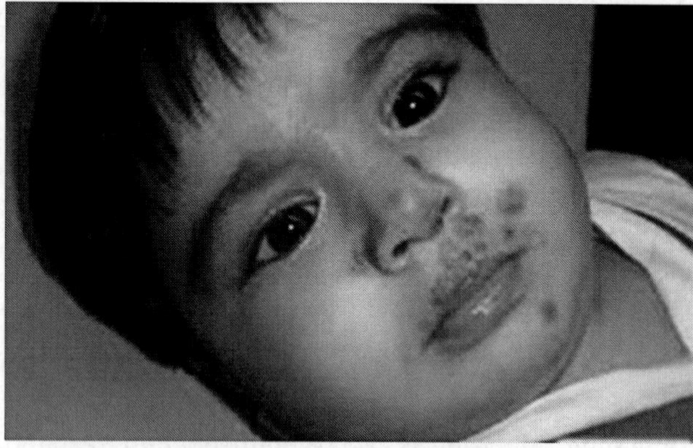

Fig. 21.2: A child with impetigo

It can either occur on its own, by bacteria entering the skin usually through a small nick in the skin, or as a complication of some other condition like eczema. Impetigo is not as common in adults. It is also known as *school sores*.

Etiology and Incidence

Impetigo is a superficial skin infection usually caused by *S. aureus* and occasionally by *S. pyogenes*. It is a contagious disease, spread by direct contact, getting too close to infected children, or by using their towels, wash cloths, etc. Toddlers and preschool children are the most commonly affected, often when recovering from upper respiratory tract infection. They are more likely to be affected if they have had other skin diseases.

> **Pathophysiology**
>
> *Impetigo starts, in an area of broken skin which allows the entry of organisms. S. aureus* produces a number of cellular and extracellular products, including exotoxins and coagulase, that contribute to the pathogenicity of impetigo, specially when coupled with preexisting tissue injury like an insect bite, scabies, or atopic dermatitis, etc. The inflammatory process results in the formation of a pustular lesion. Honey-colored fluid from this lesion becomes crusted. Impetigo commonly occurs on the face (especially around the nares in children) as nasal discharge containing the organism erodes healthy skin above the upper lip, and allows the entry of organism. It is also occurs in the extremities after trauma.

Manifestations

The nonbullous type is more common and typically occurs on the face and extremities. Smaller, crusted blisters, that pop and leave wet patches of red skin, initially with vesicles or pustules on reddened skin. The vesicles or pustules eventually rupture to leave the characteristic honey-colored (yellow-brown) crust.

Bullous impetigo, forms large, painless, fluid-filled blisters that stay longer. It is almost exclusively caused by *S. aureus*, exhibits flaccid bullae with clear yellow fluid and later become pustular, that rupture and leave a golden-yellow crust. The erosions bleed easily when crusts are removed.

Diagnosis

Diagnosis is by clinical presentation and confirmation by culture. A culture is not often done unless the child fails to respond to treatment.

Treatment

For most patients with impetigo, topical treatment is adequate. When the affected area is small it can be treated with antibiotic ointments. Treatment may involve washing with soap and warm water thrice a day, the crusts soaked and carefully removed, and letting the impetigo dry in the air. It is treated either with bacitracin (Polysporin) or mupirocin (Bactroban), applied twice daily for 7 to 10 days. If it spreads, systemic antibiotic therapy may be necessary for patients with extensive disease.

To keep the child from spreading impetigo to other parts of the body, it is recommended to cover infected areas of skin with gauze and tape or a loose plastic bandage. The child's fingernails is to kept short and clean to prevent scratching that could lead to infection.

Prevention

Keeping skin clean can help prevent impetigo. Kids should wash their hands well and often and take baths or showers regularly. Pay special attention to skin injuries (cuts, scrapes, bug bites, etc.), areas of eczema, and rashes such as poison ivy. Keep these areas clean and covered.

Anyone in family with impetigo should keep fingernails cut short and the impetigo sores covered with gauze and tape.

Prevent impetigo infection from spreading among family members by making sure everyone uses their own clothing, sheets, razors, soaps, and towels. Separate the infected person's bed linens, towels, and clothing from those of other family members, and wash these items in hot water. Keep the surfaces of your kitchen and household clean.

Candidiasis

Candidiasis, sometimes called moniliasis or a yeast infection, is an infection caused by yeast on the skin and/or mucous membranes. Fungal infections are caused by various species of a yeast-like fungus called *Candida*, particularly the species *C. albicans*. The fungus *Candida* is normally found on and in the body in small amounts. It is present on the skin and in the mouth, as well as in the intestinal tract and genital area. Most of the time, *Candida* does not cause any symptoms. It may cause an infection when the skin is damaged or when conditions are warm and humid, or when a child has a depressed immune system. In some very sick children, it can infect deeper tissues or get in the bloodstream and cause serious illness.

In infants, oral candidiasis is common (Fig. 21.3). It is a superficial fungal infection of mucous membrane, caused by overgrowth of *C. albicans*. Another most common manifestation of candidal infection is diaper dermatitis in infants, where infection passes through the intestine. Development of candida dermatitis is favored by the heat and moisture of the diaper area of the child. Persistent candidiasis suggests that the child may be immunocompromised.

Etiology and Incidence

Most times, this yeast unbalance in the intestinal flora is caused by frequent use of antibiotics or steroids. Some children, like adults, just seem to have a constitution that is susceptible to Candida yeast overgrowth and infections. It is also occur due to exposure to the mother's infected breasts, or feeding from unclean bottles and pacifiers. It is even possible for a baby to contract yeast through the birth canal of an infected mother.

Predisposing factors of candidiasis are antibiotic therapy, diabetes, and altered immune status of children (in all age groups). But, most often it occurs in infant. It is even possible for a baby to contract yeast through the birth canal of an infected mother.

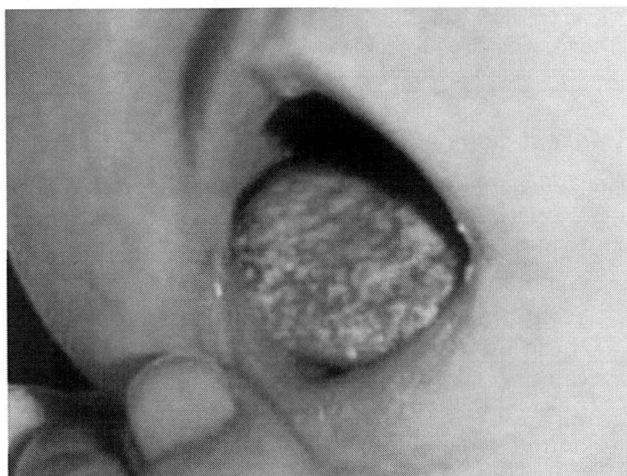

Fig. 21.3: A child with oral candidiasis

Manifestations

Candida are considered normal flora in the gastrointestinal and genitourinary tracts of humans, but invade and cause disease when there is an imbalance in their ecological niche. The clinical manifestations of infection with *Candida* species range from local mucous membrane infection to widespread multi-organ symptoms. The symptoms of candidiasis vary depending on the location of the infection.

- *Oral candidiasis:* Oral thrush causes curd-like white patches inside the mouth, on the tongue and palate and around the lips. They can be distinguished from milk curd as milk curd can be cleaned easily, but removing of plaques causes bleeding with an erythematous base. It may also cause cracked, red, moist areas of skin at the corners of the mouth. Infants with thrush may experience pain, poor feeding, or fussiness.
- Patients with cutaneous candidiasis experience itching, burning, and soreness. Most commonly affected areas are the diaper area in infants and toddlers which spreads out to the child's abdomen and thighs.

Diagnostic Evaluation

Clinical Examination

From the clinical appearance of the lesions the diagnosis of oral thrush and candidal diaper dermatitis is done.

History

To make a diagnosis, recent use of antibiotics or medications that can weaken the immune system is to be explored.

Microscopic Examination

Candidiasis is easy to identify. The yeast can be seen under the microscope after being scraped off the affected area.

Therapeutic Management

Candidiasis is not normally a dangerous disease except in rare cases when it enters the blood and spreads to vital organs of people with weakened immune systems.

For oral thrush, a suspension of antifungal medication (Nystatin 100,000 U/mL), swabbed onto the mucous membrane of the mouth is effective. Thrush may be treated with a medicated mouthwash or lozenges that dissolve in the mouth. Severe infection or infections in an immunocompromised child may be treated with oral antiyeast medications. To prevent the recurrence of infection, oral nystatin or oral fluconazole therapy is administered as Candida is present in the gastrointestinal tract.

Diaper Rash

For infection of the skin (diaper rash) (Figs 21.4A and B), an antifungal cream or powder is prescribed (e.g. nystatin or clotrimazole).

For children with diaper rash, diapers should be changed frequently and the child's skin gently cleansed with water and a mild soap, rinsed, and patted dry. Barrier creams or ointments such as Desitin or A&D are helpful. While cornstarch may be recommended for mild diaper rash, *it should not be used for children with significantly inflamed skin.*

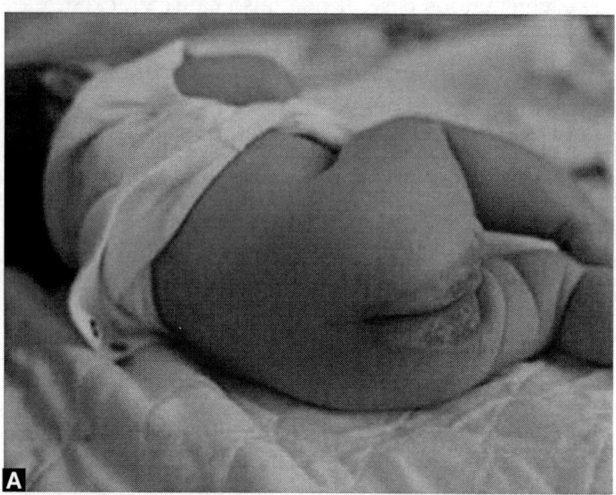

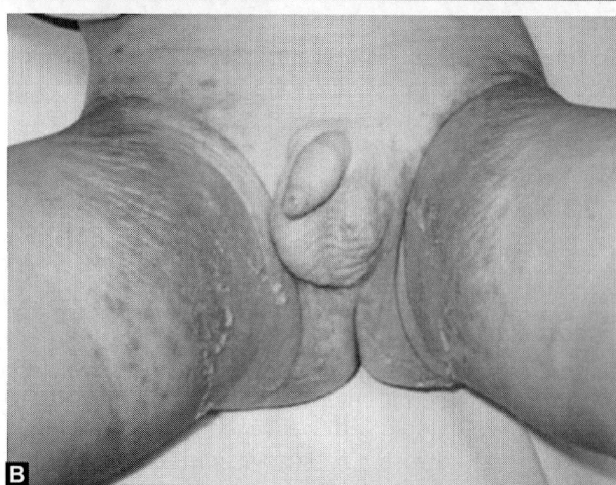

Figs 21.4A and B: Child with diaper rash

NURSING CARE OF CHILD WITH SKIN INFECTION

Tinea Infection

Tinea (ringworm) infections are fungal infections caused by dermatophytes, a group of fungi that invade and grow in dead keratin. Ringworm is a common and highly infectious fungal skin infection that causes a ring-like red rash on the skin. They tend to grow outwards on skin producing a ring-like pattern—hence the term 'ringworm'. They are very common and affect different parts of the body. These infections are designated by the word tinea followed by the Latin word for the affected part of the body. The rash can appear almost anywhere on the body, with the scalp, feet and groin being common areas.

Etiology and Incidence

Infection is very common all over the world. Some types are more common than others, tinea capitis the most common in children and with tinea pedis being most common in adults. It is a very common condition and has a higher prevalence in countries with hot humid climates. *T. rubrum* is the most common organism worldwide.

Pathophysiology

- Tinea infection is limited to the dead layers of skin, but encouraged by a damp and warm local environment. It invades hair, the stratum corneum of the skin or the nails. Clinical classification according to site can be done as *scalptinea capitis*, feet—tinea pedis, hands—tinea manuum, nail—*tinea unguium*, groin–*tinea cruris*, body including trunk and arms–*tinea corporis* (Table 21.1).
- The infection can be transmitted to humans by anthropophilic (between people), geophilic (from soil) and zoophilic (from animals) spread.

The most common organisms which invade human keratin are *epidermophyton*, *microsporum* and *trichophyton* genera.

Manifestations

Tinea is classified to the part of the body affected and symptoms depend on the affected area of the body:

- Itching, rash and nail discoloration are the most common symptoms of tinea infection.
- Scalp ringworm causes itchy, red patches on head. It can leave bald spots. Hair loss occurs with tinea capitis (mainly a disease of children).
- Ringworm is a red skin rash that forms a ring around normal-looking skin.
- Jock itch causes an itchy, burning rash in your groin area.

Table 21.1: Types of tinea-infection and its management		
Type	*Manifestations*	*Treatment*
Tinea corporis	Ring-like scaly appearance, well-defined margins, erythematous	Topical antifungal such as micanozole or clotrimazole is used. Cool compress
Tinea cruris	Well-defined scaly plaque in groin area, does not affect mucous membrane	Topical antifungal cream or lotion
Tinea pedis	Interdigital scaling and maceration	Topical antifungal cream/lotion/spray can be used
Tinea unguium	Scaliness of few nails in one hand/toe occur. Nails become brittle, broken and yellow colored	Topical application Systemic antifungal Thinning of toe nails and nail avulsion

- Complications such as secondary infection (cellulitis and impetigo) can lead to symptoms.
- It is common in people who play contact sports.
- It occurs in immunocompromised patients, particularly in adolescents who wear unventilated athletic shoes.

Diagnostic Evaluation

- Microscopy of skin and nail specimens may reveal hyphae and spores.
- Fungal culture can identify the species but is not always reliable and it can take 6 weeks to get results.
- Ultraviolet light (Wood's light) is useful for tinea capitis specially. Fluorescence is produced by the fungus. Fluorescence is not seen with tinea corporis or tinea cruris.
- Rarely, a biopsy may be needed if the case is atypical or not responding to treatment.

Therapeutic Management

For most skin infections it is sufficient to apply an imidazole cream twice daily. Treatment is continued for 1 to 2 weeks after the skin has healed. Commonly used drugs are clotrimazole, econazole, ketoconazole, miconazole.

- Systemic agents are appropriate for tinea capitis and onychomycosis. They should be used for extensive disease. They may also be used when topical treatments have failed or are inappropriate. Skin scrapings should be sent before starting oral treatment. Terbinafine 250 mg daily for 2 weeks (up to 6 weeks). Itraconazole 100 mg twice daily for 1 week (high dose for 1 week or low dose for 30 days). Itraconazole can be given in a pulsed fashion and is preferred to terbinafine.

HERPES SIMPLEX VIRUS INFECTION

See chapter 20 of this edition.

Pediculosis (Lice infestation)

The head louse is a tiny (about 2 to 4 mm in length), wingless 6-legged parasitic insect that lives among human hairs and feeds on tiny amounts of blood drawn from the scalp. Pediculosis can be explained as infestation of lice on the scalp or body. Lice are a very common problem, specially for kids (Fig. 21.5). They are contagious, annoying, and sometimes tough to get rid of. Although pediculosis is not a serious health problem, still it cause guilt and embarrassment among guardians and school personnel. The cause of worry is others will believe they are a dirty family/school with dirty kids. They do not spread disease, although their bites can make a child's scalp itchy and irritated, and scratching can lead to infection.

Etiology and Incidence

Lice live only on humans and head-to-head contact is the most common way to get head lice. The lice move from one person to the next by crawling. They cannot fly or jump. Head lice actually crawl everywhere. They

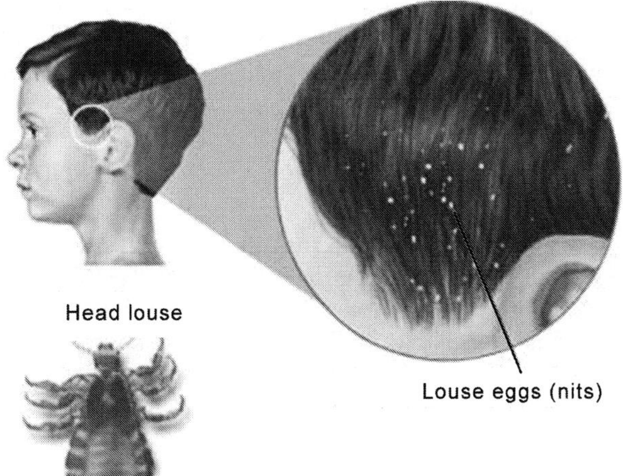

Fig. 21.5: Pediculosis capitis in child (the nits are attached to hair shaft)

crawl from person-to-person and on to objects that come into contact with human hair such as hats and towels, brushes, comb, stuffed toys.

The number of diagnosed cases of human louse infestations (or pediculosis) has increased worldwide since the mid-1960s, reaching hundreds of millions annually. Head lice infestations occur in affluent schools and underprivileged schools. All socioeconomic groups are affected. Infestations are more common in the warmer months. Girls are affected twice as often as boys. The peak incidence is in preschool and young school age children (aged 3 to 10 years).

Pathophysiology

For both head lice and body lice, transmission can occur during direct contact with an infected individual. Sharing of clothing and combs or brushes may also result in transmission of these insects. While other means are possible, in adolescents or young adults pubic lice are most often transmitted through sexual contact.

The female head louse lays egg (nits), and nits that females glue onto the base of the hair shaft near the scalp are even more difficult to spot. From each egg or "nit" may hatch one nymph (about 1 week) that will grow and develop to the adult louse (about 2 weeks). Head and pubic lice spend their life cycle on the skin of the human host, whereas body lice live in clothing, coming to the skin only to feed. Lice feed on blood once or more often each day by piercing the skin with their tiny needle-like mouthparts. While feeding they excrete saliva, which irritates the skin and causes itching. Severe itching caused by bites can predispose the child to secondary infection. Lice cannot burrow into the skin.

Manifestations

Nits (covered with gelatinous material which hardens to semiopaque, tiny, pearly whitish mass) are commonly visible behind the ears and at the nape of the neck (Fig. 21.6). It is difficult to find the adult lice as their size is small, crawl very fast to avoid light. Scattered lesions on the scalp cause intense pruritus. Posterior cervical lymph adenopathy may be associated with these lesions. Excessive scratching of the infested areas can cause sores, which may become infected.

Diagnostic Evaluation

To diagnose infestation, the entire scalp should be thoroughly combed with a louse comb. The use of a louse comb is the most effective way to detect living lice. Nits are visible in the hair shafts near the scalp. Unlike dandruff, nits are not easily removed from the hair shafts.

The most characteristic symptom of infestation is pruritus on the head which normally intensifies 3 to 4 weeks after the initial infestation. The bite reaction is very mild and it can be rarely seen between the hairs.

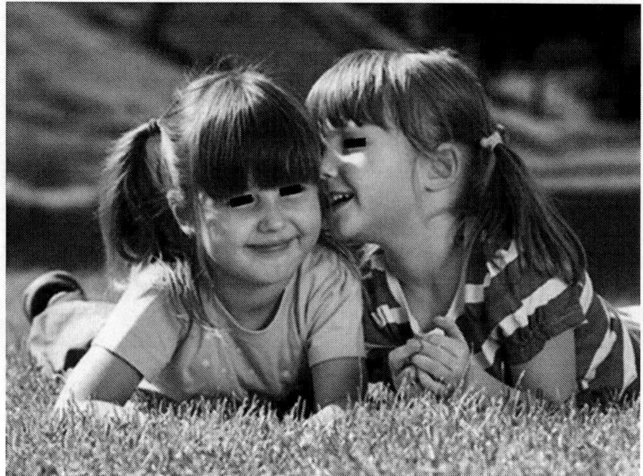

Fig. 21.6: Infected transmission of lice through head-to head-contact

Therapeutic Management

There are a number of treatment modalities that can be employed for management of child with pediculosis. The different approaches target to kill the active lice and removing nits, and preventing further spread or recurrence by managing the environment.

Killing of lice: There is no product or method which assures 100% destruction of the eggs and hatched lice after a single treatment. These methods include chemical treatments, natural products, combs, shaving, hot air, and silicone-based lotions. Medicated shampoos or cream rinses containing pyrethrins or permethrin are preferred for treating people with head lice. The pharmacological treatment of pediculosis include the use of crotamiton applied twice at 24 hour interval and washed off day after that. Retreatment after 7 to 10 days is often recommended to ensure that no eggs have survived. Benzyl benzoate also can be used when combined with lindane, it is applied once and then washed off after 24 hours.

Addressing the environment: Physical contact with infested individuals and their belongings, specially clothing, headgear and bedding, should be avoided. Health education on the life history of lice, proper treatment and the importance of laundering clothing and bedding in hot water or dry cleaning to destroy lice and eggs is extremely valuable. In addition, regular direct inspection of children for head lice, and when indicated, of body and clothing, particularly of children in schools, institutions, nursing homes and summer camps, is important. It is important to examine and treat family members and others who might be in close contact with the infested child.

Scabies (Mite Infestation)

Scabies is a contagious skin infection caused by the mite *S. scabiei*. The mite is a tiny, and usually not directly visible, parasite which burrows under the host's skin. This mite causes an intense itching sensation caused by an allergic response.

Etiology and Incidence

Direct skin-to-skin contact and close personal contact is the mode of transmission.

Scabies is widespread and seen throughout the world. Persons live in crowded condition and share beds, linen, towels are likely to transmit scabies to each other.

Pathophysiology

The linear burrows seen in the epidermis of patients with scabies are caused directly by the tunnelling mite. Female mite lays eggs into the epidermis and dies in the burrow after 4 to 5 weeks. Within 3 to 4 days the eggs hatch in and larvae migrate to the skin surface to mature and complete the life cycle.They are generally visible only once they become erythematous. The pruritus, erythema, papules, and nodules seen in affected individuals are due to the host immune response to the mite, egg and their excrement. Signs and symptoms appear 3 to 4 weeks after initial infestation but within a day upon re-infestation. Impetigo is a major complications of scabies results from scratching.

Fertilized female mites burrow for a month superficially beneath the stratum corneum of the skin where they deposit 2 or 3 eggs per day for 6 to 8 weeks. Larvae that hatches from these eggs mature in a series of molts in about 2 weeks and after that emerge to the surface of the skin, becomes adult, where they mate and subsequently reinvade the skin of the same or another host. Transmission of fertilized female mite from one person to another occurs by intimate personal contact and is facilitated by crowding, uncleanliness.

These mites cannot survive *off the human body* for more than 48 hours and cannot reproduce off the body.

Manifestations

A severe and relentless itch, specially at night is the predominant symptom of scabies.

Signs and symptoms of scabies include a skin rash composed of small red bumps and blisters that affects specific areas of the body like on the wrists, in the finger webs, the umbilicus and the axillae, on the elbows and buttocks. In infant, the head, palms and soles may be affected. Other symptoms can include tiny red burrows on the skin and relentless itching. The itch leads to frequent scratching, which may predispose the skin to secondary infections.

Diagnostic Evaluation

Diagnosis is made through history taking and clinical examination. It can also be made through microscopic examination of scrapings of the lesions.

Therapeutic Management

The medications that may be prescribed to treat scabies are:

- *5% permethrin cream:* This is the most common treatment for scabies. It is safe for children as young as 1 month old and women who are pregnant.
- 25% benzyl benzoate lotion
- 10% sulfur ointment
- 1% indane lotion.

The child/individual diagnosed with scabies and everyone who has had close contact with that one need treatment. Even people who do not have any signs or symptoms must be treated. This is the only way to prevent new infection of scabies weeks later.

Most patients may be cured with medicine that they apply to their skin. These medicines are often applied to all skin from the neck down. Infants and young children often need treatment for their scalp and face, too. A dermatologist will provide specific instructions to follow. Treating the skin more often than instructed can worsen the rash and itching. Most medicine is applied at bed time. The medicine is washed off when the patient wakes up. It may need to repeat this process 1 week later.

Scabies that covers much of the body and crusted scabies often require stronger drug. A patient with this type of scabies may receive a prescription of ivermectin. This medicine can be prescribed to children and patients who are HIV positive. Many patients need only to take 1 dose. Some patients need to take 2 to 3 doses to cure scabies. The pills are usually taken 1 week apart.

When scabies infects many people at a health care institution, extended care facility, and other institution, ivermectin may be prescribed to everyone who has a risk of catching scabies.

Other signs and symptoms: Some patients need other treatment like:

- *Antihistamine:* To control itch and help to sleep
- *Pramoxine lotion:* To control the itch
- *Antibiotic:* To combat an infection

- *Steroid cream:* To ease the redness, swelling and itch.

Treatment can get rid of mites, eliminate symptoms such as itch, and treat an infection that has developed. For the first few days to a week, the rash and itch can worsen during treatment. Within 4 weeks, skin should heal. If skin has not healed within 4 weeks, there may still have mites. Some people need to treat 2 to 3 times to get rid of the mites.

To get rid of the mites and prevent getting scabies again, people have to do more than treat the skin or take a pill. It needs to wash clothes, bedding towels to get rid of mites that may have fallen off from skin. Parents should vacuum their entire home.

Dermatitis

Atopic Dermatitis (Eczema)

Atopic dermatitis or eczema, is common chronic inflammatory condition of the skin characterized by intense itching (pruritus), hence it is commonly referred to as "the itch that rashes". The condition is associated with atopy, which refers to a predisposition toward developing hypersensitivity reactions such as eczema, asthma and allergic rhinitis. Atopic dermatitis has a strong familial association and is very common in kids, affecting 5 to 20% of children worldwide. Eczema can occur at any time in life. In most cases onset of the condition occurs before 5 years of age and may not diminish until early adulthood. Over half of the infants with atopic dermatitis grow out of the condition by age 2 years, though flare-ups can occur throughout life. The severity of the condition may wax and wane with most patients having 3 or more flare ups annually.

Etiology and Incidence

Eczema usually starts within the first 5 years of life, most often in the first 6 months. It typically lasts into childhood and adolescence. In some cases it may last into adulthood. Eczema tends to wax and wane. There are periods of time where the skin appears mildly affected or even normal, alternating with periods of moderate to severe involvement. Some children have very mild eczema and others have severe eczema (also known as atopic dermatitis). Eczema tends to be more common in families that have a history of eczema, hay fever, and asthma.

Eczema most commonly presents in early years, but adolescents and adults can also develop this condition. About 60% of patients will experience symptoms of atopic dermatitis by age 1 year, and another 30% will experience symptoms by age 5 years. Atopic dermatitis can also get worse when the skin comes into contact with irritating substances such as harsh soaps and scratchy, tight fitting clothing. Scratching can also promote infections that require treatment.

Manifestations

Pruritus is typically the most outstanding clinical feature and secondary lesions due to chronic rubbing and scratching are very common. The appearance of lesions can be varied and may present with any of these like–xerosis (dry, scaly skin), ill-defined erythema, small coalescing edematous papules or vesicles, lichenification and/or excoriations (secondary to relentless scratching), crusting (if secondarily infected). The location and appearance of eczema changes as children grow.

- In infants, red, very itchy dry patches of skin. In young babies, eczema is most prominent on the cheeks, forehead, and scalp. It may affect most of the body but usually spares the diaper area. The affected areas become erythematous, oozing and crusting occur.
- At 6 to 12 months of age, it is often worst on the crawling surfaces, the elbows and knees.
- Around the age of 2 years the distribution changes and tends to involve the creases of the elbows and knees, the wrists, ankles, and hands. It may affect the skin around the mouth and the eyelids.
- Older children and adolescents may have eczema only involving the hands. They may have red scaly rash on creases of hands, elbows, wrists and knees and sometimes on the feet, ankles and neck, thickened skin, markings, skin rash may bleed and crust after scratching.

In young babies eczema tends to be more red and weepy. In toddlers and older children it often appears more dry, and the skin may be thickened with prominent skin lines (a skin change called lichenification). *Symptoms can become worse if the child scratches the rash.*

Diagnostic Evaluation

Medical history is likely to be the most valuable diagnostic tool. A personal or family history of allergies, or asthma is often an important clue. To identify things in child's environment that may be contributing to the skin irritation, e.g. if the child started using a new soap or lotion before the symptoms appeared, etc.

Blood eosinophils and IgE level are often elevated, laboratory tests are needed. Skin testing for food allergies can identify potential food triggers.

Therapeutic Management

Unfortunately, there are no cure for eczema. Fortunately, in most children eczema becomes less severe with time. The good news is eczema can be controlled. The basics of treatment of preventing eczema flares includes, avoiding known triggers (such as harsh soaps, dust mites, food allergies), overheating and sweating (no wool and polyester clothing), and keeping child's skin well-moisturized. Since it is often hard to identify and avoid triggers, moisturizers can be the most helpful way to avoid eczema flares. Treating eczema requires treating both skin dryness and skin inflammation.

To help avoid dry skin, a daily bath using lukewarm water and a mild, moisturizing soap or soap substitute. Afterwards, cover him with a moisturizer as soon as possible to seal the moisture into his skin, are to be done. The room temperature is to be kept as regular as possible. Changes in room temperature and humidity can dry the skin. Mild laundry soap is to be used and make sure that clothes are well-rinsed.

Topical corticosteroids, also called cortisone or steroid creams or ointments, are commonly used to treat eczema. These medicines are usually applied directly to the affected areas twice a day. Continue to apply the corticosteroids for as long as it is prescribed. It is also important not to use a topical steroid prescribed for someone else. These creams and ointments vary in strength, and using the wrong strength in sensitive areas can damage the skin, specially in infants.

Nonsteroid medications are also available now in creams or ointments that can be used instead of, or in conjunction with, topical steroids.

Other prescription treatments may be recommended are antihistamines (to help to control itching). They are particularly helpful if itching is interfering with child's sleep, in which case a sedating antihistamine, like Benadryl (diphenhydramine hydrochloride) or Atarax (hydroxyzine hydrochloride), may work well.

Oral or topical antibiotics (to prevent or treat secondary infections), are common in children with eczema. Some older kids with severe eczema may also be treated with ultraviolet light under the supervision of a dermatologist to help clear it up and make them more comfortable.

In some cases, newer medications that change the way the skin's immune system reacts are also prescribed. Newer immunomodulators or steroid-free topical medications are also available to treat children with eczema. They are generally used twice a day in children over age 2 years and can be applied to all areas where your child has eczema, including his face. They may also help avoid flares if begin using them at the first sign of itching or a rash.

Cold compresses can also be effective at helping your child control his scratching when his skin itches.

Other treatments are also available for very difficult to treat cases of eczema, including using wet dressings, oral steroids, ultraviolet light therapy, and immunosuppressive drugs, like cylcosporin.

Acne Vulgaris

Acne, medically known as acne vulgaris, is a skin disease that involves the oil glands at the base of hair follicles. Acne vulgaris or simply acne is one of the most common skin problems of adolescence and is associated with a hormonal surge. *It commonly occurs during puberty when the sebaceous glands come to life—the glands are stimulated by male hormones produced by the adrenal glands of both males and females.* Acne is a chronic skin condition characterized by areas of blackheads, whiteheads, pimples, greasy skin, and possibly scarring. This problem of adolescence may results in appearance and lead to anxiety, reduced self-esteem, and in extreme cases, depression or thoughts of suicide.

Etiology and Incidence

Primary cause of acne is a rise in androgen hormone levels. Androgen levels rise when a human becomes an adolescent. Rising androgen levels make the oil glands under the skin to grow; the enlarged gland produces more oil. Excessive sebum can breakdown cellular walls (abnormal sloughing of skin cells) in pores, causing bacteria to grow. (*P. acnes*) is the anaerobic bacterium species that is widely suspected to contribute to the development of acne.

Some studies indicate heredity, hormonal influences, and emotional stress as host factors. Some medications that contain androgen and lithium may cause acne. Greasy cosmetics may cause acne in some susceptible people. Hormone changes during pregnancy may cause acne either to develop for the first time, or to recur. Poor hygiene, poor diet and stress can aggravate acne but do not cause it.

Acne usually starts during puberty and stops around 5 years later in 7 out of 10 people. It is much less common in later life. Occasionally, newborn babies can get acne in the first few weeks or months of life. It affects approximately more than 80% of adolescents and upto 20% of neonates. It is more common in boys. It flares up at winter and tends to improve in summer.

> **Pathophysiology**
>
> During puberty, an increase in sex hormones called androgens cause the follicular glands to grow larger and make more sebum. Acne starts to develop when hair follicles in the skin become blocked with the natural oil produced by skin (known as sebum) and dead skin cells. Normally each follicle is connected to a sebaceous gland that lies just underneath the surface of the skin. The sebaceous glands produce sebum to keep skin soft and supple. Normally, sebum travels up the follicle and out through small holes (pores) on the surface of skin. The earliest pathologic changes in acne are the excessive deposition of the protein keratin and oily sebum in the hair follicle resulting in the formation of a plug (microcomedo). A microcomedo may enlarge to form an open comedo (blackhead) or closed comedo (Fig. 21.7). The dark color of a blackhead occurs due to oxidation of the skin pigment melanin.
>
> Sometimes the bacterium *P. acnes*, which normally lives on the surface of skin, plays an important role in the development of acne as it causes inflammation (but not infection) and disruption of integrity of hair follicles. Deeper, inflamed lesions (nodules and cysts) can form if the inflammation is nearer the hair root. These plugged follicles can develop into swollen, red, tender pus bumps, or larger cysts or nodules that can cause temporary or permanent scarring.

Manifestations and Diagnostic Evaluation

In mild or moderate acne, the child may have greasy skin and spots (whiteheads or blackheads) on face, back and chest. Most spots will not cause any other symptoms. Sometimes, spots that have become inflamed (pustules, nodules and cysts) may be painful, tender to touch and the affected skin may feel hot.

Therapeutic Management

The goal of treatment should be the prevention of scarring so that after the condition spontaneously resolves there is no lasting sign of the affliction. The treatment must be individualized and to promote positive self-image. Prescribed acne treatments will depend on the age of the patient, skin type, and most importantly, the severity of the acne. Primary treatment starts with topical therapy with variety of agents. Here are some of the options available.

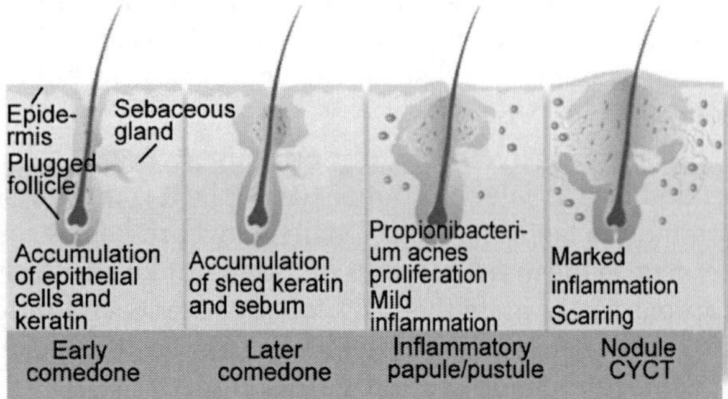

Fig. 21.7: Pathogenesis of acne

Benzoyl peroxide kills bacteria and slows down glands' production of oil. Benzoyl peroxide is a white crystalline peroxide used in bleaching (flour or oils or fats) and as a catalyst for free radical reactions. It works as a peeling agent, accelerating skin turnover and clearing pores, which in turn reduces the bacterial count in the affected area.

Retin-A

It helps unplug blocked pores and reduces comedo formation and eliminates the lesions already present. Retinoids (Retin-A) has been around for years, and preparations have become milder and gentler while still maintaining its effectiveness. Retin-A contains tretinoin, an acid from of vitamin A, also known as all-trans retinoic acid (ATRA). Tretinoin is also used for the treatment of acute promyelocytic leukemia. Retin-A has been used widely to combat aging of the skin, and it also acts as a chemical peel. Sunscreen should be used with tretinion to reduce photosensitivity.

Benzyl peroxide and tretinion, both are prescribed in case of acne. But application of the 2 drugs at a time is not effective because they have potential offsetting effect.

Salicylic acid helps to breakdown blackheads and whiteheads, also reduces shedding of cells which line the follicles of the oil glands, effective in treating inflammation and swelling. Salicylic acid is a white crystalline substance which is also used as a fungicide. It causes the epidermis to shed skin more easily, prevents pores from becoming blocked while at the same time allowing room for new cells to grow.

Depending upon the patient's age and the type of acne, *an oral antibiotic* (tetracycline, minocycline, doxycycline or erythromycin) may be beneficial. A topical antibiotic (erythromycin or clindamycin), instead of an oral antibiotic, can be very helpful.

It is important for the patient to follow the prescribed treatment for at least 6 to 8 weeks before considering changing therapy. During a follow-up visit, a re-evaluation can determine whether or not the treatment plan needs to be modified. Adolescents need support to keep from feeling of despair and discouragement. 3 to 5 months are needed for optimal result. The adolescents should be cautioned not to pick and squeeze lesions.

Other medications that have been helpful are *progestin and estrogen* pills for girl adolescents, specially when they report acne flare-ups around the menstrual period. If an individual has severe scarring acne, or if aggressive standard therapy does not improve their acne, an *oral retinoid (accutane)* may be necessary, which suppresses the sebum production and sebaceous gland activity. Because of the severity of side effects (pruritus, nose bleeds, conjunctivitis, depression) this drug is not prescribed to all adolescents. If this is dosed and monitored appropriately it can be a safe option, only if necessary.

Sexually active adolescent girls must know that isotretinoin has a high risk of inducing birth defects if taken by pregnant women. Two negative pregnancy tests before starting the drug, monthly tests during therapy, are to be done.

Treatment of acne scars: For those patients whose acne has gone away but left them with permanent scarring, several options are available. Some techniques such as dermabrasion, plastic repair, and collagen implants is done to improve appearance as scars of acne cannot be completely removed.

What products should be avoided to reduce acne?

If the acne is predominantly around the hairline, it may be associated with hair products such as conditioner, hair gels, hair mousse, oils, and grease. This type of acne can be improved by limiting hair products and pulling the hair away from the face.

Comedogenic (pore-blocking) moisturizer or cosmetics should be avoided. Try switching to a water-based noncomedogenic moisturizer and/or cosmetics.

Although diet has not been shown to influence acne, if somebody thinks certain foods cause his/her acne to flare up, then advice to avoid them.

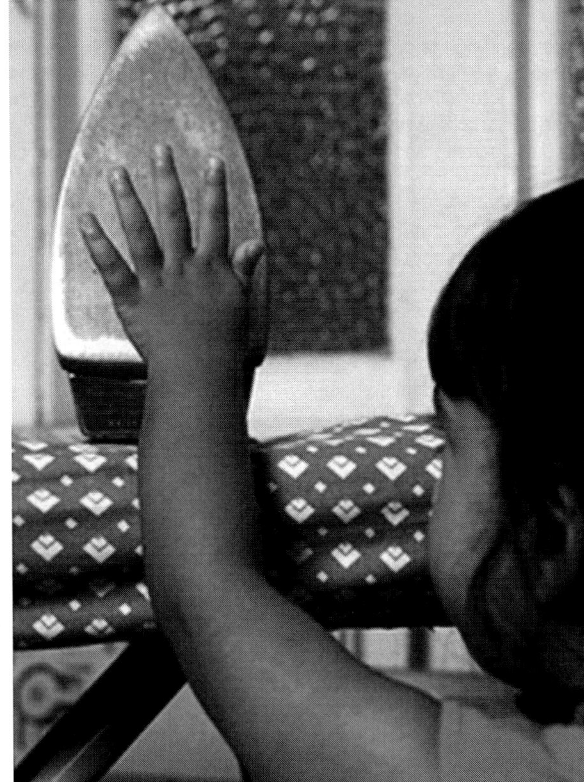

Fig. 21.8: Burns/scald due to lack of household safety

BURNS

Burns and scalds are a high injury risk for children (Fig. 21.8). A burn is a type of injury to flesh or skin caused by heat, electricity, chemicals, or radiation. A child's sensitive skin burns far more easily than adult skin. Children under 4 years are more at risk due to their increased mobility and natural curiosity, as they like to explore their surroundings. It is estimated that over half a million children are hospitalized with burn injuries per year in the world, with the majority occurring in low to middle income countries in Asia and Africa.

Burns that affect only the superficial skin are known as superficial or 1st degree burns. When damage penetrates into some of the underlying layers, it is a partial-thickness or 2nd degree burn. In a full-thickness or 3rd degree burn, the injury extends to all layers of the skin. A 4th degree burn additionally involves injury to deeper tissues, such as muscle or bone.

Etiology and Incidence

Injuries in pediatric patients are the result of behavior that can be intuitively related to developmental stages. The highest overall rate of injury exists in toddlers, who are becoming mobile and are actively searching their surroundings. They are yet, however, to learn of the dangers inherent in their behavior and readily encounter hazards in the home. When motor skill development outpaces cognitive development, disaster may result. These burns are often reported as inadequate supervision of the child by the care provider.

Burns are a global public health problem, accounting for an estimated 2,65,000 deaths annually. The majority of these occur in low-and middle-income countries and almost half occur in the South-East Asia region. According to WHO, females and males have broadly similar rates for burns. Burns are the 11th leading cause of death of children aged 1 to 9 years and are also the 5th most common cause of nonfatal childhood injuries. While a major risk is improper adult supervision, a considerable number of burn injuries in children result from child maltreatment. Other risk factors may be some occupations that increase exposure to fire, poverty, overcrowding and lack of proper safety measures; placement of young girls in household roles such as cooking and care of small children.

Pathophysiology

Understanding the pathophysiology of a burn injury is important for effective management. In addition, different injury patterns occur due to different causes of burn, which require different management. It is therefore important to understand how a burn was caused and what kind of physiological response it will induce.

Burn injuries result in both local and systemic responses. At temperatures greater than 44 °C, (due to flame, or chemical or electrical energy or ultraviolet light) cell proteins get denatured. The proteins begin to lose their three-dimensional shape, start to breakdown and destroy collagen linkages of connective tissues. This results in cell and tissue damage and leads to ultimate disruption in the normal functioning of the skin. They include disruption of the skin's sensation, ability to prevent water loss through evaporation, and ability to control body temperature. The cells lose potassium to the spaces outside the cell and to take up water and sodium due to disruption of cell membrane.

The three zones of a burn (the local responses) were described by Jackson in 1947, central necrosis, surrounded by the zones of stasis and of hyperemia. Jackson's Burn Wound Model provides a model for understanding the pathophysiology of a burn wound.

The zone of coagulation nearest the heat source is the primary injury. In this zone there is irreversible tissue loss due to coagulation of the constituent proteins. This occurs at the point of maximum damage. This zone has irreversible tissue necrosis at the center of the burn due to exposure to heat, chemicals or electricity. The extent of this injury is dependent on the temperature or concentration and the duration of exposure.

Zone of stasis— Surrounding the central zone of necrosis is a zone of ischemia in which there is a reduction in the dermal circulation. The surrounding zone of stasis is characterized by decreased tissue perfusion. The tissue in this zone is potentially salvageable. The main aim of burns resuscitation is to increase tissue perfusion here and prevent any damage becoming irreversible. This ischemic zone may progress to full necrosis unless the ischemia is reversed. If the ischemia is not relieved, for example when resuscitation and wound care are suboptimal, then persisting ischemia will worsen, and the burn depth will increase. Additional insults, such as prolonged hypotension, infection, or edema can convert this zone into an area of complete tissue loss.

Zone of hyperemia— At the periphery of the burn is a 3rd zone of hyperemia characterized by a reversible increase in blood flow and inflammation. In this outermost zone tissue perfusion is increased. The tissue here will invariably recover unless there is severe sepsis or prolonged hypoperfusion.

These 3 zones of a burn are three-dimensional, and loss of tissue in the zone of stasis will lead to the wound deepening as well as widening (Fig. 21.9).

In large burns (over 30% of the total body surface area), there is a significant inflammatory response. This results in increased leakage of fluid from the capillaries, and subsequent tissue edema. This causes overall blood volume loss, with the remaining blood suffering significant plasma loss, making the

Contd...

Contd...

blood more concentrated. Poor blood flow to organs such as the kidneys and gastrointestinal tract may result in renal failure and stomach ulcers.

Increased levels of catecholamines and cortisol can cause a hypermetabolic state that can last for years. This is associated with increased cardiac output, metabolism, a fast heart rate, and poor immune function.

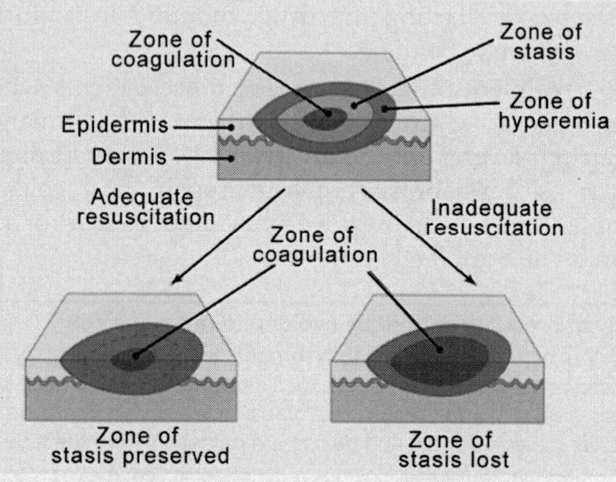

Fig. 21.9: Jackson's burns zones and the effects of adequate and inadequate resuscitation

Pediatric burns

- Thin skin
  - Increases severity of burning relative to adults
- Large surface/volume ratio
  - Rapid fluid loss
  - Increased heat loss → hypothermia
- Delicate balance between dehydration and overhydration
- Immature immunological response → sepsis
- Always consider possibility of child abuse

Fig. 21.10: Pathophysiologic response of a child in burns

A systemic effect results due to the release of cytokines and other inflammatory mediators at the site of injury once the burn reaches 30% of total body surface area. The changes may be— increased capillary permeability leads to loss of intravascular proteins and fluids into the interstitial compartment. Peripheral vasoconstriction, decreased myocardial contractility, fluid loss from the burn wound, result in systemic hypotension and end organ hypoperfusion.

Inflammatory mediators cause bronchoconstriction. The basal metabolic rate increases up to 3 times its original rate, non-specific down regulation of the immune response occurs due to burn injury.

Classification of Burn

Traditionally burns were classified as 1st, 2nd or 3rd-degree depending whether the burn was superficial, partial thickness or full thickness. The term 4th-degree was used to describe burns which involved underlying tissues such as muscle and fascia. However, since 2001, the main classification system used throughout the world is superficial, superficial partial, deep partial, or full thickness. The severity of a burn injury is determined according to the surface area affected and depth of the burn.

- *Extent of burn injury:* Although not always easy to assess in the 1st few hours, the site, depth, and extent of burns are critical factors in management, healing, and outcome. The body surface area affected is reported as a percentage of burned body surface area (% BBSA) which ranges from <1–100%. The standard "rule of nines" is not appropriate to determine extent of burn injury of child as it is well known that differences in body proportion between children and adults. The extent of surface area for pediatric burns is most accurately estimated using a chart based on the changes in body proportions commensurate with growth. The extent of surface area for pediatric burns is accurately estimated using a chart based on the Lund and Browder (Lund and Browder 1994) diagram (Figs 21.11A and B).
- *Depth of burn injury:* The depth of the burn wound relates to the layers of skin that have been affected. Skin is considered to have 2 layers namely the epidermis and dermis. The dermal layer is further classified as papillary dermis (upper layer) and the lower layer is reticular dermis.

  A classic example of a 1st-degree burn is moderate sunburn, which affect only the epidermis. Superficial burns involve only epidermis it is painful, healing usually occurs within 1 week without causing residual scarring.

  Superficial partial thickness burns (thermal, chemical, electrical injury of the skin) involve only papillary dermis and epidermis. Burns of this depth are expected to heal in 1 to 2 week. Usually no visible change to the skin is seen beyond 6 months.

  Deep dermal partial thickness burns involve epidermis and dermis to reticular dermis. The burns of this depth usually would take longer than 3 weeks to heal. This injury interferes the physiological functioning of the skin like preservation of fluid, thermoregulation, protection from infection and synthesis of vitamin D, etc. In this case skin grafting is recommended to promote early wound closure and to reduce the degree of residual scarring.

  Full thickness burns involve whole thickness of the skin and possibly subcutaneous tissue. Skin grafting

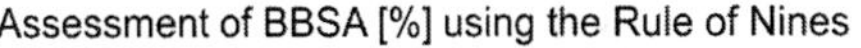

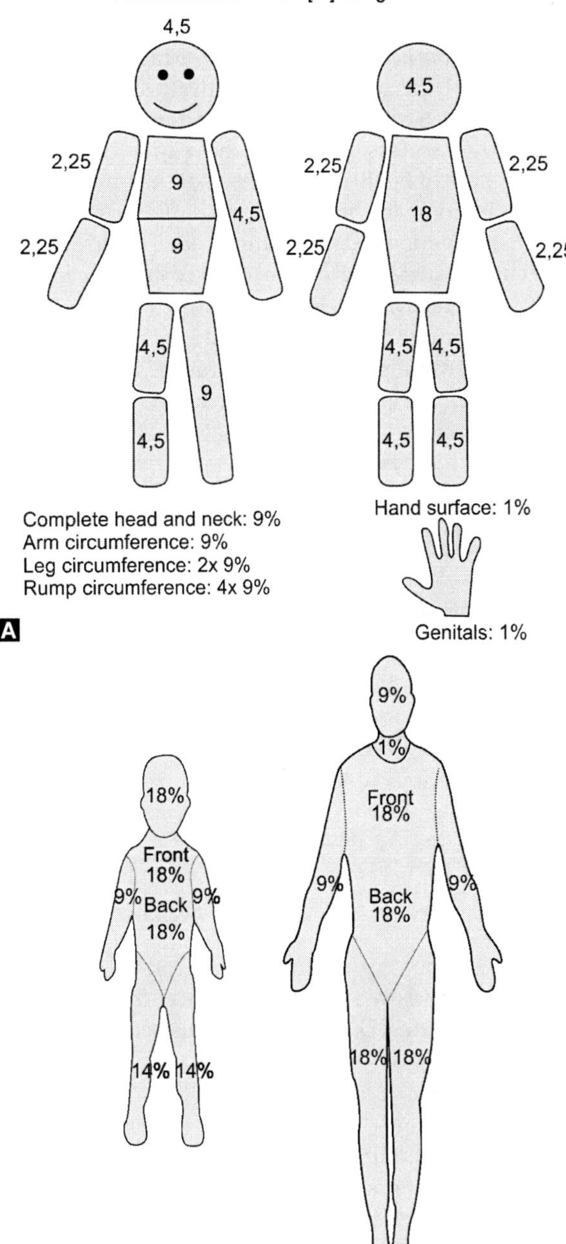

Figs 21.11A and B: Calculation of burned body surface area (% BBSA), both adult and child

is essential as there is little potential for spontaneous healing.

- *Severity of burn injury:* The severity of a burn depends largely on the depth of tissue destruction and the amount of body surface affected (Figs 21.12A and B). Other factors including the patient's age and prior state of health, the location of the burn wound (face, hands), and the seriousness of any associated injuries (concomitant trauma, like head injury, fractures, sustained at the time of burn) can also influence recovery from a burn.

Severe burns cause immediate nervous shock. The victim grows pale and is confused, anxious, and frightened by the pain and may faint. The secondary shock that comes a few hours later, is much more dangerous. This secondary shock is precipitated by loss of fluid from the circulation, not just the fluid lost in the destroyed tissue but fluid that leaks from the damaged area that has lost its protective covering of skin.

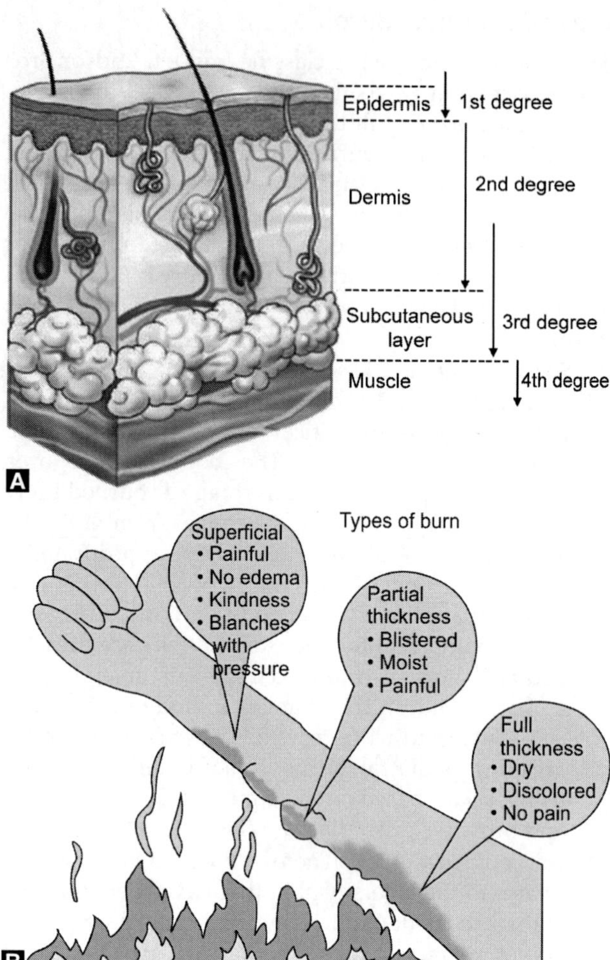

Figs 21.12A and B: Depth of the burn injury and changes in the skin and other structures

Manifestations

The following (Table 21.2) lists the clinical manifestations associated with burns of different severity.

Therapeutic Management

Therapy techniques following burn injury are focussed on minimizing impairment to body structures, as well as encouraging healthful return to activities and participation.

First Aid

Following a minor burn injury/a small 2nd-degree burn, the best first aid is to run cool tap water over the burn for 10 to 20 minutes. Do not use ice. This action will stop the burning process. The wound can be cleansed with mild soap and water and gently blotted dry.

After cleansing, the burn can be left exposed, provided it is small and will be frequently washed. Dissipate the heat energy from the wound. The injured area is to be covered with a clean, dry cloth to reduce the risk of infection.

Application of medicine or ointment is to be avoided, as it can hamper the proper assessment of the injury. Home remedies, such as butter or petroleum jelly, should *not* be applied to the wound, as these trap heat within the injury and can cause further damage. The application of antiseptics and other irritating substances should also be avoided; a good rule of thumb is to refrain from applying any substance that one would be afraid to put into one's eye.

All patients with severe burns should be hospitalized. Immediate management of a child with major burn injury includes initial assessment and establishing and maintaining the child's airway, breathing and circulation. A careful medical history is taken, and tetanus toxoid is administered. A catheter is inserted into the bladder to measure hourly urine output. A nasogastric tube is placed into the stomach to prevent aspiration.

- *Establishing and maintaining airway:* The 1st priority in treating the burn victim is to ensure that the airway remains open. Risk for smoke inhalation is greatest in victims who have injuries to the upper torso or burns of the face and in victims who cough up carbonaceous material or soot. If inhalation

Table 21.2: The clinical manifestations associated with burns of different severity

Depth	*Appearance*	*Layers involved*	*Cause*	*Surface/color*	*Texture and pain sensation*	*Healing time*
Superficial (1st degree)		Epidermis	Sun, flash, minor scald	Dry, minor blisters, erythema, brisk capillary return	Dry painful	5 to 10 days without residual scarring
Partial thickness-superficial (superficial dermal) 2nd degree		Extends into superficial (papillary) dermis	Scald	Moist, reddened with broken blister. Blanches with pressure	These wounds are typically moist and weeping painful	Less than 2 to 3 weeks
Partial thickness – deep (deep dermal) 2nd degree		Extends into deep (reticular) dermis	Scald, minor flame contact	Moist,yellow or white slough. Less blanching. May be blistering	Fairly dry painless	3 to 8 weeks
Full thickness (3rd degree burn)		Extends through entire dermis	Flame, severe scald or flame contact	Dry, charred whitish/brown. Absent capillary return	Leathery painless	Prolonged (months)
4th degree burn		Extends through entire skin, and into underlying fat, muscle and bone		Black; charred with eschar	Dry painless	

injury seems likely, a tube is to be inserted through the patient's nose or mouth into the trachea. This endotracheal tube allows the administration of high concentrations of oxygen and the use of a mechanical ventilator.

- *Shock management:* Fluid resuscitation is of paramount importance during the initial care of the burned child to combat shock. Burn shock develops after a burn injury that affects more than 15 to 20% of TBSA in children. All the capillaries of circulatory system (not only the affected areas) lose their capillary seal within few minutes of major burn injury, resulting in leakage of intravascular body fluid into the interstitial spaces. The RBCs and leukocytes remain in the circulation and produces increased hematocrit. So during the initial phase of resuscitation, adequate vascular access must be obtained. The overall objective of resuscitation is to replace fluid losses and restore euvolemia, while avoiding the detrimental effects of fluid overload.

  The fluid requirements may be calculated using several different formulae, the Parkland formula is one of them. The *Parkland formula* provides a simple and easily remembered basis for resuscitation (4 mL Ringer's lactate (RL)/kg/% BSA burned; one-half to be given during the first 8 hour after injury and the rest in the next 16 hour).

  Important points for fluid therapy in case of burn injury:
  Time for fluid replacement is calculated from the time of the injury, not the time of admission to the hospital.
  This formula is a guide to manage burns over 15 to 20%. It may be altered according to the condition of the child, urine output, lab reports.

  The type of fluid administered is generally an isotonic crystalloid, with the recommendation for the addition of dextrose to children under 20 kg to prevent the development of hypoglycemia. Thus, it is critical to monitor the endpoints of fluid resuscitation including hemodynamics, urine output-with a goal of maintenance of 1 to 2 mL/kg/h for children <30 kg and 0.5 to 1 mL/kg/h for those ≥30 kg, mental status, lactate levels, and base deficit.

- *Pain management:* Pain management is a critical piece in the overall care of the burned child. Pain is most problematic in patients with partial or deep 2nd-degree burns and is aggravated by the necessity of frequent dressing changes and physical therapy. Anxiety and depression are confounding components in a major burn and can further decrease the pain threshold. High-dose opioids are commonly used to manage acute breakthrough pain and pain associated with burn procedures. In addition, the combination of opioids and benzodiazepines (with appropriate monitoring) can be used successfully for procedural sedation, as daily wound care and dressing changes are associated with significant pain. Burn centers sometimes employ innovative measures to control pain, including the use of morphine intravenously, the administration of incomplete anesthetic drugs at the time of dressing changes, and even the use of general anesthesia during major debridements.

- *Burn wound management:* After this initial treatment of the airway and resuscitation of the burn shock, attention is directed toward burn wound management. The key elements of conservative burn wound management include cleansing, debridement, topical antimicrobial agents, and dressing changes of the burned areas. Cleansing allows better inspection of the wound surface, and debridement (removal of devitalized and necrotic tissue from the burn wound).

  Superficial burns with an intact epidermis do not require specific treatment with antimicrobial agents or dressing changes. Burn wounds are initially gently cleansed with mild soap and water, and debridement is performed using gentle mechanical techniques, such as brushing or scraping. In addition, a number of proteolytic enzymes have been used to aid debridement, although they should not be used if infection is suspected. The use of topical antimicrobial agents has reduced the incidence of invasive wound infections and sepsis.

  Hydrotherapy tank may be used to keep the burn wound under isotonic saline and cleansing done. So escher, sloughs, dead and loose skin can be removed during dressing. Regular dressing changes and aggressive wound care are instrumental toward recovery of burn injury, as it protects the wound from further infection, provides comfort, and promotes healing. There are a variety of dressings exist including standard fine mesh gauze, hydrocolloid, silver-containing dressings, biosynthetic, and biologic dressings. There is no clear evidence on which dressing provides the best coverage. This is to be noted that dressing which minimizes amount of changes may be more suitable for children.

  Grafts: Grafting is done to cover the wound where re-epithelialization is not possible, in case of deep or extensive burn wound. Grafting decreases the risk of infection, prevents further loss of protein and body fluid from the wound, minimize heat loss through evaporation, decreases contracture as it prevents the formation of hypertrophic scar. Grafts may be either temporary or permanent. It can also be categorized as biologic (homograft and heterograft), biosynthetic, synthetic and autologous or a combination of these.

- *Nutrition therapy:* Nutrition can be a particularly vexing problem because the caloric needs are often greater than the patient can consume in a normal fashion. Because in burn injury, pain leads to increased catecholamine release, which aggravates the patient's nutritional needs and energy expenditure. Glycogen stores in children are very limited to meet these increased demands. Thus, supplementary feedings administered intravenously or through a feeding tube placed into the stomach are commonplace in treating severe burns. 23% of total calories should be from proteins to maintain weight and muscle function. Addition of vitamin A and C also help to overcome the losses. One of the major advances in the treatment of the critically burned has been the use of hyperalimentation, a procedure in which total nutritional support can be provided through a catheter placed into a large central vein. Total nutritional requirement of a child with burn can be calculated by following formula :

  Davies formula

  Protein requirement—3 g/kg of body weight and 1g per percentage of TBSA.

  Calorie requirement—60 kcal/kg body weight plus 35 kcal per percentage of TBSA.

  Herndon formula

  1800 calories / m^2/24 hours + 1300 calories /m^2 BSA.

- *Maintaining position:* Maintaining position and change of position helps to prevent contracture and other complications.
- *Drug therapy:* Antibiotics, narcotic, analgesics, bronchodilator, steroids are administered as it is needed.

Complications

The use of topical antibacterial agents has reduced the incidence of postburn infection, but *infection* remains one of the most serious complications of burns. Early detection and prompt treatment of infection with antibiotics and surgical debridement can minimize its consequences.

Acute gastrointestinal ulcers are another frequent complication of burns; they appear as small, circumscribed lesions within the lining of the stomach or duodenum. These ulcers can be detected by endoscopy and are treated with antacids and drugs that reduce the amount of acid secretion.

Contractures (inability to perform full range of motion) result from factors such as limb positioning, duration of immobilization, and muscle, soft tissue and bony pathology, and place the person at risk of secondary medical and functional deficits. Contractures tend to be associated with the "position of comfort" (e.g. axillary adduction contractures, elbow and knee flexion contractures, hip flexion contractures), except for hands (claw deformity).

Hypertrophic and, to a lesser extent, *keloid-like scarring* are common and caused by proliferation of dermal tissue following skin injury. Scar is considered immature if it is red, raised and/or rigid and mature when it is avascular, flat, pliable and soft. It may create a wide range of cosmetic and functional problems. The inflexibility of the scar may limit motion of the joint or soft tissue.

Pressure ulcer is a risk due to physiological responses of postburn injury (e.g. hypovolemic shock resulting in blood flow being diverted away from the skin to preserve vital organ function). Additional injuries may add to the increased risk of pressure ulcers such as inhalation injury (requiring intubation and use of paralytic agents) and fluid resuscitation (resulting in edema that decreases the blood flow to the skin and adds weight to body parts. Careful observation of the wound as well as pressure areas and monitoring of risk areas of pressure ulcers are needed.

Nursing Management

Nursing diagnosis: Pain related to injury.

Expected outcome: Relief of pain as it will be verbalized by the child and he/she will be able to perform ADLs (activities of daily living).

Nursing interventions	*Rationale*
• Assessment of pain level through pain scale. Administration of pain relieving drug. Promote uninterrupted sleep with use of intravenous analgesics • Provide non-pharmacologic measures of pain relief • Cover burn wound as much as possible	• Objective measurement of pain can be done through pain scale and it helps in management. Pain is always present, but changes location; intensity may indicate complications. Sleep deprivation can increase pain perception • Temperature changes or movement of air causes pain

Contd...

Contd...

Nursing interventions	*Rationale*
• Assessment of pain level through pain scale. Administration of pain relieving drug. Promote uninterrupted sleep with use of intravenous analgesics • Provide non-pharmacologic measures of pain relief • Cover burn wound as much as possible • Help/encourage in change of position and range of motion exercises • Encourage verbalization of pain. Provide age appropriate play and diversional activities • Use analgesics before all dressing changes and burn care	• Objective measurement of pain can be done through pain scale and it helps in management. Pain is always present, but changes location; intensity may indicate complications. Sleep deprivation can increase pain perception • Temperature changes or movement of air causes pain • It reduces joint stiffness and prevents contracture • Provides outlet for emotion and helps the child cope. Diversional activities help lessen focus on pain • Helps to reduce pain and decreases anxiety for subsequent dressing changes

Nursing diagnosis: Altered temperature (hypothermia) related to loss of skin, microcirculation and open wound.

Expected outcome: Normal temperature of child.

Nursing interventions	*Rationale*
• Keep the child in a warm environment • Drape the child with sheet and blanket • Monitor vital signs • Provide warm drinks and feeds when oral feeding starts	• Warm environment minimizes evaporative heat loss • Minimizing exposure helps in prevention of heat loss

Nursing diagnosis: Risk for infection.

Expected outcome: Free from infection during healing process.

Nursing interventions	*Rationale*
• Keep the patient in burn unit if available or keep in a separate clean room • Ensure meticulous hand-washing before and after care • Take vital signs frequently • Follow standard precaution to handle the wound • Limit visitors • Keep burn dressing dry	• Minimizes bacterial contamination • Reduces the risk of cross contamination • Rise of temperature is an early sign of infection • Reduces risk of wound contamination • Helps reduce the number of bacteria introduced to the burn site

Nursing diagnosis: Risk for fluid volume imbalance as evidenced loss of fluid through wound.

Expected outcome: The child will maintain adequate urine output, burn site edema will be less.

Nursing interventions	*Rationale*
• Monitor vital signs, CVP, cap refill time, pulses • Administer IV and oral fluids as prescribed. Monitor strict I/O • Estimate insensible fluid losses • Weigh child daily • Insert urinary catheter, if needed • Monitor for hyponatremia and hypercalcemia	• The child is initially at risk for hypovolemic shock and needs fluid resuscitation (see above) • Careful calculation of need of fluid and its proper administration help keep the child properly hydrated. The child is at risk for fluid overload during hydration, and for edema in the tissues at the burn site • Losses are increased during the first 72 hours after burn injury; may need replacement. Plasma is lost through burn site because of capillary damage • Significant weight loss or gain can help determine fluid imbalances • Helps maintain accurate output measurement during critical care stage • Sodium is lost with burn fluid and potassium is lost from damaged cells, causing electrolyte

Nursing diagnosis: Altered nutrition: Less than body Requirements related to high metabolic needs.

Expected outcome: The child will maintain weight and demonstrate adequate serum albumin and hydration.

Nursing interventions	*Rationale*
• Provide an opportunity to choose meals. Offer a variety of foods • Provide snacks • Encourage the child to have meals with other children • Provide a multivitamin supplement • Substitute milk and juices for water • Provide nasogastric feedings as needed • Weigh the child daily	• Encourages intake. General malaise and anorexia lead to poor healing • Socialization improves intake • Vitamin C aids zinc absorption; zinc aids in healing • A child with a burn greater than 10% of BSA cannot usually meet nutrition requirements without assistance • Provides objective evaluation

Nursing diagnosis: Altered peripheral tissue perfusion related to mechanical reduction of venous and/or arterial blood flow (edema) of circumferential burns.

Expected outcome: The child will maintain adequate perfusion in burned extremities.

Nursing interventions	*Rationale*
• Elevate extremities Perform hourly distal pulse checks. Notify the physician of decreased or absent pulses • Check eschar	• Elevation helps to reduce dependent edema by promoting venous return. Dependent edema can constrict peripheral circulation • Eschar can constrict peripheral circulation in edematous extremity

Nursing diagnosis: Impaired physical mobility related to joint stiffness due to burns.

Expected outcome: The child will maintain maximum range of motion.

Nursing interventions	*Rationale*
• Arrange physical and occupational therapy twice daily for stretching and range-of-motion exercises. • Splint as ordered. Encourage independent ADLs	• Good positioning, range-of-motion exercises, and alignment prevent contractures

Nursing diagnosis: Disturbed body image related to altered look of the healing burn.

Expected outcome: The child will enter to his/her previous social settings and will feel comfortable with companions.

Nursing interventions	*Rationale*
• Be honest to answer the child's question regarding his appearance. Encourage the child to verbalize feelings about appearance and about returning to school • Encourage the family's involvement in child care and encourage the child in age appropriate self-care • Discuss ways in which the child can "cover up" any disfigurement through clothing and make up • Identify support systems and discuss child's coping strategies to face crisis	• Honesty is a building block of trusting relationship which helps the child to develop realistic expectations. Identifying the child's concern and anxieties is the primary step in developing effective coping strategies • Involvement of family in child care minimizes separation anxiety of the child • Child's participation in child care helps increase self-esteem • It can help the child to enter into his previous social settings, specially in school. School nurse can assist the child with the transition to school

Miscellaneous Skin Conditions

Warts

Warts result from an infection with a virus, and are common in children of all ages. Immunocompromised children are more susceptible to wart. Common and flat warts are caused by human papilloma virus, incubation period is 1 to 6 months. Warts commonly present as hard bumps on fingers, hands and feet.

Warts usually spread through direct contact. It is also possible to pick up the virus in moist environments.

Manifestations: Wart is hyperkeratotic papule, and it is painless. At the beginning it remains in flesh color papule then turns to brown with a rough surface. Without treatment most warts disappear in 2 to 3 years. It resolves within 2 to 3 months with treatment. Wart may spread to other areas of the body, if picking is done.

Management: Unfortunately there are no antiviral treatments that actually target the virus itself. Instead, the treatment available is targeted against the skin in which the virus is living.

Liquid salicylic acid with lactic acid is applied as it softens the abnormal skin cells and dissolves them. First, soak the wart in warm water to help the medication penetrate the skin.

Repetition of the treatment may be necessary to remove the wart. Freezing the wart with liquid nitrogen (cryotherapy) is another method.

INSECT BITES AND STINGS

Outdoor play is common for children and they come in contact with insects during play. Insect bites and stings are not serious and usually only cause minor irritation. However, some stings can be painful and trigger a serious allergic reaction due to the venom of stinging insects (Fig. 21.13). Usually bite include mosquitoes, fleas, bedbugs and, although not strictly insects, spiders, mites and ticks, which are arachnids. Insects that sting include bees, wasps and hornets. An insect bites human by making a hole in his skin to feed. Most insects sting as a defence by infecting venom into skin.

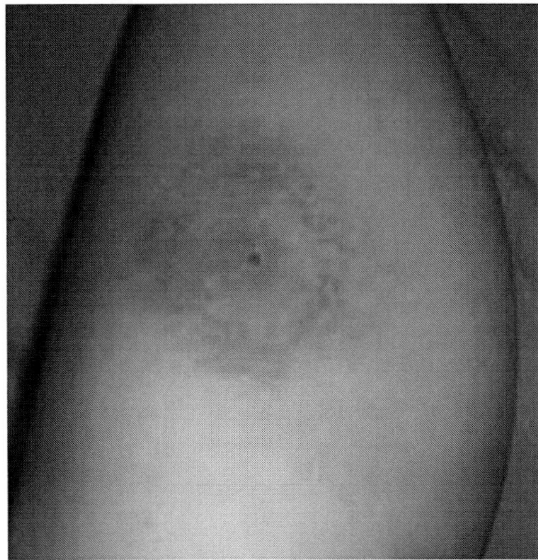

Fig. 21.13: Sting forms a wheal on the skin

Symptoms of Insect Bite or Sting

When an insect bites, it releases saliva that can cause the skin around the bite to become red, swollen and itchy.

The venom from a sting often also causes a swollen, itchy, red mark (a wheal) to form on the skin. This can be painful, but it is harmless in most cases. The affected area will usually remain painful and itchy for a few days.

The severity of bites and stings varies depending on the type of insect involved and the sensitivity of the person.

Therapeutic Management

Wash the area with soap and water, apply a cold compress. Acetaminophen or ibuprofen is given for pain. To protect against infection, antibiotic ointment is applied. Washing of child's hands is to be done.

CHAPTER 22

The Child with Sensory Alteration

Chapter Outline

- Eye and Disorders of the Eye
- Refractive Errors
- Ear and Disorders of the Ear

EYE AND DISORDERS OF THE EYE

Structure and Function of Eye

The eyes are the sense organs for vision. The orbit of the eye is a bony cavity that contains the eyeball, muscles, nerves, and blood vessels, as well as the structures that produce and drain tears. Sclera is the white layer, which covers the eyeball. Near the front of the eye, in the area protected by the eyelids, the sclera is covered by a thin, transparent membrane (conjunctiva), which runs to the edge of the cornea.

Light reflected from an object travels in all directions, some rays enter the eye. Incoming light rays are initially refracted by the cornea. Light rays enter the pupil to reach the retina (Fig. 22.1). After passing through the cornea, light travels through the pupil. The iris, circular and colored area of eye that surrounds the pupil controls the amount of light that enters the eye. The iris allows more light into the eye when the environment is dark and allows less light into the eye when the environment is bright. The size of the pupil is controlled by the action of the pupillary sphincter muscle and dilator muscle.

The lens provide fine focusing of light rays and the muscles of the ciliary body control the shape and focusing power of the lens. Retinal arteries and veins supply nutrients and remove waste from the retina. The retina contains the photoreceptor cells (rods and cones) which transform light into nerve signals. The most sensitive part of the retina is a small area called the **macula**, which has millions of tightly packed photoreceptors (the type called cones). There are two main types of photoreceptors: cones and rods. The high density of cones in makes the visual image in detailed. Cones are responsible for sharp, detailed central vision and color vision and are clustered mainly in the macula. The rods are responsible for night and peripheral vision. Rods are more numerous (about 120 million in number) than cones about 6.5 million in number and much more sensitive to light, but they do not register color or contribute to detailed central vision as the cones do.

Electrical signals from each retina pass along the optic nerves, which meet at a junction called the optic chiasm. The optic nerve from each eye divides in the optic chiasm. Half of the nerve fibers from each side cross to the other side and continue to the back of the brain. Thus, the right side of the brain receives information through both optic nerves for the left field of vision, and the left side of the brain receives information through both optic nerves for the right field of vision. The middle of these fields of vision overlaps. It is seen by both eyes (called binocular vision).

Disorders of the Eye

The eyes are complex organs, with many parts that must work together to produce clear vision. Eye development continues until a child is six years old. Vision is important in development because it allows children to interact with their environment. Vision in preschool children is uniquely important because their visual system is still developing and they are at risk of developing some problems. Disorders of the eye may develop due to systemic diseases or isolated causes like infections, vitamin deficiency, trauma, congenital disorders. If any child complains of dim vision, flashes

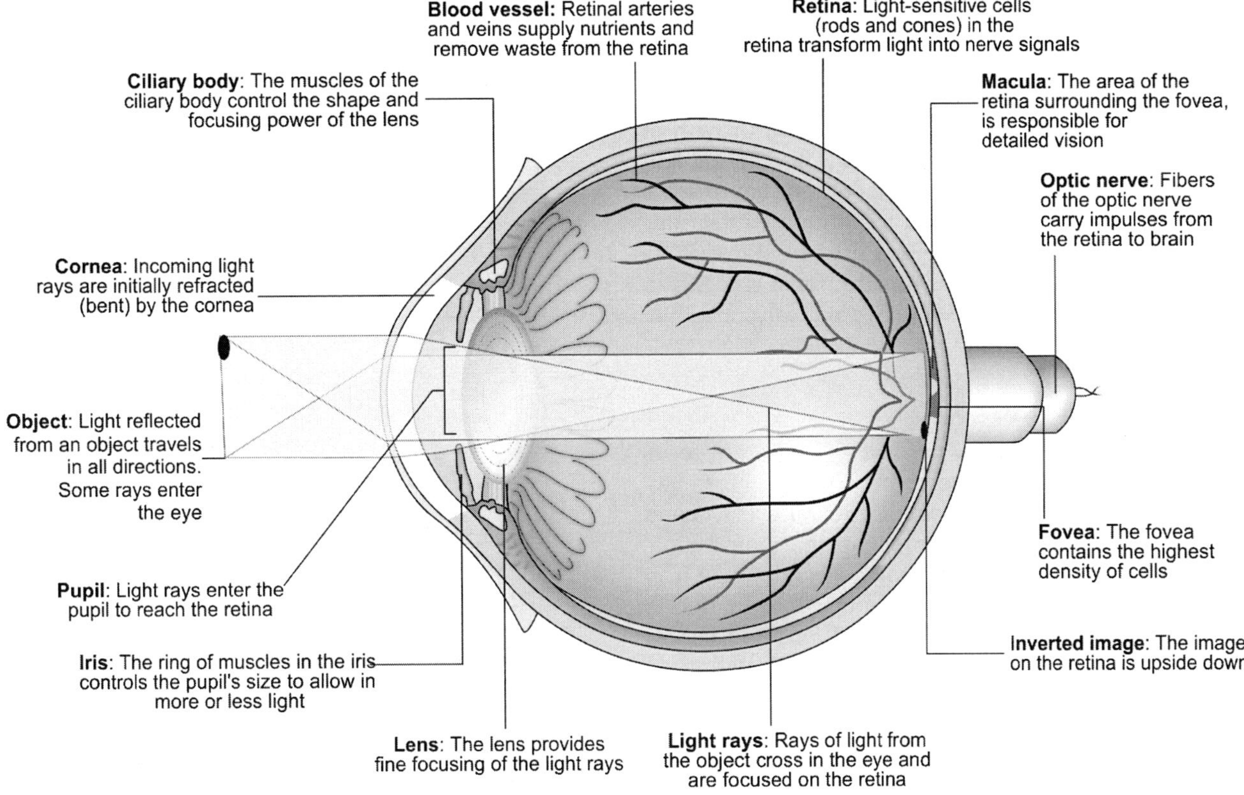

Fig. 22.1: Structure of eye

of light, pain, double vision, fluid coming from the eye, inflammation, etc. immediate professional help is to be sought for. Early detection and treatment could prevent vision loss.

Causes of visual impairment can be categorized as:

Genetic Predisposition

Vision disorders are caused due to some genetic condition like Down syndrome, Crouzon disease, Tay-sachs disease, etc. and manifested through cataract, exotropia, blindness.

Prenatal Factors

Some infections like rubella, toxoplasmosis, syphilis during pregnancy may cause cataract or blindness in children. These children may show other health problems like seizures, mental retardation and need immediate intervention.

Perinatal Factors

Prematurity and other perinatal conditions may precipitate vision problems. Respiratory distress syndrome often occurs in premature children who need high concentrations of oxygen. High concentration of oxygen for long duration causes fibrotic changes in the retinal vessels and retina may detach, called retrolental fibroplasia. This retinopathy of prematurity may lead to myopia.

Postnatal Factors

Some conditions like measles, chickenpox, trauma and infections all may cause vision changes.

Retinopathy of Prematurity (ROP) or Retrolental Fibroplasias

Normally, maturation of the retina of child starts in-utero, and at term, the medial portion of the retina is fully vascularized, while the lateral portion is only incompletely vascularized. The normal growth of the blood vessels is directed to relatively low-oxygen areas of the retina, but if excess oxygen is given, normal blood vessels degrade and cease to develop. When the excess oxygen environment is removed, the blood vessels rapidly begin forming again and grow into the vitreous humor of the eye from the retina.

Retinopathy of prematurity (ROP) or retrolental fibroplasia (RLF), is a disease of the eye affecting prematurely-born babies generally having received intensive neonatal care, including oxygen therapy. It is thought to be caused by disorganized growth of retinal blood vessels which may result in scarring and retinal detachment. ROP can be mild and may resolve spontaneously, but it may lead to blindness in serious cases. As such, all preterm babies are at risk for ROP, and very low birth weight is an additional risk factor. Both oxygen toxicity and relative hypoxia can contribute to the development of ROP.

REFRACTIVE ERRORS

A **refractive error** occurs when the eye does not focus light correctly and it causes blurry vision. Normally the cornea and lens work together to refract, to bend incoming light. Then they focus that light onto retina. The retina receives visual information and sends it to optic nerve and optic nerve carries that information to the brain. A perfectly formed, curved lens and cornea result in a perfectly focused image (Fig. 22.2). Refractive errors can usually be corrected with glasses, contacts, or surgery. They include:

- myopia (nearsightedness), which is when faraway objects look blurry
- hyperopia (farsightedness), which is when close-up objects look blurry
- astigmatism, which can result in blurry vision because the cornea is not perfectly shaped to direct light into the eye.

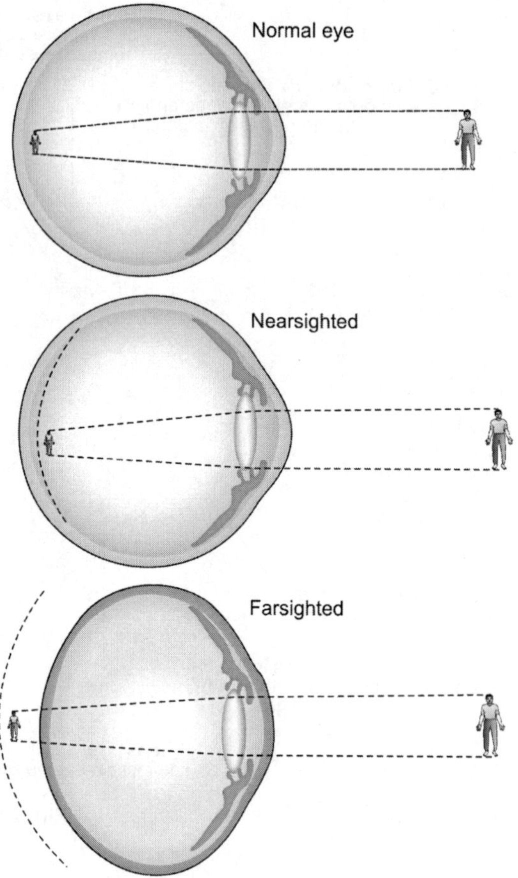

Fig. 22.2: Normal vision and different refractive errors

Myopia

Myopia is an eye condition in which near objects are seen clearly, but faraway objects appear fuzzy or blurry. In myopia, eye focuses incorrectly because its shape is slightly abnormal. A nearsighted eyeball is usually a little too long, and sometimes, its cornea is too rounded. The myopic child has excessive refractive power. In myopia, eye focuses light entering the eye in front of the retina instead of onto the retina.

According to the National Eye Institute (NEI), myopia is usually diagnosed between the ages of 8 and 12 years when eyes are growing at this age, so the shape of the eyes can change.

Blurry vision when looking at faraway objects is the most obvious symptom of nearsightedness. Children may have trouble seeing the blackboard at school.

Other signs of nearsightedness include:

- headaches
- eyes that hurt or feel tired
- squinting.

The symptoms of nearsightedness usually go away after treatment with eyeglasses or contact lenses. Eyeglasses and contact lenses are examples of corrective biconcave lenses. These devices compensate for the curvature of the cornea or the elongation of the eye by shifting the focus of light as it enters into eye.

Headaches and eye fatigue may linger for a week or two as you adjust to your new eyeglass or contact lens prescription.

Hyperopia

Hyperopia or farsightedness means it is easy to see things that are faraway, but near vision is blurry. To understand farsightedness, it is important to understand how the eye works. Two parts of the eye are responsible for focusing: the cornea and the lens. The cornea is the clear front surface of the eye. The lens is a structure inside eye that changes shape as it is focussed on objects.

A hyperopic eye is shorter than normal and it is caused by insufficient refractory power. Light from close objects cannot focus clearly on the retina. If cornea is too flat, eye cannot focus correctly. About 75% of all neonates are hyperopic; but as they have a greater accommodative ability, they overcome the error and see objects at a nearer range.

In hyperopia eyes have to work hard to see anything up close and causes eyestrain. Some symptoms of farsightedness are due to this extra eyestrain. Symptoms include:

- tension
- fatigue
- blurry vision up close
- squinting to see better
- aching or burning sensation around eyes
- headache after reading or other tasks that require to focus on something up close.

The simplest way to correct farsightedness is to get prescription eyeglasses or contact lenses. These corrective lenses are biconvex lenses which change the way light enters into eyes, helping to focus better. If one eye is hyperopic, the stronger eye is patched. Increasing the use of weaker eye increases its refractive power.

Nursing Care of a Child with Refractive Errors

Assessment

History and observation, examination, investigation and diagnostic procedure in eye. A child tilts his head, rubs eyes, squint, walks into objects, he or she holds things close to face.

Nursing Diagnosis

- Alteration in visual perception of patient, as a result of refractive error.
- Knowledge deficit, about treatment of refractive error.
- Altered comfort as a result of refractive error manifested by asthenopia.

Action

Refer for vision testing. Use corrective lenses when caring for child. As preventive measure educate parents to be aware of signs and symptoms and their meaning. Encourage vision testing at early stage.

Astigmatism

Astigmatism is a visual distortion. It distorts or blurs vision for both near and far objects. A normal cornea is round and smooth, in astigmatism, the cornea curves more in one direction than in the other. With astigmatism, the lens of the eye or the cornea, has an irregular curve. This can change the way light passes, or refracts, to retina. This causes blurry, fuzzy, or distorted vision. It is possible to have astigmatism in combination with myopia or hyperopia. It is not known what causes astigmatism, but genetics is a big factor. Visual acuity assessment test, refraction test, keratometry (to measure the curvature of cornea) are done to diagnose astigmatism. Corrective eyeglasses and contact lenses prescribed to neutralize the curvature.

Strabismus

Strabismus is a disorder in which both eyes do not line up in the same direction, so they do not look at the same object at the same time. The condition is more commonly known as 'crossed eyes.'

In normal binocular vision six different muscles surround each eye and corresponding nerves work 'as a team.' This allows both eyes to focus on the same object.

In someone with strabismus, these muscles do not have coordination and as a result, one eye looks at one object, while the other eye turns in a different direction to focus on another object resulting in double vision called diplopia.

This confuses the brain. In children, to resolve the conflicting information the brain may learn to ignore the image from the weaker eye.

If the strabismus is not treated, the eye that the brain ignores will never see well. This loss of vision is called amblyopia. Another name for amblyopia is 'lazy eye.' Sometimes amblyopia is present first, and it causes strabismus.

In most children with strabismus, the cause is unknown. In more than half of these cases, the problem is present at or shortly after birth. This is called congenital strabismus. Most of the time, the problem has to do with muscle control, and not with muscle strength.

Tests will be done to determine how much the eyes are out of alignment includes corneal light reflex, cover/uncover test, retinal exam, standard ophthalmic exam, visual acuity. A brain and nervous system (neurological) exam will also be done.

The first step in treating strabismus in children is to prescribe glasses, if needed. Next, amblyopia must be treated. A patch is placed over the better eye. This forces the weaker eye to work harder and get better vision. Eye muscle surgery may be needed if the eyes still do not move correctly. Different muscles in the eye will be made stronger or weaker. Treatment should be done before the child's self image is disturbed.

Amblyopia

Commonly referred to a 'lazy eye,' amblyopia occurs when one eye has worse vision than the other, and the brain begins to favor the better eye. This will occur if one of the eyes is blocked from producing clear images during the critical years from ages 0 to 6. One eye may be inhibited by problems such as a lid droop, tumor, or crossed eyes (strabismus) that are not fixed when a child is young.

Strabismus is classified as paralytic and non-paralytic strabismus. The earlier one is more serious where at least one of the extraocular muscles is unable to move the eye due to the damage to the muscle or to the third, fourth or sixth cranial nerve.

Glaucoma

Glaucoma is increased pressure of the fluid inside the eye, which can cause optic nerve damage. Glaucoma is a disease of eye which can cause of childhood blindness. It is usually, but not always, the result of abnormally high pressure inside the eye. Over time, the increased pressure can erode the optic nerve tissue, which may lead to vision loss or even blindness.

It is caused by disease related abnormal increase in intraocular pressure. This type of glaucoma is generally caused by increased pressure inside the eye. The abnormally high pressure is due to resistance to the flow of the normal circulation of aqueous humour. This eye fluid is needed to provide proper pressure to the eye. It also delivers nutrients to the interior parts of the eye. In a healthy eye, the fluid leaves through a network of cells and tissue that functions as a tiny drain. To replace the fluid that drains, the eye continuously makes just the right amount of more fluid. With glaucoma, something happens to this balance. In most cases, the fluid does not drain properly. The buildup of fluid causes the eye pressure to rise. Increased pressure from the excess fluid damages the fibers that make up the optic nerve.

The multiple potential causes fall into one of two categories and may be primary or secondary to some other disease process. Primary congenital glaucoma is a rare disease results from abnormal development of the ocular drainage system. This defect in the angle of the eye may slow or prevents normal fluid drainage. Congenital glaucoma usually presents with symptoms, such as cloudy eyes, excessive tearing, or sensitivity to light. Congenital glaucoma can run in families.

Secondary glaucoma results from disorders of the body or eye and may or may not be genetic. Both types may be associated with other medical diseases.

The elevated intraocular pressure (IOP) can cause the eyeball itself to enlarge and injury to the cornea. Important early symptoms of glaucoma in infants and children are poor vision, light sensitivity, tearing, and blinking. Pediatric glaucoma is treated differently than adult glaucoma. Most patients require surgery and this is typically performed early. The aim of pediatric glaucoma surgery is to reduce IOP either by increasing the outflow of fluid from the eye or decrease the production of fluid within the eye. One operation for pediatric glaucoma is goniotomy. Its rate of success is associated with the age of the child at the time of diagnosis, the type and severity of the glaucoma, and the surgery technique. Other surgical options are trabeculectomy and glaucoma drainage tubes.

If childhood glaucoma is not recognized and treated promptly more permanent visual loss will result. The treatment for glaucoma in older children is generally medical, i.e. eye drops initially and if these fail, surgery is considered. This is similar to the situation with older adults with glaucoma. Operations such as trabeculectomy or Molteno tubes are used. These procedures aim to create a controlled leak or 'fistula' by which the aqueous can bypass the trabecular meshwork and escape from the eye. As with adults anti-inflammatory and antibiotic drops are used post-operatively. When trabeculectomy is performed in children an antimetabolite such as 5-fluorouracil (5-FU for short) is very often used as children heal much more rapidly than adults.

Laser trabeculoplasty is rarely used in the treatment of glaucoma in children of any age. A cyclodestructive procedure, such as diode laser treatment of the ciliary body, is sometimes used in the treatment of aphakic glaucoma in children.

Adolescents often have difficulty accepting the need for long-term medication and regular medical review. Ensuring compliance with regular use of eye drops may be especially difficult.

Nursing Care

Assessment

Signs and symptoms like photophobia, tearing, pain and bump into objects, may be found out through taking history of patient, observation and examination. Send the patient to assess visual acuity, visual fields, IOP.

Nursing Management

Teach patient and family risks of glaucoma. Stress on importance of early detection, ophthalmologic examination. Administer medication to lower IOP. Pre- and post-operative teaching of the patient and family are to be given. Support for parents. Educate parents on use of eye medications to alleviate pain from disease and surgery.

Conjunctivitis

Conjunctivitis, is inflammation of the conjunctiva. It is most common eye condition of children, is caused due to an infection usually but sometimes bacterial, parasitic, or an allergic reaction. It is termed as ophthalmia neonatorum in neonates.

The conjunctiva is exposed to bacteria and other irritants. Tears help protect the conjunctiva by washing away bacteria. Tears also contain proteins and antibodies that kill bacteria.

Conjunctivitis is most often caused by a virus. Viral conjuctivitis is referred to as 'pink eye.' Certain forms of pink eye can spread easily among children.

Other causes include allergies, bacteria (staph aureus, S pneumoniae, H influenza, rarely N gonorrhoeae); certain diseases; chemical exposure; Chlamydia, fungi, viral (adenovirus, measles virus). Newborns can be infected by bacteria (N gonorrhoeae) in the birth canal. This condition is called ophthalmia neonatorum. It must be treated at once to preserve eyesight.

Conjunctivitis can affect one or both eyes and is the most likely diagnosis in someone with eye redness and discharge. The affected eye is often 'stuck shut' in the morning as crusts that form on the eyelid overnight. Other symptoms are blurred vision, eye pain, gritty feeling in the eyes, increased tearing, itching of the eye, sensitivity to light.

Bacterial and viral conjunctivitis are highly contagious, and are transmitted through contact with the discharge. Usually conjunctivitis goes away on its own and poses no serious health risk. Eye drops can help relieve symptoms and, for bacterial causes, likely reduce the length of the illness if given early.

Examination of eyes and swab test of the conjunctiva are sometimes done.

Treatment of conjunctivitis depends on the cause. Allergic conjunctivitis may improve when allergies are treated. It may go away on its own when triggers of allergy can be avoided. Cool compresses may help soothe allergic conjunctivitis.

Antibiotic medicines most often in the form of eye drops work well to treat bacterial conjunctivitis. Viral conjunctivitis will go away on its own. Mild steroid eye drops may help to ease discomfort. You can soothe the discomfort of viral or bacterial conjunctivitis by applying warm compresses to closed eyes.

Cataract

A cataract is a cloudy or opaque area in the lens located directly behind the iris inside the eye (Fig. 22.3). Normally, the lens is clear and allows light entering the eye to clearly focus an image on the retina. When cataracts develop, the light rays become scattered as they pass through the cloudy lens and the retinal image becomes blurred and distorted.

Cataracts can be developmental, acquired or traumatic. While the exact cause of some cataracts found in both eyes is unknown, many are hereditary. Bilateral cataracts have also been associated with a number of genetic disorders, such as Down or Turner's syndrome. Maternal viruses such as rubella, herpes zoster, or hepatitis can also cause a child to be born with cataract. Virus like rubella may remain viable in the lens of the eye for one year. Formation of cataract may be associated with excess intake of vitamin D, corticosteroids prenatally.

Cataracts found in only one eye are usually not associated with a particular disease. Acquired cataracts may develop due to metabolic diseases, like diabetes mellitus; after inflammation of eye. Retinopathy due to prematurity can also cause acquired cataract Trauma (penetrative type eye injury) is another cause of unilateral cataract.

Management

Cataracts that obscure vision should be removed as early as possible, even in the first weeks of life, to allow a clear retinal image (preserve the vision). Early intervention permits the eye to develop vision reflexes.

Surgical removal of a cataract in an infant or child is done under general anesthesia using an operating

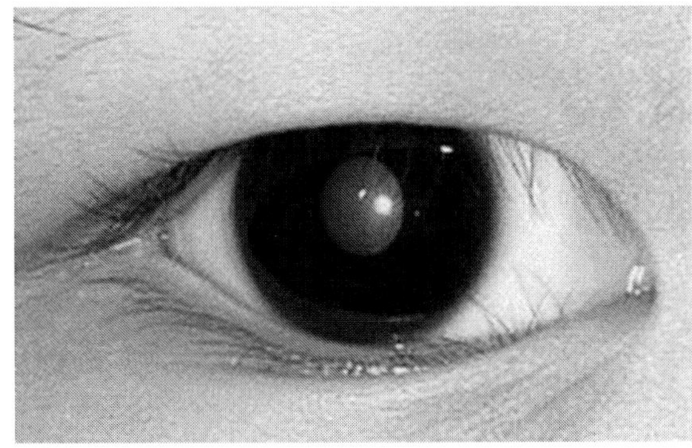

Fig. 22.3: Cataract in children

microscope. The lens is broken into small pieces with a microsurgical instrument and removed through a small incision. Once the cataract has been removed, focusing power may be restored in one of the following ways:

- *Contact lenses:* Used after surgery for bilateral or unilateral cataracts in children under two years of age. Contact lenses are recommended for this age group because the eye and focusing power change rapidly during early infancy. Contact lenses can also be used in older children.
- *Intraocular lenses:* Artificial lenses may also be implanted to replace natural lenses in children. This method is still under study for infants.
- *Glasses:* Used in selected cases when the cataract surgery involves both eyes and contact lenses have failed, or if intraocular lenses are not appropriate. Most children will also wear regular glasses even if they have a contact or an intraocular lens, as the focus needs to be managed very carefully.

The final step in the treatment process is to treat amblyopia that develops if one eye is stronger than the other, as in the case of a unilateral cataract. In patients with unilateral or asymmetric cataracts (one cataract is more severe than the other), it is necessary to patch the good eye to stimulate vision in the eye that had the cataract surgery. Antibiotic eye ointments and steroid ointment such as decadron are frequently prescribed.

Children who undergo cataract surgery generally have very little pain or discomfort. Those who receive intraocular lenses cannot feel the lens inside the eye. Children can feel the presence of contact lenses, but usually adapt to them quickly. All patients who undergo cataract surgery also require bifocal glasses to correct the residual error of refraction and to allow focusing at distance and near.

Children with congenital cataracts have a good prognosis if treated within the first two months of life. Left untreated, the prognosis is poor. Children with acquired cataract have a better visual prognosis because some visual development has occurred. With a successful surgery, long-term shielding is necessary to complete the process of restoring vision.

Nursing Care

Preoperative Phase

- History and physical assessment
- Antibiotic eye drops
- Dilating eye drops
- *Anticholinergics:* Mydriatics and cycloplegics.

Postoperative Phase

- Outpatient procedure unless complications occur antibiotic and corticosteroid eye drops discourage activities that increase IOP—week follow-up
- Glasses to correct remaining refractive error

Nursing Management Planning

Maintain level of comfort—free of infection and other complications.

Health Promotion

- Wear sunglasses
- Avoid unnecessary radiation–Adequate antioxidant vitamins
- Good nutrition.

Educate about disease process and treatment options. Teach signs and symptoms of infection.

Blindness

Blindness is defined as the state of being sightless, which spans a range from total blindness to 20/200 vision in the better eye with best correction. Blindness in children can be defined as a visual acuity of < 3/60 in the eye with better vision of a child under 16 years of age. According to Harley (1983) vision impairment can be categorized as:

- *Partial vision:* Visual acuity of 20/70 to 20/200; and the individual is able to read newsprint.
- *Low vision:* Light perception of 20/200 with corrective lens.
- *Blindness:* Visual acuity of 20/200 or less in the better eye with the best correction.
- *Total blindness:* An individual is unable to distinguish light from dark.

There are many causes of blindness in children. Blindness may be due to many causes such as genetic mutations, birth defects, premature birth, nutritional deficiencies, infections, injuries, and other causes. Severe retinopathy of prematurity (ROP), cataracts and refractive error, glaucoma, tumors are also causes. No matter what the cause, early onset blindness adversely affects psychomotor, social, and emotional development.

The prevalence of blindness is higher in developing countries because, firstly, potentially blinding conditions such as vitamin A deficiency, harmful traditional eye remedies, or cerebral malaria, which are prevalent there. Secondly, preventive measures for conditions such as measles, congenital rubella, or ophthalmia neonatorum are inadequate. Thirdly, facilities and skilled personnel for managing conditions needing surgery are lacking. Some 500,000 children become blind each year, most in developing countries, and 75% of the world's blind children live in developing countries. Almost half of all blindness in children, particularly those in the poorest communities is due to avoidable causes that are amenable to cost-effective interventions.

Types of Blindness

Congenital Blindness

If an infant is born with severe visual impairment; or unable to see, he is said to have congenital blindness. A number of different conditions can cause congenital blindness, including certain diseases and genetic factors (discussed above).

Color Deficiency

Color blindness is not actually blindness in the true sense but rather is a color vision deficiency:

Vitamin A deficiency and blindness: Vitamin A deficiency (VAD) is the leading cause of preventable blindness in children. Xerophthalmia is widely recognized as the leading cause of childhood blindness in developing countries. Current estimates are that in Asia alone, some one-half million children under six years of age develop potentially blinding corneal xerophthalmia each year. Xerophthalmia, keratomalacia, and complete blindness can also occur since Vitamin A has a major role in phototransduction. Xerophthalmia is due to vitamin A deficiency is the condition begins with night blindness and conjunctival xerosis (dryness of the eye membranes), progresses to corneal xerosis (dryness of the cornea), and in its late stages develops into keratomalacia (softening of the cornea).

Vitamin A deficiency is a nutritional disease with a primary, nutritional solution: Improve vitamin A nutrition to a physiologically acceptable level by removing the determinant of disease is done. Chronic dietary insufficiency, and/or absorption of vitamin A are taken care of. Inclusion of vitamin A oil in immunization schedule is done to prevent blindness due to malnutrition.

Nursing Management

- Emotional support
- Listening and facilitating
- Grief, anger
- Normal conversational tone
- Patient name
- Orient to surroundings start with a focal point when identifying landmarks
- Use sight guided technique to help patient around room.

Foreign Body in Eye

The eye will often flush out tiny objects, like eyelashes and sand, through blinking and tearing. The foreign body in the eye may be sharp or stuck in the eye or may sticking out of the eyelid.

Something can hit the eye at a high rate of speed or with force. The child has pain or a change in vision.

Nursing Care

In every injury, examination of the eye is important. Following areas are to be focused in caring of eye in emergency or during seeking medical help

- Do Not touch, rub or apply pressure to the eye.
- Do Not try to remove any object stuck in the eye. For small debris, lift eye lid and ask child to blink rapidly to see if tears will flush out the particle. If not, close the eye and seek treatment.
- Do not apply ointment or medication to the eye.
- A cut or puncture wound should be gently covered.
- Only in the event of chemical exposure, flush with plenty of water.

EAR AND DISORDERS OF THE EAR

Structure and Function of Ear

The ears are the sense organs for hearing. It helps in hearing and also helps to maintain the body equilibrium of the human body. The human ear consists of three parts the outer ear, middle ear and inner ear. The outer ear is called the pinna/auricle which made of ridged cartilage covered by skin. The ear canal of the outer ear meets the start of the middle ear at the eardrum or tympanic membrane. The tympanic membrane separates the outer ear from the air-filled tympanic cavity of the middle ear. The middle ear contains the three small bones, the ossicles (the malleus (hammer), incus (anvil), and the stapes (stirrup) involved in the transmission of sound. Middle ear is connected to the throat at the nasopharynx, via the pharyngeal opening of the Eustachian tube. The inner ear contains the otolith organs—the utricle and saccule and the semicircular canals belonging to the vestibular system and the cochlea of the auditory system (Fig. 22.4).

The outer ear receives sound, transmitted through the ossicles of the middle ear to the inner ear, where it is converted to a nervous signal in the cochlear and transmitted along the vestibulo-cochlear nerve.

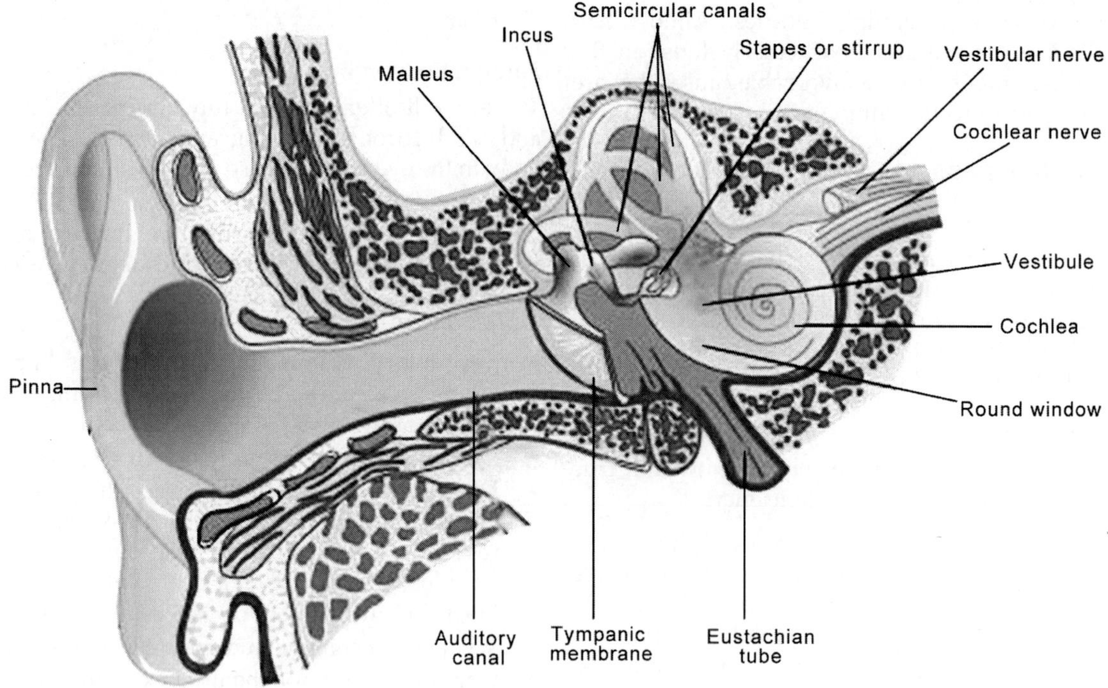

Fig. 22.4: Structures of ear

The inner ear is a very delicate mechanism. For protection, it is located deep in the skull behind the eyes. The inner ear is filled with fluid and contains two sensory systems, the balance and the hearing systems. The back section of the inner ear consists of three semicircular canals which give us our balance and help in the stabilization of eye movement. This is known as the vestibular system.

The hearing system is contained in the cochlea and the auditory nerve. The purpose of the cochlea is to change the signal from a sound message to an electrical message. The auditory nerve sends the electrical messages to the brain. The structure of cochlea is like a snail shell and it is fluid filled. There are about 30,000 tiny nerve endings called hair cells in it and all these connect to the fibers of the auditory nerve which transmits the sound message to the brain. The human ear can hear 20 to 20,000 htz.

Otitis Media

Ear infection is also known as acute otitis media (AOM) (otitis = ear, media = middle). Otitis media is an infection of the middle ear. Otitis media is the most frequently diagnosed disease in infants and young children because the Eustachian tube is smaller and more nearly horizontal in children than in adults. Therefore, it can be more easily blocked by conditions such as large adenoids and infections. Until the Eustachian tube changes in size and angle as the child grows, children are more susceptible to otitis media.

Ear infections most often develop after a viral respiratory tract infection, such as a cold or the flu. These infections can cause swelling of the mucous membranes of the nose and throat, and diminish normal host defenses such as clearance of bacteria from the nose, increasing the amount of bacteria in the nose. Viral respiratory tract infections also can impair Eustachian tube function. Fluid, called effusion may form in the middle ear and bacteria and viruses follow, resulting in inflammation in the middle ear. The increased pressure causes the eardrum to bulge, leading to the typical symptoms of pain or a perforated eardrum, often with drainage of purulent material (pus, also termed suppurative otitis media).

Fever (temperature higher than 100.4 °F or 38 °C,

- Pulling on the ear
- Fussiness or irritability
- Decreased activity
- Lack of appetite or difficulty eating
- Vomiting or diarrhea.

Examination of ear is necessary to diagnosis of an ear infection. It is done by looking at the tympanic membrane through otoscope for the typical features of an ear infection. Pneumatic otoscopy is the standard of care in the diagnosis of acute and chronic otitis media. The following findings may be found on examination in patients with AOM:

- Signs of inflammation in the tympanic membrane
- Bulging in the posterior quadrants of the tympanic membrane may bulge; scalded appearance of the superficial epithelial layer
- Perforated tympanic membrane (most frequently observed in posterior or inferior quadrants)
- Presence of an opaque serum like exudate oozing through the entire tympanic membrane
- Pain with/without pulsation of the otorrhea
- Fever.

Treatment of an ear infection may include:

- Antibiotics
- Medicines to treat pain and fever
- Observation
- A combination of the above

The 'best' treatment depends on the child's age, history of previous infections, degree of illness, and any underlying medical problems.

Surgery

Surgical management of AOM can be divided into the following three related procedures:

1. Tympanocentesis
2. Myringotomy
3. Myringotomy with insertion of a ventilating tube.

Other measures that reduce ear infection risk:

- Breastfeeding boosts baby's immune system and uses a swallowing mechanism that allows less milk to enter the Eustachian tube. Also, breast milk is less irritating to middle-ear tissue.
- Not let the baby to drink from a bottle while lying down, which may allow small amounts of formula to enter the Eustachian tube and cause blockage.
- Eliminating exposure to cigarette smoke.

Hearing Loss

Hearing loss, also known as hearing impairment, or anacusis, is a partial or total inability to hear. A child with hearing loss has trouble hearing sounds in the range of normal speech (Fig. 22.5). Hearing loss may be congenital or acquired and often is not detected until a child is 2, 3 or even 4 years old. The critical period for language development is from birth to age 3. If hearing problems get diagnosed and treated quickly, babies and children can avoid trouble with language. The failure to identify and treat hearing loss by 6 months of age can have serious implications for a child's speech. Babies born with other serious medical problems are at higher risk for hearing loss. Most deaf children are born to hearing parents. But the condition can be inherited.

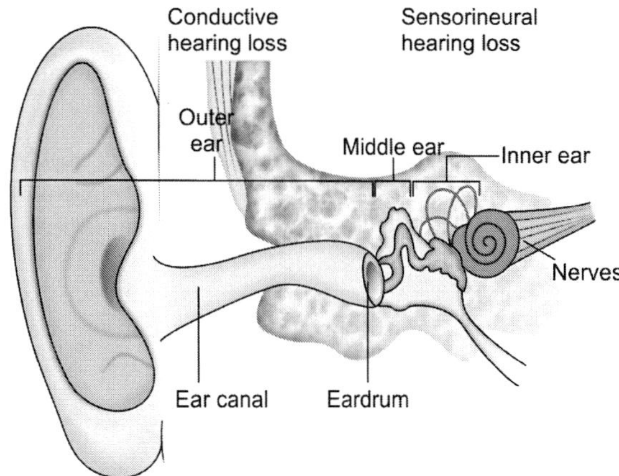

Fig. 22.5: Types of hearing loss in children

Pathophysiology

According to neurobiological perspective, there are three reasons that could cause hearing loss in an individual: either there is something wrong with the conducting system of the ear or there is something wrong with the sensory portion of the process (inner ear or cochlea and related structures) or there is something wrong with the neural portion of the process, meaning the nerves or brain.

There are two major categories of hearing loss:

- Central hearing loss involves problems with processing information in the brain.
- Peripheral hearing loss refers to problems with the ear structures. There are three types of peripheral hearing loss:
  - Conductive hearing loss is the most common type in children. It occurs when the transmission of sound through the external or middle ear is blocked (temporary or permanent) in one or both ears. Sometimes, physical abnormalities like congenital atresia of the external auditory canal; or something as simple as ear wax (cerumen) may cause this type of hearing loss. More commonly, it begins during childhood as

the result of middle ear infections, perforation of the eardrum, impacted earwax or objects in the ear canal.
   - Sensorineural hearing loss (SNHL) is a type of hearing loss, which involves problems with the transmission of sound information from hair cells deep within the ear inner ear (cochlea and associated structures), to the nerve vestibulocochlear nerve (cranial nerve VIII), or central auditory processing centers of the brain. Here, air conduction is normal but bone conduction is impaired.

It is usually a permanent condition which may affect both ears. Sensorineural hearing loss can be present at birth or it can occur later in life. Causes include prolonged exposure to loud noise, infection, severe head injury, toxic medications and some rare inherited diseases, prenatal and perinatal infections or postnatal viral or bacterial illnesses. Trauma to one side of the head can damage the cochlea on the opposite side, which is irreversible as it disrupts the hair cells of cochlea. Damage of the hair cells of inner ear may occur due to prolonged exposures to the loud noises or by a single exposure to an extremely loud noise such as an explosion.

- Mixed hearing loss is both conductive and sensorineural. Improvement of this condition depends on correction of the conductor loss
- Central auditory dysfunction means problems with auditory reception dysfunction. It may arise due to lesion in the temporal lobe and can be the result of birth trauma, toxoplasmosis, perinatal oxygen deprivation. This sensory deficit may affect the development of the child (language, speech and hearing).

A hearing impairment is usually described in terms of decibel loss. Hearing loss is measured by the volume of sounds that can be heard without amplification. It is classified as borderline or slight, mild, moderate, severe or profound.

The term 'deaf' generally applies to a person whose hearing loss is so extensive that he or she cannot communicate with another person using only voice.

Assessment

Hearing loss can show up at any age. It is often difficult to detect, especially in young children. Even slight hearing loss in one ear can impact a child's speech and language development. Indications of hearing loss in children can include:

- Listening to the television at a higher volume than other children
- Sits in close distance to the television for better listening
- Having difficulty with school adjustment
- Having speech and language problems
- Exhibiting poor behavior, irritability, temper tantrum, etc.
- Being inattentive
- Complains of difficulty hearing or blocked ears
- Complains ear ache, drainage from ear.

Various tests can be done to measure hearing loss, including:

- *Tympanogram:* This is a screening test for middle ear problems. It measures the air pressure in the middle ear and the ability of the eardrum to move. A tympanogram is the result of a hearing test with a tympanometer. It tests the function of the middle ear and mobility of the eardrum. It can distinguish conductive hearing loss from other kinds of hearing loss including SNHL.
- *Audiometry (pure tone audiometry):* This test is used to determine the volume of sound the child can hear. A relatively new refinement of pure tone audiometry is Bekesy audiometry. The child listens to sounds of various volume and frequency through earphones in a soundproof room. It charts the thresholds of hearing sensitivity at a selection of standard frequencies between 250 and 8000 Hz. There is also high frequency pure tone audiometry which tests frequencies from 8000–20,000 Hz. In children less than 2½ years old, audiometry is also used as a rough screening test to rule out significant hearing loss. An observer watches the infant's or toddler's body movements in response to sounds. This test cannot determine which ear has a problem or whether both do.
   - It can be used to differentiate between conductive hearing loss, sensorineural hearing loss, auditory processing hearing loss, and mixed hearing loss. Hearing loss which shows up as a relatively flat but lowered line on the audiogram is called 'flat loss'. It means that thresholds are higher (sounds are harder to hear) at all frequencies. A flat loss is relatively uncommon and is often caused by a conductive problem rather than a sensorineural problem. Sensorineural hearing loss is characterized by a notch or notches in the audiogram, or asymmetrical audiogram with progressively greater loss with rising frequency.

– Brainstem Auditory Evoked Response (BAE) is an auditory brainstem response test. In this test, sensors are stuck to the scalp to record electrical signals from nerves involved in hearing. The signals are studied to give information about hearing and hearing-related brain function. Using computer averaging, a characteristic pattern of brain waves is formed. The threshold is the point where the waveform is nearly diminished; it is the lowest intensity at which the ear transmits the sound to the brain. This test is used to screen newborns or to test children difficult to test. It also can be used to confirm hearing loss or to give ear-specific information after other screening tests have been done. Young children often need to be sedated during this test so that there will be very minimum muscle tensions and do not interfere with the recording.

- *Otoacoustic emissions:* Otoacoustic emissions test is a relatively quick, noninvasive test. A miniature microphone is placed in the ear which can pick up signals that normally are emitted from the hair cells in the inner ear. For all newborns, this is an excellent screening test. If a hearing problem is found, it should be confirmed with the auditory brainstem response test.

Testing is done routinely for infants and children at high-risk of hearing loss. These include children who have:

- Developmental delays, especially in speech
- Syndromes involving the head that are associated with hearing loss
- Other risk factors, such as a history of premature birth or bacterial meningitis or a family history of hearing loss.

MRI: To refine clinical findings and after audiometry, a contrast-enhanced MRI may reveal clinically unsuspected inflammatory, autoimmune or tumoral disease.

Management

Types of conductive hearing loss may be improved with amplification with a bone conduction hearing aid, or a surgically implanted, osseo-integrated device, or a conventional hearing aid, depending on the status of the hearing nerve.

Conductive hearing loss due to infection is usually treated with antibiotic or antifungal medications. Chronic ear infections, chronic middle fluid, and tumors usually require surgery. If there is no response to initial medical therapy, infectious middle ear fluid is usually treated with antibiotics. Chronic non-infectious middle ear fluid is treated with surgery wherein pressure equalizing tube is inserted. These allow fluid to drain and can help prevent infection.

Conductive hearing loss from head trauma is frequently amenable to surgical repair of the damaged middle ear structures, performed after the patient's general medical status is stabilized following acute traumatic injuries.

Sensorineural hearing loss can result from acoustic trauma (or exposure to excessively loud noise), which may respond to medical therapy with corticosteroids to reduce cochlea hair cell swelling and inflammation to improve healing of these injured inner ear structures.

Other treatments for children with hearing loss include:

Hearing Aids (HA)

Children can begin to use hearing aids when they are as young as 1 month old. A HA does not selectively amplify one source of sound in the environment; it amplifies everything. HA aids provide amplification, but do not restore hearing to normal. Two types of HA systems are:

- *Air conduction systems:* With air conduction system the acoustic signal is transmitted to the external auditory canal via a plastic tube held by a fitted ear mould. Placing microphone near to ear improves sound localization and speech discrimination ability.
- *Bone conduction system:* A bone conduction system is beneficial in case of anatomic defect of ear structure where the signal is transmitted as vibrations to the mastoid bone.

Implants

Many children may need cochlear implants. An implant is an electronic device that is put inside the inner ear to help with hearing. It is usually only for children with serious hearing problems when hearing aids have not helped.

Auditory Stimulation

Auditory stimulation is the use of focused sounds to produce an effect on the nervous system. This type of stimulation can be used as a part of sensory therapy in children with auditory or visual impairment, attention-deficit hyperactivity disorder (ADHD), etc. In case of sensorial impairment, auditory stimulation is believed to help increase their ability to process sounds. Some types of auditory stimulation allow a child to manipulate sounds using gestures or body movement while other types might relate sound to visual stimulation like pictures or colors.

Learning Language

- It is well-recognized that hearing is critical to speech and language development, communication, and learning. These children may then be at risk for other delays. Children with severe to profound hearing losses often report feeling isolated, without friends, and unhappy in school, particularly when their socialization with other children with hearing loss is limited.

Children with hearing loss have problems learning language and need extra help. Families who have children with hearing loss often need to change their communication habits or learn special skills like sign language to help their children learn language. The ideal situation is for families (parents and siblings alike) to begin learning sign language as soon as they find out their child has a hearing loss. These skills can be used together with hearing aids, cochlear implants, and other devices that help children to hear.

CHAPTER 23

Management of Selected Pediatric Surgical Problems/Disorders

Chapter Outline

- Hypospadias
- Epispadias
- Undescended Testes
- Nursing Management for Congenital Genitourinary Malformations Preoperative
- Cheilorrhaphy
- Care of the Patient with an Ostomy

Pediatric surgery is a specialty of surgery involving the surgery of fetuses, infants, children (Fig. 23.1), adolescents, and young adults. Pediatric surgery arose in the middle of the 20th century as the surgical care of birth defects required specialized techniques and methods and became more commonly based at children's hospitals. The several pediatric conditions amendable to pediatric surgical treatment are:

HYPOSPADIAS

Hypospadias repair is a surgery to fix the location of the opening in the penis when it is not in the right place at the end of the penis. Children with hypospadias may also have an abnormal bend of the penis shaft (chordate), and a partially developed foreskin, the fold of skin at the end of the penis (Figs 23.2A to C). The hypospadias repair surgery will reposition the opening and give the penis a more normal appearance. (*See* Chapter 12).

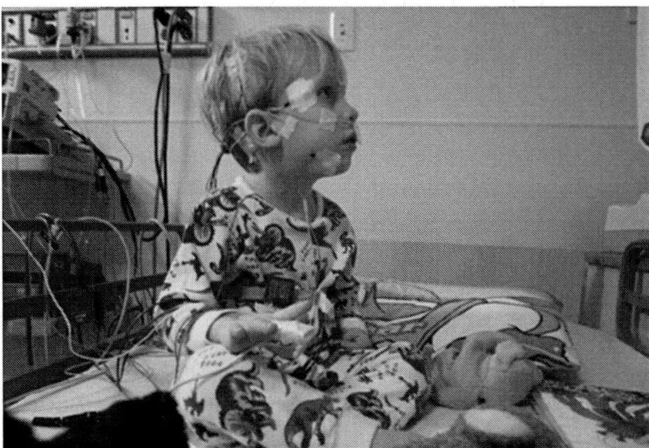

Fig. 23.1: After surgery the child is in recovery room

The surgery to repair it usually involves these steps:

- Moving the opening of the urethra to the end of the penis
- Straightening the shaft of the penis if it is curved
- Circumcising the abnormal foreskin of the penis.

After a full assessment of the penile anatomy, the shaft skin of the penis is degloved to eliminate any skin tethering, and an artificial erection is performed to rule out any curvature. Mild-to-moderate chordee may be repaired by excising any ventral fibrous tethering tissue or by plicating the dorsal tunics of the corporal bodies, compensating for any ventral-to-dorsal disproportion.

More severe chordee may require grafting of the ventral corporal bodies using synthetic, animal, cadaveric,

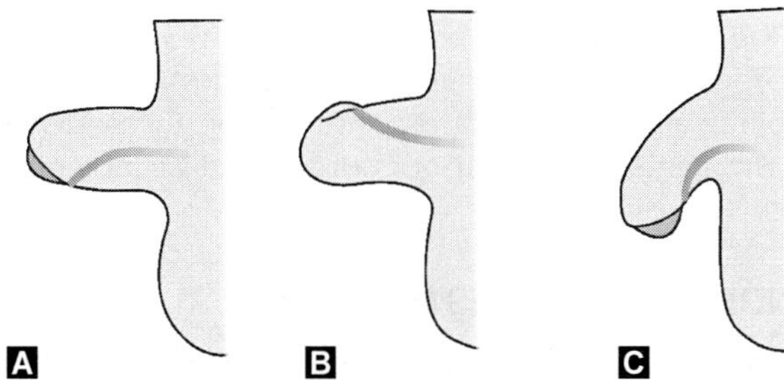

Figs 23.2A to C: Three different urethral defects. **A.** Hypospadias; **B.** Epispadias; **C.** Hypospadias with chordee

or autologous tissues (tunica vaginalis or dermal grafts) to avoid excessive shortening of penile length.

Creating the rest of the urethra or tube that did not form to the end of the penis. The urethra, the tube which carries urine out of the penis, is made of mucosal tissue. Surgeons use a flap of skin to construct or extend the urethra, the skin tube that will drain urine. Temporary urethral stents are a common adjunct to hypospadias repair and are felt to decrease the likelihood of fistula formation. Various drainage tubes have been utilized for this purpose. Often, a bulky dressing or plastic cup is placed over the penis to protect the surgical area. A urinary catheter will be put through the dressing so urine can flow into the bed or diaper.

EPISPADIAS

Epispadias represents a congenital anomaly which is characterized by short phallus with marked upward curvature (dorsal chordee). An *epispadias* is a rare type of malformation of the penis in which the urethra ends in an opening on the upper aspect (the dorsum) of the penis (discussed in Chapter 14).

Surgical Intervention

The primary goals of treatment of epispadias are to: lengthen and straighten the penis by correcting dorsal bend and chordee; and create functionality and cosmetically acceptable external genitalia with as few surgical procedures as possible. There are two popular surgical techniques that achieve these objectives. The most popular and successful technique is known as the *modified Cantwell-Ransley* approach. The first is the modified Cantwell technique, which involves partial disassembly of the penis and placement of the urethra in a more normal position. The second technique and most recent evolution of the modern epispadias repair is the complete disassembly of the penis into its separate components—two corpora cavernosa and a single corpus spongiosum. Following this disassembly surgery, the 3 components are reassembled such that the urethra is in the most functional and normal position and dorsal chordee is corrected (Figs 23.3A to F). Both techniques provide a straight urethra positioned on the underside of the penis, correction of chordee and an acceptable cosmetic result.

UNDESCENDED TESTES

Undescended testicle occurs when one or both testicles fail to move into the scrotum before birth. The testicles or 'testes' are 2 organs that hang in the scrotum below the penis. The scrotum keeps the testicles in a cooler setting than the body. This is because sperm cannot grow at body temperature. Most of the time, a boy's testicles descend by the time he is 9 months old. Undescended testicles are fairly common in infants who are born early. Some babies have a condition called retractile testes and the parent may not be able to find the testicles. In this case, the testicle is normal but is pulled back out of the scrotum by a muscle reflex. Testicles that do not naturally descend into the scrotum are considered abnormal and called cryptorchidism (Fig. 23.4).

Having surgery early may prevent damage to the testicles that can cause infertility. The main treatment is surgery, orchiopexy is done to bring the testicle into the scrotum. An orchidopexy is performed to bring the testis (testicle) down into its normal location in the scrotum. A small cut is made in the groin and the testis is freed up before placing it in a pouch in the scrotum through a second cut which is then stitched up.

Exstrophy Bladder

Bladder exstrophy repair is used to move exposed abdominal organs, such as the bladder, back into the abdomen which is necessary for development of urinary control, improvement of physical appearance prevention of infection, avoidance of future sexual function problems. Bladder exstrophy repair requires two separate surgeries. The first surgery repairs the bladder. The second repairs the attachment between the pelvic bones (*See* Chapter 14).

Treatment: Surgical reconstruction done 1st 24–48 hour after birth

- Goal:
  - Bladder/abd wall closure
  - Preserve urinary function
  - Create normal appearing of genitalia
  - Improvement of future sexual function

In the first surgery, the exposed bladder is separated from the abdominal wall. Then, the bladder is closed. The neck of the bladder and the urethra are repaired. A catheter is placed in the bladder so urine can be drained through the wall of the abdomen. Another catheter is placed to drain urine from the urethra. This promotes healing.

In the second surgery, the pelvic bone attachment is repaired. This may be done either right after the bladder repair or at a later time. More surgeries may sometimes be needed if there is a defect in the bowel.

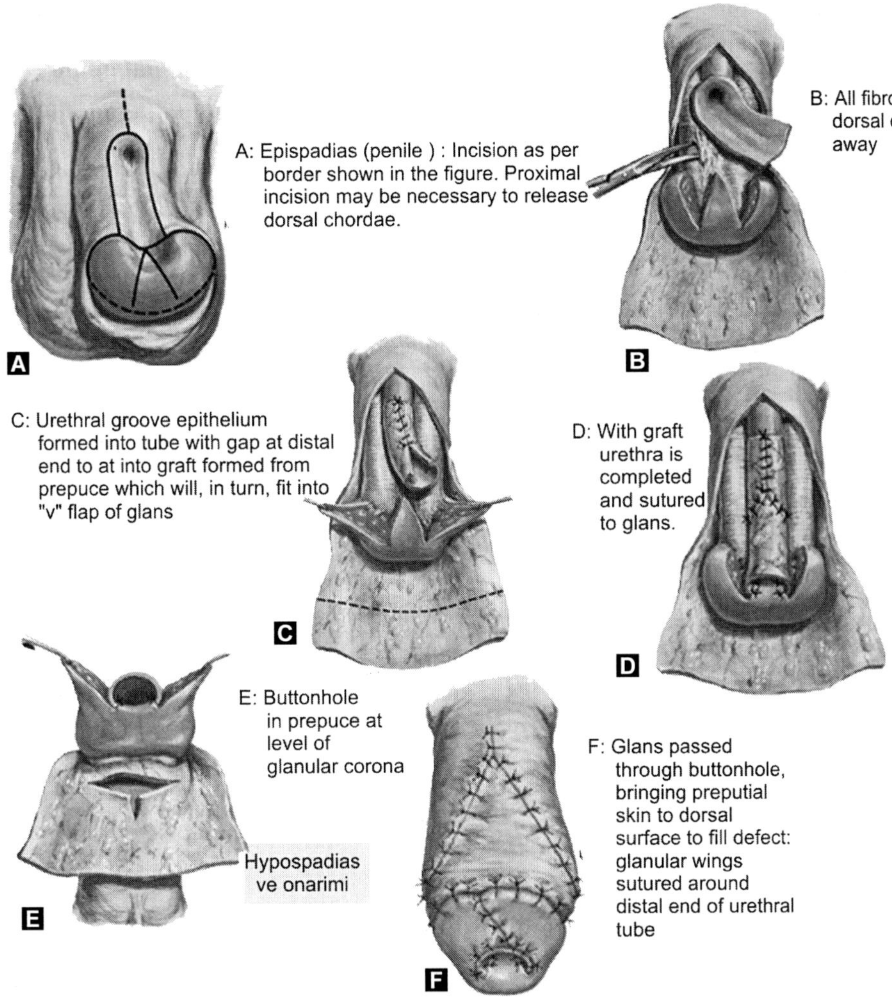

A: Epispadias (penile) : Incision as per border shown in the figure. Proximal incision may be necessary to release dorsal chordae.

B: All fibrous tissue causing dorsal curvature dissected away

C: Urethral groove epithelium formed into tube with gap at distal end to at into graft formed from prepuce which will, in turn, fit into "v" flap of glans

D: With graft urethra is completed and sutured to glans.

E: Buttonhole in prepuce at level of glanular corona

Hypospadias ve onarimi

F: Glans passed through buttonhole, bringing preputial skin to dorsal surface to fill defect: glanular wings sutured around distal end of urethral tube

Figs 23.3A to F: Steps of surgical intervention in epispadias repair

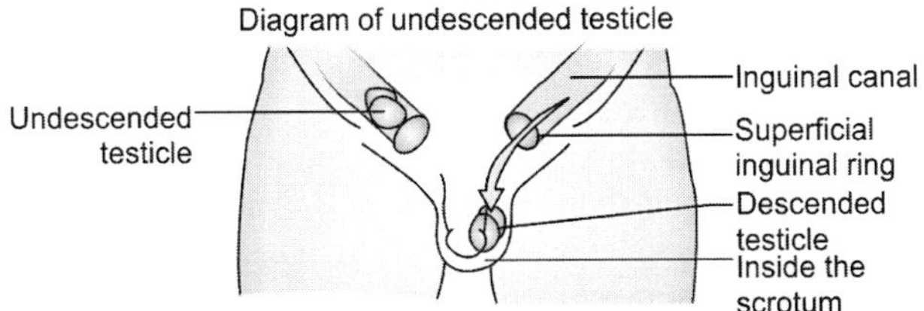

Fig. 23.4: Undescended testes (right side)

NURSING MANAGEMENT FOR CONGENITAL GENITOURINARY MALFORMATIONS PREOPERATIVE

It is important to address parents' concerns at the time of birth.

Preoperative teaching can relieve some of their anxiety about the future appearance and functioning of the penis.

Postoperative Nursing Diagnoses

- Pain (acute/chronic) related to physical factors like damage to the skin/tissue (incision)
  - Goal:
    - Reduced pain

  Expected Outcomes:
  - Saying controlled pain
  - Shows the pain disappeared, was able to sleep/ rest appropriately

  Intervention:
  - Assess pain, note the location, characteristics, intensity (scale 0-10)

- Encourage the patient to say the problem
- Provide comfort measures, if condition permits change the position
- Encourage use of relaxation techniques
- Collaboration, give medication as prescribed

Help patients to rest more effective and refocus attention thus decreasing pain and discomfort

- Impaired skin integrity related to surgical trauma
  - Goal:
    - Normal skin, no visible damage

  Expected Outcomes:
  - Demonstrate appropriate wound healing without complications
  - Intervention:
    - Protect the incision when changing position, coughing, deep breathing and ambulation
    - Observe the incision periodically
    - Provide routine maintenance incision
- Impaired urinary elimination related to surgical diversion, tissue trauma
  - Goal:
    - Elimination of urine is normal/to be like before the illness
  - Expected Outcomes:
    - Demonstrate continuous flow of urine with urine output is adequate for individual situations.
  - Intervention:
    - Record of urine output, probe reduction/ cessation of flow suddenly, decrease in urine flow may indicate a sudden obstruction/ dysfunction
  - Observe and record the color of urine
  - Show catheterization techniques
  - Encourage increased fluid intake and maintain accurate
  - Monitor vital signs
  - Postoperative management of hypospadias
  - Care of the catheter (may be foley, suprapubic or urethral stent
  - Increase fluid intake
  - Intake output. Keep records from stents and catheter separate
  - Secure stents and catheter to prevent displacement
  - Use double diapering to protect the urinary stent after surgery
  - Management of bladder spasms
  - Prophylactic medication
  - No bath until stent removed
  - Do not allow to play on straddle toys
  - Vital signs for signs of infection
  - Seek medical help for temp > 101°
  - Support and explanation on surgical intervention
    - Need to reassure that patient's genitals are intact and will function normally when the catheters are removed
    - Importance of monitoring the urine drainage from stents and urethral catheter
    - The need to assess the surgical site for bleeding or excessive drainage
    - The home care regimen that can be anticipated when patient is discharged.
- Post-operative care with surgical care of Extrophy of bladder.
  - Care of the surgical site with meticulous wound care
  - Control bladder spasms
  - Positioning: Immobilization and avoidance of abduction of legs
  - Neurovascular assessment of lower extremities
  - Monitoring renal function and obstruction of tubes
  - Promoting comfort
  - Control pain
  - Increase fluid intake
  - Do not allow to play on straddle toys
  - Prevent infection (no bathing or swimming until stents removed
  - Seek medical help if: temp >101° anorexia, pus or bleeding from stent, cloudy or foul smelling urine

  Discharge teaching
  - Need to reassure patient that his genitals are intact and will function normally when the catheters are removed
  - Importance of monitoring the urine drainage from stents and urethral catheter
  - The need to assess the surgical site for bleeding or excessive drainage
  - The home care regimen that can be anticipated when he is discharged
- Nursing care postoperative orchiopexy, correction of cryptorchidism
  - Minimal activity for few days
  - Allow opportunity to express fears about mutilation or castration
  - Prevention of infection
  - Importance of taking all medicines.

Cleft Lip and Palate

The aim of treatment of cleft lip and palate is to correct the cleft and associated problems surgically and thus hide the anomaly so that children can lead normal lives. This correction involves surgically producing a face that does not attract attention, a vocal apparatus that permits intelligible speech, and a dentition that allows optimal function and esthetics (Table 23.1).

CHEILORRHAPHY

Cheilorrhaphy is the surgical correction of the cleft lip deformity. The orbicularis oris muscle is the primary muscle of the lip and can be divided functionally and anatomically into 2 parts. The lack of continuity of this muscle allows the developing parts of the maxilla to grow in an uncoordinated manner so that the cleft in the alveolus is accentuated.

At birth the alveolar process on the unaffected side may appear to protrude from the mouth. The lack of sphincteric muscle control from the orbicularis oris will cause a bilateral cleft lip to exhibit a premaxilla that protrudes from the base of the nose and produces an unsightly appearance. Thus restoration of this muscular sphincter with lip repair has a favorable effect on the developing alveolar segments.

Cleft Palate

A cleft palate is a common congenital facial anomaly treated by plastic surgery. A cleft palate develops in a fetus when the two halves of the palate do not come together and fuse in the middle. In most cases, a cleft lip is also present. Cleft palate causes a gap in the roof of the mouth and creates problems with dental development, speech, hearing, eating, and drinking. A child may also experience frequent colds, fluid in the ears, sore throat, and problems with the tonsils and adenoids. A cleft palate is different from a *cleft lip*. A cleft lip affects the upper lip, whereas a cleft palate affects the roof of the mouth. Not all individuals with cleft palate have a cleft lip, some may have both a *cleft lip and a cleft palate*. The goals of cleft palate repair include closure of the palatal defect and attainment of normal speech, hearing, dental occlusion, and facial and palatal growth.

Palatorrhaphy is usually performed in one operation, but occasionally it is performed in two. In two operation the soft palate closure is usually performed first and the hard palate closure is performed second. The primary purpose of the cleft palate repair is to create a mechanism capable of speech and deglutition without significantly interfering with subsequent maxillary growth.

Table 23.1: Staged reconstruction of cleft lip and palate deformities

Procedure	*Timing*
Cleft lip repair	After 10 weeks
Cleft palate repair	9–18 months
Pharyngeal flap or pharyngoplastry	3–5 years or later based on speech development
Maxillary or alveolar reconstruction with bone grafting	6–9 years based on dental development
Cleft orthognathic surgery	14–16 years in girls, 16–18 years in boys
Cleft rhinoplasty	After age 5 years but preferably at skeletal maturity; after orthognathic surgery when possible
Cleft lip revision	Anytime once initial remodeling and scar maturation is complete but best performed after age 5 years

Steps followed in Z plasty cleft palate surgery are shown above:

A. Cleft of the both hard and soft from the incisive foramen to the uvula. B. Furlow double-opposing Z-plasty technique (Figs 23.5A to D); Z-plasty flaps developed on the oral and then nasal side. The cutbacks creating the nasal side flaps highlighted in blue in the graphic. C. The flaps are then transposed to lengthen the soft palate. A nasal side closure is completed in the fashion, i.e. anterior to the junction of the hard and soft palate. D. The oral side flaps are then transposed and closed in a similar fashion completing the palate closure.

Bardachand Salyer independently modified the 2-flap palatoplasty to combine elements of other operations with some innovative details (Figs 23.6A to D). The main goals are complete closure of the entire cleft without tension at an early age (< 2 months) with minimal exposure of raw bony surfaces and the creation of a functioning soft palate.

Nursing Management

Surgical Correction of Cleft Lip and/or Palate

Depending in the defect and the child's general condition, surgical correction of the cleft lip usually

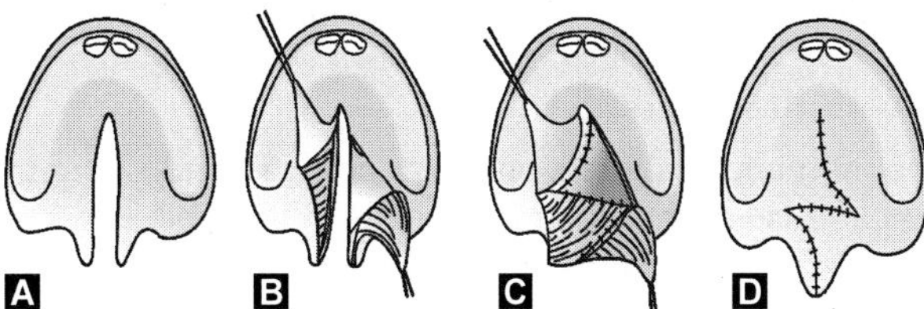

Figs 23.5A to D: Z-plasty in cleft palate surgery

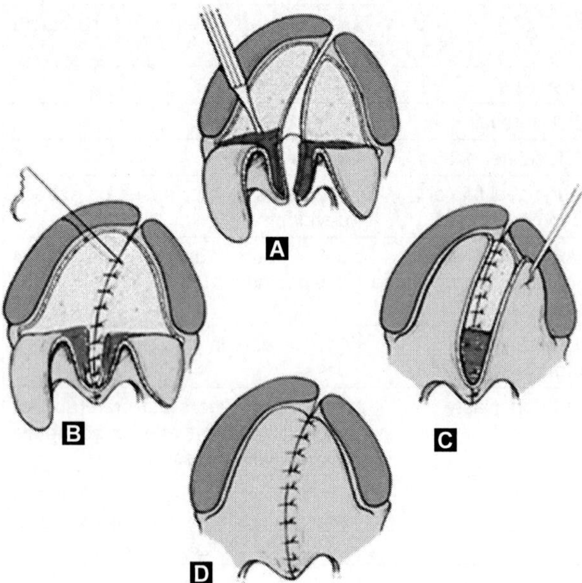

Figs 23.6A to D: Two flap palatoplasty. Closure of the nasal mucosa is shown. The muscle is repaired, and the oral mucosa is closed as a separate layer

occurs at 1 to 3 months of age; repair of the cleft palate is usually performed between 6 and 18 months of age. Repair of the cleft palate may require several stages of surgery as the child grows.

Early correction of cleft lip enables more normal sucking patterns and facilitates bonding. Early correction of cleft palate enables development of more normal speech patterns.

Delayed closure or large defects may require the use of orthodontic appliances.

Preoperative Care

Prevent Aspiration

Prior to having a cleft lip and/or palate repair it is important that the child is free from coughs and colds, any other viral infections. Explanation of surgical procedures and anesthesia to parents.

Provide mouth care to prevent infection.

Maintain Nutrition

Mention about altered child's appearance after surgery so parents and other family members will able to adapt to the fact that their child will look different after the operation.

Postoperative Care

Goal:

To prevent injury, promote healing, and maintain child's comfort.

Nursing Intervention:

- Assess airway patency and vital signs; observe for edema and respiratory distress.
- Position the child with cleft lip on her back, or propped on a side to avoid injury to the operative site; position the child with a cleft palate on the abdomen or side lying to facilities drainage.
- Clean the suture line and apply an antibacterial ointment as prescribed to prevent infection and scarring. Monitor the site for signs of infection.
- Use elbow restraints to maintain suture line integrity. Remove them every 2 hours for skin care and range-of-motion exercises.
- Feed the infant with a rubber-tipped medicine dropper, bulb syringe, breck feeder, or soft bottle-nipples, as prescribed, to help preserve suture integrity. The goal is to prevent child from having to suck hard on formula or milk, and thus protect the newly repaired lip. Expressed breast milk or formula can both be given in the feeder. Rinse mouth with water after each feed. For older children, diet progresses from clear fluids; they should not use straws or sharp objects.
- Attempt to keep the child from putting tongue up to palate sutures. Prevent the child from crying to avoid stress on the suture lines.
- Manage pain by administering analgesic as prescribed.

Provide child and family teaching.

- Show proper feeding techniques and positions
- Demonstrate wound care
- Explain that temperature of feeding formulas should be monitored closely because new palate has no nerve endings; therefore, the child can suffer a burn to the palate easily and without knowing it.
- Explain handling of prosthesis if indicated.
- Stress the importance of long-term follow up, including speech therapy, and preventing or correcting dental abnormalities.
- Discuss the need for, at least, annual hearing evaluations because of the increased susceptibility to recurrent otitis.
- Teach infection control measures.

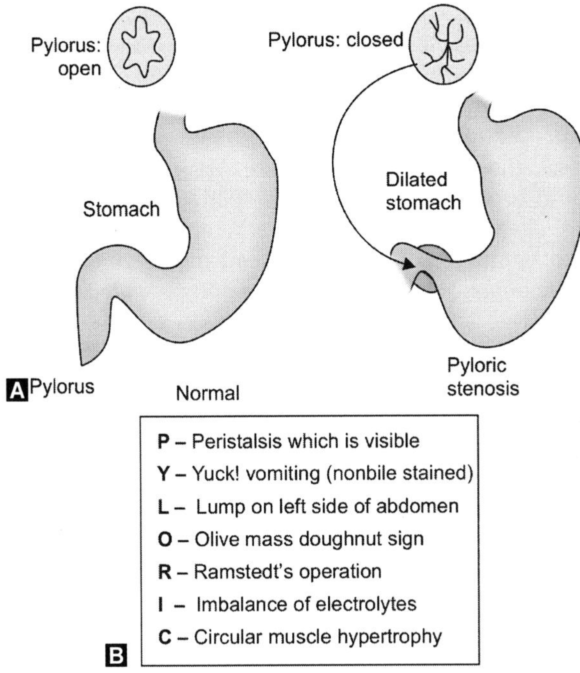

Figs 23.7A and B: Graphics of pyloric stenosis

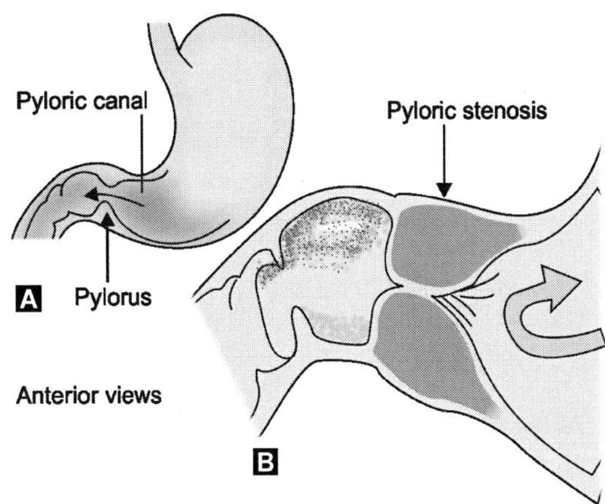

Figs 23.8A and B: Congenital hypertrophic pyloric stenosis. **A.** Normal passage through the pyloric sphincter is shown; **B.** Stoppage of flow owing to stenosis is demonstrated

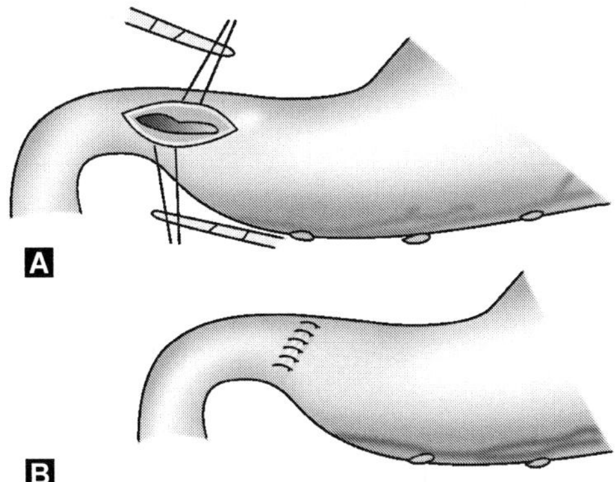

Figs 23.9A and B: Surgical steps are usually undertaken in case of pyloric stenosis

Pyloric Stenosis

Pyloric stenosis, also called infantile hypertrophic pyloric stenosis, is the most common pediatric surgical disorder of infancy (Figs 23.7A and B) that requires surgery for associated emesis (projectile vomiting). The pylorus is a muscle that opens and closes to allow food to pass through the stomach into the intestine. Pyloric stenosis involves hypertrophy of the circular muscle of the pylorus, resulting in narrowing and obstruction of the pyloric channel by compression of longitudinal folds of mucosa. When this muscle becomes enlarged, feedings are blocked from emptying out of the stomach (Figs 23.8A and B). The retained feedings cause the infant to vomit. Protracted emesis (non bilious in nature), as well as failure of the stomach to empty into the duodenum, results in progressive dehydration, electrolyte abnormalities, acid-base disorders, weight loss, and, potentially, shock.

Preoperative Management

- Directed at correcting the fluid deficiency and electrolyte imbalance.
- Most infants can have their fluid status corrected within 24 hours; however, severely dehydrated children sometimes require several days for correction.
- If necessary, administer an initial fluid bolus of 10 mL/kg with lactated Ringer's solution or 0.45 isotonic sodium chloride solution.

Surgery

Pyloric stenosis does not get better by itself and must be corrected with an operation. The definitive treatment of pyloric stenosis is with surgical pyloromyotomy known as Ramstedt's procedure (dividing the muscle of the pylorus to open up the gastric outlet). This surgery can be done through a single incision (usually 3 to 4 cm long) via a right upper quadrant transverse incision that splits the rectus muscle and fascia or laparoscopically (Figs 23.9A and B).

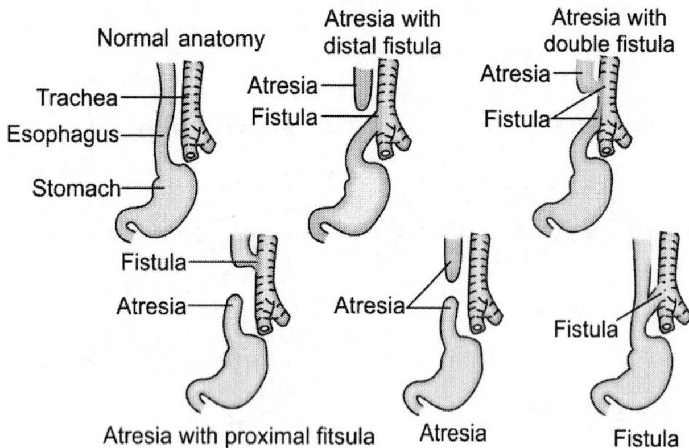

Fig. 23.10: Types of tracheo esophageal fistula (TEF)

Postoperative Management

- Continue IV maintenance fluid until the infant is able to tolerate enteral feedings.
- In most instances, feedings can begin within 8 hours following surgery.
- Graded feedings can usually be initiated every 3 hours, starting with Pedialyte and progressing to full-strength formula.

Esophageal Atresia and Tracheoesophageal Fistula/Atresia

Esophageal atresia is the failure of the esophagus to form a continuous passage from the pharynx to the stomach.

Tracheoesophageal fistula/atresia is an abnormal connection between the trachea and esophagus (Fig. 23.10).

Management

- In healthy infants without pulmonary complications, primary repair is performed within the first few days of life. Repair is delayed in patients with low birth weight, pneumonia, or other major anomalies. Initially, treat patients conservatively with parenteral nutrition, gastrostomy, and upper pouch suction until they are considered to be low risk.
- Preoperatively, a cuffed endotracheal tube is placed distal to the fistula site in order to prevent reflux of gastric contents into the lungs. The ongoing mechanical ventilation following tracheal reconstruction is associated with recurrence of TEFs or restenosis. A conservative approach is therefore used until the patient is weaned from the mechanical ventilator. A tracheostomy tube is placed distally to the TEF if possible. The head of the bed is elevated, and oral secretions are frequently suctioned. A gastrostomy tube is placed to minimize gastroesophageal reflux, and a jejunostomy feeding tube is placed for nutritional purposes. If soilage of the respiratory tract continues, esophageal diversion procedures may be required.

In the preoperative phase, risk of aspiration should be reduced. Continuous suctioning of the blind esophageal pouch with a 6–7 F catheter may decrease the risk of aspiration. The infant's head should be elevated, and he or she should be hydrated and provided energy intake (caloric intake) via intravenous dextrose solution.

If the patient develops acute respiratory failure, endotracheal intubation and mechanical ventilation are performed. Administer broad-spectrum antibiotics for patients who may have developed lower respiratory tract infection. For patients known to have pneumonia or other pulmonary problems, a gastrostomy for gastric decompression may be required to prevent further reflux of gastric contents into the trachea. The use of proton pump inhibitors may be helpful.

Operative Repair

- Timing of operation and choice of surgical approach in congenital TEFs are crucial. Make decisions based on the size and condition of the infant. Most infants are recommended to undergo primary care; however, a staged repair several weeks following birth is recommended for infants who are premature and have severe respiratory distress syndrome. The presence of other severe comorbidities, such as aspiration pneumonia, congenital cardiac disease, or other life-threatening conditions, should also delay the primary repair. Tracheostomy is required only if planning a staged repair. Infants who have severe respiratory distress syndrome may require the use of a Fogarty balloon catheter to obliterate the TEF while awaiting surgery.
- The repair is performed via right thoracotomy in the left lateral decubitus position, and the head of table is elevated to avoid gastric reflux. A posterolateral thoracotomy incision is made through the 4th intercostal space, and a retropleural exposure is obtained. During the dissection, the azygos vein is divided and the vagus nerve is identified. The distal esophagus is identified and dissected distal to the TEF. The fistula is divided and closure is performed with stay sutures. Dissection is carefully performed to avoid interruption of blood supply or the branches coming off the vagus nerve. Tracheal suture line may be covered with a flap of mediastinal pleura. Prior to esophageal anastomosis, the proximal pouch of the trachea is mobilized.

- If a fistula lies between the esophageal pouch and trachea, it is divided and closed. The esophageal anastomosis is performed in 1 to 2 layers and is covered with mediastinal pleura. A nasogastric feeding tube is placed through the esophagus into the stomach prior to the chest closure, and a chest tube is placed in the retropleural space.
- Postoperatively, the infant is ventilated as needed, nasogastric or gastrostomy feedings are resumed, and a contrast swallow radiographic examination is performed on the 7th postoperative day. If no leak is detected, oral feedings are resumed. Approximately 3 weeks later, the esophagus is dilated up to a 24F size in order to prevent future esophageal stenosis.
- The most common complications of surgery are pneumonia and atelectasis leading to respiratory failure in postoperative period. A leak at the anastomotic site and pneumothorax are other complications. Most patients who develop an anastomotic leak also develop strictures, which may be dilated later.

Nursing Care of the Child with Esophageal Atresia or Tracheoesophageal Fistula

Preoperative Care

- Maintain airway. Assess neonate for color and respiratory. Clear airway of secretions. Keep the newborn's head elevated at 30–45°. Assess the child's respiratory status correctly using a neonatal respiratory distress score.
- Oxygen therapy—Administer oxygen as prescribed. Administer humidified oxygen. Document rate of oxygen flow hourly.
- Monitor other vital signs.
- Place the child in a lateral position with the head turned to one side.
- Keep NPO–administer IV fluids. Assess hydration status of the child using clinical signs.
- Suction PRN. Use a size 6F/7F suction catheter. Gently pass the suction catheter into the esophagus until resistance is felt. Withdraw the suction catheter by 0.5 cm and apply suction, do gentle suctioning.
- Administer prophylactic antibiotics.

Postoperative Care

- Obtain advance information of the child's condition and surgical procedure from the OT prior to receiving. Maintain airway.
- Carefully handle child without hyper-extending neck. Place child's head–rest in a way that child's neck is neither flexed nor extended. Place a soft cotton roll under the head of the child to stabilize it.
- Restrain the hands of the child.
- Secure the trans – anastomotic nasogastric tube. Records the nasogastric aspirates.
- Monitor vital signs, cardiopulmonary function.
- Monitor chest tube function and drainage. Measures and records child's chest drain output every 24 hours. Documents characteristics of the chest drain exudates
- Surgical site management
- Monitor feeding tolerance, maintain nutrition by gastrostomy tube feedings. Observe nutritional status, including weight
- Assess pain/sedation level of child using neonatal pain scale and administer analgesics
- Prevent trauma
- Monitor for potential complications
- Monitor weight, growth and developmental achievements.
- Signs and symptoms of infection.
- Parent-infant interaction.

Intestinal Obstruction

Intestinal obstruction in infants typically arises from infections, organ diseases, and decreased blood flow to the intestines (Figs 23.11 and 23.12).

General principles in the medical treatment of small-bowel obstruction include the following:

- Stabilize the patient and monitor ABCs.
- Replace fluids with diligent intravenous (IV) resuscitation, using isotonic sodium chloride solution or lactated Ringer's solution.
- Early bowel decompression with an NG tube decreases the chance of bowel necrosis and perforation.
- Administer broad-spectrum antibiotics when necrosis or perforation is suspected. Bowel obstructions often require surgical interventions, but start antibiotic administration in the emergency department first. Antibiotic coverage must include gram-negative aerobic and gram-negative anaerobic organisms.

Patients who do not respond to nonoperative treatment within 12–24 hours require surgical treatment.

A possible diagnosis of adhesive small bowel obstruction requires prompt surgical consultation because delay can lead to intestinal necrosis. The most difficult part is to decide if and when the child is to undergo surgery. As a general rule, the presence of

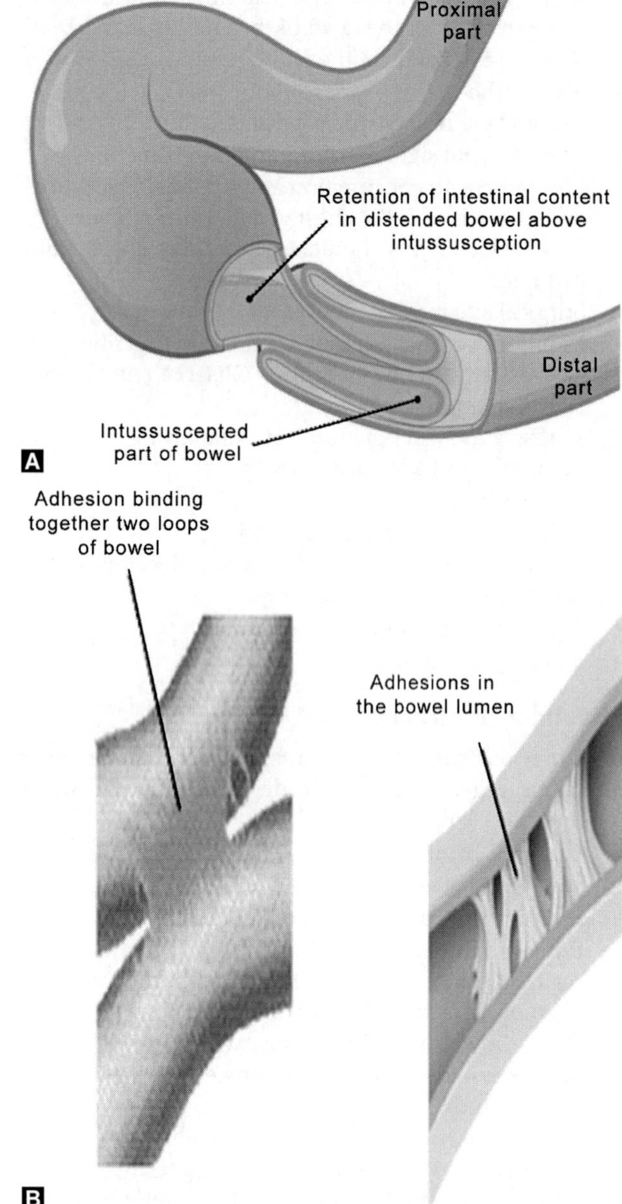

Figs 23.11A and B: A. Intestinal obstruction due to intussusception; **B.** Due to adhesions

fever, tachycardia, leukocytosis, rebound tenderness, or complete obstruction warrants surgical exploration. The options for surgical management include laparotomy with abdominal decompression, with or without resection of necrosed bowel followed by primary anastomosis or creation of an ostomy, versus peritoneal drainage alone.

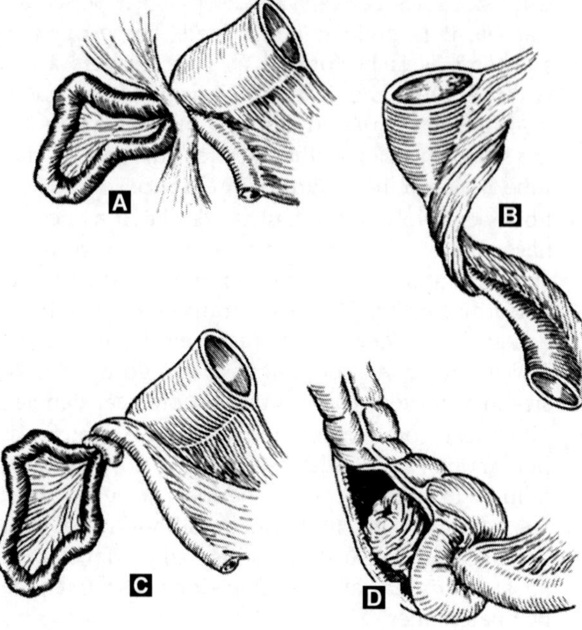

Figs 23.12A to D: Types of intestinal obstruction intussusception, adhesion, **A.** Strangulation; **B.** Jamming; **C.** Volvulus; **D.** Invagination

Surgical Management

Surgical management consists of relieving obstruction. Closed bowel procedures includes lysis of adhesions, reduction of volvulus, intussusception, or incarcerated hernia. Enterotomy is done for removal of foreign bodies.

Resection of bowel is done for obstructing lesions, or strangulated bowel with end-to-end anastomosis. Intestinal bypass around obstruction is also performed. Temporary ostomy may be indicated.

Nursing Management

Primary Prevention

Encourage well-balanced and high-fiber diet, encourage regular exercise.

Secondary Prevention

Insert an NG tube to decompress the bowel as ordered. Maintain the function of the nasogastric tube and assess and measure the nasogastric output. Maintain fluid and electrolyte balance by monitoring electrolyte, blood urea nitrogen, and creatinine levels. Begin and maintain IV therapy as ordered. Monitor nutritional status.

Continually assess his pain. Colicky pain that suddenly becomes constant could signal perforation.

Assess improvement (return of normal bowel sounds, decreased abdominal distention, subjective improvement in abdominal pain and tenderness, passage of flatus or stool). Look for signs of dehydration (thick, swollen tongue; dry, cracked lips; dry oral mucous membranes). Watch for signs of metabolic alkalosis. Report discrepancies in intake and output; worsening of pain or abdominal distention, and increased nasogastric output.

Watch for signs and symptoms of secondary infection, such as fever and chills. Administer analgesics, broad-spectrum antibiotics, and other medications as ordered. Keep the patient in semi-Fowler's or Fowler's position as much as possible. These positions help to promote pulmonary ventilation and ease respiratory distress from abdominal distention. Monitor urine output carefully to assess renal function, circulating blood volume, and possible urine retention due to bladder compression by the distended intestine. If the patient's condition does not improve, prepare patient for surgery.

Tertiary Prevention

After surgery, provide all necessary postoperative care. Care for the surgical site, maintain fluid and electrolyte balance, relieve pain and discomfort, maintain respiratory status, and monitor intake and output. Explain the rationale for NG suction, NPO status, and IV fluids initially. Advise patient to progress diet slowly as tolerated once home. Advise plenty of rest and slow progression of activity as directed by surgeon or other health care provider. Teach wound care if indicated. Encourage patient to follow-up as directed and to call surgeon or health care provider if increasing abdominal pain, vomiting, or fever occur prior to follow-up.

Medical Management

Correction of fluid and electrolyte imbalances with normal saline or Ringer's solution with potassium as required. NG suction to decompress bowel. Treatment of shock and peritonitis. Analgesics and sedatives are administered, *avoiding opiates due to GI motility inhibition*. Antibiotics are to prevent or treat infection. Ambulation for patients with paralytic ileus to encourage return of peristalsis. TPN may be necessary to correct protein deficiency from chronic obstruction, paralytic ileus, or infection.

CARE OF THE PATIENT WITH AN OSTOMY

Preoperative Nursing Responsibilities

Prepare patient by explaining the surgical procedure, stoma characteristics, and ostomy management with a pouching system.

Postoperative Nursing Responsibilities

Monitor the stoma color and amount, and color of stomal output every shift; document, and report any abnormalities. Periodically change a properly fitting pouching system over the ostomy to avoid leakage and protect the peristomal skin (Figs 23.13A and B). Use this time as an opportunity for teaching. Assess peristomal skin with each pouching system change, document findings, and treat any abnormalities (skin breakdown due to leakage, allergy, or infection) as indicated. Teach the patient and/or caregiver self-care skills of routine pouch emptying, cleansing skin and stoma, and changing of the pouching system until independence is achieved. Instruct the patient and family in lifestyle adjustments regarding gas and odor control; procurement of ostomy supplies; and bathing, clothing, and travel tips.

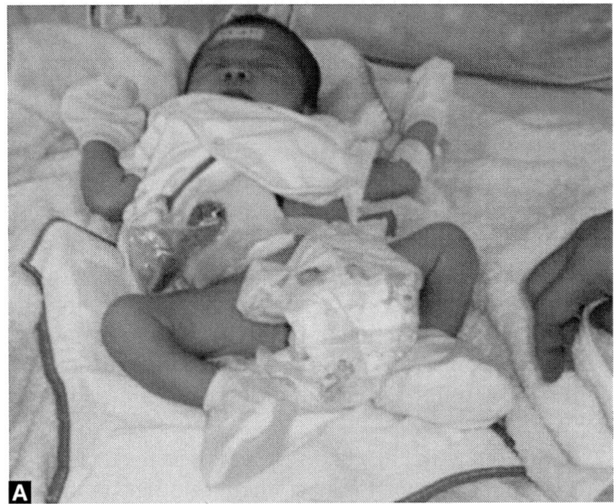

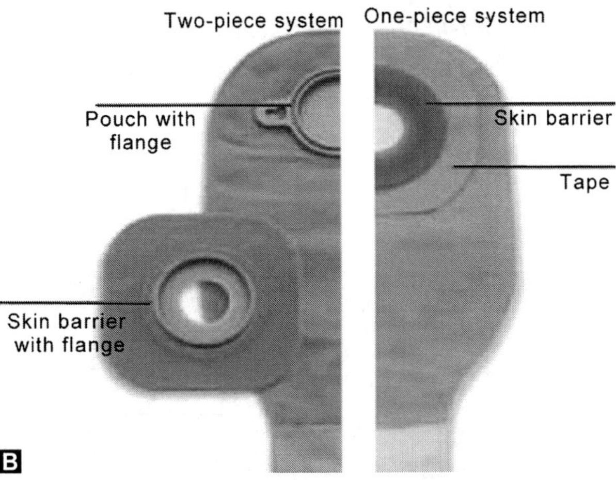

Figs 23.13A and B: A. Child with colostomy; **B.** Different systems of colostomy bag

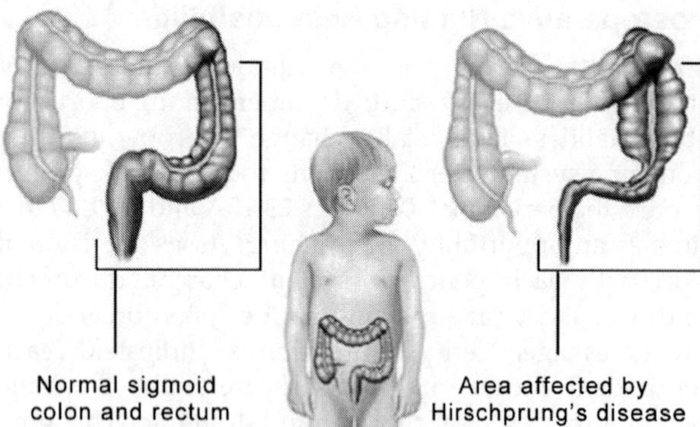

Fig. 23.14: Normal sigmoid colon and rectum and area affected by Hirschsprung's disease

Hirschsprung's Disease/Megacolon

Hirschsprung's disease, also called congenital megacolon or congenital aganglionic megacolon, is a congenital disorder of the colon in which nerve cells of the myenteric plexus in its walls, also known as ganglion cells, are absent. It is a rare disorder, with prevalence among males being four times that of females. Hirschsprung's disease develops in the fetus during the early stages of pregnancy. The exact genetic cause remains unsolved, although in familial cases, it seems to exhibit autosomal dominant transmission. The segment lacking neurons (aganglionic) in colon becomes constricted, causing the normal, proximal section of bowel to become distended with feces. Symptoms include failure to pass meconium within 48 hours of birth and abdominal distention (Fig. 23.14).

Children with Hirschsprung's disease need surgery, regular follow-up visits and sometimes other treatment.

Surgery for Hirschsprung's Disease

Treatment of Hirschsprung's disease consists of surgical removal of the abnormal section of the colon (Fig. 23.15), followed by *reanastomosis* which is also called colostomy and pull through surgery.

The first stage of treatment used to be a reversible *colostomy*. The healthy end of the large intestine is cut and attached to an opening created on the front of the abdomen and the segment of intestine that does not have ganglion cells is resected. This always includes the rectum, and it may include part of the colon. Later, when the child's weight, age, and condition are right, the 'new' functional end of the bowel is connected with the anus.

The first surgical treatment involving surgical resection followed by reanastomosis *without a colostomy* occurred as early as 1933 by Doctor Baird in Birmingham on a 1-year-old boy. Currently, there are several different surgical approaches, which include the Swenson, Soave, Duhamel, and Boley procedures. There are several ways to do a pull-through. The main ways are called the Swenson, Soave and Duhamel procedures. They differ in how much of the intestine surgeons remove and how surgeons connect the remaining intestine to the anus. There is no evidence that one procedure is better than the others. A small portion of the diseased bowel is left in the Swenson procedure. The Soave procedure leaves the outer wall of the colon unaltered. The Boley procedure is a small modification of the Soave procedure, so the term 'Soave-Boley' procedure is sometimes used. The Duhamel procedure uses a surgical stapler to connect the good and bad bowel.

Anorectal Malformations

An anorectal malformation, commonly called imperforate anus is a birth defect that affects the development of the rectum and anus. Development of the urinary structures, and genital tract may also be affected. This is accompanied by abnormal formation of muscles and nerves of the pelvic floor that control

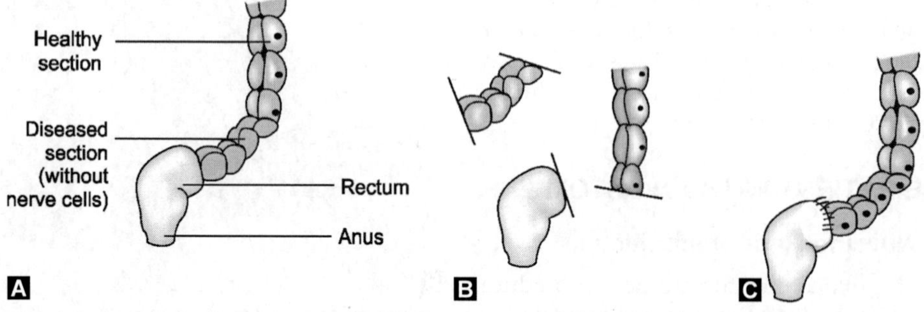

Figs 23.15A to C: A. Before surgery: The diseased section is the part of the intestine that does not work; **B.** Step 1: The diseased part is removed; **C.** Step 2: The healthy section is attached to the rectum or anus

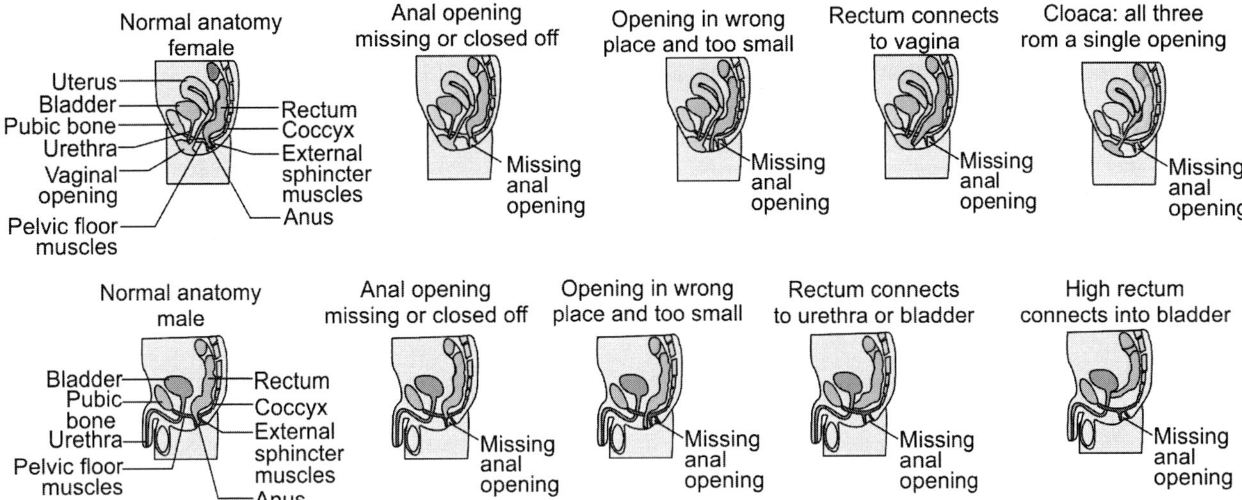

Fig. 23.16: Different types of anorectal malformations are seen in male and female children

emptying of stool. Anorectal malformations comprise a wide spectrum of disease affecting male and female and can involve malformations of the distal anus and rectum, as well as the urinary and genital tracts (Fig. 23.16).

Colostomy

- A descending colostomy with separated stomas is recommended.
- The advantages of this type of colostomy include the following:
  - It defunctionalizes only a small portion of distal colon.
  - In cases of large rectourinary fistulae in which the patient passes urine into the bowel, the urine comes out easily through the mucous fistula, avoiding problems of hyperchloremic acidosis caused by urine absorption. Urinary tract infections are also avoided.

When performing the colostomy in the newborn, the distal bowel should be irrigated to remove all the meconium. This prevents formation of a megasigmoid, which may be responsible for the future development of constipation.

Definitive repair—*Posterior Sagittal Anorectoplasty (PSARP)*

Patients are placed in the prone position with the pelvis elevated. A Foley's catheter is placed before the prone positioning.The posterior sagittal incision length varies with anorectal defect. Perineal fistulas are repaired with a minimal posterior sagittal incision that is large enough to divide the external sphincter and to mobilize the anus back to the center of the external sphincter. The sphincter mechanism is always located posterior to the fistula site. This operation can be performed in the neonatal period without a protective colostomy.

In patients with a rectourethral fistula, the Foley's catheter usually stays in place for approximately 5 to 7 days; however, occasionally, this period is longer. At 2 weeks' postoperation, anal calibration is performed, followed by a program of anal dilatations. The anus must be dilated twice daily, and the size of the dilator is increased every week. The final size to be reached depends on the age of the patient.

Once the desired size is reached, the colostomy can be closed.

Dilatations are continued afterward according to a prescribed protocol.

Dilatations are a vital part of the postoperative management to avoid a stricture at the anoplasty.

Hydrocephalus

Hydrocephalus is one of the most frequently seen problems in a pediatric surgical setting. The term hydrocephalus represents a buildup of spinal fluid inside the brain (*See* the Chapter 16).

More often the blockage cannot be removed and the fluid needs to bypass the normal circulation. Most surgeons use various types of systems called shunts to channel the fluid from the ventricles to other sites in the body such as the abdominal cavity, chest cavity or the heart. Each of these sites have various advantages and disadvantages, but by far and away the most popular for pediatrics is the abdominal cavity. Here the spinal fluid is absorbed onto the surface of the bowels to be returned to the bloodstream along with the vital salts and other products it contains.

Shunt Insertion

In most cases, a shunt is surgically inserted. The shunt is a drainage system made of a long tube with a valve. The valve helps CSF flow at a normal rate and in the right direction. The most common treatment now in use is a shunt from one lateral ventricle into the circulating blood by way of the internal jugular vein to the right atrium of the heart or superior vena cava just proximal to it. Sometimes one end of the tube is inserted in the brain, and the other end is typically inserted into the abdomen. Excess fluid then drains from the brain and out the other end of the tube, where it is more easily absorbed. The shunt is typically needed permanently and has to be monitored regularly.

Shunt and Insertion of Shunt

A shunt is a mechanical device, made up of silicone elastomer (plastic) and are often impregnated with barium, designed to transport the excess CSF from or near the point of obstruction to a reabsorption site and it is implanted under the skin. The shunt performs two functions. It allows fluid to go only in one direction and the valve allows fluid to flow out only when the pressure in the head has exceeded some value (usually referred to as the 'opening pressure'). This system regulates the amount of the CSF in the body so that not too much is taken, nor too little.

The shunt has 3 components. The first portion is called the shunt catheter or proximal portion of the shunt. This is a small narrow tube (catheter), which is implanted into the ventricle of the brain (Fig. 23.17), above where the obstruction has occurred. It is then connected to the valve and reservoir. The valve controls how much fluid is withdrawn from the brain, it is then stored in the reservoir until it is released to drain down the distal (bottom) end. The distal end is a small, narrow piece of tubing (catheter) which leads to the point where the excess CSF will drain and be absorbed by the body.

The Steps of Insertion of Shunt

- An area of hair on the head is shaved. This may be behind the ear or on the top or back of the head.
- The surgeon makes a U-shape cut behind the ear. Another small surgical cut is made in the belly.
- A small hole is drilled in the skull. A thin tube called a catheter is passed into a ventricle of the brain. This can be done with or without a computer as a guide. It can also be done with an endoscope that allows the surgeon to see inside the ventricle.
- Another catheter is placed under the skin behind the ear. It is sent down the neck and chest, and usually into the belly area. Sometimes, it stops at the chest area. The doctor may make a small cut in the neck to help position it.
- A valve is placed underneath the skin behind the ear. The valve is connected to both catheters. When extra pressure builds up around the brain, the valve opens, and excess fluid drains through the catheter into the belly or chest area. This helps lower intracranial pressure (Fig. 23.18).
- The patient is taken to a recovery area and then moved to a hospital ward.

Common complications of VP shunt include shunt malfunction or blockage, kinking, separation of shunt tube and infection. Malfunction may be related to growth and the shunt will need to be replaced with a longer catheter. Symptoms of shunt malfunction or infection

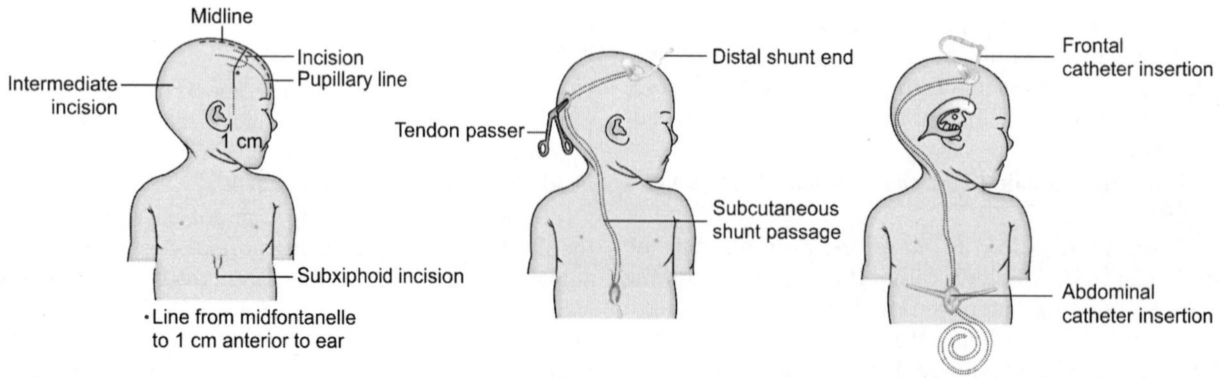

Fig. 23.17: Shunt and insertion of shunt

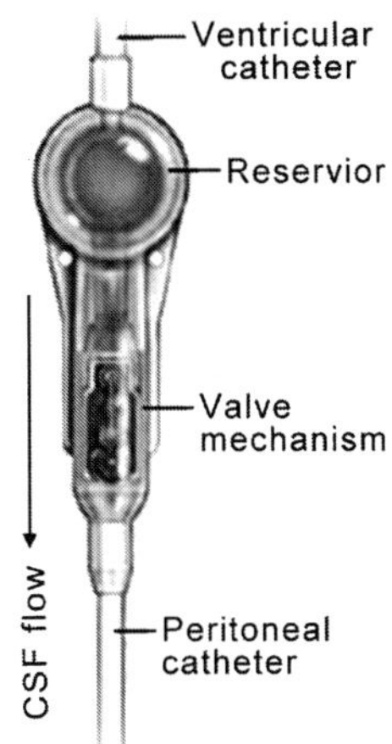

Fig. 23.18: Different parts of shunt

include headache, fever, drowsiness, convulsions, increased head circumference and bulging fontanelle.

- Antibiotics are given if there are signs of infection. Severe infections may require the shunt to be removed.

Other Treatments

Endoscopic Third Ventriculostomy (ETV)

A procedure called a ventriculostomy can be performed as an alternative to having a shunt inserted. *An endoscope being used to make a hole in the ventricle so the patient can avoid needing a shunt.*

For a small number of children, an endoscopic third ventriculostomy (ETV) surgery may be a treatment option. Most often it is done in children who have aqueductal stenosis. Depending on child's age and brain structures (typically be dilatation of the lateral ventricles, ballooning of the third ventricle, and a relatively small fourth ventricle), ETV is done instead of putting in a shunt.

The technique consists of the creation of a single burrhole in the frontal region followed by ventricular cannulation and insertion of a 3 or 4 mm wide neuroendoscope into the lateral ventricle. The third ventricle is then negotiated via the foramen of Monro and a hole is then made in the floor of the third ventricle between the infundibulum of the pituitary gland and the mammillary bodies. This creates a CSF fistula between the third ventricle and the subarachnoid space in front of the brainstem. The hole is made with a small electrode and enlarged with a balloon dilator, such that a very exciting close up view of the basilar artery is unveiled.

Choroid Plexus Cauterization (CPC)

Removing or cauterizing the parts of the brain that produce CSF.

Sometime, when child's body does not absorb CSF well, a CPC may be a treatment option. This is done during the same surgery as ETV. It is done to decrease the amount of CSF made in child's brain. This may help avoid the need for a shunt in the future.

In CPC, a flexible endoscope is used to reach the choroid plexus in the lateral ventricles each side of the brain and cauterization is done so it does not make as much CSF. CPC may lower the level of fluid enough that child's body can keep up with absorbing it.

The child will need regular checkups to make sure there are no further problems. Tests are regularly done to check the child's developmental and for intellectual, neurological, or physical problems.

Visiting nurses, social services, support groups, and local agencies can provide emotional support and assist with the care of a child with hydrocephalus who has significant brain damage (for more see the Chapter 16).

Neural Tube Defects

Neural tube defects are a group of conditions in which an opening in the spinal cord or brain remains from early in human development.

- Spina bifida
- Meningocele
- Meningomyelocele.

Cardiovascular System

Staged surgical repair and interventional cardiac catheterization have contributed to improved outcomes for children with congenital heart disease. Congenital heart disease affects 8 per 1000 live births, and 2 or 3 of these infants are estimated to have critical disease requiring cardiac catheterization or cardiac surgery.

Tetralogy of Fallot

Tetralogy of Fallot must be repaired with open-heart surgery. It is done either soon after birth or later in infancy. The goal of surgery is to repair the four defects of tetralogy of Fallot so the heart can work as normally as possible. Repairing the defects can greatly improve a child's health and quality of life. The decision of surgery depends on baby's health and weight, how severe the defects are, and how severe the baby's symptoms are. A large right ventricular incision is made for access to both the right ventricular outflow tract obstruction and ventricular septal defect (VSD). The incision usually heals in about 6 weeks.

Surgery to repair tetralogy of Fallot is done to improve blood flow to the lungs and to make sure that oxygen-rich and oxygen-poor blood flows to the right places. So the procedural steps are done as:

- *Widening the narrowed pulmonary blood vessels:* The pulmonary valve is widened or replaced, and the passage from the right ventricle to the pulmonary artery is enlarged. These procedures improve blood flow to the lungs. This allows the blood to get enough oxygen to meet the body's needs.
- *Closing the VSD:* A patch is used to cover the hole in the septum. This patch stops oxygen-rich and oxygen-poor blood from mixing between the ventricles.
- Fixing these two defects resolves problems caused by the other two defects. When the right ventricle no longer has to work so hard to pump blood to the lungs, it will return to a normal thickness. Fixing the VSD means that only oxygen-rich blood will flow out of the left ventricle into the aorta.

Temporary palliative surgery was common in the past to do temporary surgery during infancy in babies who had tetralogy of Fallot. This surgery improved blood flow to the lungs. A complete repair of the four defects was done later in childhood.

Now, most babies who have tetralogy of Fallot have their defects fully repaired in infancy. However, some babies are too weak or too small to have the full repair. They must have temporary surgery first. This surgery improves oxygen levels in the blood. It also gives the baby time to grow and get strong enough for the full repair. In the temporary surgery, a tube called a shunt is placed between a large artery branching off the aorta and the pulmonary artery. One end of the shunt is sewn to the artery branching off the aorta. The other end is sewn to the pulmonary artery. The result of this operation is that a connection is made between a systemic artery and pulmonary artery, thus increasing the blood flow to the lungs and rise of oxygen level, improving exercise tolerance, reducing cynosis. The shunt is removed when the baby's heart defects are fixed during the full repair.

Types of temporary palliative surgery are:

- In Blalock Taussig operation, a branch of aorta is anastomosed to the pulmonary artery. The innominate artery is used when the child is under 2 years, in children over 2 years the subclavion artery is preferred.
- In the Pott's operation, a direct correction is made between the aorta and the pulmonary artery.
- Direct operation for the pulmonary stenosis is called Brock operation which is done through a right ventricular approach. This operation increases the flow of blood to the lungs, but does not correct VSD.

After temporary surgery, baby may need medicines to keep the shunt open while waiting for the full repair. These medicines are stopped after the shunt is removed.

Tricuspid Atresia

Children with tricuspid atresia and too little pulmonary blood flow will require surgery to establish a connection between the systemic arteries and the arteries to the lungs. The diagnosis of tricuspid atresia with too little blood flow to the lungs or to the body requires immediate medical treatment. In a newborn, PGE_1 infusion is initiated to reopen the connection (ductus arteriosus) between the pulmonary artery and aorta, and improve blood flow to the lungs or body.

Interventional cardiac catheterization: The catheterization involves placing small IV tubes in the vein and artery of a leg, arm or the neck, which moves slowly through the circulation until it reaches the heart. In case of child with tricuspid atresia, the catheter is placed across foramen ovale, to perform balloon atrial septosomia. A balloon at the tip of the catheter is inflated and is pulled back through the foramen ovale, to tear off the septum. If the balloon procedure is not effective, a catheter blade septostomy can be performed to cut the septum.

Babies who require prostaglandin to maintain adequate oxygen level will require surgery soon after birth. The surgery involves creation of a 'shunt,' which is a tube (Gore-Tex tube) that connects one of the branches of the aorta and the pulmonary artery, and thus replaces the PDA. This operation is called the Blalock-Taussig (BT) shunt or BT shunt. Many babies with tricuspid atresia are well enough to be discharged home soon after birth. However, some of these babies may require the 'shunt' operation at a few weeks of life if the level of oxygen in their blood is decreasing.

Some babies with tricuspid atresia are too 'pink' or have too much blood-flow to the lungs, and will require an operation called 'pulmonary artery banding' to narrow the pulmonary artery and regulate blood flow to the lungs. Babies with tricuspid atresia and transposition of great arteries may require the 'Norwood operation' if the aorta is too small.

Whatever operation is necessary in the newborn period, children can expect to undergo further heart surgery by the age of 3 to 6 months. This is true whether the child has too much or too little pulmonary or systemic blood flow in the newborn period and, therefore, did not require any surgery at that time. Glen procedure, a connection between the superior vena cava and the pulmonary arteries is performed at 4 to 6 months of age, when the pulmonary vascular resistance comes to normal pressures. The superior vena cava is detached from the heart and connected directly to the pulmonary artery, and the BT shunt is removed. This allows blood from the upper body to flow directly to the lungs to pick up oxygen without having to be pumped by the heart. It also prevents blood that already has oxygen from returning to the lungs, and, thereby, keeps the heart from doing unnecessary work.

Postoperatively, pulmonary hypertension must be prevented and managed aggressively to ensure adequate pulmonary blood flow. Maintaining upright position of patient is done to encourage passive blood flow to the lungs and it will help in decreasing the degree of venous congestion in the upper body. Pleural effusion can develop as the body adjusts to the blood flow and pressure changes. Occasionally, atrial arrhythmia are noticed. After this operation, however, there is still blood returning from the body through the inferior vena cava going directly back to the body without first passing through the lungs. Because of this, some level of cyanosis will persist.

Between the ages of 2 and 5 years, children with tricuspid atresia will be ready for the third operation required to optimize their circulation. This operation is called the Fontan procedure, and involves connection of the inferior vena cava directly to the pulmonary artery, which forces all blood returning from the body to pass through the lungs and pick up oxygen before being pumped to the body. This allows a more normal color in the skin and lips as well due to a more normal oxygen saturation in the blood. Fenestration, means a connection between venous and arterial circulation is maintained. It is done in case of the pressures of pulmonary arteries is higher than normal, so that some desaturated blood can shunt right to left to the systemic circulation until the pulmonary arteries adjust to the new flow and pressures. The fenestration may be closed later.

- Ventricular septal defect
- Atrial septal defect
- Patent ductus arteriosus.

For above conditions *See* Chapter 19.

Aortic Stenosis

Aortic balloon valvoplasty is performed to treat moderate-to-severe aortic stenosis. During this procedure, a thin flexible tube called a catheter is inserted through an artery in the groin or arm and threaded into the heart. When the tube reaches the narrowed heart valve, a balloon at the end of the tube is inflated. The balloon widens the valve opening. This procedure can improve cardiac output, reduce the degree of left ventricular dysfunction and hypertrophy, and decrease the risk of sudden death.

Aortic valve replacement (AVR) may occasionally be required in infants and children. Common indications for aortic valve replacement in children include the following:

- Progressive stenosis of the aortic valve in infants and children
- Multilevel left ventricular outflow tract obstruction in association with aortic valve stenosis not amenable to aortic valve repair that requires enlargement of the outflow tract.
- Aortic insufficiency as a complication of percutaneous balloon aortic valvuloplasty
- Rheumatic aortic valve disease
- Aortic valve endocarditis.

Although no aortic valve substitute is ideal, desirable characteristics include the following:

- Excellent flow hemodynamics with reduction of left ventricular afterload and/or preload to normal values.
- Lifetime durability without need for reoperation due to structural deterioration.
- Anticoagulation will not be needed
- Absence of risk for embolic complications
- Capability of growth to avoid patient prosthesis mismatch as the child gets older.
- Resistance to infection and endocarditis
- Ease of implantation
- Appropriate size availability for all patients.

Several aortic valve repair techniques have been used in children, including pericardial leaflet extension, commissural reconstruction, annuloplasty, sinus of Valsalva reduction, sinotubular junction remodeling, and even complete leaflet replacement using autologous pericardium. Aortic valve repair in the child allows for continuing growth and eliminates the need for anticoagulation. However, long-term results have been less than satisfactory, and residual lesions (e.g. regurgitation, stenosis) are common.

Mechanical valve prostheses are not ideal valve substitutes in children. Although the incidence of structural valve deterioration is negligible, these prostheses have significant limitations at the time of implant due to the lack of appropriately sized prostheses for small children and neonates. In addition, the absence of potential for growth can result in patient-prosthesis size mismatch as the child grows and may require re-replacement. Moreover, mechanical valves require lifetime anticoagulation with associated activity limitations, difficulties with future pregnancy, and a lifetime risk of thromboembolic and bleeding complications due to potential poor compliance with anticoagulation protocol.

Homografts and bioprosthetic valves are also problematic in children. Although these biologic valves do not require anticoagulation, they do not allow growth, and their durability in the pediatric population is very limited due to the high risk of accelerated structural valve degeneration and early calcification. In addition, the availability of appropriate-sized homografts and bioprostheses can be a problem.

The Ross procedure using pulmonary autograft provides excellent hemodynamics flow characteristics, is capable of growth, and does not require anticoagulation. Despite several shortcomings of the Ross procedure, it has emerged as a popular choice for aortic valve replacement in infants and children. This review focuses on the role of the Ross procedure in the treatment of aortic valve disease in children and young adults.

Aortic valve replacement (AVR) through open-heart surgery is a common treatment for severe aortic stenosis. AVR is typically an open-heart surgery. In an aortic valve replacement surgery, the damaged valve is removed and replaced with an artificial valve (mechanical or tissue).

During surgical aortic valve replacement, the chest is opened and the patient is put on cardiopulmonary bypass while the surgeon removes the native aortic valve and replaces it with either a mechanical valve or a biological valve made from animal tissue or human tissue. Mechanical aortic valves require lifetime warfarin (Coumadin) for anticoagulation to decrease the risk of systemic thrombosis or valve failure because of thrombus. These prostheses have significant limitations at the time of implant due to the lack of appropriately-sized prostheses for small children and neonates. In addition, the absence of potential for growth can result in patient-prosthesis size mismatch as the child grows and may require re-replacement. Moreover, there is a lifetime risk of thromboembolic and bleeding complications due to potential poor compliance with anticoagulation protocol.

Sometimes aortic valve replacement can also be performed through *minimal incision valve surgery (MIVS)*. In MIVS, the surgeon can replace the diseased valve through a smaller incision. However, cardiopulmonary bypass is still used. MIVS may be an option for some patients who are suitable candidates for surgery.

For patients who have been deemed high or greater risk for traditional open-chest surgery, a procedure called transcatheter aortic valve replacement (TAVR) may be a treatment option. TAVR allows the aortic valve to be replaced, and like open-heart surgery, TAVR produces results in lengthening patients' lives.

This less invasive procedure allows a new valve to be inserted within the native, diseased aortic valve. The TAVR procedure can be performed through multiple approaches (e.g. transfemoral, transapical, or transaortic).

Pulmonary autograft replacement of the aortic valve in young patients with congenital aortic valve disease has produced excellent short-term anatomic/physiologic results and symptomatic relief with no mortality. Indices of left ventricular dilatation and hypertrophy regress after repair when the Ross operation precedes important deterioration in preoperative ventricular function. Important technical considerations include: (i) the native distal ascending aorta should be sufficiently shortened before performing the distal aortic anastomosis; and (ii) the left coronary anastomosis should be positioned relatively high on the neoaorta root with a slight amount of tension. Both of these maneuvers reduce the likelihood of coronary artery distortion. Rapid degeneration of the pulmonary homograft and the propensity towards progressive dilatation of the neoaorta are important postoperative considerations. Until more is known about the etiology and natural history of these two potential complications, postoperative anti-inflammatory and/or immunosuppressive therapy and strict control of hypertension should be strongly considered.

Intraoperative Details

All procedures are performed though midline sternotomy. Cardiopulmonary bypass is established via standard aortic and bicaval venous cannulation. The left ventricle is decompressed by venting through the right superior pulmonary vein. Mild hypothermia (32—34°) is used with a combination of antegrade and retrograde cold blood cardioplegia. Antegrade cardioplegia is initially administered through the root and then by direct coronary artery cannulation at 20-minute intervals.

Palliative Surgery—Blalock-Taussig Shunt

Pulmonary Atresia

Surgical intervention is called valvotomy, to separate fused leaflets in the pulmonary valve. Another option includes the surgical placement of a valve called a pulmonary homograft, which is a donated pulmonary valve and artery. This valve may grow with the child and blood-thinners are not required.

Ventricular Septal Defect (VSD)

Surgical repair of a ventricular septal defect usually involves open-heart surgery, which is done under general anesthesia. The surgery requires a heart-lung machine and an incision in the chest. The doctor uses patches or stitches to close the hole.

- *Catheter procedure*. This method may be used to close some ventricular septal defects. Patching during catheterization does not require opening the chest. Rather than opening the chest, the doctor inserts a thin tube (catheter) into a blood vessel in the groin and guides it to the heart. A small mesh patch or plug is used to close the hole.
- *Hybrid procedure*. A hybrid procedure uses surgical and catheter-based techniques. Access to the heart is usually through a small incision and the procedure may be performed without stopping the heart and using the heart-lung machine. A plug is delivered to close the VSD via a catheter placed through the small hole that the surgeon created. Recovery from this procedure is quicker than with standard surgery.

After repair, regular medical follow-up is necessary to ensure that the ventricular septal defect remains closed. Frequency of medical checkup depend on the size of the ventricular septal defect and the presence or absence of any other problems.

Surgery to close a ventricular septal defect generally has excellent long-term results.

Surgical Management of Coronary Heart Disease (CHD)

One surgery may be enough to repair the heart defect, but sometimes a series of procedures is needed. Three different techniques for fixing congenital defects of the heart in children are described below. In Open-heart surgery a heart-lung bypass machine is used. An incision is made through the breastbone (sternum). Tubes are used to reroute the blood through a special pump called a heart-lung bypass machine. This machine adds oxygen to the blood and keeps the blood warm and moving through the rest of the body while the surgeon is repairing the heart. Using the machine allows the heart to be stopped. Stopping the heart makes it possible to repair the heart muscle itself, the heart valves, or the blood vessels outside the heart. After the repair is done, the heart is started again, and the machine is removed. The breastbone and the skin incision are then closed.

For some heart defect repairs, the incision is made on the side of the chest, between the ribs. This is called a thoracotomy. It is sometimes called closed-heart surgery. This surgery may be done using special instruments and a camera.

Another way to fix defects in the heart is to insert small tubes into an artery in the leg and pass them up to the heart. Only some heart defects can be repaired this way.

Preoperative Preparation

Any impending open heart surgery is anxiety provoking, needs information and proper orientation. It helps in recovery and decreases postoperative complications. Introducing other families and children who have undergone similar procedures as they progress and recover from the surgery, can be an encouraging experience.

In preoperative teaching parents and child may be discussed about the sights and sounds which will be experienced, invasive lines that will be inserted, anticipated sensations from the preoperative medicines, length of the operation. The nurse should also discuss equipment that will be connected to the patient. This equipment will include the ventilator, chest tubes, nasogastric tube, invasive lines, and urinary catheter. Parents should be reassured that these tubes and lines will be removed as soon as the child's condition permits. During the preoperative teaching session, the nurse should also provide information related to post-operative expectations.

Parents should be assured that they will receive updates about the child's condition and will be permitted to visit soon after the surgery is completed. Nursing interventions important for significant others include teaching them about the expected patient appearance. The patient may appear pale, cool, and edematous.

Pulmonary care is an important part of the postoperative care of the patient after cardiothoracic surgery. Postoperative practice with the equipment (such as an incentive spirometer) that will be used postoperatively is helpful. Teaching in the preoperative period assists the patient to comprehend the necessity of coughing effectively in spite of incisional pain to achieve positive outcomes positively. Early mobilization is effective in improving postoperative pulmonary outcome.

Reassurance that pain will be managed during the postoperative period is important to communicate to the patient and others. Teaching about incision splinting and availability of effective pain medicines should be emphasized.

Postoperative Care

After surgery, infants will return to the intensive care unit (ICU) for a few days to be closely monitored during recovery. While child is in the ICU, special equipment will be used to help him or her recovery, and may include the following:

Ventilator

Nearly all children who have cardiac surgery will be 'ventilated'. Ventilator is a machine that helps child breathe while he or she is under anesthesia during the operation. The ventilator tube will be inserted through the nose or mouth into the windpipe (trachea). This tube allows air to pass from the ventilator into the lungs, which breathes for child while he or she is too sleepy to breathe effectively on his or her own. Suctioning is needed to clear secretions from the breathing tube to prevent it from blocking. Child will not be able to speak or make a noise until the ventilator tube is removed. The ventilator will be required throughout the operation and for some time while in ICU. Some children may require as little as a few hours ventilation, while the average time is about 12 to 24 hours. Other children may require ventilation for a few days. Weaning from the ventilator is done when child can breath without ventilator.

- *Intravenous (IV) catheters:* Small, plastic tubes inserted through the skin into blood vessels to provide IV fluids and important medicines that help your child recover from the operation.
- *Arterial line:* A specialized IV line is placed in the wrist or other area of the body where a pulse can be felt, that measures blood pressure continuously during surgery and while child is in the ICU. Most children will have an arterial line inserted into an artery (usually in the wrist). The arterial line appears similar to the intravenous line. Blood samples can be taken from this line via a 3-way tap. The arterial line is removed before child leaves ICU. It involves removing some tape and applying pressure to the site. A small pressure dressing will be applied.
- *Nasogastric (NG) tube:* A small, flexible tube that keeps the stomach drained of acid and gas bubbles that may build up during surgery.
- *Urinary catheter:* A small, flexible tube that allows urine to drain out of the bladder and accurately measures how much urine the body makes, which helps determine how well the heart is functioning. After surgery, the heart will be a little weaker than it was before, and, therefore, the body may start to hold onto fluid, causing swelling and puffiness. Diuretics may be given to help the kidneys remove excess fluid from the body.
- *Chest tube:* A drainage tube may be inserted to keep the chest free of blood that would otherwise accumulate after the incision is closed. Bleeding may occur for several hours, or even a few days after surgery.
- *Heart monitor:* A machine that constantly displays a picture child's heart rhythm, and monitors heart rate, arterial blood pressure, and other values.
- *Central venous line*: Most children will have an intravenous line known as a central venous line (CVC) to give fluids and medications. This is usually positioned into a large vein in one side of the neck. A vein in the groin may be used in some circumstances.

After surgery child is kept as comfortable as possible with several different medications; some of which relieve pain, and some of which relieve anxiety. The staff needs to know from the parent for their input as to how best to soothe and comfort their child.

Pain relief consists of morphine via an infusion pump into an intravenous line in the first day or so. In the early hours after surgery while the ventilator is still breathing for your child, the dose of morphine given will keep them heavily sedated. The morphine dose will be reduced before the ventilator is weaned. The reduced dose will be adequate for pain relief at this time.

When the morphine infusion ceases, Panadol and Codeine are given (by mouth or rectally) for pain relief. Eventually only Panadol will be required. It is not possible to promise 100% pain relief; however, a good level of comfort should be possible for all children. Sometimes pain management service available in the hospital to assist when necessary.

- *High-calorie formula or breast milk:* Special nutritional supplements may be added to formula or pumped breast milk that increase the number of calories in each ounce, thereby allowing baby to drink less and still consume enough calories to grow properly.
- *Supplemental tube feedings:* Feedings given through a small, flexible tube that passes through the nose, down the esophagus, and into the stomach, that can either supplement or take the place of bottle-feedings. Infants who can drink part of their bottle, but not all, may be fed the remainder through the feeding tube. Infants who are too tired to bottle-feed at all may receive their formula or breast milk through the feeding tube alone.

Health education to the parent and Family

Coping with oxygen problem—the child has 'blue spells'

- Attempt to calm the child. This is the most important thing parent can do.

- Try placing the child with his or her knees to the chest—either on the back with the knees drawn up to the chest or in a sitting position with the chest to the knees.
- Parent may need to give oxygen to the child if the spells are severe and do not improve with a change in position.
- Note when the spells occur, and plan activities to try to decrease the spells.
- Try to prevent the cyanosis by keeping the child warm, decreasing activity, and frequently feeding small meals.
- Notify to doctor when a blue spell occurs.

Point to remember: Oxygen can cause a fire to burn very rapidly, so no smoking or open flames are allowed in the room where oxygen is being used. The amount of oxygen is prescribed according to the condition of the child. Do not change the amount of oxygen which has prescribed for the child.

Giving Medicines

Parent should be sure how to give child's medicines safely. Administration of cardiac medicines to the child may be dangerous if they are not given correctly.

- Parent need to understand how much medicine to give and how to give it.
- If mother is not comfortable in giving medicine to her child, nurse should help her to learn and practice.
- Inform the mother/family member about dose, action and the most common side effects of the medicine.

Getting Child to Eat Well

Nutrition is very important for children who have heart defects. Getting child to eat right can be a challenge. Children with congenital heart defects often tire when eating, so they eat less and may not get enough calories. Feeding may take longer than expectation. Tend to use more calories (have a higher metabolic rate) than other children.

To help overcome feeding difficulties or lack of weight gain:

- Baby's feeding should start before baby starts to cry, so mother must learn to recognize her baby's first signs of hunger, such as fidgeting and sucking on a fist. Baby will have more energy to eat well if he or she is not tired from crying.
- In case of formula fed baby, use of a soft nipples make it is easier for baby to get enough formula.
- Burp baby often, specially when using a bottle. Babies who have trouble sucking take in large amounts of air when they eat, which makes them feel full before they get enough breast milk or formula.
- Feed small, frequent meals. Smaller meals do not require as much energy to eat or digest.

Prevention of Infection

A congenital heart defect can raise the risk of an infection in the heart called endocarditis. To help prevent this infection, child needs to take excellent care of his or her teeth throughout life. Good oral care can limit the growth of mouth bacteria that could get into the bloodstream and lead to infection. Medical help is to be sought for if child has signs of a skin infection or infected wound.

After surgery do not soak child's wounds in water until all of the scabs have fallen off and the area looks healed. Do not pick wound scab to make them fall off sooner. This can cause irritation and infection.

Do not put any creams on the wounds until all the scabs have fallen off and the area looks healed.

Check the wounds every day. Immediate medical attention is needed if mother finds the signs of redness, swelling, liquid draining from the wound, pain, fever.

Seeking Medical Help

Parents need to seek medical help with following concerns:

- Changes in feeding, such as decreased fluid intake; loss of appetite; weight loss; tiredness and sleeping during feeds; not waking for feeds; shortness of breath while feeding; vomiting or diarrhea; increased sweating during feeding.
- Changes in breathing, such as breathing very quickly, especially when asleep; noisy breathing or making a grunting sound; increased sweating; ongoing cough.
- Changes in behavior, such as extreme sleepiness or irritability.
- Changes in color, such as paleness; mottling of the skin (skin looks like marble); blueness of the lips and tongue or nail beds (cyanosis); rash on hands, feet, or body.
- Signs of wound infection, such as fever, redness, puffiness, increasing tenderness, or drainage from the wound.
- Signs of water retention, such as swelling or puffiness of the eyelids, face, hands, or feet; swollen genitals in boys; swollen legs or ankles in older children; less urine or fewer wet diapers.

Information Regarding Surgery

One surgery may be enough to repair the heart defect, but sometimes a series of procedures is needed. Three different techniques for fixing congenital defects of the heart in children are described below.

Open-heart surgery is when the surgeon uses a heart-lung bypass machine.

- An incision is made through the breastbone (sternum) while the child is under general anesthesia (the child is unconscious and does not feel pain).
- Tubes are used to re-route the blood through a special pump called a heart-lung bypass machine. This machine adds oxygen to the blood and keeps the blood warm and moving through the rest of the body while the surgeon is repairing the heart.
- Using the machine allows the heart to be stopped. Stopping the heart makes it possible to repair the heart muscle itself, the heart valves, or the blood vessels outside the heart. After the repair is done, the heart is started again, and the machine is removed. The breastbone and the skin incision are then closed.

For some heart defect repairs, the incision is made on the side of the chest, between the ribs. This is called a thoracotomy. It is sometimes called closed-heart surgery. This surgery may be done using special instruments and a camera.

Another way to fix defects in the heart is to insert small tubes into an artery in the leg and pass them up to the heart. Only some heart defects can be repaired this way.

Helping with Emotional Issues

Children and teens with congenital heart defects may have self-esteem issues because of how they look. They may have scars from surgery, and they may be smaller, have clubbing, or have limits on how active they can be.

Children may feel alone and have trouble coping because they have to stay in the hospital often. Most children deal well with having a heart defect. But some children with serious heart defects may have a hard time feeling 'normal'.

Emotional Support to the Parent

Dealing with a lifelong and possibly life-threatening illness in child can have a strong impact on their life as a parent. It can be hard to accept that their child has a serious illness. And it is normal to worry about the effect the condition will have on their child's future.

Help them to take good care of their own physical and emotional health. Doing so will help them and it will give them the energy needed to care for their child with special needs. Following areas need to focus:

- *Learn all you can* about your child's heart defect.
- *Stop blaming yourself:* You did not cause the heart defect. Many things occurred for the defect to happen. No single factor causes congenital heart defects.
- *Allow yourself to grieve* about having a child with a heart defect.
- *Ask questions:* Do not expect to remember everything that is involved in caring for your child. Ask questions when you don't understand. Ask your doctor for written directions on caring for your child. If directions are written, you can look at them later and call the doctor if you have questions.
- *Join a support group:* It is helpful to be in contact with organizations and people who can offer support and answer your questions. Talk with your health professional to see whether there is a local support group you might join. A support group is a good place to meet other parents who are dealing with similar issues.
- *Talk to a counselor:* It is normal to feel sad. You may grieve because your baby is not the perfectly healthy infant you imagined. If you or a family member continues to feel extremely sad, guilty, or depressed or is otherwise having trouble dealing with your child's illness, talk with a doctor.

Family counseling: Coping with a child who has a lifelong illness impacts the entire family. If you feel that you or your family needs help dealing with the condition, talk with a health professional about counseling.

CHAPTER 24

Developmental Disturbances, Challenged Child and Implications for Nursing

Chapter Outline

- Developmental Delay
- Behavior Disorder

The first three years of a child's life are an amazing time of development…

…and what happens during those years stays with a child for a lifetime. That's why it's so important to watch for signs of delays in development, and to get help if you suspect problems. The sooner a delayed child gets early intervention, the better their progress will be. ***So, if you have concerns, act early.***

DEVELOPMENTAL DELAY

Each child develops at his or her own pace and the range of normal is quite wide. Developmental delay is when the child does not reach their developmental milestones at the expected times (Fig. 24.1). However, it is helpful to be aware of red flags for potential developmental delays in children. These delays are significant lags in one or more areas of emotional, mental, or physical growth. If any child experiences a delay, early treatment is the best way to help him or her make progress or even to catch up. Developmental delays can occur in all five areas of development or may just happen in one or more of those areas. Additionally, growth in each area of development is related to growth in the other areas. So if there is a difficulty in one area (e.g., speech and language), it is likely to influence development in other areas (e.g., social and emotional).

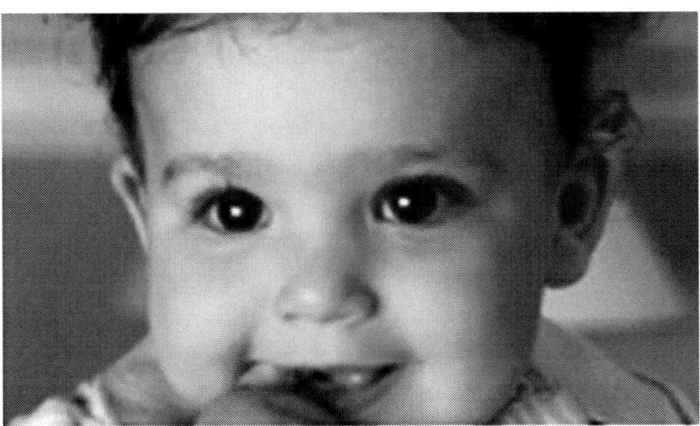

Fig. 24.1: Studying development of child is an important step in early detection of developmental disturbances

Physical	This includes gross motor skills that involve moving large muscles like arms and legs and fine motor skills that involve movement of small muscles like fingers and hands
Cognitive	Often referred to as intellectual abilities, this category covers areas such as verbal and nonverbal skills, attention and focus, hand-eye coordination and memory
Communication	Communication development refers to speech abilities and using spoken language to communicate
Social	Social development is a child's ability to cooperate and collaborate with others
Emotional	This includes abilities such as the ability to cope, control impulses, manage anger and resolve conflict

Risk Factors

Risk factors for developmental problems fall into two categories:

- Genetic
- Environmental.

Children are placed at genetic risk by being born with a genetic or chromosomal abnormality. A good example of a genetic risk is Down syndrome, a disorder that causes developmental delay because of an abnormal chromosome. Environmental risk results from exposure to harmful agents either before or after birth, and can include things like poor maternal nutrition or exposure to toxins (e.g. lead or drugs) or infections that are passed from a mother to her baby during pregnancy (e.g., measles or HIV). Environmental risk also includes a child's life experiences. For example, children who are born prematurely, face severe poverty, mother's depression, poor nutrition, or lack of care are at increased risk for developmental delays. Risk factors have a cumulative impact upon development. As the number of risk factors increases, a child is put at greater risk for developmental delay.

A developmental delay and a developmental disability sound like the same thing, but they are not. They are often confused with each other because they are both measured by the same developmental milestones. A child with a developmental disability has a life-long disadvantage. He or she could also be developmentally delayed, but a child with a delay does not necessary have a disability. A child with a developmental delay is merely in a temporary situation until he or she is able catch up with peers. Examples of developmental disabilities include autism and cerebral palsy.

Adjustment Reaction to School

Adjustment is a continual is the outcome of the individual's attempt to deal with stress and meet his needs also his efforts to maintain harmonious relationships with the environment. Psychological survival in much the same ways as biologist uses the term adaption to describe physiological survival. An adjustment disorder is an extraordinary emotional reaction to a difficult event. In children one of these events may include adjustment reaction to school. The most common challenge for most kids is saying goodbye to their parents, or trouble separating. For some children this may be their first time out of the home. Others may have separated before, but are now in a new, possibly more demanding situation.

Peter Grow wrote following lines in free to learn

'we are pushing the limits of children's adaptability. We have pushed children into an abnormal environment, where they are expected to spend ever greater portions of their day under adult direction, sitting at desk, listening to and reading about things that do not interest them, and answering questions that are not their own and are not, to them real questions. We leave them ever less time and freedom to play, explore and pursue their own interests'.

In this above contextuality most of the children try to 'adapt', at least outwardly. But parents or adults do not know what is really going on inside. So parents should be concerned if their child suddenly develops the following symptoms:

- Increased clinginess
- Withdrawing from things they usually enjoy
- Anxiety, shyness, stomach ache
- Avoiding participating in things
- Planning and organization difficulties
- Increased crying and tantrums
- Changes in eating habits
- Sleep difficulties and nightmares
- Regression to younger behaviors (e.g. bedwetting, thumb sucking, baby talk)
- Aggression
- There are a number of things parents can do to prepare their child. Prior to starting school, child can be taken to visit the classroom and meet the teacher. It would be good if there is a way of having a playdate with one of the other children who will be attending the preschool, that is great, because then the children can welcome each other when they begin school. The child can carry his or her own toy or storybook to the school, and teacher can read it. Child should be given lots of reassurance that 'Mommy's coming back,' or 'Daddy's coming back.'

Parents as 'experts' on their children, and professionals are 'experts' in their areas, such as special education or mental health. They should work together to sort out the difficulties of the child and to handle the 'separation anxiety' the basic psychological problem of the child. The problem can be worked out by talking with the child and encouraging the child for habit formation of regular school attendance, more and more play and diversional or recreational; improvement of school environment; and assessment of health condition of the child to detect any health problems for necessary interventions activities. Guidelines for parents in this regard are:

- Look for common signs of stress, irritability, lack of sleep, loss of appetite.
- Try to be patient, controlled and calm.
- Do not have unrealistic expectations.
- Be positive and reassuring, emphasize on success.
- Avoid comparison with other students.
- Do not stress on rank.
- Do not offer bribes.
- Avoid negative talk.

Habit Disorders and Speech Disorders

Habit

It is 'frequent, repetitive behaviors that cannot be explained by physiological causes and appear to serve no identifiable physiological function'. The term 'habit disorders' includes thumb sucking, nail biting, hair pulling and tics (such as shoulder, head and elbow jerks, eye blinking, twitching or squinting of the eyes and jerking of the mouth and cheek). Few habit disorders are:

Tics

Tics is 'sudden, brief, *involuntary*, rapid, nonrhythmic, repetitive movements or utterances that are purposeless and stereotypic'. Examples: eye blinking, facial grimacing, coughing, shoulder shrugging, throat clearing, growling, sniffing. Single or multiple motor and/or vocal tics occur many times a day, nearly every day for at least 4 weeks but not longer than 12 consecutive months. It causes marked distress or impairment.

It is common in school children who want to discharge tension through it. It is outlet of suppressed anger and worry for the control of aggression. A special type of chronic tics is found as 'Gilles de la Tourette's syndrome', characterized by multiple motor tics and vocal tics.

Tourette's Syndrome

In Tourette's disorder, both multiple motor and one or more vocal tics have been present but do not have to be at same time. It seems to be a genetic disorder with onset at around 11 years of age. It occurs many times a day (usually in bouts), nearly every day or intermittently for over 1 year, no more than 3 consecutive months tic free. Causes marked distress or impairment.

Bruxism

Bruxism is the forcible gnashing, grinding, clicking, or clenching of teeth. Nocturnal bruxism occurs during sleep, and the child is usually unaware of the problem. Episodes are typically brief, lasting 8 to 9 seconds, with audible grinding noises. Diurnal (daytime) bruxism is primarily associated with clenching of the teeth and generally does not produce audible noises. Diurnal bruxism is related to other oral habits, such as nail biting or lip chewing.

Spell

A breath-holding spell is a paroxysmal event in which a child stops breathing at end-expiration after crying, typically because of pain or anger. The crying may be brief or prolonged. It may occur in children between 6 months to 5 years of age. A Breath-holding spells may be divided into the following 3 categories:

- *Simple breath-holding spells:* These result when the child becomes apneic (cyanotic or pale) but then takes a deep breath; spells with loss of consciousness and muscle tone are classified by the child's color during the event.
- *Cyanotic breath-holding spells:* In these spells, which typically have an emotional precipitant (e.g. anger or frustration during disciplinary conflict) and typically last less than 1 minute, the child progresses from cyanotic to apneic and may then become limp and lose consciousness; if a seizure occurs, the results from electroencephalography (EEG) performed during rest or sleep are normal.
- *Pallid breath-holding spells:* In these spells, which are generally observed in response to pain, the child quickly becomes apneic and pale; an enhanced vagal response has been postulated to be a precursor to bradycardia or asystole; seizures rarely result. Heart rate becomes slow. The attack lasts for 1 to 2 minutes.

Trichotillomania

Trichotillomania is a recurrent pulling out of one's hair, resulting in noticeable hair loss. This habit gives pleasure, gratification, or relief when pulling out hair. Age of onset is about 13 years, more frequent in females and it often precipitated by stressful life event (incompetence, loss, academic pressures). It occurs in solitude but children do in front of family. Pulling is increased during periods of stress, relaxation, or distraction. Sometimes they may be unaware of pulling their hair and thus do not experience tension or relief.

This habit may result in total absence of hair, bald spots, or thinning of hair and most serious consequence occurs when patients eat the hair and form hairballs in the stomach. It results in all kinds of complications like anemia, loss of appetite, nausea, vomiting. Anxiety, mood disorders or OCD are the comorbid conditions, trichotillomania may present with these conditions.

Some childhood habits remain unnoticed and can persist if left untreated, even when they interfere with optimal functioning. Childhood habits can result in negative social interactions and avoidance by peers and family members. Some repetitive behaviors can cause damage. For example, bruxism (teeth grinding) can result in tooth damage. Occasional hair pulling can result in hair loss or evolve into a more severe disorder, trichotillomania.

Childhood habits that do not interfere with everyday functioning often require no treatment. However, those that cause substantial distress, social isolation, or physical injury may warrant a therapeutic intervention. Following measures may be undertaken to handle the problem:

- Physical measures (use of splints, helmets, sensory extinction: e.g., gloves, increasing effort: e.g., wrist weights).
- Behavioral therapy (mainstay of treatment).
- Pharmacotherapy.

Effective behavioral therapies for habits include the following:

- Habit reversal with differential reinforcement
- Awareness training – to practice the habit in front of mirror
- Relaxation training
- Self-monitoring
- Reinforcement
- Nocturnal biofeedback (for bruxism)
- Competing responses
- Use of bitter-tasting substances (for nail biting)
- Negative practice
- Use of aversive-tasting substances (for thumb sucking).

Most common habits in children that require treatment can be substantially improved by means of behavioral interventions, without the use of medication. Pharmacologic agents that may be considered as necessary include the following:

- Naltrexone
- Clomipramine
- Selective serotonin reuptake inhibitors (SSRIs), such as fluoxetine, sertraline, and fluvoxamine.

Isolated successes have also been reported with traditional and newer neuroleptics; however, because of their adverse effects, their use in this setting is discouraged.

When does a behavior become a problem?

When it interferes in the learning process

When it causes injury or harm to self or others

When it prevents the child from performing usual life routines and activities that are expected at his level

When the behavior results in adversely effecting the mental peace, health and the general functioning of the family members and others in the environment

Speech Problems

Speech is one of the main ways in which man communicates with those around him. It develops naturally, along with other signs of normal growth and development. To develop language, a child must be able to hear, see, understand, and remember. Children must also have the physical ability to form speech. Speech disorders are not uncommon in childhood. Intellectual disability and hearing loss make children more likely to develop speech disorders.

Disfluencies are disorders in which a person repeats a sound, word, or phrase. Stuttering may be the most serious disfluency. Usually this disorders begin between the age 3 to 5 years, probably due to inability to adjust with environment and emotional stress. The condition is characterized as repetition of sounds, words, or parts of words or phrases after age 4 years (I want...I want my doll. I...I see you); putting in (interjecting) extra sounds or words (We went to the...uh...store.); making words longer (I am Boooobbby Jones.), pausing during a sentence or words, often with the lips together, tension in the voice or sounds; head jerking, eye blinking while talking; embarrassment with speech.

Articulation disorders may have no clear cause. They may also occur in other family members. Other causes include:

- Problems or changes in the structure or shape of the muscles and bones used to make speech sounds. These changes may include cleft palate and dental malocclusions.
- Damage to parts of the brain or the nerves (such as from cerebral palsy) that control how the muscles work together to create speech.

Dyslalia is impairment of ability to speak associated with abnormality of external speech organs. It is a common speech disorder of difficulty in articulation. Dyslalia may be caused due to abnormalities of teeth, jaw and palate or due to emotional deprivation.

An unclear and hurried speech in which words tumble over each other is called cluttering. Cluttering (tachyphemia or tachyphrasia) is a speech and communication disorder characterized by a rapid rate making speech difficult to understand, erratic rhythm, poor syntax or grammar, and words or groups of words unrelated to the sentence. There may be awkward movements of hand, feet and body. Cluttering and stuttering, both communication disorders break the normal flow of speech. However, while stuttering is most often analyzed as a speech disorder, cluttering is a language disorder. In other words, a stutterer has a coherent pattern of thoughts, but cannot express those thoughts; in contrast, a clutterer has no problem putting thoughts into words, but those thoughts become disorganized during speaking. Cluttering affects not only speech, but also thought patterns, writing, typing, and conversation.

Milder forms of speech disorders may disappear on their own. Speech therapy may help with more severe symptoms or speech problems that do not improve. In therapy, the child will learn how to create certain sounds.

At-risk infants should be referred to an audiologist for an audiology exam. Audiological and speech therapy can then be started, if necessary. As young children begin to speak, some disfluency is common. Children lack a large vocabulary and have difficulty expressing themselves. This results in broken speech. If you place excessive attention on the disfluency, a stuttering pattern may develop. The best way to prevent stuttering, therefore, is to avoid paying too much attention to the disfluency.

Psychological therapy (psychotherapy, counseling, or cognitive behavioral therapy) is also recommended in case of speech problems if it is related to possible emotional or behavioral problems.

Conduct Disorders (CD)

CD is a childhood behavior disorder characterized by aggressive and destructive activities that cause disruptions in the child's natural environments such as home, school, playground, the neighborhood. CD is a psychological disorder diagnosed in childhood or adolescence that presents itself through a repetitive and persistent pattern of behavior in which the basic rights of others or major age-appropriate norms are violated. These behaviors are often referred to as 'antisocial behaviors.' It is often seen as the precursor to antisocial personality disorder, which is not diagnosed until the individual is 18-year-old. According to DSM-5 criteria for conduct disorder, there are 4 categories that could be present in the child's behavior: aggression to people and animals, destruction of property, deceitfulness or theft, and serious violation of rules. For a diagnosis, these behaviors must occur for at least a 6-month period.

The development of conduct disorder is not immutable or predetermined. In most cases conduct disorder develops due to an interaction and gradual accumulation of risk factors, i.e. cognitive variables, neurological factors, intraindividual factors, familial and peer influences, and wider contextual factors. In addition to the risk factors, several other variables place youth at increased risk for developing the disorder, including child physical abuse and prenatal alcohol abuse and maternal smoking during pregnancy. Protective factors have also been identified, and most notably include high IQ, being female, positive social orientations, good coping skills, and supportive family and community relationships.

The most effective treatment for an individual with conduct disorder is one that seeks to integrate individual, school, and family settings. Additionally, treatment should also seek to address familial conflict such as marital discord or maternal depression. In this manner, a treatment would serve to address many of the possible triggers of conduct problems. Several treatments currently exist, the most effective of which is multisystemic treatment (MST).

MST is an intensive, integrative treatment that emphasizes how an individual's conduct problems fit within a broader context. The individual is viewed functioning within a series of interconnected systems (home, school, neighborhood, etc.), that reinforces their antisocial behavior. MST seeks to break this connection through empowering the individual and family members.

The success rate of MST among severely antisocial youths has been found to be superior to other office-based therapy approaches. Adolescents that have undergone this treatment show decreased levels of aggression and improved familial relations. MST has also been found to decrease long-term rates of crime.

Cognitive Impairment

Cognitive impairment, also referred to as intellectual disability, describes the condition of a child whose intellectual functioning level and adaptive skills are significantly below the average for a child of his chronological age. Children between the ages of 6- and 12-year-old, typically experience rapid cognitive development. Cognitively, the child is learning how to solve problems and make reasonable decisions. For example, a third grader successfully memorizes his or her multiplication table and uses this new knowledge to complete math homework. With these new skills, the child develops a sense of pride in his or her accomplishments and abilities.

However, a child with a cognitive delay might not show this growing competence. Rather, these children demonstrate deficits in their intellectual and adaptive abilities. Some of the common characteristics of students with cognitive delays include lack of reasoning skills, difficulty memorizing and a rate of learning that is below grade level. In addition, a child is said to have a cognitive delay and/or a learning disability when they are performing at least two grade levels below their peers. Learning disabilities are related to difficulties in processing information:

- The reception of information
- The integration or organization of that information

- The ability to retrieve information from its storage in the brain
- The communication of retrieved information to others.

Learning Disability

- *Dyslexia, learning disability in reading: Dyslexia* is a specific reading disability due to a defect in the brain's processing of graphic symbols. It is a learning disability that alters the way the brain processes written material. It is typically characterized by difficulties in word recognition, spelling and decoding.
- *Dysgraphia, learning disability in writing:* Dysgraphia is a learning disability that affects writing abilities. It can manifest itself as difficulties with spelling, poor handwriting and trouble putting thoughts on paper (called processing disorder).
- *Dyscalculia, learning disability in reading:* Dyscalculia is a learning disability causes severe difficulty in making arithmetical calculations, as a result of brain disorder.

  It is characterized by impairments in learning basic arithmetic facts, an inability to understand the meaning of numbers, an inability to apply mathematical principles to solve problems. These difficulties must be quantifiably below what is expected for an individual chronological age (Figs 24.2A to C).
- *Learning disability in language, communication:* Children with language-based learning disabilities may have difficulty with understanding or producing spoken language, or both.

A child with a learning disability might also show the type of cognitive delay. However, the difference between a delay and a disability is that a child with a cognitive delay will require short-term assistance to catch up with his or her classmates. A child with a disability will typically need long-term assistance and will have the disability throughout his or her life. For example, a third grader who does not know his or her multiplication table is given a tutor and in a short period of time is able to learn them and thus catch up with peers. However, a child with a cognitive delay in math is different from a child who has the math learning disability known as dyscalculia. With assistance, a student with dyscalculia might be able to catch up with peers, but the condition will persist throughout his or her life.

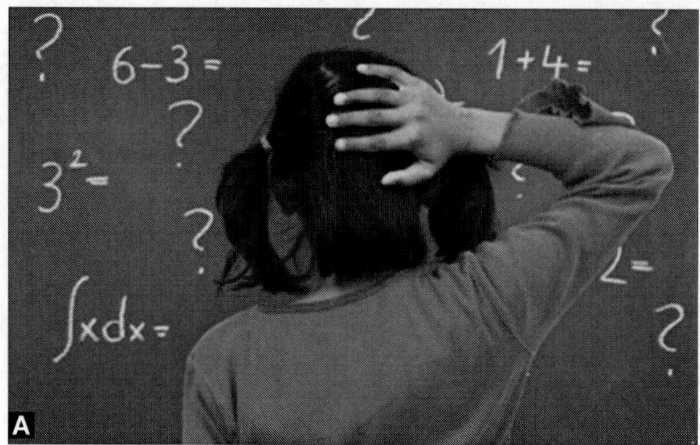

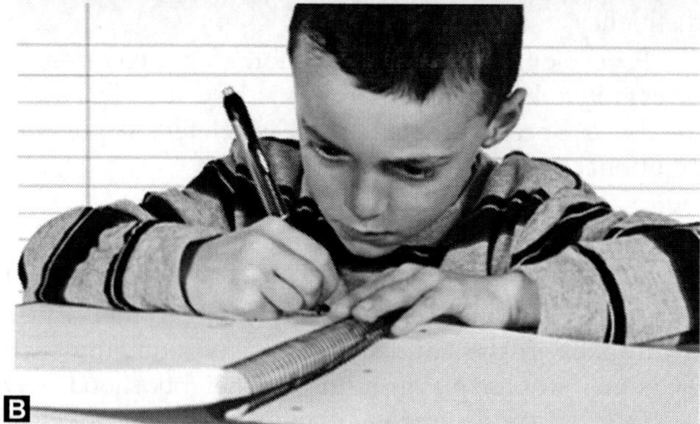

Figs 24.2A to C: **A.** The child with dyscalculia; **B.** The child with dysgraphia; **C.** Perception of word by dyslexic child

Cognitive Impairment

Cognitive impairment is a general term that denotes limitations in intellectual and functional abilities. Levels of cognitive impairment severity are defined by specific IQ ranges.

- Mild cognitive impairment—IQ of 50 to 70
- Moderate cognitive impairment—IQ of 35 to 55

- Severe cognitive impairment—IQ 20 to 40
- Profound cognitive impairment—Below 20.

Cognitive impairment can be caused by a number of factors (mentioned above).

Mental Retardation (MR) or Intellectual Disability (ID)

MR can be defined as 'a disability characterized by significant limitations both in intellectual functioning and in adaptive behavior as expressed in conceptual, social, and practical adaptive skills' (AAMR, 2002). It is defined by an IQ score below 70. Once focused almost entirely on cognition, the definition now includes both a component relating to mental functioning and one relating to individuals' functional skills in their environments.

Children with intellectual disability learn more slowly than a typical child. Children may take longer to learn language, develop social skills, and take care of their personal needs, such as dressing or eating. Learning will take them longer, require more repetition, and skills may need to be adapted to their learning levels. Nevertheless, virtually every child is able to learn, develop and become a participating member of the community.

Among children, the cause is unknown for one-third to one-half of cases. Down syndrome, velocariofacial syndrome, and fetal alcohol syndrome are the three most common inborn causes.

According to the fifth edition of the *Diagnostic and Statistical Manual of Mental Disorders* (DSM-IV), 3 criteria must be met for a diagnosis of intellectual disability:

- Deficits in general mental abilities
- Significant limitations in one or more areas of adaptive behavior across multiple environments (as measured by an adaptive behavior rating scale, i.e. communication, self-help skills, interpersonal skills).
- Evidence that the limitations became apparent in childhood or adolescence.

In general, people with intellectual disability have an IQ below 70, but clinical discretion may be necessary for individuals who have a somewhat higher IQ but severe impairment in adaptive functioning.

Autism Spectrum Disorders

Autism is known as a complex lifelong developmental disability characterized by the developmental history of these children is atypical in that the smooth, interrelated pattern of emotional, social, and intellectual development of normal children is not found (Fig. 24.3). The condition is the result of a neurological disorder that has an effect on normal brain function, affecting development of the person's communication and social interaction skills. Associated features, such as difficulties in eating and sleeping, unusual fears, learning problems, repetitive behaviors, self-injury and peculiar responses to sensory input, may or may not be present. These are the children who are unresponsive when held, withdrawn from others, and seem to live in a private inaccessible world of their own.

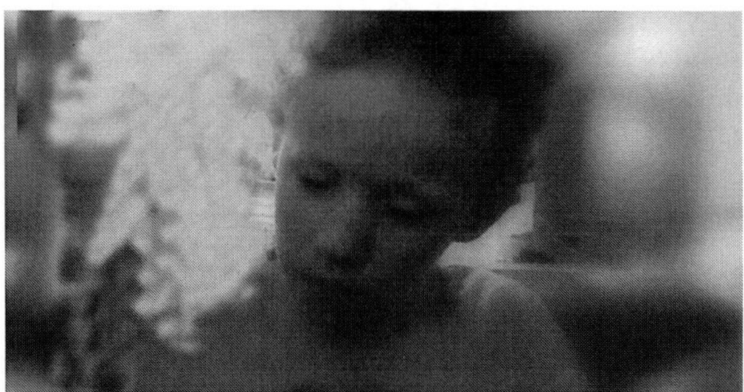

Fig. 24.3: Autistic child

An autistic parent's expression: This is Roni, my son sometimes he laughs, but we do not know what funny. Sometimes he cries and we do not know, what hurts. He has hopes, dreams, wishes and loves, but we do not know, what they are. Because he does not speak. This is autism.

If the child presents any of the following behaviors, consider this a red flag.

Social Concerns

Does not smile in response to another person, delayed imaginative play – lack of varied, spontaneous make-believe play, prefers to play alone, decreased interest in other children, poor interactive play, poor eye contact. Language is delayed, inconsistent response or does not respond to his name or instructions. Unusual language echoing other people, repetitive use of phrases, odd intonation. Poor comprehension of language, decreased ability to compensate for delayed speech by gesture or pointing. Severe repeated tantrums due to frustration, lack of ability to communicate, interruption of routine, or interruption of repetitive behavior. Narrow range of interests, he engages in repetitive activity. He has high pain tolerance and lack of safety awareness. The child shows insistence on maintaining sameness in routine, activities, clothing, etc. shows repetitive hand and/or body movements. They do not like human contacts and try to hide in places such as closet, like mouthing various objects.

BEHAVIOR DISORDER

Attention Deficit Hyperactivity Disorder (ADHD)

ADHD is a long-term chronic condition that affects millions of children and can continue into adulthood. Nevertheless, ADHD is one of the most commonly diagnosed childhood disorders and is diagnosed much more often in boys than in girls.

Symptoms of ADHD include problems with paying attention characterized by poor ability to attend to tasks (makes careless mistakes, avoids sustained mental effort, easily distracted and struggles to follow instructions), overactivity (hyperactivity like fidgets, has difficulty playing quietly, constantly touching or playing with everything in sight, talks nonstop, even when asked to be quiet) and *symptoms of impulsiveness include a* high level of impatience, blurting out inappropriate comments or answers before the question is asked, shows their emotions without restraint and acts without regard for consequences, has difficulty waiting for things they want and waiting their turn, often interrupts conversations or others' activities or some combination of the three (Figs 24.4A and B).

While it is normal for children to exhibit these behaviors on occasion, when it is out of the normal range for children of the same age and development level, a child should be evaluated. For the diagnosis to be made, the condition must be evident before age 7 years, present for >6 months, seen both at home and school and impeding the child's functioning. The condition is diagnosed in 3 to 7% of school-age children. Children with ADHD can suffer from low self-esteem, poor school performance and difficulty in relationships.

The Diagnostic and Statistical Manual (DSM-IV) lists 3 subtypes of ADHD:

1. **Predominantly hyperactive-impulsive**
   Child exhibits 6 or more symptoms of hyperactivity and impulsiveness.
   Child exhibits less than 6 symptoms of inattentiveness.
2. **Predominantly inattentive**
   Child exhibits 6 or more symptoms of inattentiveness.
   Child exhibits less than 6 symptoms of hyperactivity or impulsiveness.

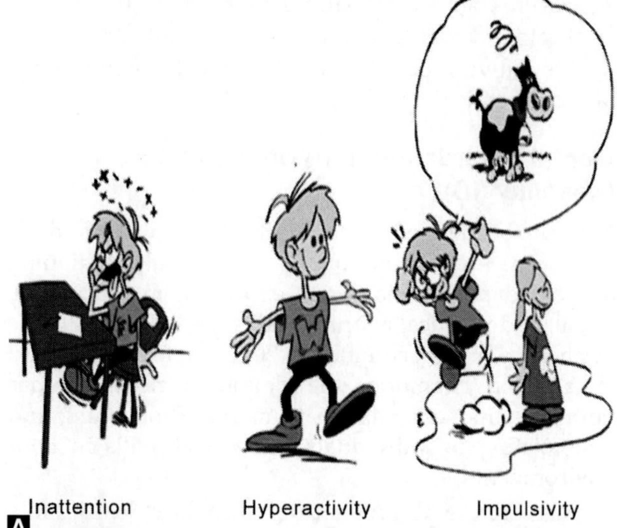

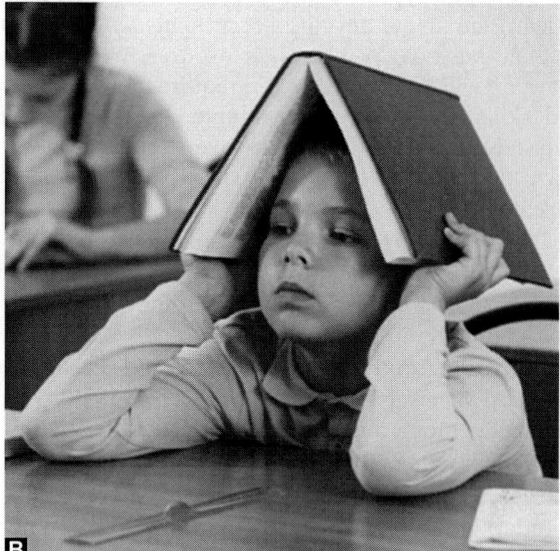

Figs 24.4A and B: Common behaviors are seen in ADHD child

3. **Combined (hyperactive-impulsive and inattentive)**
   Child exhibits 6 or more symptoms of hyperactivity and impulsiveness.
   Child exhibits 6 or more symptoms of inattentiveness.

Etiology

There is no agreement in the scientific community regarding the cause ADHD, but studies suggest it may be a combination of factors including genetics, environment, brain trauma, nutrition, and social environment that contribute to ADHD. Recent areas of study include genetics, cigaret and alcohol use during pregnancy, brain injury, and food additives such as artificial colors or preservatives. In addition, neuroimaging studies suggest that the brains of children with ADHD operate differently from their peers, specifically with their handling of neurotransmitters, such as dopamine, serotonin and adrenalin. But whatever the cause, it is set in motion early in life while the brain is still developing - between the ages of 3 and 6 years.

Diagnosis

There is currently no authoritative test to diagnose a child with ADHD.

Treatments

ADHD is a chronic condition. Treatment includes medication, psychotherapy, and behavioral training, and children can learn to manage their symptoms and lead productive lives. Methylphenidate is a stimulant medication that provides reduction of symptoms, at least in the short term. Behavioral modification and neurofeedback are the nonpharmacological treatments with the largest evidence base. Various dietary interventions have been mooted, of which the addition of essential fatty acids has the widest support.

Children with ADHD require extra guidance and understanding from their parents and educators. However, by the time a child is diagnosed, feelings of blame, frustration, even anger may have built up within a family or classroom environment. Parents and children may need to participate in family counseling or anger management therapy in order to develop new skills, attitudes, and ways of relating to one another.

Anxiety Disorders

Anxiety is a normal reaction to stress and can actually be beneficial in some situations. Anxiety is a normal part of childhood, and every child goes through phases. A phase is temporary and usually harmless. But children who suffer from an anxiety disorder experience fear, nervousness, and shyness, and they start to avoid places and activities. They will worry excessively about a variety of things such as grades, family issues, relationships with peers, and performance in sports. They tend to be very hard on themselves and strive for perfection. They may also seek constant approval or reassurance from others.

Anxiety disorders affect 1 in 8 children. Research shows that untreated children with anxiety disorders are at higher risk to perform poorly in school, miss out on important social experiences, and engage in substance abuse.

Etiology and Types

There are a wide variety of anxiety disorders, including posttraumatic stress disorder, obsessive-compulsive disorder, and specific phobias to name a few.

Posttraumatic Stress Disorder (PTSD)

Children and teens could have PTSD, if they have lived through an event that could have caused them or someone else to be killed or badly hurt. So someone who is the victim of (or threatened by) violence, injury, or harm can develop a mental health problem called *posttraumatic stress disorder (PTSD)*. PTSD is often re-experienced by the victims in the form of 'flashbacks,' memories, nightmares, or scary thoughts, specially when they are exposed to events or objects that remind them of the trauma.

Etiology and Incidence

The events may cause PTSD include sexual or physical abuse or other violent crimes; disasters such as floods, school shootings, car crashes. Other events that can cause PTSD are war, a friend's suicide, or seeing violence in the area child live. Not every child who experiences or hears about a traumatic event will develop PTSD. It is normal to be fearful, sad, or apprehensive after such events, and many children will recover from these feelings in a short time.

Children and teens that go through the most severe traumas, who directly witnessed a traumatic event, who had mental health problems before the event, and who lack a strong support network, tend to have the highest levels of PTSD symptoms. Violence at home also increases a child's risk of developing PTSD after a traumatic event. The PTSD symptoms may be less severe if the child has more family support and if the parents are less upset by the trauma. Lastly, children and teens who are farther away from the event report less distress.

Studies show that people with PTSD often have atypical levels of key hormones involved in the stress response. For instance, research has shown that they have lower-than-normal cortisol levels and higher-than-normal epinephrine and norepinephrine levels — all of which play a big role in the body's 'fight-or-flight' reaction to sudden stress. (It is known as 'fight or flight' because that is exactly what the body is preparing itself to do—to either fight off the danger or run from it).

Presenting Signs and Symptoms

People with PTSD have symptoms of stress, anxiety, and depression. Children with PTSD, may have intense fear and anxiety, become emotionally numb or easily irritable, or avoid places, people, or activities after experiencing or witnessing a traumatic or life-threatening event. The child may show signs such as sleep problems, refusal of food, isolated, anger. There may be changes in school performance and problems with friends. For many children, PTSD symptoms go away on their own after a few months. Yet some children show symptoms for years if they do not get treatment.

These children (5 to 12 years) may not have flash-backs or problems remembering parts of the trauma, the way adults with PTSD often do. They might also think there were signs that the trauma was going to happen, so they think that if they pay attention, they can avoid future traumas. Children of this age might also show signs of PTSD in their play. These games do not make their worry and distress go away. For example, a child might carry a gun to school after seeing a school shooting. PTSD symptoms in teens (12 to 18 years) begin to look like those of adults. One difference is that teens are more likely than younger children or adults to show impulsive and aggressive behaviors.

Management of PTSD

Cognitive-Behavioral Therapy (CBT)

CBT is the most effective approach for treating children. This type of therapy teaches ways to replace negative, unhelpful thoughts and feelings with more positive thinking. One type of CBT is called Trauma-Focused CBT (TF-CBT). In TF-CBT, the child may talk about his or her memory of the trauma. TF-CBT also includes techniques to help lower worry and stress at a child's own pace to help desensitize the child to the traumatic parts of what happened so he or she does not feel so afraid of them. The child may learn how to assert himself or herself. The therapy may involve learning to change thoughts or beliefs about the trauma that are not correct or true. For example, after a trauma, a child may start thinking, 'the world is totally unsafe.'

In some cases, medicine might be used to treat serious symptoms of depression and anxiety. This can help those with PTSD cope with school and other daily activities while being treated. Medicine often is used only until someone feels better, then therapy can help get the person back on track.

Finally, group therapy or support groups are often helpful because they let kids and teens know that they are not alone. Groups also provide a safe atmosphere in which to share feelings. CBT often uses training for parents and caregivers as well. It is important for caregivers to understand the effects of PTSD. Parents need to learn coping skills that will help them help their children.

Psychological first aid or crisis management—Psychological First Aid (PFA) involves in providing comfort and support, and letting children know their reactions are normal. PFA teaches calming and problem solving skills. It has been used with school-aged children and teens that have been through violence where they live. PFA can be used in schools and traditional settings. PFA also helps caregivers deal with changes in the child's feelings and behavior. Children with more severe symptoms may be referred for added treatment.

Eye movement desensitization and reprocessing (EMDR)—EMDR combines cognitive therapy with directed eye movements. EMDR is effective in treating both children and adults with PTSD, yet studies indicate that the eye movements are not needed to make it work.

Play therapy—Play therapy can be used to treat young children with PTSD who are not able to deal with the trauma more directly. The therapist uses games, drawings, and other methods to help children process their traumatic memories.

Other Treatments

The child is to be told that the traumatic event is not her fault. Encourage the child to talk about her feelings of guilt, but do not let her blame herself for what happened. Special treatments may be needed for children who show out-of-place sexual behaviors, extreme behavior problems, or that a child has thoughts of self-harm. Thoughts of suicide are serious at any age and should be treated right away.

Obsessive Compulsive Disorder

Obsessive compulsive disorder (OCD) is a type of anxiety disorder where children and adults suffer from unwanted and intrusive thoughts that they cannot seem to get out of their heads (obsessions), and often compell them to repeatedly perform ritualistic behaviors and routines (compulsions) to try and ease their anxiety.

Most people who have OCD are aware that their obsessions and compulsions are irrational, yet they feel powerless to stop them. Children with OCD also might worry about things not being 'in order' or 'just right.' Some spend hours at a time performing complicated rituals involving hand-washing, counting, or checking to ward off persistent, unwelcome thoughts, feelings, or images.

Physiologically, when the flow of serotonin (neurotransmitter) is blocked, the brain's 'alarm system' overreacts and misinterprets information. These 'false alarms' mistakenly trigger danger messages and the person experiences unrealistic fear and doubt. Predisposition for someone to develop a serotonin imbalance that causes OCD can be inherited. OCD is a disorder which child cannot stop by trying harder. Some life events (such as starting school or the death of a loved one) might worsen or trigger the onset of OCD in children who are prone to develop it.

These can interfere with a person's normal routine, schoolwork, job, family, or social activities. Several hours every day may be spent focusing on obsessive thoughts and performing seemingly senseless rituals. Trying to concentrate on daily activities may be difficult.

Once believed to be relatively rare in children and adolescents, OCD now is thought to affect as many as 2 to 3% of children. Among adolescents with OCD, the literature indicates that very few receive an appropriate and correct diagnosis, and even fewer receive proper treatment. Successful treatment of obsessive compulsive disorder (OCD) involves cognitive, behavioral, and pharmacologic treatments. The judicious use of SSRIs and structured psychotherapy designed to provide the patient with the skills to master the obsessive thoughts and accompanying compulsive behaviors. Both psychotherapy and pharmacotherapy are effective interventions for children with OCD.

Phobias

A childhood phobia is an exaggerated, intense irrational fear 'that is out of proportion to any real fear' found in children. It is often characterized by a preoccupation with a particular object, class of objects, or situation that one fears. A phobic reaction is two-fold—the first part being the 'intense irrational fear' and the second part being 'avoidance'. Common childhood phobias include animals, storms, heights, water, blood, the dark, and medical procedures.

A phobia (severe anxiety) releases adrenaline and other chemicals into blood, and these speed up heartbeat, sharpen senses and heighten physical powers. These changes prepare individual for what is called 'flight or fight'. A phobia is a disorder in which the body reacts in exactly the same way, but in situations where there is absolutely no need for 'flight or fight'. The part of the mind that controls anxiety has, to all intents and purposes, lost all sense of proportion, and screams `danger!' when the situation is not threatening in any rational way. No matter how harmless the feared creature may be, for a severely phobic person the fear reaction is every bit as real as if the cause was a major threat. People with phobias usually realize all too well that their reaction is irrational, but this makes no difference to its effect.

Children will avoid situations or things that they fear, or endure them with anxious feelings, which can manifest as crying, tantrums, clinging, avoidance, headaches, and stomach aches. Unlike adults, they do not usually recognize that their fear is irrational.

While some phobias develop in childhood, most seem to arise unexpectedly, usually during adolescence or early adulthood. Their onset is usually sudden, and they may occur in situations that previously did not cause any discomfort or anxiety. Having phobias can disrupt daily routines, limit work efficiency, reduce self-esteem, and place a strain on relationships because people will do whatever they can to avoid the uncomfortable and often-terrifying feelings of phobic anxiety.

Management

Specific phobia is highly treatable through behavior therapy. A typical method involves a gradual exposure of the child to the source of her anxiety in small, nonthreatening doses. A child afraid of cat might start treatment by looking at a picture of a cat, then work up to playing with a stuffed cat, being in the same room with a small cat, and so on. This gradual process is called *desensitization,* which should be done under the supervision of a professional.

Therapy that teaches strategies for coping with fear and anxious thought patterns is another common option for older children. Sometimes psychotherapy can also help children become more self-assured and less fearful. Breathing and relaxation exercises can assist youngsters in stressful circumstances too.

Occasionally, doctor may recommend medications as a component of the treatment program, although never as the sole therapeutic tool. These drugs may include antidepressants, which are designed to ease the anxiety and panic that often underlie these problems.

Anxiety and Depression in Children

All humans experience anxiety, it serves as a means of protection and can often enhance our performance in stressful situations. It is not uncommon for children to be diagnosed with both depression and an anxiety disorder, or depression and general anxiety. Children who are able to experience the slight rush of anxiety that often occurs prior to a math test or a big track race often can enhance their performance. However, experiencing too much anxiety or general nervousness, at inappropriate times, can be extremely distressing and interfering.

Although children have fears of specific objects, the feeling of anxiety is more general and children may feel constantly 'keyed up' or extremely alert. Given the wide range of tasks children must accomplish throughout their childhood, it is important to be sure that their level of anxiety does not begin to interfere with their ability to function. If it does, it is important that they begin to learn some skills for coping more efficiently with their anxious feelings.

Physiological effects of anxiety are fear, breathlessness, choking sensation, palpitations of the heart, restlessness, increased muscular tensions.

Depressive disorders consist of a variety of symptoms in the areas of mood, thinking, behaviors and physical reactions. Mood-related symptoms include sadness, irritability, depression and anger. Many depressed children and adolescents are also anxious and nervous. When children and adolescents are depressed their thinking may be characterized by negative thoughts about themselves (self-criticism), negative thoughts about the future and negative interpretations or thinking about ongoing events in their lives. Children with depression may display these symptoms:

- Depressed or irritable mood
- Difficulty sleeping or concentrating
- Refusing to go to school
- Change in eating habits
- Feeling angry or irritable
- Mood swings
- Feeling worthless or restless
- Frequent sadness or crying
- Withdrawing from friends and activities
- Loss of energy
- Low self-esteem
- Thoughts of death or suicide.

When symptoms last for a short period of time, it may be a passing case of 'the blues.' But if they last for more than 2 weeks and interfere with regular daily activities and family and school life, the child may have a depressive disorder. It is probably more useful to conceptualize depression along a continuum. At the mild end would be occasional feelings of sadness or misery and at the severe end would be suicidal despair to complete and persistent psychomotor retardation. What is most important is how the problem is managed. The more the child is suffering the more important it is to offer appropriate treatment, regardless of whether what is presented is a symptom, a syndrome, or a disorder. The nature and severity of depression in the younger population is determined to some extent by developmental considerations.

There are 2 types of depression—major depression and dysthymia. Major depression lasts at least 2 weeks and may occur more than once throughout the child's life. A child may experience major depression after a traumatic event such as the death of a relative or friend. Dysthymia is a less severe but chronic form of depression that lasts for at least 2 years.

Children whose parents have depression are at a greater risk of being depressed. While depression affects all ages and both genders, girls are more likely to develop depression during adolescence. Research shows that depression is also a risk factor for suicide.

Management

Depression and anxiety disorders can often be treated the same way and at the same time. Like anxiety disorders, depression can be treated with cognitive-behavioral therapy and antidepressants.

Cognitive therapy is a form of psychotherapy that has been demonstrated to be effective in the treatment of depression with children and adolescents. Cognitive therapy is an active, structured, directive form of therapy that focuses on the thoughts, beliefs and behaviors that accompany depressive disorders.

In cognitive therapy, the child learns to identify, evaluate and change the thoughts, beliefs and behaviors that accompany depression. Anxiety disorders have been shown to be highly responsive to cognitive behavioral therapy. Exposure and response prevention (ERP), is a treatment method available for a variety of anxiety disorders. The intervention is based on the idea that a child or adolescent is exposed to their fears and through repetitive exposure they learn to overcome their avoidance. In doing so the thoughts or cognitions associated with the fear are altered and the fear and avoidance lessens and ultimately is extinguished. In many cases parents are also instructed in how to help the child use CBT methods to combat their depression. CBT can lead to a significant reduction in depression symptoms , often in a brief period of time.

Childhood Schizophrenia

Longitudinal study shows that many mental disorders do not arise de novo in adult life but have roots further back in childhood (Rutter, 1984; Caspi et al, 1996). Schizophrenia is associated with significant impairments in childhood, but little work has yet been carried out on affective psychosis.

The onset of childhood schizophrenia is frequently insidious; after first exhibiting inappropriate affects or unusual behavior, a child may take months or years to meet all diagnostic criteria for schizophrenia. Children who eventually meet the criterion are often socially rejected and clingy have limited social skills. Most children who develop schizophrenia have disturbances of behavior and cognition before the onset of characteristic symptoms of psychosis. Delays in speech and language and delays in acquisition of motor milestones are noted in approximately one-half of these children. Children who develop schizophrenia have higher rates of impaired social skills and school achievement before presenting signs of schizophrenia. The signs and symptoms that may occur within the previous 12 months are:

- *Emotional:* Abnormal suspiciousness, or sensitivity (social withdrawals, relationship difficulties with peers, hostility), morbid anxiety, pathological shyness. Approximately one-third of the children develop symptoms of inattention, aggression, or rage.
- *Somatic:* Disturbance in eating, sleeping, pains of mental origin, encopresis, enuresis.

Disturbance of Relationship

Speech and language problem–Speech and language problem includes disorder of rhythm, articulation, comprehension, production; elective mutism.

Motor disturbance–Tics, other abnormal repetitive movements, clumsiness or poor coordination, restlessness or fidgetiness, gross over or under activity, habitual manipulation (rocking).

Antisocial behavior–Defiance or lying stealing, destructiveness, truancy, running away, sexual misbehavior, fighting or bullying; violent assault, cruelty to animals, etc.

Management

The child with schizophrenia who is severely impaired may need day treatment programs or hospitalization until the child is stabilized and not considered a danger to self or others.

Pharmacotherapy is essential in the treatment of individuals with childhood-onset psychosis. The first-line agents are neuroleptics. Newer atypical antipsychotic agents are generally chosen as the initial drugs of choice (DOC). Occasionally, the agitated child with new-onset schizophrenia may need a benzodiazepine to calm and alleviate the anxiety accompanying the experience of psychosis. Electroconvulsive therapy (ECT) has also been used adjunctively in rare cases.

The child with schizophrenia requires multimodal care. This should include social skills training, a supportive environment, and a structured individualized special education program. Supportive psychotherapy is used to encourage reality testing and to help the child monitor for warning symptoms of impending relapse. There are many treatment approaches that can help children with schizophrenia better adjust to their environment and increase their quality of life when used in conjunction with medications.

CHAPTER 25

Challenged Child and Implications for Nursing

Chapter Outline

- Impairment in Motor Development
- Chromosomal/Genetic Disorders

IMPAIRMENT IN MOTOR DEVELOPMENT

Knowing the motor skills children develop, and the approximate timetable on which they develop them, can help parents spot developmental delays. For example, toddlers acquire motor skills in a predictable sequence, first they walk, then run and climb, then jump with both feet. But while the sequence may be consistent, the rate at which individual children develop varies enormously. And when a toddler seems to be late on a particular milestone, such as walking, it can be difficult to tell whether the problem is just an individual quirk or a true motor development problem. Parents are in ideal position to identify first any problems their child may be having with his or her motor development or not.

Motor disorders can be categorized as qualitative and quantitative. A qualitative disorder, is something that is not normal in and of itself. For example, severe stiffness of one or both legs would signal a problem in any age range, i.e. baby, toddler, or grade-schooler. A quantitative disorder, on the other hand, is when the child's behavior is normal but the timing is off. For example, crawling is a normal developmental activity, but if the child still crawls at 18 months with no sign of walking soon, she could have a problem.

Causes

Abnormalities in Muscle Tone and Power

- *Hypertonia:* Cerebral palsy, delayed walking may be the first presentation in milder cases (hemiplegia, spastic diplegia).
- *Muscular dystrophy:* It is common to find a history of delayed walking in Duchenne muscular dystrophy (DMD) but less so in Becker's muscular dystrophy, as it has a later onset. DMD is the most common hereditary neuromuscular disease and it is progressive. Baby boys are often normal at birth and delayed walking may only be identified retrospectively, with symptoms really appearing between 4 and 6 years of age.
- *Hypotonia of any cause:* Down syndrome, Prader-Willi syndrome, Tay-Sachs disease, Williams syndrome and so on.

Environmental Factors

Environmental factors either affect brain development or directly causing delay in walking. They are antenatal infections or toxins, infections such as meningitis, encephalitis, cytomegalovirus, head injury, malnutrition, Rickets has been reported to delay walking, though this is reversible if the disease is not too advanced.

General Gross Motor Warning Signs

- Baby is unable to hold head in the middle to turn and look left and right.
- He or she has stiff arms and/or legs.
- He or she has a floppy or limp body posture compared to other children of the same age.
- He or she uses one side of body more than the other.
- He or she has a very clumsy manner compared with other children of the same age.
- Child does not walk yet.
- Child is walking on her toes.
- Child seems very clumsy.
- Child is constantly moving.
- Child has trouble grasping and manipulating objects.
- Child drools and has difficulty in eating.

Types

Motor Dyspraxia

Motor skills disorder, also called motor coordination disorder or motor dyspraxia, is a common disorder of childhood. Children with this disorder have associated problems including difficulty in processing visuo-spatial information needed to guide their motor actions they may not be able to recall or plan complex motor activities such as:

- Dancing
- Doing gymnastics
- Catching or throwing a ball with accuracy
- Producing fluent legible handwriting.
  - Often there is a history of early delay in the development of motor skills. This may present as a delay in the ability to sit up or learning to walk well.
  - Often, these children are described as clumsy or forgetful, (e.g. they may never turn the water faucet or lights off).
  - These children may have difficulty in using a cup, spoon or fork to eat.
  - They may have the tendency to drop items or run into walls/furniture and have frequent accidents due to motor planning difficulties.
  - They may have trouble with tasks requiring hand-eye coordination and dexterity (hammering a nail, connecting wires, etc.).
  - These children may also have difficulty in holding a pencil and learning to write.

Cerebral Palsy (CP)

Simply stated, 'cerebral' refers to the brain, and 'palsy' refers to muscle weakness and poor control (problems moving his or her muscles). CP is a broad diagnostic term used to describe a problem with movement and posture that makes certain activities difficult because of an abnormality in the extra-pyramidal or pyramidal motor system (motor cortex, basal ganglia, cerebellum).

These difficulties, damage to the motor system can be the result of an injury during gestation or in the first year of life, or it occurs when the brain does not develop properly during gestation. The injured or abnormal brain is unable to optimally control movement and posture, although the brain itself will not get worse.

CP causes a number of neuromuscular disabilities depending on the area of the brain has been injured (Figs 25.1A and B).

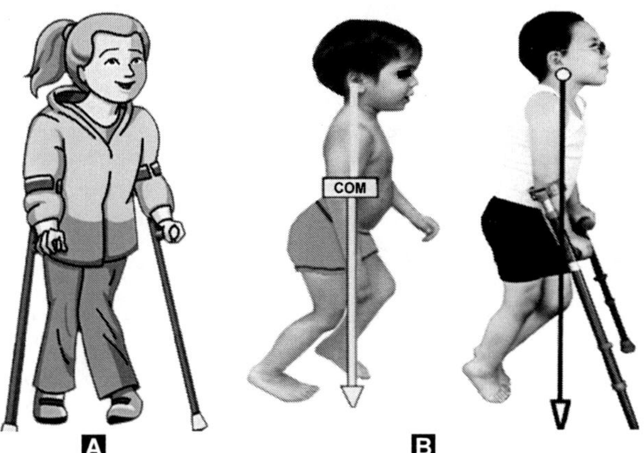

Figs 25.1A and B: Cerebral palsy (CP) causes a number of neuromuscular disabilities depending on the area of the brain has been injured

There is currently no cure for CP; however there are different treatment options for people who have cerebral palsy. These options include therapy, medications, surgery, education and support. By taking advantage of these treatments, people with CP can improve their function, minimize the development of complicating issues and optimize the quality of their lives.

Management

Most developmental screening is done by community health nurse but, if they suspect a problem, they need to bring it to the attention of the general practitioner or pediatrician. A detailed assessment of the child's motor skills, including looking at his gross and fine motor skills, his reflexes, muscle strength, range of movement, balance and postural reactions and his sensory development is done by specialist. The child may be intellectually intact, but his study may be affected because of the child's physical limitations.

On the basis of physical and mental assessment, discussion with parents with their concerns, diagnostic tests (EEG, CT, MRI, electrolyte-levels, metabolic workup), a plan is made to maximize the child in motor skills development. The treatment plan aims to:

- Assist the child to achieve physical milestones such as sitting, crawling and standing.
- Assist the child to gain improved independence in activities of daily living (Fig. 25.2).
- Improve posture, motor control, muscle strength balance and coordination.
- Improve confidence.

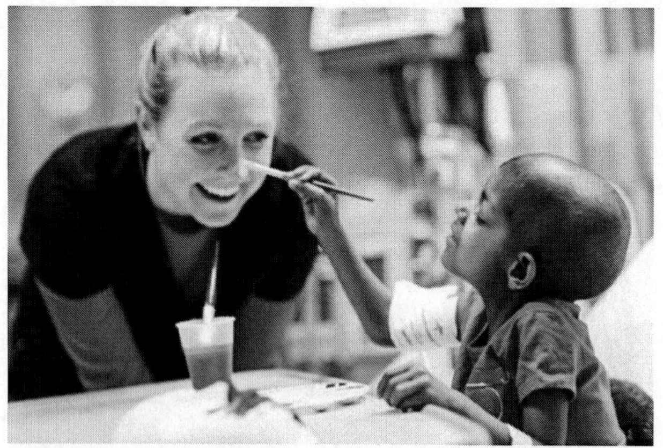

Fig. 25.2: A challenged child and nurse in care setting. The nurse encourages the child to gain improved independence in activities of daily living

- Liaise with parent/primary caregiver and teacher's to assist them to understand the child's needs and how they can assist the child with gaining motor skills and independence.

CHROMOSOMAL/GENETIC DISORDERS

Down Syndrome

Down syndrome is a genetic disorder, also known as trisomy 21, is caused by the presence of all or part of a third copy of chromosome 21. It is typically associated with abnormal cell division which results in extra genetic material from chromosome 21. This genetic disorder, which varies in severity, causes lifelong mild- to-moderate intellectual disability and developmental delays (Fig. 25.3A). The average IQ of a young adult with Down syndrome is 50, equivalent to the mental age of an 8-or 9-year-old child, but this varies widely. In some people it causes health problems like poor immune system, congenital heart disease, leukemia, thyroid disorders, and mental illness.

Etiology

Three genetic variations which cause Down syndrome are:

1. *Trisomy 21*: Most commonly Down syndrome is caused by trisomy 21. Three copies of chromosome 21 (instead of the usual 2 copies) remain in all cells. This is caused by abnormal cell division during the development of the sperm cell or the egg cell.
2. *Mosaic Down syndrome:* In this rare form of Down syndrome, children have some cells with an extra copy of chromosome 21. This mosaic of normal and abnormal cells is caused by abnormal cell division after fertilization.
3. *Translocation Down syndrome:* Down syndrome can also occur when part of chromosome 21 becomes attached (translocated) onto another chromosome, before or at conception. These children have the usual 2 copies of chromosome 21, but they also have additional material from chromosome 21 attached to the translocated chromosome.

Special Traits of Down Syndrome

Characteristic facial features, low muscle tone, short stature, upward slanting to the eyes which is unusual for the child's ethnic group. Small head, short neck, protruding tongue, broad and short hands with a single crease in the palm, relatively short fingers and small hands and feet, excessive flexibility, tiny white spots on the colored part (iris) of the eye called Brushfield spots.

Management

Intellectual disability can be distinguished in many ways from mental illness, such as schizophrenia or depression. Currently, there is no 'cure' for an established disability, though with appropriate support and teaching, most individuals can learn to do many things. Children with a cognitive impairment can be successful in school and lead fulfilling lives. They may just need individualized help in learning new skills. Extra time, repeated instruction, and appropriate modeling will help them as they master important life skills, such as appropriate hygiene, personal safety, and social manners.

In order to promote independence and developmental progress, parents and educators should be patient and give children the time they need to learn new skills by adopting different methodologies. Breaking down tasks into smaller steps can be a helpful learning tool for children with cognitive impairments. For example, getting dressed can be broken down for the child into very small simple steps: Shirt on, buttons, pants on, zipper, button, tuck in shirt, belt, socks, etc. Walk the child through each part of the task, encouraging him to do it independently and praising at success each step. This process, referred to as task analysis, can be used to teach proper hygiene techniques, household chores, or any other skills.

Core components of behavioral treatments include language and social skills acquisition. Parents can involve in child's learning and can integrate it at home. For instance, when the child is learning to tell time, periodically he/she can be asked for the time. When he is learning about money, he can be taken to the grocery

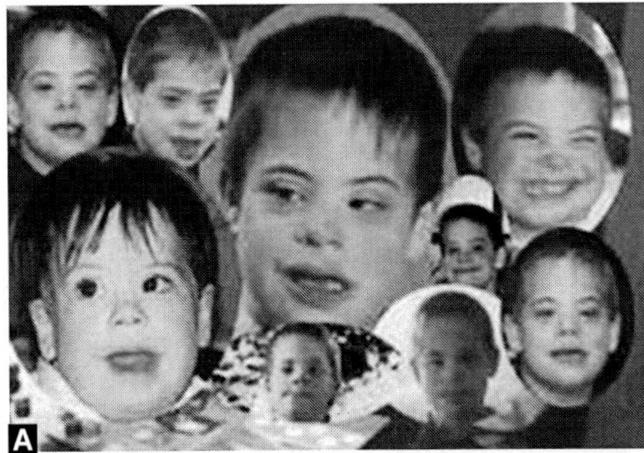

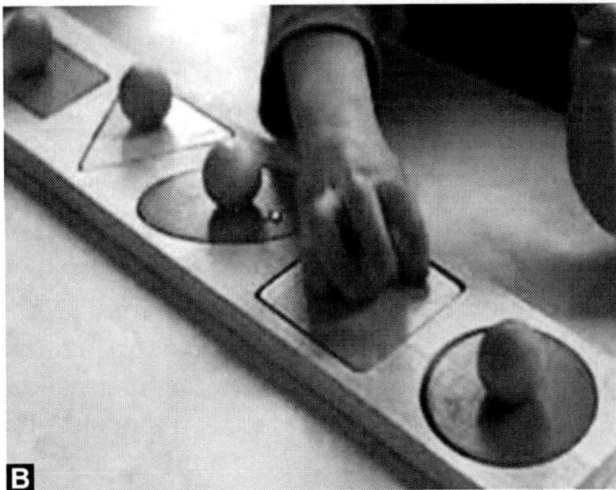

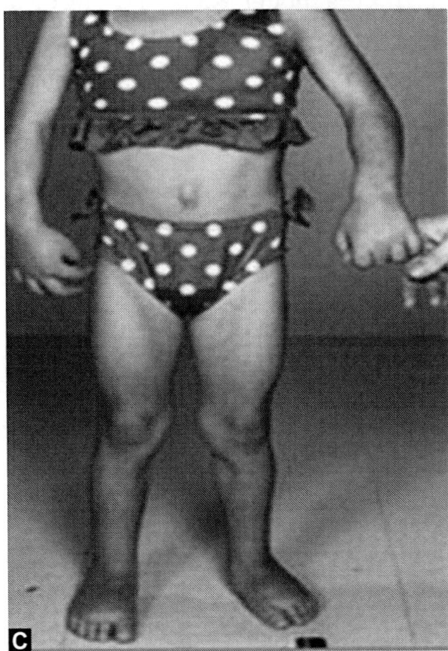

Figs 25.3A to C: **A.** Children with Down syndrome; **B.** Child with motor in-coordination (dyspraxia); **C.** Child with Turner syndrome

and can be involved in the process of buying. Activities in the community can serve as a valuable learning tool as well. Children with cognitive impairment can model the behavior of their peers, improve social skills, experience new and different settings and most importantly, have fun.

Children with delayed skills or other disabilities might be eligible for special services that provide individualized education programs in public schools, free of charge to families. In most cases, the services and goals outlined in an IEP can be provided in a standard school environment. This can be done in the regular classroom (e.g. a reading teacher helping a small group of children who need extra assistance while the other kids in the class work on reading with the regular teacher) or in a special resource room in the regular school. The resource room can serve a group of kids with similar needs who are brought together for help.

Developmental Coordination Disorder/Dyspraxia

About 6–8% of children appear to be developing in the usual way yet have difficulties with coordination and with learning new skills which affects their function and participation in their environment (home, school, playground). Developmental coordination disorder (DCD) is the internationally accepted name for this condition. DCD affects fine and gross motor abilities, balance and posture, basic motor patterns (walking, running, jumping) and in particular skilled action that require practice like drawing and handwriting, sport skills (Fig. 25.3 B).

Children with DCD can learn to perform most everyday tasks given the right opportunities and support. It just takes more practice and learning to pay attention in a special way to compensate for the way in which their brains learn new skills. Children with DCD are often referred for physiotherapy and/or an occupational therapy. Physiotherapists tend to focus on posture and gross motor skills as well as strength, flexibility, agility, endurance. Occupational therapists usually pay more attention to fine motor control, hand function, handwriting, perception and daily activities.

Turner Syndrome (TS)

TS is a genetic disorder that causes girls to be short and prevents them from maturing sexually as they grow into adulthood (Fig. 25.3C). The severity of these issues varies from girl-to-girl; in many cases, emotional challenges girls face when they have TS. Overall, TS occurs in about 1 out of 2,500 female births. About one-third of girls with TS are diagnosed as newborns, another third during childhood and the remaining third during their late teens.

Most girls are born with 2 X-chromosomes, but girls with TS are born with only one X-chromosome or they are missing part of 1 X-chromosome. The effects of TS which is caused by a missing or incomplete X-chromosome in child's genetic makeup, vary widely among affected girls. It all depends on how many of the body's cells are affected by the changes to the X-chromosome. Most girls with TS are born with poorly formed or missing *ovaries*, which can result in infertility. The occurrence of TS is not associated with the mother's age at the time of pregnancy or birth.

Besides short stature and lack of sexual development, a number of other health problems occur more often in girls with TS, including kidney and heart problems, high blood pressure, overweight, hearing difficulties, diabetes, and thyroid problems. Some girls with the condition may have learning difficulties, particularly in math. Many have a hard time with tasks that require skills such as map reading or visual organization. Some of the other physical features commonly seen in girls with TS are a 'webbed' neck, a low hairline at the back of the neck, drooping of the eyelids differently- shaped ears that are set lower on the sides of the head than usual, abnormal bone development (specially the bones of the hands and elbows), a larger than usual number of moles on the skin, edema in the hands and feet. Because TS can affect how a girl looks and develops, some girls may have problems with body image or self-esteem.

There is no cure for TS, but many of the more serious problems associated with it can be treated. This is a complicated condition that requires constant medical oversight, most girls with the disease go on to lead normal, happy lives. TS can be managed or corrected with treatment options ranging from *growth hormone therapy*, *estrogen therapy* and *progesterone therapy* to certain medications.

Treatment includes prevention and treatment of obesity, insulin resistance, and hyperlipidemia. Girls with TS need psychological interventions like:

- Coping with feelings regarding diagnosis and fertility issues.
- Teaching techniques to deal with social interactions among peers.
- Counseling for anxiety and depression.
- Approach to educational obstacles.

Klinefelter Syndrome (KS)

KS, also known as 47,XXY is the most common *chromosomal disorder*, and it occurs in 1:500 to 1:1000 live male births. It is the set of symptoms that result from 2 or more X-chromosome in males. Most males have 1 Y-and 1 X-chromosome. Having extra X-chromosomes can cause a male to have some physical traits unusual for males.

As babies and children, XXY males may have weaker muscles and reduced strength. As they grow older, they tend to become taller than average. They may have less muscle control and coordination (Fig. 25.3B) than other boys of their age. During puberty, the physical traits of the syndrome become more evident; because these boys do not produce as much testosterone as other boys, they have a less muscular body, less facial and body hair, and broader hips. As teens, XXY males may develop breast tissue and also have weaker bones, and a lower energy level than other males. Intelligence is usually normal; however, reading difficulties and problems with speech are more common. Symptoms are typically more severe if 3 or more X-chromosomes are present.

About 10% of KS cases are found by prenatal diagnosis. The first clinical features may appear in early childhood or, more frequently, during puberty, such as lack of secondary sexual characters and aspermatogenesis. The standard diagnostic method is the analysis of the chromosomes' karyotype on lymphocytes. Even though KS is a genetic disorder, it is not passed down through families.

There is no cure, but treatments are available. It is important to start treatment as early as possible. With treatment, most boys grow up to have normal lives. Treatments include testosterone replacement therapy and breast reduction surgery. Testosterone is given by injection or through a skin patch or gel. The treatment usually continues throughout a man's life but does not help infertility.

If needed, physical, speech, language, and occupational therapy may also help. Educational support can help boys who have language or learning problems. Physical therapy, speech and language therapy, counseling, and adjustments of teaching methods may be useful.

Training and Rehabilitation of Challenged Children

Training and rehabilitation of challenged children involves combined and coordinated use of medical, social, educational, and vocational measures for training or retraining the individual to the highest possible level of functional ability. The 3 main strategies for rehabilitation of challenged children are institution-based, outreach, and community-based.

In general, training and rehabilitation encompasses the following:

- Early detection, diagnosis, and intervention
- Improve, facilitate, stimulate and/or provide services for people with disabilities, their families and other caregivers
- Medical rehabilitation, i.e. management of curable disability and lessening the disability to the extent possible
- Social, psychological, and other types of counseling and assistance
- Training in self-care activities including social graces, etiquette, mobility, communication, and daily living skills with special provisions as needed.
- Provision of technical, mobility and other devices
- Specialized education services
- Vocational rehabilitation services including vocational guidance, training, open placement, and self-employment
- Certification of degree of disability and provision of available concessions/benefits
- Community awareness, advocacy, empowerment.
- Follow-up.

CHAPTER 26

Crisis and Nursing Intervention

Chapter Outline

- Four Phases of Crisis Process
- Effects of Hospitalization on Parents and the Family of Child
- Hospice Care

The hospitalization of a child often triggers a crisis that requires assistance and interventions from different sources of health care delivery system. The family's needs depend on the resources, level of adaptability, and prior experience. Crisis intervention includes treatment and education provided by physician, care and support, health education and counseling provided by nurse. Depending on the situation, different members of health care team that assists in the transition from hospital to the home or community facility. Here, nurse can play an important role in identifying and coordinating these resources to facilitate this transition, and can initiate other interventions.

DEFINITION

Crisis is an acute time limited phenomenon experienced as an overwhelming emotional reaction to a stressful event or the perception of that event. It is the struggle for equilibrium and adjustment when problems are perceived as insolvable. Crisis intervention is a short-term focuses on the solving of the immediate problem, aims to establish the former coping pattern and problem solving ability. It is usually limited to 4–6 week period after which resolution will be attained.

In western countries, family seeks services which ranges from the need for child care due to a medical emergency, to an unexpected stressful home situation (i.e. domestic violence) to a risk of abuse and neglect.

FOUR PHASES OF CRISIS PROCESS

1st phase: A person confronted by a conflict or problem that threatens the self-concept responds with increased feelings of anxiety. The increase in anxiety stimulates the use of problem solving techniques in an effort to solve the problem and lower anxiety.

2nd phase: If the usual defense response toward the crisis fails, and if the threat persists, anxiety continues to rise and produce feelings of extreme discomfort. Individual functioning becomes disorganized.

3rd phase: If the recovering attempts fail, anxiety can escalate to severe and panic levels, and the person mobilizes automatic relief behavior, such as withdrawal and flight (compromising needs or solutions should be made) (Fig. 26.1).

4th phase: If the problem is not solved; anxiety can overwhelm the person and leads to serious personality disorganization. This maladaptive response can take the form of confusion, suicidal behavior, yelling and running aimlessly.

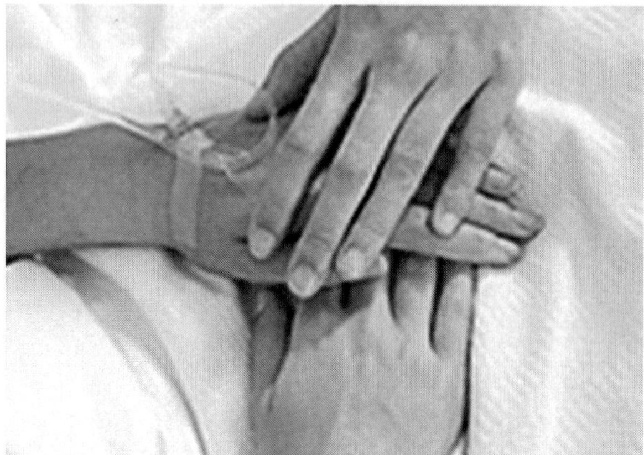

Fig. 26.1: Touch is a basic thing, people need in crisis

The Hospitalized Child

The hospitalization can be considered as a life crisis for a child, a crisis that may result in blocks or distortions in his development if not mastered properly. Maternal separation appears to be the primary stressor, but the presence of emotional disturbance prior to hospitalization and the child's level of cognitive development at the time may also be significant factors. Preparation prior to hospitalization is essential to make the transition from home to hospital as nondisruptive as possible. It has been observed that prolonged illness and hospitalization can retard growth and development and adverse reactions in the child based on stage of development. Every family should be prepared for what to expect when their child is admitted to the hospital. The child's developmental level as well as his relation with his parents determines when preparation should begin and in how much detail it should be carried out.

The Infant and Toddler

Separation Anxiety

Infants and toddlers experience separation anxiety. Separation is the major stressor to this age group and it is traumatic to both the child and the parent. Separation anxiety of infant is different from that of older child, because for the infant, the mother seems to be a part of him or her. Development of trust is disturbed when infant is separated from mother and when illness or hospitalization interferes with meeting the infant's needs and interference with development of a basic sense of trust has lifelong implications.

In case of toddler, separation represents the loss family and familiar surroundings, resulting in feeling of insecurity, grief, anxiety, and abandonment. The toddler's emotional needs are intensified by the mother's absence. Child has limited capacity to understand reality, passage of time as they are unable to communicate. Decrease in mobility—restricting mobility causes frustration. Child wants to keep moving or the pleasure it gives as well as for the feeling of independence, the opportunity to learn about the world, and the route it provides for coping with frustrations that cannot be verbally expressed. Physical interference with this freedom results in a sense of helplessness. The child passes through several stages of reaction to the separation.

Protest: Child is agitated and has urgent desire to find mother, frequently cries and shakes crib, resists caregivers, cries and inconsolable. When with mother, child shows signs of distrust with anger or tears.

Despair: Child feels increasingly hopeless about seeing mother and becomes quiet, apathetic, anorectic, listless; looks sad. He/she may cry continuously or intermittently. Use comfort measures—thumb-sucking, fingering lip, toy or own belonging like blanket, etc.

Detachment: Child becomes interested in the environment, play, and seems to form relationship with caregivers and other children, accepts care without protest. If parents reappear, the child may ignore them.

Regression: Child temporarily ceases use of newly acquired skills in an attempt to retain or regain control of a stressful situation. Regression may occur in toileting and eating.

Infants and toddler go through the different stages of separation. The older the child in this age group (infant and toddler), the more elaborate the protest. Generally child creates a scene of extreme cry, clinging to the parent, kicking, throwing, etc. Caregivers as well as parents need to understand that the behavior is a sign of healthy parent-child attachment. Parents are to be explained about the child's reactions and encourage parents to reinforce appropriate behavior while allowing the regressive behavior to occur.

Nursing Interventions

- Encourage mother to balance her responsibilities and minimize separation, staying with infant and providing care for her baby. To adjust schedule and home routines. Attempt to continue routines used at home, specially with regard to sleeping, eating, and bathing.
- Provide rooming-in, unlimited visiting, opportunity for child to express some of the feelings about the situation.
- Relieve some of tensions and loneliness with 'transference' object (i.e. blanket, toy).
- Prepare the child for procedures. The procedures should be performed in another room or a treatment room; let the mother soothe the child afterward.
- Provide for sensory stimulation and motor development appropriate for age. Provide opportunities for child to continue using acquired skills, such as feeding self and drinking from a cup.
- Obtain from parents key words in communicating with child. Find out about nonverbal behavior as well. Familiar toys, blankets, pillow cases, and family pictures can reinforce the child's sense of security.

- Allow child to make choices when possible. Arrange physical setting to encourage independence. Allow child to explore environment. Ensure an age-appropriate safe environment. No latex balloons.

Preschool Child

The preschoolers simply show similar behaviors (protest, despair, denial) to those of the toddler although the stage of protest is usually less aggressive and direct. Preschool child's cognitive capabilities have increased and the child responds less violently to separation from parents, and hospitalization. Loneliness and insecurity is experienced, fantasies and thoughts may contain vengeful wishes for other persons, for which the child expects retribution. Illness may be interpreted as punishment for thoughts. Enforced parental separation may be interpreted as loss of parental love and represents abandonment by them.

Loss of mobility due to hospitalization and intrusive procedures provide a multitude of threats, lack of self-expression and of both bodily mutilation and loss of identity, which are just beginning to develop along with the acquisition of autonomy. Separation occurs among preschoolers they show the same protest as the toddler but tends to be less direct. They show the difficulty of coping with the hospitalization through their behavior.

The preschooler has attained a good deal of independence and allowed more independence in self-care at home, day care and preschool. Hospitalization means loss of independence. He/she may like to wander about the unit and may not be happy when restricted in the bed and room. The nurse may find that child is quietly crying or may be repeatedly ask when their parent will come for a visit.

Child temporarily stops using newly acquired skills in an attempt to retain or regain control of a stressful situation. Preschooler may return to behavior of infant or toddler (regression). Child may attempt to exclude (repress) the undesirable and unpleasant stresses from consciousness and may transfer own emotional state, motives, and desires to other in environment. Preschoolers fear injury, pain and mutilation.

The preschoolers are also afraid of intrusive procedures, and fears mutilation. They may believe that their illness is somehow related to a personal deed and thought as their thinking is egocentric and magical. The nurse need to understand that this belief can lead to feelings of guilt, shame, and increased stress at a time when the child has to cope with several other stressors. Other nursing interventions include:

- Minimize stress of separation by providing for parental presence and participation in care. Strive to shorten the hospital stay. Help parents understand what hospitalization means to the child.
- Identify defense mechanisms apparent in the child and help child through the stressful situation by accepting, showing love and concern, and being alert to readiness to relinquish them.
- Set limits for the child. Let child know that someone is there. Help the child become master of something in the situation.
- Provide opportunity and encouragement for child to verbalize their unfounded fears and belief.
- Careful preparation for all procedures should be done on the child's level of development and comprehension. Provide privacy during these procedures.
- Be sure the child has opportunities for play. Play is one important medium through which the child can overcome fear and anxiety. A body outline, doll, and simple visual aids are appropriate teaching tools. Provide self-expression, role reversal through puppet, dolls, drawings.
- Encourage activities of self-care and activities with other children, to foster their independence.
- Provide consistency in nursing personnel and approach to care.
- Deal specifically with castration and mutilation fears. If the child having surgery, describe exactly which body part will be repaired.
- Whenever appropriate, reassure the child that no one is to blame for the illness or hospitalization.
- Discourage parents from reinforcing negative feelings to the child—'if you are not good, I will leave you here' or I will have the nurse give you a shot.

School-aged Children

The school age child is accustomed to periods of separation from parents. But may fear loss of recently mastered skills and may worry about separation from school and peers. They may fear loss of former roles. Mutilation and fantasies are common. Some may believe that they or their parents magically caused the illness merely by thinking that the even would occur. Often, they have increased concerns related to modesty and privacy. The imposed passivity may be interpreted as punishment for being bad. Children may feel their body no longer is their own but rather is controlled by doctors and nurses. They usually show the following reactions

- Regression
- Separation anxiety—specially early school-aged period
- Negativism
- Depression

- Tendency to be phobic (normal)
- Fears include that of the dark, doctors, hospitals, surgery, medication, and death
- Unrealistic fears are commonly attached to needles, X-ray procedures, and blood
- Suppression or denial of symptoms.

Nursing Interventions

- Help parents to prepare the child for elective hospitalizations.
- Obtain a thorough nursing history, including information regarding health and physical developments, hospitalizations, social and cultural background, and normal daily activities, use this information to plan care.
- Provide order and consistency in the environment whenever possible.
- Establish and enforce reasonable policies to protect the child and to increase sense of security in the environment.
- Arrange the environment to allow for as much mobility as possible (i.e. make sure articles are appropriately placed; move the bed if the child is immobilized).
- Respect the child's need for privacy and respect modesty during examinations, bathing, and other activities.
- Use treatment rooms whenever possible when performing painful or intrusive procedures. Keep the room as 'safe' territory.
- Help young children identify problems and questions (often through play). Then help them find the answers.
- Provide information about the illness and hospitalization based on assessment of what facts the child needs and wants, and how this information can be made readily understandable.
- View all nursing care activities as teaching situations. Explain the function of equipment, and allow the child to handle it. Teach scientific terminology for body parts, procedures and equipment.
- When explaining a procedure make sure that the child knows its purpose, what will be done, and what will be expected. Reassure the child during the procedure by continuing the explanations and support.
- Reassure the child having surgery; explain where the organ to be removed or repaired is located and that no other body part will be removed.
- Carefully assess pain, and provide appropriate relief.
- Use play whenever appropriate to provide information about the hospital experience and to identify and decrease the child's fantasies and fears.
- Reassure the child that he or she or parents are not to blame for illness.
- Facilitate discharge of energy and aggression through appropriate play activities or through sharing aspects of ward management.
- Encourage the child's participation in care and self-hygiene.
- Support intellectual potential through the use of games, puzzles, school work, and drawings.
- Assist the family to understand the child's reactions to illness and hospitalization so family members can facilitate positive coping patterns.
- Let the child know that his or her normal status as a family member remains intact during hospitalizations. Encourage a consistent visiting pattern and allow sibling visits.
- Help parents to deal with their own anxieties about hospitalization and assist them to help their child cope with the situation.
- Encourage parental participation in the child's care when appropriate.
- Encourage written communication with peers, and allow peer visiting when appropriate.
- Begin discharge planning early, including plans for physical and emotional needs. Alert families to possible behavioral changes, including phobias, nightmares, regression, negativism, and disturbances in eating and learning.

Adolescents

- Physical illness, exposure and lack of privacy may cause increased concern about body image and sexuality.
- Separation from security of peers, family, and school may cause anxiety.
- Interference with struggle for independence and recognition from parents is a concern.
- The adolescent may be threatened by helplessness and may see illness as a punishment for feelings not mastered or for breaking rules imposed by parents or physicians.
- Illness and hospitalizations may interfere with peer associations, self-concept, sexuality, and independence.
- Anxiety or embarrassment related to loss of control
- Insecurity in strange environment

- Intellectualization about disease details to avoid addressing actual concerns. They may know other with the same chronic type of illness who have died; may fear the future or feel guilty they have survived.
- Rejection of treatment measures, even if previously accepted
- Anger (may be directed toward parents or staff) because goals are being thwarted.
- Depression
- Increased dependency on parents, staff
- Denial or withdrawal
- Demanding or uncooperative behaviors (usually an attempt to assert control)
- Capitalization on gains from illness or pain.

Nursing Interventions

- Help parents to prepare the adolescent for elective hospitalization.
- Assess the impact of illness on the adolescent by considering factors such as timing, nature of illness, new experiences imposed changes in body image, and expectations for the future. Be aware of misconceptions.
- Introduce the adolescent to the hospital staff and to the regular routines soon after admission.
- Obtain a thorough nursing history that includes information about hobbies, school, family, illness, hospitalization, food habits, sexuality, and recreation.
- Encourage adolescents to wear their own clothes, and allow them to decorate their beds or rooms to express themselves.
- Have drawers and closets available to store personal items.
- Allow the adolescent access to a telephone.
- Allow adolescents control over appropriate matters (i.e. timing of bath, selection of food and so forth).
- Respect their need for periodic isolation and privacy.
- Have a supervised recreational and activity program available that is planned by a professional child care worker.
- Accept adolescent's level of performance. Allow regression with expectation of growth.
- Involve adolescent patients in planning care so they will be more accepting restrictions and receptive to health teaching. Focus on capabilities rather than limitations. Adolescent should be accepted as a vital member of the health care team. The adolescent's consent should be obtained for procedures and surgery.
- Explain clearly all procedures, routines, expectations, and restrictions imposed by illness. If necessary clarify the adolescent's interpretation of illness and hospitalization. Plan separate teaching sessions for parents.
- Facilitate verbal rejection of treatment measure to protect the adolescent from harming himself physically by stopping treatment.
- Assess the adolescent's intellectual skills, and provide necessary information to allow for problem solving to deal with illness and hospitalization.
- Recognize positive and negative coping behaviors attempts to adjust to a threatening situation. Attempt to deal with feeling that caused the behaviors as well as with the behavior itself.
- Be a good listener. Maintain a sense of humor. Be honest and respectful with the adolescent and family.
- Provide opportunities such as writing, art work, and recreational activities to allow nonverbal adolescents to express themselves.
- Foster interaction with other hospitalized adolescents and continuation of peer relationship with outside friends.
- Establish regular group meetings to allow patients to meet with staff members and with each other to comment and ask questions about their hospital experiences.
- Set necessary limits to encourage self-control and ensure the rights of others.
- Help adolescents work through sexual feelings. Avoid behavior that could be interpreted as provocative or flirtatious. Masturbation, unless excessive, may be considered a psychologically healthy way to discharge sexual tension.
- Describe and interpret the needs and reactions of hospitalized adolescents to parents. Emphasize the adolescents need to be respected as a unique individual, separate form parents.
- Assist parents to cope with illness and hospitalization as well as to deal effectively with the adolescent's response to related stress.
- Encourage continuation of education.
- Stress the confidential nature of conversations.

EFFECTS OF HOSPITALIZATION ON PARENTS AND THE FAMILY OF CHILD

Illness and hospitalization are often critical events that a child is faced with and the stress of it can affect all family members. Parents become upset, helpless, mentally and physically exhausted, and experience loss of sleep and disruption of daily routine during the hospitalization of their child. Hospitalization of young children has considerable emotional impact and creates significant distress, in addition to causing significant financial burden for parents.

Stressors

- Strange environment in the hospital
- *Separation from the child:* The hospitalization/ separation of a child is a stressful time for parents/ family, and more so if the hospitalization is for life-threatening or chronic illnesses. The emotional impact of a child's physical illness on parents either concentrated on severe life-threatening illnesses such as leukemia, brain tumor, etc. Parents may complaint some symptoms like shock, guilt and regret, powerlessness and frustration, grief, fear and anxiety, emotional and physical exhaustion, health problems out of stress.
- *Unknown events and outcomes:* Feelings of stress and anxiety are often associated with the lack of information on diseases and medical procedures. The stress is caused by the imposed treatments, unfamiliarity with the hospital rules and regulations, unfriendly staff and being afraid of asking questions.
- The suffering of the child
- Spread of infections to other members in family
- Unbearable financial obligations
- Parents show reactions like anxiety, anger, fear, disappointment, self-blame, guilt. The anxiety interferes with the parent's ability to care the child, support. This anxiety could be recognized by the trembling, coarse voice, restlessness, irritability and withdrawal.

Nursing Implications

Nurse should begin to build a working relationship with the patients and the child from the first contact with them.

Nurse should be aware that all behavior is meaningful.

Nurse should accept the parents and the child exactly as they are, show empathy for parents and children.

Nurse should let them know that their problems are of importance, the nurse is there to aid their solutions. Encourage to perform the tasks.

Nurse must be willing to acknowledge the parents rights to their own decisions concerning their children. Introduce them with parent support group and care by parent unit.

Nurse permits the parents and the child to express even negative emotions. Recognize the need of the parent for support, encourage to obtain help from other family members or friends. Nurse should speak the language understandable to parents and the child.

Health team members should help the parents to feel that there is unity among them.

Terminal Illness and Death During Childhood

A terminal illness of child: It is a disease that is incurable and untreatable, and that is reasonably expected to result in the death of the child within a short period of time is termed as terminal illness. A child who has a terminal illness has been diagnosed with a disease or illness that has no expectation of cure. This term is more commonly used for progressive diseases such as cancer or advanced heart disease than for trauma. It indicates a disease which will eventually end the life of the sufferer. Terminally-ill children, now more than ever, need love, support, and honesty from their family and friends.

Parental Decision Making

When the death is unexpected, the confusion of emergency services and possibly an intensive care setting presents challenges to the parents as they are asked to make difficult choices. If the child has experienced a life-threatening illness that has now reached its terminal phase, parents are often unprepared for the reality of their child's impending death. The emotional, physical, and spiritual impact a dying child has on a family and community cannot be measured. Nurses should ensure the families that there are options. The nurse's first responsibility is to explore the family's wishes.

The Dying Child

It is the natural instinct of parents want to shield their children from any unpleasant news. When a child is diagnosed as being permanently ill, this urge is intensified.

Almost all children need honest information about their illness, treatment and prognosis. An open conversation early in the course of illness can be done and provide appropriate literature. Children are amazingly perceptive and will pick up on the fact that things are not okay, that they are not going to be okay. Find ways to be honest and open with the child.

It is natural for parents, relatives, and friends to want to protect a dying child from the impact of a diagnosis. What and how much to tell a child depends on many variables, including culture and social background, the family structure and available support, and the individual characteristics of the child and family.

Decisions regarding involving child in care during their dying process and death, is an individual matter. The child's age or developmental stage is considered. A shared decision making is important to the child's and family's emotional health. Parents require professional support and guidance in this. Adolescents have autonomy in decision making with regard to care and treatment.

Perceptions of death (according to developmental stage of child):

- *Infants:* Death has least significance to them specially < 6 months of age.
- *Toddler:* Instead of understanding death they will be more affected by the change in lifestyle. They are also affected by the loss of comfort measures, such as when they experience pain and cold. Infant and toddlers may react to the dying process based on the sadness, anger and anxiety conveyed by their parents.
- *Preschooler:* They believe their thoughts and actions are sufficient to cause death; the consequence is the burden of guilt, shame and punishment. They see death as departure, and believe it to be only temporary, a kind of sleep. They may recognize the fact of physical death but do not separate it from living abilities. They have no understanding of inevitability of death.

  Their self-imposed guilt may cause them to believe them that parents and others see them as 'bad' and are angry with them. Feelings are kept inside and the child withdraws him/her from everyone, sometimes they also show acute discharge of anger.
- *Schooler:* School children understand death as a sad and irreversible event, yet it still may be considered inevitable only for adults. They associate misdeeds or bad thoughts with causing death and feel intense guilt and responsibility for the event. As there is increased cognition, they respond well to the logical explanations about death. They have a deeper understanding about death. They personify death as devil, monster, etc. By age of 9 to 10 years they have an adult concept of death, realizing it is inevitable, universal and irreversible.
- *Adolescents:* They have a mature understanding of death, i.e. it is inevitable and irreversible. They accept it logically but view death as a distant event and may consider themselves invincible to death. They are still influenced by the remnants of magical thinking and are subject to guilt and shame. They are likely to see deviations from accepted behavior as reasons for their illness. Adolescents become isolated from caring adults, may feel lonesome and fear that they will die without the love and support that they need and desire.

Care of Terminally-ill Child

Caring for dying children involves certain potential stressors for all involved, including the nurse. Providing nursing care to the child with fatal disease, and nearing to death as well as to the family members need a heightened level of understanding, compassion and support. The goal of nursing care is to provide comfortable, peaceful time for the child and family with minimum disruptions.

Some families prefer to take child home. Children are usually less upset when they are cared for at home than in hospital and their long-term outcome is better; children's hospices can provide specialist and respite care if it is needed.

Families may choose to remain in the hospital to provide care in his unstable condition and home care is not an option. Then the setting should be made homelike as possible. Familiar items of child are encouraged to bring. There should be a consistent, coordinated care plan for the family's comfort. When this happens, the primary aim of a child's care shifts from seeking a cure to making the child more physically and emotionally comfortable and as free from pain as possible. This is known as palliative care.

- *Fear of pain and pain management:* The presence of unrelieved pain in a terminally-ill child can have effects on the quality of life of child and family. Nurses can alleviate the fear of pain and suffering by providing interventions aimed at treating the pain and symptoms associated with the terminal process in children. Educate the child and family regarding pain control and then provide constant, consistent reassurance that everything possible and appropriate will be done for the comfort of the child.

Pain control for children in the terminal stages of illness or injury must be given the highest priority. Limit unnecessary painful procedures to perform for the child, if it is necessary, administer sedation and giving pre-emptive analgesia prior to a procedure.

The current standard for treating children's pain follows the WHO analgesic stepladder, which promotes tailoring the pain interventions to the child's level of reported pain. Pain should be assessed frequently and medications adjusted as necessary. Opioid drug such as morphine should be given for severe pain. Along with drug therapy, distraction, relaxation techniques and guided imagery should be used.

- *Sleep routine:* The child is sick and being in the hospital can be exhausting. Make sure that child gets as much sleep and rest as they can manage, as there are constant interruptions and visitors; it is also a new and unfamiliar situation. Keep the room friendly and softly lit in case the child wakes up confused about where he or she is.
- *Nutrition:* This can be a difficult subject to tackle given that the child may be nauseated, vomiting, experiencing reduced appetite, or upset GI depending on the nature of the illness and treatment. In addition to regular meals, high-protein shakes may help supplement the child's diet. Additionally a feeding tube may be placed to help ensure that the child gets the nutrition that he or she needs.
- *Waste:* The child's system is likely in a state of havoc, and with that they may experience incontinence, diarrhea, constipation, or other voiding issues. Make sure that the child is clean and taken care of. Never let the child be embarrassed by anyone, he or she cannot help it.
- *Playtime:* Despite the severity of the circumstances, child is still young. He or she still needs time to play and be a child. Setting aside time to play with them can go a long ways toward making both child and parents more comfortable.
- *Mental health:* Address coincident depression, anxiety, sense of fear or lack of control of child. Consider guided imagery, relaxation, hypnosis, art/pet therapy, acupuncture/acupressure, biofeedback, massage, heat/cold, yoga, transcutaneous electric nerve stimulation.

  Communication and exploring feelings can be challenging. Depending on his or her emotional development, your child may not express his or her emotions in an easily understood way. Be patient with your child and make sure that he or she knows you are there to listen and be supportive.
- *Symptom management:* Symptoms during their terminal course as a result of their disease process or as side effect of medication. The symptoms include fatigue, nausea and vomiting, constipation, anorexia, dyspnea, congestion, seizures, anxiety, depression, restlessness, agitation and confusion. The symptoms should be managed with appropriate medications or treatments and with non-pharmacologic interventions such as repositioning, relaxation, massage and other measures to maintain comfort and quality of life.

HOSPICE CARE

Once a word that evoked shelter for tired and ill religious pilgrims; the term hospice has come to describe a concept of end-of-life care centered on quality of life. Hospice care, encompasses physical, emotional, and spiritual needs. It may take place at home or at a nursing home, assisted living center, or hospice residence. When a cure is not possible and aggressive treatment is not desired, hospice care offers symptom relief, pain control, and a great deal of support.

Hospice care, sometimes called end-of-life palliative care, comprehensive and compassionate in nature, and is designed for patients who are in the final stages of a terminal illness. Hospice care focuses not only on dying as peacefully, comfortably, and with as much dignity as possible, but also on living as fully as possible until death occurs.

Usually, hospice care is offered to those who are expected to live no longer than 6 months and have stopped receiving curative treatments. The goal of hospice care is *not* to speed up the process of dying or to slow it down—but rather, to provide the best possible quality of life for dying patients and their families. It focuses on preventing and relieving pain and suffering and easing the fear and anxiety associated with the end of a person's life.

Hospice is a community health care organization that specializes in the care of dying patients by combining the hospice philosophy with principles of palliative care. Management of physical, psychological, social and spiritual needs of child and family. Care is provided by a multidisciplinary group of professionals in the patient's home.

In hospice care, family members are the principle caregivers and are supported by team of professional and volunteer staff who provide information and advice and support. Keeping families involved in the decision-making allows them to feel more in control of their child's care. The priority of care is comfort. The child's needs are considered. Pain and symptom control are primary concerns and no extraordinary efforts are taken to prolong life. Family's needs are considered to be as important as child's needs. It is considered with the family's postdeath adjustment and care may continue for 1 year or more. They are helped in spiritual care, such as exploring the meaning of death and helping with religious ceremonies or rituals. Hospice care includes grief counseling and support, which helps parents and other family members through the bereavement process.

CHAPTER 27

Drugs used in Pediatrics

Chapter Outline

- Review of Anatomical and Physiological Features of Pediatric Patients that Influence Drug Administration
- Guidelines of Rational Drug Therapy
- Guidelines on the Use of Drugs in Children
- Different Methods of Drug Calculation
- Administration of Drug and Fluid—Nursing Responsibilities
- Pediatric Pain Management
- Adverse Drug Interaction

Infants and children have frequent but not usually serious illnesses. A child's frequent illnesses in the early years are part of a natural process which develops his or her immature immune system. These generally mild infections help to build immunity against common diseases. Nutritious food, cleanliness and vaccinations are three important bodyguards that protect children against many diseases.

Drug treatment in children differs from that in adults, most obviously because it is usually based on weight or surface area. Doses differ because of age-related variations in drug absorption, distribution, metabolism, and elimination. The main reason for children being more prone to adverse sideeffects of drugs is that children are not just small adults. The way a child's body deals with drugs is completely different from that of an adult body.

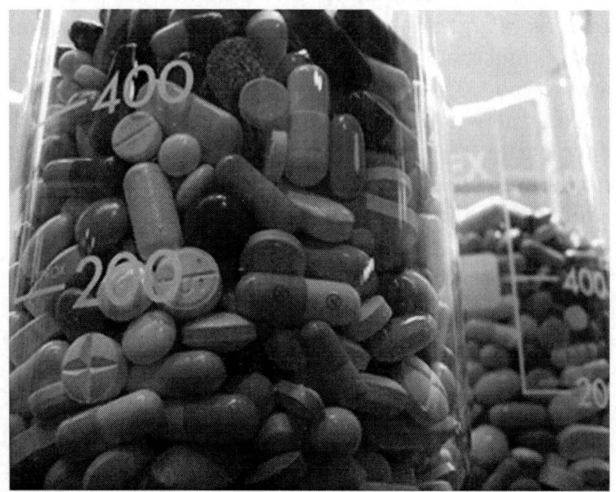

Review of anatomical and physiological features of pediatric patients that influence drug administration.

The administration of medicines to infants, children and teenagers requires a complex set of skills that must be grounded in a sound understanding of child development, not only in terms of biophysiological changes but also changes that occur from a psychological perspective. Why does a child need a special dose? How is their body different from an adult's? Knowledge regarding these points and special considerations are needed before administration of pediatric drug.

Children's bodies are a world apart from adults'. One of the easiest ways to understand why drugs may have different actions and different effects in children is to take a system-by-system approach to pediatric anatomy.

NEUROLOGIC SYSTEM

A large amount of blood circulates oxygen, nutrients and other chemicals into the brain. Because brain cells are very sensitive to harmful substances and cannot be reproduced, it is important to keep harmful chemicals out of brain matter. For this reason, the epithelial cells, or outermost brain cells that connect with circulating blood at the capillary level, have grown very tightly together. The blood-brain barrier is the layer of tightly

Table 27.1: Pediatric vital signs							
Age	*Premature*	*Newborn*	*1–12 months*	*1–3 years*	*3-5 years*	*6–12 years*	*13+ years*
Weight	1 to 2 kg	2 to 3 kg	4 to 10 kg	10 to 14 kg	14 to 18 kg	20 to 42 kg	>50 kg
Pulse	140+	120 to 160	80 to 140	80 to 130	80 to 120	70 to 110	60 to 90
Respirations	30 to 40	30 to 50	30 to 60	20 to 40	20 to 30	20 to 30	12 to 20
Systolic BP	40+10	60+10	85+15	90+15	95+15	100+15	115+15
Skin	Pink, warm moist						
Temperature	98.6 °F						

packed epithelial cells, which prevents most proteins and polarized molecules from entering the brain. While lipid-soluble molecules can pass through the blood-brain barrier easily, most other chemicals are kept out.

Drugs with known side effects that include neurological impairment require careful administration. These side effects are more common in the pediatric patient. For example, morphine is known to cause respiratory depression and sedation by slowing responses in the central nervous system. This effect can be seen more dramatically and at lower doses in children.

CARDIOVASCULAR SYSTEM

A child's cardiovascular system is weaker than an adult's, and cardiac output is significantly lower. The heart is less developed and cannot increase the strength of contraction as a result the pediatric heart compensates best by increasing its rate instead of its contractile force. Peripheral vasoconstriction occurs earlier in pediatric patients and is less effective at increasing circulating blood volume. Tachycardia, or rapid pulse rate, needs to be recognized as a compensation mechanism. It is usually okay if it persists until the underlying problem can be corrected.

Child tries to compensate for hypovolemia, which he cannot do as well as an adult patient with the same problem. Adults compensate to maintain a normal cardiac output (stroke volume times heart rate [SV × HR]). While adults can increase preload to maintain a high stroke volume and increase heart rate, child can only effectively increase heart rate. The pediatric patient's stroke volume decreases as blood volume decreases.

Since pediatric patients have a much smaller blood volume than adults, they must vasoconstrict earlier and more dynamically. Pale, cool, clammy skin can develop very rapidly. Consider a 150 mL blood loss: In a small pediatric patient, this loss can trigger decompensated shock, while an adult patient can handle the loss well. Tachycardia is a common but nonspecific response to any increase in the child's metabolic needs, including increased oxygen demand, cardiac output or energy for physical activity.

Seek out the cause of any tachycardia to determine what the child is compensating for. A persistently bradycardic heart rate is a serious finding in children and is most often triggered by hypoxemia. Children also compensate with tachypnea, or fast breathing.

Children have a much higher basal metabolic rate than adults. To adjust for this, they need higher cardiac output and higher oxygen consumption. Because of the relatively small size of their heart and lungs, the child's heart rate and respiratory rate are both higher (Table 27.1). Blood pressure is lower because children do not have the same peripheral vascular resistance as adults. The specific vital sign numbers are not as important as noting how the patient's vital signs change, or trend, over time. Rather than focusing on a single set of vitals, or a single number obtained, note whether the patient's vital signs change with interventions. Determine if they are returning toward normal or becoming more abnormal and adjust nursing intervention or treatment accordingly.

BODY COMPOSITION

Relative to their size, neonates and newborns consist of up to 70% water, by adulthood it comes down to about 55%. This means water-soluble drugs, such as acetaminophen, will be relatively more dilute in a child than an adult. Because the child's circulating blood volume is very small, dehydration can quickly affect how well drugs are transported by the bloodstream throughout the body.

As individual grows through childhood, circulating blood volume is determined by weight. Neonates have a blood volume of 85 to 90 mL/kg, infants 75 to 80 mL/kg, children 70 to 75 mL/kg, and, during the adolescent years, 65 to 70 mL/kg. While the mL/kg are decreasing as a child grows, the weight increases so dynamically that the total fluid volume increases drastically. Thus, older children can more easily tolerate fluid and/or blood losses and have a much greater total volume in which to dilute drugs. Comparing a 4 kg infant and a 40 kg child, how much blood does each have available to dilute a given drug volume?

Half of the pediatric patient's fluid is in the extracellular space, whereas the adult patient's extracellular fluid is only 20%. This means that fluid loss in the pediatric patient can very rapidly affect more of the total body fluid reservoir than with an adult. Intracellular fluid reserves available to the adult patient are not readily available to the pediatric patient. As a result, dehydration has a more dynamic effect on the patient's ability to compensate.

RESPIRATORY SYSTEM

A significant difference in pediatric patients is their relatively small airway size, which means excessive secretions and inflammation can easily compromise the airway. In respiratory distress, an early administration of drugs is required to dry airway secretions and promote bronchodilation.

Supplemental oxygen is also a key therapy for pediatric patients, in whom oxygen consumption is almost twice that of adults. Oxygen consumption is measured in milliliters (mL) of oxygen per gram of weight for each organ in the body. The typical adult brain requires 3 mL of oxygen for every 100 g (grams) to function for 1 minute; a child's brain requires twice that, or 6 mL of oxygen for every 100 g. The higher oxygen consumption rate results from the child's rapidly growing organs. Pediatric patients do not tolerate hypoxemia, or low blood-oxygen saturation levels. A major sign of significant hypoxemia is bradycardia.

GASTROINTESTINAL SYSTEM

A child's stomach is extremely small compared to an adult's (capacity of adult stomach 2 to 3 L, a 1-year-old's stomach capacity is 360 mL, while a 30-day-old term infant's stomach capacity is only 90 mL). Administering multiple oral drugs to young children can potentially reduce the amount of food they are capable of consuming. Fortunately, children process food more than twice as fast as an adult. This means that orally administered (PO) drugs can be absorbed and enter the circulatory system faster than in an adult patient.

There are two key considerations about stomach size that directly affect drug administration. The rapid absorption rate is a benefit when administering PO medications, such as liquid PCM for fever or pain; however, ingested toxins will also enter circulation twice as fast, leading to a more rapid onset of deleterious effects. In case of poisoning adults generally can receive oral activated charcoal up to one hr after toxin ingestion and the charcoal will inhibit absorption, but in case of children earlier administration is necessary. Knowing the patient's stomach size can be a benefit when considering toxin and poison ingestion, as it can help predict the maximum amount ingested, specially if the patient vomits a measurable amount of liquid. Stomach size importance is to be considered in drug administration as it should not over fill the stomach.

ENDOCRINE SYSTEM

Child's body contains much smaller glycogen than adults, but their large brain-to-body mass ratio increases their glucose demand. This predisposes children to hypoglycemia and suggests that glucagon may be less effective than for an adult. Another endocrine difference is in metabolism. Metabolism, in regard to drugs, refers to the body's changing the drug from its original form into another chemical structure or form. Some drugs must be metabolized to be utilized by the body. All drugs must be metabolized to be converted into a product the body can eliminate as waste.

The newborn baby's metabolism is significantly slower than an adult's, meaning the neonate's body will convert and remove drugs much more slowly. However, within a few short years, their metabolic rate accelerates to three times that of an adult's, leading to faster drug metabolism (biotransformation). Throughout childhood, metabolism remains elevated to facilitate growth as a gradual rate decline occurs. By onset of adolescence, a child's metabolism is roughly that of an adult.

RENAL SYSTEM

The renal system is immature in young children. Normal urine output is 2 mL/kg/h, compared to ½ to 1 mL/kg/hr for adolescents and adults. This indicates that children cannot concentrate urine as well as adults, meaning they cannot conserve fluids as well. Waste production rate of children is high, meaning metabolized drugs will be eliminated more quickly than in an adult. However, this same rate of waste production with a higher urine production rate also predisposes pediatric patients for dehydration.

Infants and children have frequent but not usually serious illnesses. A child's frequent illnesses in the early years are part of a natural process which develops his or her immature immune system. These generally mild infections help to build immunity against common diseases. Nutritious food, cleanliness and vaccinations are three important bodyguards that protect children against many diseases.

Drug treatment in children differs from that in adults, most obviously because it is usually based on weight or surface area. Doses differ because of age-related variations in drug absorption, distribution, metabolism, and elimination.

An important question which arises is that should children be given so many drugs for their illness? The answer is 'No'. However, the fact remains that too many drugs are being given to infants and children although most of them have very little or no value. Moreover; subjecting children to lot of drugs means subjecting them to lot of adverse effects.

RATIONAL DRUG THERAPY (RDT)

Some general guidelines of RDT are:

- There should be a genuine indication for the use of drug in the patient.
- A minimum number of appropriate familiar and inexpensive drugs of good quality should be used.
- Drugs should preferably be prescribed by generic name.
- The dosage of the drug should be optimum to achieve the desired chemical benefits.
- It is desirable to administer drugs as far as possible through oral route in children.
- Adverse drug reactions should be anticipated, monitored and appropriately monitored.

The main reason for children being more prone to adverse side effects of drugs is that children are not just small adults. The way a child's body deals with drugs is completely different from that of an adult body.

The organs responsible for the breakdown and elimination of drugs, that is, the liver and the kidney respectively, are less efficient in a child's body than in an adult body. Hence if adult doses of a drug are given to children, drugs get accumulated in their body and produce harmful effects. This is why it is important that accurate doses be calculated for children taking into consideration both their age and weight.

Certain drugs are harmful to children even in therapeutic doses and should be completely avoided, e.g., loperamide, tetracycline. Parents should always determine if a drug is really necessary for their child's condition and check if there is any nondrug alternative. They should avoid giving unnecessary drugs to their children who may grow up believing that medicines are solutions to many of life's health problems.

There are many drugs which are commonly misused in children. Some examples are:

- Antibacterials for viral upper respiratory infections.
- Decongestants for colds, resulting in unacceptable adverse effects.
- Drugs to treat diarrhea.
- Oral antiemetics for vomiting.
- Antipyretic agents for fever.
- Tricyclic antidepressants for bed wetting.
- Sedatives for sleepless children or those labelled hyperactive.
- Spasmolytics for abdominal pain.
- Appetite stimulants, vitamins and tonics.

Guidelines on the Use of Drugs in Children

While administering drugs to children, particularly neonates, special care is always needed because they differ from adults in their response to drugs. Doses should invariably be calculated on the basis of weight till 50 kg or puberty is reached. In the neonatal period, the risk of toxicity is higher due to inefficient renal clearance, relative deficiencies of various enzymes, heightened sensitivity and inadequate detoxifying mechanism.

If possible, painful intramuscular injections should be avoided. It is always a good practice to state the age of child patient while writing prescriptions. Even though liquid preparations are more easily accepted by children, many contain sucrose which can lead to dental decay.

Dosage

Children's doses are usually stated in the following age ranges: Neonate (first month), infant (upto 1 year), 1 to 5 years and 6 to 12 years. Where a single dose is given, it applies to the middle of the age range. Hence adjustment would need to be made for lower and upper limits of the stated range.

Dose Calculation

The dosage for children can be calculated from adult doses by using either age, or body weight or body surface area or by a combination of these factors (Table 27.2). Even though body surface area provides the most reliable method of determining dosage, in practice it is exceedingly difficult.

Body weight can be easily used to calculate doses and are generally expressed in mg/kg. Because of their higher metabolic rate, children generally require higher dose per kilogram than adults.

Table 27.2: The *percentage method* to calculate doses for children as per body weight or body surface area

	Body weight	*Length/ Height*	*BSA*	*Adult dose*
Newborn	3.4 kg	50 cm	0.23 m	12.5%
1 month	4.2 kg	55 cm	0.26 m	14.5%
3 months	5.6 kg	59 cm	0.32 m	18%
6 months	7.7 kg	67 cm	0.40 m	22%
1 year	10 kg	76 cm	0.47 m	25%
3 years	14 kg	94 cm	0.62 m	33%
5 years	18 kg	108 cm	0.73 m	40%
7 years	23 kg	120 cm	0.88 m	50%
12 years	37 kg	148 cm	1.25 m	75%

$$\text{Young's formula of child dose} = \frac{\text{Age of the child} \times \text{adult dose}}{\text{Age} + 12}$$

$$\text{Dilling's formula} = \frac{\text{Age of the child} \times \text{adult dose}}{20}$$

This method can pose problems while calculating dose for obese children since they are liable to be given higher than required dose. Under such circumstances, it is better to calculate dose based on ideal body weight of the child in that particular age.

Body Surface Area (BSA): It is technically a better and more accurate method since many physical phenomenon are more closely related to body surface area. The average body surface area of a 70 kg adult is about 1.7 to 1.8 square meter. Thus to calculate the dose for a child the following formula is used:

$$\text{Approximate dose for child} = \frac{\text{Surface area of child (m}^2) \times \text{adult dose}}{1.8}$$

The *Percentage method* as given below can be conveniently used to calculate doses for children when there is wide margin between therapeutic and toxic dose:

Dose Frequency: Doses of antibiotics are usually stated as every 6 hrs. In the case of children, some flexibility may be allowed so that they are not woken up at night.

Administration of Drug

Before determining the route of drug administration, several questions need to be addressed such as:

Which is the most convenient route for the patient?

How quickly does the drug need to reach its site of action?

How long the drug dose need to remain in the body?

Where is the drug to act? (skin/heart/kidney).

Which organs is the drug to be kept away from?

Selection of the route of drug administration is important as it can have profound effects on the (a) onset of drug action, (b) the plasma concentration achieved, and (c) the duration of drug action.

Topical application of drug: The term topical application of medicines means the application of drugs directly to the surface where its action is wanted.

The oral route: The oral route is a systemic route. It is the oldest and commonest mode of drug administration.

Mixture: A mixture is a liquid that contains several ingredients dissolved or diffused in water or some other solvent. Example of mixture is alkali mixture, carminative mixture. A mixture dispensed in a single dose is called a 'draught' or a 'haustus'.

Emulsion: An emulsion is a mixture of two immiscible liquids (i.e. oil and water) in which one is dispersed through the other in a finely divided state viz. milk of magnesia.

Syrup: Syrup is a 66% solution of sucrose in water. It is used as a vehicle for active ingredient. It is used to mask the bitter taste of ingredient viz. syrup chloroquine. *Advantages*—Syrup is convenient to administer. The GI tract provides a huge surface area for absorption and drug are absorbed by diffusion.

Inhalation: The inhalational route of administration is used to give gaseous anesthetics and other therapeutic gases. This route is also used to apply drugs directly to the lungs to treat for example asthma. Because of the very large surface area of the alveolar membrane and the high blood flow through the lungs, gases of suitable solubility are rapidly absorbed from the lungs. Steroids such as beclomethasone are inhaled, as are the β_2 adrenoceptor agonist bronchodilator drugs.

When drugs must be given by injection, several options are available (Fig. 27.1).

Intravenous (IV) injections: The drug is injected directly into a vein, usually in the arm or hand. The IV route is the most direct and bypasses the absorption barriers. It is also the most hazardous, because a very high concentration of drug is delivered to the target organs very rapidly.

Intramuscular (IM) injection: The drug is injected in one of the large skeletal muscles—deltoid, triceps,

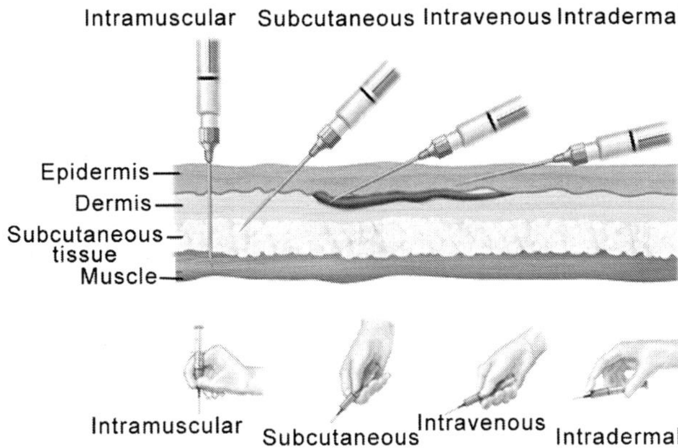

Fig. 27.1: Types and techniques of injection

gluteus maximus, rectus femoris, etc. Muscle is less richly supplied with sensory nerves and mild irritant drugs can be given by this route. Muscle is more vascular and absorption of aqueous solution drug is faster. Absorption is variable, depending on which muscle is used, being most efficient from the deltoids of the arms, and least from the buttocks. Easier to administer, the GI tract and first pass metabolism are avoided, a long-term effect from a single dose can be achieved.

Intradermal injection: The drug is injected into the skin raising a bleb (BCG vaccine sensitivity test). The aim is to localize the injection as much as possible in order to minimize more general effects and maximize the local effect (used in dentisty).

Subcutaneous route: The drug is administered in the loose subcutaneous tissue which is richly supplied by nerves (irritant drugs cannot be given) but is less vascular (absorption is slower than IM injection). Common sites for injection include the thigh or upper arm. The skin is pinched and the needle inserted so that the drug is administered under the layer of skin. Self injection is possible because deep penetration is not needed, i.e., insulin, local anesthesia, etc. This route should be avoided in shock patients who are vasoconstricted – absorption will be delayed.

Intrathecal injection: To achieve a high local concentration of a chemotherapeutic or antibacterial drug intrathecal injections can be given. It can be used for acute or intermittent treatment. In this method drug is directly administered into the CNS, thus by-passing blood-brain barrier. For example, sometimes epidural injection is used to alleviate the pain in labor.

CALCULATION OF DRUGS IN PEDIATRICS

Metric Units

- 1 g (g) = 1000 mg (milligrams)
- 1 mg (mg) = 1000 mcg (micrograms)
- 1 mcg = 1000 ng (nanograms)
- 1 lit = 1000 mL (milliliter)

Q. 1. Answer the following decimal unit questions.

i. 5 g = how many mg?
ii. 2575 mcg = how many mg?
iii. 800 mg = how many g?
iv. 0.25 mcg = how many nanograms?
v. 0.075L = how many mL?
vi. 850 mL = how many l?
vii. 0.05 mg = how many mcg?

Dosage Calculations

Pediatric dosage calculation is done by the child's body weight, i.e. mg/kg or mcg/kg.

Q. 2. A 5-year-old baby requires cefotaxime. The dosage is 50 mg/kg, the baby weighs 3.5 kg, what dose is required?

Calculation of Volume of Drug

Once the prescription is received the volume of drug is to be worked out for administration. Often the concentration of the drug is stated in fraction on the label of the drug. The straightforward for working this out is

$$\text{Volume needed} = \frac{\text{Desired dose} \times \text{The volume it is in}}{\text{Dose in hand}}$$

Example: A child requires PCM as pain relief. The dosage prescribed as 180 mg. The PCM comes as oral suspension 120 mg/5 mL.

- 180 mg = desired dose
- 120 mg = dose in hand
- 5 mL = the volume it is in

So the child needs the dose = 180/120 × 5 = 7.5 mL PCM

Q. 3. Ibuprofen 130 mg is to be given orally for pain relief. The stock mixture contains 100 mg in 5 mL.

i. What is the volume to be given?
ii. Prescription is oral phenobarbitone 45 mg. It is available as 50 mg/mL. What is the volume required?
iii. Metrogyl comes as 500 mg in 100 mL bottle. The child is prescribed 75 mg IV. What is the drug volume required?
iv Prescription was 200 mcg, and the drug comes as 5 mg in 5 mL. What volume is required?

(v) Postoperative child requires 0.5 mg drug. The IV drug is available as 250 mcg per mL. What volume is required?

Percentage of Drug Calculation

Drug calculations are not always stated as mg or mcg/mL, drug doses can also be prescribed in % (w/v).

Percentage means the weight of drug in gram dissolved in 100 mL of solution.

For example 1% (w/v) = 1 g in 100 mL.

Glucose 5% (w/v) means that 5 g of glucose is contained in 100 mL solution.

Prescription—A child is prescribed 5 g of mannitol; the supply of mannitol in the ward is 20% (w/v), how many mL is to be given to the child?

20% (w/v) = 20 g in 100 mL

The dose will be = 5 / 20 × 100 mL = 25 mL.

Q. 4.

i. What volume of 20% (w/v) potassium chloride injection contains 3 g of potassium chloride?
ii. Prescription is 2 g potassium chloride, which is to be added to a liter bag of NaCl 0.9%. The ampoules are 20% (w/v). What volume of potassium chloride will need to add to the bag?
iii. What concentration in mg/mL is 8.4% (w/v) sodium bicarbonate.
iv. What concentration in mcg/mL in 4.2% (w/v)?

Ratio Calculations

Ratio calculations are essential for measuring the concentration of drugs such as adrenaline. The dose of this drug is stated as 1 in 100, 1 in 10,000, etc.

One in something concentration means grams in mL.

It means 1 in 100 – 1 g in 100 mL
1 in 1000 – 1g in 1000 mL
1 in 10,000 – 1g in 10,000 mL

Prescription—Give 1 mg of adrenaline using 1 in 10,000 injection

1 in 10,000 = 1 g in 10,000 mL
= 1000 mg in 10,000

Desired dose = 1 mg
What in hand = 1000 mg
Volume it is in = 10,000 mL
1/1000 × 10,000 = 10 mL injection is to be administered

Q. 5.

i. Give 5 mg of adrenaline using 1 in 1000 injection.
ii. Give 0.5 mg of adrenaline using 1 in 10,000 injection.
iii. A newborn weighing 2 kg requires 30 mcg/kg of 1 in 10,000 mL of adrenaline.
iv. A child weighing 12 kg requires 10 mcg/kg of 1 in 10000 of adrenaline injection.
v. A child weighing 19 kg requires 100 mcg/kg of 1 in 1000 of adrenaline injection.

Normal Fluid Requirement of Child (Table 27.3)

Body weight	Fluid requirement for 24 hrs
10 kg	100 mL/kg/24 hrs
Next 10 kg	50 mL/kg/24 hrs
Further weight in kg	20mL/kg/24 hrs

Fluid requirement of a child of 30 kg

10 kg at the rate 100 mL = 1000 mL
10 kg at the rate 50 mL = 500 mL
10 kg at the rate 20 mL = 200 mL.

So total prescribed fluid in mL /hr = 1700/24 = 70 to 71 mL.

- If a child weighs below 5 kg (normally 1 month of age); the equation changes
  - For those below 5 kg full maintenance is 150 mL/kg/day.
- Full maintenance fluid over 24 hrs should not exceed 2 liter for girls or 2.5 liter for boys.
- In emergency situation, where weight of the child is unknown.
  - more than one year (age + 4) × 2 = estimated weight.
  - age less than one year (age in months +9) / 2 = estimated weight.

Q. 6.

i. A child weighing 15 kg requires full maintenance fluid, what would their fluid requirement be for 24 hrs?
ii. Calculate full maintenance fluid for 24 hrs for a child weighing 4 kg.
iii. A child weighing 28 kg requires full maintenance fluids, what would their fluid requirement be for 24 hrs?
iv. A child aged 4 years is admitted and requires full maintenance fluid, how much fluid is required over 24 hrs?
v. A child aged 8 months requires full maintenance fluid over 24 hrs. How much is required?
vi. For each of the above questions work out the child's maintenance fluid per hr.

Administration of Restricted Fluid

Sick child and administration of fluid is a most important aspect of pediatric nursing, delay in fluid therapy can be fatal. However, in some cases a smaller percentage of the full maintenance amount is required to prevent fluid overload. This is often the case of cardiac or neurological cases.

Example: A child with heart disease requires 75% of her full maintenance fluid. The child weighs 16 kg. What is her fluid requirement over 24 hrs?

- 10 kg at the rate × 100 mL = 1000 mL
- 6 kg at the rate × 50 mL = 300 mL.
- 1300 mL over 24 hrs. We need to work out 75% of 1300 mL.
- Multiply full maintenance fluid by the % asked for; then divide by 100.
- 1300 × 75 = 97500; then 97500/100 = 975 mL over 24 hrs.

Q. 7.

i. A child weighing 24 kg requires 60% of her full maintenance fluid, what is the amount required over 24 hrs?
ii. A child weighing 19 kg requires 80% of her full maintenance fluid, what is the amount required over 24 hrs?
iii. A child weighing 4 kg requires 75% of her full maintenance fluid, what is the amount required per hr?

Rehydrating the Sick Child

When children are admitted to hospital they have the potential to become, or are already dehydrated. Rehydration needs to be commenced quickly to prevent further problems.

When children are dehydrated they always receive full maintenance fluid over 24 hrs + the deficit (% of dehydration) over 48 hrs.

Deficit = % dehydration × child's weight × 10.

Example: A child weighing 18 kg is admitted with the history of diarrhea and vomiting for last 24 hrs, the child is very sick and is 10% dehydrated. What volume of fluid does this child require ?

Step one: Normal fluid requirement of 18 kg child is 1400 mL over 24 hrs (follow the basic rule).

Step two: Work out of child's deficit

- Dehydration = 10%
- Child's weight = 18 kg
- Deficit = 10 × 18 × 10 =1800 mL over 48 hrs.

Step three: Volume required per hr over 48 hrs

- Maintenance = 58.3 mL/hr
- Rehydration = 37.3 mL/hr
- Total = 95.6 mL/hr

It is important to note, if the child is acutely ill and needs emergency fluids then bolus 20 mL/kg can be given immediately. In cases of trauma it would be 10 mL/kg.

Answers of the above calculations are given below.

ADMINISTRATION OF DRUG AND FLUID: NURSING RESPONSIBILITIES

Nurses, because they administer the drugs directly to patients, are the last links in the safe medication administration chain. Because of the climate of health care today, nurses need to become cognizant of their practice's vulnerability and vigilant about protecting their practice. Before administration of drug nurses must :

- Have the knowledge (indications, contraindications, dose, interactions, adverse effects, route and knowledge of how to administer drug safely) skill, and judgement to assess the appropriateness of the medication for a particular patient.
- Know patient drug allergies.

Nurses Need to Assess

- The developmental stage of the infant or child or adolescent patient.
- Any alterations in the infant or child or adolescent's condition or functional status which interferes with the physical capacity to take oral medications.
- The child and family's level of understanding, knowledge of each medication and their readiness to assume self or parent medication administration.
- As precaution nurses should inspect prescription medication carefully. All prescription medications should be in their original, include the following:
  - The child's first and last name
  - The physician's signature
  - The date of expiry on the container.

All nurses have been taught the five 'Rights' of medication administration. The right patient, the right drug, the right dose, the right route and the right time form the foundation from which nurse practices safely when administrating medications to all patients in all health care settings. Five more 'R's have been added recently by the hospitals and medical groups which includes:

1. The rights of the parents and child to know
2. The right to monitor
3. The right to documentation

4. The right in evaluation
5. The right to refuse.

Pediatric drug administration means drugs are administered in smaller, but more frequent doses as there is physiological difference between adult and child. Dosages are weight-based in milligrams, micrograms or milli-equivalents per kilogram, which allows for much safer drug administration. Thus, as part of nurses' assessment, determine the patient's weight. When the child's weight is unknown and cannot be reasonably estimated, use a height-based scale to make an estimate.

Once the child's weight has been determined, multiply the weight by the dose per kilogram for the drug you need to administer. Pediatric doses for commonly given drugs are to be listed in the nurses' station. If nurses do not have the doses memorized, be sure to confirm them prior to administration with an accurate source like a drug reference, pocket guide, Broselow tape or online medical control can also be availed.

Based on the simple, visual system of Dr James Broselow, invented a medication reference tool that eliminates errors in medication preparation and administration. The Broselow tape and Pedi-Wheels are tools to estimate patient weight based on age and height. Both also provide calculated dosages for common drugs administered to critically-ill pediatric patients. A reference at each color bar on the tape informs you of the proper equipment sizes to perform emergency resuscitation on a child. A reference at each weight zone on the tape shows pre-calculated medication dosages. The doctors and nurses can access standard procedures and algorithms (PALS).

Fluid Administration

Pediatric physicians prefer IV fluids containing dextrose, such as D5 in one-half normal saline, for fluid maintenance. When volume resuscitation is required, fluid boluses are determined by administering 20 mL of an isotonic crystalloid per kilogram of body weight. In addition to any needed fluid bolus, double the infusion rates when dehydration is suspected. If an isolated brain injury is suspected, cut the infusion rate by one-half. rule of 6s in administering IV fluid.

Most IV drug infusions come in standardized concentrations and are available in premixed bags. However, the need may occasionally arise when a premixed infusion is not available and nurses need to mix their own. In that case, consider using the rule of 6's to prepare administration of any IV infusions, particularly with vasoactive drugs like dopamine. The rule of 6s has 6 steps and 1 multiplication by 6.

1. First, determine the patient's body weight in kilograms. For this example, say the patient weighs 20 kilograms and dopamine is the drug to be administered.
2. Determine the amount of drug needed by multiplying the patient's weight in kilograms by 6 (this 6 is what creates the rule of 6's). For example, 20 times 6 is 120, so you need 120 mg of drug.
3. Mix the quantity of drug determined in Step 2 in a 100 mL bag of normal saline or D5W. Label the bag with the name of the drug you added, the quantity and the resulting concentration.
4. Connect a 60-drop infusion set to the mixed bag, so every 1 drop per minute, or 1 mL per hr, administered is exactly 1 mcg/kg/min for the patient.
5. Determine the drug dose to be administered. The starting dose for dopamine is 5 mcg/kg/min. With this mixed infusion set, five drops per minute administers 5 mcg/kg/min.
6. For each microgram per kilogram per minute increase in drug dose, increase the drip rate by 1 drop/min. Remember, each drop per minute equals 1 mL/hr.

Pediatric Pain Management

Children do not always, and sometimes cannot, tell that they are experiencing pain, yet ill children are at high risk for pain. Management of pediatric patient pain is not only difficult , but is unfortunately complicated by failing to assess or under assessing pediatric patient pain, which has led to many myths, including:

- Infants cannot feel pain.
- Children experience less pain than adults.
- Children will tell you when they feel pain.
- Children recover more quickly than adults from pain.
- Narcotics are dangerous and always cause respiratory depression in children.

A few guides have been developed to help identify pain in children. The Wong-Baker faces scale is a reliable tool to evaluate pain in children older than age 3 years. Use the scale to ask the child, 'Can you show me which face looks like how you are feeling right now?' Observe the child to see which face he or she selects and document the corresponding number beneath each face as the patient's pain level.

Table 27.3: Pediatric IV fluid calculation

Body weight (kg)	*Daily fluid requirement*	*Fluid administration rate*
<10	100 mL/kg	4 mL/kg/hr
10 to 20	1000 mL + 50 mL/kg for each kg over 10	40 mL/hr + 2 mL/hr for each kg over 10
>20	1500 mL + 20 mL/kg for each kg over 20	60 mL/hr + 1 mL/kg/hr for each kg over 20

Table 27.4: FLACC pain scale

Behavioral observation pain rating scale			
Categories	*Scoring*		
	0	1	2
Face	No particular expression or smile; disinterested	Occasional grimace or frown, withdrawn	Frequent to constant frown, clenched jaw, quivering chin
Legs	No position or relaxed	Uneasy, restless, tense	Kicking, or legs drawn up
Activity	Lying quietly normal position, moves easily	Squirming, shifting back and forth, tense	Arched, rigid, or jerking
Cry	No crying (awake or asleep)	Moans or whimpers, occasional complaint	Crying steadily, screams or sobs, frequent complaints
Consolability	Content, relaxed	Reassured by occasional touching, hugging, or talking to, Distractable	Difficult to console or comfort

Each of the 5 categories (F) Face; (L) Legs; (A) Activity; (C) Cry; (C) Consolability is scored from 0 to 2, which results in a total score between 0 and 10.

The FLACC scale is an objective way to measure a child's pain when he is unable to verbally tell you the amount of pain he is in (Table 27.4). FLACC stands for face, legs, activity, cry and consolability. Each component is evaluated and scored 0 to 2. By totaling each category, the scale gives a score of 0 to 10, with 10 being the worst pain and zero the least. Another pain rating scale is Wong-Baker faces pain rating scale, which can be used to assess pain of a child (Fig. 27.2).

There are many nonpharmacologic tools available to manage pain and always document the pain control measures provided. Pharmacologic pain control begins with oxygen. Acetaminophen is a centrally acting analgesic that is safe and easy to administer to children. Acetaminophen is given in a dose of 10 to 15 mg/kg, with noticeable effects usually seen within about 15 to 20 minutes. It is available in both tablet and liquid-drop form. Another benefit of acetaminophen is that it can be administered via rectal suppository if there is concern the patient should not have anything by mouth, such as when surgery may be necessary.

Aggressive pain management is recommended for any wound, fracture or dislocation, and burns. Opioids are a good and acceptable first-line drug for pediatric pain

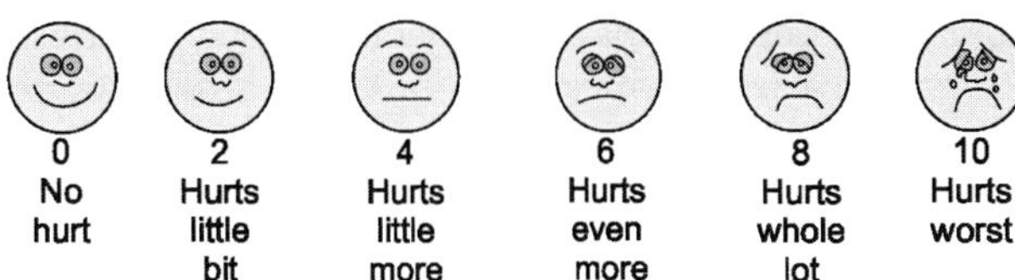

Fig. 27.2: Wong-Baker faces pain rating scale

management. Fentanyl and morphine are 2 commonly administered prehospital pain drugs. Fentanyl is dosed at 1 to 2 mcg/kg and can be given every 20 minutes. Morphine is administered 0.1 to 0.2 mg/kg and can be given every 5 minutes. Both have side effects. Fentanyl can cause chest rigidity when given too rapidly, and morphine can cause respiratory depression in high doses.

Following administration of any medication, -especially analgesics, careful ongoing monitoring is essential. Close attention to the child's pulse oximetry and level of consciousness is important. Sedation may occur, presence of which is to be documented. Vital signs should be documented at least every 15 minutes, and more frequently for unstable patients and those with mental status changes. As part of vital signs, document the patient's pain level.

Adverse Drug Reaction

Adverse drug reactions (ADRs) are a major health problem to the individual as well as for society. Adverse drug reaction is an event that is noxious and unintended and occurs at doses in humans for prophylaxis, diagnosis, therapy or for the modification of physiologic function (WHO). This definition excludes intentional or deliberate overdose and drug abuse. Adverse drug reactions impose significant burdens on hospitals through prolonging patient stay, increase admission rates and financial burden of family.

A wide range of drugs has been reported as being involved in ADRs in children. These include antibiotics, NSAIDs, glucocorticoids, anti-tuberculosis drug, immunosuppressive agents, antituberculosis, vaccines.

Age—Infants and very young children are at high risk of developing adverse drug reactions than adults as their drug metabolizing capacity is not fully developed like adult. Gray baby syndrome, a serious/fatal reaction is developed if chloramphenicol is administered to newborn; who cannot metabolize and eliminate this drug.

Drug-disease interaction refers to the worsening of a disease by a drug. Most drugs exert most of their effects on a specific organ or systems; however, because most drugs circulate throughout the body, they may also affect other organs and systems. A drug taken for a lung disease may affect the heart, and a drug taken to treat a cold may affect the eyes. Because drugs can affect diseases other than the one being treated, parents or caregivers should inform their doctor all diseases the child has before he prescribes new drug.

A greater understanding about predictors and management systems is needed to institute quality assurance procedures to ensure ADR incidence is minimized. Adverse drug reactions are global problems affecting children in both developing and developed countries. A higher level of clinical suspicion and vigilance, good knowledge of the predisposing factors, and proper monitoring of at-risk drugs in at-risk patients may help prevent ADRs, thus reducing its global incidence.

CONCLUSION

Administering drugs to pediatric patients is safe when their unique physiological and anatomical differences are considered. Use weight-based dosing to administer smaller, more frequent doses. Also remember that pediatric patients do indeed feel pain, and they deserve the same aggressive pain management as adults. Utilize both pharmacologic and nonpharmacologic techniques when providing pain management.

Answers of above mentioned drug calculations

Q. 1	Q. 2	Q. 3	Q. 4	Q. 5	Q. 6	Q. 7
i. 5000 mg ii. 2.575 mg iii. 0.8 g iv. 250 nanogram v. 75 mL vi. 0.85 L vii. 50 mcg	175 mg	i. 6.5 mL ii. b. 0.9 mL iii. c. 15 mL iv. 0.2 mL v. e. 2 mL	i. 15 mL ii. 10 mL iii. 84 mL iv. 42000 mcg	i. 15 mL ii. 5 mL iii. 0.6 mL iv. 1.2 mL iv. 1.9 mL	vi. 1250 mL to 52 mL/hr vii. 600 mL to 25 mL/hr viii. 1660 mL to 69.2 mL/hr ix. 1300 mL to 54.2 mL/hr x. 850 mL to 35.4 mL/hr	i. 948 mL ii. 1160 mLs iii. 18.75mLs/hr

CHAPTER 28

High-risk Newborn

Chapter Outline

- Concept, Goal, Assessment, Principles of High-risk Newborn Care
- Apnea

CONCEPT, GOAL, ASSESSMENT, PRINCIPLES OF HIGH-RISK NEWBORN CARE

According to medical dictionary, high-risk infant can be defined as any neonate, regardless of birth weight, size, or gestational age, who has a greater than average chance of morbidity or mortality, specially within the first 28 days of life. Risk factors include preconceptual, prenatal, natal, or postnatal conditions or circumstances that interfere with the normal birth process or impede adjustment to extrauterine growth and development.

In most cases, the infant is the outcome of a pregnancy involving one or more predictable risk factors, including the following:

- Low socioeconomic level of the mother, poor nutrition.
- Exposure to poor environmental conditions such as toxic chemicals.
- Preexisting maternal morbidity such as heart disease, diabetes.
- Obstetric factors such as age or parity, other premature births.

Goals

The goals of care of high-risk newborn are:

- Perinatal prevention
- Resuscitation and stabilization
- Evaluate and manage
- Monitoring and therapeutic modalities
- Family-centered care.

The ultimate aim of the nursing care of the high-risk newborn is to ensure a physiologically stable infant, and to prepare the family who can provide the necessary care with appropriate support services in the community.

Assessment

Following birth, the average healthy newborn undergoes three predictable periods of responsiveness:

- *A period of reactivity:* In the first 15–60 minutes after birth, the normal infant will be highly responsive to many different stimuli. There is a lot sniffing, grimacing, sucking, chewing, crying, hiccupping and trembling.
- *A relatively unresponsive interval:* The next 60 minutes are characterized by a lack of responsiveness and a lower rate of metabolism although there may be a few spontaneous jerks during sleep.
- *A second period of reactivity:* Between 2–6 hours, responsiveness returns and there may be periods of rapid respiration, gagging and vomiting and the passing of meconium. Newborns continue to be very responsive during this period.

Initial assessment (first period of reactivity and second period of reactivity); clinical assessment; transitional assessment; behavioral assessment; physical assessment; reflexes [discussed in new born chapter 5].

Understanding these distinct periods of reactivity will help nurse with initial expectations. Early identification and prompt management are imperative in treating newborns with complications. Medical conditions related to pregnancy such as PIH, premature rupture of membranes, infection, etc. are to be explored and prompt management to be done.

Classification of High-risk Infants

- Classification according to gestational age:
  - *Preterm:* Infants born before completion of 37 weeks gestation.

- *Term:* Infants born between the 38 and 42 weeks gestation.
- *Postterm:* Infants born after 42 weeks gestation.

- Classification according to gestational age and birth weight:
  - *Large for gestational age (LGA):* Infant at any week the weight is above the 90th percentile.
  - *Appropriate for gestational age (AGA):* Infant at any week the weight is between the 10th and 90th percentile.
  - *Small for gestational age (SGA):* Infant at any week the weight is below the 10th percentile.

Nursing Management of Premature Infant

The preterm infant must travel the same complex pathway from intrauterine to extrauterine life as the term infant. The preterm neonate is unable to make this transition as smoothly, because of immaturity.

Small for Gestational Age (SGA)

Body weight of the baby is < 10th percentile compared to others of same gestational age. There is IUGR and failure to thrive viz. 38 week. weighs 5 lbs. Most common cause is placental anomaly; placenta not receiving sufficient nutrition from uterine arteries or placenta. Severe diabetic mellitus, preeclampsia, poor nutrition, smoking, cocaine; decreases blood flow to placenta. Fundal height is lower than expected for gestational age. General appearance in SGA infant: wasted look, in SGA, neuro responses are mature. Despite their size, SGA infants have physical characteristics (e.g. skin appearance, ear cartilage, sole creases) and behavior (e.g. alertness, spontaneous activity, zest for feeding) similar to those of normal-sized infants of like gestational age. However, IUGR child (Fig. 28.1) may appear thin with decreased muscle mass and subcutaneous fat tissue and excess skin folds on the buttocks and thighs. Facial features may appear sunken, resembling those of an elderly person ('wizened facies'). Other features are dull hair, small liver, poor skin turgor, low glucose, low temperature and the umbilical cord can appear thin.

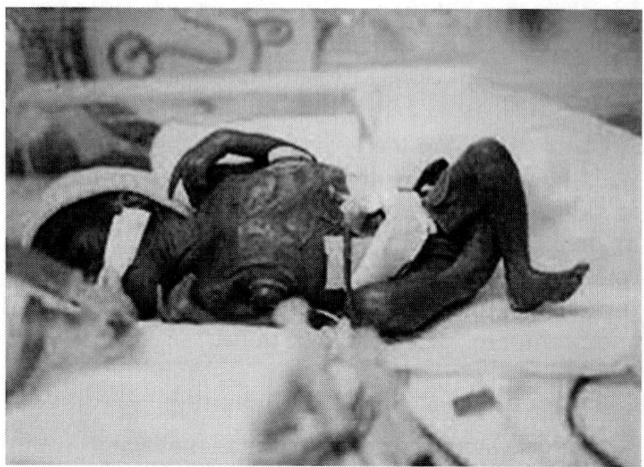

Fig. 28.1: Intrauterine growth retardation (IUGR) baby

Asymmetrical IUGR

- Probably it occurs during last part of gestation.
- Head circumference is more (generally about 3 cm) than chest circumference.
- Growth restriction due to placental insufficiency.
- Prognosis is good with nutritional intervention.

Symmetrical small fetus

- These neonates are constitutionally small fetus.
- It occurs due to genetic syndrome or chromosomal abnormalities.
- Very early onset of IUGR.
- Prognosis is poor, with permanent mental and physical growth retardation.

Ponderal Index

Ponderal index (PI) (fetal weight in grams × 100 / (fetal length in centimeters). PI is one of the anthropometric methods used to diagnose impaired fetal growth. Irrespective of the infant's position on the growth-weight-for-gestational age charts, PI is low in malnourished infants and high in obese ones. In asymmetric IUGR, PI lies in less than 2. PI more than 2 indicates symmetric IUGR. PI more than 2.5 indicates term AGA neonate.

Lab Findings

High hematocrit level (polycythemia): It causes thicker blood making heart work harder; increased chance of thrombosis. Prolonged acrocyanosis. Monitoring fetal growth scan (biometry), measure the amniotic fluid, evaluate the blood flows, Dopplers (notching indicates a high-risk pregnancy).

Management

Care should either be provided for in a nursery at a temperature greater than 24 °C or, for very small babies, in an incubator at a temperature of 26 to 32 °C and humidity 65 to 75%.

Hypoglycemia is common in asymmetrical SGA babies because their larger brains burn calories at a faster rate than their usually limited fat stores hold. Hypoglycemia is treated by frequent feedings and fluid or additions of cornstarch-based products (such as Duocal powder) to the feedings.

90% of babies born SGA catch up in growth by the age of 2 years. However, all SGA babies should be watched for signs of failure-to-thrive (FTT).

Underlying conditions and complications are treated. There is no specific intervention for the SGA state, but prevention is aided by prenatal advice on the importance of avoiding alcohol, tobacco, and illicit drugs.

Preterm Infant (24 to 36 Weeks)

Preterm is defined as babies born alive before 37 weeks of pregnancy are completed. According to WHO, preterm birth is the most common direct cause of newborn mortality. Preterm birth and being small for gestational age (SGA), which are the reasons for low-birth-weight (LBW), are also important indirect causes of neonatal deaths. LBW contributes to 60 to 80% of all neonatal deaths. The global prevalence of LBW is 15.5%, which amounts to about 20 million LBW infants born each year, 96.5% of them in developing countries. About 10 to 12% of Indian babies are born before 37 weeks of gestation. They are vulnerable to various physiological limitations with high mortality rate due to their anatomical and functional immaturity.

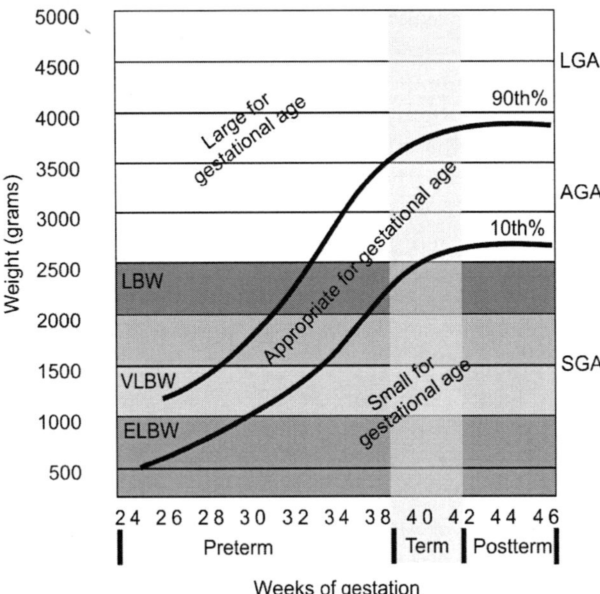

Fig. 28.2: Growth chart

Category of Preterm

There are subcategories of preterm birth, based on gestational age (Fig. 28.2):

- Extremely preterm (<28 weeks).
- Very preterm (28 to <32 weeks).
- Moderate to late preterm (32 to <37 weeks).

Induction or cesarean birth should not be planned before 39 completed weeks unless medically indicated. (WHO).

Characteristics

Small, underdeveloped, head disproportionately large with large fontanelles; skin thin and ruddy [little subcutaneous fat]; veins noticeable; prolonged acrocyanosis. Vernix depends on gestational age.

- < 24 weeks vernix not formed.
- None or few sole creases.
- Ear cartilage immature; no quick rebound of pinna.
- Extensive lanugo.
- Suck or swallow absent, weak cry < 33 weeks. Ballard gestational scale to estimate age.
- Poor general activity, with sluggish or incomplete neonatal reflexes. Extended limbs due to hypotonia.
- Eyes remain closed and protruding as due to shallow orbits.
- *Infection:* Decreased maternal antibodies.
- Skin is shiny, fragile; edema may present.
- Breast nodules are absent or less than 5 mm and nipples and areola are flat.
- Abdomen is full, round with prominent veins.
- *Genitalia:* In female baby the labia minora is exposed due to poorly developed labia majora and clitoris hypertrophied and prominent. In male baby undescended testes, poorly pigmented with less rugosities.

Physiological Characteristics of Preterm Neonates

- Respiratory system
  - Insufficient production of surfactant -incomplete aeration of lungs.
  - Immaturity of alveolar system—smaller lumen, greater collapsibility of respiratory passages.
  - Immaturity of musculature and insufficient calcification of bony thorax.
  - This condition leads to respiration like rapid, shallow, irregular with cyanosis and periods of apnea in preterm child. Breathing is mostly diaphragmatic, respirations 40 to 60/min. Prone to respiratory distress.
- Central nervous system
  - Poor muscle tone—muscles appear limp, flaccid, assumes frog-like position at rest. Muscles weak and underdeveloped.

- Cry—weak and feeble.
- Reflexes—weak and immature, slow to respond to stimulation.
- Susceptibility to brain damage.

- Impaired thermoregulation

  The preterm babies are prone to develop hypothermia due to poorly developed heat regulating center.
  - Body temperature may be normal but it fluctuates; small muscle mass; absent sweat or shiver response.
  - Large body surface in proportion to body weight.
  - Lack of subcutaneous fat.
  - Poor capillary response to environmental changes.
- Digestive system
  - Gag and suck reflexes may be weak and poorly developed may lead to poor intake of feeds. Hypotonic cardiac sphincter. Increase chance of regurgitation and aspiration. These neonates are prone to malnutrition, iron deficiency anemia and deficiency of vitamin A, D, E, K due to poor absorption of nutrients.
  - Suck and swallow reflexes may be uncoordinated.
  - Small stomach capacity—2mL In 1200 g. 15 mL in 2000 g baby.
  - Vomiting more likely to occur.
  - Digestion of protein and carbohydrate is adequate but fat is poorly absorbed.
  - Immature absorption, decreased amounts of HCl.
  - Abdominal distension and functional intestinal obstruction are found due to hypotonia.
- Integumentary system
  - Skin thin and capillaries easily seen, reddened and translucent.
  - Little subcutaneous fat.
  - Lanugo plentiful, widely distributed.
  - Vernix may cover body is born between 31 and 33 weeks.
  - Ears—minimal cartilage, pliable, folded over.
- Immune system

  Preterm neonates are 3 to 10 times more vulnerable to infection due to following reasons:
  - They lack of passive immunity from mother; deficient placental transmission.
  - Inability to produce own antibodies—immature system.
  - Skin is thin and offers little protection from disease causing organisms.
  - Inefficient cellular immunity. Number of WBCs is decreased and therefore have decreased ability to phagocytize bacteria. Low IgG antibody level make them more susceptible to infections.
- Hepatic system
  - Poor glycogen stores—increased susceptibility to hypoglycemia.
  - Inability to conjugate bilirubin—increase hyperbilirubinemia.
  - Decrease ability to produce clotting factors, low plasma prothrombin levels leads to hemorrhagic disease.
- Circulatory system
  - Capillary fragility increases susceptibility to hemorrhage, specially intracranial. Leads to increase bilirubin levels.
  - The closure of ductus arteriosus may be delayed.
  - Intracranial hemorrhage may occur due to poor autoregulation of cerebral blood flow.
  - Prone to anemia—poor iron stores.
- Renal system
  - Renal function immature due to poor GFR and poor ability to concentrate urine.
  - Fluid and electrolyte and acid-base balance precarious.
  - Dehydration may occur due to inability to conserve water.
- Drug toxicity
  - Impaired renal clearance and poor hepatic detoxification lead to toxic effects of drugs unless proper precautions are followed during administration.
  - Oxygen administration in preterm neonates needs special precaution as higher concentration of oxygen with prolong administration constrict the retinal arteries results anoxic damage and retinal detachment, termed as retrolental-fibroplasias.

Management

Preterm birth is a risk factor for cardiorespiratory maladaptation and the need for resuscitation.

The lower the gestational age, the greater the need for assistance and the skill required of the staff who manage the neonate.

Births at less than about 34 weeks should be attended by someone with up-to-date skills in endotracheal intubation.

For births at less than 32 weeks this should ideally be attended by neonatologist for prompt management.

The equipments and procedures that can be used to monitor the physiological status of the high-risk neonates include the following:

Thermoregulation: These should aim at maintaining body temperature with minimal increased energy consumption by the infant. Maintenance of a controlled thermal environment is to be done by the use of radiant warmers or incubators.

Monitoring of heart rate, respiratory rate and blood pressure is to be done. Sometimes a pulse rate indicator is used that signals when pulse rate goes beyond predetermined limit (usually above 160 beats/min or below 80 beats/min).

Maintenance of respiration: Apnea monitors are used to register respiratory activity. This equipment can monitor both heart rate and respiratory activity through alarm system. Assess respiratory effort, respiration rate, rhythm, signs of distress, chest retraction, nasal flaring. Apnea, cyanosis, oxygen saturation, etc. are to be monitored at frequent interval. Child may need intubation to maintain respirations. Oxygen therapy should be given when it is indicated. Concentration of oxygen is to be maintained to have SaO_2 between 90 to 92% and PaO_2 between 60 to 80 mmHg.

Collection of specimens is needed for continuous monitoring of the physiological state of the high-risk neonate. The tests include blood glucose, hematocrit, bilirubin, calcium and blood gases.

Urinary elimination: Children have high insensible water loss due to large body surface compared with total body weight. Lower GFR occurs in high-risk neonates due to immature kidneys. Strict I/O is needed to avoid fluid overload or dehydration.

Immature kidneys secrete glucose slowly > hyperglycemia can result.

Insensible water loss [Approximate water loss in body]	
• Age group	Water
• Premature infant	90%
• Newborn infant	70 to 80%
• 12 to 24 months	64%
• Adult	60%

General Nursing Management

Maintenance of Body Temperature

The high-risk newborn whose weight is less than normal has difficulty in maintaining normal body temperature because:

- Risk for hypothermia related to large surface in relation to body weight.
- Limited stores of brown fat.
- Decreased or absent reflex control of skin capillaries.
- Immature temperature regulation in brain.
- Lack of flexion of the extremities increases the exposure of the total body surface to the environment.

Due to these above reasons, the infant cannot physiologically respond with cold stress by shivering. Instead, heat is produced by nonshivering thermogenesis, i.e. through increased metabolic activity. The external thermal gradient is the difference between the environmental temperature and the infant's skin temperature. Heat is transferred between the infant's body and the environment by evaporation, radiation, conduction, and convection. So to conserve the body heat of neonates is one of the most important nursing responsibilities.

The provision of neutral thermal environment is important in high-risk newborn care as it permits the maintenance of a normal core temperature in an infant whose oxygen consumption and metabolic rate at rest are minimal. The child without clothing is placed in neutral thermal environment, generally in an incubator. The thermal environment is adjusted so that an abdominal skin temperature over the epigastrium is maintained at 36.5 °C (97.7 °F). The high-risk infant may be cared for in a radiant warmer if incubator is not available. But the maintenance of normal core temperature may be difficult to maintain because of airflow in the nursery, heat is lost through convection. Moreover, a problem may arise because insensible water loss is much greater when a radiant heat unit is used than when the infant is in an incubator. Water losses are most significant in the tiniest infant (discussed above), and intravenous fluids may be necessary to maintain the required level of hydration. Sometimes thermal environment is created with any one of the methods like hot water bag, use of plastic sheet, use of plastic bubble wrap, goose neck lamp, etc.

Prevention of Infection and Injury

Nosocomial infection, that could spread to the nursery can be prevented by:

- Meticulous and thorough hand washing by all persons entering into the nursery is must.
- Complete sterilization or disinfection of equipment and supplies.

The rules concerning hand washing may vary in institutions. In general, during entering into the nursery the hands should be washed for at least 2 minutes to above the elbows. Washing for at least 15 seconds should also be done between caring for different infants.

Usually soap or iodinated solution is used for hand wash. Iodinated preparation is active against gram-negative rods and gram-positive cocci, but they may cause sensitivity reactions to some persons. The containers of this lotion are also to be sterilized periodically. All equipment and linens that come in contact with the infants must be scrupulously clean and sterile.

Nutrition

Promote normal growth and development:

- Tries to maintain rapid rate of intrauterine growth.
- Lack of cough reflex: can aspirate formula.
- Have weak sucking, swallowing, gag reflexes
- Weak abdominal muscles; weak gag reflex
- Aspiration risk is high
- High BMR—High caloric needs but small stomach capacity
- Limited store of nutrients
- Decreased ability to digest proteins and absorb nutrients, and immature enzyme systems.
- TPN, PPN, Gavage, or IV feedings.

Feeding

- Caloric requirement of preterm: 95 to 130 kcal/kg/day.
- Term infant: 100 to 110.
- Smaller stomach capacity: Small, frequent feedings (2 to 3 hourly).
- *Formula:* Calories for preterm 24 cal/oz. Term: 20 cal/oz.
- Breast milk good due to immunologic properties.
- *Gavage:* Nasogastric/orogastric. Gag reflex not intact till infant 32 weeks; avoid over filling stomach; may cause respiratory distress.
- *Fluid requirement of newborn child:* Requirement of fluid of LBW neonates depends on body weight of the baby (Table 28.1).

Developmentally Supportive Activities

Kangaroo care/skin-to-skin care is important for these children.

Nonnutritive Sucking: Nonnutritive at the breast (pacifer) improves milk production; provides sucking experience; prepares infant for breastfeeding. Long-term effects: increased length of exclusive breastfeeding; increased length of total breastfeeding.

Skin care: Limit alcohol; rinse with water. Adhesives cause skin tearing. Use skin barriers to protect skin. Tegaderm tape. Hand washing is must.

Table 28.1: Requirement of fluid of LBW neonates (mL/kg/day)

Day	*Less than 1000 g*	*1000 to 1500 g*	*More than 1500 g*
1st and 2nd	100 to 120	80 to 100	60 to 80
3rd and 4th	130 to 140	110 to 120	90 to 100
5th and 6th	150 to 160	130 to 140	110 to 120
7th and 8th	170 to 180	150 to 160	130 to 140
9th onwards	190 to 200	170 to 180	150 to 160

Parent and family education and support: The involvement of family members other than the mother in establishing relationships with an infant in the NICU is recommended.

Large for Gestational Age (LGA)/ Postmature Infant

LGA newborns are those whose weights are above 90th percentile in intrauterine growth chart. By far, maternal diabetes is the most common cause of LGA babies. Diabetes during pregnancy causes the mother's increased blood glucose (sugar) to circulate to the baby. In response, the baby's body makes insulin. All the extra sugar and the extra insulin production can lead to excessive growth and deposits of fat, thus, a larger baby. Elective cesarean section is intended to prevent several of the complications associated with fetal macrosomia, specially brachial plexus injuries and maternal perineal lacerations. Appears healthy; may be gestationally immature (immature neuro responses and respiratory effort).

Assessment

Larger than average uterine size for gestational age, possible flexed clavicles; facial/head bruising, facial/neck palsy, caput, cephalohematoma. Observe: hypoglycemia, polycythemia, irregular heart rate, cyanosis [in transposition].

Symptoms and Complications

Symptoms depend on which complications occur. Common complications include the following:

- *Polycythemia:* LGA newborns may have a ruddy complexion because too many red blood cells are produced. As the excess red blood cells are broken down, bilirubin is formed, which, along with poor feeding, results in jaundice.

- *Hypoglycemia:* In newborns of mothers with diabetes, the oversupply of glucose from the placenta stops abruptly at delivery when the umbilical cord is cut and the continuing rapid production of insulin by the newborn's pancreas leads to hypoglycemia. Often hypoglycemia causes no symptoms. Sometimes, newborns are listless, limp, or jittery.
- *Lung problems:* Lung development is delayed in newborns whose mothers have diabetes. When these newborns are delivered by cesarean, they are at risk of developing lung problems. Newborns born prematurely are more likely to have immature lungs and to develop respiratory distress syndrome, even when born only a few weeks before full term.
- *Increased risk of birth injuries:* Newborns who are LGA are at increased risk of birth injuries such as stretching of the nerves in the shoulder (brachial plexus injuries) and collarbone (clavicle) fractures. Therefore, such a fetus may have to be delivered by cesarean.

Infants whose mother has diabetes also have a higher rate of birth defects than other newborns. LGA newborns born to mothers with diabetes are likely to be significantly overweight later in childhood and as adults.

Management

To treat hypoglycemia in newborns, glucose given intravenously or frequent feedings by mouth or by tube into the stomach are often needed. Treatment of respiratory distress syndrome may require supplemental oxygen through a tube placed in the nose or intense intervention, such as respiratory support with a ventilator. Other complications may also require treatment, such as phototherapy for jaundice.

Respiratory Conditions

Asphyxia Neonatorum

WHO–Birth asphyxia: A failure to initiate and sustain breathing at birth.

NNF–Moderate asphyxia: Slow gasping breaths or an Apgar score of 4 to 6 at 1 minute of age.

Severe asphyxia: No breathing or an Apgar score of 0 to 3 at 1 minute of age.

Asphyxia neonatorum is also known as perinatal asphyxia, hypoxic-ischemic encephalopathy, or birth asphyxia. It can be fatal. Causes of asphyxia neonatorum include:

Antepartum: Mother's age is below 16 years or more than 40 years.

Maternal illnesses, such as diabetes, hypertension, Rh-sensitization, severe anemia, poor obstetrical history, placental malformations, maternal drug therapy (with lithium, reserpine, magnesium), drug abuse by mother.

Intrapartum

- Compromised fetus who cannot tolerate transient, intermittent hypoxia of normal labor.
- The baby's airway becomes blocked. The umbilical cord becomes improperly wrapped around the baby.
- The baby is anemic and his or her blood cells do not carry enough oxygen.
- Delivery that lasts too long or is very difficult.
- The mother does not get enough oxygen before or during birth.
- The placenta separates from the uterus too quickly, resulting in loss of oxygen.

Babies who lose oxygen before, during, or after delivery can experience asphyxia neonatorum in one of two ways. The first is immediate damage due to lack of oxygen, which can happen within minutes. The second is when the cells recover from lack of oxygen and the damaged cells release toxins into the body. Asphyxia neonatorum is characterized as progressive hypoxia, hypercapnia and hypoperfusion and metabolic acidosis (pH less than 7).

Pathophysiology

Birth asphyxia is described as a condition that occurs when a baby fails to initiate and maintain respiration; which leads to hypoventilation, aerobic to anaerobic metabolism, glycolysis and lactic acidosis. Baby fails to cry, an attempt is made to breathe, but there is primary gasps and subsequent raise in heartbeat and blood pressure. After 1 minute there is primary apnea. It there is no resuscitation, there will be secondary gasps, a flat heartbeat and a rapid drop in blood pressure and in 5 to 8 minutes slight brain damage begins. there will be long gasps and long apneas and the baby will be acidotic due to low levels of pH in the blood, hypoxia and hypercapnea. Brain damage becomes more severe, there is cerebral edema and rupture of small blood vessels resulting in cerebral hemorrhage. There is ischemia of brain cells resulting in severe brain damage. Signs are convulsions, inability to suck, baby is more flaccid, cerebral palsy. Death then follows as a result of failure to resuscitate.

Clinical Features

The symptoms of asphyxia neonatorum are:

- Bluish or gray skin color (cyanosis).
- Slow heartbeat.
- Apnea or bradycardia. Altered respiratory pattern - gasping and grunting.
- Stiff or limp limbs (hypotonia), and a poor response to stimulation.

Management

The need for neonatal resuscitation at birth cannot always be anticipated or predicted. At every birth, no matter how 'low-risk', suitable equipment and staff must be available and prepared to resuscitate the newborn infant. Considering every birth is high-risk, neonatal resuscitation skills are essential for all health care providers who are involved in the delivery of newborns. Newborn resuscitation is a critical skill that requires constant practice. 10% of newborns require resuscitation. Perinatal asphyxia and extreme prematurity are the 2 complications of pregnancy that most frequently necessitate complex resuscitation by skilled personnel. Effective ventilation is the key to successful resuscitation.

Basic resuscitation of newborn is called TABC's of resuscitation which includes:

T. provide warmth. Wrap the child with warm towels under heat source. The steps are drying the baby and removing the wet linens and place the baby under radiant heat source.

- Establishment of an open airway. Position the baby, suction mouth, nose. In case of meconium stained liquor, trachea is suctioned and endotracheal tube is inserted to ensure open airway.
- Initiation of breathing. Tactile stimulation is given to initiate respiration. PPV (positive pressure ventilation), using either bag and mask or bag and ET tube.
- Maintenance of circulation. Stimulate and maintain blood circulation by chest compression and or medications (Fig. 28.3).

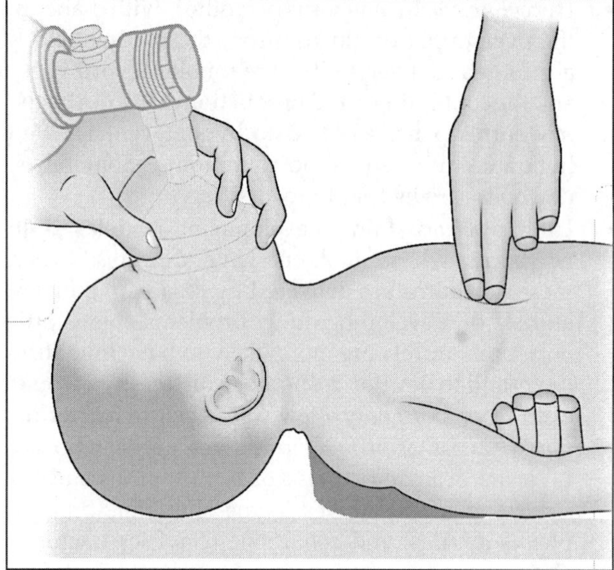

Fig. 28.3: Cardio pulmonary resuscitation of asphyxiated baby

Clear Airway

- Dry, stimulate, reposition.
- Evaluation includes.
- Signs: Respiration, heart rate, color.
- *Apgar score is not a prerequisite.*
- Resuscitation success.
- Anticipation.
- Adequate preparation.
- Timely evaluation.
- Quick and correct action.
- Preparation—warm towels, suction devices, self-inflating bags, masks, radiant heater, clock.
- Meconium aspiration syndrome.

Prevention

- Oropharyngeal suctioning of infant > delivery.
- Laryngoscopic visualizaiton of vocal cords > intubation.
- Additional suctioning of trachea.
- *Amnioinfusion:* Dilutes meconium. Thins out particulate meconium. Do sepsis workup; CBC, bl.cx., chest X-ray. AB therapy to prevent pneumonia.

Meconium Aspiration Syndrome

- Present in fetal bowel as early as 10 weeks. Infant may aspirate meconium in utero or with 1st breath.
- Can cause severe respiratory distress, inflammation or blockage of small bronchioles by mechanical plugging.
- Ductus arteriosus may remain open; causes blood to shunt from pulmonary artery to aorta instead of passing through lungs [high pulmonary resistance], causing high hypoxia.

Symptoms

- Retractions
- SOB and expiratory grunting
- Nasal flaring

- Periods of apnea
- Bluish color of skin and mucous membranes
- Arms or legs puffy or swollen.

Nursing Management

Management of the neonate with meconium stained amniotic fluid is done in following way:

- Oropharyngeal suctioning of infant after delivery.
- Laryngoscopic visualizaiton of vocal cords after intubation.
- Additional suctioning of trachea.
- Stomach of the child may be suctioned in order to remove swallowed meconium that could be vomited and aspirated.
- Amnioinfusion: Dilutes meconium. Thins out particulate meconium.
- Prevention of sepsis is done through CBC, bl.cx., chest X-ray.
- Antibiotic therapy to prevent pneumonia.

In term infant

- Sepsis [GBS].
- Persistent pulmonary hypertension of newborn (PPHN) – ductus arteriosus does not close.
- Meconium aspiration due to oligoamnion, uteroplacental insufficiency, and fetal distress.
- Infants of diabetic mothers.
- May need resuscitation after birth.

Idiopathic Respiratory Distress Syndrome (IRDS)

Idiopathic respiratory distress syndrome (IRDS), formerly known as respiratory distress syndrome or hyaline membrane disease; is an acute disorder, most common disorder of premature infants. It is a syndrome in premature infants caused by developmental insufficiency of surfactant production and structural immaturity in the lungs. Most alveolar surfactant is produced after 30 weeks of gestation. Inadequate surfactant production causes air sacs to collapse on expiration and greatly increases the energy required for breathing. The development of interstitial edema makes the lung even less compliant. This leads to hypoxia and retention of carbon dioxide. The syndrome is also frequent in infants of diabetic mothers and in the second born of premature twins.

Pathophysiology

The lungs of infants with IRDS are developmentally deficient in a material called surfactant, which has the property of lowering surface tension. It is a complex system of lipids, proteins and glycoproteins that are produced in specialized lung cells called Type II pneumocytes. It helps prevent collapse of the terminal air-spaces (the future site of alveolar development) throughout the normal cycle of inhalation and exhalation. In premature infant insufficient surfactant in alveoli:

- Causes lungs to collapse; not enough O_2.
- Immature lungs have increased pulmonary vascular resistance. High resistance causes fibrous tissue in bronchioles and alveoli.
- Poor O_2/CO_2 exchange.
- Hypoxia and hypercapnia occur owing to progressive atelectasis and pulmonary hypoperfusion.
- Self-limiting within 72 to 96 hrs in most late preterm or full term.
- If hypoxia and hypercapnia persists; causes metabolic acidosis and drop in blood pH.
- RDS can persist days or weeks due to immature lungs, noncompliance, and low surfactant levels in VLBW (ELBW).

Extremely immature in neonates (between 1000 to 1500 g) may develop apnea and/or hypothermia. Progressive signs of respiratory distress are noted soon after birth and include the following:

- Tachypnea.
- Cyanosis.
- Expiratory grunting (from partial closure of glottis).
- Subcostal and intercostal retractions.
- Nasal flaring.
- Can progress to loss of effort, fatigue → apnea → hypoxia and the need for assisted ventilation.

Management

- The use of antenatal steroids to enhance pulmonary maturity. RDS is prevented if mothers who are about to deliver prematurely can be given glucocorticoids. This speeds the production of surfactant.
- Appropriate resuscitation facilitated by placental transfusion and immediate use of continuous positive airway pressure (CPAP) for alveolar recruitment. The use of gentler modes of ventilation, including early use of 'bubble' nasal CPAP to minimize damage to the immature lungs.

Oxygen is given with a small amount of continuous positive airway pressure (CPAP), the use of gentler modes of ventilation, including early use of 'bubble' nasal CPAP to minimize damage to the immature lungs.

Ventilation

Most babies born with IRDS will require assisted ventilation. Most will initially be intubated and ventilated (partly to administer surfactant and partly to adequately oxygenate the infant).

Caffeine should be started as early as possible to help reduce apnea and facilitate earlier extubation.

- Intravenous fluids are administered to stabilize the blood sugar, blood salts, and blood pressure. An endotracheal tube is inserted into the trachea and intermittent breaths are given by a mechanical device, if the baby's condition get worsen.
- *Surfactant administration*: A baby develops RDS when the lungs do not produce sufficient amounts of surfactant. This is a substance that keeps the tiny air sacs in the lung open. Surfactant can be administered as an adjunct to oxygen and ventilation therapy. Before 34 weeks of gestation, most infants do not produce enough surfactant to survive extrauterine life. As a result, lung compliance is decreased, and not enough gas exchange occurs as the lungs become atelectatic and require greater pressures to expand. An exogenous preparation of surfactant is given through the breathing tube into the lungs, respiratory compliance is improved until the infant can generate enough surfactant on his or her own.
  Systematic reviews of randomized, controlled trials confirmed that exogenous surfactant administration in preterm infants with established respiratory distress syndrome (RDS) reduces mortality, decreases the incidence of pulmonary air leak (pneumothoraces and pulmonary interstitial emphysema), and lowers the risk of chronic lung disease. Moreover, secondary surfactant deficiency also contributes to acute respiratory morbidity in late-preterm and term neonates with meconium aspiration syndrome, pneumonia/sepsis, and perhaps pulmonary hemorrhage; surfactant replacement may be beneficial for these infants.
- *Extracorporeal membrane oxygenation therapy*: Infants older than 34 weeks of gestation having severe pulmonary dysfunction may be candidates for extracorporeal membrane oxygenation therapy. The purpose of ECMO is to allow time for intrinsic recovery of the lungs and heart; a standard cardiopulmonary bypass to oxygenate the infant's blood outside the body through a membrane oxygenator. The membrane oxygenator serves as an artificial lung while the infant's lungs heal. Because of the massive systemic anticoagulation therapy required in the pump tubing and the increased risk for hemorrhage, the criteria for its use are very strict, and the use of this therapy is therefore limited.

  The risk for intraventricular hemorrhages in preterm infants is particularly high, and for this reason, ECMO therapy cannot be used in them. This therapy has been successful in the treatment of various acute and chronic lung diseases, including meconium aspiration syndrome and persistent pulmonary hypertension of the newborn.
- Supportive therapies, such as the diagnosis and management of patent ductus arteriosus (PDA), fluid and electrolyte management, trophic feeding and nutrition, and the use of prophylactic fluconazole.

Supportive therapy includes the following:

- Gentle and minimal handling.
- *Temperature regulation:* Prevent hypothermia.
- *Fluids, metabolism and nutrition:* Closely monitor and maintain blood glucose, electrolytes, acid balance, calcium, phosphorous, renal function and hydration.
- Pulse oximetry is used as a noninvasive tool to monitor oxygen saturation, which should be maintained at 90 to 95%.
- Once the infant is stable, intravenous nutrition with amino acids and lipid. Gavage feeding is a method for providing nourishment to the infant who is compromised by respiratory distress, the infant who is too immature to have a coordinated suck-and-swallow reflex, or the infant who is easily fatigued by sucking. Breast milk or formula is given to the infant through a nasogastric or orogastric tube. This spares the infant the work of sucking.
- After the respiratory status is stable, initiate small-volume gastric feeds (preferably breast milk) via a tube initially to stimulate gut development.
- *Circulation and anemia:* Monitor heart rate, peripheral perfusion and blood pressure. Blood or volume expanders may be required.
- *Antibiotics:* Start antibiotics in all infants who present with respiratory distress at birth, after obtaining blood cultures. Discontinue antibiotics after 3 to 5 days if blood cultures are negative.
- *Support of parents and family:* Keep the parents well-informed. Encourage parents to visit frequently and stay with their baby.

APNEA

Apnea is a 'pause in breathing of longer than 10 to 15 seconds, often associated with bradycardia, cyanosis, or both.' Apnea of prematurity is defined as cessation of breathing by a premature infant that lasts for more than 20 seconds and/or is accompanied by color change, bradycardia. Apnea in premature infants can result in a failure of the mechanisms that protect cerebral blood flow, resulting in ischemia and eventually leukomalacia. The frequency and severity of symptoms is inversely proportional to gestational age, and almost all extremely low birth weight infants (birth weight below 1000 g) are affected. A much more serious condition may lead to hypoxia, cyanosis, brain damage and death.

Apnea is traditionally classified as either obstructive, central, or mixed.

Pathophysiology

Central Apnea

Central apnea means there is no signal to breathe being transmitted from the CNS to the respiratory muscles. It occurs when there is a lack of respiratory effort due to either a cessation of output from the central respiratory centers or the inability of the efferent peripheral nerves and respiratory muscles required for oxygenation and ventilation to receive or process the signals from the brain. This is due to immaturity of brainstem control of central respiratory drive, is seen in certain premature infants, who have a decreased response to hypercapnia. Patients with central apnea have no respiratory effort. This can be seen by a lack of chest wall movement and no breath sounds will be appreciated on auscultation.

The premature infant also manifests an immature response to peripheral vagal stimulation. For example, stimulation of laryngeal receptors in the adult results in coughing. However, stimulation of these same receptors in the premature infant results in apnea. As this reflex apnea can be induced by gavage feeds, aggressive pharyngeal suctioning and gastroesophageal reflux, caregiver should be cautious about that.

Obstructive Apnea

Obstructive apnea, as the name suggests, a pause in alveolar ventilation due to obstruction of airflow within the upper airway, particularly at the level of the pharynx. The pharynx collapses from negative pressure generated during inspiration, because the muscles responsible for keeping the airway open (the genioglossus and geniohyoid) are too weak in the premature infant. Once collapsed, the mucosal adhesive forces of the area tend to prevent the reopening of the airway during expiration. Neck flexion is to be avoided as it worsens this form of apnea. Excessive secretions in the nasopharynx and hypopharynx may also cause obstructive apnea.

Mixed Apnea

A combination of both types of apnea representing as much as 50% of all episodes. A premature infant with central apnea who has an obstruction due to nasal congestion brought on by a viral illness. Gastroesophageal reflux is thought to cause this mixed picture as regurgitated gastric contents may occlude the airway and block laryngeal chemoreceptors to send signals for dilation to the brain.

During apneic episodes, in an attempt to protect cerebral blood flow, cardiac output is diverted away from the mesenteric arteries resulting in intestinal ischemia and possibly necrotizing enterocolitis (NEC).

Management

Premature infants with a low gestational age (less than 35 weeks) should be monitored for apnea because of the high prevalence of apnea in this neonates. Cardiac monitors, pulse oximeters, and pneumography are used to monitor for apnea of prematurity and its associated bradycardia and hypoxemia in NICU.

Sensory stimulations and positioning—Extension of the neck 15° from the prone position is referred to as the head elevated tilt position, which has been reported to improve apnea, bradycardia. Several studies suggest that sensory stimulants, including tactile and olfactory stimulation, are useful in the treatment or prevention of apnea of prematurity. Cutaneous stimulation often arouses the infant and markedly affects breathing pattern in premature infants.

If the infant does not respond, resuscitation procedure must be carried out immediately, i.e. bag and mask ventilation (at about 60 respirations/min), along with suctioning and airway positioning, may be needed. After the baby's color improves an orogastric tube is inserted to decompress the stomach. If bradycardia continues, the child may need mechanical ventilation.

Noninvasive respiratory support is a means of providing ventilatory support to children with either upper airway obstruction or respiratory failure. Respiratory failure constitutes either failure of ventilation or failure of lung function, noninvasive respiratory support encompasses CPAP (Fig. 28.4), continuous bi-level positive airway pressure (BiPAP) and negative pressure ventilation (NPV).

Continuous positive airway pressure (CPAP)—CPAP is effective in treating both obstructive and mixed apnea, but not central apnea. CPAP splints the upper airway with positive pressure during both inspiration and expiration, thereby preventing pharyngeal collapse.

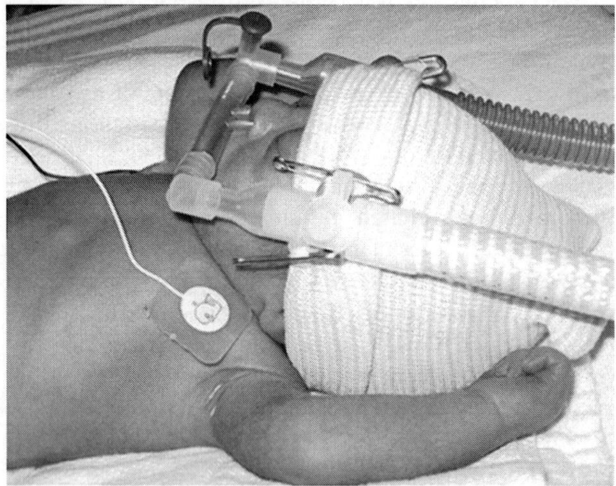

Fig. 28.4: Child is on CPAP system

Bi-level positive airway pressure (BiPAP)—*CPAP machines can only be set to a single pressure* that remains consistent throughout the period. The main difference between BiPAP and CPAP machines is that BiPAP machines have two pressure settings: the prescribed pressure for inhalation (IPAP), and a lower pressure for exhalation (EPAP). The dual settings allow the patient to get more air in and out of their lungs.

CPAP/BiPAP may be used to treat preterm infants whose lungs have not fully developed, e.g. respiratory distress syndrome or bronchopulmonary dysplasia.

Weaning from Respiratory Assistance

Respiratory assistance is weaned slowly as the infant's status improves means the ABG and oxygen saturation levels are maintained within normal limits. A spontaneous, adequate respiratory effort must be present, and the infant must show improved muscle tone during increased activity. It is done in a stepwise and gradual manner. This may consist of the infant being extubated, placed on CPAP, and then weaned to oxygen by means of a hood or mask. Throughout the weaning process, the infant's oxygen levels are monitored by pulse oximetry, transcutaneous tissue oxygen pressure ($TcPO_2$) monitoring, and blood gas levels. The goal of weaning is the withdrawal of all oxygen support. Throughout the weaning period, the infant is assessed for signs and symptoms indicating poor tolerance of the process. These include an increased pulse, respiratory distress, or cyanosis, or a combination of these. If these occur, the amount of oxygen being delivered is increased, and weaning proceeds more slowly while further assessments are done. Underlying causes of intolerance of weaning may be bronchopulmonary dysplasia (BPD), a PDA, or CNS damage.

Thermoneutral Range

A mild increase in body temperature in infants enhances the instability of the breathing pattern. It has been observed, less apnea was found at an incubator temperature of 30.4 °C than at 32.5 °C. Of course, a number of factors play a role in incubator and baby temperature, but overheating may be a factor in apnea in prematurity. Cold stress may also cause apnea. Extended periods of cold stress can lead to harmful side effects which include hypoglycaemia, respiratory distress, hypoxia, metabolic acidosis, necrotizing enterocolitis and failure to gain weight. So premature infants are to be kept in thermoneutral environment. Following interventions are needed in this situation:

Place a neonate of < 1.5 kg in an incubator at the upper range, i.e. > 37 °C. Increase the set temperature by 0.5 °C every 15 minutes according to the neonate's response. Neonate's temperature is to be taken every 30-60 minutes until warmed to an acceptable temperature. Identify and eliminate any environmental causes, e.g. wet bed, over exposure, handling. Promote a flexed position. Ensure ventilator gases are adequately warmed to 37 °C. One of the popular method of thermoregulation of infant is **Kangaroo care (skin-to-skin holding)**.

In this technique, the infant dressed only in a diaper, is placed directly on the parent's bare chest and then covered with the parent's clothing or a warmed blanket. In this way, the parent's body temperature also functions as an external heat source that enhances the infant's temperature regulation. Moreover it helps infants to interact directly with their parents.

Severe apnea or apnea of unknown cause is treated with following medicines:

Drug Therapy

The most common drugs used to treat apnea are the methylxanthines: Caffeine (1,3,7-trimethylxanthine) and theophylline (1,3-dimethylxanthine).

Methylxanthines block adenosine receptors. Adenosine inhibits the respiratory drive, thus by blocking inhibition, the methylxanthines stimulate respiratory neurons resulting in an enhancement of minute ventilation.

Caffeine citrate is also used to improve ventilation and to establish more regular breathing patterns through central nervous system stimulation.

- Theophylline is a bronchodilator and in neonates with bronchopulmonary dysplasia (BPD) it offers the advantage of treating both apnea and bronchospasm.

Blood Transfusion

Anemia correction is done in case of apnea, which increases the oxygen carrying capacity. Apnea associated with hypoglycemia and hypocalcemia may be relieved by treating sepsis with antibiotic.

Icterus Neonatorum

Icterus neonatorum means jaundice in a newborn infant. Neonatal jaundice is the yellowish discoloration of the skin and/or sclerae of newborn infants caused by tissue deposition of bilirubin. In neonates, jaundice tends to develop because of 2 factors—the breakdown of fetal hemoglobin as it is replaced with adult hemoglobin and the relatively immature metabolic pathways of the liver, which are unable to conjugate and so excrete bilirubin as quickly as an adult (Flowchart 28.1). This causes an accumulation of bilirubin in the blood called hyperbilirubinemia, leading to the symptoms of jaundice. Physiological jaundice is mild, unconjugated (indirect-reacting) bilirubinemia, and affects nearly all newborns.

Causes of Neonatal Jaundice

Infants with severe hyperbilirubinemia are at risk for developing kernicterus as bilirubin is a potential neurotoxin (Fig. 28.5). Unconjugated bilirubin that is not bound to albumin can enter the brain and cause focal necrosis of the neurons and glia, resulting in bilirubin encephalopathy, which is known as kernicterus.

Prevention and Management

Assessment and Counseling

Infants should be assessed for jaundice at 24 to 48 hrs of age and prior to hospital discharge. Counseling regarding jaundice and breastfeeding should be provided before discharge of the child from hospital where the importance of frequent feedings should be emphasized.

Flowchart 28.1: Pathway of icterus neonatorum

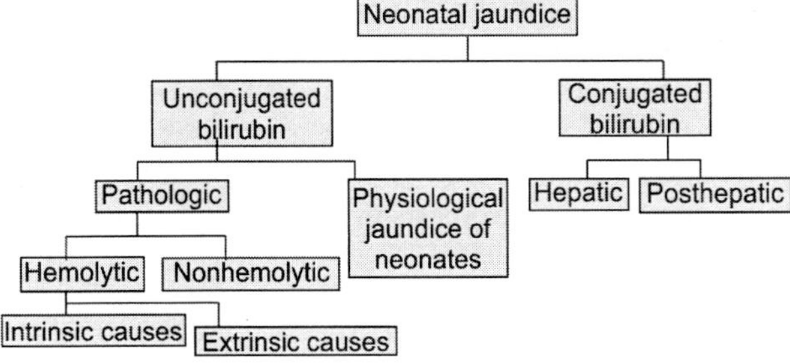

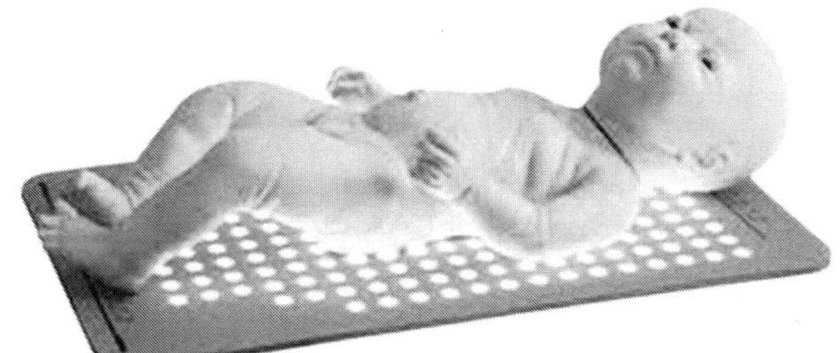

Fig. 28.5: Phototherapy is the standard treatment for pathologic unconjugated hyperbilirubinemia

Feeding of the Child

Providing adequate breast milk is an important part of preventing and treating jaundice because it promotes elimination of the yellow pigment in stools and urine. Mother will know that her child is getting enough milk or formula if she or he has at least 6 wet diapers per day, the color of the bowel movements changes from dark green to yellow, and she or he seems satisfied after feeding.

Phototherapy is the standard treatment for pathologic unconjugated hyperbilirubinemia. Rare cases of extremely high TSB levels (>25 mg/dL) require an exchange transfusion.

Exchange Transfusion

Exchange transfusion is used to remove bilirubin from the circulation when intensive phototherapy fails. It is specially useful for infants with increased bilirubin production from immune-mediated hemolysis because the circulating antibodies and the sensitized red blood cells also are removed. This procedure is done urgently to prevent or minimize bilirubin-related brain damage. The transfusion replaces an infant's blood with donated blood in an attempt to quickly lower bilirubin levels. Exchange transfusion may be performed in infants who have not responded to other treatments and who have signs of or are at significant neurologic risk of bilirubin toxicity.

ABO incompatibility and hemolytic disease of newborn (*See* chapter 15 of this edition).

Birth Injuries

Birth injury is defined as an impairment of the neonate's body function or structure due to an adverse event that occurred as a result of physical pressure or trauma during childbirth. The term also encompasses the long-term consequences, often of a cognitive nature, of damage to the brain or cranium.

The birth process is a blend of compression, contractions, torques, and traction. When fetal size, presentation, or neurologic immaturity complicates this event, such intrapartum forces may lead to tissue damage, edema, hemorrhage, or fracture in the neonate. There is a wide spectrum of birth injuries ranging from minor and self-limited problems, e.g. laceration or bruising to severe injuries that may result in significant neonatal morbidity or mortality (i.e. spinal cord injuries). The overall incidence of birth injuries has declined with improvements in obstetrical care and prenatal diagnosis. The use of obstetric instrumentation may further amplify the effects of such forces or may induce injury alone.

However, there are often clear distinctions to be made between brain damage caused by birth trauma and that induced by intrauterine asphyxia. It is also crucial to distinguish between 'birth trauma' and 'birth injury'. Birth injuries encompass any systemic damages incurred during delivery (hypoxic, toxic, biochemical, infection factors, etc.), but 'birth trauma' focuses largely on mechanical damage. Caput succedaneum, subcutaneous hemorrhages, small subperiosteal hemorrhages, hemorrhages along the displacements of cranial bones, intradural bleedings, subcapsular hematomas of liver, are among the more commonly reported birth injuries. Birth trauma, on the other hand, encompasses the enduring side effects of physical birth injuries, including the ensuing compensatory and adaptive mechanisms and the development of pathological processes (pathogenesis) after the damage.

Risk Factors

- *Macrosomia:* The incidence of birth injuries rises as the fetal size increases viz. more than 4 kg. Different studies compared with normosmic neonates, the incidence of birth injury was two-fold greater in infants weighing 4 to 4.5 kg. Maternal obesity – Maternal obesity (defined as a body mass index greater than 40 kg/m^2) is associated with an increased risk of birth injuries. This may be due to the greater use of instrumentation during delivery and/or these mothers having an increased risk of delivering a large for gestational age infant with shoulder dystocia .
- *Abnormal fetal presentation:* Fetal presentation other than a vertex position, particularly breech presentation, is associated with an increase in the risk of birth injury with vaginal delivery. Deep, transverse arrest of descent of presenting part of the fetus.
- *Operative vaginal delivery:* Operative vaginal delivery refers to a delivery in which the clinician uses forceps or a vacuum device to assist the mother in delivering the fetus to extrauterine life. The instrument is applied to the fetal head, and then the clinician uses traction to extract the fetus, typically during a contraction while the mother is pushing. Both forceps and vacuum delivery are associated with an increase in birth injury .
- *Cesarean delivery:* Cesarean delivery is generally found to have a lower risk of birth trauma compared with vaginal deliveries.
- *Other factors:* One study reported an increased incidence of birth trauma to the head and neck in male infants and in babies born to primiparous mothers. Additionally, small maternal stature and the presence of cephalopelvic disproportion, maternal pelvic anomalies. Maternal pelvic anomalies are associated with an increased risk of birth injuries.

Cephalhematoma

Cephalhematoma is a subperiosteal collection of blood secondary to rupture of blood vessels between the skull and the periosteum; suture lines delineate its extent. Most commonly parietal, cephalhematoma may occasionally be observed over the occipital bone.

Sometimes cephalohematoma is confused with subdural hematomas, which are less common. A subdural hematoma is a collection of blood inside the skull, while a cephalohematoma is a collection of blood under the skin of the scalp. Because of the connections of the tissues there, a cephalohematoma stays on top of one of the skull bones; it does not cross the midline. They are usually caused from the events surrounding birth. They can come from the head banging against the pelvic bone during labor, a prolonged second stage of labor or instrumental delivery, particularly ventouse.

The extent of hemorrhage may be severe enough to cause anemia and hypotension, although this is uncommon. The resolving hematoma predisposes to hyperbilirubinemia. Rarely, cephalhematoma may be a focus of infection that leads to meningitis or osteomyelitis.

No laboratory studies are usually necessary. Skull radiography or computed tomography (CT) scanning is performed if neurologic symptoms are present. Usually, management solely consists of observation. Transfusion for anemia, hypovolemia, or both is necessary if blood accumulation is significant. Aspiration is not required for resolution and is likely to increase the risk of infection.

Management

Cephalohematomas generally do not present any problem to babies, except for an increased risk of jaundice in the first days. The lump of a cephalohematoma goes away on its own with no treatment needed. It can take weeks or months, with 3 months being pretty common. No laboratory studies usually are necessary.

Vitamin C deficiency has been reported to possibly be associated with development of cephalohematomas. Skull X-ray or CT scanning is used if neurological symptoms appear. Usual management is mainly observation. Phototherapy may be necessary if blood accumulation is significant leading to jaundice. Rarely anemia can develop needing blood transfusion. Do not aspirate to remove accumulated blood because of the risk of infection and abscess formation. The presence of a bleeding disorder should be considered but is rare. Skull radiography or CT scanning is also used if concomitant depressed skull fracture is a possibility. It may take weeks and months to resolve and disappear completely.

Caput Succedaneum

Caput succedaneum is a serosanguineous, subcutaneous, extraperiosteal fluid collection with poorly-defined margins; it is caused by the pressure of the presenting part against the dilating cervix. Caput succedaneum extends across the midline and over suture lines and is associated with head molding. Caput succedaneum does not usually cause complications and usually resolves over the first few days. Management consists of observation only.

Difference Between Caput Succedaneum and Cephalohematoma

A caput succedaneum is an edema of the scalp at the neonate's presenting part of the head. It often appears over the vertex of the newborn's head as a result of pressure against the mother's cervix during labor. The edema in caput succedaneum crosses the suture lines. It may involve wide areas of the head or it may just be a size of a large egg. Cephalhematoma is a collection of blood between the periosteum of a skull bone and the bone itself. It occurs in one or both sides of the head. It occasionally forms over the occipital bone. The swelling with cephalhematoma is not present at birth rather it develops within the first 24 to 48 hours after birth.

Congenital Anomalies

According to WHO congenital anomalies can be defined as structural or functional *anomalies* (e.g. metabolic disorders) that occur during intrauterine life and can be identified prenatally, at birth or later in life.

- Congenital anomalies are important causes of childhood death, chronic illness and disability in many countries. An estimated 276,000 babies die within 4 weeks of birth every year, worldwide, from congenital anomalies.
- Congenital anomalies can result in long-term disability, which may have significant impacts on individuals, families, health care systems and societies.
- The most common severe congenital anomalies are heart defects, neural tube defects and Down's syndrome.
- Although congenital anomalies may be genetic, infectious, nutritional or environmental in origin, most often it is difficult to identify the exact causes.
- Some congenital anomalies can be prevented. For example, vaccination, adequate intake of folic acid or iodine through fortification of staple foods or provision of supplements, and adequate antenatal care are keys for prevention.....WHO.

Treatment and Care

Many structural congenital anomalies can be corrected with pediatric surgery and early treatment can be administered to children with functional problems such as thalassemia (inherited recessive blood disorders), sickle cell disorders and congenital hypothyroidism (*See* chapters 15 and 18).

Neonatal Seizures

(*See* chapter 16 of this edition).

Neonatal Hypoglycemia

Low blood sugar level in newborn babies is also called neonatal hypoglycemia. It refers to low blood sugar (glucose) in the first few days after birth. Hypoglycemia is a serum glucose concentration < 40 mg/dL (< 2.2 mmol/L) in term neonates or < 30 mg/dL (< 1.7 mmol/L) in preterm neonates. It can occur from an excessive rate of removal of glucose from the blood or from decreased secretion of glucose into the blood.

Etiology and Incidence

In some babies glucose level can drop if there is too much insulin in the blood (hyperinsulinism). Congenital hyperinsulinism is a genetic conditions transmitted in both autosomal dominant and recessive fashion. Insulin is a hormone that pulls glucose from the blood. The baby develops hypoglycemia when he or she is not producing enough glucose, the baby's body is using more glucose than is being produced, the baby is not able to feed enough to keep glucose level up. Neonatal hypoglycemia may be transient or persistent and its causes are given in the box.

Risk Factors for Hypoglycemia in the Neonate

- *Transient Hypoglycemia in Neonates*—It is caused due to inadequate substrate, and immature enzyme function leading to deficient glycogen stores. The conditions include severe respiratory distress, asphyxia or other birth stress, prematurity, SGA babies (<2.5kg), infant with Rh incompatibility, baby of diabetic mother, maternal toxemia.
- *Persistent Neonatal Hypoglycemia*—It causes of persistent hypoglycemia include hyperinsulinism, adrenal insufficiency.
- *Underlying Disorder/Cause*—Hypoglycemia in neonates is caused due to inherited disorders of metabolism (e.g. glycogen storage diseases, disorders of gluconeogenesis), maternal medication use (such as propranolol, ritodrine, terbutaline).

Hypoglycemia may also occur if an IV infusion of D/W is abruptly interrupted. Finally, hypoglycemia can be due to malposition of an umbilical catheter or sepsis.

Pathophysiology

The baby gets glucose from the mother through the placenta before birth. This sugar is used to support the rapid growth taking place in the fetus. In the last weeks of gestation, excess glucose is stored in the liver and skeletal muscle as glycogen or converted to fatty acids and then stored as triglycerides in fat cells. Insulin is not transferred through placenta, so fetus needs to produce insulin.

After birth, the glucose supply from mother ceases, and newborn has to rely on own hepatic glycogen stores and glucoregulatory mechanism to mobilize and use glucose. When the steady supply of glucose from mother stops, the glucose level of newborn comes down to a lowest level within 1 to 3 hrs of postnatal age. Babies need blood sugar for energy and this requirement of sugar is relatively high because of several factors. Most of that glucose is used by the brain as it is larger in proportion to body size. Baby needs more energy as they have increased metabolic and motor activity, but access to glucose is limited because of the newborn's immature liver enzyme system. The function of glucagon, the hormone which promotes the release of glucose from the glycogen stores decreases due to immature liver enzyme system of the newborn.

Deficiency of glycogen stores at birth is common in very low-birth-weight preterm infants, infants who are small for gestational age (SGA) because of placental insufficiency, and infants who have perinatal asphyxia. Anaerobic glycolysis consumes glycogen stores in these infants, and hypoglycemia may develop at any time in the first few days, specially if there is a prolonged interval between feedings or if nutritional intake is poor. A sustained input of exogenous glucose is therefore important to prevent hypoglycemia.

Contd...

Contd...

Transient hyperinsulinism most often occurs in infants of diabetic mothers and is inversely related to the degree of maternal diabetic control. It also commonly occurs in physiologically stressed infants who are SGA. Hyperinsulinemia characteristically results in a rapid fall in serum glucose in the first 1 to 2 hrs after birth when the continuous supply of glucose from the placenta is interrupted.

Manifestations

Infants with low blood sugar may not have symptoms. Many infants remain asymptomatic. Prolonged or severe hypoglycemia causes both adrenergic and neuroglycopenic signs. Adrenergic signs include diaphoresis, tachycardia, lethargy or weakness, and shakiness. Neuroglycopenic signs include seizure, coma, cyanotic episodes, apnea, bradycardia or respiratory distress, and hypothermia. Listlessness, poor feeding, hypotonia, and tachypnea may occur.

Diagnosis

Newborns at risk for hypoglycemia should have a blood test to measure blood sugar level every few hrs after birth, even if there are no symptoms. This will be done using a heel stick. The health care provider should continue taking blood tests until the baby's glucose level stays normal for about 12 to 24 hrs. Babies with the following symptoms may require test for blood sugar:

- Bluish-colored or pale skin
- Breathing problems, such as apnea, rapid breathing, or a grunting sound
- Irritability or listlessness
- Loose or floppy muscles
- Poor feeding or vomiting
- Problems keeping the body warm
- Tremors, shakiness, sweating, or seizures.

Other Possible Tests

- Newborn screening for metabolic disorders – other tests may be done to rule out underlying metabolic disorders.
- Urine tests may be performed to test for ketones. In case of child with hyperinsulinism, ketones are not present.

Therapeutic Management

- Administration of IV dextrose for prevention and treatment of hypoglycemia.
- Enteral feeding.
- Sometimes IM glucagon.

Infants with low blood sugar level will need to receive extra feedings with breast milk or formula or 5% dextrose in water. Gavage feeding may be given to the children who are lethargic and not sucking breast milk well. Intravenous glucose is given in bolus at first then and then by continuous drip when blood glucose level comes down to 20 to 25 mg/dL. The goal is to maintain blood glucose level in the range of 50 mg/dL or greater.

Most high-risk neonates need preventive treatment. Those children are baby of diabetic women who have been using insulin are often started at birth on a 10% D/W infusion IV or given oral glucose, as are those who are sick, are extremely premature, or have respiratory distress. Other at-risk neonates who are not sick should be started on early, frequent breast milk feedings to provide carbohydrates.

Any neonate whose glucose falls to ≤ 50 mg/dL (≤ 2.75 mmol/L) should begin prompt treatment with enteral feeding or with an IV infusion of up to 12.5% D/W, 2 mL/kg over 10 min. Dextrose with higher concentrations can be infused if necessary through a central catheter. Serum glucose levels must be monitored to guide adjustments in the infusion rate. The infusion should then continue at a rate that provides 4 to 8 mg/kg/min of glucose (i.e. 10% D/W at about 2.5 to 5 mL/kg/hr). Once the neonate's condition has improved, IV infusion may be replaced to enteral feedings gradually while the glucose concentration continues to be monitored. IV dextrose infusion should always be tapered, because sudden discontinuation can cause hypoglycemia.

Glucagon 100 to 300 μg/kg IM, (maximum, 1 mg) is given to hypoglycemic neonates, where immediate administration of an IV infusion is difficult. Glucagon usually raises the serum glucose rapidly, an effect that lasts 2 to 3 hrs, except in neonates with depleted glycogen stores. Diazoxide may be given to suppress pancreatic insulin secretion in children with hyperinsulinism. Hypoglycemia refractory to high rates of glucose infusion may be treated with hydrocortisone. Steroids may be used to stimulate gluconeogenesis from non-carbohydrate sources.

Treatment will be continued until the baby can maintain blood sugar level. This may take hours or days. Infants who were born early, have an infection, or were born at a low weight may need to be treated for a longer period of time.

If the low blood sugar continues, in rare cases the baby may also receive medicine to increase blood sugar level. In very rare cases, newborns with very severe hypoglycemia who do not improve with treatment may need surgery to remove part of the pancreas (to reduce insulin production).

Possible Complications

Severe or persistent low blood sugar level may affect the baby's mental function. Babies with more severe symptoms are more likely to develop learning problems. This is more often true for babies who are at a lower-than-average weight or whose mother has diabetes. In rare cases, heart failure or seizures may occur.

Hypocalcemia

Hypocalcemia is a condition in which there is too little calcium in a baby's blood. A common form of hypocalcemia in babies is called neonatal hypocalcemia. In children, hypocalcemia is defined as a total serum calcium concentration less than 7.0 mg/dL. In term infants, hypocalcemia is defined as total serum calcium concentration less than 7 mg/dL or ionized fraction of less than 4.4 mg/dL.

Neonatal hypocalcemia occurs in 2 forms, i.e. early onset (in the first 2 days of life), late onset (> 3 days), which is rare. Some infants with congenital hypoparathyroidism have both early and late hypocalcemia. Normally, parathyroid hormone helps maintain normal Ca levels when the constant infusion of ionized Ca across the placenta is interrupted at birth. A transient, relative hypoparathyroidism may cause hypocalcemia in preterm and some small-for-gestational-age neonates, who have parathyroid glands that do not yet function adequately. Other risk factor for early-onset hypocalcemia is history of diabetes or hyperparathyroidism of mothers. Because these women have higher-than-normal ionized Ca levels during pregnancy it may cause early-onset hypocalcemia after delivery, perinatal asphyxia may also increase serum calcitonin, which inhibits calcium release from bone and results in hypocalcemia.

Symptoms of hypocalcemia may not be obvious in newborn babies. They may experience irritability, muscle twitches, jitteriness, tremors, poor feeding, lethargy, changes in ECG and, rarely seizures.

Initiation of feedings is often the only treatment to correct early hypocalcemia. Many babies with this problem receive essential fluids and electrolytes through intravenous (IV) fluids. Some babies may need a special preparation called parenteral nutrition, which contains nutrients they need until they are able to take milk feedings. The contents of IV fluids and parenteral nutrition should be carefully calculated for each baby. Calories, protein, fats and electrolytes, including sodium, potassium, chloride, magnesium and calcium are all important components.

Calcium supplementation oral or parenteral is administered in children who have significant hypoglycemia, or low enteral intake. Late onset hypocalcemia is treated with oral calcitriol or Ca.

Oral supplementation is given with food as it may cause gastric irritation. Oral Ca preparations have a high sucrose content, which may lead to diarrhea in preterm infants.

Those term infants with levels < 7 mg/dL and preterm infants with Ca < 6 mg/dL should be treated with 2 mL/kg of 10% Ca gluconate (200 mg/kg) by slow IV infusion over 30 min. IV supplementation of calcium may be given in bolus doses or in continuous infusion. Too-rapid infusion can cause bradycardia, so heart rate should be monitored during the infusion. The IV site should also be watched closely because tissue infiltration by a Ca solution is irritating and may cause local tissue damage or necrosis. Manifestations of Ca infiltration include skin redness, calcification, and necrosis or slough; there can be radial nerve damage at the wrist. The infusion site is to be checked for signs of infiltration, and hyaluronidase is used to treat infiltrates. Many drugs (such as sodium bicarbonate) may precipitate with calcium ions, so it should not be mixed in the IV lines. Evaluation of calcium level is necessary in case of persistent hypocalcemia.

Neonatal Infections or Neonatal Sepsis

Neonatal sepsis is invasive infection, usually bacterial, occurring during the neonatal period. Neonatal sepsis may be categorized as early-onset or late-onset. Onset of neonatal sepsis can be early (≤ 3 days of birth) or late (after 3 days). Of newborns with early-onset sepsis, 85% present within 24 hrs, 5% present at 24 to 48 hrs, and a smaller percentage present within 48 to 72 hrs. Onset is most rapid in premature neonates.

Early-onset sepsis is associated with acquisition of microorganisms from the mother. Transplacental infection or an ascending infection from the cervix may be caused by organisms that colonize the mother's genitourinary (GU) tract; the neonate acquires the microorganisms as it passes through the colonized birth canal at delivery. The microorganisms most commonly associated with early-onset infection include the following:

- Group B *Streptococcus* (GBS)
- *Escherichia coli*
- Coagulase-negative *Staphylococcus*
- *Haemophilus influenzae*.

Signs are multiple, nonspecific, and include diminished spontaneous activity, less vigorous sucking, apnea, bradycardia, temperature instability, respiratory distress, vomiting, diarrhea, abdominal distention, jitteriness, seizures, and jaundice.

Diagnosis is Clinical and based on Culture Results

Treatment is initially with ampicillin plus either gentamicin or cefotaxime, narrowed to organism-specific drugs as soon as possible (*See* chapter 5 of this edition).

CONCLUSION

Modern technology and expert nursing care have made important contributions in improving the health and overall survival of high-risk infants. The birth of any high-risk infant can cause profound parental stress. They are fearful of the possible eventual outcomes for the infant. They also must deal with the technological world surrounding their infant, and amid all the equipment, it is sometimes difficult for them to perceive the infant and respond to its needs. Hence, pediatric nurses play an important role to minimize some of these concerns by involving the family in the infant's care, providing privacy, answering questions, and preparing them for the inevitability of the outcome of the infant's condition.

CHAPTER 29

Intensive Care for Pediatric Patients

Chapter Outline

- Resuscitation, Stabilization, and Monitoring of Pediatric Patients
- Bili Lights
- Bili Blanket

Children who require intensive care are usually critically ill as a result of an accident, acute medical illness or life-threatening surgical condition. Timely and appropriate management can save the lives. Child may require intensive care when they are low birth weight baby or an acute illness is superimposed on a chronic condition or congenital anomaly. During postoperative period, children need intensive care when they undergo complex surgical procedure.

RESUSCITATION, STABILIZATION, AND MONITORING OF PEDIATRIC PATIENTS

Most children with respiratory or cardiovascular compromise can be easily recognized during a rapid initial assessment. Obvious examples include children with respiratory conditions such as severe asthma exacerbations, or inadequate perfusion, such as hypovolemic shock. The resuscitation and stabilization of ill and injured children is a stressful affair for parents and members of medical team alike. The initial evaluation of critically-ill children must quickly identify those with respiratory or circulatory compromise. Early recognition and treatment of a patient with deficiencies in oxygenation, ventilation, or perfusion frequently prevents deterioration to respiratory or cardiac arrest. Outcomes for children who develop cardiopulmonary arrest are poor.

Resuscitation and stabilization will generally commence where at the bedside of the child. First line equipment and drugs are to be kept on the nearest pediatric resuscitation trolley. Printed guidelines, inotrope and infusion doses are made to be available in the emergency set up. At the earliest opportunity, the pediatrician, anesthetist (ICCU on call or otherwise) and senior pediatric nurse should be informed and should attend. If possible, the child should be transferred to emergency management set up where stabilization can continue (Fig. 29.1). The advanced pediatric resuscitation equipment and portable ventilator should be brought to the patient. This includes equipment for further resuscitation and stabilization—lines, transducers, catheters and drains, etc. Pediatric intensive care team should be available 24 hrs a day to assist in the treatment of critically-ill children, both before and during transfer to intensive care.

Signs and Symptoms

Cardiovascular: a. Bradycardia, b. tachycardia, c. hypertension, d. hypotension, e. dysrhythmias, f. poor capillary perfusion, and g. cardiopulmonary arrest.

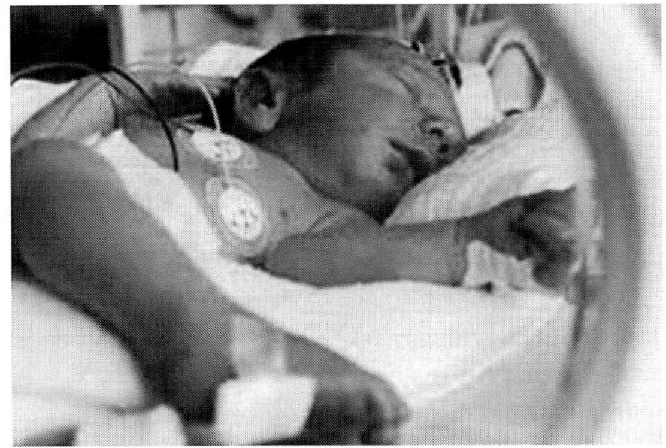

Fig. 29.1: The child is kept in emergency management set up for intensive care

Respiratory: a. Tachypnea, b. dyspnea, c. apnea, d. cyanosis/hypoxemia, e. increased work of breathing, f. decreased air movement, g. stridor, h. wheezing, and i. pulmonary edema.

Neurologic: a. Altered mental status, b. seizures, c. encephalopathy, d. altered thermoregulation, e. decorticate/decerebrate posturing, f. acute paresis, and g. coma.

Renal: a. Anuria, b. hematuria, c. oliguria, and d. polyuria.

Hematologic: a. Petechiae, b. purpura, c. anemia, d. neutropenia, and e. thrombocytopenia.

Gastrointestinal: a. Abdominal distension, b. hematemesis, c. hematochzia, d. melena, and e. peritoneal signs.

Common conditions: a. Injury, b. shock, c. acute d. respiratory distress syndrome, respiratory distress/ failure status asthmaticus, e. upper airway obstruction, f. acute head injury, g. increased intracranial pressure, h. cerebral edema status epilepticus, i. disseminated intravascular coagulation, j. gastrointestinal bleeding, k. abdominal trauma acute abdomen, l. sepsis, m. septic shock, n. toxic shock syndrome, o. meningitis, p. encephalitis, q. dehydration hypovolemic shock, r. diabetic ketoacidosis, etc.

Respiratory Conditions

Assessment of respiration and intervention:

- Tired appearance/decreased or altered LOC.
- Children have thin chest walls that make it relatively easy to hear their lung sounds. If it cannot be heard them, means something is wrong!
- Anxiety, air hunger
- Cyanosis does not become clinically apparent until < 88%.
- Stridor/snoring respirations
- Head bobbing
- Prolonged expiration.

Interventions: Administer 100% oxygen via non-rebreather (NRB) mask, the *NRB* allows for the delivery of higher concentrations of oxygen.

- Wean O_2 as patient stabilizes using face mask or nasal cannula
- Provide bag valve mask ventilation for children who are not breathing effectively
- Unable to maintain O_2 saturations on oxygen
- Cyanosis
- Unable to protect airway
- Bag with enough force to make chest rises
- One breath every 3 seconds.

Rapid Intubation

Procedure Includes

- Oxygenation with FiO_2 of 1.0.
- Administration of atropine which prevents vagally induced bradycardia and minimizes secretions.
- Administration of an opiate and benzodiazepine helps in sedation.
- Administration of paralytic relaxes all muscles allowing ease of opening airway and controlling breathing.
- Then intubation procedure starts.

Management of Shock

- *Venous access*: Ideally 2 large bore IV's.
- *Fluid resuscitation:* 20 mL/kg bolus of NS or LR.
- Reassess patient after each bolus.
- Convert to blood bolus if patient is bleeding.
- Inotropic support for hypotension that persists despite fluid resuscitation. Be careful about catecholamine resistant shock!
- Treat hypothermia
- Correct fluid and electrolyte imbalances
- Find the cause and fix it!

Stabilization Goals on Transport

Neonatal Intensive Care Unit (NICU)

The neonatal intensive care unit (NICU) is where newborn is kept for days, weeks, or possibly longer, depending on the baby's degree of prematurity. This department or area in the hospital is where hospital staff care for newborns who have medical complications, or babies who have been born prematurely.

The long-term outlook for premature babies saved by NICUs has always been a concern. Neonatology and NICUs have greatly increased the survival of very low birth-weight and extremely premature infants. In the era before NICUs, infants of birth weight less than 1400 g (about 30 weeks gestation) rarely survived. Today, infants of 500 g at 26 weeks have a fair chance of survival (Fig. 29.2). Besides prematurity and extreme low birth-weight, common diseases cared for in a NICU include perinatal asphyxia, major birth defects, sepsis, neonatal jaundice, and infant respiratory distress syndrome due to immaturity of the lungs.

A Level III NICU provides advanced care for premature, low birth-weight and critically-ill infants.

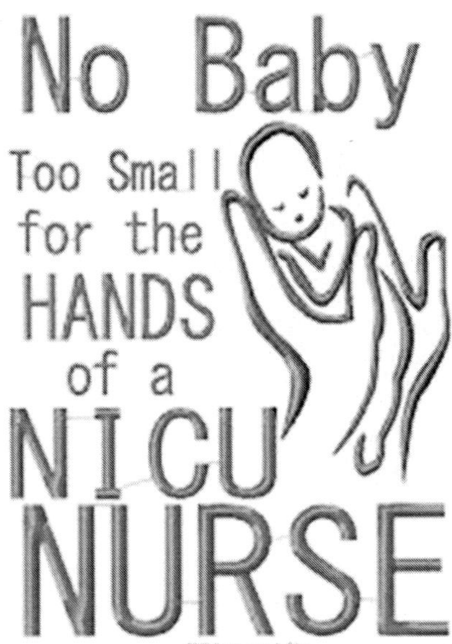

Fig. 29.2: Neonatal nurses render care in different levels of NICU

NICUs are categorized into Level I (normal newborn infants requiring additional nursing care), Level II (moderately ill infants) and Level III, for the most complex and severely ill babies.

India has 3-tier system, based on weight and gestational age of neonate.

Level I Care

Neonates weighing more than 1800 g or having gestational maturity of 34 weeks or more are categorized under Level I care. The care consists of basic care at birth, provision of warmth, maintaining asepsis and promotion of breastfeeding. This type of care can be given at home, subcenter and primary health center.

- Basic neonatal care; minimum requirement for a facility that provides inpatient maternity care.
- Able to perform neonatal resuscitation.
- Evaluate healthy newborns; provide standard care.
- Stabilize newborns till transfer to intensive care.

Level II Care

Neonates weighing 1200 to 1800 g or having gestational maturity of 30 to 34 weeks are categorized under Level II care and are looked after by pediatric specialized personnel. The equipment and facilities used for this level of care are include equipment for resuscitation, maintenance of thermoneutral environment, intravenous infusion, gavage feeding, phototherapy and exchange blood transfusion. This type of care can be given at first referral units, district hospitals, teaching institutions and nursing homes.

- Basic care to moderately ill infants; ~ 32 to 42 weeks
- Step down from Level III NICU; infants recover.

Level III Care

Neonates weighing less than 1200 g or having gestational maturity of less than 30 weeks are categorized under Level III care. The care is provided at apex institutions and regional perinatal centers equipped with centralized oxygen and suction facilities, servo-controlled incubators, vital signs monitors, transcutaneous monitors, ventilators, infusion pumps, etc. This type of care is provided by specialized professionals.

- Newborns <32 weeks critical illness, needing surgical intervention.

NICU nurses: Neonatal nurses work in Level I nurseries, where most healthy infants are brought for transitional (from the mother's womb into the outside environment) care and observation immediately after delivery and for the next 24 to 48 hrs.

Neonatal nurses assigned to Level II nurseries care for premature or sick babies who may need extra time in the hospital for oxygen, medication or special feedings, and neonatal nurses work at Level III nurseries. These units are designed for the most premature and/or ill babies who need high-tech medical and nursing care (Fig. 29.2).

Anatomical and physiological basis of critical illness in infancy and childhood

Children are not small size adults. There are various anatomical and physiological differences between adult and child. Neonates have large head, short trachea, large tongue, the cricoids cartilage which is a full ring of cartilage, anterior larynx which is at higher level.

Basic airway management, intubation is difficult in child. During basic airway management the head needs to be in the neutral position. A straight bladed laryngoscope is needed to lift the epiglottis in child up to 2 years of age to give a better view of the vocal cord. To reduce the risk of subglottic edema or stenosis, uncuffed ET tubes are used up to about 10 years of age.

Alveoli increase mainly in numbers in infants and in size in older children. Structurally bronchi have more cartilage, less muscles, and more glands. Muscle spasm is more likely in older children and small airway obstruction is in infants due to inflammation and edema. Ribs of children are horizontal, breathing is diaphragmatic. Greater elasticity of chest wall causes intercostals, subcostal recession. As there is fewer type 1 muscle fibers in diaphragm and intercostals muscles which needs for sustained activity; leads to earlier tiring of the muscles. Neonates have higher oxygen consumption. Chemoreceptors have a more effective response to CO_2 rise than oxygen fall, surfactant production is reduced in premature babies. 50% of airway resistance is in the nasal passages tend to have respiratory failure or arrest when critically ill.

Cardiovascular

Normally foramen of ovale closes during first 48 hrs of life with pulmonary vascular resistance and arterial pressure comes to normal by 2 to 4 weeks of age. In neonates cardiac output is heart rate dependent. There is relatively less intracellular calcium in neonates. Central capillary refill time normally less than 2 seconds and core peripheral temperature difference is less than 2 °C. Longer capillary refill may results due to hypothermia. Response to fluid loss is tachycardia and vasoconstriction, leading to increased capillary refill time and sometimes mottling and air hunger. Assessment of fluid in infants can be done by palpation of anterior fontanelle. Systolic blood pressure can be estimated by the formula, i.e. **80 + (age in years × 2).**

Central Nervous System (CNS)

Newborns and infants have relatively larger brain and larger portion of cardiac output goes to brain. Myelination of nerve fibers increases during first 2 years of life. So there is slower nerve conduction due to low myelin sheath.

So problem arises as there is greater passage of some drugs specially opiates and barbiturates across blood-brain barrier. There is also more sensitivity to sedative and analgesic drugs.

Renal

Rrenal bed is immature at birth and rapid improvements occur after birth. The proportion of cardiac output to the kidneys increases from 4 to 6% at birth to 20 to 25% when mature. Children have difficulty in excreting sodium. Low blood flow is the cause of low GFR (about one-third that of adults) and therefore reduced excretion of some drugs. They have difficulty to cope with water load, unable to concentrate urine efficiently.

Temperature Control

Head of children has a greater surface area leading to heat loss, also fluid losses greater in premature infants compared to term babies. They have greater surface area to volume ratio than in adults. In addition the greater surface area to weight ratio of infants over children leads to greater fluid loss. Heat production of children is occurred by nonshivering thermogenesis by increasing brown fat metabolism in the first few hours of life. This leads to increased oxygen consumption. Infants easily become hyperthermic as sweat glands cannot function efficiently. In colder environmental temperatures heat loss of child occurs by radiation, conduction and convection. Prematurity of the baby aggravates the condition of heat loss. As they cool down easily if left exposed, need to keep warm by wrappings or heating devices. Neonates need more fluid relative to older children.

Blood

Hemoglobin F (Hb F) predominant at birth, only small remain by 6 months of age. This hemoglobin has greater affinity for oxygen than hemoglobin A. physiological anemia is maximal at 3 months and tends to be lower the smaller the infant at birth. Blood volume is increased in neonates (90 mL/kg).

Gastrointestinal System

In a mature infant, sucking usually precedes swallowing, which in turn inhibits respiration. Since the infant, specially critically-ill child cannot coordinate this activity, aspiration may occur. Sometimes, periodic breathing may occur soon after a feeding is completed in sick child. The immature infant also has poor muscle tone of the cardiac sphincter and feeding is regurgitated easily into the esophagus.

Nutritional Needs of Critically-ill Child

Adequate nutritional and metabolic support of the critically-ill child under different conditions is a daunting task. It involves an accurate calculation of caloric delivery with a precise mixture of carbohydrates, proteins, lipids and micronutrients, which needs periodic review. The type of feeding to be given, the amount of feeding, and the position in which the infant is held during and after the feeding are important nursing concerns. The route of nutrient delivery also needs contemplation with increasing popularity of enteral feeding in the critically-ill child. The emptying time of the stomach is more rapid after tube feeding than after bottle feeding. The Emerging knowledge of the non-nutritional functions of nutrients has added another dimension to critical care nutritional support.

Critical illness is associated with increased energy demands related to stress. In sick children, stress due to illness or healing process is an additional factor affecting energy requirements. In order to ensure that optimal calories are provided to the sick child, while calculating energy requirements, the basal energy expenditure (kcals) should be multiplied by a stress factor, which is specific for that particular ailment. This pattern of requirement will vary according to the disease and from patient-to-patient and needs to be considered while formulating individual diets, which must be modified from time-to-time. Therefore, no one routine can be established for feeding all such infants.

In order to provide successful parenteral nutrition, clinical and biochemical monitoring is essential. Clinical monitoring includes vital parameters recording, checking IV sites and rates, daily weight record and maintaining an intake output chart meticulously. Biochemical monitoring entails measurements of blood electrolytes, sugar, creatinine, calcium, phosphates, lipid profile and serum protein levels every third day during the initial unstable phase and weekly and SOS thereafter. Urine should be checked for sugar and ketone bodies 3 to 4 times daily. It is essential to use micro methods for biochemical monitoring and the blood loss due to sampling must be replenished to prevent anemia. Complications relating to metabolic derangement, infection and mechanical line problems should be looked for and judiciously attended to. It must be realized that successful parenteral nutrition requires constant vigilance, dedicated personnel and specialized facilities in order to achieve maximum benefits and minimum complications. However this form of therapy is neither as nebulous nor as difficult as it may appear, and its benefit should therefore not be denied to the patient who needs it most.

Nutrition in Special Situations

In burns, sepsis and trauma the type of protein and amino acid given is most important in maintaining optimal nutrition. In these conditions formulas rich in branched chain amino acids up to 35 to 50% of amino acids administered need to be provided. Moreover, immature infants need some amino acids that are not required by full-term neonates. In liver failure, increased branched chain amino acids and lower concentration of aromatic amines should be used. In addition fiber, lactulose and lactilol are effective. In renal failure, a high concentration of essential amino acids with a greater nonprotein caloric concentration needs to be provided.

Nutritional management is an integral and vital part of critical care support. The stress of severe illness complicates the delivery of adequate nutrients. Enteral feeding has several advantages. However there are specific instances when parenteral nutrition as an adjunctive or as sole therapy becomes mandatory to meet nutritional needs. Whatever the modality, with meticulous attention to nutrient requirements along with rigorous monitoring, it is possible to provide full nutritive support to the critically-ill child.

Care of a Child with Long-term Ventilation

Ventilatory support can be provided noninvasively through a mask, or invasively through a tracheostomy. Long-term ventilation refers to ventilatory support for those who are unable to breathe on their own, for part or all of the day, on an on-going basis. Two main groups of children need long-term ventilation; those with respiratory failure who require ventilatory support and those with diagnoses that might eventually lead to respiratory failure. In the intensive care unit, some patients become medically stable but cannot be weaned from the ventilator. For such individuals, the transition to a level of care that promotes more independence is an important step in improving their quality of life.

Nursing of the child on ventilator includes:

- Patients should receive a complete nursing respiratory assessment at least once at the commencement of each shift where the patient's respiratory status changes or CPAP/NIV settings are adjusted – respiratory rate, heart rate, chest rise and fall, work of breathing, oxygen requirement, pulse oxymetry, compliance with therapy, synchronization between patients respiratory effort with ventilator support.
- Auscultation of lungs frequently is needed to assess for abnormal sounds, suction as needed, turn and reposition two hourly, secure ETT properly, pulse oximetry value and ABG values are to be monitored.
- Suctioning of artificial airway is to keep it patent and to increase gas exchanges (it is important to oxygenate before and after suctioning).
- Monitoring for signs of respiratory distress of the child includes restlessness, apprehension, irritability and increase heart rate.
- Assessment for possible early complication like rapid electrolyte changes, severe alkalosis is needed.
- Prevention of infection. Maintain sterile technique in suctioning. Infection is a risk; replacement of the tube and regular suction of the airway is a must. Monitor color, amount and consistency of sputum.
- Increased need for regular oral hygiene, increased need for pressure area assessment and skin care.

- Enteral feeds can be administered during periods of ventilation (CPAP/NIV). Begin tube feeding as soon as it is evident the patient will remain on ventilation for a long time. However nurses should be mindful of the increased risk of abdominal distension and need for increased venting or aspiration of nasogastric tube or other gastrostomy tubes. Daily weighing of the baby and maintaining intake and output are needed.
  Increased risk of overfeeding with intubation/ sedation are impair liver function by inducing steatosis/cholestasis, increase risk of infection, hyperglycemia, prolonged mechanical ventilation.
- Assess signs and symptoms of rupture of lungs (barotrauma). It can be identified by increasing dyspnea, less or absent of breathing sounds, tracheal deviation, away from affected side, decreasing PaO_2 level.

Ventilator assisted children can live in the community, in complex continuing care facilities or in acute care hospitals. Medical advances mean that these children can now survive intensive care and become well enough to go home. Some remain dependent on technology, such as a breathing machine, to keep them alive, and ventilator assisted individuals can live in the community.

Legal and Ethical Issues in Pediatric Intensive Care

Due to rapid advances in medical technology over the years, the care of critically-ill children with life-threatening disorders in the pediatric intensive care unit (PICU) has unfolded complex medical, social, ethical, philosophical, moral and legal issues. The critical care nurses are often confronted with ethical and legal dilemmas related to various ethical principles and it has increased dramatically since the early 1990s. Many dilemmas are byproducts of advanced medical technologies and therapies developed over the past several decades. Common legal and ethical issues are informed consent, cardiopulmonary resuscitation decisions, withholding or withdrawal of life support, use of restraints, medicolegal cases, etc.

Consent problem arises because children experiencing acute, life-threatening illness that interfere with parents ability to make decisions on treatment or surgical intervention. The informed consent is based on the principle of autonomy. Consent denotes voluntary agreement, permission or compliance. Consent obtained from a minor, or given under fear, fraud or misrepresentation is not valid. Consent obtained from the distant relation, or consent obtained in language not understood by the person is not correct. Moreover, consent obtained without providing adequate information on the possible risks are invalid under law.

Withholding or withdrawal of life support—'withholding' refers to never initiating a treatment, whereas 'withdrawing' refers to stopping a treatment once started. The distinction between not starting a treatment and stopping it is not itself of ethical significance; what is whether the decision is consistent with the patient's interests and preferences.

Decisions about treatment at the end of life are often difficult and best made after careful discussions between the health care professional and the patient and family members. The nurse ensures that the patient or others understand the information by clarifying technical terms and helping the patient and family members weigh treatment options. The parents then consider their own wish and decision in the context of prognoses and realistic options. The final decision reflection the patient or family's wishes should be supported by the nurse and other members of the health care team. The nurse is morally permitted to refuse to participate in withholding or withdrawing treatment from the patient as stated.

A medicolegal case (MLC) is any case where the discipline of medicine comes to help the legal fraternity in its discharge of duties. Health care professionals have to be very cautious in dealing with the medicolegal cases. Request of the patient or relatives or friend for not registering the case as medicolegal should not be accepted. The MLC should be registered as soon as physician suspect's foul play or case brought several days after the incident. The MLC is received in hospital by; any case brought by police for the purpose of examination and reporting and any case referred for expert management and advice. Cases of suspected abuse, self-inflicted injuries or attempted suicide are to be considered in MLC and notification to police, collection and preservation of samples, recording of dying declaration, etc. are needed.

Medical Documentation

The proper medical documentation is legal necessity. A good record should be correct, clear, comprehensive, chronological and contemporaneous. It is the fact that good records are indispensible for proper care and treatment of patients. Consent from patients before carrying out any procedure is mandatory legal, ethical and moral requirement. Similarly the document once prepared has also to be preserved for specified period of time (at least 3 to 5 years from the date of commencement of treatment).

If any request is made for medical records either by patient to authorized attendant to legal authorities, the documents shall be issued within period of 72 hrs and refusal to do so would be misconduct. The following medical documents are almost important as for as legalities are concerned: specialist consultations and referral slips, nurses record, treatment record, TPR chart, BP monitoring chart, IO chart, operative notes, anesthetists notes, progress report, final diagnosis, discharge summary and follow up notes, etc. as for as medicolegal issues are concerned, e.g. death certificate, medicolegal reports, medicolegal investigation reports, all are of immense important and have to be very specific.

Few frequently cited ethical issues reported by the nurses are protecting patients' rights and human dignity, providing care with possible risk to her health (e.g. TB, HIV, violence), respecting/not respecting informed consent to treatment, staffing patterns that limit patient access to nursing care, use/nonuse of physical/chemical restraints, etc. Reports reveal the following as being the most personally disturbing issues faced by the nurses in the PICU are:

- Is there a reasonable chance of survival of the child with the available technology or are the efforts going to be futile?
- Would the quality of life be worthwhile if the child survives with aggressive management?
- Can the family afford expensive management?
- In what clinical situations intensive life support therapy should be withheld?
- Should they prolong the dying process with inappropriate measures?
- Should an unsalvageable child be hooked off the ventilator when a relatively better risk child who needs assisted ventilation is admitted to the PICU?

However, whatever final decision is taken jointly by the multidisciplinary medical team of experts and parents, it should be without any ambiguity and recorded in the case file with full justifications. PICU should be staffed with skillful, dedicated and trained people. But above all, they should be enthused and equipped with qualities of human warmth, compassion and consideration. The general atmosphere of PICU should show overall optimism rather than the gloom of hopelessness despite all the odds.

The ethical and legal responsibility of nurse working in critical care areas has increased since 1990s. Nurses must maintain and continually update their knowledge base and clinical competence. Failure to do so could not only cause harm to patients but could also put nurses and their employer at risk for allegations and professional negligence. As a registered nurse working within the health care industry it is important to consider all sides of the ethical debate and to always act within the law and with the best interests of the patient in mind.

Equipments

The neonatal intensive care unit (NICU) contains many machines and other types of equipment used to care for sick babies with many different problems. These machines seem less intimidating when parents and family members understand how they can help the baby. The nurse on duty of the unit is expected to have knowledge and skill to determine whether the monitoring devices are set at the required limits and the tracings are within normal expectations. Functioning of the assisted ventilation, oxygen therapy, infusion pump, suction apparatus, phototherapy is okay or not that to be checked daily in each shift. Any malfunctioning of the apparatus or electrical connection is to be reported on time to get the work done.

Incubator (Fig. 29.3)

An incubator is an apparatus used to maintain environmental conditions suitable for a neonate. It is used in preterm births or for some ill full-term babies. It is a rigid box-like enclosure in which a baby can be kept in a controlled environment for observation and care (Tables 29.1 to 29.3). The device may include a heater, a fan, a container forz water to add humidity, a control valve through which oxygen may be added, and access ports for nursing care. Incubators may be described as bassinets enclosed in plastic, with climate control equipment designed to keep them warm and limit their exposure to microorganisms.

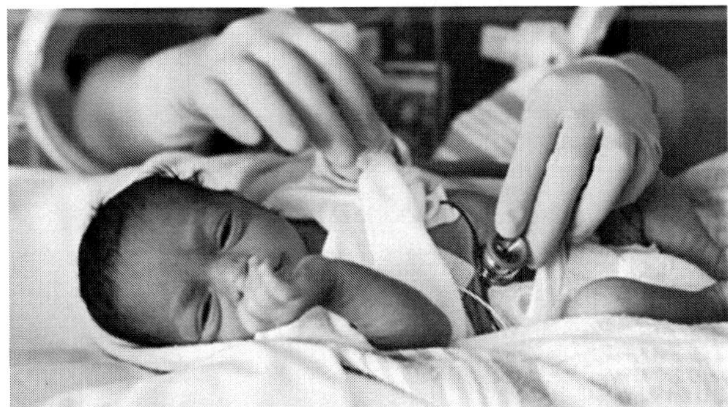

Fig. 29.3: A nurse looks after a premature baby inside an incubator

Table 29.1: Nursing care of a child in incubator

Step	*Action*
1	Preparation of incubator before receiving baby Set the temperature (prewarmed) appropriate to the infant's age, size and condition Use in air mode and must always be switched on with the motor running if in use for a baby Hourly temperature monitoring of the incubator Place the incubator away from draughts or direct sunlight Do not routinely use on the humidity function while in use for babies Test the functioning of the incubator, specially its alarm system
2	Care of baby • Maintain axilla temperature between 36.5 °C and 37.2 °C • Access baby by using the portholes, limit opening of large door as this interferes with air temperature • Ensure baby is nursed only with a nappy • Position baby utilizing rolled towels or baby sheet to provide boundaries that support 'nesting' and flexion of limbs but keeping face clear Maintain a quiet environment • There is no tapping on the canopy • No equipment is placed on top of the canopy • Careful opening and closing of doors • Educate parent how to access baby and to touch him/her
3	Adjusting incubator temperature • Default incubator temperature in NICU is 35° • Adjust the incubator temperature by no more or less than 0.5 of a degree at a time • Recheck the temperature within half an hour of making any adjustment
4	Monitoring • Check axilla temperature on admission into the incubator and recheck in the first hour • Temperature is documented 4 to 6 hourly as condition dictates
5	Use of humidification Maintain humidification as indicated Important to know: • A stressed baby is less able to maintain thermo-neutrality • Surgical babies are prone to stress both before, during and after surgery

Possible functions of a neonatal incubator are:

- Oxygenation, through oxygen supplementation by head hood or nasal cannula, or even continuous positive airway pressure (CPAP) or mechanical ventilation.
- Observation includes measurement of temperature, respiration, cardiac function, oxygenation, and brain activity.

Table 29.2: Weaning incubator temperature in preparation for cot care

Step	*Action*
1	When the decision is made to remove the infant from the incubator The incubator temperature should be weaned by 0.5 degree's until 30 degree's is achieved For term infants being cared for in an incubator in for observation purposes—weaning is NOT required. As long as baby is clothed and wrapped adequately he/she may be transferred to a cot when clinically safe to do so check temperature within 1 hr of transfer.

Table 29.3: Care of the incubator

Step	*Action*
1	Wipe down daily using minimal soap/water Do not use alcohol
2	Incubator is changed every 7 days Incubators are cleaned with hot soapy water; all inserts are removed and thoroughly washed and dried. Filters are changed every 3 months (label to indicate the due date)

- Protection from cold temperature, infection, noise, drafts and excess handling. Provision of nutrition, through intravenous catheter or nasogastric tube.
- Administration of medications.
- Maintaining fluid balance by providing fluid and keeping a high air humidity to prevent too great a loss from skin and respiratory evaporation.

A *transport incubator* is available, which is used when a sick or premature baby is moved, e.g. from one hospital to another. A miniature ventilator, cardio-respiratory monitor, IV pump, pulse oximeter, and oxygen supply built into it.

An infant may require an incubator for the following reasons:

Children are unable to maintain their own temperature with clothing and wrapping.

They are small for gestational age:

- When they are acutely ill and close observation is required.
- When they are at risk of abnormal heat loss.
- They have a known infection or the potential to develop sepsis.

BILI LIGHTS

The effect of light on jaundice in neonates, and the ability of light to decrease serum bilirubin levels, was first described by Cremer et al. in 1958. This observation led to the development of light sources for use in the treatment of infants with hyperbilirubinemia, a treatment now referred to as phototherapy.

The bright blue fluorescent lights placed over a baby's incubator are used to treat jaundice. Bili lights are a type of light therapy (phototherapy) that is used to treat newborn jaundice. Phototherapy treatment in the hospital has been provided by a row of lights or a spotlight suspended at a distance form a baby. Babies with jaundice usually receive this phototherapy treatment for 3 to 7 days. Narrow band ultraviolet B (UVB) light is the most common type of *phototherapy.* This uses a special machine to emit UVB light at 311 to 312 nm, which is the most beneficial portion of natural sunlight for skin diseases. Blue-green light in the range of 460 to 490 nm is most effective for phototherapy. At its most basic, phototherapy refers to the use of light to convert bilirubin molecules in the body into water -soluble isomers that can be excreted by the body.

Phototherapy involves shining fluorescent light from the bili lights on bare skin.

The newborn is placed under the lights without clothes or just wearing a diaper.

The eyes are covered to protect them from the bright light.

The baby is turned frequently.

The health care team carefully notes the infant's temperature, vital signs, and responses to the light. They also note how long the treatment lasted and the position of the light bulbs.

The baby may become dehydrated from the lights. Fluids may be given through a vein during treatment.

Blood tests are done to check the bilirubin level. When the levels have dropped enough, phototherapy is complete.

Some infants receive phototherapy at home. In this case, a nurse visits daily and draws a sample of blood for testing.

Treatment depends on three things:

- Gestational age
- Concentration of bilirubin in the blood
- Newborn's age (in hours).

In severe cases of increased bilirubin in a low birth weight newborn that is younger than 24 hours old, an exchange transfusion may be done instead. When the bilirubin level is very high, an exchange transfusion may be the best option.

BILI BLANKET

A Bili blanket is a portable phototherapy device for the treatment of neonatal hyperbilirubinemia. Bili Blanket is a colloquial term for a range of similar products and the term used in the medical professions. The name is a combination of bilirubin and blanket. Other names used are home phototherapy system, bilirubin blanket, or phototherapy blanket.

Bili blankets can be used for treating some degrees of jaundice at home as long as the baby is otherwise healthy.

This system uses fiber optics and represents advanced technology in phototherapy treatment given in the hospital or at home.

The bili blanket provides the highest level of therapeutic light available to treat baby. This form of light is also found in sunlight. The strength of light form the bili blanket is about the same, as it would get in the shade on a sunny day, yet is safer because the biliblanket filters out potentially harmful ultraviolet and infrared energy.

A pad of woven fibers is used to transport light from a light source to baby. This covered fiberoptic pad is placed directly against baby to bathe the skin in light. Absorption of this light leads to the elimination of bilirubin (Fig. 29.4).

The bili blanket can be used 24 hrs a day to provide continuous treatment. Blood may be drawn and tested during treatment to check bilirubin levels and determine when normal levels are reached and phototherapy is no longer needed. With this convenient form of phototherapy the child can be diapered, clothed, held, and nursed during treatment.

Central Line

A central venous line (CVL) is a special intravenous (IV) line that is used in children who need IV therapy for a long time. A CVL is a long, soft, thin, flexible tube that is inserted into one of the large veins leading to the heart.

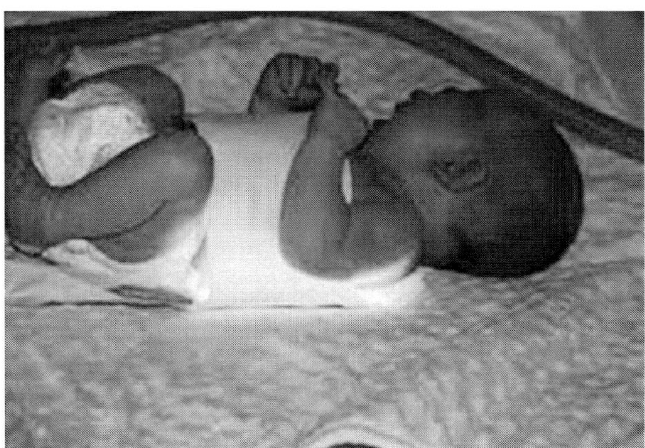

Fig. 29.4: The child is on bili blanket

Children's veins may become damaged by frequent, painful needle insertions. A CVL makes it easier and more comfortable for child to receive medicines such as chemotherapy and IV fluids, or to have blood samples taken. Some treatments like dialysis also need a CVL. Central venous lines are essential in anesthesia for major surgical procedures, for treatment in the ICU as well as for nutrition and drug administration in patients with enteral malnutrition or malignancy.

An interventional radiologist or surgeon inserts child's CVL in the OT or in the image guided therapy (IGT) department. Under general anesthesia CVL tube is inserted through a vein in the neck and places it in the large vein leading to the heart, where the blood flow is fast. This placement allows for better mixing of medicines and IV fluids. Equipment such as ultrasound and fluoroscopy, a special X-ray machine, may be used during the procedure. A chest X-ray may be taken after the procedure to ensure the CVL is in the correct position. It will take about 1 hr to insert the CVL.

Maintenance problems of CVL may be catheter-related infection/sepsis, central venous thrombosis, catheter obstruction, mechanical lesions during long-term use. So is to be kept under close watch and immediate measure is to be taken if the child has fever or chills, bleeding, redness, or swelling around the CVL or neck, leaking or drainage at the CVL site, or the child's CVL is hard to flush or will not flush at all, he/she has pain when the CVL is being used or child's CVL is dislodged or comes out a little or all the way.

CPAP (continuous positive airway pressure)

Air is delivered to a baby's lungs either through small tubes in the baby's nose or through a tube that has been inserted into her windpipe. The tubes are attached to a ventilator (respirator), which helps the baby breathe but does not breathe for her.

Endotracheal Tube

A small plastic tube, which is inserted through a baby's nose or mouth down into the trachea. The tube is attached to a ventilator (respirator), which can either help a baby breathe (as in CPAP) or breathe for her.

Nasal Cannula or Nasal Prongs

Small plastic tubes that fit into your baby's nostrils and deliver oxygen. They often are used with a treatment called continuous positive airway pressure (CPAP), which uses a ventilator to deliver pressurized air to a baby's lungs.

Oxygen Hood

A clear plastic box that fits over the baby's head and supplies her with oxygen. This is used for babies who can breathe on their own but still need some extra oxygen.

Pulse Oximeter

A small U-shaped device that's wrapped around a baby's foot or hand and secured with a stretchy bandage. It uses a light sensor to help determine whether the baby has enough oxygen in her blood. This sensor does not hurt your baby at all. It helps doctors and nurses determine whether your baby needs more or less oxygen, while reducing the need for painful blood tests.

Radiant Warmer

Radiant warmer is an open bed with an overhead heating source that provides heat to a baby. A warmer may be used instead of an incubator if a baby needs to be handled frequently. Incubators and radiant warmers are used to maintain the body temperature of newborn infants and in order to prevent morbidities and minimize the mortalities associated with hypothermia. Infants are cared for on radiant warmer beds in order to provide accessibility for resuscitation or procedures without jeopardizing thermal stability. This is best done so that the energy expended for metabolic heat production is minimized. As long as an infant remains critically ill and is likely to require resuscitation or frequent procedures, he should be kept on a warmer bed. Very small infants (<1000 g) can be kept warm more easily on a radiant warmer, if a very small infant has difficulty maintaining normal body temperature on a radiant warmer, plastic wrap can be stretched across the bed (from side-to-side). This reduces the movement of cool air over the baby's body surface.

The heat output of these devices is usually regulated by servo-control to keep the skin temperature constant at a site on the abdomen where a thermostat probe is attached. The most serious complication of radiant warmers is extreme hyperthermia, which may occur from improper use or from dislodgement of the sensor probe. Hyperthermia may result in death or permanent neurological damage.

If baby is having fever, examine the baby carefully. A baby who is overheated due to warmer will have his skin red flushed, the temperature of sole/palms will be warm to touch by dorsum of hand in addition to warm abdomen. Malfunction of equipment, i.e. probe getting disconnected or keeping baby in manual mode with high heater output can explain this situation. On the other hand fever due to illness will result in warm abdomen to touch but palms/soles will be cold to touch (gradient between abdomen and palms/soles temperature). In addition clinical examination will reveal features that point towards sepsis in the baby.

The infant's eyes should be protected from prolonged exposure to the light emitted by the observation lamp in this unit. Intravenous tubing systems for delivery of blood components to infants occupying a warmer, should be covered with aluminum foil. When using a radiant warmer, change the patient's diapers frequently. Radiant energy causes more rapid urine evaporation, and may lead to inaccurate urine diagnostic test/ analysis and inaccurate weight measurements.

Few Important Points Need to Consider

Ensure that the temperature of the room is 22 °C, place the warmer away from air currents.

Turn on the warmer at least 20 minutes prior to pre-warm the linen and mattress so that the baby does not lie on a cold surface initially.

Adjust the temperature in following way:

- *High:* If baby's temperature is below 36 °C
- *Medium:* If baby's temperature is between 36 to 36.5 °C
- *Low:* If baby's temperature is between 36.5 to 37.5 °C

Once the baby's temperature is between 36.5 to 37.5 °C, switch on the servo mode/skin mode.

If baby is in supine position place the skin probe on the right hypochondrium, when in prone position, place the probe on the loin area. To prevent skin injury, place tegaderm and fix the probe on it with an adhesive. Ensure that the baby's head is covered with cap and feet secured in socks and the baby is clothed or covered unless it is necessary for the baby to be naked or partially undressed for observation or for a procedure.

Place only one baby under each radiant warmer.

Turn the baby frequently while under the warmer, if possible.

Check the temperature of the warmer and of the room every hour, and adjust the temperature setting accordingly.

Record the heater output in each shift (every 6 hours). Any sudden increase in heater output is an early indicator of sickness.

Move the baby to be with the mother as soon as the baby no longer requires frequent procedures and treatment.

For disinfection—i. For daily cleaning of front panel use damp cloth soaked in mild detergent, ii. do not use spirit or other chemical, and, iii. cot should be disinfected daily using mild detergent solution or disinfection solution.

Umbilical Line

An umbilical line is a catheter that is inserted into one of the two arteries or the vein of the umbilical cord. Generally the UAC/UVC is used in NICU as it provides quick access to the central circulation of premature infants. Umbilical cord of newborn has two arteries and one vein, which end in her belly button. A catheter can be inserted into one of these vessels and threaded to the aorta, the largest artery supplying oxygen to the body. An umbilical artery catheter (UAC) allows blood to be taken from an infant at different times, without repeated needle sticks.

An umbilical artery catheter is most often used if:

- The baby needs breathing help.
- The baby needs blood gases and blood pressure monitored.
- The baby needs emergency management like fluid and ionotropic drugs.

Fluids and medicines are given through umbilical venous catheter (UVC) without frequently replacing an intravenous (IV) line. UVC may used when the baby is very premature, the baby needs prolong drug and fluid therapy, the baby has bowel problems that prevent feeding, the baby needs exchange transfusion.

After choosing the blood vessel a catheter is placed into the blood vessel, and an X-ray is taken to determine the final position. Once the catheter is in the right position, they are held in place and is fixed on baby's abdomen with a suture.

Through this catheter, blood can be drawn painlessly, so they do not have to repeatedly stick the baby with needles. The child can be given fluids, blood, nutrients, and medications through this tube. A small device can be attached to the catheter to continuously monitor a baby's blood pressure. An UVC allows fluids and medicines to be given without frequently replacing an IV line.

Ventilator

A ventilator (also called a respirator) is a mechanical breathing machine that delivers warmed and humidified air to a baby's lungs. The sickest babies receive mechanical ventilation, meaning that the ventilator temporarily breathes for him/her, it is so designed to mechanically move breathable air into and out of the lungs. A ventilator does not treat a disease or condition. It is used only for life support. These machines mainly are used in hospitals to

- Get oxygen into the lungs
- Remove carbon dioxide from the body
- Help to breathe easier
- Breathe for child/dult who have lost all ability to breathe on their own.

A modern positive pressure ventilator consists of a compressible air reservoir or turbine, air and oxygen supplies, a set of valves and tubes, and a disposable or reusable "patient circuit". The air reservoir is pneumatically compressed several times a minute to deliver room-air, or in most cases, an air/oxygen mixture to the patient. The air is delivered to the baby's lungs through an endotracheal tube (inserted through a baby's nose or mouth). If a turbine is used, the turbine pushes air through the ventilator, with a flow valve adjusting pressure to meet patient-specific parameters (amount of oxygen, air pressure, and number of breaths per minute can be regulated to meet each baby's needs).

Monitor ventilator device each shift or when resuming treatment.

Check Ventilator Setting

Inspiratory pressure, expiratory pressure, mode, rate, inspiratory time, the minimum time spent in inspiration (TiMin), the maximum time spent in inspiration (TiMax), trigger, ramp, cycle, its alarm settings, battery backup. Synchronization of device with patient's respiration when on bi-level NIV, in S, T and ST mode are to be checked before use. About oxygen therapy careful observation is necessary like oxygen supply appropriately connected or not, circuit patency, FiO_2/ oxygen flow rate, nasal prong oxygen for patients receiving NPV, mask fit and leak, pressure areas from mask and strapping, exhalation port present and patent, antiasphyxiation port is patent and in situ. Humidifier setting is also important, i.e. its water level, its alarm system, etc.

CHAPTER 30

Rights of Children in India

Chapter Outline

- Homes
- The Right of Children to Free and Compulsory Education Act, 2009
- The Child Labor (Prohibition and Regulation) Act, 1986
- Some Salient Features of Some Acts Related to Children Welfare and Rights

'I am child
All the world waits for my coming.
Civilization hangs in the balance
For what I am, the world of tomorrow will be.'

–The Child's Appeal by Mamie Gene Cole

From the 20th century, there has been a great awakenings around the world over the issue of recognition and implementation of Child Rights. The parliament of India had signed and ratified a number of international mechanisms/instruments, adopted by United Nations over the years and the Supreme Court of India created some important case laws for the care and protection of child rights.

The government and law makers as a part of their responsibility towards children, have enacted a number of rules and laws of juvenile justice like 'The Juvenile Justice (care and protection a children) Act, 2000'. This act changed from the concept of welfare of children to the recognition rights of children.

Subsequently, the supreme court and various high court have been maintain vigilance over the proper implementation of the said law regimes. In the famous 'Bachpan Bachao Andolan' Case *[(2010) 12 SCC 1803]*, the supreme court designated the national commission for protection of child rights (constituted under the child right's act) to act as the nodal prime agency to keep watch as the implementation of the direction passed by the court from time to time.

Not only that, the Indian Parliament have enacted some other significant laws to meet the issues of children in 21st century. These are: The right of children to free and compulsory education Act, 2009; Commission for Protection of Child Rights Act, 2005; Protection of children from sexual offences act 2012; Prohibition of Child Marriage Act, 2006, and child labor (Prohibition and Regulation Act, 1986).

The word 'Juvenile' originated from the Latin word 'Juvenis' meaning young. Over the years, word has came to be associated with delinquency. The above noted Act of 2000 has introduced the concept of children in conflict with law and children in need of care and protection as an effort to move away from this kind of labelling. Instead of the words 'Delinquent juvenile' and 'neglected juvenile' mentioned in 1986 Act the terms employed in the 2000 Act are 'Juvenile in conflict with law', Child in need of care and protection.

In recent years, not only in India, in other countries too, juvenile justice system has received significant attention. Children who come in conflict with the law are often from the most vulnerable and marginalized segments of society. Both the Convention on the rights of the child (CRC) and the UN guidelines encourage good practice that aims to ensure the dignity of child and processes that promote reintegration into the community. Hence, rule 3 (VIII) of the Juvenile justice rules, 2007 prohibits that use of adversarial, accused, charge sheet, trial and prosecution, warrant, conviction, etc. In fact, the new act is based on two philosophical objectives: The *parens patriae* and individualized treatment. The *parens patriae* doctrine allows the court to conduct the proceedings principally to determine what should be done in the best interests of the child and not as trials to determine criminal guilt and give sentence. The individualized treatment doctrine views the disposition decision in view to inherently rehabilitate. It seeks to prescribe a treatment program fitting the needs, personality, psychological development and social circumstances of a youth.

This act of 2000 provides for a wide range of reformative measures under SS.15 and 16 for children in conflict will law—from simple admonition to maximum 3 years of institutionalization is a special home.

Hence, undoubtedly now India has for the care and protection of children, uniform and comprehensive regime distinct from the regular judicial system for the adults, in the form of new act of 2000.

Recently, however, the Government at Centre and the parliament made certain amendments to this Act of 2000. These amendments on certain aspects are complete deviation from the concept of juvenile justice. Various organizations and many members of the parliament did register protest and opposed the amendments. They had pointed out that the Standing Committee of the parliament raised objections to amend the Act, there are observations and orders of apex court which held that the Act of 2000 rightly define the age of juvenile as 18 years and under no circumstances, it should be lowered to 16 years.

Ignoring all these observations, the majority members of the Parliament, as a knee jerk reaction to the release from the Home of one of the convicted persons of the NIRVAYA case amended the section of the Act in December 2015 to the extent that the event of various heinous acts, such as murder, rape, the age of juvenile will be lowered from 18 to 16 and he will be tried under criminal justice system. The Quantum of punishment is also enhanced from 7 years to 10 years imprisonment under this new amendments, few juveniles who accused of conflict in law, were already sent to jail custody and booked under criminal justice system. They would face trial in adult criminal courts.

It is pertinent to note that there were amendments to the act of 2000 in 2006, 2011 to include the definition of adoption and to include mandatory provisions for registration of homes/institutions, either run by government or NGOs.

HOMES

There are some changes incorporated in the Act in terms of treatment and of rehabilitation of children in conflict with law and children in need of care and protection.

Children's Homes

Under Section 34, it has been provided that the State Government may establish and maintain either by itself or in association with voluntary organizations, children's homes in every district or group of districts for the reception of children in need of care and protection during the pendency of any inquiry and subsequently for their care, treatment, education, training and rehabilitation. The State Government may provide for the management of children's homes including the standards and the nature of services to be provided by them. The Government may also appoint inspection teams for children's home (Under section 35).

Shelter Homes

The State Government under Section 37 may recognize reputed and capable voluntary organizations and provide them assistance to set up and administer as many shelter homes for juveniles or children as may be required. These shelter homes shall function as drop-in-centers for children brought in need of urgent support.

Rehabilitation and Social Reintegration

It has been provided under Section 40 of the Act that the rehabilitation and social reintegration of his/her child shall begin during stay of the child in a children's or special home. There are three ways mentioned in which the rehabilitation and social reintegration of children shall be carried out, alternatively, by

- Adoption
- Foster care
- Sponsorship
- *Adoption:* The primary responsibility for providing care and protection to a child shall be that of his family but adoption shall be resorted to for children orphaned, abandoned, neglected and abused, in accordance with the guidelines for adoption issued by the Government.
- *Foster care:* Section 42 provides that foster care may be used for temporary placement of those infants who are ultimately to be given for adoption. In foster care, the child may be placed in another family for a short or extended period of time. The State Government may make rules for carrying out foster care programs for children.
- *Sponsorship:* The sponsorship program may provide supplementary support to families, to children's homes and to special homes to meet medical, nutritional, educational and other needs of children according to rules made by State Government.

THE RIGHT OF CHILDREN TO FREE AND COMPULSORY EDUCATION ACT, 2009

Article 21A of the Constitution, as inserted by the Constitution (Eighty-sixth Amendment) Act, 2002 provides that the State shall provide free and compulsory education to all children in the 6–14 years age group in such manner as the State may, by law, determine. The manner in which this obligation will be discharged by the State have been left to the State to determine by law. The Right of Children to Free and Compulsory Education (RTE) Act, 2009 was enacted to give effect to the above constitutional mandate enshrined under Art. 21A.

The Act provides that every child of the age of 6—14 years shall have a right to free and compulsory education in a neighborhood school till completion of elementary education. In accordance with the Act, child shall not be liable to pay any kind of fee or charges or expenditure which may prevent him or her from pursuing and completing the elementary education.

THE CHILD LABOR (PROHIBITION AND REGULATION) ACT, 1986

In accordance with the Article 24 of the Constitution of India, no child below the age of fourteen years shall be employed to work in any factory or mine or engaged in any other hazardous employment. There are a number of Acts which prohibit the employment of children below 14 years or 16 years in certain specified employments. The Child Labor (Prohibition and Regulation) Act, 1986 provides for a general provision for the employment of children, i.e. those who have not completed that fourteenth year, in the scheduled occupations and processes. The Act authorized the Central Government to add any occupation or processes to the Schedule by a Notification in the Official Gazette and thereupon the Schedule shall be deemed to have been operative accordingly. The Act also provides for regulation of work conditions in employments where children are not, prohibited from working. The Act prescribes enhanced penalties for employment of children in violation of the provisions of the Child Labor (Prohibition and Regulation) Act as well as other Acts which forbid the employment of children. It is pertinent to note that much before this act of 1986, immediately after independence, the factories Act of 1948 prohibited employment of young children. In addition, Injuries Act, 1912; Motor Transport Workers Act, 1961; the Apprentice Act, 1961; The Beedi and Cigar Workers Act, 1966; Merchant Shipping Act of 1958, Plantation Labor Act, 1951; Shops and Commercial Establishment, 1969 prohibited the care and employment of child labor.

SOME SALIENT FEATURES OF SOME ACTS RELATED TO CHILDREN WELFARE AND RIGHTS

Notwithstanding this plethora of progressive laws to uplift the welfare of children as well as the protection of rights of children, nobody would agree that the creditable provisions of these laws and rules have fully accomplished their objectives in India. Still in our country, we have deserted street children; neglected children are exploited by trafficking rackets; despite stringent legislation children are found in industries, including hazardous avocations. L Misra, who served secretory to Govt. of India, ministry of labour, made a thorough study on child labor. In foreword to his work, Justice MN Venkatachaliah wrote succinctly: 'So laws as child labor persists, child education will be impossible. It is a vicious circle, if not broken, will entrap and immobilize India to the position of a near Lysander, watching the great excitement of the new transformation of the world pass nearly.' Long ago, Justice VR Krishna Iyer, while talking about Juvenile Justice, wrote in his superb literary language: *The hallmark of culture and advance of civilization consists Lakshmidhar Misra, Child Labour in India: (Oxford, 2000) P. 338 in the fulfillment of our obligation to the young generation by opening up all opportunities for every child to unfold its personality and rise to its full stature, physical, mental, moral and spiritual. It is the birth right of every child that cries for justice from the world as a whole.*

The implementation of anti-child labor laws in India is pathetic. To quote again L Misra in extensor will reveal the actual state of affairs and remedy. It is now admitted fact that children instructions have not risen to the level of standard reformation centers even. Adoption as a mode of rehabilitation has not gained prevalence even though there are huge numbers of children couples desiring to adopt and despite the fact that the law forward adoption over institutionalization for the purpose of rehabilitation of children who are orphaned, abandoned or surrendered.

'The enforcement of the law relating to the prohibition of children in hazardous employment would continue to be the primary responsibility of the state. The track record of state's performance in the area of child labor law enforcement has not been very encouraging. Few prosecutions are filed and fewer still end in conviction. The prosecutions are often poorly conducted and the penalties in the event of conviction are generally in the shape of paltry fines that do not act as a deterrent. Also, the labor law machinery is inadequately manned and there is often collusion between it and the accused. It is, therefore, essential that measures need to be taken to sensitize all government functionaries, including the child labor law enforcement machinery and judiciary with the help of individuals who are themselves fully committed to the cause of elimination of child labor and are skilled communicators and trainers.

To overcome rigid and pre-conceived notions and inculcate the right attitude and approach, it is necessary to create a conducive environment with the involvement of all the ministries, departments, departmental undertakings, public sector undertakings and other agencies, including NGOs, both at the central and state levels, as part of a continuing process rather than a one-time exercise. The central theme should be child survival, child protection and child development, taking into its ambit the elimination of child labor. It should be repeatedly reinforced through songs, slogans, paintings, elocution and essay competitions, and state and street theater that child labour is one of the worst forms of deprivation and ensure through environment building exercises that all policy formulators, planners and implementers responsible for the enforcement of the Child Rights Convention (CRC), 1989 are fully committed to the issue.

Child Marriage

Bengal is among the top four states in the country when it comes to child marriage. A nation-wide survey by the Center has revealed that of the total marriages that take place in Bengal, 54.7% are of minor girls, taking the state to the fourth place with Uttar Pradesh in the National Family Health Survey.

The findings of the study were recently shared with breakthrough, an NGO, that is partnering with the Center to sensitize the states against child marriage.

According to the survey, that is based on 2007–08 data, of the total marriage that take place in Bengal at least 54.7% are of underage children.

Bihar has topped the list with 68.2% minor marriages percent followed by Rajasthan with 57.6% and Jharkhand 55.7% child marriages. The figures of Bengal and UP tally.

A further break-up or simplification of the data shows that the number of child marriages in the rural areas is much higher than in the urban areas. While 57.9% of the rural marriages in Bengal are child marriages, the figure of minor marriage– 36.1%–is much lower in case of total urban marriages and stands at only 36.1%.

The total number of underage married girls, who have also become mothers before attaining the age of 15 in Bengal, stands at a whopping 27,082, which is the second highest in the country after Bihar where the number is 31,665.

The findings of survey are backed by the data collected by government agencies. The National Crime Records Bureau, that has recently released data for 2012, has mentioned how a total of 88 arrests, related to child marriage, where carried out by the cops in Bengal this state between 2008–12. And this figure, incidentally, is the highest in the country.

While a total of 21 persons were arrested in connection with child marriage in 2011, a phenomenal 35 persons were held in 2012. Both Malda and Murshidabad have recorded seven arrests each in 2012. A year earlier, 10 persons were arrested from Murshidabad and six from Malda.

North Dinajpur, topped the list in 2012 with 21 cases and eight arrests. Incidents of child marriages and subsequent arrests were also reported from the districts of North 24-Parganas, Burdwan Cooch Behar, Howrah City, West Midnapore and East Midnapore in 2012.

Police said that all crime against children were somewhat linked to child marriage. 'Take the example of Murshidabad. In 2012, when over 17 cases were officially acted upon by the police, also registered 209 cases of kidnapping and 80 cases of procuration of minor girls. This is a larger social malaise where daughters are yet to equal sons,' said a CID official who did not wish to be named.

'Malda is one of the top three districts in terms of child marriage. In a survey conducted by the Burdwan University using police findings, it was revealed that 42% of the total child marriages in Bengal took place at Malda.' Said a CID officer. Cops confirmed that in Malda, a total of 24 child marriages were prevented since July, 2012. However, of this at least six girls child brides were later married off by their families.

'A 10-year-old student of class 3 of Laxmighat village under Narhatta gram panchayat was married off by her family after her first marriage was thwarted on 2 November, 2012. Rozina Khutun, daughter of Abdul Khaleq of Manikchak was also married to the groom chosen by her family after her marriage was prevented by child line on 1 November. In both cases FIRs were asked to be lodged by the district social welfare officer but no arrests have been made so far. 'The entire village gets united and it gets difficult to even get a proper eyewitness to the case,' claimed a cop. (*Source*—Times of India).

CHAPTER 31

The Child with a Musculoskeletal Alteration

Chapter Outline

- Review of the Musculoskeletal System
- Disorders of Musculoskeletal System

REVIEW OF THE MUSCULOSKELETAL SYSTEM

The musculoskeletal system provides form, support, stability, and movement to the body. It is made up of the bones of the skeleton, muscles, cartilage, tendons, ligaments, joints, and other connective tissues that supports and binds tissues and organs together. There are 206 bones in the adult body. The bones of the body perform five main functions such as:

- Provide support for the body
- Store minerals and lipids
- Produce blood cells
- Protect body organs
- Provide leverage and movement.

Bones begin to form in a mother's womb about six weeks after fertilization, and portions of the skeleton do not stop growing until about the age of 25. Most bones originate as hyaline cartilage and converted to bone through a process called ossification. Bone growth begins at the center of the cartilage. As bones enlarge, bone growth activity shifts to the ends of the bones called the growth plate (epiphysis) which results in an increase in bone length. Long bones grow primarily by elongation of the diaphysis, with an epiphysis at each end of the growing bone.

The outer shell of the long bone is made of solid compact bone. This is covered by a membrane of connective tissue called the periosteum. There is a layer of spongy cancellous bone beneath the cortical bone. Inside this is the medullary cavity which has an inner core of bone marrow made up of yellow marrow in the adult and red marrow in the child (Fig. 31.1). The proportion of compact and spongy bone varies with the shape of the bone. Spongy bone is much lighter than compact bone, which helps in reducing the weight of the body.

- *Joints:* Joints are structures that connect individual bones and may allow bones to move against each other to cause movement. Each joint reflects a compromise between stability and range of motion. For example, the bones of the skull are very stable but with little motion, whereas the shoulder joint allows for a full range of motion but is a relatively unstable joint (Fig. 31.2).
- *Tendons:* A tendon is a tough, flexible band of fibrous connective tissue that connects muscles to bones. As muscles contract, tendons transmit the forces to the relatively rigid bones, pulling on them and causing movement (Fig. 31.2).
- *Ligaments:* Ligaments attach bone to bone. A ligament is a small band of dense, white, fibrous elastic tissue. Ligaments connect the ends of bones together in order to form a joint (Fig. 31.2). Most ligaments limit dislocation, or prevent certain movements that may cause breaks.

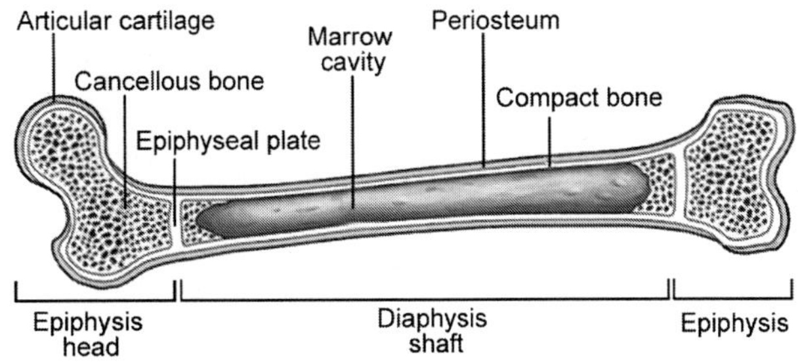

Fig. 31.1: Description of a long bone

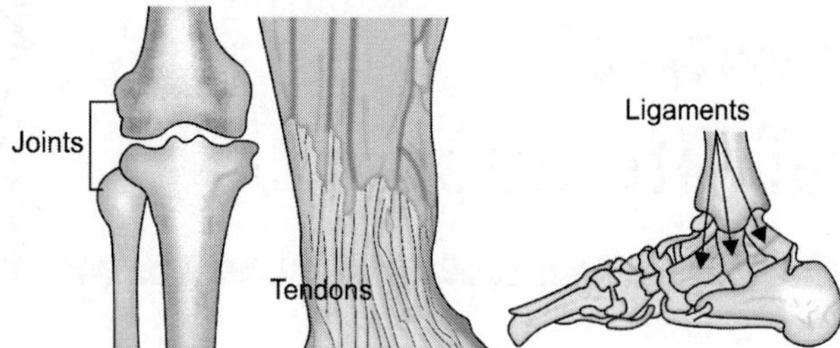

Fig. 31.2: Other elements of the musculoskeletal system

- *Skeletal muscles:* These muscles contract to pull on tendons and move the bones of the skeleton. In addition to producing skeletal movement, muscles also maintain posture and body position, support soft tissues, guard entrances and exits to the digestive and urinary tracts, and maintain body temperature.
- *Nerves:* Nerves control the contraction of skeletal muscles, interpret sensory information, and coordinate the activities of the body's organ systems.
- *Cartilage:* This is a type of connective tissue. It is a firm gel-like substance. The body contains three major types of cartilage: hyaline cartilage, elastic cartilage, and fibrocartilage.

DISORDERS OF MUSCULOSKELETAL SYSTEM

Limb Defects

Congenital Club Foot

Club foot or clubfoot, also called congenital talipes equinovarus (CTEV), is a congenital deformity of lower extremity that affects the lower leg, ankle and foot (Fig. 31.3). It involves one foot or both. The affected foot appears to have been rotated internally at the ankle.

Etiology and Incidence

In most cases the cause of clubfoot is unknown. There may be a genetic link because it can run in families but environmental factors that are not well-understood. In a small number of cases, clubfoot occurs as part of a more serious underlying neuromuscular condition affecting the baby's development, such as spina bifida, meningomyelocele. The incidence of clubfoot in newborns is 1 in 1000, and boys are commonly affected than girls.

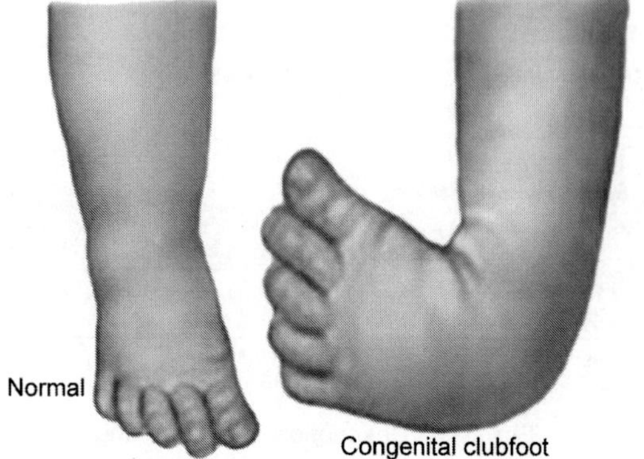

Fig. 31.3: Congenital talipes equinovarus

Manifestations and Diagnostic Evaluation

A range of unusual positions of the foot are given below. Each of the following characteristics may be present, and each may vary from mild to severe:
- The foot (especially the heel) is usually smaller than normal.
- The foot may point downward.
- The front of the foot may be rotated toward the other foot.
- The foot may turn in, and in extreme cases, the bottom of the foot can point up.

Clubfoot is painless in a baby, but it can eventually cause discomfort and a noticeable disability may be seen. Left untreated, clubfoot does not straighten itself out. The foot will remain twisted out of shape, and the affected leg may be shorter and smaller than the other.

Without treatment, people with clubfeet often appear to walk on their ankles or on the sides of their feet.

Therapeutic Management

Treatment for clubfoot should ideally start within a week or two of the baby being born, but it can still be effective if started later in childhood and includes orthopedic surgical approaches. The goal of the treatment is to stretch tighten ligaments and tendons gently and return the foot to a maximal anatomic position and being put in cast. This technique is known as the Ponseti method which is repeated weekly for around five to eight weeks.

After this stage, it is likely that the baby may need a minor procedure to make a small cut in their Achilles tendon. This can help to release their foot into a more natural position.

The baby with club foot will need to wear special boots attached to each other with a bar, to prevent club foot returning. These are only worn full-time for the first three months, then overnight until the child is four or five years old.

Developmental Dysplasia of the Hip

Developmental dysplasia of the hip (DDH), previously known as *congenital hip dysplasia* is a common disorder affecting infants and young children. The change in name reflects the fact that DDH is a developmental process that occurs over time. It develops either in the uterus or during the first year of life. It may or may not be present at birth.

DDH is defined as partial or complete displacement of the femoral head from the acetabular cavity since birth. The condition varies in severity from a spectrum of disorders including acetabular dysplasia without displacement, subluxation and dislocation. DDH can be congenital, but in some children it develops after birth, hence, it termed developmental.

Etiology and Incidence

DDH appears to be multifactorial in origin. According to genetic theory generalized joint laxity and shallow acetabulum develops due to hereditary predisposition.

In other cases the infant's position may affect how the hip joint forms, either during growth inside the mother or after birth. For example, a breech position in utero limits movement. It also puts the hips in a position with the hips bent, knees straight, and legs together. This position puts abnormal stresses on the joint that do not foster normal development.

Hip position and free hip movement remain important during the first months after birth. This is when the hip continues to develop and forms a deep socket and stable joint. An infant carried on a parent's body with the hips bent and open wide is less likely to develop DDH. Infants in some cultures are swaddled or wrapped with the legs together and extended out straight on papoose board. An infant that spends a good deal of time in this position is at greater risk for DDH.

DDH is much more common in girls than boys. This may be linked with hormonal differences. Estrogens and a hormone called relaxin present during development in uterus and still present at the time of birth may cause generalized laxity or looseness of the ligaments.

The left hip is affected more than the right hip. Again, this is probably linked with position before birth. The most common position in utero places the child's left hip next to the mother's spine and limits hip motion.

Children with developmental disabilities who do not move normally or who cannot stand up and walk are also at risk for DDH.

Pathology

Normal hip joint is a multi-axial ball and socket joint designed for stability and weight bearing (Fig. 31.4). Head of femur covered with hyaline cartilage articulates with acetabulum of hip bone to form hip joint. Different ligaments like iliofemoral, pubofemoral, ischiofemoral and transverse ligament hold this ball and socket joint

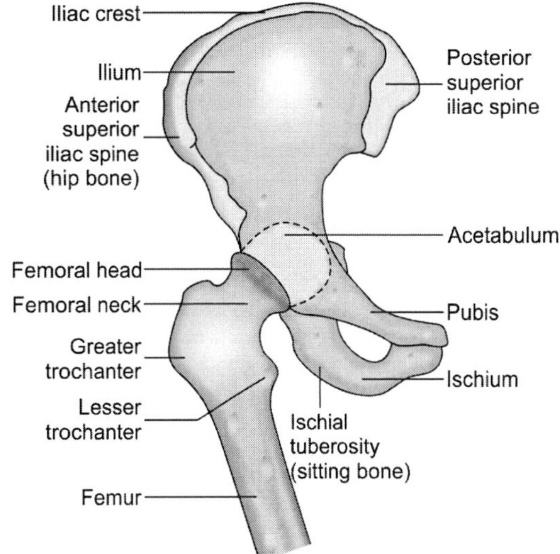

Fig. 31.4: Bones of the hip and pelvis

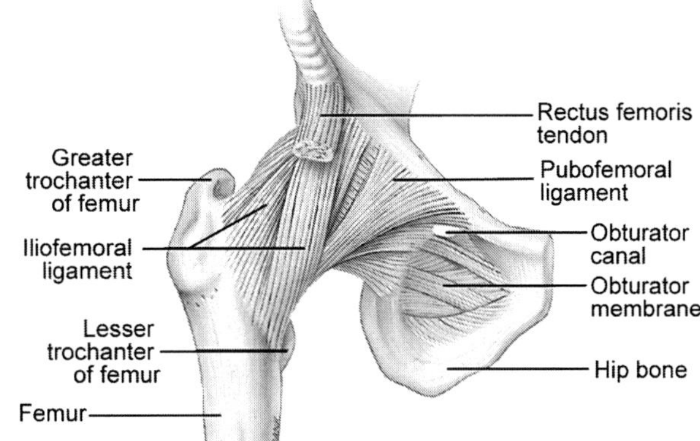

Fig. 31.5: Ligaments of the hip joint

(Fig. 31.5). Movements at the joint include flexion, extension, abduction, adduction, medial and lateral rotation, and circumduction.

In DDH there is a disruption in the normal relationship between the head of the femur and the acetabulum. It can affect one or both hips and may be mild to severe. In mild cases called unstable hip dysplasia the hip is in the joint but easily dislocated. More involved cases are partially dislocated or completely dislocated. A partial dislocation is called subluxation. In classic DDH (dislocated at birth) or dislocated after birth (underlying laxity) shows changes like the head of the femur is located in the acetabulum but may be subluxated (partially dislocated), femoral head is displaced or lying upwards and laterally, epiphysis is small and ossifies late (Fig. 31.6). Femoral neck excessively anteverted.

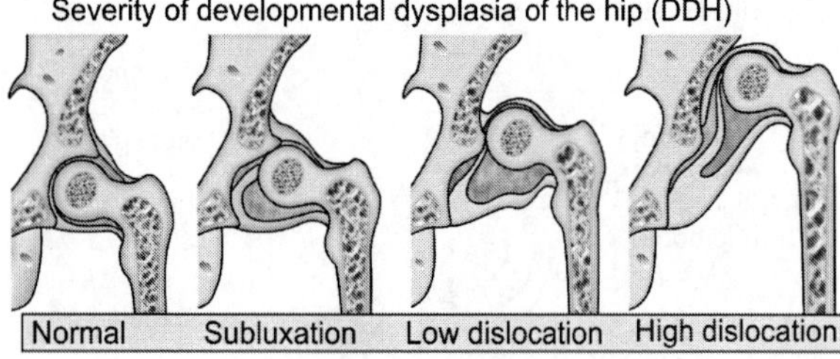

Fig. 31.6: Developmental dysplasia of the hip

Acetabulum shallow, hip ligaments are lax, capsule is stretched, hip muscles undergo adaptive shortening.

Clinical Features

The clinical features vary according to age, means detected at birth or soon after when child starts walking. The newborn, infant, or young child may not have any symptoms such as pain to signal a problem. There may be some differences in how the legs and buttocks look from side to side.

Birth: Routine screening for suggestive signs in every newborn especially those at high-risk. Due to laxity of the ligaments around the hip allows the femoral head to be displaced from the acetabulum on manipulation.

Early childhood: Asymmetry of groin fold, click, limitation of movement and asymmetric abduction is present when the child is placed supine with the knees and hips flexed.

Older child: The symptoms change from lax ligaments to contractures and stiffness in affected hip joint. It results in peculiar gait, with lurching toward the affected side, no pain.

Diagnosis

Examination of infant: It includes checking asymmetry of groin crease, limitation of movement or audible click and special tests like Barlow's and Ortolani's (Figs 31.7A and B).

Barlow's Test: To assess DDH in neonate the Barlow maneuver identifies the unstable hip that is in a reduced position that the clinician can passively dislocate. Here, the hip is started reduced and the test will dislocate the hip.

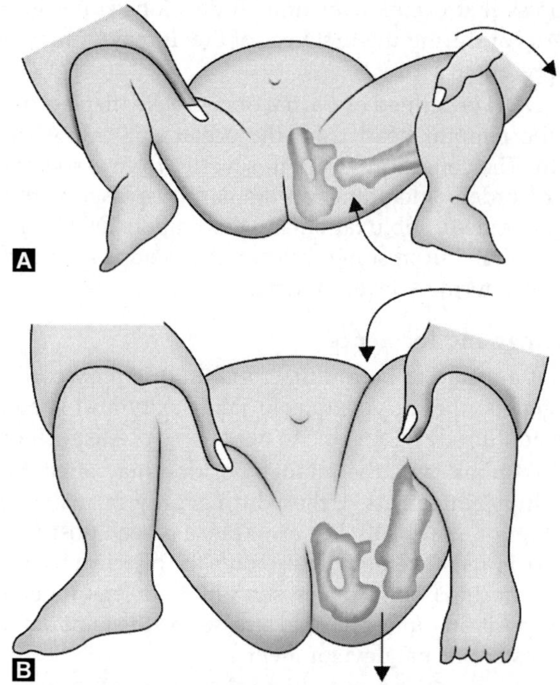

Figs 31.7A and B: Examination of infant to assess DDH in neonate. **A.** Barlow's test; **B.** Ortolani's test

Ortolani's Test: Ortolani maneuver is performed following Barlow's test to determine if the hip is actually dislocated. Here, the hip is started dislocated and the test will reduce the hip.

For the infant three months or older, *Galeazzi's* or *Allis'* test can be performed (Figs 31.8A and B). The child is placed in the supine position with the hips and knees bent and the feet flat. The examiner looks for any unevenness between the knees. If one knee is lower than the other, there may be a dislocated hip on the lower side.

Since DDH can develop over time, repeated exams are advised. Well-baby check-ups should include repeated hip examination. This is done until the child begins to walk normally with no sign of a limp or altered gait pattern. The clinic nurse should look for changes in hip range of motion, uneven skin folds around the thighs and buttocks, and a difference in leg length from side to side.

X-rays are not reliable in infants because bony ossification is not complete but may be of some diagnostic value in the older child. Ultrasonography (USG) and physical examination of the child are more accurate in the first six months of life. CT scan and MRI may be helpful in difficult cases, but use of these studies is limited.

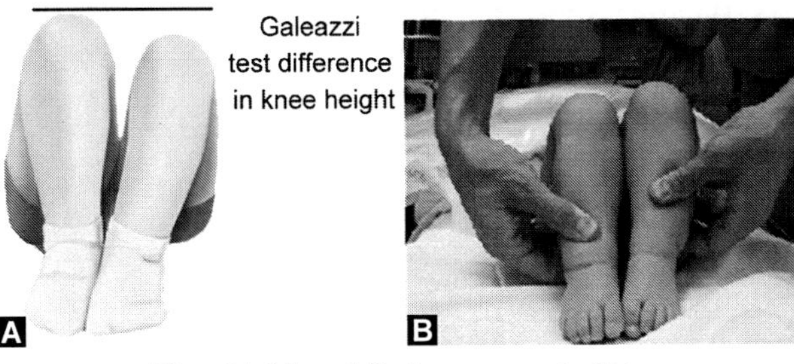

Figs 31.8A and B: Assessment of hip

Hip USG is most important investigation for detection and management of DDH in newborns and young infants. By using high frequency sound waves, there is no risk of radiation to the baby. Because many of the bones making up the hip joint are made of soft cartilage, not hard bone, plain X-rays are generally not helpful until the baby is 5–6 months old. USG enables direct imaging of the cartilaginous portions of the hip that cannot be seen on plain radiographs.

Therapeutic Management

Once the diagnosis of DDH has been made, the treatment will depend on the age of the child and the degree of instability. The goal of treatment of DDH, regardless of age, is to keep the femoral head in good contact with the acetabulum. A stable hip encourages the development of a normally shaped socket and rounded head of the femur.

Birth to 6 months: If hip is reduced and has a normal cartilaginous outline, no treatment is required, the child is observed for 3–6 months. If acetabular dysplasia or hip instability, the hip is splinted in a position of flexion and abduction and USG done at intervals. The proper hip position must be maintained for enough time to stabilize the joint. The hip should be flexed to 95 degrees and abducted at least 90 degrees. This position keeps the femoral head in the best position and allows the ligaments and joint capsule to tighten up.

In case of unavailability of ultrasound the child is nursed in double napkins or an abduction pillow for the first 6 weeks and observed for first 6 months for development of acetabular roof.

In newborns and older and infants younger than six months, reduction of the hip joint by using several braces is the method of treatment. The hip is reduced preferably by closed methods but if necessary by operation and held reduced until acetabular development is satisfactory. If the ultrasound shows that the hip is subluxating, dislocated, or that the acetabulum is shallow, the initial

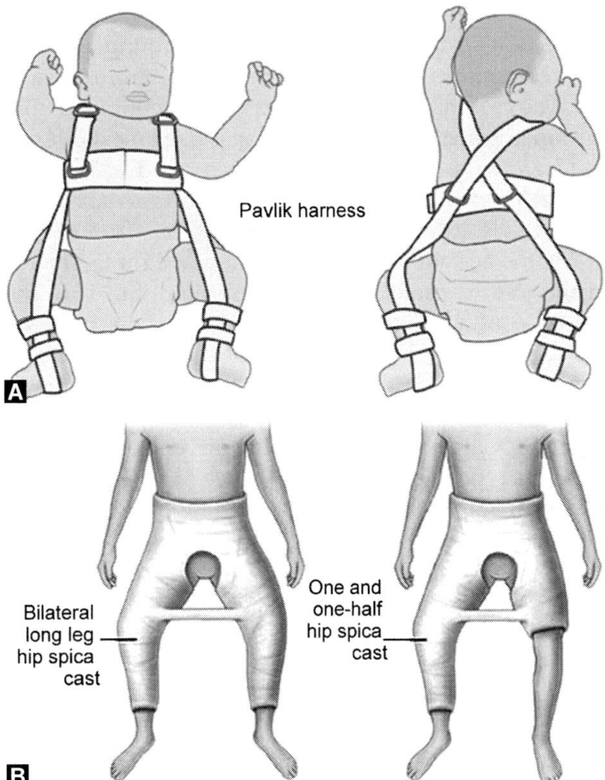

Figs 31.9A and B: Pavlik harness for early correction of hip dysplasia in infants

treatment may consist of a Pavlik harness. The Pavlik harness is often used as the initial treatment of hip dysplasia in infants. Treatment involves a special soft dynamic harness called the *Pavlik harness, initially which* can be used for six to twelve weeks. The harness keeps the hip in flexion and abduction and external rotation. Pavlik harness consists of chest and shoulder straps and foot stirrups (Figs 31.9A and B). This position maintains the proper position of the femoral head and allows for 'tightening up' of the ligamentous structures as well as for stimulation of normal formation and deepening of the hip socket.

Too much force into abduction can block the blood supply to the femoral head causing a condition called avascular necrosis. In the older child, X-rays may be used to confirm that the hip is stable. The Pavlik harness is successful in approximately 90–95% of infants with hip dysplasia. If there is no improvement seen, the Pavlik harness will be discontinued, and it will be necessary to proceed with closed reduction and spica body casting.

Surgery may be needed for children (above 18 months) when the hip cannot be stabilized and kept in the socket. Before the surgery, the child may be placed in traction to loosen the soft tissues around the hip. Then the child is put in a full hip spica cast from waist to toe. The cast may be needed for several months to hold the hip in place. An open reduction is used most often in children two years old or older when hip dysplasia has not been corrected. During this operation, any abnormal tissues that are keeping the femoral head from fitting inside the acetabulum are removed any tight ligaments in the joint capsule around the hip joint are cut. The tightly contracted tendons or muscles in the hip area may also be cut. This relaxation of the tight structures around the hip joint and allows the hip to be placed in the socket. These tissues grow back with scar tissue as the child heals. The child is usually placed in a spica cast after this type of surgery and will need to wear this cast for several months.

For profoundly affected children, traction is often followed by osteotomy (Salter's osteotomy, Chiar osteotomy) and repositioning of the femur. The spica cast is necessary after surgery for long-term immobilization to hold the hip in place and to achieve healing. The progress achieved with the treatment is assessed by radiograph and it is necessary for further modification of treatment.

Complications

Failed reduction: The acetabulum remains undeveloped, the femoral head may be deformed, the neck is usually anteverted and the capsule is thickened and adherent.

Avascular necrosis (AVN): Ischemia of the immature femoral head. It may occur at any age and any stage of treatment and is probably due to vascular injury or obstruction due to forceful reduction and hip splintage in abduction.

Nursing Management of a Child with Musculoskeletal Impairment

Nursing diagnosis related to musculoskeletal impairment:

- Risk for disproportionate growth related to congenital disorders.
- Impaired physical mobility related to musculoskeletal impairment.
- Impaired skin integrity related to musculoskeletal impairment.
- Disturbed body image related to developmental changes.
- Social isolation related to alterations in physical appearances.

Assessment: Abnormal position of foot and ankle, ball and socket joint of pelvis.

Nursing Diagnosis: Impaired physical mobility due to musculoskeletal disorders.

Intervention: Detection of the abnormality after birth by head to foot assessment. Nurses need to record the type and degree of deformity in the musculoskeletal system at the time of birth and early reporting for intervention.

Help in early treatment: Application of cast or appliances to hold the musculoskeletal part in the corrected positions are important. It should be continued after discharge.

Assessment: Parental anxiety.

Nursing Diagnosis

- Knowledge deficit related to condition and treatment.
- Potential for physiologic injury, due to failure to provide appropriate care to the child.

Nursing Action

- Allow parents to verbalize their concerns
- Explain to the parents the effect of the device being used
- The need to change the device as child grows
- If the device is in effective, surgery may be performed
- Care of a child with plaster cast.

Preparation

- Discuss pathology/deformity and expected treatment in terms the parents can understand and rule out misconceptions and to provide information about the deformity.
- Review the pathology, prognosis and future expectations to mothers to provide knowledge base from which parents can make informed choice.
- Casting means immobilization of the body part, maintaining correct position, etc. Explain to the child what to expect with casting.
- Allow the parent to accompany the child to the cast room to hold the baby and talk to them during application.
- Stretch a tube stockinet over the area to be casted and place soft cotton sheets over the bony prominences.
- Inform the child the cast feels cool when it is applied wet but, will feel warm when it starts drying.

Nursing diagnosis: Risk for altered peripheral tissue perfusion due to pressure from cast.

Interventions

- Check every 1–2 hours for temperature, pulse, color, sensation, motion, and capillary refill time of the casting limb (fingers/toes). Elevate the extremity to promote venous return and prevents edema. Check circulation frequently (Every 15 min for the first 1 h, hourly for 24 hours and 4 hourly thereafter). Assess for warmth, presence of pedal pulses (plaster in the lower limb) and sensations of numbness or tingling.
- Signs of impaired neurovascular function are pain, pallor, pulselessness and paresthesia. In that case reviewing of the cast area is to be done by making window or cutting the plaster cast.
- Edema that is not improved by elevation indicates also neurovascular impairment.
  - The cast may be removed and replaced only if the child grows and there are signs that the cast is too small or if there is evidence of skin breakdown. The child should be checked several times (as mentioned above). Leg or foot pain, cool or numb toes, or loss of motion in the feet must be reported to the physician right away.

Nursing diagnosis: Risk for impaired tissue integrity due to pressure from cast.

Interventions

- Move the child in a wet cast cautiously, always use open palms to move the cast.
- Pressing with fingers in dent the cast and cause pressure points which can lead to an ulcer.
- The child is to be turned every 2 hour to allow the under surface of the cast to dry.
- Use of external heat or use of fans to dry the cast is to be avoided as it causes uneven drying.
- When the cast is dry if the edges are hard and uneven, smooth the edges by applying adhesive tape strips.
- Special care must be taken not to get the cast wet with water or urine. If casted area covers the genitalia, cover the edges of the cast covering the genital area with a plastic or waterproof material. Younger children remain in diapers. A special hole is cut open to allow the older child to go to the bathroom.
- Teach the child nothing to put between the cast and skin.

Nursing diagnosis: Parental health seeking behaviors to render care of the child with cast at home.

Interventions

- Assess and teach parent to assess for signs of excessive pressure on skin, redness, excoriation because these signs require immediate evaluation and intervention.
- Parents are to be explained about immobilization and maintenance of the position of cast limb. If the cast is for the lower extremity discuss how much weight bearing is allowed and the use of crutches if prescribed. Crutch walking demonstration is to be done.
- Discuss with the parents how the child will be comfortable with the cast.
- Demonstrate how to move or position the child and allow return demonstrations.
- If an abduction bar is used with the cast the parents should know the purpose of the bar. They should not use it as a handle to move or lift the child.
- Encourage providing touch stimulation to the remaining body parts of the child.
- Instruct parents to apply a hand lotion or massage the area gently if it is reachable, in case of itching problem.
- If not reachable blow cool air through the cast using a fan.
- Aware parents not to put anything inside to scratch.
- Encourage parents to hold and play with child and participate in care to promote bonding.
- Discuss the importance of physical therapy to enhance mobility maintain appropriate muscle tone
- Parents are to be aware about prevention of urinary stasis and constipation. Introduction of adequate fluid and proper diet are two important areas need to be focused adequately.
- Physical and occupational therapy is important during the postoperative period in the cast. Opportunities to move and develop gross motor skills are limited. The therapist will closely monitor overall gross and fine motor skills normally occurring during this time.

Scoliosis

Scoliosis is derived from the Greek term meaning curvature. People with scoliosis have a sideways curve in their spine that makes an 'S' or 'C' shape. Scoliosis is a sideways curve of the spine that causes stiffness and pain. The vertebrae can rotate at the thoracic level of the spine causing this curve and resulting in a hump near the rib cage (Figs 31.10A and B). Scoliosis is a painful condition wherein the spine has a sideway curvature. The majority of the scoliosis cases are reported before puberty, during the growing years. The exact cause for scoliosis is still unknown, however; it can result due to 'cerebral palsy' or 'muscular dystrophy'.

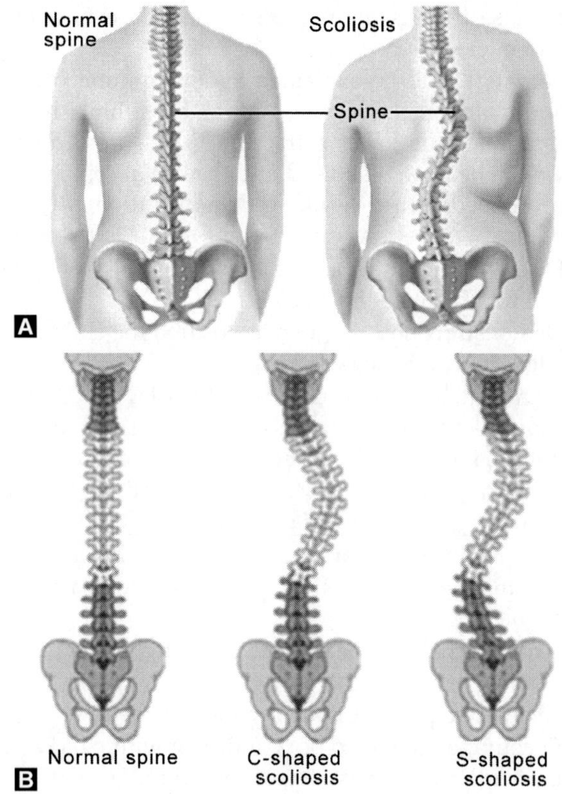

Figs 31.10A and B: Normal spine and its curvature due to scoliosis

Incidence and Causes

It is called an idiopathic disease because the cause of it is unknown. Scoliosis is more common in females and begins in childhood. If it is detected early, scoliosis treatment will prevent it from worsening over time.

There are many types and causes of scoliosis, including:

- *Congenital scoliosis:* Caused by a bone abnormality present at birth.
- *Neuromuscular scoliosis:* A result of abnormal muscles or nerves. Frequently seen in people with spina bifida or cerebral palsy or in those with various conditions that are accompanied by or result in paralysis.
- *Degenerative scoliosis:* This may result from traumatic bone collapse, previous major back surgery or osteoporosis.
- *Idiopathic scoliosis:* The most common type of scoliosis. It has no specific identifiable cause.

The one or more of the following signs of scoliosis are observed:

- One shoulder is higher than the other (Fig. 31.11).
- One shoulder blade sticks out more than the other.

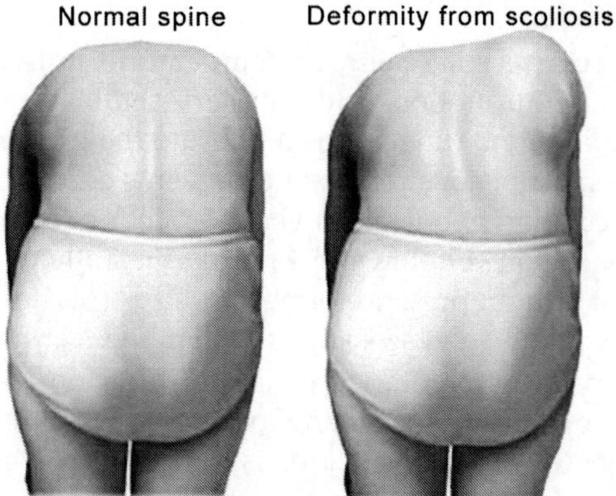

Fig. 31.11 : The Adam's forward bend test

- One side of the rib cage appears higher than the other.
- One hip appears higher or more prominent than the other.
- The waist appears uneven.
- The body tilts to one side.
- One leg may appear shorter than the other.

Pathophysiology

Scoliosis is defined as a deviation of the normal vertical line of the spine, consisting of a lateral curvature with rotation of the vertebrae within the curve. Scoliosis can be the result of a neuromuscular condition. One sided muscle weakness of the spinal column results in shortening of the muscles and ligaments on the opposite side. The curvature of the spinal column is developed due to tightening of the ligaments. Moreover this tightness compresses the vertebrae on that side on a concave curve. As growth spurt is high during adolescence, spinal curvature exacerbates during this period (may be more than 50 degrees), and may cause in spinal instability. The curvature of spine is measured by Cobb method.

For using the Cobb method of measuring the degree of scoliosis, the most tilted vertebrae above and below the apex of the curve are chosen (Fig. 31.12). The angle between intersecting lines drawn perpendicular to the top of the top vertebrae and the bottom of the bottom vertebrae is the Cobb angle. Less than 10° is considered as normal, less than 20° is mild, 25–45° is moderate and more than 45° of curvature is called severe scoliosis.

Signs of Scoliosis

The vast majority of patients with idiopathic scoliosis initially present because of a perceived deformity.

Without an **X-ray of the spine**, there are several common physical symptoms that may indicate scoliosis.

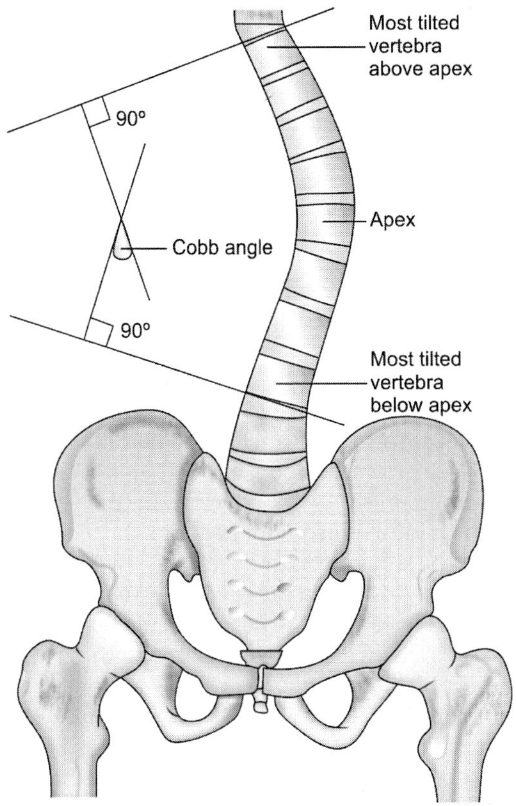

Fig. 31.12: Spinal curvatures are usually determined using a standard measurement called the Cobb angle

One of the most common tests for detecting scoliosis is called the Adam's forward bend test, in which the individual bends from the waist as if touching the toes. Then one or more signs of scoliosis are observed.

If a scoliosis curve gets worse, the spine will also rotate or twist, in addition to curving side to side. This causes the ribs on one side of the body to stick out further than on the other side. Severe scoliosis can cause back pain and difficulty breathing.

Lateral curvature—scoliosis

Front to back curvature—Kyphosis

Exaggerated curvature of the spine in lumbar region–lordosis (Figs 31.13A to C).

Diagnostic Evaluation

The clinical evaluation will usually include a physical exam, during which the curvature of the spine is assessed. Adam's test, the spinal curvature is measured by Cobb method are done as specific tests to identify scoliosis. A complete neurological examination should evaluate

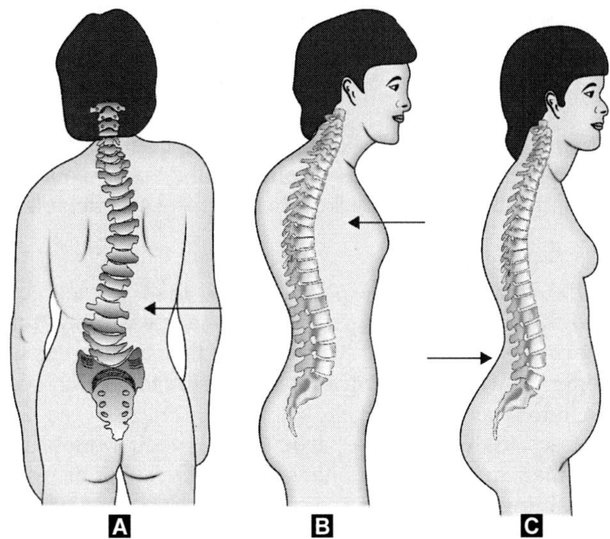

Figs 31.13A to C: Most spinal abnormalities in children are abnormal curvatures. A. Scoliosis; B. Kyphosis; C. Lordosis

balance, reflexes and motor testing in all muscle groups, and sensory testing of the lower extremities, back and chest. Rapid assessment of strength and balance can be made by observing gait, toe-walking, heel-walking, heel-to-toe walking along a straight line and hopping on one foot.

The X-ray is ordered to both confirm the scoliosis diagnosis and check on the magnitude of the spinal curvature. The X-ray will also give some indication as to the skeletal maturity of the patient which may influence treatment decisions.

Therapeutic Management

Scoliosis treatment decisions are primarily based on two factors:

- The age of the child and his/her *skeletal maturity* (or rather, how much more growth can be expected).
- The *degree of spinal curvature.*
- The presence or absence of associated complications.

Although the cause of idiopathic scoliosis is unknown, the way scoliosis curves behave is well-understood.

- Generally no treatment is necessary in case of a small degree of curvature in a patient nearing skeletal maturity.
- On the other hand, a younger patient with a bigger curve is likely to have a curve will continue to advance and will need treatment.

There are three main scoliosis treatment options for adolescents:

- Observation
- Back braces
- Scoliosis surgery.

No exercises for scoliosis have proved to reduce or prevent curvature. However, exercise is highly recommended for both scoliosis and non-scoliosis patients alike to keep back muscles strong and flexible.

Bracing

If the curvature of the spine is less than 25 degrees and the patient is still growing, he/she is examined for every 4 to 6 months and wait to see if the curvature gets better or worse. Bracing is the usual treatment choice for adolescents who have a spinal curve between 25 degrees to 40 degrees—particularly if their bones are still maturing and if they have at least 2 years of growth remaining.

The purpose of bracing is to halt progression of the curve; it does not resolve the exiting curve. It may provide a temporary correction, but usually the curve will assume its original magnitude when bracing is eliminated.

Surgery

Those who have curves beyond 40 degrees to 50 degrees are often considered for scoliosis surgery. Surgical correction of idiopathic scoliosis is considered for curves greater than 45° in immature patients and for curves greater than 50° in mature patients. The goal is to make sure the curve does not get worse, but surgery does not perfectly straighten the spine. During the procedure, metallic implants are utilized to correct some of the curvature and hold it in the correct position until a bone graft, placed at the time of surgery, consolidates and creates a rigid fusion in the area of the curve. Scoliosis surgery usually involves joining the vertebrae together permanently called spinal fusion.

The treatment of scoliosis is complex. It needs regular and periodic observation with radiographic evaluation. The goals for surgical treatment are to prevent progression and to improve spinal alignment and balance.

Fracture

A fracture is a partial or complete break in the bone. Fractures occur when there is more force applied to the bone than the bone can absorb.

A child's bone differs from adult bone in a following ways:

- Healing of child's bone is much faster than an adult's bone. The younger the child, the faster the healing occurs.
- Bones are softer in children and tend to bend rather than completely break.
- Growth plates, called epiphysis are located at the end of the long bones of children. Injury to the growth plate can lead to limb length discrepancies or angular deformities.

Etiology and Incidence

Breaks in bones can occur from falls, trauma, or as a result of a direct blow or kick to the body. Bones are weakest when they are twisted.

Pathophysiology

In a fracture the injured bone and surrounding tissues start to bleed, forming a fracture hematoma. The blood coagulates to form a blood clot situated between the broken fragments. As blood clots at the site, fibrin strands provide a network for healing. The blood vessels grow into the jelly-like matrix and the new blood vessels bring phagocytes to the area, which gradually remove the non-viable material. The blood vessels also bring fibroblasts in the walls of the vessels and these multiply and produce collagen fibers. In this way the blood clot is replaced by a matrix of collagen. Calcium salt are deposited in the new bone matrix and callus is formed. This mineralization of the collagen matrix stiffens it and transforms it into bone.

When a fracture occurs, it is classified as either open or closed:

- *Open fracture (compound fracture):* The bone exits and is visible through the skin, or a deep wound that exposes the bone through the skin.
- *Closed fracture (simple fracture):* The bone is broken, but the skin is intact.

Below is a listing of the common types that may occur in children (Fig. 31.14):

- *Greenstick:* Incomplete fracture. A portion of the bone is broken, causing the other side to bend.
- *Transverse:* The break is in a straight line across the bone.
- *Spiral:* The break spirals around the bone; common in a twisting injury.
- *Compression:* The bone is crushed, causing the broken bone to be wider or flatter in appearance.
- *Comminuted:* The break is in three or more pieces.
- *Avulsion:* An avulsion fracture occurs when a small chunk of bone attached to a tendon or ligament gets pulled away from the main part of the bone.
- *Stress:* A stress fracture is a tiny crack in a bone that usually happens from overuse. Putting repetitive strain on bones can break them down.

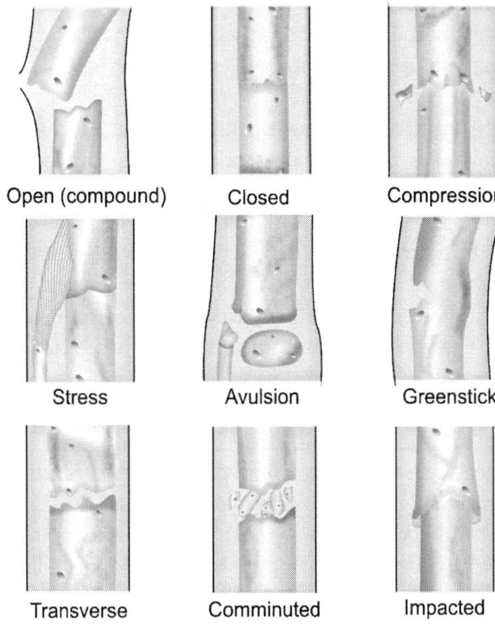

Fig. 31.14: The common types of fracture that may occur in children

Children's bones also have growth plates (epiphyseal plate), which are bands of softer cartilage near the end of the bone that allow the bone to elongate as it grows. Since the bone is softer in the area of the growth plate, it is common to see fractures in this zone and injury to the growth plate may affect that bone's growth. If the germinal cells remain with the epiphysis and no injury occurs in it, healing is rapid and growth is seldom affected. Many of these fractures of the growth plates in the hand and wrist heal well without later deformity.

Salter-Harris Fracture Classification (Fig. 31.15)	Description
Type I	The epiphyseal plate is completely separated from the metaphysis without fracture.
Type II	Transverse fracture through the separated epiphyseal plate.
Type III	fracture through the epiphysis and physis.
Type IV	fracture through the metaphysis, physis and epiphysis.
Type V	Crush injury involving part or all of the growth plates and causes cell death in the growth plate.

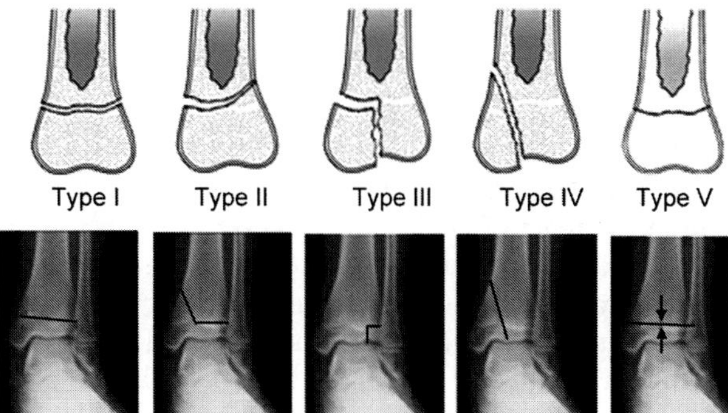

Fig. 31.15: Salter-Harris fracture classification

Signs and Symptoms

The following are the most common symptoms of a fracture. However, each child may experience symptoms differently. Symptoms may include:

- Pain in the injured area
- Swelling in the injured area
- Obvious deformity in the injured area
- Difficulty using or moving the injured area in a normal manner
- Warmth, bruising, or redness in the injured area
- Other signs and symptoms include crepitus, muscle spasm, erythema, ecchymosis and inability to bear weight.

Diagnostic Evaluation

The diagnosis is done with physical examination and diagnostic tests. During the examination a complete medical history of the child is obtained and asks how the injury occurred. X-rays are usually used to confirm if a bone is broken and, to find the locations of any loose bony pieces. Imaging of suspected fracture usually begins with plain radiography. Although X-ray will reveal most fractures, subtle fractures, including those in skeletally immature children and some stress fractures may not be visible immediately on X-ray. If symptoms of fracture persist, an occult fracture is suspected. Follow-up X-rays may show a fracture due to loss of bone around the fracture site during the healing process. However, if plain X-rays continue to be negative but clinical suspicion remains, further imaging tests like MRI, CT are warranted.

This test is done to rule out any associated abnormalities of the spinal cord and nerves.

Therapeutic Management

The goal of treatment is to control the pain, promote healing, prevent complications, and restore normal use of the fractured area.

Broken fingers, wrists, and hands are mostly commonly treated in children with casting or splinting. If the broken bone is not lined up, the bone may need to be 'set' or 'reduced' with a manual manipulation. In more severe fractures, surgery may be needed to reset the fracture and a metal plate, screws, pins, or rods placed in order to keep the bone in proper position while it is healing. Specific treatment for a fracture is determined by the

- age of the child, overall health, and medical history
- extent of the fracture
- tolerance for specific medications, procedures or therapies
- expectations for the course of the fracture
- opinion or preference of the parents.

Treatment may include

The human body is very good at repairing itself after an injury, and it comes equipped with all the tools it needs to fix fractures. Medical professionals work together with the body by creating the best possible conditions for healing. After that, it is just a matter of standing back and giving the body to do its job.

Non-surgical steps

- Many stable fractures heal successfully with cast or splint immobilization. Splint or cast immobilizes the injured area to promote bone alignment and healing to protect the injured area from motion or use. Splints provide less support than casts; however, they can be easily adjusted to accommodate swelling from injuries. In many cases, a splint is applied to a fresh injury first. As swelling subsides, a full cast may replace the splint.

In some stable elbow fractures, the bones may need to be repositioned before applying a splint or cast. In a closed reduction doctor gently moves the arm to manipulate the bones back into place. Some form of sedation or anesthesia is given for this procedure.

As the fracture heals, additional X-rays are schedule to make sure the bones stay in place.

- *Medication:* For pain management
- *Traction:* Traction is the application of a force to stretch certain parts of the body in a specific direction. Traction consists of pulleys, strings, weights, and a metal frame attached over or on the bed. Stretching of the muscles and tendons around the broken bone to allow the bone ends to align and heal is the main purpose of the traction.
- *Surgery:* Surgery may be required to put certain types of broken bones back into place. Occasionally, internal fixation (metal rods or pins located inside the bone) or external fixation devices (metal rods or pins located outside of the body) are used to hold the bone fragments in place to allow alignment and healing.
- If the bone fragments are displaced, surgery may be required to ensure that the fracture heals fully.
- *Closed reduction and percutaneous pinning:* In this procedure, the displaced bone fragments are repositioned during closed reduction and held in place with metal pins. The pins are inserted through the skin, into the bone and across the fracture. A splint is applied to protect the area for the first week, then is typically replaced with a cast. The pins and cast are removed after healing has begun, a few weeks after surgery.
- *Open reduction and internal fixation:* Open fractures, fractures that cannot be repositioned during a closed reduction, and fractures that are accompanied by nerve or vascular injuries require open surgery or open reduction and internal fixation.
- Traction has been used for the management of fractures and dislocations that cannot be treated by means of casting. With the advancement of orthopedic implant technology and operative techniques, traction is rarely used for definitive fracture/dislocation management. Two types of traction exist: skin traction and skeletal traction. A number of pins, plates, wires and screws, external fixation are commonly used to promote fracture healing. These include Steinmann pin, Kirschner wires, buttress plate, etc. The other biologic agents such as hydroxyapatite, tricalcium phosphate have been recognized as stimulators of fracture healing molecules

Children heal quickly and many fractures heal in as little as in one month. In children with a growth plate fracture, immediate diagnosis is important so that if the bone is displaced and needs to be realigned, it can be reset while the fracture is still pliable before it starts to heal.

Children are able to 'remodel' (the specific process of bone resorption and formation) a broken bone after it heals and as the child grows. Certain breaks may not have to be re-aligned perfectly because of this ability to remodel with growth. Younger children have greater potential for remodeling with growth. Fractures that disrupt the surface of a joint usually need to be realigned as precisely as possible. Fractures that are rotated or twisted, or angled out to the side also need to be realigned more precisely as they have less potential to remodel.

Nursing Intervention

Nursing diagnosis

Loss of bone integrity.

Intervention

Immediate support and immobilization of the limb is necessary. Maintain bed rest/limb rest and provide support to joints of both below and above of the affected limb, especially during movement or turning. It gives stability and reduces the possibility of disturbing the alignment.

The distal neurologic and vascular status must be clinically assessed and documented before and after realignment and splinting. If a patient sustains an open fracture, helping physician for achieving hemostasis as rapidly as possible at the injury site is essential; this can be achieved by placing a sterile pressure dressing over the injury site.

Care of children with plaster cast

Preparation of the child on cast application

- Casting means immobilization of the body part, maintaining correct position, etc. Explain to the child what to expect with casting.
  - Place bed board under the mattress. Sagging mattress may deform a wet plaster cast, crack a dry cast, or interfere with pull of traction.
- Allow the parent to accompany the child to the cast room to hold the baby and talk to them during application.
- Stretch a tube stockinet over the area to be casted and place soft cotton sheets over the bony prominences.

Nursing diagnosis

The child is on traction.

Intervention

- Maintain the position of traction which permits pull on the long axis of the fractured part and overcomes muscle tension.
- Make sure that all clamps are functional; lubricate pulleys and check ropes for fraying, to avoid interruption of fracture approximation.

Nursing diagnosis

Impaired physical mobility related to loss of integrity of bone structures (fracture).

Intervention

- The degree of immobility in relation to suggested scale is to be determined.
- Determine presence of complications related to immobility (pneumonia, elimination problems, decubitus, foot drop).
- Physical therapy like chest expansion therapy, range of motion exercises, muscle tightening exercises are to be done to prevent complication. Physiotherapy can help patients to recover from joint stiffness and to maintain and restore ROM.

Nursing diagnosis

Risk for infection related to wound secondary to fracture. Complications of external fixation include pin tract infection.

Intervention

- Note risk factor for occurrence of.infection
- Observe for signs for localized infection
- Dress hand hygiene by all caregivers
- Change surgical or other wound dressings, as indicated, using proper technique for changing or disposing of contaminated materials.
- Maintain individual nutritional need.

Nursing diagnosis

Patient is on plaster/traction.

Intervention

- The patient is to be educated and assisted in performing proper body mechanics in sitting, assisted walking as indicated. It provides an avenue for the child to develop a sense of self-reliance and would guide him/her appropriately within precautionary measures.
- Review X-rays of the child is necessary to assess the healing process (ossification). It provides visual evidence of proper alignment/healing process of the fractured bone; the need for continued therapy.

Osteomyelitis

Osteomyelitis is inflammation of the bone caused by an infecting organism. Although bone is normally resistant to bacterial colonization, events such as injury, surgery, the presence of foreign bodies, may disrupt bony integrity and lead to the onset of bone infection. Bone infections in children are primarily hematogenous in origin, usually occur in the long bone metaphysis. In children, the long bones are usually affected. Acute osteomyelitis almost invariably occurs in children.

Pathophysiology

Approximately 50% of osteomyelitis cases occur in preschool-aged children. Acute hematogenous osteomyelitis is caused due to the rich vascular supply in the growing bones of the children. Circulating organisms tend to start the infection in the metaphyseal ends of the long bones because of the sluggish circulation in the metaphyseal capillary loops. Once the bone is infected, leukocytes enter the infected area and in their attempt to engulf the infectious organisms release enzymes that lyse the bone. The blood flow of the bones get impaired as pus spreads into it and areas of devitalized bone known as *sequestra*, is formed as a result of a chronic infection.

In infants, the infection can spread to a joint and cause arthritis. The presence of vascular connections between the metaphysis and the epiphysis make infants particularly prone to arthritis of the adjacent joint (shoulder joint or hip joint). In children, large subperiosteal abscesses can form because the periosteum is loosely attached to the surface of the bone.

Signs and Symptoms

Osteomyelitis is often diagnosed clinically with nonspecific symptoms such as fever, chills, fatigue, lethargy, or irritability. The classic signs of inflammation, including local pain, swelling, or redness and guarding the affected body part are common. It may also occur and normally disappear within 5–7 days. Long bones, including the femur, tibia and humerus are most commonly affected. Inability to support weight and asymmetric movement of extremities are often early signs in newborns and infants. It is important to note whether the adjacent joint is involved by assessing the range of motion of the joint and signs of inflammation. Often, patients are able to localize the infected bone on examination, owing to pain.

Causes

- *Staphylococcus aureus* is the most common pathogen, followed by *Streptococcus pneumoniae* and *Streptococcus pyogenes*.
- Gram-negative bacteria and group B streptococci are frequently seen in newborns.
- *Pseudomonas aeruginosa* is often associated with osteomyelitis following penetrating wounds.
- Children who are immune-compromised are prone to infection with various fungi and bacteria, in addition to common pathogens.

Diagnosis

The diagnosis of osteomyelitis is complex and relies on a combination of clinical suspicion and indirect laboratory markers such as a high white blood cell count and fever, although to confirm a clinical diagnosis of osteomyelitis, adequate radiologic and laboratory data are necessary.

Except in small bones infections, the C-reactive protein and ESR are almost always elevated. To recover the organism causing the bone infection, such as blood, bone, or joint aspirate cultures can be done. It is important to obtain these cultures before any antibiotics are given. A bone biopsy may be needed if the patient does not respond to standard therapy.

Confirmation is most often by MRI. This test remains the criterion standard, especially in early infections. On T2-weighted images, increased marrow intensity with surrounding inflammation is suggestive of osteomyelitis.

Treatment

The objective of treating osteomyelitis is to eliminate the infection and prevent the development of chronic infection. Chronic osteomyelitis can lead to permanent deformity, possible fracture, and chronic problems, so it is important to treat the disease as soon as possible.

Optimal antibiotic selection, adequate dosing and a sufficiently prolonged antibiotic course with monitoring for clinical response and for the toxicity of therapy are essential. Studies have reported successful treatment of acute uncomplicated osteomyelitis with 3–5 days of intravenous antibiotics and 16–18 days of oral antibiotics.

For successful treatment, high-dose antimicrobials are used for an optimal period and provide close follow-up care throughout treatment with weekly measurements of ESR, C-reactive protein levels, liver function tests, and CBC counts to monitor response and diagnose antibiotic-related neutropenia. In treatment oral antibiotic dosages may need to be increased to keep peak serum-cidal levels of 1:8 or greater. If serum-cidal levels are not adequate with oral antibiotics, the patient is given parenteral treatment. Once the pathogen is identified and antibiotic susceptibility results are available, narrowing of antibiotic therapy is considered.

The usual choice is an antistaphylococcal antibiotic; nafcillin, vancomycin, clindamycin, and cefazolin are the preferred agents. Use of third-generation cephalosporins alone to treat osteomyelitis is not recommended because they are not optimal for treating serious *S aureus* infections.

Neonatal osteomyelitis is treated with nafcillin and tobramycin or vancomycin and gentamicin combinations to provide coverage of bacteria from the *Enterobacteriaceae* family, in addition to group B streptococci and *S aureus*.

Antipseudomonal treatment is considered after surgical debridement in children and adolescents with penetrating trauma of the foot. History taking is very vital to the diagnosis, as infection can occur days to weeks before initial presentation.

Splinting or cast immobilization: Splinting or cast immobilization may be necessary to immobilize the affected bone and nearby joints in order to avoid further trauma and to help the area heal adequately and as quickly as possible. These are frequently done in children, although motion of joints after initial control is important to prevent stiffness and atrophy.

Surgery

Most well-established bone infections are managed through open surgical procedures during which the destroyed bone is scraped out. Surgery is not performed in the case of spinal abscesses unless there is compression of the spinal cord or nerve roots. After surgery, antibiotics against the specific bacteria involved in the infection are then intensively administered during the hospital stay and for many weeks afterward.

Nursing Intervention

Nursing intervention focuses care on controlling infection, protecting the bone from injury, and providing support. It also encourages the patient to verbalize his concerns about his disorder.

Nursing diagnosis	*Nursing intervention*
Acute pain related to inflammation and swelling	Immobilization of the affected area with a splint to reduce pain and muscle spasms. Moreover protection of bones by means of immobilization and avoiding stress on the bone are needed because bones become weak due to the infection process.
	Application of pain management techniques such as massage, distraction, relaxation, hypnosis to reduce pain perception and providing analgesic.
Impaired physical mobility related to pain	Weight bearing and aggressive physical activity should be restricted until the infection and treatment course are completed.
	Support the affected limb with firm pillows which reduces swelling and discomfort.
	Joints above and below the affected area should be made so that still can be moved according to the range yet gently. The wound itself is sometimes very painful and must be handled carefully and slowly.
	Encourage the patient to perform as much self-care as his conditions allows.
	Help the patient identify care techniques and activities that promote rest and relaxation and encourage him to perform them.
Impaired skin integrity related to the effects of surgery; immobilization and chances of infection	Monitor the affected extremity neurovascular status.
	Assess vital signs, observe wound appearance, and note any new pain which may indicate secondary infection.
	Use strict aseptic technique when changing dressings and irrigating wounds.
	Provide a well-balanced diet to promote healing.
	Provide thorough skin care.
	Provide complete cast care.
	Watch for signs of pressure ulcer formation.
	Look for sudden mal-positioning of the affected limb, which may indicate fracture.

Complications

Despite adequate treatment and appropriate surgical intervention, 5–10% of patients may experience recurrence.

Possible complications from osteomyelitis include disturbances in bone growth, limb-length discrepancies, arthritis, abnormal gait, and pathologic fractures. In patients with chronic osteomyelitis, bone necrosis and fibrosis can occur.

Health Education

It is important to discuss age-appropriate care with the patient and his/her family to ensure compliance with medical therapy.

Juvenile Rheumatoid Arthritis

Also known as juvenile idiopathic arthritis (JIA), is the most common type of arthritis in children under the age of 17. It is not a single disease but a group of diseases what they all have in common is joint pain, swelling and stiffness. Some children may experience symptoms for only a few months, while others have symptoms for the rest of their lives.

Some types of juvenile rheumatoid arthritis can cause serious complications, such as growth problems and eye inflammation. Treatment of juvenile rheumatoid arthritis focuses on controlling pain, improving function and preventing joint damage.

Etiology and Types

Juvenile rheumatoid arthritis occurs when the body's immune system attacks its own cells and tissues. It is unknown why this happens, but both heredity and environment seem to play a role. Certain gene mutations may make a person more susceptible to environmental factors such as viruses, that may trigger the disease.

Juvenile rheumatoid arthritis can be categorized as:

Pauciarticular disease: This is the most common form of JIA. It is common in children younger than 8 years and only a few joints (may be fewer than five joints) get affected. The large joints, such as the shoulder, elbow, hip, and knee, are most likely to be affected. These children require frequent eye examinations as they have a 20–30% chance of developing inflammatory eye problems and that can be serious. Children with this problem have a higher than normal risk of developing an adult form of arthritis. Children can outgrow the arthritis.

Polyarticular type disease affects five joints or more, sometimes many more. Hands and feet's small joints are most likely to be affected. This type can begin at any age. In some cases, the disease is identical to adult-type rheumatoid arthritis.

- Systemic disease affects many systems throughout the body. Children may have high fevers, skin rash, and problems caused by inflammation of the internal organs such as the heart, spleen, liver, and other parts of the digestive tract. It usually, but not always, begins in early childhood. Medical professionals sometimes call this Still's disease.
- Spondyloarthropathy: In the form of JIA where the inflammation of the spine occurs, is often referred to as a spondyloarthropathy. Enthesitis-related disease involves inflammation of the ligaments and tendons at their attachment points to adjacent bone.
- Psoriatic arthritis disease is characterized by joint inflammation and inflammatory skin disease called psoriasis. There may be a history of psoriasis in other family members. The features such as patches of inflamed scaly skin, pitting and lifting of fingernails and toenails as well as inflamed, swollen digits are seen in psoriatic arthritis.

Signs and Symptoms

The most common signs and symptoms of juvenile rheumatoid arthritis are:

- *Pain:* While child might not complain of joint pain, parents may notice that he or she limps especially first thing in the morning or after a nap.
- *Swelling:* Joint swelling is common but is often first noticed in larger joints like the knee.
- *Stiffness:* Parent might notice that their child appears clumsier than usual, particularly in the morning or after naps.

Juvenile rheumatoid arthritis can affect one joint or many. In some cases, juvenile rheumatoid arthritis affects the entire body causing swollen lymph nodes, rashes and fever.

Diagnosis

Diagnosis of juvenile rheumatoid arthritis can be difficult because joint pain can be caused by many different types of problems. Different tests can help to rule out some other conditions that produce similar signs and symptoms.

Some of the most common blood tests for suspected cases of juvenile rheumatoid arthritis include:

- Erythrocyte sedimentation rate (ESR): An elevated rate can indicate inflammation.
- C-reactive protein: This blood test also measures levels of general inflammation in the body but on a different scale than the ESR.
- Antinuclear antibody: Antinuclear antibodies are proteins commonly produced by the immune systems of people with certain autoimmune diseases, including arthritis.

- Rheumatoid factor: This antibody is commonly found in the blood of children who have rheumatoid arthritis.
- Cyclic citrullinated peptide (CCP): Like the rheumatoid factor, the CCP is another antibody that may be found in the blood of children with rheumatoid arthritis.

In many children with juvenile rheumatoid arthritis, no significant abnormality will be found in these blood tests.

X-rays or MRI may be taken to exclude other conditions, such as, fractures, tumors, infection, congenital defects.

Periodic imaging may be used from time to time after the diagnosis to monitor bone development and to detect joint damage.

Management

For some children, pain relievers may be the only medication needed. Other children may need help from medications designed to limit the progression of the disease.

Typical medications used for juvenile rheumatoid arthritis include:

- *Nonsteroidal anti-inflammatory drugs (NSAIDs):* These medications, such as ibuprofen and naproxen sodium (Aleve), reduce pain and swelling. Stronger NSAIDs are available by prescription. Side effects include stomach upset and liver problems.
- *Disease-modifying antirheumatic drugs (DMARDs):* Doctors use these medications when NSAIDs alone fail to relieve symptoms of joint pain and swelling.

  It may be taken in combination with NSAIDs and are used to slow the progress of JRA. Commonly used DMARDs for children include methotrexate and leflunomide.

  Side effects may include nausea and liver problems.
- *Biologic agents:* Also known as biologic response modifiers, this newer class of drugs includes tumor necrosis factor (TNF) blockers, such as etanercept (Enbrel) and adalimumab. These medications can help reduce pain, morning stiffness and swollen joints.

  But these types of drugs increase the risk of infections. There may also be a mild increase in the chance of getting some cancers, such as lymphoma. Other biologic agents work to suppress the immune system, including abatacept (Orencia), rituximab (Rituxan), anakinra (Kineret) and tocilizumab (Actemra).
- *Corticosteroids:* Medications such as prednisone may be used to control symptoms until a DMARD takes effect or to prevent complications, such as inflammation of the sac around the heart (pericarditis).

  Corticosteroids may be administered by mouth or by injection directly into a joint. But these drugs can interfere with normal growth and increase susceptibility to infection, so they generally should be used for the shortest possible duration.

Other Therapies

Physiotherapy: The child can work with a physical therapist to help keep joints flexible and maintain range of motion and muscle tone. They can also recommend for the use of joint supports or splints to help protect joints and keep them in a good functional position.

Nursing Management

Nursing diagnosis

- Impaired physical mobility related to pain and restricted joint movement, skeletal deformity and decreased muscle strength
- Acute pain may be due to distension of tissues by accumulation of fluid/inflammatory process, destruction of joint
- Disturbed body image.

Nursing action with rationale

Assess pain of the patient by using pain assessment scale. Precipitating factors and nonverbal pain cues are to be assessed.

Patient needs firm mattress or bed-board, small pillow. Elevation of linens with bed cradle, as needed, can be done. Soft and sagging mattress, large pillows prevent maintenance of proper body alignment, placing stress on affected joints. Pressure on inflamed or painful joints can be minimized by placing bed linens on cradle it also reduces pain.

Place the patient at bed rest as needed. Place and monitor use of pillows, sandbags, trochanter rolls, splints, braces which rests painful joints and maintains neutral position. Use of splints can decrease pain and may reduce damage to joint. However, prolonged inactivity can result in loss of joint mobility and function.

Frequent changing of position of the patient is important. The patient may be assisted to move in bed, supporting affected joints above and below, avoiding jerky movements.

Monitoring of the duration, not the intensity of morning stiffness is to be done, as it more accurately reflects the disease's severity.

Warm bath and applying warm, moist compresses to affected joints several times a day are needed. Heat promotes muscle relaxation and mobility, decreases pain, and relieves morning stiffness. Cold may relieve pain and swelling during acute episodes.

Appropriate play and diversional therapy for the child enhances self-esteem and feelings of general well-being.

Prescribed drugs are to be administered. Analgesics and anti-inflammatory drugs are given to control mild to moderate pain and inflammation by inhibition of prostaglandin synthesis. Corticoids drugs modify the immune response and suppress inflammation. Disease-modifying antirheumatic drugs (DMARDs): methotrexate (Rheumatrex), hydroxychloroquine are administered to reduce pain and swelling, lessening arthritic symptoms rather than eliminating them.

Physical therapy like whirl pool bath, range of motion exercises of the unaffected parts are also important interventions.

Encourage patient to verbalize about self. Acknowledge and accept feelings of grief, hostility, dependency, it provides feedback that feelings are normal.

Note withdrawn behavior, use of denial, or over concern with body changes. Early detection of the behavior and psychological support of the patient is necessary. Patient may anti-anxiolytic or anti-depressive drugs.

Encourage patient to involve in planning care and scheduling activities. Enhances feelings of competency and self-worth, encourages independence and participation in therapy.

Children with JIA may experience complications

The most common complications in children with JIA relate to adverse effects of medications taken to treat the disease, particularly nonsteroidal anti-inflammatory drugs, such as ibuprofen. When taken frequently, these drugs can cause irritation, pain, and bleeding in the stomach and upper intestine. They also can cause problems in the liver and kidneys that often have no symptoms until they are very severe. In some cases, the child must undergo frequent blood tests to screen for these problems.

- Some children with JIA have emotional or psychological problems. Repeated depression and problems functioning in school are the most common.
- The death rate in children with JIA is somewhat higher than in healthy children. The highest death rate in children with JIA occurs among patients with systemic JIA who develop systemic symptoms (such as pleural and pericardial disease). JIA can also evolve into other diseases, such as systemic lupus erythematosus (SLE) or scleroderma, which have higher death rates than pauciarticular or polyarticular JIA.

Appendices

Appendix 1

BIRTH REGISTRATION OF NEWBORN

Birth Registration: Right from the Start

'The child shall be registered immediately after birth and shall have the right from birth to a name, the right to acquire a nationality and as far as possible, the right to know and be cared for by his or her parents.'

1989 United Nations Convention on the Rights of the Child (CRC), Article 7.

Human rights standards and Birth Registration.

The Convention on the Rights of the Child

While many CRC articles have links to birth registration, the following (paraphrased) are of particular relevance. In some cases, such as the right to family reunification, the proof of identity offered by birth registration and birth certificates is critical.

Article 1: A child means every human being below the age of 18 years unless, under the law of the country, majority is attained earlier.

Article 2: All rights shall be respected and ensured to every child within the State's jurisdiction without discrimination of any kind.

Article 3: The best interests of the child shall be a primary consideration in all actions regarding children.

Article 4: The State shall take all appropriate legislative, administrative and other measures for the implementation of children's rights.

Article 7: The child shall be registered immediately after birth and has the right to a name and nationality and to know and be cared for by his or her parents. The State shall ensure the implementation of these rights in accordance with national law and its obligations under the relevant international instruments in this field, in particular where the child would otherwise be stateless.

Article 8: The State will respect the child's right to preserve his or her identity, including nationality, name and family relations, and will intervene in cases where a child is illegally deprived of any of these elements of identity with a view to re-establishing it.

Article 9: The State shall ensure that a child shall not be separated from his or her parents against their will.

Innocenti Digest no. 9
Innocenti Research Centre
Florence, Italy

Appendix 2

STEPS OF NEWBORN RESUSCITATION

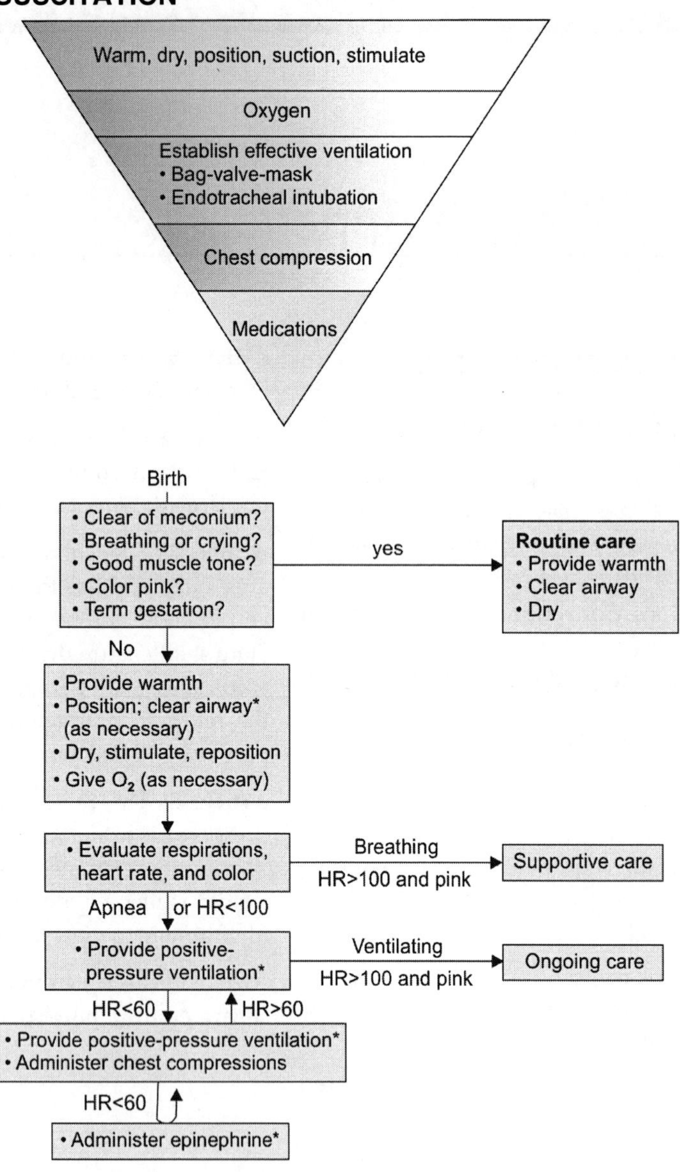

* Endotracheal intubation may be considered at several steps

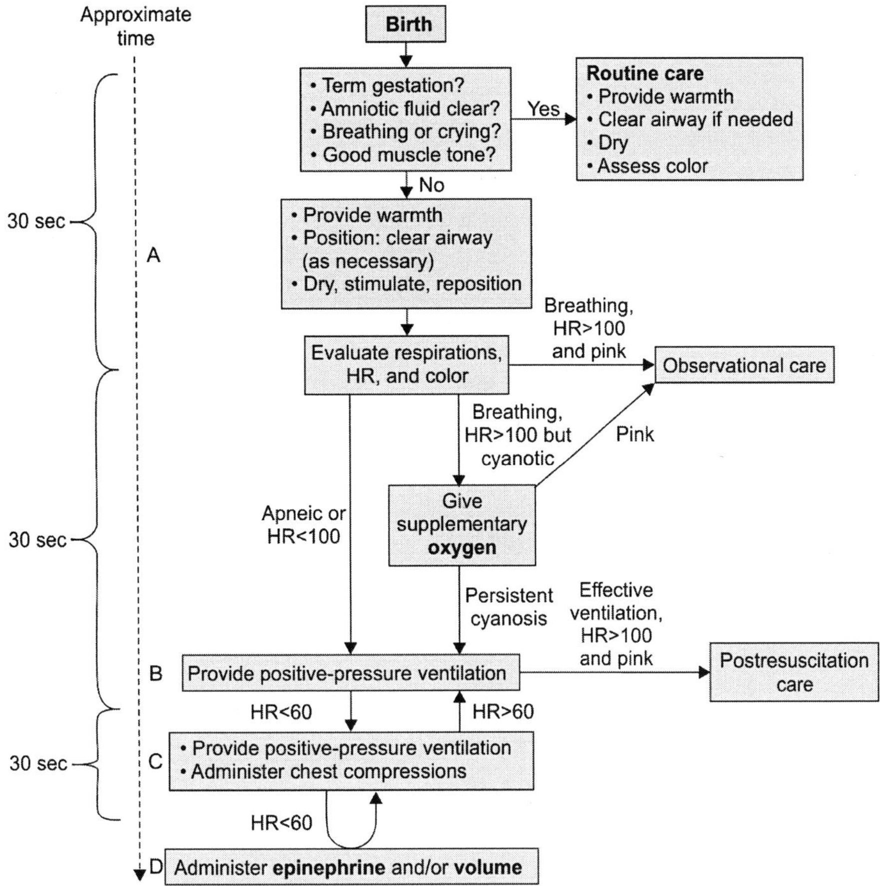

Algorithm: Newborn resuscitation

Appendix 3

HEIGHT AND WEIGHT CHART OF CHILDREN

Average Height and Weight of Girls at Different Ages		
Age	*Weight (kg)*	*Height (cm)*
Birth	3.2	49.9
3 Months	5.4	60.2
6 Months	7.2	66.6
9 Months	8.6	71.1
1 Year	9.5	75.0
2 Years	11.8	84.5
3 Years	14.1	93.9
4 Years	16.0	101.6
5 Years	17.7	108.4
6 Years	19.5	114.6
7 Years	21.8	120.6
8 Years	24.8	126.4
9 Years	28.5	132.2
10 Years	32.5	138.3
11 Years	33.7	142.0
12 Years	38.7	148.0
13 Years	44.0	150.0
14 Years	48.0	155.0
15 Years	51.5	161.0
16 Years	53.0	162.0
17 Years	54.0	163.0
18 Years	54.4	164.0

Average Height and Weight of Boys at Different Ages		
Age	*Weight (kg)*	*Height (cm)*
Birth	3.3	50.5
3 Months	6.0	61.1
6 Months	7.8	67.8
9 Months	9.2	72.3
1 Year	10.2	76.1
2 Years	12.3	85.6
3 Years	14.6	94.9
4 Years	16.7	102.9
5 Years	18.7	109.9
6 Years	20.7	116.1
7 Years	22.9	121.7
8 Years	25.3	127.0
9 Years	28.1	132.2
10 Years	31.4	137.5
11 Years	32.2	140.0
12 Years	37.0	147.0
13 Years	40.9	153.0
14 Years	47.0	160.0

Ideal Height - Weight Chart for Adults		
Height in ft' inches"	*Weight in kg*	
	Female	*Male*
5'0" (152 cm)	45–51	50–56
5'1" (154 cm)	47–52	52–57
5'2" (157 cm)	48–53	53–58
5'3" (160 cm)	49–55	54–60
5'4" (162 cm)	51–57	56–62
5'5" (165 cm)	52–58	57–63
5'6" (167 cm)	54–61	59–66
5'7" (170 cm)	56–63	61–68
5'8" (172 cm)	58–64	63–69
5'9" (175 cm)	59–66	64–71
5'10" (177 cm)	61–68	66–74
5'11" (180 cm)	63–70	68–74
6'0" (182 cm)	65–72	70–77

(Nutrient Requirements and Recommended Dietary Allowances for Indians, I.C.M.R. 1990)

Appendix 4

MATURATIONAL ASSESSMENT OF GESTATIONAL AGE (NEW BALLARD SCORE)

Name .... Sex ....

Hospital No. ....

Date of birth .... Length..

Head circumference ....

Date/time of examination...

Age when examined ....

Examiner ....

Neuromuscular Maturity Sign	Score							Record Score Here	**Score** Neuromuscular: Physical: Total:
	–1	0	1	2	3	4	5		
Posture									
Square windows (wrist)	>90°	90°	60°	45°	30°	0°			
Arm recoil		180°	140° -180	110° -140	90° -110	<90°			
Popliteal angle	180°	160°	140°	120°	100°	90°	<90°		
Scarf Sign									
Heel to ear									
Total neuromuscular maturity score									

Physical Maturity

Physical Maturity Sign	Score						
	–1	0	1	2	3	4	5
Skin	Sticky, friable, transparent	Gelatinous, red, translucent	Smooth pink, visible veins	Superficial peeling and/ or rash, few veins	Cracking, pale areas, rare veins	Parchment, deep cracking, no vessels	Leathery, cracked, wrinkled
Lanugo	none	Sparse	Abundant	Thinning	Bald areas	Mostly bald	
Plantar Surface	Heel-toe 40-50 mm: –1 <40 mm: –2	>50 mm no crease	Faint red marks	Anterior transverse crease only	Creases ant. 2/3	Creases over entire sole	
Breast	Imperceptible	Barely perceptible	Flat areola no bud	Stippled areola 1–2 mm bud	Raised areola 3–4 mm bud	Full areola 5–10 mm bud	
Eye/Ear	Lids fused loosely: –1 tightly: –2	Lids open pinna flat stays folded	Slightly curved pinna; soft; slow recoil	Well-curved pinna; soft but ready recoil	Formed and firm instant recoil	Thick cartilage ear stiff	
Genitals (Male)	Scrotum flat, smooth	Scrotum empty, faint rugae	Testes in upper canal, rare rugae	Testes descending, few rugae	Testes down, good rugae	Testes pendulous, deep rugae	
Genitals (Female)	Clitoris prominent and labia flat	Prominent clitoris and small labia minora	Prominent clitoris and enlarging minora	Majora and minora equally prominent	Majora large, minora small	Majora cover clitoris and minora	
Total physical maturity score							

Maturity Rating

Score	Weeks
–10	20
–5	22
0	24
5	26
10	28
15	30
20	32
25	34
30	36
35	38
40	40
45	42
50	44

Ballard score is used to assess extremely premature infant.

Appendix 5

PEDIATRIC VITAL SIGNS

Age	*Premature*	*Newborn*	*1–12 mo.*	*1–3 yr.*	*3–5 yr.*	*6–12 yr.*	*13+ yr.*
Weight	1–2 kg	2–3 kg	4–10 kg	10–14 kg	14–18 kg	20–42 kg	>50 kg
Pulse	140+	120–160	80–140	80–130	80–120	70–110	60–90
Respirations	30–40	30–50	30–60	20–40	20–30	20–30	12–20
Systolic BP	40+10	60+10	85+15	90+15	95+15	100+15	115+15
Skin	Pink, warm moist						
Temp	{98.6 ° F}						

Body Temperature Conversion formula:
Conversion of Fahrenheit temperature to Celsius scale
$C = (F - 32) \times 5/9$
Conversion of Celsius scale to Fahrenheit scale
$F = C \times 9/5 + 32$

Appendix 6

SOME IMPORTANT CALCULATIONS

I. Formula for calculation of expected weight

a. For age 1 month to 12 months.

$$\text{Body weight} = \frac{\text{age in months} + 9}{2}$$

b. For age 1 to 6 years

Body weight = (age in years × 2) + 8

c. For age 6 to 12 years

$$\text{Body weight} = \frac{(\text{Age in years} \times 7) - 5}{2}$$

II. Formula for calculation of expected height

a. At birth = 50 cm

b. At one year of age = 75 cm

c. At 2 to 12 years of age

Height = Age in years × 6 + 77 cm

or

Height = Age in years × 7 + 66 cm

III. Approximate Body Surface Area Calculation

Weight (kg)	*Approximate surface area (m^2)*
1– 5	(0.05 x weight) + 0.05
6–10	(0.04 x weight) + 0.10
11–20	(0.03 x weight) + 0.20
21–40	(0.02 x weight) + 0.04
Costeff's formula: surface area (m^2)	$\frac{4W + 7}{W + 90}$

IV. Calculation of Body Mass Index (BMI)

Body Mass Index (BMI) uses a mathematical formula and calculates individual's weight according to his/her height.

BMI is calculated as weight in Kilograms divided by square of height in meters

BMI = weight in kg/m^2

Normal Range : 8.5 – 24.9

Over Weight : 25.0 – 29.9

Obese : 30.0 – 39.9

Morbidly Obese : 40.0 and above

V. **Pediatric Fluid Calculations**

Body weight (kg)	*Daily fluid requirement*	*Fluid administration rate*
<10	100 mL/kg	4 mL/kg/hr
10–20	1000 mL+ 50 mL/kg for each kg over 10	40 mL/hr + 2 mL/hr for each kg over 10
>20	1500 mL + 20 mL/kg for each kg over 20	60 mL/hr + 1 mL/kg/hr for each kg over 20

VI. Calculating Flow Rate

$$\text{Drop/minute} = \frac{\text{Total volume} \times \text{Drop factor}}{\text{Time in minutes}}$$

VII. Infusion Time Calculation

$$\text{Infusion Time} = \frac{\text{Total volume of infusion}}{\text{ML per hour being infused}}$$

VIII. Estimation of Child Drug Dose Calculation

Young's formula according to Age

$$\text{Child dose} = \frac{\text{Age of Child} \times \text{Adult dose}}{\text{Age of Child}}$$

[Detailed fluid and drug calculations—discussed in Drug chapter in this edition]

IX. Fluid Replacement Formula in Burn Injury

Parkland formula

a. For first 24 hours

Total amount of fluid requirement = 4 mL of ringer's lactate × body weight × percentage of TBSA (total body surface area) burnt

- One half of fluid is to be given in first 8 hours (start from the time of accident)
- Remaining half of fluid is to be given in next 16 hours.

b. For next 24 hours

c. Total amount of fluid requirement = 2 mL of ringer's lactate per kg of body weight × percentage of burns

This formula is used when the burn is 15 to 20 percent total body surface area (TBSA)

X. Percentage of malnutrition

$$\text{Malnutrition} = \frac{\text{Actual weight} \times 100}{\text{Expected weight}}$$

Appendix 7

TOOTH ERUPTION OF CHILD

Tooth Eruption Times ....
....

Teeth	*Number*	*Age at Eruption**
Baby Deciduous Teeth (20 Total)		
Lower front teeth (lower central incisors)	2	5–9 months
Upper front teeth (upper central incisors)	2	8–12 months
Upper side teeth (upper lateral incisors)	2	10–12 months
Lower side teeth (lower lateral incisors)	2	12–15 months
First back teeth (first molars)	4	10–16 months
Eye teeth or cuspids (canines)	4	16–20 months
Second back teeth (second molars)	4	20–30 months
Adult Permanent Teeth (32 Total)		
First back teeth (first molars)	4	5–7 years
Front teeth (incisors)	8	6–8 years
Bicuspids (premolars)	8	9–12 years
Eye teeth or cuspids (canines)	4	10–13 years
Second back teeth (second molars)	4	11–13 years
Wisdom teeth (third molars)	4	17–25 years

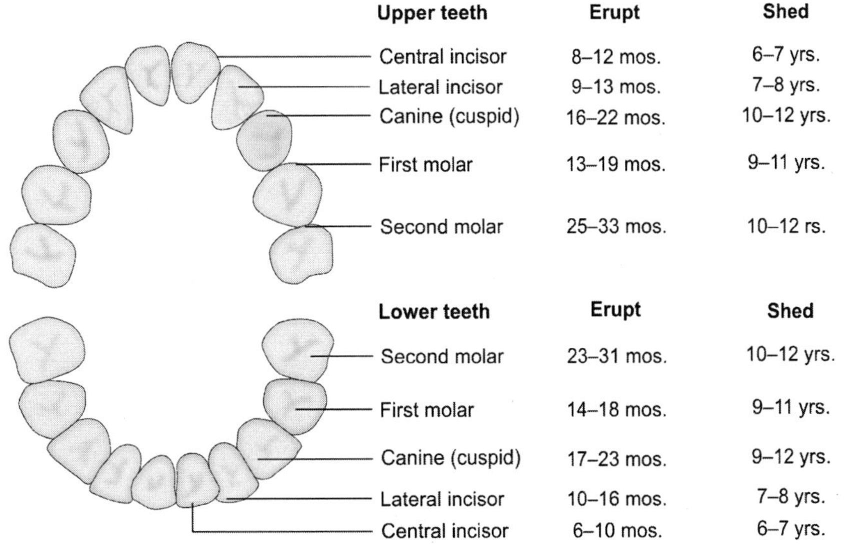

Appendix 8

MOTOR REFLEXES

Table 1: Common infant motor reflexes

Reflex	*Stimulus/Action*
Blinking	In response to a puff of air, the infant closes both eyes.
Babinski	in response to stroking the side of its foot, the infant twists its foot inward and fans out its toes.
Grasping	In response to an object pressed against its palm, the infant attempts to grasp the object.
Moro	In response to a shock or loud noise, the infant arches its back and throws its arms outward.
Rooting	In response to stroking its cheek, the infant turns its head toward the touch and attempts to suck.
Stepping	In response to holding the infant so that its feet barely touch a surface, the infant 'walks'.
Sucking	In response to inserting a finger or nipple into its mouth, the infant begins rhythmically sucking.
Babkin	In response to stroking its forehead, the infant turns its head and opens its mouth.
Plantar	In response to touching the ball of the foot, the infant curls its toes under.

Appendix 9

NORMAL DEVELOPMENT OF CHILD

Developmental Milestones*

Age	*Behavior*
Birth	• Sleeps much of the time • Sucks • Clears airway • Responds with crying to discomforts and intrusions
4 weeks	• Brings hands toward eyes and mouth • Moves head from side to side when lying on stomach • Eyes follow an object moved in an arc about 15 cm above face to the midline • Responds to a noise in some way (e.g. startling, crying, quieting) • May turn toward familiar sounds and voices • Focuses on a face
6 weeks	• Regards objects in the line of vision • Begins to smile when spoken to • Lies flat on abdomen • Head lags when pulled to a sitting position
3 months	• Lifts head up when held at parents shoulder, Lifts head up when on tummy 45° • Opens and shuts hands • Pushes down when feet are placed on a flat surface • Swings at and reaches for dangling toys • Follows an object moved in an arc above face from one side to the other • Watches faces intently • Smiles at sound of caretaker's voice • Vocalizes sounds
4 months	• Keeps head in midline and brings hands to chest when lying on back, lifts head and supports self on forearms on tummy, holds head steady when supported in sitting position
5–6 months	• Holds head steady when upright • Sits with support • Rolls from back to stomach or stomach to back, pushes up on hands when on tummy, reaches for objects • Recognizes people at a distance • Listens intently to human voices • Smiles spontaneously • Squeals in delight • Babbles to toys,
7 months	• Sits without support • Bears some weight on legs when held upright • Transfers objects from hand to hand • Holds own bottle • Looks for dropped object • Responds to own name • Responds to being told 'no' • Combines vowels and consonants to babble • Moves body with excitement in anticipation of playing • Plays peekabo
9 months	• Sits on floor without support, Moves self forward on tummy or rolls continuously to get item, stands with support • Crawls or creeps on hands and knees • Pulls self up to standing position • Works to get a toy that is out of reach; objects if toy is taken away • Gets into a sitting position from stomach • Says 'mama' or 'dada' indiscriminately

Contd...

Contd...

Age	*Behavior*
12 months	• Gets up to a sitting position on own, pulls to stand at furniture, walks holding onto hands or furniture • May walk 1 or 2 steps without support • Stands for a few moments at a time • Says 'Dada' and 'Mama' to the appropriate person • Drinks from a cup • Claps hands and waves bye-bye • Speaks several words
18 months	• Walks alone, crawls up stairs, pushes or pulls toys or other objects when walking • Can climb stairs holding on • Draws a vertical stroke • Makes a tower of 4 cubes • Turns several book pages at a time • Speaks about 10 words • Pulls toys on strings • Partially feeds self
2–2½ years	• Walks backwards or sideways pulling a toy, Plays in a squat position, Kicks a ball, Runs well/with coordination, Climbs on furniture • Jumps • Climbs up and down stairs without help • Handles a spoon well • Turns single book pages • Makes a tower of 7 cubes • Opens doors • Scribbles in a circular pattern • Puts on simple clothing • Makes 2- or 3-word sentences • Verbalizes toilet needs
3 years	• Stands on one foot briefly, climbs stairs with minimal or no support, kicks a ball forcefully • Mature gait in walking • Favors using one hand over the other • Copies a circle • Dresses well except for buttons and laces • Counts to 10 and uses plurals • Recognizes at least 3 colors • Questions constantly • Feeds self well • Can take care of toilet needs (in about half of children)
4 years	• Alternates feet going up and down stairs, stands on one foot for one to three seconds without support, goes up stairs alternating feet, rides a tricycle using foot paddles, walks on a straight line without stepping off • Throws a ball overhand • Hops on 1 foot • Copies a cross • Dresses self • Washes hands and face
5 years	• Skips, catches a bounced ball, copies a triangle, draws a person in 6 parts, knows 4 colors, dresses and undresses without help
6 years	• Walks along a straight line from heel to toe • Writes name

*The sequence is fairly consistent, but the timing of milestones varies; times above represent median values.

Problem signs... if a child is experiencing any of the following, consider this a red flag: 1. Baby is unable to hold head in the middle to turn and look left and right. 2. Unable to walk with heels down four months after starting to walk. 3. Asymmetry (between two sides of body; or body too stiff or too floppy).

Appendix 10

RECOMMENDED DIETARY ALLOWANCES (RDA)

The Recommended Dietary Allowances (RDA) provide the essential-nutrient intake levels required to meet the known nutritional needs of most (97–98%) healthy persons in specific age and gender groups. The RDA has been developed by the Food and Nutrition Board of the National Academy of Sciences.

Recommended daily allowances (RDA), 1989										
Life-stage Group	*Energy (kcal)*	*Protein (g)*	*Vitamin A (mcg RE)*	*Vitamin E (mg)*	*Vitamin K (mcg)*	*Vitamin C (mg)*	*Iron (mg)*	*Zinc (mg)*	*Iodine (mcg)*	*Selenium (mcg)*
Infants										
0–6 months	650	13	375	3	5	30	6	5	40	10
7–12 months	850	14	375	4	10	35	10	5	50	15
Children										
1–3 years	1300	16	400	6	15	40	10	10	70	20
4–6 years	1800	24	500	7	20	45	10	10	90	20
7–10 years	2000	28	700	7	30	45	10	10	120	30
Males										
11–14 years	2500	45	1000	10	45	50	12	15	150	40
15–18 years	3000	59	1000	10	65	60	12	15	150	50
19–24 years	2900	58	1000	10	70	60	10	15	150	70
25–50 years	2900	63	1000	10	80	60	10	15	150	70
>50 years	2300	63	1000	10	80	60	10	15	150	70
Females										
11–14 years	2200	46	800	8	45	50	15	12	150	45
15–18 years	2200	44	800	8	55	60	15	12	150	50
19–24 years	2200	46	800	8	60	60	15	12	150	55
25–50 years	2200	50	800	8	65	60	15	12	150	55
>50 years	1900	50	800	8	65	60	10	12	150	55
Pregnancy										
	+300	60	800	10	65	70	30	15	175	65
Lactation										
1st 6 months	+500	65	1300	12	65	95	15	19	200	75
2nd 6 months	+500	62	1200	11	65	90	15	16	200	75

NB: The RDA are currently under revision; values for certain nutrients have been released periodically over the past few years. The new recommendations are called Dietary Reference Intakes (DRI), and include four levels of values: (1) Recommended Dietary Allowances (RDA); (2) Adequate Intakes (AI); (3) Tolerable Upper Intake Level (UL); and (4) Estimated Average Requirement (EAR)

Appendix 11

IMPORTANT MATERNAL AND CHILD HEALTH INDICATORS—CURRENT STATUS VS GOALS

Indicator	*Target by 2015*	*MDG goal*	*At present*
Infant Mortality Rate	<30/1000 live births	<30/1000 live births by 2015	40/1000 live births (SRS 2013)
Neonatal Mortality Rate	<20	<20	26 (SRS 2000)
Under five mortality	42/1000 live birth by 2015	42/1000 live birth by 2015	49/1000 live births in 2013 (SRS)
Maternal Mortality Ratio	As per the MDGs, it is 109 by 2015.	<100	167 per 100,000 live births in 2011–13
Institutional deliveries			47%
Crude Birth Rate (Per 1000 Population)			21.4
Crude Death Rate (Per 1000 Population)			7.0
Total Fertility Rate (Per women)			2.3 (2013)

Appendix 12

COMMON PEDIATRIC MEDICINES AND DOSES

Drugs	*Doses*
Atropine sulfate	0.01 mg/kg SC or IV
Acetaminophen Forms: Liquid, tablet, capsule, rectal suppository	Children < 12 years: 10–15 mg/kg/dose every 4–6 hours as needed. Do not exceed 5 doses (2.6 g) in 24 hours Children > 12 years and adults: 325–650 mg every 4–6 hours as needed not to exceed 4g/day
Aspirin	10–15 mg/kg/dose q4-6h 75–100 mg/kg/day for rheumatic fever 5 mg/kg/day antiplatelet dose Watch use in children and adolescents (Reye's Syndrome)
Acetazolamide (Diamox)	10–30 mg/kg/day 3–4 divided doses
Acyclovir	10 mg/kg/over in 1 hour in NS or DS
Adrenaline	0.01 mL/kg SC. Do not exceed 0.5 mL/dose
Albendazole	1–2 years–200 mg single dose 2 years and above–400 mg single dose
Albuterol	2–6 years up to 0.1 mg/kg/dose 6–8 hourly 6–12 years: 2 mg q 6 h
Amikacin	7.5 mg/kg/dose × 2–3 doses/day
Amoxicillin Forms: Liquid, tablet, capsule	Children > 3 months of age up to 40 kg: 20–40 mg/kg/day in divided doses every 8 hours, or 25–45 mg/kg/day in divided doses every 12 hours Children > 40 kg and adults: 250–500 mg every 8 hrs or 500–875 mg every 12 hours
Amoxicillin clavulanate (Augmentin) Forms: Liquid, tablet	Usual oral dosage 1: Children > 3 months of age up to 40 kg: 25–45 mg/kg/day in divided doses every 12 hours. Children > 40 kg and adults: 500–875 mg every 12 hours
Aminophylline	5 mg/kg/dose IV with double volume dextrose
Ampicillin	50–100 mg/kg/day 4 doses a day
Ascorbic acid	10 mg/kg/day
Atenolol	1 mg/kg
Azithromycin	10 mg/kg up to 500 mg on first day 5 mg/kg up to 250 mg for 2–5 days
Cephalexin Forms: Liquid, tablet, capsule	Children: 25–50 mg/kg/day in divided doses Adults: 250 mg every 6 hours
Cefotaxime (claforan), third generation cephalosporin	Neonates 0–7 days old > 2000 g *Dose:* 100–150 mg/kg/day IM/IV divided q8–12h; Info: dose, duration varies with infection type, severity Infants/children < 50 kg *Dose:* 75–200 mg/kg/day IM/IV divided q6–8h
Ceftazidime third generation cephalosporin (Fortum)	Neonates > 7 days old, > 1200 g *Dose:* 150 mg/kg/day IM/IV divided q8h child 1 mo–12 years *Dose:* 90–150 mg/kg/day IM/IV divided q8h; Max: 6 g/day
Ceftriaxone	Neonates, > 7 days old > 2000 g *Dose:* 50–75 mg/kg IM/IV q24h; Info: dose, duration vary with infection type, severity Infants/children *Dose:* 50–100 mg/kg/day IM/IV divided q12–24h; Max: 4 g/24h; Information : dose, duration vary with infection type, severity

Contd...

Contd...

Drugs	*Doses*
Cefuroxime 3 months to 12 years: • Oral suspension: 10 to 15 mg/kg orally twice a day • Maximum dose: 1 g/day • Tablets: 250 mg orally every 12 hours **Parenteral:** 3 months or older: 50 to 100 mg/kg/day IV or IM in equally divided doses every 6 to 8 hours • Maximum dose: 1.5 g/dose	Oral: 3 months to 12 years: • Oral suspension: 10 to 15 mg/kg orally twice a day • Maximum dose: 1 g/day • Tablets: 250 mg orally every 12 hours **Parenteral:** 3 months or older: 50 to 100 mg/kg/day IV or IM in equally divided doses every 6 to 8 hours • Maximum dose: 1.5 g/dose
Chloramphenicol, second–generation cephalosporin antibiotic (AFUROX–250 tab, altacef tab)	Infants/children Dose: 50–75 mg/kg/day IV divided q6h; Max: 4 g/day; Important: adjust dose based on levels
Chloroquine	According to WHO Total dose: 25 mg/kg given over 3 days. Day 1: 10 mg/kg, followed by 5 mg/kg 6–8 hours later. Days 2 and 3: 5 mg/kg in a single dose.
Ciprofloxacin	The dose is usually 10 to 20 milligrams (mg) per kilogram (kg) of body weight every 12 hours. However, the dose is usually not more than 750 mg per day.
Cloxacillin	Oral: Children ≤20 kg: 25 to 50 mg/kg/day in divided doses every 6 hours Children and Adolescents >20 kg: Refer to adult dosing.
Clarithromycin	Children 6 months to 12 years of age: The recommended dose is 7.5 mg/kg twice a day.
Dopamine	The hemodynamic effects of dopamine are dose dependent: Low dosage: 1 to 5 mcg/kg/minute, increased renal blood flow and urine output Intermediate dosage: 5 to 15 mcg/kg/minute, increased renal blood flow, heart rate, cardiac contractility, cardiac output, and blood pressure High dosage: greater than 15 mcg/kg/minute, alpha-adrenergic effects begin to predominate, vasoconstriction, increased blood pressure
Dobutamine	2–20 mcg/kg/min IV Start: 0.5–1 mcg/kg/min IV; Max: 40 mcg/kg/min
Erythromycin	30–60 mg/kg/day
Frusemide	*Dose:* 1–6 mg/kg PO qd-bid; Start: 2 mg/kg PO x 1, increase 1–2 mg/kg q6–8h; Max: 6 mg/kg/dose; Information: for patients with CHF, hepatic or renal disease; poor bio-availability when given PO [IM/IV route, infants/children] *Dose:* 0.5–2 mg/kg IM/IV q6–12h; Start: 1 mg/kg IM/IV x 1, increase 1 mg/kg q2h; Max: 6 mg/kg/dose
Gentamicin	Children up to two years 2 mg–2.5 mg /kg TDS
Ibuprofen	4–10 mg/kg/dose every 6–8 hours, Children > 12 years 200–400 mg every 4–6 hours as needed (maximum 1200 mg/24 hrs)
Mannitol	0.25–0.5 g/kg IV q4–6h Start: 0.2 g/kg IV test dose, then 0.5–1 g/kg IV x1; Max: 12.5 g/dose; Info: discontinue if no response within 2h

Contd...

Drugs	*Doses*
Metoclopramide	Metoclopramide is not approved for postoperative nausea and vomiting in pediatric patients; however, the following doses have been studied: IV injection—Children less than or equal to 14 years: 0.1 to 0.2 mg/kg/dose (maximum dose: 10 mg/dose); repeat every 6 to 8 hours as needed in case of prevention of delayed chemotherapy induced nausea and vomiting (CINV) as a second line option
Penicillin V	Children < 12: 25–50 mg/kg/day in 3–4 divided doses Children > 12 and adults: 125–500 mg q 6–8 hrs
Phenobarbitone	*Dose:* Up to 8 mg /kg/day IV: 5–10 mg/ kg IV at a rate of not more than 30 mg /min (dilution of injection 1 in 10).
Phenytoin sodium (Eptoin)	Initially 3–5 mg/kg daily in 2 divided doses. Increase dose according to clinical response and plasma concentration. Maintenance dose: 4 to 8 mg/ kg daily (maximum 300 mg daily).
Vancomycin	1 mo–11 years 10–15 mg/kg IV q6–8h; Max: 1 g/dose 12–16 years *Dose:* 1000 mg IV q12h; Alt: 10–15 mg/kg IV q12h; Information: adjust dose based on serum levels.

Children: Treatment of Shock

Drug	*Receptor*	*Action*	*Dose*
Dopamine	Dopamine, β, α	Chronotropy, inotropy, vasoconstriction	3–20 mcg/kg/min
Dobutamine	β	Chronotropy, inotropy, vasodilatation	5–20 mcg/kg/min
Epinephrine	β, α	Chronotropy, inotropy, vasoconstriction	0.05–0.2 mcg/kg/min
Norepinephrine	α, β	Vasoconstriction, chronotropy, inotropy	0.01–2 mcg/kg/min
Milrinone	PDE inhibitor	Inotropy, lusitropy, vasodilatation	0.25–4 mcg/kg/min
Nitroprusside	NO donor, smooth muscle relaxation	Vasodilatation	0.5–10 mcg/kg/min
Vasopressin	V1 vascular receptors	vasoconstriction	0.3–4 mU/kg/min

Appendix 13

DRUGS AND BREASTFEEDING

A. Drugs Usually Safe to Take in Usual Doses

Name of drug	*Brand name*	*Used to treat*
Acetaminophen	Tylenol	Pain
Acyclovir	Zovirax	Herpes infections
Antacids	Maalox, Mylanta	Upset stomachs
Cephalosporins	Ceclor, Ceftin, Omnicef, Suprax	Lung, ear, skin, urinary tract, throat, and bone infections
Clotrimazole	Lotrimin, Mycelex	Yeast and fungal infections
Contraceptives (progestin-only)	Micronor, Norplant, Depo-Provera	Birth control
Corticosteroids	Prednisone	Inflammation of joints and other conditions
Decongestant nasal sprays	Otrivin	Treat stuffy noses
Digoxin	Lanoxin	Treat heart problems
Erythromycin	Erythrocin	Skin and respiratory infections
Fexofenadine	Allegra	Allergies and hay fever (antihistamine)
Fluconazole	Diflucan	Treat yeast infections
Heparin		Used to keep blood from clotting
Ibuprofen	Motrin, Brufen	Pain relief
Inhalers, bronchodilators, and corticosteroids	Albuterol, becolate	Asthma
Insulin		Diabetes; dosage required may drop up to 25 percent during lactation
Laxatives, bulk-forming and stool softening	Metamucil, Colac	Treat constipation
Lidocaine	Xylocaine	A local anesthetic
Loratadine	Claritin	As antihistamine for allergies and hay fever
Low molecular weight heparins (enoxaparin, dalteparin, tinzaparin)	Lovenox, Fragmin, Innohep	Anticoagulants
Magnesium sulfate		Preeclampsia and eclampsia
Methyldopa	Aldomet	High blood pressure
Methylergonovine (short courses)	Methergine	Prevent or control bleeding after childbirth
Metoprolol	Lopressor	Treat high blood pressure (a beta-blocker)
Miconazole	Monistat 3	Treat yeast infections
Nifedipine	Adalat, Procardia	Used for high blood pressure and raynaud's syndrome of the nipple
Penicillins	Amoxicillin, Dynapen	Treat bacterial infections
Propranolol	Inderal	Heart problems, and high blood pressure (a beta-blocker)
Theophylline	Theo-Dur	Asthma and bronchitis
Tretinoin	Retin A	Acne. Avoid contact of cream with infant.

Contd...

Contd…

Name of drug	*Brand name*	*Used to treat*
Thyroid replacement	Eltroxin	Thyroid problems
Vancomycin	Vancocin	An antibiotic
Verapamil	Calan, Isoptin, Verelan	Used for high blood pressure
Warfarin	Coumadin	Prevent blood clots

B. Probably Safe in Usual Doses: Breastfeeding

Little is known about the effects of these drugs on a breastfeeding infant, but if there is an effect, it will probably be mild. In rare cases, a child might have allergic reaction.

Name of drug	*Brand name*	*Use*
ACE inhibitors	Enalapril (Vasotec), Benazepril	Used to treat high blood pressure
Anticholinergic agents	Pro-Banthine	Used to treat intestinal and gallbladder spasms; may reduce milk supply
Anticonvulsants	Depakote, Dilantin, Tegretol (avoid ethosuximide, phenobarbital, and primidone)	Used for seizures and mood disorders
Antihistamines, First-generation	Benadryl, Chlor-Trimeton	May reduce milk supply and cause infant drowsiness or fussiness
Antituberculars	INH	Used to treat tuberculosis
Azathioprine (low doses)	Imuran	Used to suppress the immune system following organ transplants
Barbiturates (except phenobarbital)	Fiorinal, Fioricet	For sedation and tension headaches
Bupropion	Wellbutrin	For depression
Clindamycin	Cleocin	Used to treat abdominal and vaginal infections
Oral decongestants	Sudafed, Entex PSE	Used to treat congestion associated with colds or allergies; often reduces milk supply
Ergonovine (short course)		Used to treat uterine bleeding. May reduce milk supply.
Fluconazole	Diflucan	Antifungal
Gadolinium	Magnevist, Omniscan	Contrast agent for MRI studies
Histamine H2 blockers	Cimetidine (Tagamet), ranitidine (Zantac), nizatadine (Axid), and famotidine (Pepcid — preferred)	Used to treat stomach problems
Labetalol	Normodyne, Trandate	Used for high blood pressure; caution with preterm babies
Hydrochlorothiazide (low doses)	Hydrodiuril	Diuretic for high blood pressure
Lorazepam	Ativan	Used to treat anxiety
Methimazole	Tapazole	Used for hyperthyroidism; less than 20 mg/day is probably safe
Metoclopramide	Reglan	Used for gastrointestinal problems and to increase milk supply. Limit to 2 weeks.
Midazolam		Sedative used in anesthesia
Naproxen	Naprosyn, Anaprox, Aleve	Used for pain relief; okay if baby is at least 1 month old

Contd…

Contd...

Name of drug	*Brand name*	*Use*
Omeprazole	Prilosec	Used to treat stomach problems
Oxazepam	Serax	Used to treat anxiety
Paroxetine	Paxil	Used to treat depression
Propofol	Diprivan	Sedative used in anesthesia
Quinidine		Used to treat heartbeat irregularities
Quinolone antibacterials	Cipro and Levaquin; Noroxin is preferred	Treatment of urinary tract infections
Salicylates (occasional use)	Aspirin	Used for pain relief
Sertraline	Zoloft	Used to treat depression
Spironolactone	Aldactone, Aldactazide	Used to treat high blood pressure
Sumatriptan	Imitrex	Used to treat migraines
Tetracyclines < 14 days	tetracycline, doxycycline	Used to treat acne and urinary tract infections
Trazodone		Used for depression and sleep
Tricyclic antidepressants (avoid doxepin)	Elavil, Tofranil, Pamelor	Used to treat depression; nortriptyline preferred
Verapamil	Calan, Isoptin, Verelan	Used for high blood pressure

C. Drugs Potentially Hazardous: Breastfeeding

Mothers should avoid or use these drugs with caution, particularly while breastfeeding a newborn or premature infant.

Name of drug	*Brand name*	*Use*
Atenolol	Tenormin	A beta blocker used to treat high blood pressure and abnormal heart rhythms.
Antihistamine/decongestant combinations	Contac, Dimetapp	Used to treat colds and allergies; may reduce your milk supply
Benzodiazepines, Long-Acting	Librium, Valium, Dalmane	Used to treat anxiety and for sleep (lorazepam, oxazepam preferred)
Chlorthalidone		Diuretic used to treat high blood pressure; may reduce milk supply
Contraceptives (estrogen-containing)	Lo-Ovral, Loestrin	Used for birth control; may reduce milk supply
Doxepin	Sinequan	Used to treat depression
Egotamine	Cafergot	Used to treat migraines
Escitalopram	Lexapro	Used to treat depression
Ethosuximide	Zarontin	Used to treat epilepsy
Fluoxetine	Prozac, Serafem	Used to treat depression
Iodinated contrast media		Used to examine kidneys; withhold breastfeeding temporarily
Lithium (monitor infant serum levels)	Lithosun	Used to treat bipolar disorder
Metronidazole	Flagyl	An antibiotic used to treat some intestinal and genital infections
Narcotics, especially meperidine in addicts and high doses with newborns	Tylenol , Vicodin	Used for pain (one tablet every six hours maximum; watch for drowsiness)
Nicotine		Smoking can reduce milk supply
Nitrofurantoin	Macrobid	Used to treat urinary tract infections (safe if the baby is at least 1 month old)
Phenobarbital, anticonvulsant doses		Sedative and anticonvulsant
Piroxicam	Feldene	Used to treat arthritis and pain

Contd...

Contd...

Name of drug	*Brand name*	*Use*
Sotalol	Betapace	Used to treat heart problems
Thiazide diuretics, long-acting or high doses	Aquatensin, Enduron, Lozol, Renese	For high blood pressure or edema; high dose may reduce milk supply
Venlafaxine	Effexor	Used to treat depression

D. Drugs Not Safe to Take: Breastfeeding

These drugs are not safe for breastfeeding mothers. If these drugs are prescribed for health reasons, breastfeeding should be stopped—either temporarily or permanently—depending on how long mother needs to take them. To keep milk supply up mother can 'pump and dump'—until she is ready to breastfeed again.

Name of drug	*Brand name*	*Use*
Amantadine	Symmetrel	Used to treat the flu or Parkinson's disease; may reduce milk supply
Antilipemics (excluding resins)	Lescol, Lipitor, Zocor	Used to lower the level of cholesterol in the blood
Antineoplastic agents		Used to treat cancer
Aspirin (large doses)		Used to treat arthritis
Chlorampenicol		Used to treat serious infections
Clozapine	Clozaril	Schizophrenia
Gold Salts	Myochrysine	Used to treat arthritis
Iodide products	Betadine, potassium iodide	Douching or as an expectorant
Iodine, radioactive		Diagnose and treat hyperthyroidism
Salicylates, large doses	Aspirin	Treat arthritis

Appendix 14

NATIONAL HEALTH MISSION (NHM)

The National Health Mission (NHM) encompasses its two Sub-Missions, the National Rural Health Mission (NRHM) and the National Urban Health Mission (NUHM). The main programmatic components include health system strengthening in rural and urban areas, Reproductive Maternal-Neonatal-Child and Adolescent Health (RMNCH+A) and Communicable and Noncommunicable Diseases. The NHM envisages achievement of universal access to equitable, affordable and quality health care services that are accountable and responsive to people's needs.

Major Initiatives Under NRHM/NHM

ASHA: More than 9.15 lakh Accredited Social Health Activists (ASHAs) are in place across the country and serve as facilitators, mobilizers and providers of community level care. ASHA is the first port of call in the community especially for marginalized sections of the population, with a focus on women and children.

Rogi Kalyan Samiti/Hospital Management Society is a simple yet effective management structure. This committee is a registered society whose members act as trustees to manage the affairs of the hospital and is responsible for upkeep of the facilities and ensure provision of better facilities to the patients in the hospital. The **Untied Grants to Sub-Centers (SCs)** has given a new confidence to our ANMs in the field. The SCs are far better equipped now with blood pressure measuring equipment, hemoglobin (Hb) measuring equipment, stethoscope, weighing machine, etc. This has facilitated provision of quality antenatal care and other health care services.

The Village Health Sanitation and Nutrition Committee (VHSNC) is an important tool of community empowerment and participation at the grassroots level to address issues of environmental and social determinants. **Health care service delivery requires intensive human resource inputs**. NHM has attempted to fill the gaps in human resources by providing nearly 1.88 lakh additional health human resources to States including 7,263 GDMOs, 3,355 Specialists, 73,154 ANMs, 40,847 Staff Nurses on contractual basis. NHM has also focused on multiskilling of doctors at strategically located facilities identified by the States, e.g. MBBS doctors are trained in Emergency Obstetric Care (EmOC), Life Saving Anesthesia Skills (LSAS) and Laparoscopic Surgery. Due importance is also being given to capacity building of nursing staff and auxiliary workers such as ANMs. NRHM also supports co-location of AYUSH services in health facilities such as PHCs, CHCs and DHs. A total of 24,890 AYUSH doctors have been deployed in the States with NRHM funding support.

Janani Suraksha Yojana (JSY) aims to reduce maternal mortality among pregnant women by encouraging them to deliver in government health facilities. Under the scheme, cash assistance is provided to eligible pregnant women for giving birth in a government health facility. Since the inception of NRHM, 8.55 crore women have benefited under this scheme.

Janani Shishu Suraksha Karyakram (JSSK): Launched on 1st June, 2011, JSSK entitles all pregnant women delivering in public health institutions to absolutely free and no expense delivery, including cesarean section. This marks a shift to an entitlement based approach. The free entitlements include free drugs and consumables, free diagnostics, free diet during stay in the health institutions, free provision of blood, free transport from home to health institution, between health institutions in case of referrals and drop back home and exemption from all kinds of user charges. Similar entitlements are available for all sick infants (up to 1 year of age) accessing public health institutions.

Facility Based Newborn Care: A continuum of newborn care has been established with the launch of home based and facility based newborn care components ensuring that every newborn receives essential care right from the time of birth and first 48 hours at the health facility and then at home during the first 42 days of life. Newborn Care Corners (NBCCs) are established at delivery points to provide essential newborn care at birth, while Special Newborn Care Units (SNCUs) at District Hospital/Medical College and Newborn Stabilization Units (NBSUs) at FRUs provide care for sick newborns. As on June 2015, a total of 14,441 NBCCs, 2,020 NBSUs and 575 SNCUs have been made operational across the country.

National Mobile Medical Units (NMMUs): Support has been provided in 333 out of 672 districts for 1107 Mobile

Medical Units (MMUs) under NHM in the country. To increase visibility, awareness and accountability, all Mobile Medical Units (MMUs) have been repositioned as 'National Mobile Medical Unit Service' with universal color and design.

National Ambulance Services (NAS): As on date, 31 States/UTs have the facility where people can dial 108 or 102 telephone number for calling an ambulance. Presently, 7358 Dial-108, 400 Dial-104 and 7836 Dial-102 Emergency Response Service Vehicles are operational under NHM, besides 6290 empaneled vehicles for transportation of patients, particularly pregnant women and sick infants from home to public health facilities and back.

Up to 33% of NHM funds in High Focus States can be used for infrastructure development.

Mainstreaming of AYUSH: Mainstreaming of AYUSH has been taken up by allocating AYUSH facilities in 10042 PHCs, 2732 CHCs, 501 DHs, 5714 health facilities above SC but below block level and 421 health facilities other than CHC at or above block level but below district level.

Launch of National Quality Assurance Framework for Health facilities: To improve quality of healthcare in over 31000 public facilities.

Launch of Kayakalp: An initiative for Award to Public Health facilities: Kayakalp initiative has been launched to promote cleanliness, hygiene and infection control practices in public health facilities.

Free Drugs Service Initiative: An incentive of up to 5% additional funding (over and above the normal allocation of the state) under the NHM is provided to those States that introduce free medicines scheme.

Free Diagnostics Service Initiative: The NHM—Free Diagnostics Service Initiative was launched in 2013 to provide free essential diagnostic services at public health facilities under which substantial funding was provided to States within their resource envelope.

Biomedical Equipment Maintenance: States have been asked to plan interventions for comprehensive equipment maintenance for all functional medical equipment/machinery.

Comprehensive Primary Health care: Primary health care including preventive and promotive health care enables early detection and prompt treatment and serves a gatekeeping function to secondary and tertiary care and also reduces the cost of care.

Kilkari: To create proper awareness among pregnant women, parents of children and field workers about the importance of Antenatal Care (ANC), Institutional Delivery, Postnatal Care (PNC) and Immunization, it was decided to implement the Kilkari and Mobile Academy services across India in phased manner. In the first phase Kilkari would be launched in 6 States viz. Uttarakhand, Jharkhand, Uttar Pradesh, Odisha, Rajasthan High Priority Districts (HPDs) and Madhya Pradesh High Priority Districts (HPDs). The Mobile Academy would be launched in 4 States viz. Uttarakhand, Jharkhand, Rajasthan and Madhya Pradesh. Kilkari is an Interactive Voice Response (IVR) based mobile service that delivers time-sensitive audio messages (Voice Call) about pregnancy and child health directly to the mobile phones of pregnant women, mothers of young children and their families. The service covers the critical time period where the most maternal/infant deaths occur from the 4th month of pregnancy until the child is one year old. Families which subscribe to the service receive one pre-recorded system generated call per week. Each call will be 2 minutes in length and serve as reminders for what the family should be doing that week depending on woman's stage of pregnancy or the child's age. Kilkari services will be available to states in regional dialect too.

Mobile Academy is an anytime, anywhere audio training course on interpersonal communication skills that the ASHA can access from her mobile phone. It gives ASHAs tips on how to convince families to adopt priority RMNCH behaviors, while refreshing her existing knowledge. The course is 240 minutes long and consists of 11 chapters with 4 lessons each. At the end of each chapter, there is a quiz for them the ANM/ASHAs who pass the course will be provided with a certificate.

Launch of Nationwide Anti-TB drug resistance survey: Drug resistance survey for 13 anti-TB drugs was launched to provide a better estimate on the burden of Multi-Drug Resistant Tuberculosis within the community. This is the biggest ever such survey in the world with a sample size of 5214 patients. Results are expected by 2016.

Kala Azar Elimination Plan: To reduce the annual incidence of Kala-azar to less than one per 10,000 population at block PHC level by the end of 2015.

Criteria for incentives to States under the NHM were revised. States that show improved progress made on key Outcomes/Outputs such as IMR, MMR, Immunization, number and proportion of quality certified health facilities, etc. will be able to receive additional funds as incentives.

RMNCH+A: National Health Mission

Following the Government of India's ***'Call to Action (CAT) Summit' in February, 2013,*** the Ministry of Health and Family Welfare launched 3 years National Campaign focusing on **Reproductive, Maternal, Newborn Child and Adolescent** health and health related system strengthening (including Nutrition) to influence key interventions for prevention and treatment of diseases that result in unacceptable levels of morbidity and mortality in the high risk and vulnerable communities.

The ***12th Five Year Plan*** has defined the National Health outcomes and the 3 goals that are relevant to RMNCH +A strategies approach as follows:

- Reduction of Infant Mortality Rate to 25/1000 live birth by 2017.
- Reduction in Maternal Mortality Ratio to 100/100000 live birth by 2017.
- Reduction in Total Fertility Rate to 2.1 by 2017.

The RMNCH+A strategic approach has been developed to provide an understanding of 'continuum of care' to ensure equal focus on various life stages. Priority interventions for each thematic area have been included in this to ensure that the linkages between them are contextualized to the same and consecutive life stage. It also introduces new initiatives like the use of **Score Card** to track the performance, National **Iron + Initiative** to address the issue of anemia across all age groups and the **Comprehensive Screening and Early interventions for defects at birth, diseases and deficiencies among children and adolescents**. The RMNCH+A appropriately directs the States to focus their efforts on the most vulnerable population and disadvantaged groups in the country. It also emphasizes on the need to reinforce efforts in those poor performing districts that have already been identified as the high focus districts.

'Beti Bachao Beti Padhao' Scheme by Govt of India, the scheme has three primary objectives:

1. Prevent female infanticide.
2. Devise new schemes and work cohesively to ensure that every girl child is secured and protected.
3. Ensure every girl child gets quality education.

5 × 5 Matrix for RMNCH+A				
Let's make every mother and child healthy, **Transformational Leadership can do it**				
Reproductive Health	**M**aternal Health	**N**ewborn Health	**C**hild Health	**A**dolescent Health
• Focus on spacing methods, particularly PPIUCD at high case load facilities • Interval IUCD at sub-centers on fixed days • Doorstep delivery of contraceptives by ASHA • Strengthening safe abortion services • Maintaining sterilization services	• Use MCTS to ensure early registration of pregnancy and provide full ANC • Detect high risk pregnancies and line list and manage severely anemic mothers • Equip delivery points with trained HR and other infrastructure • Review maternal, infant and child deaths for corrective actions • Notify sub-centers with less institutional delivery load, distribute mesoprostol and incentivize ANMs for domiciliary deliveries	• Early initiation and exclusive breastfeeding • Home based newborn care through ASHA • Essential newborn care and resuscitation services at all delivery points • Equip special newborn care units with highly trained HR and other infrastructure • Empower ANM for community level use of gentamycin	• Complementary feeding, IFA supplementation and focus on nutrition • Diarrhea management at community level using ORS and Zinc • Management of pneumonia • Full immunization coverage • Rashtriya Bal Swasthya Karyakram (RBSK) screening of children for 40 (birth defect, development delays, deficiencies and disease) and its management	• Community based services through peer educations • Delay in age of marriage • Strengthen ARSH clinics • Weekly IFA Supplementation (WIFS) under national iron plus initiative • Promote menstrual hygiene
Health Systems		**Cross cutting**		
• Case load based deplopment of HR at all levels • Ambulances, drugs, diagnostics, reproductive health commodities • Behavior change communication • Supportive supervision and use of scorecards based on HMIS • Public grievances redressal mechanism		• Equip nurses to provide specialized and quality care • Address social determinants of health through convergence • Introduce difficult area and performance based incentives • Focus on un-served and underserved villages, urban slums and blocks • Bring down out of pocket expenses		

Appendix 15

THE NATIONAL POLICY FOR CHILDREN, 2013

1. INTRODUCTION

1.1. India is home to the largest child population in the world. The constitution of India guarantees fundamental rights to all children in the country and empowers the State to make special provisions for children. The directive principles of state policy specifically guide the State in securing the tender age of children from abuse and ensuring that children are given opportunities and facilities to develop in a healthy manner in conditions of freedom and dignity. The State is responsible for ensuring that childhood is protected from exploitation and moral and material abandonment.

1.2. Declaring its children as the nation's 'supremely important asset' in the National Policy for Children, 1974, the Government of India reiterated its commitment to secure the rights of its children by ratifying related international conventions and treaties. These include the declaration of the rights of the child, Universal declaration of human rights and its covenants, the convention on the rights of the child and its two optional protocols, the United Nations Convention on the rights of persons with disabilities, the United Nations Conventions against transnational organized crime, the protocol to prevent, suppress and punish trafficking in women and children, the Hague Convention on protection of children and cooperation in respect of inter-country adoption, and the convention on the elimination of all forms of discrimination against women.

1.3. The National Policy for Children, 1974 recognized that programs for children should find prominent place in national plans for the development of human resources, so that children grow up to become robust citizens, physically fit, mentally alert and morally healthy, endowed with the skills and motivations provided by society. The policy also laid emphasis on equal opportunities for the development of all children during the period of growth.

1.4. The National Charter for Children 2003 adopted on 9th February 2004, underlined the intent to secure for every child its inherent right to be a child and enjoy a healthy and happy childhood to address the root causes that negate the healthy growth and development of children, and to awaken the conscience of the community in the wider societal context to protect children from all forms of abuse, while strengthening the family, society and the nation.

1.5. To affirm the Government's commitment to the rights-based approach in addressing the continuing and emerging challenges in the situation of children, the Government of India hereby adopts the resolution on the National Policy for Children, 2013.

2. PREAMBLE

2.1. *Recognizing that:*
- A child is any person below the age of eighteen years
- Childhood is an integral part of life with a value of its own
- Children are not a homogenous group and their different needs need different responses, especially the multidimensional vulnerabilities experienced by children in different circumstances
- Long-term, sustainable, multi-sectoral, integrated and inclusive approach is necessary for the overall and harmonious development and protection of children.

2.2. *Reaffirming that:*
- Every child is unique and a supremely important national asset
- Special measures and affirmative action are required in diminish or eliminate conditions that cause discrimination
- All children have the right to grow in a family environment in an atmosphere of happiness, love and understanding
- Families are to be supported by a strong social safety not in caring for and nurturing their children
- The Government of India reiterates its commitment in safeguard, inform, include, support and empower all children within its territory and jurisdiction, both in their individual situation and as a national asset. The State is committed in take affirmative measures—

legislative, policy or otherwise to promote and safeguard the right of all children to live and grow with equity, dignity, security and freedom, especially those marginalized or disadvantaged; to ensure that all children have equal opportunities; and that no custom, tradition, cultural or religious practice is allowed to violate or restrict or prevent children from enjoying their rights.

2.3. This policy is to guide and inform all laws, policies, plans and programs affecting children. All actions and initiatives of the national, state and local government is all sectors must respect and uphold the principles and provisions of this policy.

3. GUIDING PRINCIPLES

i. Every child has universal, inalienable and indivisible human rights
ii. The rights of children are interrelated and interdependent, and each one of them is equally important and fundamental to the well-being and dignity of the child
iii. Every child has the right to life, survival, development, education, protection and participation
iv. Right to life, survival and development goes beyond the physical existence of the child and also encompasses the right to identity and nationality
v. Mental, emotional, cognitive, social and cultural development of the child is to be address in totality
vi. All children have equal rights and no child shall be discriminated against on grounds of religion, race, caste, sex, place of birth, class, languages, and disability, social, economic and any other status
vii. The best interest of the child is a primary concern in all decisions and actions affecting the child, whether taken by legislative bodies, courts of law, administrative authorities, public, private, social, religious or cultural institutions
viii. Family or family environment is most conductive for the all around development of children and they are not to be separated from their parents, except where such separation is necessary in their best interest
ix. Every child has the right to a dignified life, free from exploitation
x. Safety and security of all children is integral to their well-being and children are to be protected from all forms of harm, abuse, neglect, violence, maltreatment and exploitation in all settings including care institutions, schools, hospitals, crèches, families and communities
xi. Children are capable of forming views and must be provided a conducive environment and the opportunity to express their views in any way they are able to communicate, in matters affecting them
xii. Children's views, especially those of girls, children from disadvantaged groups and marginalized communities, are to be heard in all matters affecting them, in particular judicial and administrative proceedings and interactions, and their views given due consideration in accordance with their age, maturity and evolving capacities.

4. KEY PRIORITIES

Survival, health, nutrition, development, education, protection and participation are the undeniable rights of every child and are the key priorities of this policy.

Survival, Health and Nutrition

4.1. The right to life, survival, health and nutrition is an inalienable right of every child and will receive the highest priority.

4.2. The State stands committed to ensure equitable access to comprehensive, and essential, preventive, promotive, curative and rehabilitative health care, of the highest standard, for all children before, during and after birth, and throughout the period of their growth and development.

4.3. Every child has a right to adequate nutrition and to be safeguarded against hunger, deprivation and malnutrition. The State commits to securing this right for all children through access, provision and promotion of required services and supports for holistic nurturing, well-being with nutritive attainment of all children, keeping in view their individual needs at different stages of life in a life cycle approach.

4.4. The State shall take all necessary measures to:
   i. Improve maternal health care, including antenatal care, safe delivery by skilled health personnel, postnatal care and nutritional support
   ii. Provide universal access to information and services for making informed choices related to birth and spacing of children
   iii. Secure the right of the girl child to life, survival, health and nutrition
   iv. Address key causes and determinants of child mortality through interventions based on continuum of care, with emphasis on nutrition, safe drinking water-sanitation and health education

v. Encourage focused behavior change communication efforts to improve newborn and childcare practices at the household and community level
vi. Provide universal and affordable access to services for prevention, treatment, care and management of neonatal and childhood illnesses and protect children from all water-borne, vector-borne, blood-borne, communicable and other childhood diseases
vii. Prevent disabilities, both mental and physical, through timely measures for prenatal, perinatal and postnatal health and nutrition care of mother and child, provide services for early detection, treatment and management, including interventions to minimize and prevent further disabilities, prevent discrimination faced by children with disabilities (mental and physical), and provide service for rehabilitation and social support
viii Ensure availability of essential services, supports and provisions for nutritive attainment in a life cycle approach, including infant and young child feeding (IYCF) practices, special focus on adolescent girls and other vulnerable groups, and special measures for the health, care and nutrition, including nutrition education, of expectant and nursing mothers
ix. Provide adolescent access to information, support and services essential for their health and development, including information and support on appropriate life style and healthy choices and awareness on the ill effects of alcohol and substance abuse
x. Prevent HIV infections at birth and ensure infected children receive medical treatment, adequate nutrition and after-care, and are not discriminated against in accessing their rights
xi. Ensure that only child safe products and services are available in the country and put in place mechanisms to enforce safety standards for products and services designed for children
xii. Provide adequate safeguards and measures against false claims relating to growth, development and nutrition.

Education and Development

4.5. Every child has equal right to learning, knowledge and education. The State recognizes its responsibility to secure this right for every child, with due regard for special needs, through access provision and promotion of required environment, information, infrastructure, services and supports, towards the development of the child's fullest potential.

4.6. The state take all necessary measures to:
i. Provide universal and equitable access to quality early childhood care and education (ECCE) for optimal development and active learning capacity of all children below six years of age
ii. Ensure that every child in the age group of 6–14 years is in school and enjoys the fundamental right to education as enshrined in the constitution
iii. Promote affordable and accessible quality education up to the secondary level for all children
iv. Foster and support interschool networks and linkages to provide vocational training options including comprehensively addressing age-specific and gender-specific issues of children's career choices through career counseling and vocational guidance
v. Ensure that all out of school children such as child laborers migrant children, trafficked children, children of migrants labor, street children, child victims of alcohol and substance abuse, children in areas of civil unrest, orphans, children with disability (mental and physical), children with chronic ailments, married children, children of manual scavengers, children of sex workers, children of prisoners, etc. are tracked, rescued, rehabilitated and have access to their right to education
vi. Address discrimination of all forms in schools and foster equal opportunity, treatment and participation irrespective of place of birth, sex, religion, disability, language, region, caste, health, social, economic or any other status
vii. Priorities education for disadvantaged groups by creating enabling environment through necessary legislative measures, policy and provisions
viii. Ensure physical safety of the child and provide safe and secure learning environment
ix. Ensure that all process of teaching and learning are child-friendly
x. Ensure formulation and practice of pedagogy that engages and delights children, with a special focus on mental health, from a social and gender just, life skills and age appropriate perspective

xi. Provide access to ICT tools for equitable, inclusive and affordable education for all children especially in remote, tribal and hard to reach areas

xii. Promote safe and enjoyable engagement of children's experiences with new technology in accordance with their age and level of maturity, even as there is respect for their own culture and roots

xiii. Review, develop and sustain age-specific initiatives, services and programs for safe space for play, sports, recreation, leisure, culture and scientific activities for children in neighborhoods, schools and other institutions

xiv. Enable children to develop holistically, bringing out their aspirations, with focus on their strengths, empowering them to take control of their lives, bodies and behaviors

xv. Ensure no child is subjected to any physical punishment or mental harassment. Promote positive engagement to impart discipline so as to provide children with a good learning experience

xvi. Ensure that children's health is regularly monitored through the school health program an arrangements are made for health and emergency care of children

xvii. Provide services to children with special needs in regular schools and ensure that these are inclusive and have all facilities such as trained teachers and special educators appropriate pedagogy and education material, barrier-free access for mobility, functional toilets and co-curricular activities towards the development for child's fullest potential and anatomy and sense of dignity and self-worth

xviii. Promote engagement of families and communities with schools for all round development of children, with emphasis on good health, hygiene and sanitation practices, including sensitization on ill-effects of alcohol and substance abuse

xix. Facilitate concerted efforts by local governments, nongovernmental organizations/community-based organizations to map gaps in availability of educational services, especially in backward, child labor intensive areas, areas of civil unrest, and in situations of emergency, and efforts for addressing them

xx. Identify, encourage and assist gifted children, particularly those belonging to the disadvantaged groups, through special programs

xxi. Provide and promote crèche and day care facilities for children of working mothers, mothers belonging to poor families, ailing mothers and single parents

xxii. Promote appropriate baby feeding facilities in public place and at workplaces for working mothers in public, private and unorganized sector.

Protection

4.7. A safe, secure and protective environment is a precondition for the realization of all other rights of children. Children have the rights to be protected wherever they are.

4.8. The State shall create a caring protective and safe environment for all children to reduce their vulnerability in all situations and to keep them safe at all places, especially public spaces.

4.9. The State shall protect all children from all forms of violence and abuse, harm, neglect, stigma, discrimination, deprivation, exploitation including economic exploitation and sexual exploitation, abandonment, separation, abduction, sale or trafficking for any purpose or in any form, pornography, alcohol and substance abuse, or any other activity that takes undue advantage of them, or harms their personhood or affects their development

4.10. To secure the rights of children temporarily or permanently deprived of parental care, the State shall endeavor to ensure family and community-based care arrangements including sponsorship, kinship, foster care and adoption, with institutionalization as a measure of last resort, with due regard to the best interests of the child and guaranteeing quality standards of care and protection.

4.11. The State commits to taking special protection measures to secure the rights and entitlements of children in need of special protection, characterized by their specific social, economic and geopolitical situations, including their need for rehabilitation and reintegration, in particular but not limited to, children affected by migration, displacement, communal or sectarian violence, civil unrest, disasters and calamities, street children, children of sex workers, children force into commercial sexual exploitation, abused and exploited children, children forced into begging, children in conflict and contact with the law, children in situations

of labor, children of prisoners, children infected/affected by HIV/AIDS, children with disabilities, children affected by alcohol and substance abuse, children of manual scavengers and children from any other socially excluded group, children affected by armed conflict and any other category of children requiring care and protection

4.12. The State shall promote child friendly jurisprudence, enact progressive legislation, build a preventive and responsive child protection system, including emergency outreach services, and promote effective enforcement of punitive legislative and administrative measures against all forms of child abuse and neglect to comprehensively address issues related to child protection

4.13. The State shall promote and strengthen legislative, administrative and institutional redressal mechanisms at the National and State level for the protection of child rights. For local grievances, effective and accessible grievance redressal mechanisms shall be developed at the program level.

Participation

4.14. The State has the primary responsibility to ensure the children are made aware of their rights, and provided with an enabling environment, opportunities and support to develop skills, to form aspirations and express their views in accordance with their age, level of maturity and evolving capacities, so as to enable them to be actively involved in their own development and in all matters concerning and affecting them

4.15. The State shall promote and strengthen respect for the views of the child, especially those of the girl child, children with disabilities and of children from minority groups or marginalized communities, within the family; community; schools and institutions; different levels of governance; as well as in judicial and administrative proceedings that concern them

4.16. The State shall engage all stakeholders in developing mechanisms for children to share their grievances without fear in all settings; monitor effective implementation of children's participation through monitorable indicators; develop different models of child participation; and undertake research and documentation of best practices.

5. ADVOCACY AND PARTNERSHIPS

5.1 The State shall encourage the active involvement, participation and collective action of stakeholders such as individuals, families, local communities, nongovernmental organizations, civil society organizations, media and private sector including government in securing the rights of the child.

5.2 The State shall make planned, coordinated and concerted efforts to raise public awareness on child rights and entitlements amongst the parents and caregivers/guardians as well as functionaries and duty bearers. All stakeholders are to promote the use of rights-based and equity-forced strategies, platforms, programs, communications and other tools to generate awareness on child rights and the commitment to their achievement.

5.3 This policy is to be given wide publicity and supported by focused advocacy measures to ensure that children's best interests and rights are accorded the highest priority in areas of policy, planning, resource allocation, governance, monitoring and evaluation, and children's voice and views are heard in all matters and actions which impact their lives.

5.4 The State shall ensure that service delivery and justice delivery mechanisms and structures are participatory, responsive and child-sensitive, thereby enhancing transparency and ensuring public accountability. Synergistic linkages will be created with other progressive and successful experiments to learn from best practices across regions.

6. COORDINATION, ACTION AND MONITORING

6.1. Addressing the rights and needs of children requires programming across different sectors and integrating their impact on the child in a synergistic way. Rights-based approach to survival, development and protection calls for conscious, convergent and collateral linkages among different sectors and settings, with indicators for tracking progress.

6.2. Community and local governance play a significant role in ensuring the child's optimum development and social integration. Ensuring coordination among Central Government Ministries/Departments, between Central and State Governments, between different levels of governance and between government and civil society is crucial for effective implementation of this policy.

6.3. The Ministry of Women and Child Development (MWCD) will be the nodal ministry for overseeing and coordinating the implementation of this policy. A National Coordination and Action Group

(NCAG) for children under the minister in charge of the Ministry of Women and Child Development will monitor the progress with other concerned ministries as its member. Similar coordination and actions groups will be formed at the state and district level.

6.4. The Ministry of Women and Child Development, in consultation with all related ministries and departments, will formulate a national plan of action for children. Similar plans at the state, district and local level will be formulated to ensure action on the provisions of this policy. The national, state and district coordination and action groups will monitor the progress of implementation under these plans.

6.5. The National Commission for Protection of Child Rights and State Commissions for Protection of Child Rights will ensure that the principles of this policy are respected in all sectors at all levels in formulating laws, policies and programs affecting children.

7. RESEARCH, DOCUMENTATION AND CAPACITY BUILDING

7.1. The implementation of this policy will be supported by a comprehensive and reliable knowledge based on all aspects of the status and condition of children. Establishing such a knowledge base would be enabled through child focused research and documentation, both quantitative as well as qualitative. A continuous process of indicator-based child impact assessment and evaluation will be developed, and assessment and evaluation will be carried out on the situation of children in the country, which will inform policies and programs for children.

7.2. Professional and technical competence and capability in all aspects of programming, managing, working and caring for children at all levels in all sectors will be ensured through appropriate selection and well planned capacity development initiatives. All duty bearers working with children will be sensitized and oriented on child rights and held accountable for their acts of omission and commission.

8. RESOURCES ALLOCATION

8.1. The State commits to allocate the required financial, material and human resources, and their efficient and effective use, with transparency and accountability, to implement this policy

8.2. Child budgeting will track allocation and utilization of resources and their impact on outcomes for children with regard to budgets and expenditure on children by all related ministries and departments.

9. REVIEW OF POLICY

9.1. A comprehensive review of this policy will be taken up once in five years in consultation with all stakeholders, including children. The Ministry of Women and Child Development will lead the review process.

Index

Page numbers followed by *f* refer to figure and *t* refer to table, respectively.

A

Abatacept 685
Abdomen 190, 195
  acute 286, 287
  flat plate of 255
  lower 324
  pain 253*f*
Abdominal distension 253
Abdominal examination 270
Abortive poliomyelitis 511
Abuse 22
Accident prevention 165
Accredited social health activist 231
ACE inhibitors 705
Acetabular dysplasia 671
Acetaminophen 704
Acetazolamide 390, 701
Acid
  indigestion 261
  reflux 252
  regurgitation 252
Acid-base
  disturbances 245*t*
  equilibrium 236
  management 321
  status, disturbances in 242
Acidosis 236, 237
  correction of 244
Acne
  pathogenesis of 552*f*
  vulgaris 551
Acrocyanosis 471
  in newborn 87*f*
Actinomycin D 439, 440
Acts to Children Welfare and Rights 667
Acyanotic heart diseases 470, 475
Acyclovir 383, 701, 704
Adam's forward bend test 676*f*
Adenoiditis 296
Adenovirus 567
Adequate nutrition 204
Adjuvant therapy 381
Admission assessment 184
Adolescence 155
  developmental issues in 159
  early 157, 158
  late 157, 159
  theories of 163
Adolescent 183, 184, 220, 221
  health 208
  identity crises 58*f*
  reactions of 222
  reproductive and sexual health 209
Adoptive families 18
Adrenal gland 444, 452
  disorder of 445
Adrenal hyperplasia, congenital 447, 450, 452
Adrenaline 701
Adrenocorticotropic hormone 448
Adriamycin 440
Aggressive behavior 172
Air contrast barium enema 256
Airway
  care of 383
  management, basic 655
  obstruction, treatment of 312
Albendazole 540, 701
Albuminuria 340
Albuterol 701
Aldosterone, production of 452
Alkalosis 236, 237
Allergic disorders 315
Allis' test 672
Allogeneic stem cell transplant 430
Allogenic type of transplant 417
Allopurinol 423
All-transretinoic acid 552
Alopecia 415
Amantadine 707
Amaurotic Cat's eye reflex 441
Amblyopia 565, 566
American Academy of Pediatrics 97, 337
American Nurses Association Code for Nurses 8
Amikacin 701
Amino acids, essential 657
Aminophylline 701
Amniocentesis 75*f*, 378
Amoebicidal drugs 275
Amoxicillin clavulanate 701
Ampicillin 701
Amputation 436
Anal stage 55
Anaphylactic shock 501
Ancylostoma duodenale 538
Ancylostomiasis 538
Androgens 453
  cause 552
Andvanillymandelic acid 432
Anemia 174, 328, 351, 354, 366, 534, 599, 644
  acute 352
  mild microcytic 352
  severe 352, 534
Anganwadi workers 207
Angiotensin-converting enzyme 339, 343, 498
Anomalies, congenital 649
Anorectal malformations 586
  types of 587*f*
Anorectoplasty, posterior sagittal 587
Anorexia 488, 623
Antacids 262, 704
Antenatal care 199
Antenatal health 199
Antenatal preventive pediatric 198
Antibiotic 272, 273, 307, 549, 644
  drugs 275
  medicines 567
  therapy 337, 506
Anti-child labor laws 667
Anticholinergic 568
  agents 705
Anticonvulsant 265, 427, 705
  medications 491
Antidiarrheals 264
Antidiuretic hormone 447
Antiemetics 272
Antiglobulin 351
Antihistamine 549, 705
Antihypertensive agents 343
Anti-inflammatory treatment 491
Antilipemics 707
Antimotility agents 273
Antineoplastic agents 414, 707
Antinuclear antibody 684
Antipseudomonal treatment 683
Antirheumatic drugs, disease-modifying 685
Antiseizure 383
Antispasmodics 264
Antithyroid drugs 459
Antitoxin therapy 506
Antituberculars 705
Antiviral medications 383
Anxiety 391, 431, 508, 599, 607, 623
  disorders 605, 608
    etiology 605
    types 605
  severe 607
  signs of 224

Aortic
  balloon valvoplasty 591
  coarctation 482
  insufficiency 492
  stenosis 481, 591
  valve 591
    replacement 591, 592
Apgar scoring system 87
Apheresis machine 417
Aplastic anemia 352, 353
Apnea 644
  central 645
  management 645
  mixed 645
  pathophysiology 645
Appendicitis 286
Appetite, loss of 599
Arm circumference 188
Arm strength 191
Arnold-Chiari malformation 389, 395
Arousal, changing states of 105
Arrhythmia 494
  symptoms of 494
Arterial blood gas 243, 245
Arterial duct 80
Arterial oxygen tension 290
Arterial pressure 80
Arterial switch 473
Artery 290
Arthritis 492, 682
Ascaris-lumbricoides 538
Ascites 285
Ascorbic acid 701
Asphyxia
  moderate 641
  neonatorum 641
  severe 641
Asphyxiated baby 642*f*
Aspirin 293, 359, 369, 499, 701, 707
Asthma 319*f*
  action plan 320
  bronchial 315
  cycle 316*f*
  management
    acute 318
    long-term 320
  severe acute 318
Astigmatism 565
Astrocytes 425
Astrocytoma 427
Atenolol 701, 706
Atonic seizure 400
Atopic dermatitis 550
Atraumatic care 5, 6*f*
Atresia 480, 582
  congenital 571
Atrial arrhythmia 496
Atrial fibrillation 495
Atrial flutter 495
Atrial septal defect 473, 476, 477, 477*f*
Atrioventricular septal defect 479
  treatments 479
Atropine sulfate 701
Attention deficit hyperactivity disorder 153, 175, 573, 604
Audiometry 572
Augmentin 701
Augmenting myocardial contractility 487
Authoritarian child-rearing emphasizes 19
Autism spectrum disorders 603
Autistic child 603*f*
Autoantibody testing 464
Autoimmune hepatitis 283
Autosomal dominant inheritance 72, 73, 73*f*, 74*f*
Avascular necrosis 674
Avian influenza 294
Axial skeleton 373
Azathioprine 705
Azithromycin 701

B

Babinski reflex 92
Bacillary dysentery 274
Bacille calmette-guerin 528
Bacteria 35
Bacterial gastroenteritis 263
Bacterial illnesses 572
Bacterial infection 337, 379, 523, 543
  secondary 304
Bacterial meningitis 378, 379, 533
Bacterium *Bordetella pertussis* 506
Bacteroides 322
Balanced diet for children 32, 32*f*
Balloon valvuloplasty 482
Barium 255
  enema 256
Barlow's test 672
Basal fracture 403
Becker's muscular 610
Bedtime routine 141
Behavior disorder 604
Behavioral pediatric 167
  principles, basic 169
Behavioral problem 170
  causes of 171
  management of 170
Behavioral tests 401
Bekesy audiometry 572
Bell's palsy 497
Benzodiazepines 525, 706
Benzoyl peroxide 552
Benzyl benzoate lotion 549
Berger's disease 337
Beta-hemolytic streptococci 296
Bicuspid aortic valve 482
Bile ducts obstruction 283
Bili blanket 661, 661*f*
Bili lights 660
Bilirubin 366
  encephalopathy 369
Binocular vision 562
Biological stress 223
Biomedical equipment maintenance 709
Biopsy 411, 435, 438
  excisional 431
  incisional 431
  of tumor 435
  open
    excisional 412
    incisional 412
Birth asphyxia 79, 460, 641
Birth defects 71
Birth injuries 100, 641, 647
Birth of child, registration of 102
Birth registration of newborn 687
Biting fingernails 175
Bladder 324, 331
  dysfunction 384
  exstrophy repair 576
  infection, symptoms of 336
Blalock-Taussig shunt 474, 590, 592
Blastoma 431
Bleeding 406
Blended families 18
Blindness 568, 569
  types of 569
Blood 255, 290, 656
  capillaries 284
  cells 430*f*
  coagulation 82
  count 351
  culture 493
  electrolyte 438
  eosinophils 550
  examination, routine 533
  flow 81
  gas analysis 290
  hormone testing 451
  in urine 336
  occult 255
  oxygen level 300
  pressure 185
    decrease 488
    low 494
  smear 358
  studies 354
  supply 325

test 278, 290, 300, 314, 345, 401, 413, 435, 446, 453, 486, 528
transfusion 522, 647
volume 80
Blurred vision 497
Body
composition 625
fluid 97, 235
balance 349
hair 157
image 159, 160
proportions, changes in 104
surface area 628
temperature, maintenance of 639
water, regulation of 236
Bone
cancer 409, 434
density 278
growth, abnormal 415
long 669*f*
marrow
aspiration 435, 438
biopsy 351, 353
depression 414
suppression 416
transplant 417
of hip 671*f*
of pelvis 671*f*
scans 413
Boosts cognitive development 36
Bordetella pertussis 35, 506
Boston children's hospital 2
Botryoid type 438
Bowel biopsy, small 279
Bowel disorder 245
Bowel movement 254
Brachytherapy 416, 442
Bracing 678
Brain 374, 424
development 104, 136
function 404
plasticity 105
scans 378, 401
tumor 398, 424, 425
symptoms of 426
types of tumor in 424*f*
Brain-gut signal problems 263
Brainstem
gliomas 425, 427
upper 373
Breast milk 93, 97, 594
composition of 93, 96
production mechanism 95
Breastfed infants 367
Breastfeeding 28, 93, 94*f*, 95, 99, 704-706
benefits of 97
jaundice 369
promotion of 198
to twin babies 94*f*
Breastmilk jaundice 367
Breath-holding spell 599
Breathing 289
trouble 289
Brock operation 590
Bronchial tree 305*f*
Bronchiectasis 312, 321
diagnosis 322
etiology of 321
signs 321
symptoms 321
treatment 322
Bronchiolitis 301
airways in 301*f*
severe 303
Bronchitis 304
acute 304
chronic 305
Bronchodilators 704
Bronchopulmonary dysplasia 646
Bronchoscopy 291, 311
Brudziński sign 381
Brushfield spots 612
Bruxism 599, 600
Bulbospinal poliomyelitis 512
Bull neck 505
Bullous impetigo 543, 544
Bupropion 705
Burn 134, 553
classification of 555
complication of 558
etiology 553
incidence 553
injury 556*f*
depth of 555
extent of 555
first aid of 556
minor 556
severity of 556
wound management 558

C

Calcium 152, 346
loss of 278
Calories 27, 152
Campylobacter 255, 286
Canadian Nurses Association Code for Nurses 8
Cancer 409, 414, 415
cells 350, 410*f*
in children, signs of 411
pathophysiology of 410
related fatigue 427
Candida 545
Candida albicans 545
Candidiasis 544
Capsule endoscopy 278
Caput succedaneum 649
Carbohydrate 93
low 401
Carbon dioxide 289
in arterial blood, partial pressure of 245
tension 290
Carcinogens 410
Cardiac catheterization 472, 473, 480
Cardiac conditions 495*t*
Cardiac demands, decrease 489
Cardiac diseases, congenital 483
Cardiac examination 480, 482, 483
Cardiac function 489
Cardiac monitoring 387
Cardiac output 80, 503
Cardiac problems 484*t*
Cardiac work, reducing 487
Cardio pulmonary resuscitation 642*f*
Cardiomyopathy
dilated 500
in children 500
etiology 500
symptoms of 501
types of 500
Cardiorespiratory monitoring 5
Cardiovascular
assessment 484
problems, signs of 484
system 106, 195, 468, 589, 625
disorders of 470
Caries spine 527*f*
Cartilage 670
Cataract 567
in children 567*f*
Catecholamine-induced tachycardia 502
Catheter
ablation 496
based procedure 479
procedure 476, 593
Causative organisms 322
Ceftriaxone 369, 701
Cefuroxim 702
Celiac disease 277, 277*f*
Cell
growth, abnormal 409*f*, 410
normal 410*f*
Cellular respiration 289
Central nervous system 253, 372, 637, 656
disorders of 378
infection of 378
tumors 409, 424
Central pontine myelinolysis 238

Central social welfare board 214
Central venous line 594
Cephalohematoma 648, 649
Cephalopelvic disproportion 100
Cephalosporins 337, 704
Cerebellar function 192
Cerebellum 374
Cerebral blood flow 375, 406
Cerebral cortex 105
Cerebral hemispheres 137
Cerebral malaria 533
Cerebral palsy 611, 675
causes 611*f*
management 611
Cerebral perfusion pressure 405, 406
Cerebrospinal fluid 375, 513
aspiration of 413*f*
Cerumen 571
Cesarean delivery 648
Cheilorrhaphy 579
Chemotherapy 414, 435
effects of 415
Chest 189, 195
circumference 119, 188
cold 304
drainage 315, 315*f*
pain 313
radiograph 480
tube 594
tumors 432
Chiar osteotomy 674
Chickenpox 113, 516, 517*f*
Child
abuse 22
and family health services 24
development, principles of 50
guidance clinic 176, 211
head 583
health 1-3, 41, 202, 208
care 9
initiatives in 204
nurse 25*f*
nurse, qualities of 25
nursing 1, 3, 7, 10, 37
nursing, trends in 4
promotion 26, 41, 198
promotion and prevention of diseases, role of family in 24
illness, reactions to 222
immune system 297
in burns 554*f*
Labor (Prohibition and Regulation) Act, 1986 667
marriage 668
terms of 668
movement 333
neurons 137
physical limitations 611
short stature 455
survival and safe motherhood 201
Welfare Programs 215
Childhood
cancers, causes of 411
development 53*f*
glaucoma 566
illness, management of 206, 228, 229
lymphoma, treatment of 429
schizophrenia 608
management 609
Children's
development 50, 51
diseases 3
health 4
homes 666
Chlamydia pneumoniae 297
Chlorampenicol 707
Chloroquine 702
sensitive malaria, treatment in 534*t*
Cholecystokinin 252
Cholesterol 454
Chondroblastoma 431
Chorion villi 70
Chorionic villi 68
sampling 378
Choroid plexus 390
cauterization 393, 589
Chromosomal disorder 72, 74, 612, 614
Chromosome 75*f*
abnormal 597
Chvostek's sign 242
Ciprofloxacin 702
Cirrhosis 283
of liver 283
Clarithromycin 702
Cleft lip 259, 579
types of 259*f*
Cleft palate 259, 579
surgery 579*f*
Clindamycin 552, 705
Clofazimine 531
Closed-heart surgery 593, 596
Clostridium tetani 35, 523, 524
Clotrimazole 704
Cloxacillin 702
Clozapine 707
Club foot, congenital 670
Coagulopathy 280, 285, 351
Coarctation of aorta 483*f*
Coats' disease 441
Cobb method 676
Cognitive development 45, 59, 61, 65, 106, 117, 151, 157
milestones 118
theory 58
Cognitive impairment 601, 602
Cognitive jean piaget 163
Cognitive-behavioral therapy 606
Cold 288, 292
treatment for common 293
Colonoscopy 258
Colostomy 585*f*, 587
Colostrum 96
feeding 96
Coma 521
Common cold 293*f*
Common pediatric disorders 71
Communicable diseases 504, 504*f*
in children 504
Communicate with kindness 164
Communicating hydrocephalus 389
Communication 623
development 36
method 163
with adolescents 163
Comorbidities, severe 582
Complementary feeding 30, 30*f*, 31*f*
Complete blood count 317, 352, 357, 435, 438, 493
Complex focal seizures 399
Compylobacter 269
Concrete operation 60
Conduct disorder 172, 601
development of 601
Congenital abnormalities 328, 331, 486
Congenital adrenal hyperplasia, cause of 452
Congenital cardiac anomalies, classification of 470
Congenital disorders 562
Congestion 623
Congestive cardiac failure 485, 486
etiology 485
Congestive heart failure 478
Conjunctivitis 567
treatment of 567
Consciousness, loss of 471
Constipation 253, 262, 286, 623
Contact lenses 568
Contagious bacterial disease 35
Continuous positive airway pressure 645, 662
Contrecoup head injury 403*f*
Contrecoup injury 403
Contusion 403
Cool extremities 488
Cooley anemia 356
Coombs' test 351, 366
Core biopsy 431, 435
Corynebacterium diphtheriae 35
Coronary heart disease, surgical management of 593

Corticosteroids 318, 427, 685, 704
Cost containment 6
Cough 486, 507
 up blood 312
Cow's milk 29
Cranial nerve 375, 384, 572
 functioning 192*t*
 functions of 375*t*
 types of 375*t*
Craniopharyngioma 426, 454
C-reactive protein 684
Creatinine clearance test 328
Cryotherapy 442
Cryptorchidism 336
Cushing's syndrome 445, 453
Cyanosis 187, 470-472, 480, 484, 595
 central 470
Cyanotic breath-holding spells 599
Cyanotic heart diseases 470, 471
Cyberknife therapy 435
Cycloplegics 568
Cystic fibrosis 311
Cysts 274
Cytokines 274
Cytomegalovirus 71
Cytotoxin 269

D

Dactinomycin 439
Dalteparin 704
Dandy-Walker syndrome 389
Dapsone 531
Dash eating plan 498
Death during childhood 621
Decidua 68
Decongestant nasal sprays 704
Deep tendon reflexes 384
Defibrillators 496
Deficit fluid needs 247
Degenerative scoliosis 676
Dehydration 244, 246, 247, 253, 270, 463
 causes of 245
 classification for 232*t*
 in children 246
 mild 270
 moderate 270
 pathophysiology of 245
 severe 247, 270
 signs of 253, 270, 270*f*, 508
 symptoms of 270*f*
 types of 246*t*
Delivery, type of 460
Denatonium benzoate 175
Dendrites synapses 105
Dengue 518
 fever 518
  symptoms of 518*f*
 hemorrhagic fever 518
 infection, diagnosis of 518
 shock syndrome 518
Dental care 145
Dental health 128, 165
Dental problems 260, 415
Depression 608, 623
 in children 607
Depressive disorders 608
Dermatitis 550
Detruser muscles 325
Developmental disturbances 597
Developmental-behavioral pediatrics 167
Diabetes 461, 462
 insipidus 447
 mellitus 326, 459, 461
 symptoms of 463
Diabetic ketoacidosis 463
Dialysis 348
Diamox 701
Diaper rash 103, 546, 546*f*
Diarrhea 245, 253, 268, 272, 458, 509
 nonspecific 263
Diarrheal diseases 208, 308*f*
Diascopy 351
Diazepam 525
Dietary allowance 193
Dietary guideline 126
Dietary interventions 272
Diethylstilbestrol 71
Digestive enzymes 251
Digestive system 638
Digestive tract 255
Digoxin 704
Diphenhydramine 517
Diphtheria 35, 113, 505, 505*f*, 525
 diagnosis of 505
 disease, causes of 505
 symptoms of 505
Diplopia 565
Discharge teaching 578
Disseminated intravascular coagulation 364
Diuretic 343, 427
 therapy 346
Dizziness 494
Dobutamine 702, 703
Dopamine 702, 703
Double contrast barium enema 256
Down syndrome 72, 75*f*, 612, 613*f*
 etiology 612
 management 612
Doxepin 706
Doxorubicin 440
Doxycycline 552
Drug 283
 administration of 628, 631
 antirheumatic 686
 application of 628
 calculation 634
  of volume of 629
  percentage of 630
 corticosteroid 408
 disease interaction 633
 illicit 522
 in children 627
 in pediatrics 624
  calculation of 629
 potentially hazardous 706
 reaction, adverse 633
 safety during breastfeeding 99
 service initiative, free 709
 therapy 646
 toxicity 638
 treatment 624
 withdrawal 398
Duchenne muscular dystrophy 610
Ducts, collecting 325
Ductus arteriosus 80, 81, 473, 478
Duodenal ulcer 265
Duodenum 265
Dying child 621
Dyscalculia 602*f*
 learning disability in reading 602
Dyselectrolytemias 237
Dysentery 274
 treatment of 275
 types 274
Dysfunctional swallowing 254
Dysgraphia, learning disability in writing 602
Dyslalia 600
Dyslexia, learning disability in reading 602
Dysphagia 254
Dysplasia of hip, developmental 670
Dyspnea 472, 623
Dysrhythmia 494
Dysuria 327, 337

E

Ear 90, 189, 194, 569
 disorders of 569
 function of 569
 infection 260, 570
 structure of 569, 570*f*
Eating disorder 174
Eating problems 259
Ecchymoses 518
Echinococcosis 539
Echinococcus granulosus 539
Echinococcus multilocularis 539

Echinococcus oligarthrus 539
Echinococcus vogeli 539
Echocardiography 503
Echovirus 381
Ectodermal tissue 541
Ectopia vesicae 331
Eczema 550
Edema 326, 341
  triad of 338
Education 179
  and development 713
Educational guidance 177, 178
Egotamine 706
Electroconvulsive therapy 609
Electroencephalogram 376
Electrolyte 235, 236
  balance 237, 237*t*, 248
  in children 235
Electromyography 376
Electrosurgical tonsillectomy 298
Embryonal rhabdomyosarcoma 438
Emotional development 45, 64, 138, 158
  in school child 147
Emotional disorders 172
Encephalitic poliomyelitis 512
Encephalitis 381
Encephalopathy 381
Endemic cretinism 457
Endocarditis 595
Endocrine
  diseases 444
  disorder 443, 459
    in children 444
    symptoms of 444
  glands 444, 444*f*
  system 443, 626
    disorders in 445
Endoscopic third ventriculostomy 392, 589
Endoscopy 257, 278
Endotracheal intubation 525
Endotracheal tube 662
Energy metabolism 82
Energy, amount of 27
Engraftment 418
Enourein 175
Enoxaparin 704
Entamoeba histolytica 274
Enterobacteriaceae 683
Enterobacter sakazakii 100
Enteroinvasive 269
  with cytotoxin 269
Enuresis 141, 175, 328
Environment, safe 124
Environmental diseases 457
Environmental stress 223
Enzyme phenylalanine hydroxylase 446
Ependymomas 425, 427
Epidural hematomas 404, 404*f*
Epiglottis, examination of 300
Epiglottitis 300
  cardinal
    signs of 300
    symptoms of 300
  etiology 300
Epilepsy 396, 398
  neurotransmitters in 398*f*
  seizures 401
Epinephrine 703
Epiphyseal plate 679
Epispadias 332, 575*f*, 576
  treatment of 576
Epistaxis 497, 518
Epstein-Barr virus infection 385
Eptoin 703
Ergonovine 705
Ergosterol 542
Erickson's psychosocial stages 106
Erikson's theory 56, 57
Erythema 416
Erythrocyte sedimentation rate 351, 684
Erythromycin 262, 552, 702, 704
Escherichia coli 255, 286
  infections 270
Escitalopram 706
Esophageal atresia 582, 583
Esophageal electrophysiologic study 496
Esophageal sphincter, lower 261
Estimated glomerular filtration rate 339
Estrogen therapy 614
Ethical dilemmas 8
Ethosuximide 706
Euvolemic hyponatremia 237
Ewing's sarcoma 409, 436, 437*f*
Ewing's tumors 437
Exstrophy bladder 331, 332*f*, 576
  treatment of 332
Extended families 16
Extracellular fluid 235, 235*f*, 245
Extracorporeal membrane oxygenation therapy 644
Extremities 190
Eye 90, 128*f*, 189, 194, 562
  crossed 565
  disorders of 562
  enucleation of 442
  function of 562
  hyperopia 565
  movement, rapid 39
  structure of 562, 563*f*

F

Face 189
Facial nerve 192
Family 53, 147
  and child health nurse 12
  coping with stress 23
  disorder, counseling of 484
  planning 200, 205
  roles, altered 223
  rules 40
  types of 16
Family-centered care 4, 5*f*, 12
Fasting blood glucose level 463
Fat 94, 152
  cells 542
Fatigue 416, 488, 497
  mild 294
Faulty parental attitude 171
Feeding 91, 113, 303, 640
  formula 28, 29, 99
  of child 647
  problems 31
  technique 31
Female genitalia 191
Fertilization 67, 68*f*
Fetal
  alcohol syndrome 71
  circulation 469, 469*f*
  development 67
  growth and development 70
  heart tone 70
  maturity 75*f*
  membranes 69, 69*f*
  period of development 70*f*
  presentation, abnormal 648
Fetus inside womb 69*f*
Fever 246, 327
  control 303
Fexofenadine 704
Fiber 152
  supplements 264
Fiber-optic laryngoscopy 292
Fibrotic liver 279
Filariasis 536
Fine motor skills 121, 136
Fine-needle aspiration biopsy 431
Fingers and toes, clubbing of 472
Finger-to-nose test 192
Fissure 255
Flaccid paralysis, acute 383, 384*t*
Flaccidity 384
Flank pain 327, 337
Fluconazole 704, 705
Fluid 237, 247
  administration of 631, 632
  and electrolyte therapy 247
  balance 82

electrolyte balance 383
imbalance 244
maintenance requirements 248*t*
therapy 407
volume deficit 309
Fluorometric 446
Fluoxetine 706
Focal segmental glomerulosclerosis 340
Focal seizures, simple 399
Foley's catheter 587
Folic acid 76, 199, 255, 358, 370
Follicle-stimulating hormone 448, 451
Follicular glands 552
Fontan procedure 591
Food
groups 28*f*
hygiene 31
preparation 31
Foramen ovale 80, 81
Forebrain 374*f*
Foreign body
aspiration 309
in eye 569
Foremilk 96
Foreskin, inflammation of 333
Formal operations 60
Foscavir 383
Fracture 678
compound 403, 678
depressed 403
linear 403
open 678
types of 679*f*
Frusemide 702
Fungal meningitis 380
Fusobacterium 322

G

Gadolinium 705
Galeazzi's test 672
Gallbladder 250
Gallium
citrate 413
scan 413
Gastric inhibitory peptide 252
Gastric regurgitation 261*f*
Gastric ulcer 265
Gastrin 252
Gastroenteritis 273, 275, 286
Gastroesophageal reflux 260
disease 254, 261, 295
Gastrointestinal bleeding 254
Gastrointestinal disorder 250
signs of 252
symptom of 252, 253*f*
Gastrointestinal system 83, 106, 250, 250*f*, 251, 626, 656
Gastrointestinal tests, lower 256
Gastrointestinal tract 245
Gastrointestinal ulcers, acute 558
Gemcitabine 337
Gene
mono 72
single 72
Genetic
blood tests 453
counseling 76
disorder 75*f*, 283, 612
prevention of 76
information 68
inheritance 72, 360*f*
studies 438
test 77, 312, 377, 446
trait of thalassemia 356*f*
Genital stage 55
Genital touching 162
Genitalia 191, 637
Genitourinary disorders 324, 326
Genitourinary system 326
disorders of 336
Genotropin 454
Gentamicin 702
German measles 113
Gestational age 89, 635, 691
large for 640
small for 79, 636
Giardia lamblia 269
Gland 443
Glans penis, infection of 333
Glasgow coma scale 405, 405*t*
Glaucoma 566
secondary 566
Glial cell tumors 425
Gliomas 425
low-grade 425
Glomerular filtration rate 83, 328, 345
Glomerulonephritis 338, 345
acute 337
causes, acute 337
postinfectious 337
primary 338
secondary 338
types, acute 338
Glomerulus 325
Glossopharyngeal nerve 193
Glucagon 651
Glucocorticoids 452
Gluten free diet 278
Glycosylated hemoglobin test 464
Goat's milk 276
Gonadotropin-releasing hormone 451, 452
Gonads, disorder of 445
Graft disease
acute 418
chronic 418
Gram-negative
aerobic 583
anaerobic organisms 583
bacteria 682
Grand mal seizure 400
Grasp reflex 92
Graves' disease 458, 458*f*, 459
Great arteries 472
Greenstick 678
Gross motor
skills 136
development of 121
warning signs 610
Growth and development 43, 46, 52, 116, 135
concepts of 43
stages of 46
Growth chart 49, 637*f*
of toddler 120*f*
Growth hormone 448
deficiency 453
dysfunction 453
disorders 455*t*
therapy 614
Growth monitoring 36, 49
and growth chart 48
and nutrition
education 49
surveillance 49
and nutritional status 48
chart 49*f*
Growth of intelligence 124
Growth retardation 327
Guillain-Barré syndrome 384, 385, 388
Guthrie test 446

H

Habit disorders 599
Hemophilia
mild 361
moderate 361
severe 361
symptoms of 361
Haemophilus influenzae 113, 295, 297, 300, 305, 322, 379, 380, 567
vaccine 359
Hair 194
cells 570
Hand strength 191
Handicapped child care 208
Handicapped conditions 171
Head 194
and neck 188
injury 402

internal 403
severity of 405
trauma 404*f*
Headache 497
Health
care 217*f*
check-up 153, 206
education 210, 248, 268, 594, 684
of preschool child 144
of school child 151
problems during school-age 154
promotion 4, 26, 26*f*, 112, 163, 568
status 53
supervision 146
Health-promoting initiatives 41
Healthy
cognitive development 158
environment 23
nutrition 145*f*
Hearing 86
aids 573
loss 260, 415, 571
types of 571*f*, 573
Heart 189, 468*f*
and circulation 468
changes in 81
disease
acquired 489
congenital 470, 589
failure 352, 480
digoxin in 487*t*
signs of 477
symptoms of 477
function 481
monitor 594
murmur 472, 475, 494
muscle
damage to 493
function 469
problems 415
rate 91, 185
sounds 190, 477
transplantation 501
valve disease 480
Heart-lung bypass machine 593, 596
Helicobacter pylori 265, 362
infection 266*f*
Helium-oxygen mixture 318
Helminthiasis 361, 538, 538*t*
Helminths, lifecycle of 539
Hemarthrosis 361*f*
Hematemesis 518
Hematocrit 352
Hematogenous osteomyelitis, acute 682
Hematologic alteration 349
Hematologic disorders 370
Hematologic system 349, 349*f*
Hematological malignancies 351
Hematology, classification of 351
Hematopoietic stem cells 349
Hematuria 326, 338
Hemodialysis 348*f*
Hemodynamics, altered 472, 473, 475, 476, 482
Hemoglobin 656
Hemoglobinopathy 351
Hemolytic anemia, chronic 354
Hemolytic disease 365
cause of 365
of newborn 365, 647
Hemolytic uremic syndrome 274, 345
Hemophilia 360, 360*f*, 361, 361*f*, 362
A 360
B 360
Hemophilus inflenzae type B 525
Hemopoietic system 350*f*, 420*f*
Henoch-Schonlein purpura 342
Heparin 704
Hepatic disorders 279
Hepatic system 638
Hepatitis 280
A 281, 282
virus 281
B 113, 281, 282, 362
surface antigen 342
C 281, 282
virus infection 283
causes of 283
acute 281
D 282
E 282
prognosis for 283
symptoms of 281
treatment for 283
Hepatopulmonary syndrome 280
Hepatorenal syndrome 280
Hepatosplenomegaly 279, 366
Herpes simplex
encephalitis 381
virus infection 547
High-calorie formula 594
High-risk infants, classification of 635
Hindbrain 374*f*
Hindmilk 96
Hip 673*f*
dysplasia of 672*f*
congenital 670
joint, normal 671
Hirschsprung's disease 586, 586*f*
treatment of 586
Histamine H_2 blockers 705
Hodgkin's disease 434
Hodgkin's lymphoma 428, 430, 430*f*
Holistic nursing care 179
Holter monitor 470, 496
Homovanillic acid 432
Hookworm 538
Hormonal change 543
Hormone 251, 443
secretion of 445*f*, 448*t*
Horse shoe kidney 329, 330*f*
Hospice care 623
Hospital care 303
Hospital Management Society 708
Hospital stressors 219, 220
Hospitalized child 217, 617
care of 220
Host disease 418
chronic 418
Household safety, lack of 553*f*
Human chorionic gonadotropin 68
Human fertilization, dynamics of 67
Human immunodeficiency virus 362, 521
infected mothers 200
infection 521
etiology 521
Human lymphocyte antigens 417
Humatrope 454
Hyaline cartilage 669
articulates 671
Hybrid procedure 476, 593
Hydatid disease 539
Hydrocephalus 388, 390*f*, 587
causes 388
symptoms of 389
types 389
Hydrochloric acid 267
Hydrochlorothiazide 705
Hydrogen breath test 258
Hydrophobia 519
Hydrops fetalis 366
Hydroxychloroquine 686
Hydroxyzine 517
Hyperactive bowel sounds 254
Hyperbilirubinemia 367, 647
unconjugated 647*f*
Hypercalcemia 242
causes of 242
management 242
signs of 242
symptoms of 242
Hypercapnia 243
Hypercarbia 288
Hyperemia, zone of 554
Hyperglycemia 464*t*, 466
Hyperinsulinism 649
congenital 649
Hyperkalemia 240, 240*f*, 241, 346
management 241
treatment of 241

Hyperkinetic disorders 172
Hyperlipidemia 340, 341
Hypernatremia 238, 239*f*, 245
  diagnosis 238
  management 239
Hypernatremic dehydration 271
Hyperopia 564
Hyperosmolar dehydration 271
Hyperparasitemia 533
Hyperparathyroidism 326
Hyperpyrexia 533
Hypersensitivity 263
Hypertension 326, 327, 497
  causes of secondary 498
  portal 280
  secondary 498
Hyperthyroidism 458
Hypertonia 610
Hypertrophic cardiomyopathy 500
Hypertrophic pyloric stenosis, congenital 581*f*
Hypervolemic hyponatremia 237
Hypnotherapy 265
Hypoalbuminemia 338, 340, 341
Hypocalcemia 241, 367, 651
  causes of 242
  management 242
  symptoms of 651
Hypoglossal nerve 193
Hypoglycemia 367, 463, 464*t*, 466, 533, 636, 641
  causes, severe 650
  in neonate 650
  neonatal 649
  refractory 651
  symptoms of 463
Hypokalemia 239, 240*f*
  causes of 239
  management 240
Hyponatremia 237, 346
  acute severe 238
  etiology 237
  hypovolemic 237
  management 238
  signs of 238, 238*f*
  symptoms 238
Hypoosmolar dehydration 271
Hypopituitarism 454
  acquired 454, 457
  congenital 454, 456
Hypoplasia 329
Hypospadias 332, 333, 575, 575*f*
  classification of 332
  signs of 333
  symptoms of 333
Hypotension 502
Hypothalamic hamartoma 450
Hypothalamus 374, 443
Hypothermia 407, 559, 639
Hypotonia 610
Hypovolemia 352, 625
Hypoxemia 280, 288, 307
Hypoxia 352, 484

I

Ibuprofen 702, 704
Icterus neonatorum 647
Idiopathic disease 676
Idiopathic respiratory distress syndrome 643
Idiopathic scoliosis 676
Idiopathic thrombocytopenic purpura 363*f*
Immature eccrine glands 543
Immune
  disorders 337
  system 84, 106, 418, 638
    problems 321
  thrombocytopenic purpura 362
Immunity 526
Immunization 34, 35, 113, 198, 205
  active 520
  coverage 34
  of children 34*f*
  passive 520
Immunocompromise 274
Immunological superiority 95
Immunosuppressive therapy 344, 353
Immunotherapy 418
  active 419
  passive 419
Impetigo 544*f*
Inappropriate antidiuretic hormone 449
Indane lotion 549
Indian Academy of Pediatrics 207
Indian Council for Child Welfare 214
Indian Red Cross Society 214
Infant 182, 183, 219, 221
  mortality rate 7, 700
  normal 103
  postmature 640
  preterm 637
  reactions of 221
Infantile colic 286
Infantile eczema 446
Infantile hypertrophic pyloric stenosis 581
Infection 418, 422
  chronic 312
  meningeal 378
  neonatal 652
  parasitic 297, 532
  prevention of 347, 595, 639
Infectious croup 298
Infectious disease 504
Infectious disorders 265
Infectious gastroenteritis 268, 269*t*
Infectious hepatitis 281
Infectious mononucleosis 385
Infective endocarditis 493
Infective polyneuritis 384
Inflammation 305*f*
  signs of 571
Influenza 113, 294
  prevention 295
Inguinal hernia 336
Inhaled steroids 317
Inhalers 704
Inherited disorder 283
Injection
  techniques of 629*f*
  types of 629*f*
Injury 402
  causes of 132
  prevention of 40, 41, 131, 466, 639
  prevention strategies 132
Insect bite 561
  symptoms of 561
Insulin 464, 704
  like growth hormone 454
  rapid-acting 465
  resistance 461
  short-acting 465
  types of 465
Integumentary system 638
Intellectual disability 603
Intensive care unit 481
  neonatal 654
International and National Welfare Organizations 211
International Council of Population Development 201
Interstitial fluid 235
Interventional cardiac catheterization 590
Interventional health services 197
Intestinal bacterial overgrowth, small 263
Intestinal obstruction 286, 583, 584*f*
  causes of 286
  intussusception, types of 584*f*
Intestinal villus atrophy 277*f*
Intestine
  part of 586*f*
  small 250
Intracellular fluid 235*f*
Intracranial hemorrhage 404
Intracranial pressure 403
Intradermal injection 629
Intramuscular injection 628
Intramuscular regimens 520

Intraocular lenses 568
Intrathecal injection 629
Intrauterine growth retardation 454, 636*f*
Intravenous catheters 594
Intravenous fluid 239
  administration of 346
Intravenous immunoglobulin 499
Intravenous injections 628
Intrinsic renal failure 345
Intubation, rapid 654
Iodide products 707
Ipratropium 318
Iron 199, 370
  deficiency anemia 351
    classification 352
    etiology 351
Irritable bowel syndrome 263, 273
Isonatremic dehydration 271

J

Jackson's burns zones 554*f*
Janani Shishu Suraksha Karyakram 708
Janani Suraksha Yojana 708
Japanese encephalitis 382
Jaundice 102, 254, 279, 281, 366, 367
  from hemolysis 367
  neonatal 368
    physiologic 368
  physiologic 83, 367, 368
  severe 368
  symptoms of 647
Joint 191
  destruction 361, 361*f*
  mobility 89
Jugular venous pressure 503
Juvenile delinquency, problems of 176
Juvenile rheumatoid arthritis 684
  diagnosis 684
  etiology 684
  management 685
  signs 684
  symptoms 684
  types 684
Juxtamedullary cortex 325

K

Kala-azar 535
  elimination plan 709
  epidemiology 535
Kangaroo care 646
Kasturba Gandhi Balika Vidyalaya 215
Kaushika sutra 3
Kawasaki disease 499, 500
Kawasaki syndrome 499*f*
Keloid like scarring 559
Keratin 541
Keratometry 565
Kernicterus 369
Kernig's sign 381
Ketoacidosis 464*t*
Kidney 236, 245, 324, 328
  causes, absence of 329
  damage, severe 336
  dialysis 339
  disease
    chronic 327, 347
    end stage 347
  dysfunction 339
  function 345
  inflammation, type of 337
  normal 330*f*
  problem 415
  structure of 324*f*, 325
  test 412
  transplant 339
Kishori Balika Scheme 209
Klebsiella pneumoniae 322
Klinefelter syndrome 72, 72*f*, 614
Knees, deformed 514*f*
Kohlberg's stages 62

L

Labetalol 705
Lactase deficiency 276
Lactose intolerance 273, 275, 276
Lagophthalmos 530
Langerhans cells 542
Language development 45, 50, 121
Language problem 609
Laryngoscopy 291*f*
Latent tuberculosis infection 528
Laxatives 264
Learning development 46
Learning disability 415, 602
  in language 602
Learning growth 46
Leg strength 191
Leishmania bodies 535
Leishmania donovani 535
Leishmania parasites 535
Leishmaniasis 535, 536
  infection 535*f*
Lepromatous leprosy, borderline 530
Leprosy 529, 530*f*
  classification of 529
  treatment 531, 531*t*
Leukemia 419, 420, 422*t*
  etiology 419
Leukocoria 441
Lice
  infected transmission of 548*f*
  infestation 547
  killing of 548
Lichenification 550
Lidocaine 704
Ligaments 669
  of hip joint 671*f*
Ligamentum
  arteriosum 80
  venosum 80
Limb defects 670
Limbic system 157*f*
Lipodystrophy 522
Live attenuated vaccine 294
Live-born 78
Liver 250, 415
  disease 279
  function 367, 438
    test 412, 438
Loratadine 704
Lorazepam 705
Low-birth-weight 78, 637
Lugol's solution 459
Lumbar puncture 377, 412
Lung 189, 236, 415
  abscess 322, 323
    complications 323
    diagnose 323
    diagnostic evaluation 323
    management 323
    prognosis 323
    types 322
  baby's 662
  collapsed 312
  function 481
    test 312
  problems 641
Luteinizing hormone 448, 451
Lymph node 188, 428*f*
  biopsy 431
Lymphadenopathy 536
Lymphatic filariasis 535*f*, 536
  diagnosis of 537
  infection 537
Lymphatic system 428*f*
Lymphocytes 429
Lymphocytic leukemia, acute 421
Lymphoma 409, 431, 432*t*
  malignant 428

M

Macrosomia 648
Macula 562
Magnesium sulfate 318, 704
Malabsorption disorders 275
Malaise 337
Malaria 532, 534
  malignant 533
Male genitalia 191
Male sex hormones 453

Malnutrition 274, 278, 508*f*
 disorders of 230*f*
Mannitol 702
Mantoux test 342
Mass drug administration 537
Mass media, influence of 171
Masturbation 162
Maternal age 76
Maternal and child health indicators 700
Maternal health 199
Maternal mortality ratio 700
Maternal varicella 517
Maturation 44
McCune-Albright syndrome 450, 451
Mean corpuscular volume 352
Measles 113, 508
 complications 509
 cycle of 508*f*
 rash 509*f*
 vaccination, routine 510
 virus 509, 567
Mebendazole 540
Meconium 84
 aspiration syndrome 84, 642
Medical dryness 244
Medical termination of pregnancy 201
Medroxyprogesterone 452
Medulloblastomas 425, 427
Megacolon, congenital 586
Melanocytes, lack of 543
Membrane, inner 69
Membranoproliferative glomerulonephritis 338, 340
Membranous glomerulonephritis 338
Mendelian disorders 72
Meninges 373
Meningitis 378
Meningocele 394*f*, 395, 395*f*, 397*t*, 589
Meningococcal disease 113
Meningococcal meningitis 379
Meningomyelocele 395*f*, 589
Menstrual periods 156
Mental
 development 59, 138, 149
 disorders 603
 health 467, 623
  problems 263, 265
 retardation 603
Mesenteric lymphadenitis 286
Metabolic acidosis 243, 243, 346, 472
 diagnosis 243
 management 243
 mild 243
Metabolic alkalosis 244
 management 244
 signs of 585
Metabolic disorder 443
Metabolic rate, reducing 347
Metabolic screening 76
Metabolism, inborn errors of 447
Metacognition 151
Metanephric blastema 439
Methimazole 705
Methyldopa 704
Methylergonovine 704
Methylxanthines 318
Metoclopramide 703, 705
Metoprolol 704
Miconazole 704
Micronutrient 273
Microtubercles 380
Microvascular perfusion 502
Micturition, abnormalities of 326
Midazolam 705
Mid-borderline leprosy 530
Midbrain 374*f*
Mid-day Meal Scheme 215
Migration 22
Milk, preterm 96
Millennium development goals 127
Milrinone 703
Mineral 94
 supplementation 278
Minimal change nephropathy 338
Minimal incision valve surgery 592
Minocycline 552
Miscarriage 71
Missile injury 403
Mite infestation 549
Mitomycin 337
Moisture retention 542
Molecular weight heparins, low 704
Moniliasis 544
Monocytes 350
Mood disorders 599
Moodiness 159
Moral development 61, 65
 theory of 61
Moraxella catarrhalis 295
Moro reflex 92
Mortality rate, neonatal 7, 700
Mosaic down syndrome 612
Mosquitoes 519
Mother and child health 199
Mother and Child Health Programs 202
Mother cells 541
Motilin 252
Motility disorders 260
Motor ability 47, 48
Motor coordination disorder 611
Motor development 106, 136
 causes 610
 impairment in 610
Motor dyspraxia 611
Motor reflexes 696
Motor skills 119
 disorder 611
Motor vehicle accidents 134
Mouth 189, 195
Mucous membranes, dry 449
Mucus sucker after delivery 87*f*
Multicystic dysplastic kidney 330
Multicystic kidney 330
Multifactorial disorders 72, 75
Multigenerational families 17, 17*f*
Mumps 113, 515
Muscle 191
 relaxation 407
 tone 89, 384
Muscular dystrophy 610
Musculoskeletal alteration 669
Musculoskeletal impairment 674
Musculoskeletal system 195, 669, 670*f*
 disorders of 670
Mycelex 543
Mycobacterium leprae 529
Mycobacterium tuberculosis 35, 526
Mycoplasma 297
Myelin sheath 373
Myelination of nerve fibers 656
Myelogenous leukemia, diagnosis of acute 421
Myelomeningocele 394*f*, 395, 397*t*
Myoclonic seizure 400
Myopia 564

N

Nail biting 175
 severe 175
Naproxen 705
Nasal
 cannula 303, 662
 cavity 288
 polyps 312
 prongs 662
Nasogastric tube 594
National Ambulance Services 709
National Health Mission 708, 710
National Immunization Schedule 35, 36*t*
National Institute for Play 38
National Mobile Medical Units 708
National Neonatology Forum 229
National Nutrition Policy 33
National Policy for Children, 2013 711
National Rural Health Mission 215
National Society of Genetic Counselors 76
Nausea 252, 389, 599
Necator americanus 538

Neck 194
 stiffness 380
Neisseria gonorrhoeae 297, 567
Neisseria meningitidis 379
Neonatal and childhood illness, management of 203, 206, 207, 228
Neonatal jaundice, causes of 647
Neonatal period, early 398
Neonatal reflexes 92
Neonatal resuscitation 79, 642
Neonatal seizures 649
Neonatal sepsis 652
Neonate's ductus arteriosus 478
Neonates
 preterm 637
 reactions of 221
Neoplasia 409
Neoplasms, benign 409
Nephritis, chronic 326
Nephrogenic diabetes insipidus 447
Nephrogenic rests 439
Nephron 325
 structure of 325*f*
Nephrotic syndrome 340, 341*f*
 cause of 341
Nephrotoxic substances 345
Nerve 670
 abducent 192
 accessory 193
 conduction velocity test 376
 enlarged 531
 oculomotor 192
 pairs of 375
 trigeminal 192
 trochlear 192
Nervous habits 175
Neural system 373*f*
Neural tube
 defects 75*f*, 388, 589
 development, disorder of 394
Neuroblastoma 409, 431
 cause of 431
Neurofibromatosis 425
Neurogenic shock 502
Neurologic alterations 372
Neurologic system 85, 196, 624
Neurological assessment 192
Neurological diagnostic tests 376
Neurological problem 376, 398
Neurological tests 401
Neuromuscular scoliosis 676
Neuron, structure of 373*f*
Neurosurgical management 406
Neurotransmitters 398
Neutralizing unbound toxin 525
Newborn
 assessment 90*f*
 baby at birth 91
 care 708
  high-risk 635
  of high-risk 635
 high-risk 635
 identification 101
 respirations 87
 resuscitation 689
  steps of 688
 skin 85
  characteristics of 85
 thermal regulation of 92
 with jaundice 83*f*
Nicotine 706
Nifedipine 704
Night blindness 285
Nitrofurantoin 706
Nitroprusside 703
Nonalcohol-based lotion 343
Nonbullous impetigo 543
Noncompaction cardiomyopathy 500
Non-Hodgkin's lymphoma 429
Noninfectious meningitis 380
Nonnutritive sucking 640
Nonparalytic poliomyelitis 511
Nonsteroid medications 551
Nonsteroidal anti-inflammatory drugs 685
Nontraditional families 17
Norepinephrine 703
Normocytic anemia 328, 352
 severe 533
Nose 189, 194, 303
Nuclear families 16
Nuclear medicine scans 413
Numerical disorder 74
Nurse
 advocacy role of 25*f*
 in nutritional counselling, role of 33
 perspective 181
 render care, neonatal 655*f*
 role in preventive pediatrics 214
 role of 37
 to child health 115
Nursing action 488
Nursing care of child 223
 with refractive errors 565
 with shunt 392
Nursing diagnosis 225
Nursing ethics 8
Nursing management 264
Nutrient 152
Nutrition 26, 34*f*, 53, 53*f*, 113, 125, 144, 165, 165*f*, 224, 264, 580, 623, 640
 altered 488
 counseling for 33
 parenteral 651
 therapy 558
Nutritional assessment 193
Nutritional guidance 178
Nutritional management 657
Nutritional policy 33
Nutritional Programs 210
Nutritional services 210
Nutritional status 33, 193
 of hospitalized child, effects on 221
Nutritional supplementation 199
 safe 387
Nutritional support 285
Nutritional surveillance 198

O

Obsessive compulsive disorder 606
 treatment of 607
Obstructive apnea 645
Obstructive disorders 275
Obstructive heart diseases 479
Olfactory nerve 192
Oliguria 327
Omalizumab 318
Omeprazole 706
Oncogenes 410
Oncovin 421
Ongoing Child Welfare Programs 214
Onychophagia 175
Ophthalmia neonatorum 567
Optic chiasm 562
Optic nerve 192
 damage 566
 gliomas 425
 hypoplasia 454
Optimum dental health 145*f*
Oral
 antibiotics 307
 candidiasis 102, 545, 545*f*
 decongestants 705
 glucose tolerance test 464
 rehydration 198
  therapy 203, 247, 271
 route 628
 stage 54
 trimethoprim 337
Organ
 function tests 312
 toxicity 418
Oropharyngeal dysphagia 254
Orthodontic treatment 140
Orthotic treatment 513
Ortolani's test 672
Osteogenic sarcoma 434
 cancer cells 434

Osteomyelitis 682
causes 682
diagnosis of 682
neonatal 683
pathophysiology 682
signs 682
symptoms 682
treatment 682
Osteosarcoma 434
cause of 434
Osteotomy 674
Ostium primum 477
Ostium secundum 477
Otitis media 296, 570
acute 570
Otoacoustic emissions 573
Outpatient treatment 232
Ovum 67*f*
Oxazepam 706
Oxygen 289, 662
in arterial blood, partial pressure of 245
saturation 185
supplemental 626
therapy 485, 583
treatment of 508
Oxygenated blood 80, 375
Oxygenation, signs of poor 354
Oxyuriasis 538
vermicularis 539

P

Pacchioni's granulations 389
Pacemaker, artificial 497
Pain
abdominal 253, 268, 273, 328
acute 391
fear of 622
management 622
severe 354
Palatoplasty, two flap 580*f*
Palliative care, end-of-life 623
Pallid breath-holding spells 599
Palmar erythema 280
Pancreas 250, 444
disorder of 444
Paralysis
ascending 385
progression of 384
Paralytic polio myelitis 512
Paramyxovirus 515
Parasites 255
Parathyroid gland 444
Parent unit, care by 218
Parent-child relationship 168
Parenteral corticosteroid therapy 299
Paroxetine 706
Paroxysmal atrial tachycardia 495
Paroxysms 507
Pasteurella multocida 322
Patent ductus arteriosus 478, 478*f*
Pauciarticular disease 684
Paucibacillary 529
Pediatric
care, integral part of 2*f*
difference 326, 543
hospitalization 217
intensive care 658
intensive care unit 5, 658
life, stages of 66, 67*f*
medicines and doses 701
nurse 8*f*, 178
advanced preparation of 10, 10*f*
in genetic testing, role of 78
independent 11
practitioners 10
researcher 10
specialist 10
nursing 3, 4, 167
care 5
pain management 632
patient 180, 184, 653
population, vaccination in 294
postnatal preventive 198
shock, types of 503*t*
surgery 575
surgical problems, management of 575
vital signs 625*t*, 693
Pediculosis 547
capitis 547*f*
Peer group, attributes of 160
Pelvic ultrasound 451
Penicillin 704
V 703
Pentavalent vaccines 35
Peptic ulcer
disease 265, 266
etiology of 265
Peptostreptococcus 322
Percutaneous balloon valvuloplasty 482
Percutaneous needle biopsy 412
Percutaneous pinning 680
Perinatal mortality rate 6
Periosteum 669
Peripheral nervous system 372
Peripheral pulses 488
Peritoneal dialysis 348*f*
Permethrin cream 549
Persistent neonatal hypoglycemia 650
Persistent truncus arteriosus 475
Pertussis 113, 506, 507*f*, 525
diagnosis of 507
pH in digestion 252
Pharyngeal tonsils 296
Pharyngitis 296
acute 297
signs of 297
symptoms of 297
Pharyngotonsillitis 297
Phenobarbitone 703
Phenylalanine 447
Phenylketonuria 445
Phenytoin 383, 407
sodium 703
Phimosis 333, 334*f*
diagnosis of 334
physiologic 333, 334
treatments for 334
Phobia 607
management 607
Phobic anxiety 607
Photophobia
signs 566
symptoms 566
Physical care 144, 152
Physical development 44, 119, 123, 136
Physical examination 164
of newborn 91
Physical growth 119
Physical maturity 89, 692
Piaget's theory 59, 64, 106
Pica
complications of 174
treatment for 174
Pineal gland 444
Piroxicam 707
Pituitary deficiencies 454
Pituitary gland 374, 443
anterior 448*t*
disorder of 445, 447
release hormones 450
Pituitary tumors 455
Placenta acts 69
Placental development 69
Plantar creases 90
Plasma exchange 339
Plasmapheresis 387
Plasmodium 532
Plasmodium falciparum 532, 533
Plasmodium ovale 532
Plasmodium species 534
Plasmodium vivax 532
infection 533
Platelet 351
count 351
Playtime 623
Pleomorphic type 438
Pleural effusion 313, 313*f*
sign of 280
Pleural fluid, analysis of 314

Pneumococcal disease 113
Pneumococcal meningitis 379
Pneumocystis jiroveci 305, 522
Pneumocytes 643
Pneumonia 208, 305, 306*f*, 681
  management of 308*f*
Pneumothorax 312
Poisoning 133
Polio 35, 113
  vaccine 514*f*
Poliomyelitis 384, 510, 514*f*
  types of 511
Poliovirus 511
  isolation 513
  vaccine 514
Polycystic kidney 330, 330*f*
  disease 330, 347
Polycythemia 640
Polysomnogram 377
Ponderal index 636
Portacaval anastomosis 284
Postnatal respiratory changes 288
Postneonatal mortality rate 7
Postpartum family planning 201
Postpolio syndrome 515
Postrenal failure 345
Poststreptococcal glomerulonephritis 339
  acute 338
Post-term baby 79
Post-traumatic amnesia 405
Post-traumatic stress disorder 605
  etiology 605
Potassium 241
  supplementation 498
Prader-Willi syndrome 72, 73*f*
Pramoxine lotion 549
Precipitate cardiac arrhythmia 346
Precocious puberty 450
  in boys, signs of 451
Prednisolone 343
Premature atrial contractions 495
Premature infant 636
Premature supraventricular contractions 495
Premature ventricular contractions 495
Prenatal development, disorders of 259
Prenatal pediatrics 67
  focuses 67
Prenatal respiratory development 288
Prenursery education 206
Preputial hygiene 334
Prerenal failure 344, 345
Preschool child 135, 141*f*, 183
  development of 138*f*
  play of 138
  problems of 140
  reactions of 222
Preschoolers 183, 221
Pre-schoolers, diet of 144*f*
Preventive pediatrics 197, 198
Primary health care 49
  comprehensive 709
Probiotics 265
Progesterone therapy 614
Prokinetics 262
Prolactin 448
Propofol 706
Propranolol 704
Prostaglandin 80, 473
Protect child health 204*f*
Protein 94, 152
  substitute 447
Proteinuria 341
  compensate 343
Proteus mirabilis 322
Prothrombin time 351
Proximodistal growth 50*f*
Pruritus 279
Pseudomonas aeruginosa 322, 682
Pseudomonas infection 381
Psoriasis 684
Psoriatic arthritis disease 684
Psychoanalytic theory 54, 64
Psychological stress 223
Psychosocial development 56, 64
Psychosocial problem 260
Pubertal hormones, production of 452
Pubic bones, widening of 331
Pulmonary artery banding 474, 590
Pulmonary atresia 474, 480, 592
Pulmonary blood
  flow 475
  vessels, narrowed 590
Pulmonary function 347
  test 291, 291*f*, 312, 412
Pulmonary homograft 475, 592
Pulmonary stenosis 480, 481
Pulse oximeter 291, 470, 473, 662
Pure tone audiometry 572
Pyelonephritis 336, 345
Pyloric stenosis 581, 581*f*

Q

Quinidine 706
Quinine 337
Quinolone antibacterials 706

R

Rabies 519
  pathogenesis 519
Radioactive iodine 459
Radiology tests 377
Ramstedt's procedure 581
Random blood sugar 463
Rapid strep tests 297
Rational drug therapy 627
Reactive airway diseases 315
Rectus femoris 629
Red cell indices 358
Reed-Sternberg cell 430
Refraction test 565
Refractive errors 564, 564*f*
Regular physical activity 129*f*
Regurgitation 252, 480
Rehydrating sick child 631
Rehydration therapy 271, 275
Remission induction therapy 342
Renal agenesis 329
Renal bed 656
Renal colic 327
Renal disease 328
  end stage 347
Renal dysplasia 330
Renal ectopia 329
Renal failure 347
  acute 344
  chronic 344, 347
  symptoms of acute 345
Renal function 438
  test 412, 438
Renal parenchyma 336
Renal system 106, 324, 626, 638
Reproductive and Child Health Program 201, 203
Reproductive health 200
Reproductive tract infection 201
Residual paralysis, treatment of 514
Respiration
  external 289
  internal 289
  maintenance of 639
Respiratory acidosis 243
  management 243
Respiratory alkalosis 244
Respiratory alveoli 306*f*
Respiratory conditions 641, 654
Respiratory difficulties 384
Respiratory disorders 288
Respiratory distress syndrome 563, 643, 644
Respiratory function 529
Respiratory infections, acute 292
Respiratory noises 290
Respiratory rate 91, 185
Respiratory symptoms 289
Respiratory syncytial virus 316
Respiratory system 79, 105, 288, 289*f*, 626, 637
  of child 288*f*
Respiratory therapy 386
Respiratory tract 245
  disorders, lower 298

Responsible parenthood 14
Restlessness 488, 623
Restrictive cardiomyopathy 500
Resulting circulatory changes 81
Retinoblastoma 425, 441
Retinopathy of prematurity 563, 564
Retractile testes 576
Retrolental fibroplasia 563
Reye syndrome 517
Rhabdomyosarcoma 409, 437
  tumors 438
Rheumatic fever 485, 489, 490, 491*t*, 534
Rheumatic heart disease 485, 492
  treatment 492
Rheumatoid factor 685
Ridley-Jopling system 529
Rifampicin 531
Rights of children 208, 665, 687
Ringer's lactate 407
Ringworm 546
Rogi Kalyan Samiti 708
Romberg test 193
Root reflex 92
Rotavirus 113, 269
Roundworm 538
Rubella 71, 113, 563

S

Salicylates 706
Salicylic acid 552
Salivary glands 250
Salk vaccine 514
Salmonella 255, 286
Salter's osteotomy 674
Salter-Harris fracture classification 679, 679*f*
Sarva Shiksha Abhiyan 215
Scabies 549
  signs of 549
  symptoms of 549
Scalds 134
School child 147
  and family 148*f*
School environment, healthful 210
School health 198, 209
School Health Committee 210
School health nurse, role of 211
School Health Program 203, 210, 210*f*, 211*f*
School nurse 211*f*
School-age child 183, 184, 618
  reactions of 222
Scoliosis 675, 676
  causes of 676
  congenital 676
  severe 676
  signs of 676
  treatment 677
  types of 676
Seeking medical help 595
Segmental glomerulosclerosis 338
Seizure 623
  absence 400
  classification 399
  control 407
  disorder 396
  management of 381
Sensation 542
Sense of
  autonomy 116
  identity 159
    developing 159
Sensorineural hearing loss 572
Sensory
  alteration 562
  capacities 47
  development 86, 107, 121
    hearing/speech 121
    sight 121
    tactile 121
  integration 121
  sign 384
  stimulation 111, 645
  symptoms 384
Separation anxiety 617
Sertraline 706
Serum
  albumin 341, 368
  cholesterol 341
  tumor marker test 426
Sex characteristics, secondary 156
Sex determination 68
Sexual behaviors 162
Sexual development, delayed 415
Sexual identity 161
Sexual maturation, sign of secondary 450
Sexual orientation 162
Sexual transmission 522
Sexuality in school-age child, development of 151
Sexually transmitted infection 201
Shelter homes 666
Shigella 255, 269, 286
Shingles 516
Shock 352, 501
  cardiogenic 501, 503
  classification of 502
  compensated 502
  early signs of 503
  hypovolemic 502
  irreversible 502
  management of 557, 654
  signs of 503, 503*t*
  treatment of 703
  types of 501, 503
  uncompensated 502
Shunt 391, 392*f*, 588, 588*f*
  insertion 390, 391, 392*f*, 588, 588*f*
  parts of 392*f*, 589*f*
  steps of insertion of 588
Siblings reactions 222
Sickle cell anemia 354
  diagnosis 354
  etiology 354
  management 354
Sickle cell crisis 354
Sickness 21
Sinus 288
  arrhythmia 494, 495
  cultures from 296
  tachycardia 495
  venosus 477
  X-rays 296
Sinusitis 295
  acute 296
  chronic 296
  etiology 295
Six killer diseases 205
Skeletal muscles 670
Skin 85, 90, 186, 188, 194, 245, 518, 531
  care 113, 285 347, 640
  conditions 541, 561
    examination of 187*t*
  cross-section of 541*f*
  dry 103
  function of 541, 542
  immune system 551
  infection of 543, 546
  patches 531
  rashes 446
  smear test 531
  structure of 541
  test 528
  turgor, diminished 449
Skin-to-skin holding 646
Skull fractures 403
Sleep 38, 91
  and activity 127
  routine 623
  tests 377
  tips for toddlers 127
Smallpox 517*f*
Social and emotional development 37
Social change, influence of 171
Social cognitive albert bandura 163
Social development 63, 122, 138, 150, 158
  theory 63, 65
Social interaction, role of 65
Social reintegration 666
Social worker 226
Sodium 346, 487, 489
  concentrations 346
  nitroprusside 346

Solid food, consumption of 272
Sore throat 294, 296
Sotalol 707
Sounds 47
Spasmodic croup 299
Speech
 disorders 599
 problem 260, 600, 609
Sperm 67*f*
 to ovum, travel of 67*f*
Spermatozoon 67
Spina bifida 394, 589
 cystica 394*f*
 malformations 394
 meningocele 395
 occulta 394*f*, 395, 395*f*
 types of 394*f*
Spinal cord 375, 407
 injury 407, 408
Spinal curvature 677, 677*f*
Spinal fusion 678
Spinal type 512
Spine 190
Spironolactone 706
Spleen 428*f*
 nonpalpable 363
Splenectomy 359
Spondyloarthropathy 684
Sputum culture 312
Staphylococcal meningitis 379
Staphylococcus aureus 305, 322, 544, 682
 bacteremia 494
 infections 683
Steady growth stage 48
Stem cell transplant 417, 422
Stenosis 480
Steroid 383
 cream 550
 treatment by 342
Stillborn 79
Stomach 268
 flu 268
 ulcer 266*f*
Stool investigations 270
Strabismus 441, 565, 566
 congenital 565
Streptococcus agalactiae 300
Streptococcus pneumoniae 295, 300, 305, 322
Streptococcus pyogenes 322, 544
Stress
 of hospitalization 221
 physiological 223
 signs of 598
Stressors of family affect child care 21
Stridor 299
Subconjunctival hemorrhages 507
Subcutaneous route 629
Subdural hematomas 404, 404*f*
Subtotal thyroidectomy 459
Suck reflex 92
Sucking pleasure 111
Sudden vision changes 463
Sulfamethoxazole 337
Sulfisoxazole 369
Sulfur ointment 549
Sumatriptan 706
Supplemental tube feedings 594
Supplementary nutrition 206
Suppress immune system 339
Supraventricular tachycardia 494, 495
Sushruta samhita 3
Sweat glands 542
Sweat test 312
Swollen glands 420
Synaptic pruning 105
Syphilis 563
Systemic chemotherapy 442
Systemic diseases 341
Systemic lupus erythematosus 342, 686
Systemic steroids 317
Systemic vascular resistance 502
Systemic venous resistance 503

T

Tachycardia 449, 486, 488
Tachyphemia 600
Tachyphrasia 600
Tachypnea 486
Tactile stimulation 288
Talipes equinovarus, congenital 670, 670*f*
Talk therapy 265
Tantrum 131, 173
Tape-worm 538
Target cells 445*f*
Teeth 105, 250
 baby 105*f*
 clean child's 145
 eruption of child 695
 first 105*f*
 grinding 599
Temper tantrums 173
 causes 173
 management 173
 severe 174
 types 173
Temporary palliative surgery 590
 types of 590
Tendons 669
Teniasis 538
Teratogens 71
Terminally-ill child, care of 622
Testes, undescended 576
Testosterone 453
Tetanus 113, 523, 525, 526
 toxoid 199
Tetracycline 552, 706
Tetralogy of Fallot 471, 589, 590
Thalamus 374
Thalassemia 356, 358*f*
 alpha 356
 beta 356
 etiology 356
 major 356
 management of beta- 359
 minor 356
 splenomegaly in 359*f*
 type of 358
Thalidomide 71
Theophylline 704
Therapeutic management 247, 264, 267, 284, 299, 339, 342, 457, 472, 670, 673
Thermoneutral range 646
Thermoregulation 82, 639
Thermotherapy 442
Thoracotomy 593
Threadworm 538
Throat 189
 culture 300
 infection 490
Thrombocytopenia 363
Thumb sucking 140, 140*f*, 219, 598, 600
Thymus 444
Thyroglobulin proteins 458
Thyroid
 dysgenesis 456
 gland 443, 456*f*
  disorder of 445, 455
 hormone deficiency 457
 peroxidase 458
 problems 415
 scan 459
 stimulating
  hormone 448
  immunoglobulins 458
Thyroxine 455
Tick-borne encephalitis 382
Tilt table test 496
Tinea 546
 corporis 547
 cruris 547
 infection 546
  management of 547*t*
 pedis 547
 unguium 547
Tinea-infection, types of 547*t*
Tinzaparin 704
Tobacco smoke, prevention from 498
Toddlers
 accidents in 132
 reactions of 221

Toilet training 125, 126*f*
difficulties 176
process of 142
Tolerable upper intake level 193
Tongue 250
Tonic neck reflex 92
Tonic-clonic seizures 399
Tonsillectomy 298
Tonsillitis 296
Total body weight 235
Tourette's disorder 599
Tourette's syndrome 599
Toxin 283
production, elimination of 525
removal of 542
Toxoplasmosis 563
Tracheoesophageal fistula 582, 583
types of 582*f*
Tracheolaryngobronchitis 299*f*
acute 298
Transcatheter aortic valve replacement 592
Transcatheter device closure 479
Transcutaneous monitoring 292
Transient hypoglycemia 650
Trauma 460
abdominal 286
Trazodone 706
Trendelenburg position 87
Tretinoin 704
Trichotillomania 599
Trichuris trichiura 538
Tricuspid atresia 473, 474, 590
symptoms 474
Trihydroxymethyl aminomethadone 244
Triiodothyronine 455
Tripod sign 512, 512*f*
Trismus 524
Trousseau's sign 242
Tuberculoid leprosy 529
borderline 529
Tuberculosis 526
disease 528
signs of 527
symptoms of 527
infection 526
Tuberculous meningitis 380
Tubular hypoplasia 482
Tubular necrosis, acute 345
Tubule 325
Tumor lysis syndrome, management of 419
Tumor necrosis factor 685
Turner syndrome 72, 483, 613, 613*f*
Tympanogram 572

U

Ulcer 530*f*
pressure 559
Ultrasound, abdominal 451
Umbilical arteries 69, 81
Umbilical cord 91, 102
Umbilical venous catheter 663
Under five clinic 203, 204
United Nations International Children's Emergency Fund 212
Universal Immunization Program 34, 35, 203
Unstable hip dysplasia 671
Upper respiratory
infections 103
tract, disorders of 292
Upper urinary tract 328
Ureter 324
duplication of 331, 331*f*
Urethra 324
anterior 333
Urethral defects 575*f*
Urethral valve
posterior 335
types of 335
Urinalysis 438
Urinary bladder 324
Urinary catheter 594
Urinary elimination 639
Urinary tract 328, 336
infection 328, 336
etiology 336
incidence 336
lower 331
Urine 255
catecholamines levels 432
examination 328
for protein 343
output, decrease 488
test 345, 453, 486
Uterine
fibroids 409
tube, ampulla of 67
wall 68

V

Vaccine prevented diseases 34, 35, 113
Vaginal delivery, operative 648
Vagus nerve 193, 402
stimulation 402
Valve
ablation 335
artificial 493
disease
acquired 479
congenital 479
regurgitation 492
stenosis 492
Valvoplasty 493
Valvotomy 475, 592
Valvular heart disease 480
Vancomycin 703, 705
Varicella 113, 516
Varicella-Zoster virus 516
Vasculitis 337
Vasopressin 703
Ventilation 643
care of child with 657
Ventilator 304, 594, 663
Ventricular fibrillation 495
Ventricular septal defect 473, 475, 475*f*, 476, 589, 593
Ventricular tachycardia 495
Verapamil 705, 706
Vesicostomy 335
Vesicoureteral reflux 331, 336
Vestibulocochlear nerve 192
Vestibulo-cochlear nerve 569
Village Health Sanitation and Nutrition Committee 708
Vincristine 421, 439, 440
Viral
conjunctivitis 567
croup 299
hepatitis 281, 282*t*
pathophysiology of 281
infection 35, 340, 505
meningitis 379
Vision
disorders 563
low 568
normal 564*f*
partial 568
problems 415
Visual
distortion 565
impairment 573
Vital signs 185, 344
Vitamin 94, 278
A 285, 510, 525
deficiency 569
supplements 509
B_{12} 255, 370
C deficiency 649
D 542
production 542
deficiency 562
K 279
deficiency 285
support 285
Vomiting 102, 245, 246, 252, 268, 389, 534, 599, 623
of hydatid membranes 540
projectile 253
Vygotsky 63*f*, 64*f*

W

Warfarin 705
Warning signs 171
Warts 561
Waste products 349
Water
 and electrolytes 94
 bag of 70
Watery eyes 103
Weakness 488
Weaning foods 31
Weight loss 458
West Nile encephalitis 382
West Nile virus 381
Wheezing 289, 486
Whirlpool emotion 161
White blood cells 298, 350
Whooping cough 35, 506, 506*f*
Wilms tumor 409, 438
 symptoms of 439
Wolff-Parkinson-White syndrome 495
Wong-Baker faces pain 633*f*
 rating scale 633
World Health Organization 211, 531
Wound
 care 332, 585
 treatment 520
Wuchereria bancrofti 537

X

Xanthomas 280

Y

Yersinia 255

Z

Zanamivir 294
Zinc supplementation 272
Zovirax 383
Zygote 67
Zyloprim 423